Pediatric Hematology and Oncology

This book is dedicated to all past, present and future children with cancer and the people who care for them.

FINES PAYABLE
IF OVERDUE

This book is due for return on or before the last date shown below.

1 4 FEB 2011

- 7 JUN 2011

WITHDRAWN

Pediatric Hematology and Oncology

Scientific Principles and Clinical Practice

EDITED BY

EDWARD J. ESTLIN BSc (Hons), PhD, MRCP, FRCPCH
Macmillan Consultant in Paediatric Oncology
Department of Paediatric Oncology
Royal Manchester Children's Hospital
Manchester, UK

RICHARD J. GILBERTSON B.Med.Sci (Hons), MRCP, PhD
Co-Leader, Neurobiology and Brain Tumor Program
Director, Molecular Clinical Trials Core
Departments of Developmental Neurobiology and Oncology
St Jude Children's Research Hospital
Memphis, TN, USA

ROBERT F. WYNN BA, MD, MRCP, FRCPath
Consultant Paediatric Haematologist and
Programme Director, Blood and Marrow Transplant Unit
Royal Manchester Children's Hospital
Manchester, UK

WILEY-BLACKWELL
A John Wiley & Sons, Ltd., Publication

This edition first published 2010, © 2010 by Blackwell Publishing Ltd

Blackwell Publishing was acquired by John Wiley & Sons in February 2007. Blackwell's publishing program has been merged with Wiley's global Scientific, Technical and Medical business to form Wiley-Blackwell.

Registered office: John Wiley & Sons Ltd, The Atrium, Southern Gate, Chichester, West Sussex, PO19 8SQ, UK

Editorial offices: 9600 Garsington Road, Oxford, OX4 2DQ, UK
The Atrium, Southern Gate, Chichester, West Sussex, PO19 8SQ, UK
111 River Street, Hoboken, NJ 07030-5774, USA

For details of our global editorial offices, for customer services and for information about how to apply for permission to reuse the copyright material in this book please see our website at www.wiley.com/wiley-blackwell

The right of the author to be identified as the author of this work has been asserted in accordance with the Copyright, Designs and Patents Act 1988.

Library of Congress Cataloging-in-Publication Data

Pediatric hematology and oncology : scientific principles and clinical practice / edited by Edward J. Estlin, Richard J. Gilbertson, Robert F. Wynn.

  p. ; cm.
 Includes bibliographical references.
 ISBN 978-1-4051-5350-8
 1. Pediatric hematology. 2. Tumors in children. I. Estlin, Edward J. II. Gilbertson, Richard J.
III. Wynn, Robert F.
 [DNLM: 1. Hematologic Diseases. 2. Child. 3. Neoplasms. WS 300 P3702 2010]
 RJ411.P37 2010
 618.92′15—dc22

         2009018585

ISBN: 978-14051-5350-8

A catalogue record for this book is available from the British Library.

Set in 9.25pt/12pt Minion by Toppan Best-set Premedia Limited
Printed in Singapore by Markono Print Media Pte Ltd

1 2010

Contents

Contents

Contributors

John Anderson BA MRCP PhD
Senior Lecturer in Paediatric Oncology
Honorary Consultant Paediatric Oncologist
Institute of Child Health and Great Ormond Street
Hospital
London, UK

Sue Ablett BA, PhD, MRCPCH
Executive Director
Children's Cancer and Leukaemia Group (CCLG)
Leicester, UK

Ute Bartels MD
Pediatric Brain Tumor Program
The Hospital for Sick Children
Toronto, Ontario, Canada

Gianni Bisogno MD, PhD
Consultant Paediatric Oncologist
Division of Hematology and Oncology
Department of Paediatrics
University Hospital of Padua
Padua, Italy

Eric Bouffet MD, FRCP(C)
Director of the Paediatric Brain Tumour Program
Professor of Paediatrics
Division of Haematology and Oncology
The Hospital for Sick Children
Toronto, Ontario, Canada

Bernadette Brennan MBChB,
FRCPCH, MD
Consultant Paediatric Oncologist
Royal Manchester Children's Hospital
Manchester, UK

Penelope Brock MD, PhD, FRCPCH
Consultant Paediatric Oncologist
and Honorary Senior Lecturer
Great Ormond Street Hospital for Children NHS
Trust
and Institute of Child Health
London, UK

Lynda Brook MBChB, MRCP, MSc
Macmillan Consultant in Paediatric Palliative Care
Alder Hey Children's Hospital Specialist Palliative
Care Team
Department of Pediatric Oncology
Alder Hey Children's Hospital
Liverpool, UK

Steven C. Clifford PhD
Professor of Molecular Paediatric Oncology
Northern Institute for Cancer Research
Newcastle University
The Medical School
Newcastle-upon-Tyne, UK

Wolfgang Dörffel MD
Hospital for Children and Adolescents
HELIOS-Klinikum Berlin-Buch
Berlin, Germany

François Doz MD
Department of Pediatric Oncology
Institute Curie;
University René Descartes
Paris, France

Michael Dyer PhD
Department of Developmental Neurobiology
St Jude Children's Research Hospital;
Department of Ophthalmology
Howard Hughes Medical Institute
University of Tennessee Health Science Center
Memphis, TN, USA

R. Maarten Egeler MD, PhD
Professor of Pediatrics
Head, Division of Immunology, Hematology,
Oncology, Bone Marrow Transplantation and
Auto-immune Diseases
Department of Pediatrics
Leiden University Medical Center
Leiden, The Netherlands

Edward J. Estlin BSc(Hons), PhD,
MRCP, FRCPCH
Macmilllan Consultant in Paediatric Oncology
Department of Pediatric Oncology
Royal Manchester Children's Hospital
Manchester, UK

Amar Gajjar MD
Director, Division of Neuro Oncology
Co-Leader, Neurobiology and Brain Tumor
Program
Co-Chair, Department of Oncology
St Jude Children's Research Hospital
Memphis, TN, USA

Richard J. Gilbertson MD, PhD
Co-Leader
Neurobiology and Brain Tumor Program
Director
Molecular Clinical Trials Core
Departments of Developmental Neurobiology
and Oncology
St Jude Children's Research Hospital
Memphis, TN, USA

Richard Gorlick MD
Associate Professor of Pediatrics and Molecular
Pharmacology
Albert Einstein College of Medicine;
Vice Chairman
Division Chief of Pediatric Hematology and
Oncology
Department of Pediatrics
The Children's Hospital at Montefiore
Bronx, New York, USA

Norbert Graf MD
Department of Paediatric Haematology and Oncology
University Hospital of Saarland
Homburg, Germany

Annie Huang MD, PhD, FRCP(C)
Pediatric Brain Tumor Program
The Hospital for Sick Children
Toronto, Ontario, Canada

Contributors

Dieter Körholz MD
Chairman, Department of Pediatrics
Martin Luther University Halle/Wittenberg
Halle/Saale, Germany

Ged Lalor BA (Hons), CQSW
Social Worker
Department of Paediatric Oncology and
Haematology
Royal Manchester Children's Hospital
Manchester, UK

Thomas E. Merchant DO, PhD
Member and Chief
Division of Radiation Oncology
St Jude Children's Research Hospital
Memphis, TN, USA

Lara Mussolin, PhD
Clinica di Oncoematologia Pediatrica
Azienda Ospedaliera-Università di Padova
Padova, Italy

James Nicholson DM, MA, MB, BChir,
MRCP, FRCPCH
Consultant Paediatric Oncologist
Addenbrooke's Hospital
Cambridge, UK

Roger Palmer BSc (Hons), PhD MB, BChir,
MRCP(UK), MRCPCH
MRC Career Development Fellow
MRC Cancer Cell Unit
Cambridge, UK

Andrew D. J. Pearson MD, FRCP,
FRCPCH, DCH
Chairman of Paediatric Oncology
The Institute of Cancer Research & Royal
Marsden Hospital
Sutton, Surrey, UK

Martha Perisoglou MD
Richard Scowcroft Research Fellow
Department of Oncology
University College Hospital
London, UK

Bob Phillips MA, BM BCh, MMedSci,
MRCPCH
Consultant in Paediatric Oncology,
Leeds Teaching Hospitals Trust, Leeds
UK;
MRC Research Fellow, Centre for Reviews
and Dissemination,
University of York,
York, UK

Jack Plaschkes MD, FRCS
Senior Pediatric Surgeon and Consultant for
Pediatric Surgical Oncology (Ret.)
University Children's Hospital
Bern, Switzerland

Ian F. Pollack, MD, FACS, FAAP
Chief, Pediatric Neurosurgery
Children's Hospital of Pittsburgh
Walter Dandy Professor of Neurosurgery
Vice Chairman for Academic Affairs
Department of Neurological Surgery
Director, UPCI Brain Tumor Program
University of Pittsburgh School of Medicine
Pittsburgh, PA, USA

Derek J. Roebuck MRCPCH FRCR FRANZCR
Consultant Interventional Radiologist
Department of Radiology
Great Ormond Street Hospital for Children
NHS Trust
London, UK

Angelo Rosolen MD
Clinica di Oncoematologia Pediatrica
Azienda Ospedaliera-Università di Padova
Padova, Italy

Roderick Skinner BSc (Hons), MB ChB
(Hons), PhD, FRCPCH, DCH, MRCP(UK)
Consultant and Honorary Clinical Senior Lecturer
in Paediatric and Adolescent Oncology / BMT
Children's BMT Unit
Newcastle General Hospital
Newcastle upon Tyne, UK;
Department of Paediatric and Adolescent Oncology
Royal Victoria Infirmary
Newcastle upon Tyne, UK

Helen Spoudeas DRCOG, FRCPCH,
FRCP, MD
Consultant in Neuro-Endocrine and Late Effects of
Childhood Malignancy
Honorary Senior Lecturer in Paediatric
Endocrinology
London Centre for Paediatric and Adolescent
Endocrinology Neuroendocrine Division
University College London & Great Ormond Street
Hospital for Children NHS Trust
London, UK

Charles Stiller MSc
Senior Research Fellow
Childhood Cancer Research Group
University of Oxford
Oxford, UK

Louise Talbot D.Clin.Psy., BSc (Hons)
Macmillan Clinical Psychologist
Paediatric Psychosocial Department
Royal Manchester Children's Hospital
Manchester, UK

Michael D. Taylor MD, PhD, FRCS
Assistant Professor
Department of Neurosurgery
The Hospital for Sick Children
Toronto, Ontario, Canada

Sucheta J. Vaidya MBBS, DCH, MB, MD
Consultant in Paediatric Oncology
Royal Marsden Hospital
Sutton, Surrey, UK

David K.H. Webb MD, FRCP, MRCPath,
MRCPCH
Consultant Haematologist
Department of Haematology and Oncology
Great Ormond Street Hospital for Children
NHS Trust
London, UK

Adrienne Weeks MD
Department of Neurosurgery
The Hospital for Sick Children
Toronto, Ontario, Canada

Sheila Weitzman MB BCh, FCP (SA),
FRCP (C)
Senior Staff Oncologist
Associate Director Clinical Affairs
The Division of Haematology and Oncology
The Hospital for Sick Children
Professor, Department of Pediatrics
University of Toronto
Toronto, Ontario, Canada

Jeremy Whelan MD, FRCP
Consultant Medical Oncologist
Department of Oncology
University College Hospital
London, UK

Robert F. Wynn BA, MD, MRCP, FRCPath
Consultant Paediatric Haematologist
and Programme Director
Blood and Marrow Transplant Unit
Royal Manchester Children's Hospital
Manchester, UK

1 Introduction

Edward J. Estlin[1], Richard J. Gilbertson[2] and Robert F. Wynn[3]

[1] Department of Pediatric Oncology, Royal Manchester Children's Hospital, Manchester, UK, [2] Departments of Developmental Neurobiology and Oncology, St Jude Children's Research Hospital, Memphis, TN, USA and [3] Blood and Marrow Transplant Unit, Royal Manchester Children's Hospital, Manchester, UK

Scope and aims

The aim of this textbook is to provide the reader with a focused but comprehensive overview of the clinical and scientific principles that guide current treatments for childhood cancer. For this purpose, the book is divided into four sections, namely central nervous system tumors, hematological malignancies, non-central nervous system (CNS) solid tumors of childhood, and a final section which covers psycho-social support, palliative care and survivorship issues.

For each of the disease specific chapters, our aim is to present the reader with information that is visually distinctive and should allow easy access to key factual information that relates to the epidemiology, presentation, diagnosis, treatment, and prognosis for individual categories of childhood malignancy, along with a brief overview given of the history of therapeutic developments for any given disease type. To facilitate this, the paragraphs will contain regular bullet points to highlight the presentation of key factual information, tables and fact boxes which we hope will enable any reader to quickly pick out important information in relation to the disease type they are interested in.

Progress for the treatment of children's cancers has traditionally involved advances at the scientific interface such as the recognition of the importance of chromosomal abnormalities, oncogene amplification and aberrations of tumor suppressor gene functions. In more recent times, advances in our understanding of the cellular biological characteristics of cancers is leading towards new insights that can enable a more rational treatment stratification and is also leading towards the development of specific and targeted therapies. Therefore, each of the disease-specific chapters will focus on an integration of the scientific and clinical principles that guide the treatment for these individual cancer types, and introduce the reader to advances in the field that are at the level of the clinical interface. Therefore,

Pediatric Hematology and Oncology, 1st edition. Edited by Edward J. Estlin, Richard J. Gilbertson, and Robert F. Wynn. © 2010 Blackwell Publishing Ltd.

in order to help orientate the reader with the scientific information that is incorporated into individual chapters in the rest of the text book, the aim of this introduction is to help define those key scientific principles that pertain to the contemporary management of children with cancer, and which are currently informing novel therapies that are now close to or actually at the clinical interface.

For the descriptions that will be presented below, our aim is not to provide an exhaustive text and reference resource for the reader, but really to highlight the key terms and scientific principles that will serve as a glossary for the main body of the text book to follow, and which will involve referencing against contemporary textbooks and review articles that act as a starting point for further reading.

The epidemiology of childhood cancer

When compared with the adult population, cancer in children is rare and comprises less than 1% of the national cancer burdens of industrialized countries [1]. Moreover, whereas most adult cancers are carcinomas, the cancers that occur in childhood are histologically very diverse and comprise [2]:

- Leukemia, myeloproliferative diseases and myelodysplastic diseases.
- Lymphomas and reticuloendothelial neoplasms.
- CNS tumors.
- Neuroblastoma and other peripheral nervous cell tumors.
- Retinoblastoma.
- Renal tumors.
- Hepatic tumors.
- Malignant bone tumors.
- Soft tissue and other extra osseous sarcomas.
- Germ cell tumors, trophoblastic tumors, and neoplasms of the gonads.
- Other malignant epithelial neoplasms and malignant melanoma.
- Other unspecified malignant neoplasms.

Thus, for children, carcinomas are rare, and the majority of cancers present as acute leukemia, lymphoma (non-Hodgkin's lymphoma, Hodgkin's disease), sarcoma (osteogenic sarcoma, rhabdomyosarcoma), germ cell tumor and embryonal malignancies (neuroblastoma, nephroblastoma, medulloblastoma, hepatoblastoma). Embryonic tumors, which are thought to arise during intra-uterine or early post-natal development from an organ rudiment or immature tissue, and form structures that are characteristic of the affected part of the body, are rare in adults.

The age-standardized incidence of all cancers in children under the age of 15 years is between 70 and 160 per million children per year, corresponding to a risk of 1 in 100 to 1 in 400, and an annual worldwide incidence of approximately 160 000 new cases per year [2]. The epidemiology of childhood cancers is characterized by [1, 2]:

• The incidence is highest in the first 5 years of life, reaches a nadir at 9–10 years of age and then rises thereafter.

• Boys are affected more than girls.

• While total incidence rates vary only modestly between world regions, there is more marked variation for diagnostic subgroups. For example, among children of North America and Europe, acute leukemia forms the largest diagnostic sub-group, accounting for one-third of the total number of cases, with a lower incidence seen for sub-Saharan Africa, where lymphomas predominate as the most frequent childhood cancer.

• Within geographical regions, there are indications that racial influences may form a part in the susceptibility of children to cancer. For example, whereas in the USA, the incidence rates for acute lymphoblastic leukemia are highest for children of Hispanic origin, and lower for those of Afro-American ethnicity, the incidence of Wilms' tumor is lowest for this latter ethnic group.

• Brain and spinal cord tumors are second only to leukemia in industrialized countries, where they account for 20–25% of childhood cancer. The lower recorded incidence in developed countries may represent under diagnosis.

• Neuroblastoma and nephroblastoma have a fairly constant incidence rate worldwide.

• Environmental influences play a part in the variations of the incidence rate for individual cancers types found worldwide.

• Embryonal tumors and common acute lymphoblastic leukemia tend to affect younger children, osteogenic sarcoma and Hodgkin's disease are more a diagnosis of adolescence, and rhabdomyosarcoma has bi-modal peaks with both younger children and adolescents being affected.

However, for the great majority (>95%) of cases of childhood cancer the causation is unknown, but those factors that are known to increase the risk of childhood are indicated in Box 1.1, and can be generally categorized as:

• Genetic causes – The largest contributions here come from heritable retinoblastoma, neurofibromatosis type 1 (NF1), tuberous sclerosis and the Li-Fraumeni syndrome. For example, children with NF1 have a relative risk for glioma and soft tissue sarcoma of 40, and germline mutations of the tumor suppressor gene TP53 (Li-Fraumeni genetic abnormality) are present in

---

Box 1.1 The epidemiology of childhood cancer.

• Genetic causes – retinoblastoma, neurofibromatosis type 1, tuberous sclerosis, Li-Fraumeni cancer family syndrome

• Constitutional chromosomal disorders – Down's syndrome, Turners syndrome

• Inherited immunodeficiency and bone marrow failure syndromes

• Irradiation

• Infection

---

most children with adrenocortical carcinoma and about 10% of children with rhabdomyosarcoma.

• Infection – associated with Epstein-Barr virus (Hodgkin's lymphoma & nasopharyngeal carcinoma), hepatitis B (hepatocellular carcinoma) and Human Herpes Virus 8 (Kaposi sarcoma), a phenomenon that at least in part explains some of the worldwide differences for the incidence rates of these diseases.

• Although the subject of extensive investigation, the influence of other environmental factors such as ultraviolet light, electromagnetic fields is uncertain, although the Chernobyl nuclear disaster has seen an associated increase in thyroid cancer in children of the affected geographical region.

Genetics in relation to children's cancers

The study and investigation of the genetics of children's cancers has led to important advances in the understanding of the epidemiology and causation of certain malignancies such as retinoblastoma; the recognition of karyotypic abnormalities provides a vital part of the diagnosis and risk stratification for therapy of many children's cancers. Some examples are described as follows:

• Philadelphia chromosome, which represents translocation between chromosomes 9 and 22 [t(9;22)], confers an adverse prognosis when this is associated with the diagnosis of acute lymphoblastic leukemia in children [3].

• Other translocations such as the translocation involving chromosomes 11 and 22 [t(11;22)] can help define disease entities such as Ewing's tumor and malignant peripheral neuroectodermal tumor from their differential diagnoses [4].

• Chromosome losses from 1p and 11q and gain of chromosomal material for 17q for neuroblastoma are associated with an adverse outcome for this cancer type [5].

The chromosomal translocations described for acute lymphoblastic leukemia (ALL) and Ewing's tumor above promote the malignant phenotype of these cancers. For example, the Ewing's tumor gene translocation results in an oncogenic transcription factor, EWS-Fli-1, and the Philadelphia translocation results in production of a constitutively active receptor kinase, bcr-abl, which has influences on proliferation, cell cycle control, and cell death. The recognition of the links between the genetics of cancer and subsequent cellular biological functions are leading to advances in therapy with mechanism-based compounds, such as imatinib in the case of bcr-abl positive leukemia [3].

Cellular and molecular biology in relation to children's cancers (Box 1.2)

Receptor kinases and intracellular signalling
Although underlying genetic abnormalities such as loss of tumor suppressor function and gain of oncogenic gene activity may underlie the pathogenesis of individual cancers in children, science is now bringing us insights into the processes that are important as biological determinants of the malignant phenotype in cancer cells. For example, extracellular growth factor/cytokines or mitogens can bind to receptors on the cell surface that are linked to receptor kinases, or these cell surface receptors can be constitutively active [6]. Such ligand/receptor interactions can lead to:
• The activation of intercellular signalling pathways such as Akt/PI3, mTOR and MAP kinases, which in turn leads to:
• The dysregulation of various cellular activities such as gene expression, mitosis, differentiation, cell survival/apoptosis and motility, and invasiveness.

Moreover, genetic mutations can also lead to dysregulation of intracellular signalling, as in the example of loss of the inhibitory effect of PTEN function on Akt/PI3 signalling by gene deletion [7], or the loss of tumor suppressor gene function by gene promoter methylation as in the example of Ras-association domain family 1. Proteins in the ras family are very important molecular switches for a wide variety of signal pathways that control such processes as cellular skeletal integrity, proliferation, cell adhesion, apoptosis and migration. Ras-related proteins are often deregulated in cancers, leading to increased invasion and metastases, and decreased apoptosis. Ras activates a number of pathways, but especially an important one seems to be the mitogen-activated protein kinases, which themselves transmit signals downstream to other protein kinases and gene-regulatory proteins. Inappropriate activation of the gene can occur when tumor

suppressor genes are lost, such as the tumor suppressor gene NF1, and ras oncogenes can be activated by point mutations to be constitutively activated [8].

The biological characteristics of cancers are also influenced by their environment. For example, tissue hypoxia is known to contribute to the pathogenesis and maintenance of the malignant phenotype, and interaction between the physicochemical properties of cancers and biological systems that control cellular proliferation, migration, and survival is now increasingly well understood. As a particular example of this, the vascular endothelial growth factor family of ligands and receptors are modulated by hypoxia, and has now been extensively studied for both children's and adult malignancies. This in turn is bringing forward the rational introduction of novel mechanism-based therapies that aim to disrupt specific processes important for the pathogenesis of cancer [9], rather than attempting to cause cancer cell death by non-specific DNA damage as in the case of most conventional cytotoxic agents as will be discussed below.

Cell cycle control
Cell cycle progression is monitored by surveillance mechanisms, or cell cycles checkpoints, that ensure that initiation of a later event is coupled with the completion of an early cell cycles event. Dysregulation of the progression of cells through the cell cycles is also a feature of malignant cells, and defects in certain molecules such as p53, the retinoblastoma protein (pRb) and cyclin kinase inhibitors (e.g. p15, p16, p21) that control the cell cycle have been implicated in cancer formation and progression [10]. Virtually all human tumors degregulate either the retinoblastoma (pRb/p16(INK4a)/cyclin D1) and/or p53 (p14 (ARF)/mdm2/p53) control pathways [10].

One of the most studied control systems in cancer involves p53, otherwise known as protein 53, a transcription factor that regulates the cell cycle, and hence functions as a tumor suppressor [11].
• p53 has many anti-cancer mechanisms in that it can activate DNA repair proteins when DNA has sustained damage, it can hold the cell cycle at the G1/S regulation point upon DNA damage recognition, and it can initiate apoptosis if the DNA damage proves to be irreparable [11].
• In normal cells, p53 is usually inactive, bound to the protein MDM2, which prevents its action and promotes its degradation by acting as a ubiquitin ligase. Upon DNA damage or other stress, various pathways will lead to the association of P53 and the MDM2 complex [12].

Once activated, P53 will either induce cell cycle arrest to allow repair and survival of the cell or apoptosis to discard the damaged cell. How p53 makes this choice is currently unknown.

If the p53 gene is damaged, then tumor suppression is severely impaired. People who inherit only one functional copy of the p53 gene, TP53, are at risk of developing tumors in early adulthood, a disease known as the Li-Fraumeni cancer family syndrome. Indeed, more than 50% of human tumors contain a mutation or deletion of the TP53 gene [2]. The occurrence of retinoblastoma

Box 1.2 Cancer biology and immunology.

• Loss of tumor suppressor function or amplification of oncogenic function promotes malignant phenotype
• Dysregulation of cellular signalling
• Deregulation of cell cycle control
• Disordered proliferation, metastases and survival
• Knowledge informing treatment stratifications and novel therapies
• Immunological properties exploited in diagnosis and therapy.

serves as a paradigm for the effects of loss of the tumor suppressor function of pRb, and this will be discussed in Chapter 18 of the textbook.

Cancer biology and risk stratification

Advances in our understanding of the biology of childhood cancer are providing new insights into prognosis and will serve to underpin rational approaches to the stratification of treatments. For example, whereas an adverse prognosis for childhood medulloblastoma is found to relate to the growth factor receptor erb-b2 expression [13], nuclear accumulation of beta-catenin is associated with the activation of the Wnt/Wg signalling pathway and a more favorable prognosis [14]. This information may allow a staged reduction in the radiotherapy burden for the treatment of medulloblastoma, and also promote the development of specific mechanism-base therapies [15].

Cancer immunology

Knowledge of the immunology of childhood cancer is important for the diagnosis of childhood leukemias and can also be exploited for the therapy of childhood cancers. For example, the cluster of differentiation (CD nomenclature) has been developed to characterize the monoclonal antibodies that have been generated against epitopes on the surface molecules of leucocytes.
• The CD system is commonly used as cell markers; this allows cells to be defined based on what molecules are present on their surface.
• CD molecules are utilized in cell sorting using various methods, including flow cytometry, and can be used for the recognition of stem cells (CD34+, CD31−): all leukocyte groups, (CD45+): T lymphocytes, (CD3+) and B leukocytes, (CD19+).

The immune system can also be utilized to direct therapy against the cancers themselves. For example, dendritic cell-based immunotherapy utilizes dendritic cells, which are antigen-presenting cells that are harvested from patients to activate a cytotoxic response towards an antigen. Briefly, the dendritic cells are harvested from patients, these cells are then either incubated with an antigen or infected with a viral vector, and the activated dendritic cells are then transfused back into the patient. These cells then present the tumor-associated antigens to the effector lymphocytes, namely CD4+ T-cells and CD8+ T-cells, and some classes of B lymphocyte also. A similar procedure exists for T cell-based adoptive immunotherapy, which sees T-cells that have a natural or genetically-engineered reactivity to a patient's cancer expanded *in vitro* and than adoptively transferred into the cancer patient [16].

In the situation of bone marrow transplantation, in particular in the case of allogeneic bone marrow transplantation, a balance is sought between rejection of the transplanted graft, eventual immune tolerance of the graft and maintenance of a controlled degree of graft versus host disease in order to maximize anti-leukemic effect [17].

The general principles of pharmacology in relation to childhood cancer

Radiotherapy continues to form an important part of the treatment of many childhood cancers, and this will be discussed further in the subsequent disease-specific chapters of this textbook. The cornerstone for the treatment of many cancers of childhood remains conventional chemotherapy agents, and a summary of these is presented below. Although a detailed description of the properties of anticancer agents in terms of their pharmacokinetic profiles, and a description of the cellular and molecular pharmacological processes that can limit or potentiate their effectiveness in cancer cells, is beyond the scope of this chapter, the reader is referred to the excellent reference text by Chabner and Longo for further information [18]. Basically, conventional chemotherapy agents usually act to promote DNA damage in all cells of the body, and the cure for cancer thus relies on there being a therapeutic index allowing eradication of the tumor at acceptable toxicity to the patient. The conventional cytotoxic agents commonly employed in the therapy of children's cancer include the following classes of agent:
• Alkylating agents that cross-link DNA – examples include ifosfamide, cyclophosphamide, cisplatin, carboplatin, busulphan, melphalan, and temozolomide.
• Anti-metabolites that cause fraudulent incorporation of bases into DNA – examples include methotrexate, 6-mercaptopurine and cytarabine.
• Anti-tumor antibiotics that have variety of actions such as free radical formation, DNA intercalation, topoisomerase II inhibition – examples include doxorubicin, daunorubicin and actinomycin-D.
• Topoisomerase inhibitors that prevent normal conduct of DNA relaxation to facilitate repair and replication – examples include etoposide (topoisomerase II inhibitor) and topotecan and irinotecan (topoisomerase I inhibitor).
• Vinca alkyloids that promote microtubular instability and inhibit the polymerization of tubulin – examples include vincristine and vinorelbine.
• Miscellaneous agents – examples include prednisone, dexamethasone and L-asparaginase.

The science of pharmacology has contributed to the progress of the cure of children's cancers over the years, and also the pharmacokinetic profiles (how the drug is handled by the body) and pharmacodynamic effects (the effect the drug has on the body) remains important for the rational selection of treatment schedules for existing and novel therapies. These concepts have been extensively studied, mainly in relation to acute lymphoblastic leukemia, and in particular in an elegant series of studies performed at St Jude Children's Research Hospital in Memphis, USA.

When considering the pharmacological properties of anticancer agents, the plasma concentration-versus-time profile is important as this allows a measurement of peak, maximum, or steady-state drug concentrations, the half-life of decline of drug concentration, measures of system exposure, and the volume of distribution found. Pharmacological studies also define the routes of elimination and metabolism of chemotherapeutic agents [18].

When studied, pharmacological parameters have generally been shown to be important for the prognosis of childhood cancers. For example, the dose intensity (amount of chemotherapy received over a period of time) of chemotherapy agents has been shown to be important for diseases as diverse as infant ependymoma [19] and acute lymphoblastic leukemia [20]. The clinical pharmacological studies performed at St Jude's Children's Research Hospital with methotrexate, in the context of the treatment of acute lymphoblastic leukemia, serve as a paradigm for the investigation of the relationship between pharmacokinetics, cellular pharmacology, and the cellular determinants of chemosensitivity and prognosis.

- Over a series of studies performed in the 1980s up to the present day, successive investigations have demonstrated the importance of high-dose methotrexate steady-state concentration and systemic exposure, and also the relationships of these to the optimal intracellular metabolism of methotrexate in leukemic blasts for children with ALL. They have led to therapeutic strategies that have improved survival for children with this disease [20].
- Similar findings for dose intensity and systemic exposure have been described for the metronomic/maintenance chemotherapy phase of treatment of childhood ALL, where the influence of genetic polymorphisms that related to the metabolism of this thiopurine agent have been related to factors such as toxicity and survival [21].

Pharmacological studies are an essential part of the structure of Phase I studies and also, in many cases, Phase 2 studies where relationships between the pharmacokinetic profiles of new agents and pharmacodynamic effects, such as toxicity and disease response, could be identified at as early a stage as possible in order to inform rational scheduling, and even in some cases, adaptive dosing.

The conduct of clinical studies in children with cancer (Box 1.3)

At a national and increasingly international level, the various phases of clinical trials in children with cancer are conducted as multicenter or even multinational collaborations [22]. New drug development is performed through the auspices of multicenter collaborations, such as the Innovative Therapies for Children's Cancers in Europe, or the Children's Oncology Group Early Clinical Studies Committee or the Pediatric Brain Tumor Consortium in North America. International guidelines have been established for the prioritization of new agents and also for the methodological considerations involved in Phase I trials.

- Upon completion of developmental pre-clinical studies in adults and children, which would include efficacy, toxicity, and pharmacokinetic information, a new drug can enter a Phase I

Box 1.3 Key facts – clinical trials and pharmacology in childhood cancer.

- International collaborations are now the norm
- Phase I studies define the safe dose to take forward for phase II studies of efficacy
- Phase III trials compare first-line treatments
- Pharmacokinetic and pharmacodynamic studies now embedded in phase I/II trial process
- Pharmacogenetics, dose intensity, pharmacokinetics and cellular pharmacology guides the rational use of chemotherapy agents

---

study to assess the safety, tolerability, pharmacokinetics, and pharmacodynamics of the agent.

- These studies are usually dose-ranging and involve escalation of cohorts of patients, and children who have no other hope of cure or significant palliation are eligible for such studies, which are designed to describe dose limit and toxicities that prevent further dose escalation and thereby establish the maximum-tolerated dose to take forward for Phase II study.

Once the initial safety of this new drug is confirmed in the Phase I trial, Phase II trials are performed, usually in children with relapsed disease, to assess how well the drug works at the prescribed dose and schedule. Such studies involve an initial cohort of patients to determine that some clinical activity could be expected and Phase II trials in pediatric oncology usually follow a two-stage design, which allows early termination of studies if the efficacy level is too low or is adequately high, and in general objective response rates of 20–30% are deemed as interesting enough to take a new agent forward.

Phase III trials are the staple activity of the national and international study groups in pediatric oncology. Phase III trials compare the effectiveness of an experimental therapy with that of a standard or control therapy and are only feasible in a collaborative group or multicenter setting. Phase III clinical trials usually include a randomization between treatment times and are commonly based on sequential or factorial designs, and generally require the recruitment of hundreds of children with a given disease type in order to answer questions of statistically significant differences between different treatments.

Summary

The treatment of children with cancer in the western industrialized world has been long held as a model for multicenter collaborations involving a wider multidisciplinary team. Over the past 40 years, the survival for many children's cancers has improved markedly, and the overall survival rates are now in the area of 75–80%. However, diseases such as diffuse intrinsic pontine glioma, metastatic sarcoma in adolescence, and high-risk neuroblastoma are still associated with a poor prognosis and new therapies will be needed to improve this for the future.

The early clinical trial study groups for Europe and North America are increasingly working with the pharmaceutical industry to develop new compounds of interest. A major challenge ahead will be to prioritize their introduction into upfront treatment protocols for high risk diseases and to design study methodologies that optimize the scientific information gained for each clinical trial. In addition, our discipline has traditionally held a strong interest in the late physical and psychological effects of the treatment of children's cancer, and this also will be important as new therapies are introduced and perhaps more children survive, but maybe in difficult circumstances following treatment with modalities such as cranial radiotherapy. Having introduced the scientific terminologies that the reader may encounter in the various disease-specific chapters of this textbook, we hope that the integration of the clinical and scientific principles that follow for the different tumor types will reflect our practice in terms of where we have come from, where we are at present, and where we might be going for the future.

References

1 Stiller CA. Epidemiology and genetics of childhood cancer. Oncogene 2004; 23: 6429–44.

2 Stiller CA. Pediatric Cancers. In: Kris Heggenhougen K, Quah S (Eds), International Encyclopaedia of Public Health, Vol. 5. San Diego: Academic Press, 2008: 28–40.

3 Kolb EA, Pan Q, Ladanyi M, et al. Imatinib mesylate in Philadelphia chromosome-positive leukaemia of childhood. Cancer 2003; 98: 2643–50.

4 de Alva E. Molecular pathology in sarcomas. Clin Trans Oncol 2007: 9; 130–44.

5 Park JR, Eggert A, Caron H. Neuroblastoma, biology, prognosis and treatment. Pediatr Clin North Am 2008; 55: 97–120.

6 Steelman LS, Abrams SL, Whelan J, et al. Contributions of the Raf/MEK/ERK, PI£K/PTEN/Akt/mTOR and Jak/STAT pathways to leukaemia. Leukaemia 2008; 22: 686–707.

7 Carnero A, Blanco-Aparicio C, Rener O, et al. The PTEN/PI3K/AKT signalling pathway in cancer, therapeutic implications. Curr Cancer Drug Targets 2008; 8: 187–98.

8 Agatthanggelou A, Cooper WN, Latif F. Role of the Ras-association domain family 1 tumor suppressor gene in human cancers. Cancer Res 2005; 65: 3497–508.

9 Adamski JK, Estlin EJ, Makin GWJ. The cellular adaptations to hypoxia as novel therapeutic targets in childhood cancer. Cancer Treat Rev 2008; 34: 231–46.

10 Macaluso M, Montanari M, Cinti C, et al. Modulation of cell cycle components by epigenetic and genetic events. Semin Oncol 2005; 32: 452–7.

11 Vasquez A, Bond EE, Levine AJ et al. The genetics of the p53 pathway, apoptosis and cancer therapy. Nat Rev Drug Discov 2008; 7: 979–87.

12 Hambardzumyan D, Becher OJ, Holland EC. Cancer stem cells and survival pathways. Cell Cycle 2008; 7: 1371–8.

13 Gajjar A, Hernan R, Kocak M, et al. Clinical, histopathologic and molecular markers of prognosis: toward a new disease risk stratification system for medulloblastoma. J Clin Oncol 2004; 22: 984–93.

14 Ellison DW, Onilude OE, Lindsey JC, et al. beta-Catenin status predicts a favourable outcome in childhood medulloblastoma: the United Kingdom Children's Cancer Study Group Brain Tumour Committee. J Clin Oncol 2005; 23: 7951–7.

15 Ihle NT, Powis G. Take your PIK: phosphatidylinositol-3-kinase inhibitors race through the clinic and toward cancer therapy. Mol Cancer Ther 2009; 8: 1–9.

16 Rousseau RF, Brenner MK. Vaccine therapies for paediatric malignancies. Cancer J 2005; 11: 331–9.

17 Feig SA, Lampkin B, Nesbit ME, et al. Outcome of BMT during first complete remission of AML: a comparison of two sequential studies by the Children's Cancer Group. Bone Marrow Transplant 1993; 12: 65–71.

18 Collins J, Supko JG. Cancer Chemotherapy and Biotherapy – Principles and Practice, 4th Edn. Chabner BA, Longo DL (Eds). Philadelphia: Lippincott Williams & Wilkins, 2006: 31–44.

19 Grundy RG, Wilne SA, Weston CL, et al. Primary postoperative chemotherapy without radiotherapy for intracranial ependymoma in children: the UKCCSG/SIOP prospective study. Lancet Oncol 2007; 8: 696–705.

20 Estlin EJ, Rongue M, Burke GAA, et al. The clinical and cellular pharmacology of vincristine, corticosteroids, L-asparaginase, anthracyclines and cyclophopsphamide in relation to childhood acute lymphoblastic leukaemia. Br J Haematol 2000; 110: 780–90.

21 Estlin EJ. Continuing therapy for childhood acute lymphoblastic leukaemia – the clinical and cellular pharmacology of methotrexate, 6-mercaptopurine and 6-thioguanine. Cancer Treat Rev 2001; 27: 351–63.

22 Estlin EJ, Ablett S. The practicalities and ethics of running clinical trials in paediatric oncology – The UK experience. Eur J Cancer 2001; 37: 1394–401.

I Central Nervous System Tumors of Childhood

2 Low- and High-Grade Glioma

Ian F. Pollack

Department of Neurosurgery, Children's Hospital of Pittsburgh, University of Pittsburgh School of Medicine, Pittsburgh, PA, USA

Introduction

Gliomas account for more than half of childhood central nervous system neoplasms [4, 5]. On a regional basis, they comprise at least 60% of supratentorial hemispheric tumors, 50% of supratentorial midline tumors and 40% of infratentorial tumors. The majority of such lesions are World Health Organization Grade I or II (i.e. low-grade) astrocytomas [4, 5] or other low-grade glial and glioneuronal neoplasms, such as oligodendrogliomas, oligoastrocytomas, gangliogliomas, and a number of less common lesions, such as pleomorphic xanthoastrocytoma, dysembryoplastic neuroepithelial tumor, and desmoplastic infantile ganglioglioma [6–11]. In contrast to the situation in adults, grade III or IV (i.e. high-grade or malignant) gliomas account for a minority of glial neoplasms in children in all locations within the neuraxis, with the notable exception of the brainstem, in which so-called diffuse malignant gliomas are substantially more frequent than lower grade lesions [3]. Given the diversity in the types of gliomas that arise in children, there are a wide range of therapeutic approaches, based both on histology and tumor location, and a correspondingly diverse profile of outcomes, incorporating the prognostically most favorable (e.g. cerebral and cerebellar pilocytic astrocytoma) and least favorable (e.g. diffuse brainstem glioma) tumor subtypes in pediatric neuro-oncology.

Epidemiology

For the vast majority of gliomas, contributory environmental or genetic factors have yet to be elucidated. However, there are a handful of genetic syndromes that predispose children to the development of gliomas. The most common of these is type 1 neurofibromatosis (NF1), which is caused by inactivation of the neurofibromin gene on chromosome 17q11.2 [12] that encodes

Pediatric Hematology and Oncology, 1st edition. Edited by Edward J. Estlin, Richard J. Gilbertson, and Robert F. Wynn. © 2010 Blackwell Publishing Ltd.

a protein with GTPase-activating properties, loss of which may promote G-protein-mediated signaling [13]. Although the most characteristic intracranial tumors in children with NF1 are low-grade visual pathway gliomas, many patients develop glial neoplasms in other locations, which can occasionally be malignant [14].

A second genetic syndrome that predisposes to glial tumor development is tuberous sclerosis (TS). This syndrome has been linked to mutations in another member of the GTPase-activating protein family [15], loss of which promotes downstream signaling via the mTOR pathway. Subependymal giant cell astrocytomas are the characteristic intracranial neoplasm in patients with TS; conversely, these tumors are seen almost exclusively in patients with this syndrome. Affected children characteristically have seizures, mental retardation, and adenoma sebaceum in addition to non-neoplastic cortical and subependymal tubers, and various systemic manifestations.

Other, much less common, syndromes that have been associated with an increased incidence of gliomas are Turcot's and Li-Fraumeni. The former is associated with mutations in the mismatch repair or adenomatosis polyposis genes and affected patients typically have multiple intestinal polyps [16]. Affected patients generally have malignant gliomas or primitive neuroectodermal tumors (PNETs) [17]. The latter is associated with mutations in the p53 gene [18], and affected patients can have neoplasms in a variety of systemic locations.

Histopathology classification (Box 2.1)

Low-grade gliomas can be broadly separated into distinct histological groups, based on their microscopic appearance and presumed cell of origin [6]. These are: (1) astrocytic tumors, including pilocytic and non-pilocytic astrocytoma, pleomorphic xanthoastrocytoma, and subependymal giant cell astrocytoma; (2) oligodendroglial tumors; (3) mixed gliomas; and (4) benign neuroepithelial tumors, such as ganglioglioma, desmoplastic infantile ganglioglioma, and dysembryoplastic neuroepithelial

---

Box 2.1 Histological subgroups of low-grade glial and glioneuronal tumors of childhood.

Low-Grade Astrocytomas

Pilocytic

Non-pilocytic (fibrillary)

Low-Grade Astrocytoma variants:

    Pilomyxoid astrocytoma

    Pleomorphic xanthoastrocytoma

    Subependymal giant cell astrocytoma

Low-Grade Oligodendroglial Tumors

Oligodendroglioma

Mixed oligoastrocytoma

Low-Grade Neuroglial Tumors

Ganglioglioma

Desmoplastic infantile ganglioglioma

Dysembryoplastic neuroepithelial tumor

Malignant Gliomas

Anaplastic astrocytoma

Anaplastic mixed glioma

Anaplastic oligodendroglioma

Anaplastic ganglioglioma

Glioblastoma multiforme

Gliosarcoma

---

tumor. Malignant gliomas are subdivided into anaplastic (grade III) astrocytoma, mixed glioma, and oligodendroglioma; and glioblastoma multiforme (grade IV).

The grading of non-pilocytic astrocytomas has evolved significantly over time from the classification scheme of Bailey and Cushing [19]. Kernohan [20] proposed a four-tiered classification that was further simplified by several groups into a three-tiered system [21]. Because both approaches incorporated a large number of subjectively determined features, neither entirely resolved difficulties with tumor categorization. To provide a more straightforward classification schema, Daumas-Duport *et al.* proposed a relatively simple grading system based on a limited number of histological features [22]. Lesions were given one point for each of the following: nuclear atypia, mitoses, endothelial proliferation, and necrosis. Grade 1 lesions had none of these characteristics, grade 2 had 1, grade 3 had 2, and grade 4 had 3 or 4. Because these features often appeared in sequence, grade 2 tumors were generally characterized by nuclear atypia, grade 3 by mitotic activity, and grade 4 by the presence of either necrosis or endothelial proliferation. More recently, the revised World Health Organization classification guidelines [6] have incorporated a modified four-tier classification scheme, which has seemed to reduce (although not eliminate) the frequency of discordance between reviewers examining individual tumor samples [23–25].

The categorization of other types of glial tumors is somewhat more straightforward, particularly in the appropriate clinical setting. Pilocytic astrocytomas characteristically have areas of compact bipolar astrocytes alternating with loosely packed areas containing microcysts. Eosinophilic granular bodies and Rosenthal fibers are also commonly observed.

Pleomorphic xanthoastrocytomas contain cells with nuclear atypia, pleomorphism and multinucleation with abundant lipid-rich cells and pronounced reticulin reactivity. Most lesions arise in the temporal or parietal lobes and often incorporate an underlying cyst. Some of these tumors also exhibit more malignant features with pronounced mitosis, necrosis, and endothelial proliferation [26, 27].

Subependymal giant cell astrocytomas almost exclusively occur in the setting of tuberous sclerosis in the region of the foramen of Monro. These tumors are comprised of large cells resembling astrocytes with immunoreactivity for both glial and neuronal markers [6, 28].

Oligodendroglial tumors are composed of spherical cells with a 'fried egg' appearance, resulting from hyperchromatic nuclei and pale cytoplasm surrounded by a well-defined plasma membrane. Some lesions include a major astrocytic component, and are classified as mixed oligoastrocytomas. Oligodendroglial tumors can exhibit features of anaplasia with mitoses, necrosis, and vascular proliferation, and such cases are referred to as anaplastic oligodendroglioma or oligoastrocytoma.

Gangliogliomas are classified as benign neuroglial tumors, and exhibit binucleated neurons in a background of neoplastic astrocytes [29]. Desmoplastic infantile ganglioglioma is characterized by the young age of affected patients and by the presence of a pronounced desmoplastic component that incorporates neoplastic astrocytes and neurons [10, 11]. Finally, dysembryoplastic neuroepithelial tumors are cortically based lesions that exhibit a characteristic multinodular architecture that incorporates neoplastic oligodendrocytes, neurons, and astrocytes, with an internodular neuroglial component comprised of neurons that appear to be suspended in a background of oligodendroglial cells [6, 9, 30].

Molecular biology

Although tremendous energy has been directed at unraveling the steps in the development of adult astrocytomas, comparatively little work has been focused on pediatric tumors, particularly lower grade lesions. Although pilocytic astrocytomas have been noted to exhibit deletions of chromosome 17q [31], the site of the neurofibromin gene that is commonly mutated in patients with NF1, an association with neurofibromin mutations has not been confirmed for most sporadic lesions. More recently, pilocytic astrocytomas have been noted to have characteristic alterations in the BRAF gene, characterized by duplications, activating mutations, and translocations to produce a constitutively active variant [1–3]. Studies of other pediatric low-grade gliomas have not demonstrated a consistent pattern of genetic abnormalities. For example, mutations of the p53 gene are uncommon in low-grade pediatric astrocytomas [32], in contrast to the situation in adult low-grade gliomas [33], which suggests that tumors in these two age groups arise from different molecular events.

Pediatric high-grade gliomas also appear to differ from their adult counterparts in terms of their molecular abnormalities. Our analysis of three cohorts of childhood malignant gliomas found p53 mutations in approximately 40% of tumors, comparable to the frequency in adult secondary malignant gliomas, which begin as low-grade non-pilocytic lesions, evolve into anaplastic astrocytomas, and ultimately become glioblastomas [33–37]. However, because this evolution is infrequently observed in pediatric gliomas, it is doubtful whether such tumors are analogous to the secondary adult subgroup. Moreover, a worse prognosis has been noted in childhood malignant gliomas with p53 mutations than those without, which contrasts with the lack of such an association in adult lesions [37]. In addition, studies in adult primary malignant gliomas indicate that this group of tumors may well encompass several molecularly defined subsets of lesions, and the relevance of these categories to the pediatric context remains to be defined [135]. A second molecular pathway in adult gliomagenesis involves so-called 'de novo' or primary development of a glioblastoma, which is characterized by loss of a portion of chromosome 10 in and around the region of the PTEN gene [36, 38], in association with amplification and/or rearrangement of the epidermal growth factor receptor gene, but without mutation of the p53 gene [33, 35]. Recent studies by our group and others indicate that EGFR amplification and PTEN deletion occur in less than 10% of pediatric malignant gliomas, suggesting that this pathway is less commonly implicated than in adults [39–42]. In addition, secondary adult malignant gliomas have also been observed to commonly have mutations in the IDH1 gene, and such changes are relatively uncommon in pediatric malignant gliomas (1,2), further calling into question the similarities of these groups [136, 137]. A third group of adult malignant gliomas arise by a distinct pathway, with characteristic deletions of chromosomes 1p and 19q [43]. Such tumors typically have oligodendroglial morphology, and carry a better prognosis than other groups of malignant gliomas [43]. Although such changes are observed in about 20% of childhood gliomas, a favorable association between 1p/19q loss and outcome has not been observed [44].

In contrast to the above markers, which indicate molecular differences between childhood and adult malignant gliomas, other biological factors associated with drug resistance mechanisms have been reported to similarly influence prognosis in both adult and pediatric malignant gliomas. In particular, several studies have noted that the response of malignant gliomas to alkylating agents may be strongly influenced by expression of proteins that contribute to drug resistance, such as methylguanine methyltransferase (MGMT) and mismatch repair (MMR) [45–47]. In several independent studies in adults, tumors with MGMT overexpression had a significantly worse prognosis for event-free survival after treatment with nitrosoureas [45, 46] and temozolomide [47]. Recent studies have identified a comparable association in childhood malignant gliomas, in independent blinded analyses of two cooperative group cohorts, one involving treatment with a nitrosourea and a second involving use of temozolomide [48, 49]. Because nitrosoureas, such as lomustine, and temozolomide have each formed an important element in the therapy of malignant gliomas, an evaluation of their combined activity in the context of MGMT status is being undertaken in a prospective fashion in the recently completed ACNS0423 high-grade glioma study, which administers temozolomide in conjunction with irradiation and lomustine.

Clinical presentation

The mode of presentation of a glioma is influenced by the age of the child, tumor histology, and the location of the lesion. Tumors in infants often manifest with non-localizing signs of increased intracranial pressure, such as lethargy, irritability, failure to thrive, macrocephaly, and a bulging fontanel [50, 51]. Tumors in older children more commonly present with localizing symptoms and signs that suggest the site as well as the histological grade of the tumor [4]. For example, cerebral hemispheric gliomas often produce seizures, headaches, and focal neurological deficits, such as hemiparesis. Symptoms generally progress insidiously with low-grade tumors, and more rapidly with malignant gliomas. Low-grade lesions are more likely than high-grade tumors to present with seizures as an isolated finding [4], whereas high-grade gliomas tend to present with headaches and focal neurological deficits. Chiasmatic-hypothalamic gliomas often present with visual loss, eye movement abnormalities, neuroendocrine dysfunction, behavioral and appetite disturbances, and failure to thrive.

Infratentorial tumors manifest in a variety of ways, depending on tumor type. Cerebellar astrocytomas often exhibit a several-month, and occasionally several-year, history of ataxia and headaches resulting from increased intracranial pressure due to obstruction of the fourth ventricle. In contrast, diffuse intrinsic brainstem gliomas characteristically manifest with rapidly progressive cranial neuropathies and long-tract signs, such as hemiparesis or quadriparesis.

Diagnostic investigation and staging

Either computed tomography (CT) or magnetic resonance imaging (MRI), performed with and without intravenous contrast, may be employed to establish the diagnosis of a brain tumor. MRI, if feasible to obtain, better delineates the location and anatomical relationships of the tumor, and is preferred in most circumstances. For certain types of gliomas, such as diffuse intrinsic brainstem glioma [52] and chiasmal gliomas in patients with NF1 [14], the MRI appearance is often sufficiently characteristic to establish the diagnosis without the need for biopsy confirmation. For tumors in which a resection has been attempted, post-operative imaging provides an objective measure of the amount of residual tumor, which is of major prognostic significance for several types of childhood glial tumors, guiding subsequent therapy. Ideally, such studies should be performed within 48 hours of surgery to minimize post-surgical enhancement, which complicates assessment of disease status. Staging evaluations are generally not warranted for childhood glial tumors, unless the patient manifests symptoms or signs suspicious for tumor dissemination, or suggestions of multifocal disease are apparent on the cranial MRI.

Treatment and outcome (Box 2.2)

Cerebral hemispheric low-grade gliomas

Surgical resection is typically the initial management approach for superficially situated low-grade hemispheric gliomas. Pilocytic tumors are often well circumscribed and amenable to complete removal in most cortical locations (Figure 2.1a). In comparison, non-pilocytic lesions often have less distinct margins and a greater tendency to infiltrate normal brain, and can be challenging to safely remove in functionally significant cortical regions

Box 2.2 Summary of treatment options.

Tumors in which extent of resection has been associated with progression-free survival

Low-grade cerebral and cerebellar astrocytomas

Oligodendrogliomas

Subependymal giant cell astrocytoma

Glioneuronal tumors

Malignant non-brainstem gliomas

Tumors in which chemotherapy plays a role in management

Unresectable/progressive low-grade gliomas and oligodendroglial tumors in young children

Non-brainstem malignant gliomas

Tumors in which radiotherapy plays a role in management

Unresectable/progressive low-grade gliomas and oligodendroglial tumors in older children and selected younger children

Non-brainstem malignant gliomas

Diffuse brainstem gliomas

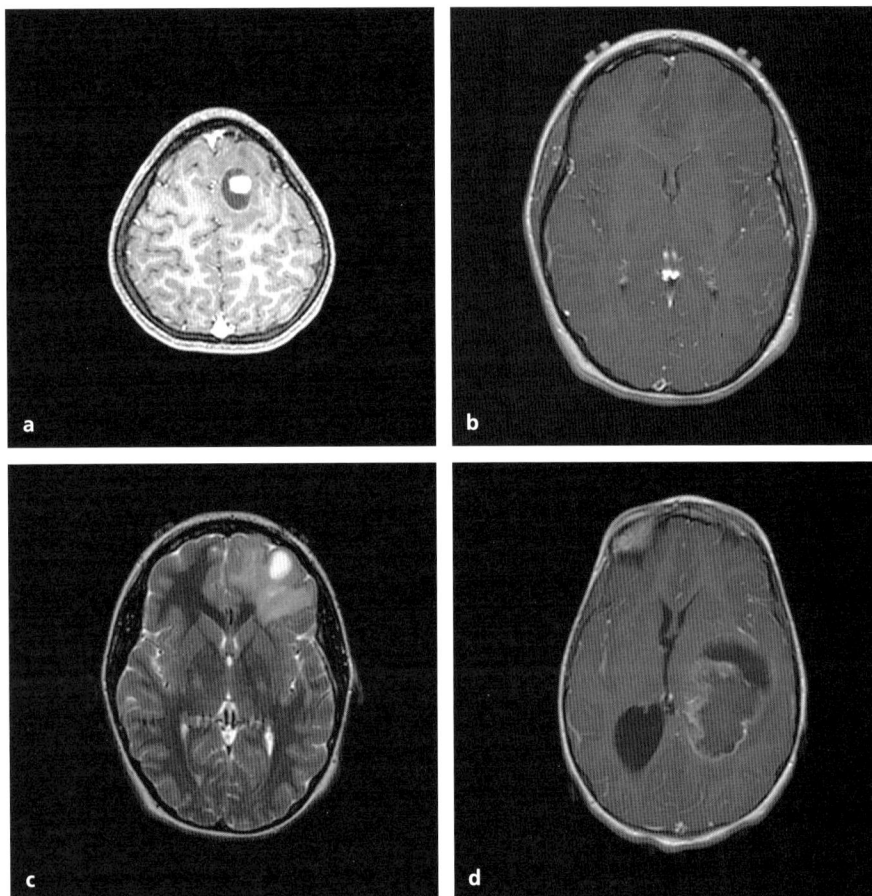

Figure 2.1 Cerebral hemispheric astrocytomas. (a), This superficial pilocytic astrocytoma incorporated a cyst with a well circumscribed mural nodule. (b), The margins of this low-grade non-pilocytic astrocytoma are poorly circumscribed on T1-weighted images. (c), The T2-weighted image of this tumor highlights the lesion's infiltrative nature. (d), This malignant glioma demonstrates irregular enhancement, significant mass effect, and a large area of central necrosis.

(Figure 2.1b, c). Because several studies, including an analysis of a large pediatric cooperative group natural history cohort, indicate that extent of resection is the most important predictor of outcome for these tumors [53, 54], there has been increasing interest in applying cortical mapping strategies (e.g. functional MRI and magnetoencephalography) and neuronavigational techniques to enhance the percentage of tumors amenable to gross total resection.

After a gross total resection, 5-year overall and progression-free survival rates exceed 90% [53–55]; as a result, adjuvant therapy is generally not used. In contrast, following incomplete resection, there is at least a 50% risk of disease progression within 5 years [53, 54]. Although children with pilocytic tumors seem to have a better prognosis than those with non-pilocytic lesions [53], a confounding factor is that pilocytic tumors are more likely to be well circumscribed and amenable to resection. Defining a prognostic effect of histology that is independent of resection extent has been difficult, even in large studies [54].

Management for patients with post-operative residual disease is controversial. Although at least half of such patients will progress within 5 years, overall 5-year survival for children with subtotally resected low-grade gliomas exceeds 90% [54], which is substantially better than results observed in adults [56–58], and provides some rationale for managing small amounts of residual disease in high-risk locations expectantly, particularly if the patient is asymptomatic. This prognostic difference reflects that progressive low-grade gliomas in adults commonly exhibit malignant transformation [56–59], whereas the vast majority of pediatric low-grade gliomas remain histologically benign at progression [53].

Although an attempt was made to define the role of radiotherapy for children with subtotally resected low-grade gliomas in the CCG9891/POG8930 study, this aim was not feasible because of persistent difficulties in accruing randomized patients. In a non-randomized institutional series, the use of radiotherapy after an initial incomplete resection significantly improved the frequency of progression-free survival, but had no influence on overall survival [53], reflecting that irradiated patients were more likely to develop malignant lesions within the treatment fields, a change that was not observed in the non-irradiated patients. Other groups have also noted an improvement in progression-free survival with irradiation, without a discernible advantage in terms of overall survival [56, 58, 60]. New methods of delivering fractionated radiotherapy using three-dimensional image-based treatment planning and delivery, coupled with the use of narrow peritumoral margins (i.e. stereotactic radiotherapy, conformal irradiation, intensity-modulated radiation therapy (IMRT)) have been developed in an effort to minimize treatment-induced morbidity [61–63]. This approach has been applied in a recent pilot study involving 47 children with progressive low-grade gliomas, in whom the target included the pre-operative tumor volume with a 2 mm margin, and doses ranged from 5000 to 5800 cGy in standard fractions. After a median follow-up of 3.4 years, there was only one local recurrence and no marginal failures [61].

Recent observations in a series of 17 patients indicated that cognitive function was unaffected in all but one patient with a four-year follow-up, suggesting that sequelae may be less than with conventional irradiation [63]. A conformal irradiation strategy is currently being evaluated in further detail in a cohort of 100 children in the Children's Oncology Group ACNS0221 study for children older than 10 years of age with progressive or high-risk residual low-grade gliomas, and for children younger than 10 years of age who have progressive disease after previous chemotherapy.

An alternative strategy, particularly in young children, involves the administration of chemotherapy to treat the unresectable residual disease [64, 65], thereby avoiding or delaying the risks of radiation to the developing nervous system [66–68] and the potential for radiation-induced malignancies [69], which together may counterbalance any improvements in progression-free survival that are potentially achieved by up-front irradiation [53]. This approach has been extensively evaluated in children with visual pathway gliomas (discussed below), but separate studies in children with hemispheric gliomas have not been performed. A third alternative is expectant management, since it is clear that a subset of incompletely resected lesions will show long-term stability without additional intervention. Because malignant degeneration of non-irradiated childhood low-grade gliomas is uncommon, lesions that progress after initial operation can potentially be treated with repeat resection [53, 70].

An additional consideration in the management of hemispheric low-grade gliomas is that many of these lesions manifest with seizures, which in some cases can prove intractable. In such instances, surgical strategies for tumor removal are coupled with extra- and intraoperative techniques, such as cortical mapping and electrocorticography, and functional imaging to enhance the likelihood of seizure control post-operatively, which is an important element of long-term quality of life in affected patients.

Supratentorial malignant (high-grade) gliomas

Current therapy for children older than three years of age with supratentorial malignant gliomas (Figure 2.1d) consists of maximal safe resection followed by irradiation to the tumor bed and a margin of surrounding brain to a dose of 5000–6000 cGy in 180 cGy/day fractions, in conjunction with some form of chemotherapy. This follows from the results of the Children's Cancer Group (CCG)-943 study, in which the use of adjuvant chemotherapy with lomustine (CCNU), vincristine, and prednisone was shown to enhance survival in comparison with treatment with irradiation alone [71]. An attempt to further improve outcome using the '8-in-1' regimen in the subsequent CCG-945 study was unsuccessful [72]. This provided the impetus for a series of subsequent studies by the CCG, the Pediatric Oncology Group, and European cooperative groups, which examined the efficacy of administering more intensive chemotherapy regimens in a neoadjuvant (pre-irradiation) setting [73–75]. Unfortunately, the results with several strategies were disappointing. For example, the CCG-9933 study compared the use of three different alkylating agents (carboplatin, ifosfamide, and cyclophosphamide) with etoposide, before irradiation. Each of these combinations was associated with a high rate of early disease progression, and progression-free survival was only in the range of 15% at 2 years [75]. In addition, the POG 9135 study examined the use of neoadjuvant cisplatin-BCNU *versus* cyclophosphamide-vincristine. The cisplatin-BCNU arm was associated with a 20% 5-year event-free survival, which was comparable to the results with adjuvant CCNU and vincristine, *versus* less than 5% for cyclophosphamide-vincristine ($P < 0.05$). Similarly, POG 9431 noted relatively poor activity of neoadjuvant procarbazine and topotecan [74].

A parallel strategy that attempted to enhance the efficacy of chemotherapy involved administering highly intensive myeloablative regimens coupled with autologous bone marrow or peripheral blood stem cell rescue. Although some studies suggested an improvement in outcome with this approach [76], the results were severely discouraging in others, and the potential for significant treatment-induced morbidity and mortality with some highly intensive regimens was a deterrent to further cooperative group application [77]. Although CCG-9922 noted an encouraging 2-year progression-free survival rate of 46% among 11 patients with newly diagnosed high-grade glioma who were treated with a highly intensive regimen that included carmustine (BCNU), thiotepa, and etoposide, there was a substantial incidence of significant pulmonary and/or neurologic toxicity, and an 18% toxic death rate, which limited enthusiasm for further exploration of this regimen [77].

As an alternate approach, more recent studies have attempted to enhance the efficacy of chemotherapy by administering active agents concurrently with, as well as after, irradiation [25], following up on the results of a trial for adults with malignant gliomas conducted by the EORTC in which treatment with radiation and concurrent as well as adjuvant temozolomide improved outcome compared to treatment with irradiation alone [78]. This study was not, however, designed to demonstrate that results with temozolomide were superior to those achieved with adjuvant nitrosourea therapy. In that context, a recently completed study of the Children's Oncology Group (ACNS0126), which evaluated the activity of administering temozolomide on a daily basis during irradiation and on a standard five-day schedule after irradiation, found that initial results were no better than those achieved in CCG-945 with adjuvant CCNU and vincristine [25]. An important observation of both the ACNS0126 and CCG-945 studies was that patients who had tumors that overexpressed MGMT, as assessed by immunohistochemistry, had a 2-year survival rate approaching 0%, significantly worse than those with non-overexpressing tumors [48, 49]. This mirrored the observations of the adult temozolomide study, in which MGMT status was assessed by promoter methylation, using methylation-specific PCR [47]. The impact of MGMT status on outcome was also examined in a follow-up study, which built upon the ACNS0126 backbone by adding CCNU in conjunction with temozolomide, based on promising results in the COG ADVL0011 study that

incorporated both agents in children with high-grade glioma who had bulky post-operative residual disease [79]. It is conceivable that subsequent studies will further extend these results by administering temozolomide with other chemotherapeutic and biologically targeted agents, by incorporating stratification based upon MGMT status, and by expanding on current pilot studies of the Pediatric Brain Tumor Consortium that are combining temozolomide with 06-benzylguanine as a way of reversing MGMT overexpression.

Another factor that has been associated with outcome in children with high-grade glioma, and has therefore constituted a stratification factor in a number of more recent studies, is the extent of post-operative residual disease. Patients who have undergone extensive tumor removal have had a significantly better outcome than those undergoing more limited surgery or biopsy alone [72, 80]. Although it impossible to exclude the possibility that certain tumors with more favorable biological characterics are inherently more amenable to radical resection [80], molecular studies that have attempted to control for biologically important factors have nonetheless noted a strong independent association between resection extent and outcome [24].

A second clinical factor associated with outcome is tumor histology [71]. Children with glioblastoma seem to fare worse than those with anaplastic astrocytoma, in agreement with data derived from adults [71, 72], although the trend is less striking. In addition, high-grade gliomas with an oligodendroglial component have a better prognosis than purely astrocytic malignant gliomas [72], possibly reflecting that oligodendroglial lesions are often more sensitive to adjuvant therapies [43]. Although in adults, this sensitivity correlates with 1p and 19q chromosomal deletions [43], no such association has been noted in childhood lesions [44].

Optic-hypothalamic glioma

Although optic-hypothalamic gliomas, also commonly referred to as visual pathway gliomas, are generally low-grade neoplasms histologically, they can vary widely in behavior between patients. Accordingly, their management is typically individualized. In patients with NF1, who are commonly found to have asymptomatic or minimally symptomatic lesions on screening imaging, management is often conservative initially, with intervention deferred until there is clear evidence of disease progression, because many such lesions will never progress. Accordingly, it warrants emphasis that not all chiasmal gliomas in children with NF1 require treatment [14]. Moreover, in rare cases, lesions have been observed to regress spontaneously. In those NF1 patients with symptomatic tumors, the etiology of the lesion is rarely in question and biopsy strictly for histological confirmation is usually not required [14, 81]. In contrast, biopsy confirmation is often prudent in patients with non-NF1-related suprasellar masses to rule out other histologies. In both the NF1 and non-NF1 subgroups, resection is generally limited to tumors that are exophytic and causing mass effect or hydrocephalus [82] (Figure 2.2a). Although complete resection is not safely feasible because

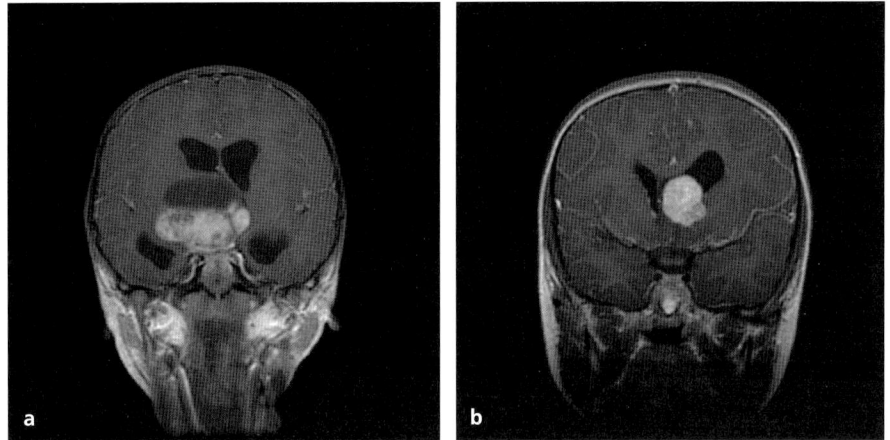

Figure 2.2 Supratentorial midline gliomas. (a), This exophytic, partially cystic chiasmatic hypothalamic glioma was amenable to debulking, which avoided the need for shunt insertion to treat the associated hydrocephalus. (b), This subependymal giant cell astrocytoma also presented with obstructive hydrocephalus, which resolved following tumor removal.

these lesions infiltrate the optic chiasm and hypothalamus, substantial cytoreduction can sometimes be achieved [82, 83]. An alternate strategy in such cases is to obtain a histological diagnosis by stereotactic or endoscopic biopsy and then give chemotherapy or irradiation initially, reserving resection for lesions that fail to respond.

The behavior of optic hypothalamic gliomas after treatment varies widely [84]. Whereas some lesions regress substantially, others enlarge rapidly despite treatment. Jenkin *et al.* [85] observed that survival was significantly better in patients with NF1 than in those without this diagnosis. A similar observation has been made in the recently completed Children's Oncology Group A9952 study, in which patients with NF1 had a significantly better prognosis than those without this diagnosis [86]. It has also been suggested that chiasmal gliomas that extend into the hypothalamus carry a worse prognosis than lesions situated exclusively in the chiasm [84]. In addition, tumors tend to behave more aggressively in infants than in older children [82–84, 86]. Recently, a histological subset of these tumors with 'pilomyxoid' features has been identified, and this group has been noted to have a more aggressive behavior than typical pilocytic lesions [87].

Radiation therapy has historically been the initial adjuvant treatment for these lesions and yields 5-year survival rates of 75–90% [84, 88]. However, because this modality, as administered in the past to young children with these midline tumors, has been associated with potentially disabling late effects of cognitive deterioration, endocrinopathy, moya moya syndrome, and second malignancies [66–69], chemotherapy has become the preferred approach in recent years in patients younger than 5–10 years [64, 65, 86]. A variety of regimens have been employed (e.g. carboplatin/vincristine and 6-thioguanine/procarbazine/CCNU/vincristine), with response or stabilization rates in excess of 75% [64, 65]. These two regimens were compared in terms of activity and tolerability in the A9952 study, the results of which are currently pending [86]. Another agent that has demonstrated activity against low-grade gliomas is temozolomide [89, 90], and the

feasibility of adding this agent to the carboplatin/vincristine backbone is being examined in the ACNS0223 study. More recently, studies have also been conducted using vinblastine, which has a lower incidence of neurological toxicity than vincristine and appears to exhibit promising independent activity [91]. Although some patients initially treated with chemotherapy later require radiotherapy for disease control, the deferral of irradiation for several years is probably beneficial in improving functional outcome. As a way to potentially minimize late effects from this modality, the ACNS0221 study is examining the efficacy of three-dimensional image-based conformal radiotherapy treatment planning and delivery in children who require irradiation for these tumors [92].

Ganglioglioma and benign neuroepithelial tumors

As with pilocytic astrocytomas, gangliogliomas are generally well circumscribed lesions amenable to complete resection with >90% 10-year survival rates in the absence of adjuvant therapy [93]. The role of radiotherapy for incompletely resected benign gangliogliomas remains unclear [93], and is generally reserved for tumors that progress after resection and are not deemed appropriate for repeat resection [94]. Notwithstanding the generally benign nature of these tumors, there is clearly a subgroup in which malignant progression and even dissemination can occur, calling attention to the need for close surveillance of lesions that are not amenable to complete removal.

Several other uncommon benign neuroepithelial tumors of childhood, such as desmoplastic infantile ganglioglioma [10, 11] and dysembryoplastic neuroepithelial tumor (DNET) [9] are also typically managed surgically. DNETs are indolent lesions that generally present with seizures and exhibit a favorable long-term outcome, although late recurrences have been reported [9, 30]. These tumors are often well circumscribed and amenable to complete resection. Accordingly, adjuvant therapy is commonly deferred [9, 30]. As with low-grade gliomas, post-operative seizure control is an important element in evaluating long-term functional outcome, and measures to localize and resect epileptogenic foci in the vicinity of the tumor have a role in improving ultimate seizure control.

In contrast to the above groups of tumors, desmoplastic infantile gangliogliomas often present with signs and symptoms of increased intracranial pressure. Although complete resection is the operative goal for these tumors and is associated with a favorable prognosis [10, 11, 95, 96], their size and vascularity in an infant with a limited blood volume may preclude a safe complete tumor removal in some cases. Several groups have examined administering adjuvant chemotherapy to patients with residual tumor [11] to prevent disease progression and induce tumor shrinkage, although this has not been systematically examined. This approach may provide a temporizing measure to allow a second-stage complete tumor resection, where clinically warranted. Other groups advocate expectant management and re-exploration in the event of tumor progression, because spontaneous regression of the residual tumor has sometimes been observed [97, 98].

Pleomorphic xanthoastrocytoma

Although these tumors have histological features that can sometimes be misinterpreted as malignant, they have a reasonably good prognosis, with survival rates in the range of 70–80 % at 10 years [26]. However, tumors with evidence of necrosis and increased mitotic activity or proliferation labeling have been noted to have a higher risk of progression than those without these features [27, 99–101]. As with other gliomas of childhood, extent of resection appears to have a strong association with outcome, with long-term survival in approximately 90% of patients after gross total resection versus only 65% after incomplete resection [99, 102]. The observation that tumors that recur often show evidence of necrosis at reoperation suggests that incompletely resected lesions exhibit a potential for malignant progression. However, the role of adjuvant radiotherapy in the treatment of such cases remains uncertain [27, 99].

Subependymal giant cell astrocytoma

These tumors arise almost exclusively in children with tuberous sclerosis in the vicinity of the foramen of Monro. As with tumors in children with NF1, many lesions are indolent and do not require treatment. Indications for operative intervention are large size or obstruction of the ventricular system. These tumors can be quite vascular and their juxtaposition to deep venous drainage can complicate attempts at complete removal [103]. The prognosis for long-term disease control is excellent after total or near total resection [104, 105] (Figure 2.2b). After less extensive resections, the residual tumor can enlarge slowly over time [103], although such lesions can be radically resected at a subsequent operation. Radiotherapy or stereotactic radiosurgery has on occasion been used for the management of unresectable recurrent lesions, although the efficacy of this strategy remains uncertain. More recently molecularly targeted therapy using inhibitors of mTOR have demonstrated promise in inducing disease regres-

sion, and these data suggest a potential alternative to surgery or radiation in the management of these lesions [138].

Oligodendroglioma and mixed oligo-astrocytoma

Oligodendrogliomas and mixed oligoastrocytomas of childhood are similar to low-grade astrocytomas in terms of their frequent presentation with seizures and their favorable response to surgical therapy. Lesions that are amenable to complete resection have an excellent long-term prognosis in children, with a 5-year survival rate in the range of 90%, which is superior to results reported in adults [53, 106, 107]. The adjuvant management of subtotally resected lesions remains controversial. Several groups have reported that incompletely resected childhood oligodendrogliomas show a low incidence of disease progression with several years of follow-up [106]. In that context, it has been noted that one of the strongest predictors of outcome among patients with oligodendrogliomas is the mode of presentation [107], and manifestation with seizures (the most frequent presenting symptom of these lesions during childhood) has been noted to be a favorable prognostic feature. However, our own experience suggests that many lesions will eventually progress slowly over time. Data from some adult cohorts have suggested that long-term disease control in patients with residual disease is favored by the use of involved field radiotherapy [108–110], although others have obtained contradictory data [111, 112]. In the absence of conclusive data for childhood oligodendroglial tumors, it is common to follow children with known residual disease expectantly, reserving further surgery or adjuvant therapy for those with tumor progression.

In recent years, there has been a trend for adult oligodendroglial tumors and to some extent in childhood lesions to treat patients with residual disease using chemotherapy, based on the observation that many tumors are chemosensitive [43]. In particular, adult low-grade and anaplastic oligodendroglial tumors with deletions of chromosomes 1p and 19q frequently have a favorable response to chemotherapy [43]. However, a similar association has not been detected in childhood lesions [44].

Cerebellar astrocytoma

Cerebellar pilocytic astrocytomas (Figure 2.3) are similar to cerebral cortical lesions in having an excellent prognosis after gross total surgical resection, with 10-year survival rates exceeding 95% [113, 114]. Non-pilocytic astrocytomas also generally have a favorable outcome if an extensive resection can be achieved [114]. As with other low-grade gliomas, prognosis is strongly affected by the extent of resection determined by post-operative imaging, and some surgeons advocate re-exploration if the post-operative MRI demonstrates accessible residual disease. However, in cases in which the residual tumor is deeply embedded in the vermis or adherent to the brainstem, expectant management is often advisable with intervention reserved for tumor remnants that eventually progress. In recent years, we have treated selected patients with small foci of deep-seated recurrent disease with stereotactic radiosurgery, with rates of disease regression and control that seem comparable to those achieved by reoperation

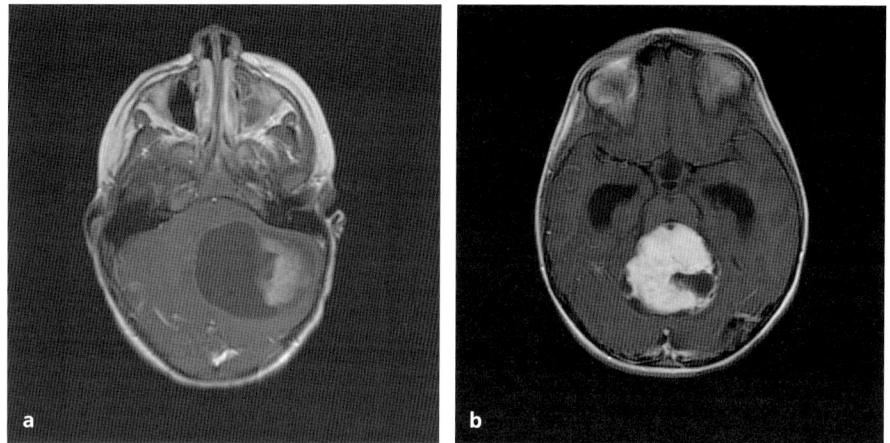

Figure 2.3 Cerebellar low-grade astrocytomas. (a), A cerebellar hemispheric pilocytic astrocytoma. (b), Histologically similar lesions can arise in the vermis.

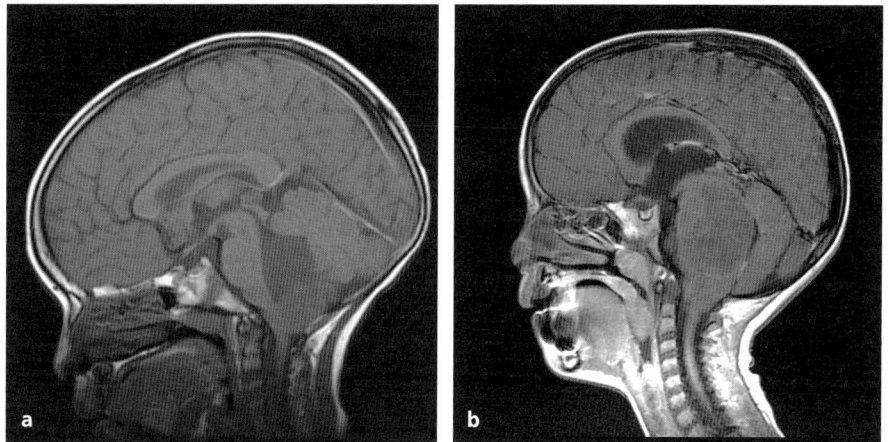

Figure 2.4 Brainstem gliomas. (a), A dorsally exophytic medullary glioma that was amenable to extensive resection. (b), A diffuse intrinsic brainstem glioma.

[115]. Alternatively, patients may be treated with conventionally fractionated radiotherapy or chemotherapy. Although histologic features suggestive of malignancy (e.g. vascular proliferation, leptomeningeal invasion, or occasional mitotic figures) in pilocytic astrocytomas do not necessarily indicate a poor prognosis [116], the same does not apply to non-pilocytic tumors, in which features of anaplasia are an adverse prognostic factor. Such lesions are treated identically to cerebral high-grade gliomas, with adjuvant radiotherapy and chemotherapy.

Brainstem gliomas

Brainstem gliomas have historically been considered to have an extremely poor prognosis, but reports during the MR era have highlighted the wide range of outcomes that characterize such lesions, depending on the growth characteristics of the tumor (i.e. focal or diffuse) [52]. On the most benign end of the spectrum are the intrinsic tectal tumors [117], which usually present with obstructive hydrocephalus, and are generally managed by cerebrospinal fluid (CSF) diversion, typically a third ventriculostomy, and expectant follow-up for the tumor. In our series of more than 40 such lesions managed without specific treatment for the

tumor, less than 25% have exhibited progression with a median follow-up in excess of 5 years. Dorsally exophytic brainstem gliomas are less indolent than the tectal tumors (Figure 2.4a), but nonetheless have an excellent prognosis with extensive resection, which is usually feasible [118–120]. Most prove histologically to be pilocytic astrocytomas or other low-grade glial lesions. Focal intrinsic midbrain, pontine, medullary, and cervicomedullary tumors are also histologically benign in most cases, although their removal carries higher risks because of the greater potential for brainstem injury [118, 119]. In some cases, such lesions have been effectively treated with biopsy or limited debulking in conjunction with focal radiotherapy or radiosurgery.

In contrast to the above groups of benign brainstem gliomas, diffuse intrinsic brainstem gliomas are biologically and generally histologically malignant lesions, and have a dismal prognosis with a median survival of less than one year [121–125]. The diagnosis is made based on a characteristic imaging appearance (Figure 2.4b) in the appropriate clinical setting, characterized by rapidly progressive cranial neuropathies and long-tract signs. Treatment is non-operative, apart from the need for CSF diversion in about 20% of cases, and has typically consisted of external beam irradiation to a dose of 5400–6000 cGy, administered to the tumor and a margin of surrounding brain. Radiotherapy frequently produces transient disease regression and symptomatic improvement, although the salutary effects are generally brief. To improve on these results, numerous studies have examined the efficacy of pre- and post-irradiation chemotherapy, although to date no regimen has been found to improve prognosis. In an early CCG study comparing irradiation alone versus irradiation plus adjuvant CCNU, vincristine, and prednisone, there was no survival benefit in patients who received chemotherapy [122], and subsequent studies using intensive pre- or post-irradiation chemotherapy have been equally disappointing [123–125].

Based on the ability of radiotherapy to promote at least transient tumor regression, there has been a rationale to examine approaches to enhance the efficacy of irradiation as a way to increase survival. Unfortunately, studies from both CCG and POG that attempted to escalate the dose of irradiation to as high as 7800 cGy using hyperfractionated delivery observed no improvement in survival [121, 123, 125, 126], even when combined with chemotherapy [123, 125], which dampened enthusiasm for further evaluating this approach.

A more recent strategy to potentially enhance the efficacy of irradiation has involved administering radiosensitizing or conventional chemotherapeutic agents concurrently with irradiation in order to potentiate the effect of this modality. This approach has been examined in studies of the SIOP and CCG involving topotecan, POG studies of cisplatin, phase I and II COG studies involving gadolinium texaphyrin and phase II studies of temozolomide. In addition, ongoing studies by the Pediatric Brain Tumor Consortium are exploring the efficacy of combining irradiation with molecularly targeted agents (see below – Novel Therapies) [127]. A limitation in validating the biological rationale for such therapies has been the lack of evaluable tissue for molecular characterization, which has necessitated a conjectural approach to agent selection based on assumptions that molecular data from non-brainstem high-grade gliomas in children and adults apply to diffuse brainstem gliomas. Although some studies have been conducted on archival material from the pre-MR era, during which brainstem gliomas still underwent biopsy [128], it is difficult in the absence of MR imaging to be certain what percentage of these cases were diffuse brainstem gliomas versus more benign brainstem tumors. The lack of contemporary tissue specimens for biological analysis clearly represents an additional challenge to making progress in the management of these tumors.

Strategies for follow-up and late effects

In terms of surveillance for tumor recurrence, there are no clear-cut guidelines for imaging or clinical follow-up in children with gliomas, and practices vary widely between institutions. Clearly, the frequency of monitoring needs to be tailored to the aggressiveness of the glioma being treated. For patients with benign intrinsic tectal tumors, annual or biennial follow-up visits and imaging are often sufficient. For completely resected cerebral and cerebellar astrocytomas, a follow-up scan and visit 3–6 months after surgery may be appropriate followed by a scan 1 year postoperatively and periodically thereafter. On the other hand, in patients with malignant gliomas or diffuse intrinsic brainstem tumors, follow-up should occur every 2–3 months because of the high risk of early progression.

Another aspect of follow-up relates to monitoring for late effects among long-term survivors, a particular issue in children who have received irradiation. Many of the most troubling sequelae in this regard are detected several years after diagnosis, which highlights the need for long-term multidisciplinary follow-up. Young children who have received whole brain irradiation have been noted to have a gradual decline in intelligence during the first 2 years after treatment [66, 67]. This may be mitigated by the use of focal irradiation, particularly if the medial temporal lobes and hypothalamus are outside the treatment volume.

Children who have received cranial irradiation also have an increased incidence of vasculopathy, particularly in those treated for chiasmatic-hypothalamic gliomas, presumably because of irradiation to the circle of Willis. Endocrine dysfunction is also common in children with these tumors [68], even in the absence of irradiation. As noted earlier, second neoplasms are also observed in up to 5% of children with brain tumors [69, 129]. The most common lesions in this regard are malignant gliomas, meningiomas, and sarcomas that occur within radiotherapy treatment fields 5–20 years after irradiation. In addition, the use of alkylating chemotherapy agents has been associated with an increased incidence of hematological malignancies.

Novel therapeutic approaches

Given the emergence of a variety of platforms to characterize tumors based on their protein expression, genotypic abnormalities and gene transcription, it is likely that future treatment will increasingly incorporate molecular phenotype into treatment planning [48]. Efforts to unravel the molecular pathways of tumor development have identified a number of genomic alterations and expression patterns that are commonly observed in malignant gliomas [130]. The involvement of transmembrane tyrosine kinases, such as EGFR and PDGFR, in tumorigenesis has fostered a series of studies of receptor inhibitors, such as erlotinib, gefitinib, and imatinib, in both the Children's Oncology Group and the Pediatric Brain Tumor Consortium. In parallel with these efforts, studies have examined the effect of interfering with downstream signaling transduction, by blocking Ras, Raf, PI3K and mTOR signaling.

An alternative approach for targeting cellular receptors that are overexpressed in brain tumors has involved the use of immunotoxin conjugates, in which binding to a cell surface receptor by a ligand or antibody conjugated to an immunotoxin provides a basis for toxin internalization and cell killing [131, 132]. Because such agents are large molecular weight molecules, drug administration typically involves convection-enhanced delivery in which the conjugates are delivered to the tumor and peritumoral brain by interstitial infusion and bulk flow.

A third experimental approach involves the use of immunotherapy in which tumor-specific antigens are delivered to the host immune system in the setting of dendritic cells or immunoadjuvants to promote antitumor immunoreactivity. Anecdotal reports of such studies suggest the potential for some activity [133, 134]. Finally, recent studies have begun to examine the effect on outcome of interfering with tumor-induced angiogenesis. Because this approach is predominantly considered cytostatic, rather than cytotoxic, ongoing studies are examining how best to combine such agents with conventional therapeutic approaches.

Summary and future directions for management

The management and outcome for children with gliomas varies widely as a function of tumor type. For low-grade gliomas, the factor that has the strongest impact on outcome is resection extent. For tumors that are amenable to extensive resection, outcome is excellent without the need for adjuvant therapy. Survival results appear to be significantly better than for similar lesions in adults. For unresectable midline low-grade gliomas, disease control can often be achieved with a combination of chemotherapy and irradiation, with the preferred option in part determined by the age of the patient. The optimal chemotherapy regimen remains to be defined as does the efficacy and activity of conformally directed irradiation. Despite these approaches, a percentage of children exhibit intractably progressive disease that ultimately proves fatal. For children with high-grade gliomas, the prognosis is even more discouraging, despite numerous studies over the last two decades. In view of the recently identified associations between molecular and biological markers and treatment response, it is likely that stratification of therapy based on such features will occur in future studies. Unfortunately, even in the best biological subgroups of high-grade gliomas, survival is less than 40%, calling attention to the need to continue to explore novel therapeutic approaches, as outlined above. The necessity for such approaches is even more strikingly demonstrated in children with diffuse intrinsic brainstem gliomas, for which prognostically useful biological information has been lacking. The outcome for children with such tumors has shown no improvement during the last two decades, highlighting the need for radically different treatment strategies and innovative therapies for these challenging neoplasms.

Acknowledgment

This work was supported in part by NIH grants P01NS40923 and R01NS37704.

References

1 Bar EE, Lin A, Tihan T, Burger PC, Eberhart CG. Frequent gains at chromosome 7q34 involving BRAF in pilocytic astrocytoma. J Neuropathol Exp Neurol 2008; 67: 878–87.

2 Jones DT, Kocialkowski S, Liu L, et al. Tandem duplication producing a novel oncogenic BRAF fusion gene defines the majority of pilocytic astrocytomas. Cancer Res 2008; 68: 8673–77.

3 Korshunov A, Meyer J, Capper D, et al. Combined molecular analysis of BRAF and IDH1 distinguishes pilocytic astrocytoma from diffuse astrocytoma. Acta Neuropathol 2009; 118: 401–5.

4 Pollack IF. Brain tumors in children. N Engl J Med 1994; 331: 1500–7.

5 Young JL. Cancer incidence, survival, and mortality for children younger than 15 years. Cancer 1986; 58: 561–8.

6 Kleihues P, Burger PC, Scheithauer BW, et al. World Health Organization Histological Typing of Tumours of the Central Nervous System. New York: Springer-Verlag, 1993.

7 Berger MS, Keles GE, Geyer JR. Cerebral hemispheric tumors of childhood. Pediatr Neuro-Oncol 1992; 3: 839–52.

8 Giannini C, Scheithauer BW, Burger PC, et al. Pleomorphic xanthoastrocytoma: what do we really know about it. Cancer 1999; 85: 2033–45.

9 Daumas-Duport C, Scheithauer BW, Chodkiewicz J-P, et al. Dysembryoplastic neuroepithelial tumor (DNT): a surgically curable tumor of young subjects with intractable partial seizures: report of 39 cases. Neurosurgery 1988; 23: 545–56.

10 VandenBerg SR, May EE, Rubinstein LJ, et al. Desmoplastic supratentorial neuroepithelial tumors of infancy with divergent differentiation potential ('desmoplastic infantile gangliogliomas'). Report on 11 cases of a distinctive embryonal tumor with a favorable prognosis. J Neurosurg 1987; 66: 58–71.

11 Duffner PK, Burger PC, Cohen ME, et al. Desmoplastic infantile gangliogliomas: an approach to therapy. Neurosurgery 1994; 34: 583–9.

12 Xu G, O'Connell P, Viskochil D, et al. The neurofibromatosis type 1 gene encodes a protein related to GAP. Cell 1990; 62: 599–608.

13 Basu TN, Gutmann DH, Fletcher JA, et al. Aberrant regulation of ras proteins in malignant tumors cells from type 1 neurofibromatosis patients. Nature 1992; 356: 713–15.

14 Pollack IF, Mulvihill JJ. Special issues in the management of gliomas in children with neurofibromatosis 1. J Neuro-oncol 1996; 28: 257–68.

15 The European Chromosome 16 Tuberous Sclerosis Consortium. Identification and characterization of the tuberous sclerosis gene on chromosome 16. Cell 1993; 75: 1305–15.

16 Hamilton SR, Lui B, Parsons RE, et al. The molecular basis of Turcot's syndrome. N Engl J Med 1995; 332: 839–47.

17 Kikuchi T, Rempel SA, Rutz H-P, et al. Turcot's syndrome of glioma and polyposis occurs in the absence of germ line mutations of exons 5 to 9 of the p53 gene. Cancer Res 1993; 53: 957–61.

18 Kyritsis AP, Bondy ML, Xiao M, et al. Germline p53 gene mutations in subsets of glioma patients. J Natl Cancer Inst 1994; 86: 344–9.

19 Bailey P, Cushing H. A Classification of Tumors of the Glioma on a Histogenetic Basis with a Correlated Study of Prognosis. Philadelphia: JB Lippincott, 1926.

20 Kernohan J, Mabon RF, Svien JH, et al. A simplified classification of gliomas. Proc Staff Meet Mayo Clin 1949; 24: 71–5.

21 Burger PC, Vogel FS. Surgical Pathology of the Nervous System and its Coverings. 2nd edn. New York: John Wiley and Sons, 1982: 226–66.

22 Daumas-Duport C, Scheithauer B, O'Fallon J, et al. Grading of astrocytomas: a simple and reproducible grading method. Cancer 1988; 62: 2152–65.

23 Gilles FH, Sobel EL, Leviton A, Tavaré CJ, Hedley-Whyte ET. Histological feature reliablity in childhood neural tumors. J Neuropath Exp Neurol 1994; 53: 559–71.

24 Pollack IF, Boyett JM, Yates AJ, Burger PC, Gilles FH, Davis RL, Finlay JL. The influence of central review on outcome associations in childhood malignant gliomas: results from the CCG-945 experience. Neuro-Oncology 2003; 5: 197–207.

25 Cohen KJ, Heideman R, Zhou T, et al. Should temozolomide be the standard of care for children with newly diagnosed high grade gliomas? Results of the Children's Oncology Group ACNS0126 study. Neuro-Oncology 2007, in press.

26 Kepes JJ, Rubinstein LJ, Eng LF. Pleomorphic xanthoastrocytoma: a distinctive meningocerebral glioma of young subjects with relatively favorable prognosis; a study of 12 cases. Cancer 1979; 44: 1839–52.

27 Macauley RJ, Jay V, Hoffman HJ, et al. Increased mitotic activity as a negative prognostic indicator in pleomorphic xanthoastrocytoma. J Neurosurg 1993; 79: 761–7.

28 Nakamura Y, Becker LE. Subependymal giant cell tumor: astrocytic or neuronal? Acta Neuropathol (Berl) 1983; 60: 271–7.

29 Miller DC, Lang FF, Epstein FJ. Central nervous system ganglioglio-mas. Part 1. Pathology. J Neurosurg 1993; 79: 859–66.

30 Taratuto AL, Pomata H, Sevlever G, Gallo G, Monges J. Dysembryoplastic neuroepithelial tumor: morphological, immuno-cytochemical, and deoxyribonucleic acid analyses in a pediatric series. Neurosurgery 1995; 36: 474–81.

31 von Deimling A, Louis DN, Menon AG, et al. Deletions on the long arm of chromosome 17 in pilocytic astrocytoma. Acta Neuropathol 1993; 86: 81–5.

32 Lang FF, Miller DC, Pisharody S, et al. High frequency of p53 protein accumulation without p53 gene mutation in human juvenile pilocytic, low grade and anaplastic astrocytomas. Oncogene 1994; 9: 949–54.

33 Rasheed BKA, McLendon RE, Herndon RE, et al. Alterations of the TP53 gene in human gliomas. Cancer Res 1994; 54: 1324–30.

34 Pollack IF, Finkelstein SD, et al. Age and TP53 mutation frequency in childhood gliomas. Results in a multi-institutional cohort. Cancer Res 2001; 61: 7404–7.

35 Sidransky D, Mikkelsen T, Schwechheimer K, et al. Clonal expansion of p53 mutant cells is associated with brain tumor progression. Nature 1992; 355: 846–7.

36 Collins VP. Progression as exemplified by human astrocytic tumors. Cancer Biol 1999; 9: 267–76.

37 Pollack IF, Finkelstein SD, Woods J, et al. Expression of p53 and prognosis in malignant gliomas in children. N Engl J Med 2002; 346: 420–7.

38 Sung T, Miller DC, Hayes RL, Alonso M, Yee H, Newcombe EW. Preferential inactivation of the p53 tumor suppressor pathway and lack of EGFR amplification distinguish de novo high grade pediatric astrocytomas from de novo adult astrocytomas. Brain Pathol 2000; 10: 249–59.

39 Bredel M, Pollack IF, Hamilton RL, James CD. Epidermal growth factor receptor (EGFR) expression in high-grade non-brainstem gliomas of childhood. Clin Cancer Res 1999; 5: 1786–92.

40 Raffel C, Frederick L, O'Fallon JR, et al. Analysis of oncogene and tumor suppressor gene alterations in pediatric malignant astrocyto-mas reveals reduced survival for patients with PTEN mutations. Clin Cancer Res 1999; 5: 4085–90.

41 Pollack IF, Hamilton RL, James CD, et al. Rarity of PTEN deletions and EGFR amplification in malignant gliomas of childhood: results from the Children's Cancer Group 945 cohort. J Neurosurg: Pediatr 2006; 105: 3431–7.

42 Cheng Y, Ng, H-K, Zhang S-F, Ding M, Pang JC-S, Zheng J, Poon W-S. Genetic alterations in pediatric high-grade astrocytomas. Hum Pathol 1999; 30: 1284–90.

43 Ino Y, Betensky RA, Zlatescu MC, et al. Molecular subtypes of ana-plastic oligodendroglioma: implications for patient management at diagnosis. Clin Cancer Res 2001; 7: 839–45.

44 Pollack IF, Finkelstein SD, Burnham J, et al. The association between chromosome 1p loss and outcome in pediatric malignant gliomas: results from the CCG-945 cohort. Pediatr Neurosurg 2003; 39: 114–21.

45 Esteller M, Garcia-Foncillas J, Andion E, et al. Inactivation of the DNA-repair gene MGMT and the clinical response of gliomas to alkylating agents. N Engl J Med 2000; 343: 1350–4.

46 Belanich M, Pastor M, Randall T, et al. Retrospective study of the correlation between DNA repair protein alkyltransferase and sur-vival of brain tumor patients treated with carmustine. Cancer Res 1996; 56: 783–8.

47 Hegi ME, Diserens A-C, Gorlia T, et al. MGMT gene silencing and benefit from temozolomide in glioblastoma. N Engl J Med 2005; 352: 997–1003.

48 Pollack IF, Hamilton RL, Sobol RW, et al. O⁶-methylguanine-DNA methyltransferase expression strongly correlates with outcome in childhood malignant gliomas: results from the CCG-945 cohort. J Clin Oncol 2006; 24: 3431–7.

49 Pollack IF, Hamilton RL, Burnham J, et al.. Molecular predictors of outcome in childhood malignant gliomas. The Children's Oncology Group Experience. Neuro-Oncology 2007; 9: 188.

50 Albright AL. Brain tumors in neonates, infants, and toddlers. Contemp Neurosurg 1985; 7: 1–8.

51 Reed UC, Rosenberg S, Gherpelli JLD, et al. Brain tumors in the first two years of life: a review of forty cases. Pediatr Neurosurg 1993; 19: 180–5.

52 Albright AL, Packer RJ, Zimmerman R, et al. Magnetic resonance scans should replace biopsies for the diagnosis of diffuse brain stem gliomas: a report from the Children's Cancer Group. Neurosurgery 1993; 1026–30.

53 Pollack IF, Claassen D, Al-Shboul Q, et al. Low-grade gliomas of the cerebral hemispheres in children: an analysis of 71 cases. J Neurosurg 1995; 82: 536–47.

54 Sanford A, Kun L, Sposto R, et al. Low-grade gliomas of childhood: impact of surgical resection. A report from the Children's Oncology Group. J Neurosurg 2002; 96: 427–8.

55 Hirsch J-F, Rose CS, Pierre-Kahn A, et al. Benign astrocytic and oligodendroglial tumors of the cerebral hemispheres in children. J Neurosurg 1989; 70: 568–72.

56 Laws ER Jr, Taylor WF, Clifton MB, et al. Neurosurgical manage-ment of low-grade astrocytoma of the cerebral hemispheres. J Neurosurg 1984; 61: 665–73.

57 Vertosick FT Jr, Selker RG, Arena VC. Survival of patients with well-differentiated astrocytomas diagnosed in the era of computed tom-ography. Neurosurgery 1991; 28: 496–501.

58 Philippon JH, Clemenceau SH, Fauchon FH, et al. Supratentorial low-grade astrocytomas in adults. Neurosurgery 1993; 32: 554–9.

59 Muller W, Afra D, Schroder R. Supratentorial recurrences of gliomas. Morphological studies in relation to time intervals with astrocytomas. Acta Neurochirurgica 1977; 37: 75–91.

60 Shaw EG, Daumas-Duport C, Scheithauer BW, et al. Radiation therapy in the management of low-grade supratentorial astrocytomas. J Neurosurg 1989; 70: 853–61.

61 Dutton SC, Goumnerova L, Billett AL, et al. Fractionated stereotactic radiotherapy for localized pediatric brain tumors: results of a prospective study. Int J Radiat Oncol Biol Phys 1999; 45(Suppl 1): 234 (Abst).

62 Nishihori T, Shirato H, Aoyama H, et al. Three-dimensional conformal radiotherapy for astrocytic tumors involving the eloquent area in children and young adults. J Neuro-Oncol 2002; 60: 177–83.

63 Vigliani MC, Sichez N, Poisson M, Delattre JY. A prospective study of cognitive functions following conventional radiotherapy for supratentorial gliomas in young adults: 4-year results. Int J Radiat Oncol Biol Phys 1996; 35: 527–33.

64 Packer RJ, Ater J, Allen J, et al. Carboplatin and vincristine chemotherapy for children with newly diagnosed progressive low-grade gliomas. J Neurosurg 1997; 86: 747–54.

65 Petronio J, Edwards MSB, Prados M, et al. Management of chiasmal and hypothalamic gliomas of infancy and childhood with chemotherapy. J Neurosurg 1991; 74: 701–8.

66 Ellenberg L, McComb JG, Siegel S, Stowe S. Factors affecting intellectual outcome in pediatric brain tumor patients. Neurosurgery 1987; 21: 638–44.

67 Radcliffe J, Packer RJ, Atkins TE, et al. Three- and four-year cognitive outcome in children with noncortical brain tumors treated with whole-brain radiotherapy. Ann Neurology 1992; 32: 551–4.

68 Livesey EA, Hindmarsh PC, Brook CGD, et al. Endocrine disorders following treatment of childhood brain tumors. Br J Cancer 1990; 61: 622–5.

69 Dirks PB, Jay V, Becker LE, et al. Development of anaplastic changes in low-grade astrocytomas of childhood. Neurosurgery 1994; 34: 68–78.

70 Bowers DC, Krause TP, Aronson LJ, et al. Second surgery for recurrent pilocytic astrocytoma. Pediatr Neurosurg 2001; 34: 229–34.

71 Sposto R, Ertel IJ, Jenkin RDT, et al. The effectiveness of chemotherapy for treatment of high-grade astrocytoma in children: results of a randomized trial. J Neuro-oncol 1989; 7: 165–77.

72 Finlay J, Boyett J, Yates A, et al. Randomized phase III trial in childhood high-grade astrocytoma comparing vincristine, lomustine, and prednisone with the eight-drugs-in-1-day regimen. J Clin Oncol 1995; 13: 112–23.

73 Pollack IF, Boyett J, Finlay JL. Chemotherapy for high-grade gliomas of childhood. Child's Nerv Syst 1999; 15: 529–44.

74 Chintagumpala MM, Friedman HS, Stewart CF, et al. Pediatric Oncology Group Study. A phase II window trial of procarbazine and topotecan in children with high-grade glioma: a report from the Children's Oncology Group. J Neuro-Oncol 2006; 77: 193–8.

75 MacDonald TJ, Arenson EB, Ater J, et al. Phase II study of high-dose chemotherapy before radiation in children with newly diagnosed high-grade astrocytoma: final analysis of Children's Cancer Group Study 9933. Cancer 104: 2862–71.

76 Wolff JE, Gnekow AK, Kortmann RD, et al. Preradiation chemotherapy for pediatric patients with high-grade glioma. Cancer 2002; 94: 264–71.

77 Grovas AC, Boyett JM, Lindsley K, et al. Regimen-related toxicity of myeloablative chemotherapy with BCNU, thiotepa, and etoposide followed by autologous stem cell rescue for children with newly diagnosed glioblastoma multiforme: report from the Children's Cancer Group. Med Pediatr Oncol 1999; 33: 83–7.

78 Stupp R, Dietrich PY, Ostermann-Kraljevic S, et al. Promising survival with newly diagnosed glioblastoma multiforme treated with concomitant radiation plus temozolomide followed by adjuvant temozolomide. J Clin Oncol 2002; 20: 1375–82.

79 Jakacki R, Yates A, Zhou T, et al. A phase I trial of temozolomide and lomustine in newly diagnosed high-grade gliomas of childhood. 2008; 10(4): 569–76.

80 Campbell JW, Pollack IF, Martinez AJ, Shultz BL. High-grade astrocytomas in children: radiologically complete resection is associated with an excellent long-term prognosis. Neurosurgery 1996; 38: 258–64.

81 Listernak R, Charrow J, Greenwald MJ, Esterly NB. Optic gliomas in children with neurofibromatosis type 1. J Pediatr 1989; 114: 788–92.

82 Wisoff JH, Abbott R, Epstein F. Surgical management of exophytic chiasmatic-hypothalamic tumors of childhood. J Neurosurg 1990; 73: 661–7.

83 Hoffman HJ, Humphreys RP, Drake JM, et al. Optic pathway/hypothalamic gliomas: a dilemmna in management. Pediatr Neurosurg 1993; 19: 186–95.

84 Alvord E Jr, Lofton S. Gliomas of the optic nerve and chiasm. Outcome by patient's age, tumor site, and treatment. J Neurosurg 1988; 68: 85–98.

85 Jenkin D, Angyalfi S, Becker L, et al. Optic glioma in children: surveillance, resection or irradiation? Int J Rad Oncol Biol Phys 1993; 25: 215–25.

86 Ater J, Holmes E, Zhou T, et al. Treatment of young children with progressive or symptomatic low-grade glioma with chemotherapy: Preliminary report from the Children's Oncology Group (COG) Phase 3 protocol A9952. Neuro-Oncology 2006; 8: 465.

87 Komotar RJ, Burger PC, Carson BS, et al. Pilocytic and pilomyxoid hypothalamic/chiasmatic astrocytomas. Neurosurgery 2004; 54: 72–9.

88 Pierce SM, Barnes PD, Loeffler JS, et al. Definitive radiation therapy in the management of symptomatic patients with optic glioma. Survival and long-term effects. Cancer 1990; 65: 45–52.

89 Quinn JA, Reardon DA, Friedman AH, et al. Phase II trial of temozolomide in patients with progressive low-grade glioma. J Clin Oncol 2003; 21: 646–51.

90 Kuo DJ, Weiner HL, Wisoff J, et al. Temozolomide is active in childhood, progressive, unresectable, low-grade gliomas. J Pediatr Hematol Oncol 2003; 25: 372–8.

91 Lafay-Cousin L, Holm S, Qaddoumi I, et al. Weekly vinblastine in pediatric low-grade glioma patients with carboplatin allergic reaction. Cancer 2005; 103: 2636–42.

92 Nishihori T, Shirato H, Aoyama H, et al. Three-dimensional conformal radiotherapy for astrocytic tumors involving the eloquent area in children and young adults. J Neuro-Oncol 2002; 60: 177–83.

93 Lang FF, Epstein FJ, Ransohoff J, et al. Central nervous system gangliogliomas. Part 2: Clinical outcome. J Neurosurg 1993; 79: 867–73.

94 Matsumoto K, Tamiya T, Ono Y, Furuta T, Asari S, Ohmoto T. Cerebral gangliogliomas: clinical characteristics, CT and MRI. Acta Neurochir 1999; 141: 135–41.

95 Sugiyama K, Arita K, Shima T, et al. Good clinical course in infants with desmoplastic cerebral neuroepithelial tumor treated by surgery alone. J Neuro-Oncol 2002; 59: 63–9.

96 Mallucci C, Lellouch-Tubiana A, Salazar C, et al. The management of desmoplastic neuroepithelial tumors in childhood. Childs Nerv Syst 2000; 16: 8–14.

97 Bachli H, Avoledo P, Gratzl O, Tolnay M. Therapeutic strategies and management of desmoplastic infantile ganglioglioma: two case reports and literature overview. Childs Nerv Syst 2003; 19: 359–66.

98 Tamburrini G, Colosimo C Jr, Giangaspero F, Riccardi R, Di Rocco C. Desmoplastic infantile ganglioglioma. Childs Nerv Syst 2003; 19: 292–7.

99 Papahill PA, Ramsay DA, Del Maestro RF. Pleomorphic xanthoastrocytoma: case report and analysis of the literature concerning the efficacy of resection and the significance of necrosis. Neurosurgery 1996; 38: 822–9.

100 Prayson RA, Morris HH 3rd. Anaplastic pleomorphic xanthoastrocytoma. Arch Path Lab Med 1998; 122: 1082–6.

101 Sugita Y, Shigemori M, Okamoto K, Morimatsu M, Arakawa M, Nakayama K. Clinicopathological study of pleomorphic xanthoastrocytoma: correlation between histological features and prognosis. Pathol Internat 2000; 50: 703–8.

102 Fouladi M, Jenkins J, Burger P, et al. Pleomorphic xanthoastrocytoma: favorable outcome after complete surgical resection. Neuro-Oncol 2001; 3: 184–92.

103 Sinson G, Sutton LN, Yachnis AT, et al. Subependymal giant cell astrocytomas in children. Pediatr Neurosurg 1994; 20: 233–9.

104 Cuccia V, Zuccaro G, Sosa F, Monges J, Lubienieky F, Taratuto AL. Subependymal giant cell astrocytoma in children with tuberous sclerosis. Childs Nerv Syst 2003; 19: 232–43.

105 Torres OA, Roach ES, Delgado MR, et al. Early diagnosis of subependymal giant cell astrocytoma in patients with tuberous sclerosis. J Child Neurol 1998; 13: 173–7.

106 Tice H, Barnes PD, Goumnerova L, et al. Pediatric and adolescent oligodendrogliomas. Am J Neuroradiol 1993; 14: 1293–300.

107 Celli P, Nofrone I, Palma L, et al. Cerebral oligodendroglioma: prognostic factors and life history. Neurosurgery 1994; 35: 1018–35.

108 Shaw EG, Scheithauer BW, O'Fallon JR, et al. Oligodendrogliomas: the Mayo Clinic experience. J Neurosurg 1992; 76: 428–34.

109 Wallner KE, Gonzales M, Sheline GE. Treatment of oligodendrogliomas with or without postoperative irradiation. J Neurosurg 1988; 68: 684–8.

110 Lindegaard K-F, Mork SJ, Eide GE, et al. Statistical analysis of clinicopathological features, radiotherapy, and survival in 170 cases of oligodendroglioma. J Neurosurg 1987; 67: 224–30.

111 Westergaard L, Gjerris F, Klinken L. Prognostic factors in oligodendrogliomas. Acta Neurochirurg 1997; 139: 600–9.

112 Bullard DE, Rawlings CE III, Phillips B, et al. An analysis of the value of radiation therapy. Cancer 1987; 60: 2179–88.

113 Garcia DM, Latifi HR, Simpson JR, et al. Astrocytomas of the cerebellum in children. J Neurosurg 1989; 71: 661–4.

114 Schneider JH, Raffel C, McComb JG. Benign cerebellar astrocytomas of childhood. Neurosurg 1992; 30: 58–63.

115 Somaza SC, Kondziolka D, Lunsford LD, Flickinger JC, Bissonette DJ, Albright AL. Early outcomes after stereotactic radiosurgery for growing pilocytic astrocytomas in children. Pediatric Neurosurg 1996; 25: 109–15.

116 Tomlinson FH, Scheithauer BW, Hayostek CJ, et al. The significance of atypia and histologic malignancy in pilocytic astrocytoma of the cerebellum: a clinicopathologic and flow cytometric study. J Child Neurol 1994; 9: 301–10.

117 Pollack IF, Pang D, Albright AL. The long-term outcome in children with late-onset aqueductal stenosis resulting from benign intrinsic tectal tumors. J Neurosurg 1994; 80: 681–8.

118 Abbott R, Coh KYC. Brainstem gliomas. In: Albright AL, Pollack IF, Adelson PD (Eds), Principles and Practice of Pediatric Neurosurgery. New York: Thieme, 1999; 629–40.

119 Epstein FJ, Constantini S. Practical decisions in the treatment of pediatric brain stem tumors. Pediatr Neurosurg 1999; 24: 24–34.

120 Pollack IF, Hoffman HJ, Humphreys RP, Becker L. The long-term outcome after surgical treatment of dorsally exophytic brain-stem gliomas. J Neurosurg 1993; 78: 859–63.

121 Packer RJ, Boyett JM, Zimmerman RA, et al. Outcome of children with brain stem gliomas after treatment with 7800 cGy of hyperfractionated radiotherapy. Cancer 1994; 74: 1827–34.

122 Jenkin RDT, Boesel C, Ertel I, et al. Brain-stem tumors in childhood: a prospective randomized trial of irradiation with and without adjuvant CCNU, VCR, and prednisone. J Neurosurg 1987; 66: 227–33.

123 Kretschmar CS, Tarbell NJ, Barnes PD et al. Pre-irradiation chemotherapy and hyperfractionated radiation therapy 66Gy for children with brain stem tumors. Cancer 1993; 72: 1404–13.

124 Dunkel IJ, Garvin JH, Goldman S, et al. High dose chemotherapy with autologous bone marrow rescue for children with diffuse pontine brain stem tumors. J Neurooncol 1998; 37: 67–73.

125 Jennings MT, Sposto R, Boyett JM, et al. Pre-radiation chemotherapy in primary high risk brain stem tumors: CCG-9941, a phase II study of the Children's Cancer Group. J Clin Oncol 2002; 20: 3431–7.

126 Freeman CR, Krischer JP, Sanford RA, Cohen ME, et al. Final results of a study of escalating doses of hyperfractionated radiotherapy in brain stem tumors in children, A Pediatric Oncology Group study. Int J Radiat Oncol Biol Phys 1993; 27: 197–206.

127 Pollack IF, Jakacki RI, Blaney SM, et al. Phase I trial of imatinib in children with newly diagnosed brainstem and recurrent malignant gliomas: A Pediatric Brain Tumor Consortium Report, Neuro Oncology 2007; 9: 145–60.

128 Gilbertson RJ, Hill A, Hernan R, et al. *ERBB1* is amplified and overexpressed in high-grade diffusely infiltrative pediatric brain stem glioma. Clin Cancer Res 2003; 9: 3620–4.

129 Peterson KM, Shao C, McCarter R, MacDonald TJ, Byrne J. An analysis of SEER data of increasing risk of secondary malignant neoplasms among long-term survivors of childhood brain tumors. Pediatric Blood Cancer 2006; 47: 83–8.

130 Pollack IF. Growth factor signaling pathways and receptor tyrosine kinase inhibitors. In: Newton HB (Ed), Handbook of Brain Tumor Chemotherapy. Philadelphia: Elsevier, 2006; 155–72.

131 Laske DW, Youle RJ, Oldfield EH. Tumor regression with regional distribution of the targeted toxin TF-CRM107 in patients with malignant brain tumors. Nature Med 1997; 3: 1362–8.

132 Sampson JH, Akabani G, Archer GE, et al. Progress report of a phase I study of the intracerebral microinfusion of a recombinant chimeric protein composed of transforming growth factor (TGF)-α and a mutated form of the *Pseudomonas* exotoxin termed PE-38 (TP-38) for the treatment of malignant brain tumors. J Neuro-Oncol 2003; 65: 27–35.

133 Kikuchi T, Akasaki Y, Irie M, Homma S, Abe T, Ohno T. Results of a phase I clinical trial of vaccination of glioma patients with fusions

of dendritic and glioma cells. Cancer Immunology Immunother 2001; 50: 337–44.

134 Okada H, Lieberman FS, Edington HD, et al. Interleukin-4 gene transfected autologous tumor cell vaccine in the treatment of recurrent glioblastoma: preliminary observations in a patient with a favorable response to therapy. J Neuro-Oncol 2003; 64: 13–20.

135 Verhaak RGW, Hoadley KA, Purdom E, et al. Integrated genomic analysis identifies clinically relevant subtypes of glioblastoma characterized by abnormalities in *PDGFR, IDH1, EGFR,* and *NF1.* Cancer Cell 2010; 17: 98–110.

136 Parsons DW, Jones S, Zhang X, et al. An integrated genomic analysis of human glioblastoma multiforme. Science 2008; 321: 1807–12.

137 Hartmann C, Meyer J, Balss J, et al. Type and frequency of IDH1 and IDH2 mutations are related to astrocytic and oligodendroglial differentiation and age: a study of 1,010 diffuse gliomas. Acta Neuropathol 2009; 118: 469–74.

138 Lam C, Bouffet E, Tabori U, Mabbott D, Taylor M, Bartels U. Rapamycin (sirolimus) in tuberous sclerosis associated pediatric central nervous system tumors. Pediatric Blood Cancer 2010; 54: 476–9.

3 Ependymoma

Thomas E. Merchant[1] and Richard J. Gilbertson[2]

[1] Division of Radiation Oncology and [2] Departments of Developmental Neurobiology and Oncology, St Jude Children's Research Hospital, Memphis, TN, USA

Introduction

Ependymomas are one of four types of ependymal tumor that originate throughout the central nervous system (CNS) from the wall of the ventricular system and the spinal canal [1]. These tumors display moderate cellularity, ultrastructural properties of ependymal cells and express markers of glial differentiation [1]. Ependymomas arise in all age groups, but children and adults are predisposed to develop these tumors in different parts of the CNS [2]. Posterior fossa ependymoma presents most often in patients aged less than 10 years, while spinal tumors are largely a disease of adults [3]. The variable patterns of histology and clinical presentation of ependymoma, and the separation of pediatric and adult oncology services, have hindered efforts to coordinate clinical trials in this disease. As a result, no new therapeutic approaches have been identified to treat ependymoma during the last 20 years and up to 40% of patients' tumors remain incurable [4, 5]. Current treatments for ependymoma include aggressive surgical resection and radiation therapy. No effective conventional chemotherapy regimens to treat ependymoma have been identified, although clinical trials for novel therapies that target specific cell signal pathways are being undertaken by the Pediatric Brain Tumor Consortium (PBTC) and the Children's Oncology Group (COG).

Ependymoma remains a challenging disease to treat, but laboratory and clinical research conducted during the last decade has resulted in important discoveries that are likely to provide a new direction for the management of this disease. Translating these discoveries into curative combinations of conventional and novel treatments for all patients with ependymoma will require close collaboration between clinicians and scientists.

Pediatric Hematology and Oncology, 1st edition. Edited by Edward J. Estlin, Richard J. Gilbertson, and Robert F. Wynn. © 2010 Blackwell Publishing Ltd.

Epidemiology

Ependymoma is the third most common CNS tumor in children, accounting for 6–12% of brain tumors in this age group. The disease is characterized by the following epidemiological features:

- Most often found in children aged less than 4 years [3].
- Male:female ratio, 1.6:1 [3, 6].
- No apparent variation in the incidence of ependymoma by geographic region or socioeconomic class, but the disease might be more common in Caucasians [6, 7].
- Around 50–60% of pediatric cases occur within the posterior fossa (floor or roof of the IV ventricle or cerebellopontine angle) (Figures 3.1 and 3.2). The tumor can arise also from the III and lateral ventricles or within the parenchyma of the cerebral hemispheres (30–40% of pediatric cases). Although ependymoma is the most frequent form of spinal tumor in adults, this tumor rarely arises in the spine of children [1].

Histology

Ependymomas are characterized by pseudorosettes of tumor cells that surround a central blood vessel and that punctuate fields of tumor cells that display a glial immunophenotype and ultrastructural properties of ependymal cells (Plate 3.1). A number of ependymoma histologic subtypes are recognized:

- Myxopapillary and sub-ependymomas occur almost exclusively in the cauda equina and are relatively benign tumors (WHO grade I).
- Classic ependymomas can display papillary or clear cell features (WHO grade II).
- Anaplastic ependymoma display increased cellularity, cytologic atypia, and microvascular proliferation (WHO grade III).

Prior attempts to correlate ependymoma histologic grade with prognosis have proved controversial; although more contemporary studies of relatively large cohorts suggest that anaplastic histology predicts a poor clinical outcome [8].

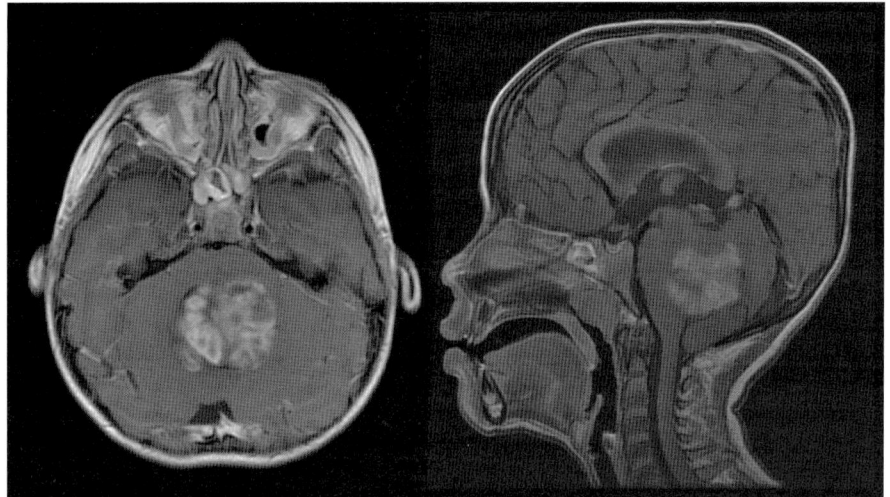

Figure 3.1 Transverse and sagittal pre- and post-operative T1- and T2-weighted MR imaging of a IVth ventricular ependymoma.

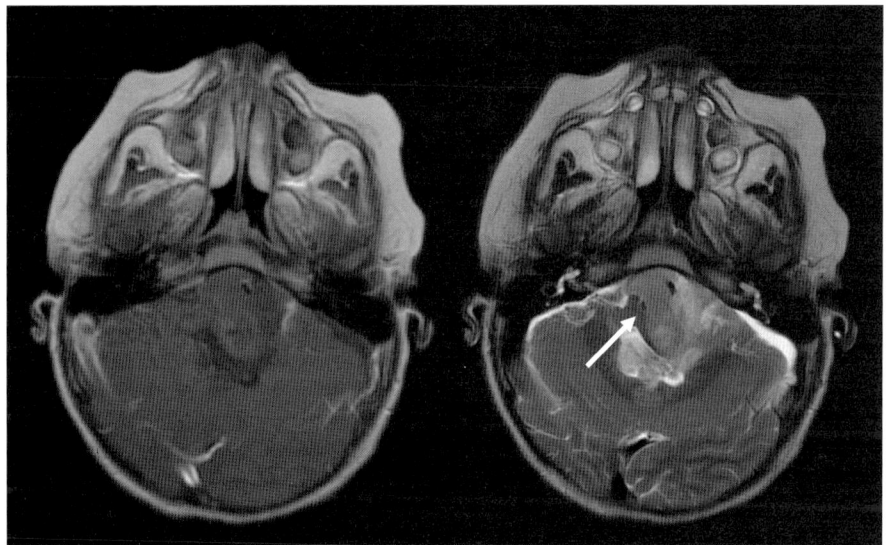

Figure 3.2 Transverse T1- and T2-weighted MR images demonstrating a left cerebellopontine angle ependymoma. Arrows shows position of the displaced medulla.

Genetics and tumor biology

Until recently, knowledge of the genetic alterations in ependymoma was limited to lists of large chromosomal gains and losses, e.g. +1q, −6q, +7p, −9p, −16q, and −22q [9–16] and a very small number of tumor suppressor genes (TSG) identified by studies of heritable tumors. Ependymoma is associated with certain tumor predisposition syndromes:

• Patients with neurofibromatosis type 2 are predisposed to spinal ependymoma [17] and around 25% of sporadic forms of this tumor contain somatic mutations in *neurofibromin 2* (*NF2*, 22q12.2) [18, 19].

• Ependymomas have also been reported in two patients with Turcot's syndrome (germline mutation in *APC*) [20, 21], and in one patient with Li-Fraumeni syndrome (germline mutation in

TP53) [22]. However, mutations in *CTNNB1*, *APC* or *TP53* occur in less than 1% of sporadic ependymomas [23–25].

More recently, genomic tools that detect genome-wide patterns of gene expression and chromosomal alteration have provided some key insights into the biology of ependymoma. Of particular note, these studies have shown that ependymomas from the different regions of the CNS are molecularly distinct diseases [26–30]. For example, while the great majority of cerebral ependymomas activate the NOTCH signal pathway and delete the *INK4A/ARF* TSG locus, spinal ependymomas express high-levels of members of the HOX gene family [26, 29]. Efforts are now underway to apply technologies of higher resolution (500 K single nucleotide polymorphism mapping arrays) to pinpoint specific oncogenes and TSG among large cohorts of ependymoma.

Studies of the gene expression profiles of ependymoma have also provided considerable clues to the cellular origin of the

disease. A recent analysis of over 100 ependymomas, demonstrated that ependymomas share the gene expression profiles of neural progenitor cells, termed radial glia, in the corresponding region of the CNS [26]. These studies suggest:
• Radial glia in different parts of the CNS are predisposed to acquire distinct genetic abnormalities that transform these cells into ependymoma cancer stem cells (CSC).
• Ependymomas arise from radial-glia and ultimately contain radia glia-like CSC that are both required and sufficient to generate tumors *in vivo*.
• More recently, CSC in ependymoma were shown to reside in aberrant vascular stem cell niches, reminiscent of those observed in the normal brain, providing further evidence that ependymomas are maintained by stem-like cancer cells [31, 32].

Clinical presentation

The symptoms and signs caused by ependymoma vary with tumor site. Symptoms and signs of ependymomas of the posterior fossa relate to raised intracranial pressure (headache worse in the morning, vomiting, lethargy, papilledema) and cerebellar dysfunction (ataxia, nystagmus).

Ependymomas of the cerebrum cause hemiparesis, visual field defects, seizures and cognitive impairment depending upon the affected lobe.

Ependymomas are generally slow growing tumors and therefore symptoms may be present up to a year prior to diagnosis and may wax and wane in severity. Although very rare, ependymomas may metastasize to extraneural tissues including lymph nodes, liver and lung [33].

Investigation and staging

Neuroimaging
Ependymomas appear as densely cellular and sometimes calcified lesions when imaged.

Magnetic resonance imaging (MRI) of posterior fossa ependymomas:
• Often reveals extension of the tumor through the foramen magnum into the upper cervical spinal canal and involvement of other structures in the posterior fossa including cranial nerves, brainstem, basilar, and vertebral arteries.
• Rostral extension along the brainstem to the level of the tentorial incisura is considered extensive disease and presents a particularly difficult therapeutic challenge.

MRI of cerebral ependymomas:
• Often reveals large and cystic tumors that may mimic some features of malignant glioma; but ependymomas lack the invasive features of these high-grade tumors (Figure 3.5).
• Ependymomas of the suprasellar region, diencephalon, thalami, and brainstem appear similar on MRI to the more common tumors that arise at these sites.

Staging
There is no official staging classification of ependymoma, but the diagnosis of metastatic disease is important for assigning appropriate treatment. Disseminated disease is detected using neuraxis MRI and cerebrospinal fluid (CSF) cytology; however, for a number of reasons these modalities are rather inaccurate and unreliable:
• Spinal MRIs often contain movement artifacts as a consequence of inadequate patient preparation, sedation, or anesthesia.
• Metastatic ependymomas do not manifest the clear linear enhancement observed in embryonal tumors, and non-specific transient enhancement along the surface of the brainstem and spinal cord can be observed in patients with non-metastatic disease [34].
• CSF cytology is a poor predictor of disease dissemination since patients with surgically confirmed neuraxis dissemination after focal irradiation often contain no tumor cells in the CSF [33].
The development of reliable methods to detect metastatic ependymoma is remains an important challenge. Such tests are likely to become more important since improvements in surgery and radiation therapy have shifted patterns of disease failure from local to disseminated relapse.

Treatment of ependymoma

A historical perspective
Surgery and radiation have been used as treatments for ependymoma for more than 40 years [35]. Twenty years ago, less emphasis was placed on the extent of surgery; but it is now recognized that complete removal of ependymoma is critical if the disease is to be treated successfully [36–38]. Previous methods of delivering radiation to children with ependymoma were also suboptimal. Investigators often treated all patients with craniospinal irradiation on the erroneous assumption that many tumors were disseminated at the time of diagnosis. This exposed patients to the risk of debilitating side-effects for the sake of the minority with disseminated tumors. Further, conventional techniques for delivering radiation restricted doses to the primary tumor site of 54 Gy and irradiated large volumes of normal tissue. Consequently, many patients developed early local tumor recurrence and only 20% achieved long-term event-free survival.

In the early 1990s investigators began to explore the possibility of increasing the dose of radiation to the primary tumor bed as well as the efficacy of systemic chemotherapy. However, event-free and overall survival rates remained largely unchanged since many patients continued to receive only partial tumor resections and chemotherapy proved ineffective [39, 40]. Concerns associated with irradiating the brains of very young children meant that most children with ependymoma aged less than 3 years experienced early tumor recurrence and inferior outcomes when compared with older patients.

The results of clinical studies conducted in the last 10 years have led to a general consensus in the US regarding the treatment

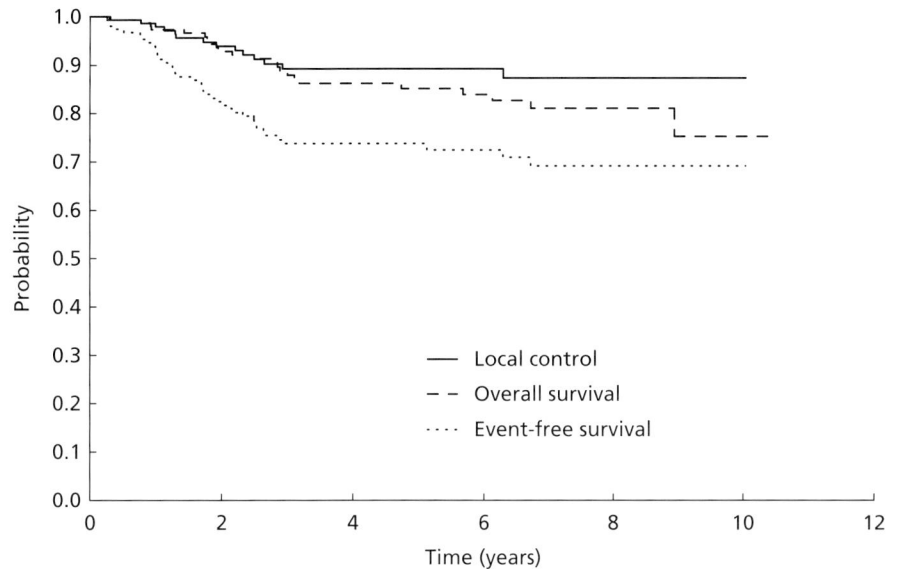

Figure 3.3 Disease control data from the St Jude Children's Research Hospital Experience. Local control, solid line. Overall survival, dashed line. Event-free survival, dotted line [72].

of non-disseminated ependymoma. A landmark prospective phase II trial of conformal radiation therapy (RT-1) was conducted at St Jude Children's Research Hospital (SJCRH) between 1997 and 2003 [41]. RT-1 accrued 88 patients including 48 children aged less than 3 years at the time of irradiation. Importantly, over 85% of children enrolled on RT-1 achieved a gross-total tumor resection, since patients with residual disease were referred routinely for second surgery prior to radiation therapy. Consequently, local disease control was achieved in 80% ± 6% and 95% ± 4% of children with anaplastic and differentiated ependymoma, respectively, and the overall event-free survival rate was 75% ± 4% at 3 years (Figure 3.3). Importantly, longitudinal prospective assessment of neurologic, endocrine and cognitive function among children treated on RT-1 has shown that most function within the normal range following therapy [75]. The encouraging survival rates associated with RT-1 have been attributed to a combination of factors that include better tumor imaging, the high-rate of gross-total tumor resection and improved radiation planning and delivery methods. The Children's Oncology Group (COG) subsequently conducted a clinical trial (ACNS0121) with more than 350 subjects that used the same methods of irradiation and strongly encouraged second surgery. This trial was completed in 2007 and the results are expected in 2011.

Surgery

Total tumor resection remains the most important treatment for patients with localized ependymoma [36–38]. Resection of tumors arising in the supratentorial brain follows the same principles as those used to remove other supratentorial tumors. Tumors in the infratentorial brain, especially those involving the lateral aspect of the brainstem and lower cranial nerves, often present a particular challenge to the neurosurgeon. A two step

approach is often required based on the configuration of the tumor (Figure 3.4) Operative mortality is rare for these patients; however morbidity remains high and includes cranial nerve dysfunction, deficits of coordination and fine motor skills and, less commonly, swallowing dysfunction with vocal cord paralysis [42, 43]. Tracheostomy and gastrostomy are temporarily required in a small subset of patients, but the great majority of these recover with almost normal function [73, 74].

Surgical planning and evaluation has benefited greatly from improvements in neuroimaging and the absence of detectable tumor on post-operative imaging remains a core component of the definition of a gross-total resection. However, the trial divided these cases further between those that did or did not contain evidence of residual tumor by intraoperative microscopy. Patients who displayed no evidence of detectable disease by either imaging or intraoperative microscopy were managed with observation alone following surgery. This approach was based on data, albeit limited, that these patients did not require adjuvant therapy [44].

Patients who undergo less than gross-total resection have been classified as receiving either near-total or sub-total resection in an attempt to determine if residual disease burden correlates with survival. However, these terms are inexact. For example, sub-total resection is used in an all encompassing manner to describe anything from a limited volume of residual tumor to a large residual mass after tumor biopsy. Some investigators have applied to ependymoma the same definitions used to define subtotal ($>1.5\,cm^2$ residual of tumor on a single cross sectional image) and near-total (residual tumor $<1.5\,cm^2$) resection of medulloblastoma [36]. The COG trial ACNS0121 defined residual tumor by 'thickness' on serial image slices rather than tumor area: near-total resection was defined as $\leq0.5\,cm$ residual tumor thickness and sub-total as $>0.5\,cm$ thickness. Thin linear enhancement

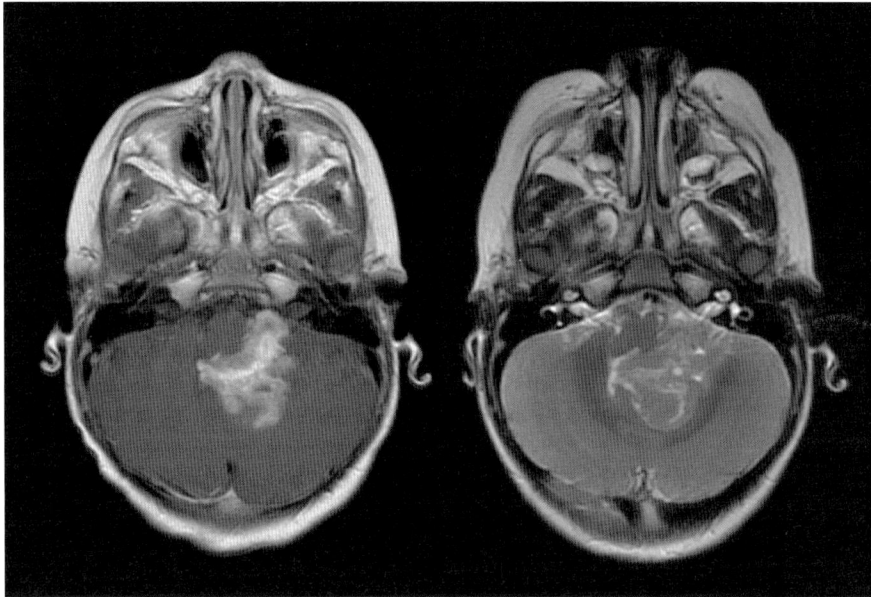

Figure 3.4 Cerebellopontine angle tumor that required two surgical approaches.

<0.5 cm, regardless of the area involved, was regarded as near-total resection. It remains to be determined which, if any, classification of surgical resection is useful for predicting prognosis.

Second surgery

If a gross-total resection is not achieved at first surgery, careful consideration needs to be given to the use of additional or second surgery. There are a number of reasons why gross-total resection may not be achieved at a first attempt, e.g. patients *in extremis* at presentation, or tumors that require two different surgical approaches. Second surgery may be accomplished safely and in most cases has been shown to be effective at achieving a gross-total resection ([45] and [76]. Second surgery should be performed as soon as possible. Chemotherapy might be helpful in reducing further the size of the primary tumor in between first and second look surgery and improving the chance of achieving a complete resection [46]. This strategy was studied in the ACNS0121 trial. Although, a gross-total resection is an important goal for all patients, radiation is an effective therapy and aggressive surgery should not be conducted at the expense of damaging the cranial nerves or brainstem that could result in devastating side-effects.

Chemotherapy

Although ependymoma is sensitive to conventional chemotherapy, there is no convincing evidence that this treatment improves overall patient survival:

• Cisplatin is the most active agent against ependymoma, with reported response rates of 30% [47–49].
• Carboplatin [50, 51], ifosfamide [52] and etoposide [53, 54] have each demonstrated modest activity against the disease; but

combination chemotherapy regimens have proved ineffective at improving the cure rates achieved with surgery and radiation therapy alone.

• Combination regimens have proved equally ineffective.
• A randomized trial of lomustine (CCNU), vincristine and prednisone, versus no chemotherapy for one year following surgery and radiation conducted by the Children's Cancer Group (CCG), failed to show any added benefit of the chemotherapy [55].
• A second CCG study of children aged ≥2 years with newly diagnosed ependymoma that randomized patients to receive either CCNU, vincristine and prednisone or the eight-drugs-in-1-day regimen, also demonstrated no advantage of chemotherapy relative to historical controls [36]. The German HIT 88/89 and 91 trials failed to show any benefit of chemotherapy for patients with newly diagnosed anaplastic ependymoma [56].
• Very young patients with ependymoma have shown responses to chemotherapy and this modality may have a role in delaying radiation of the brains of very young patients. The role of dose intensive chemotherapy in this age group, however, is unclear.
• Pediatric Oncology Group 8633 reported a 48% response rate to a combination of vincristine, cyclophosphamide, cisplatin and etoposide among 25 children with post-operative residual tumor [57].
• The French Society of Pediatric Oncology reported a 4 year overall survival rate of 23% among patients aged <5 years receiving seven cycles of adjuvant alternating 'procarbazine and carboplatin'-'etoposide and cisplatin'-'vincristine and cyclophosphamide' and no radiation, [58]. Early reports that dose intensification of chemotherapy might improve survival rates among young children with ependymoma have not been validated. More recent studies suggest that myeloablative chemotherapy and autologous stem cell rescue does not improve survival of patients with ependy-

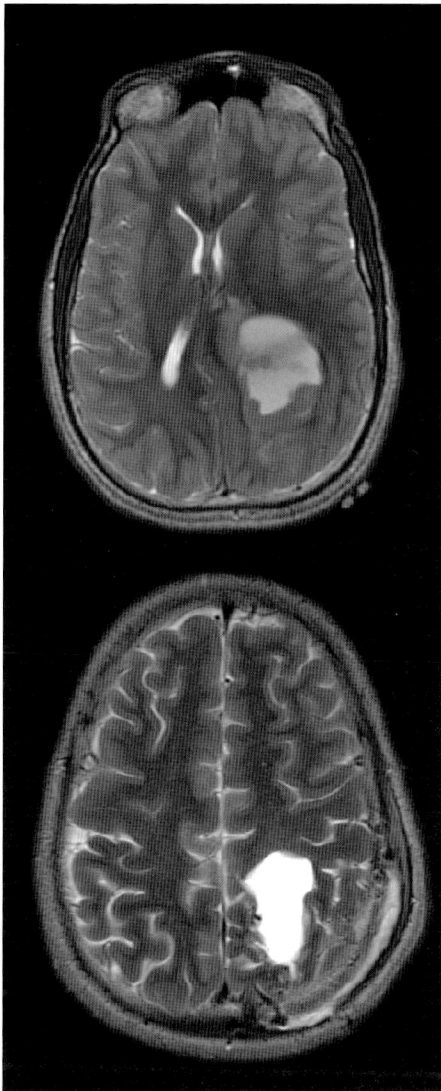

Figure 3.5 Supratentorial ependymoma before (upper) and after (lower) gross-total resection. MR T2-weighted imaging of cystic and solid anaplastic ependymoma in the left parietal region.

moma but is associated with unacceptable toxic death-rates [40, 59, 60]. The current strategy in COG is to test the ability of post-irradiation chemotherapy to improve event-free and overall survival in children with ependymoma after gross- or near-total resection. This trial known as ACNS0831 was opened in 2010. It will randomize patients between observation after radiation therapy and treatment with four cycles of chemotherapy including the followingt agents: vincristine, cyclophosphamide, etoposide and cisplatin.

Radiation therapy
Focal irradiation
Most children with ependymoma present with localized disease and may be treated with post-operative focal irradiation directed to the primary tumor site. This has been made possible by technological improvements in radiation planning and delivery. The volume of irradiation required to treat patients adequately, while sparing normal tissue, is one of the primary questions under investigation by radiation oncologists. The ability of new treatment systems to limit the highest dose of radiation to the tumor bed and spare surrounding normal tissues has been demonstrated in the RT-1 trial [41]. Patients enrolled on RT-1 were treated with 54–59.4 Gy of conformal radiation with a 1 cm clinical target volume margin targeted to the post-operatively-defined tumor bed. Serially evaluation of patients using a variety of objective measures of cognitive function identified no decline in cognitive function [77].

Craniospinal irradiation
Although rare, ependymoma can disseminate throughout the neuraxis, and craniospinal irradiation is required treatment for these patients. In pediatric neuroradiotherapy, craniospinal irradiation is defined as irradiation of the entire neuraxis with additional focal or 'boost' treatments of the primary tumor and metastatic sites. Historically, all patients were treated with this extensive volume based on the erroneous assumption that a large proportion of ependymomas are disseminated throughout the neuraxis at diagnosis. Retrospective studies have since shown that neuraxis irradiation does not improve the survival of patients with adequately staged disease compared with focal irradiation [61, 62]. Craniospinal irradiation continues to be employed for the less than 7% of patients who present with metastatic ependymoma. Doses in excess of 36 Gy, and typically 39.6 Gy, are prescribed prior to boost treatment of the primary (59.4 Gy) and metastatic sites (>54 Gy). Radiosurgery (high-dose single fraction radiation therapy) to small intracranial or spinal lesions has been used with limited success as a supplement to craniospinal irradiation or focal fractionated irradiation [63, 64]. Despite aggressive surgery and radiation therapy, disseminated ependymoma is extremely difficult to cure. Long-term survival rates for this population are unknown but are likely to be in the 20–30% range when measured at 5 years.

Radiation therapy has contributed increasingly to the contemporary care of children with ependymoma. This has been made possible by the advent of more sophisticated planning and delivery methods that can reduce the radiation dose to normal tissues (Plate 3.2). The dosimetric and theoretical safety advantages of proton beam therapy should be explored among children with ependymoma now that it is becoming increasingly available. It is important to note that proton radiotherapy has commanded the attention of parents and caregivers and will have a significant effect on future protocol development and will likely concentrate patients in centers with this capability.

Long-term side effects
The side effects of ependymoma therapy depend on the age of the patient and tumor location, as well as the impact of specific treatments on normal tissues.

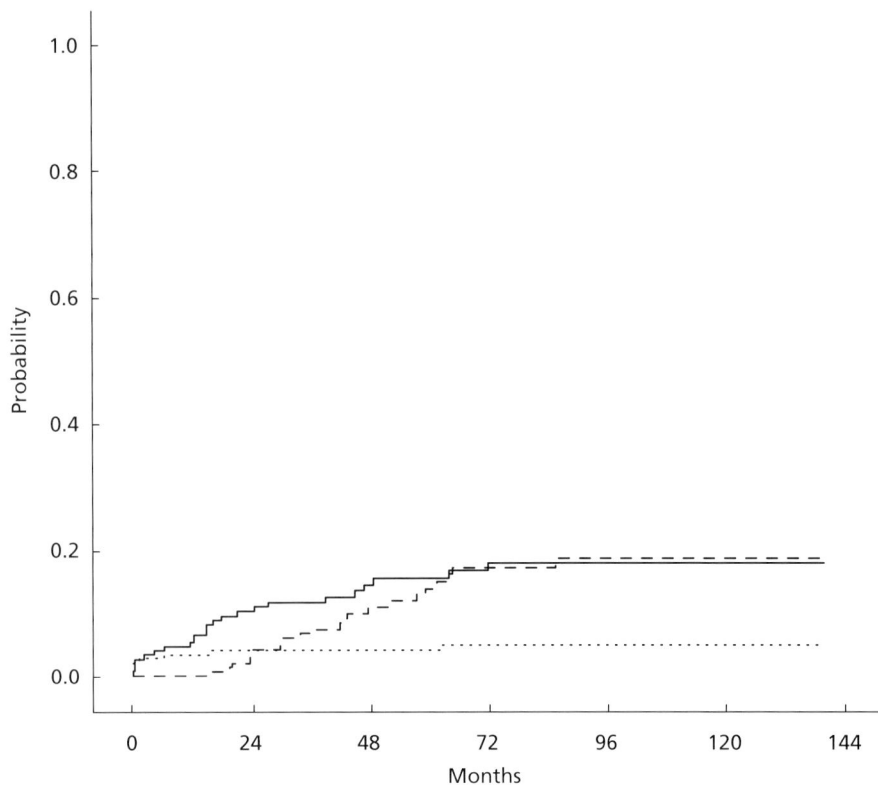

Figure 3.6 Incidence of hormone replacement after conformal radiation therapy. Thyroid (solid line), growth (dashed line) and glucocorticoid (dotted line) replacement based on 148 patients with a median follow-up of 71 months.

• Surgery (including cerebrospinal fluid shunting) and chemotherapy are both associated with relatively rare treatment complications, e.g. incidental infections.

• Exposure of the brain to radiation results in long-term endocrine and cognitive deficits (including learning, memory attention, and behavior disorders).

• In addition to damaging the hypothalamic–pituitary axis (Figure 3.6), radiation therapy can disrupt normal growth by impacting directly bone and soft tissues within the field of treatment.

• Rare but devastating complications of radiation therapy include symptomatic vasculopathy, brain and spinal cord necrosis, and secondary malignancies. Some patients show changes on MRI in brain tissues that receive the highest doses of radiation. These changes may be more apparent in children who receive chemotherapy and may indicate tissue damage or treatment effects that do not necessarily result in serious complications and often resolve with time.

• Recent data suggest that IQ after radiation therapy may be predicted on the basis of 3-dimensional radiation dosimetry [65]. If validated, these models should prove useful for designing the next generation of clinical trials and in particular implementing intensity-modulated radiation therapy.

When parents and caregivers seek information about ependymoma, their interest alternates between the effectiveness of treatment and the potential for side effects. The balance of concern about disease control and side effects is modulated by the age of the patient and time after diagnosis. With younger patients tolerating aggressive surgery and newer methods of radiation therapy, concerns about treatment-related effects give way to fears of disease progression and the lack of effective therapy in patients who fail frontline treatment. Improving our understanding about side effects of treatment, especially radiation therapy, and appreciating that limited objective and prospective data has been published about radiation-related side effects, will help patients, parents and caregivers make important decisions. Proactive surveillance for side effects, regardless of their attribution, will also serve to improve functional outcomes for all children.

Future strategies
Continued improvements in the use of conventional therapies
In the future, risk-adapted strategies for the treatment of ependymoma may be developed with knowledge from ongoing clinical trials and tumor biology research. The ACNS0121 trial results will provide more information about patients who might be observed after microscopic complete resection, the value of chemotherapy to improve gross-total resection rates, and the feasibility of conformal radiation therapy administered in a cooperative group setting. Other important findings will include correlation of functional outcomes with the effects of therapy and important information about tumor pathology, the value of medical imaging and the follow-up care provided to these patients. Current data

indicate that local tumor control is greatest among patients with differentiated ependymoma who receive 59.4 Gy after gross-total resection. Indeed, all patients treated with gross-total resection have relatively high rates of local tumor control but distant metastatic spread has become a more common mode of failure. New methods are required to define residual disease at the primary site or evidence of metastatic dissemination. There are patients who might benefit from craniospinal irradiation or chemotherapy or delays in the administration of adjuvant therapy. Differences in outcome need to be determined with optimally treated patients; prognostic factors from the past may be less relevant when state of the art therapy is administered.

Development of novel therapies

While improvements have been made in the use of conventional treatments, these will not cure all patients with ependymoma. There is therefore a great need for new treatments of ependymoma. Seminal studies of a variety of hematologic and solid tumors have identified gene mutations as targets of effective new anti-cancer therapies [66–70]. Thus, the characterization of oncogenic mutations in ependymoma could lead to the development of new treatments. Further, the recent discovery that ependymomas are derived from radial glia-like cancer stem cells that reside in perivascular niches [26, 31] has identified a series of completely new potential drug targets to treat this disease [71].

References

1 Kleihues P, Louis DN, Scheithauer BW, et al. The WHO classification of tumors of the nervous system. J Neuropathol Exp Neurol 2002; 61: 215–25; discussion 26–9.

2 Moynihan TJ. Ependymal tumors. Curr Treat Options Oncol 2003; 4: 517–23.

3 CBTRUS. Statistical Report: Primary Brain Tumors in the United States, 1995–1999. Hinsdale, IL: Central Brain Tumor Registry of the United States, 2002: 2006.

4 Merchant TE, Fouladi M. Ependymoma: new therapeutic approaches including radiation and chemotherapy. J Neurooncol 2005; 75: 287–99.

5 Brandes AA, Cavallo G, Reni M, et al. A multicenter retrospective study of chemotherapy for recurrent intracranial ependymal tumors in adults by the Gruppo Italiano Cooperativo di Neuro-Oncologia. Cancer 2005; 104 :143–8.

6 Gurney J, Smith M, Bunin G. CNS and miscellaneous intra-cranial and intraspinal neoplasms. SEER Pediatric Monograph, National Cancer Institute 2001: 51–63.

7 Alston RD, Rowan S, Eden TO, Moran A, Birch JM. Cancer incidence patterns by region and socioeconomic deprivation in teenagers and young adults in England. Br J Cancer 2007; 96: 1760–6.

8 Merchant TE, Jenkins JJ, Burger PC, et al. Influence of tumor grade on time to progression after irradiation for localized ependymoma in children. Int J Rad Oncol Biol Phys 2002; 53: 52–7.

9 Dyer S, Prebble E, Davison V, et al. Genomic imbalances in pediatric intracranial ependymomas define clinically relevant groups. Am J Pathol 2002; 161: 2133–41.

10 Hirose Y, Aldape K, Bollen A, et al. Chromosomal abnormalities subdivide ependymal tumors into clinically relevant groups. Am J Pathol 2001; 158: 1137–43.

11 Jeuken JW, Sprenger SH, Gilhuis J, Teepen HL, Grotenhuis AJ, Wesseling P. Correlation between localization, age, and chromosomal imbalances in ependymal tumors as detected by CGH. J Pathol 2002; 197: 238–44.

12 Grill J, Avet–Loiseau H, Lellouch–Tubiana A, et al. Comparative genomic hybridization detects specific cytogenetic abnormalities in pediatric ependymomas and choroid plexus papillomas. Cancer Genet Cytogenet 2002; 136: 121–5.

13 Koschny R, Koschny T, Froster UG, Krupp W, Zuber MA. Comparative genomic hybridization in glioma: a meta-analysis of 509 cases. Cancer Genet Cytogenet 2002; 135: 147–59.

14 Ward S, Harding B, Wilkins P, et al. Gain of 1q and loss of 22 are the most common changes detected by comparative genomic hybridisation in paediatric ependymoma. Genes Chromosomes Cancer 2001; 32: 59–66.

15 Carter M, Nicholson J, Ross F, et al. Genetic abnormalities detected in ependymomas by comparative genomic hybridisation. Br J Cancer 2002; 86: 929–39.

16 Reardon DA, Entrekin RE, Sublett J, et al. Chromosome arm 6q loss is the most common recurrent autosomal alteration detected in primary pediatric ependymoma. Genes Chrom Cancer 1999; 24: 230–7.

17 Rouleau GA, Merel P, Lutchman M, et al. Alteration in a new gene encoding a putative membrane-organizing protein causes neuro-fibromatosis type 2. Nature 1993; 363: 515.

18 Ebert C, von Haken M, Meyer–Puttlitz B, et al. Molecular genetic analysis of ependymal tumors. NF2 mutations and chromosome 22q loss occur preferentially in intramedullary spinal ependymomas. Am J Pathol 1999; 155: 627–32.

19 Rubio MP, Correa KM, Ramesh V, et al. Analysis of the neurofibromatosis 2 gene in human ependymomas and astrocytomas. Cancer Res 1994; 54: 45–7.

20 Mullins KJ, Rubio A, Myers SP, Korones DN, Pilcher WH. Malignant ependymomas in a patient with Turcot's syndrome: case report and management guidelines. Surg Neurol 1998; 49: 290–4.

21 Torres CF, Korones DN, Pilcher W. Multiple ependymomas in a patient with Turcot's syndrome. Med Pediatr Oncol 1997; 28: 59–61.

22 Metzger AK, Sheffield VC, Duyk G, Daneshvar L, Edwards MS, Cogen PH. Identification of a germ-line mutation in the p53 gene in a patient with an intracranial ependymoma. Proc Natl Acad Sci USA 1991; 88: 7825–9.

23 Onilude OE, Lusher ME, Lindsey JC, Pearson AD, Ellison DW, Clifford SC. APC and CTNNB1 mutations are rare in sporadic ependymomas. Cancer Genet Cytogenet 2006; 168: 158–61.

24 Ohgaki H, Eibl RH, Wiestler OD, Yasargil MG, Newcomb EW, Kleihues P. p53 mutations in nonastrocytic human brain tumors. Cancer Res 1991; 51: 6202–5.

25 Gaspar N, Grill J, Geoerger B, Lellouch–Tubiana A, Michalowski MB, Vassal G. p53 pathway dysfunction in primary childhood ependymomas. Pediatr Blood Cancer 2006; 46: 604–13.

26 Taylor MD, Poppleton H, Fuller C, et al. Radial glia cells are candidate stem cells of ependymoma. Cancer Cell 2005; 8: 323–35.

27 Ammerlaan AC, de Bustos C, Ararou A, et al. Localization of a putative low–penetrance ependymoma susceptibility locus to 22q11 using a chromosome 22 tiling-path genomic microarray. Genes Chromosomes Cancer 2005; Epublication ahead of print.

28 Mendrzyk F, Korshunov A, Benner A, et al. Identification of gains on 1q and epidermal growth factor receptor overexpression as independent prognostic markers in intracranial ependymoma. Clin Cancer Res 2006; 12: 2070–9.

29 Modena P, Lualdi E, Facchinetti F, et al. Identification of tumor–specific molecular signatures in intracranial ependymoma and association with clinical characteristics. J Clin Oncol. 2006; 24: 5223–33.

30 Korshunov A, Neben K, Wrobel G, et al. Gene expression patterns in ependymomas correlate with tumor location, grade, and patient age. Am J Pathol 2003; 163: 1721–7.

31 Calabrese C, Poppleton H, Kocak M, et al. A perivascular niche for brain tumor stem cells. Cancer Cell 2007; 11: 69–82.

32 Gilbertson RJ, Rich JN. Making a tumor's bed: glioblastoma stem cells and the vascular niche. Nature Reviews Cancer:in press.

33 Kumar P, Rastogi N, Jain M, Chhabra P. Extraneural metastases in anaplastic ependymoma. J Cancer Res Therap 2007; 3: 102–4.

34 Butler WE, Khan A, Khan SA. Posterior fossa ependymoma with intense but transient disseminated enhancement but not metastasis. Pediatr Neurosurg 2002; 37: 27–31.

35 Kricheff, II, Becker M, Schneck SA, Taveras JM. Intracranial ependymomas: factors influencing prognosis. J Neurosurg 1964; 21: 7–14.

36 Robertson PL, Zeltzer PM, Boyett JM, et al. Survival and prognostic factors following radiation therapy and chemotherapy for ependymomas in children: a report of the Children's Cancer Group. J Neurosurg 1998; 88: 695–703.

37 Rousseau P, Habrand JL, Sarrazin D, et al. Treatment of intracranial ependymomas of children: review of a 15–year experience. Int J Radiat Oncol Biol Phys 1994; 28: 381–6.

38 Duffner PK, Krischer JP, Sanford RA, et al. Prognostic factors in infants and very young children with intracranial ependymomas. Pediatr Neurosurg 1998; 28: 215–22.

39 Bouffet E, Foreman N. Chemotherapy for intracranial ependymomas. Childs Nerv Syst 1999; 15: 563–70.

40 Grill J, Kalifa C, Doz F, Schoepfer C, et al. A high-dose busulfan-thiotepa combination followed by autologous bone marrow transplantation in childhood recurrent ependymoma. A phase-II study. Pediatr Neurosurg 1996; 25: 7–12.

41 Merchant TE, Mulhern RK, Krasin MJ, et al. Preliminary results from a phase II trial of conformal radiation therapy and evaluation of radiation-related CNS effects for pediatric patients with localized ependymoma. J Clin Oncol 2004; 22: 3156–62.

42 Pollack IF, Polinko P, Albright AL, Towbin R, Fitz C. Mutism and pseudobulbar symptoms after resection of posterior fossa tumors in children: incidence and pathophysiology. Neurosurgery 1995; 37: 885–93.

43 Doxey D, Bruce D, Sklar F, Swift D, Shapiro K. Posterior fossa syndrome: identifiable risk factors and irreversible complications. Pediatr Neurosurg 1999; 31: 131–6.

44 Hukin J, Epstein F, Lefton D, Allen J. Treatment of intracranial ependymoma by surgery alone. Pediatr Neurosurg 1998; 29: 40–5.

45 Korshunov A, Golanov A, Sycheva R, Timirgaz V. The histologic grade is a main prognostic factor for patients with intracranial ependymomas treated in the microneurosurgical era: an analysis of 258 patients. Cancer 2004; 100: 1230–7.

46 Foreman NK, Love S, Gill SS, Coakham HB. Second-look surgery for incompletely resected fourth ventricle ependymomas: technical case report. Neurosurgery 1997; 40: 856–60; discussion 60.

47 Khan AB, D'Souza BJ, Wharam MD, et al. Cisplatin therapy in recurrent childhood brain tumors. Cancer Treat Rep 1982; 66: 2013–20.

48 Sexauer CL, Khan A, Burger PC, et al. Cisplatin in recurrent pediatric brain tumors. A POG Phase II study. A Pediatric Oncology Group Study. Cancer 1985; 56: 1497–501.

49 Walker RW, Allen JC. Cisplatin in the treatment of recurrent childhood primary brain tumors. J Clin Oncol 1988; 6: 62–6.

50 Gaynon PS, Ettinger LJ, Baum ES, Siegel SE, Krailo MD, Hammond GD. Carboplatin in childhood brain tumors. A Children's Cancer Study Group Phase II trial. Cancer 1990; 66: 2465–9.

51 Friedman HS, Krischer JP, Burger P, et al. Treatment of children with progressive or recurrent brain tumors with carboplatin or iproplatin: a Pediatric Oncology Group randomized phase II study. J Clin Oncol 1992; 10: 249–56.

52 Chastagner P, Sommelet-Olive D, Kalifa C, et al. Phase II study of ifosfamide in childhood brain tumors: a report by the French Society of Pediatric Oncology (SFOP). Med Pediatr Oncol 1993; 21: 49–53.

53 Needle MN, Molloy PT, Geyer JR, et al. Phase II study of daily oral etoposide in children with recurrent brain tumors and other solid tumors. Med Pediatr Oncol 1997; 29: 28–32.

54 Davidson A, Lewis I, Pearson AD, Stevens MC, Pinkerton CR. 21-day schedule oral etoposide in children – a feasibility study. Eur J Cancer 1993; 29A: 2223–5.

55 Evans AE, Anderson JR, Lefkowitz-Boudreaux IB, Finlay JL. Adjuvant chemotherapy of childhood posterior fossa ependymoma: cranio-spinal irradiation with or without adjuvant CCNU, vincristine, and prednisone: a Childrens Cancer Group study. Med Pediatr Oncol 1996; 27: 8–14.

56 Timmermann B, Kortmann RD, Kuhl J, et al. Combined postoperative irradiation and chemotherapy for anaplastic ependymomas in childhood: results of the German prospective trials HIT 88/89 and HIT 91. Int J Radiat Oncol Biol Phys 2000; 46: 287–95.

57 Duffner PK, Horowitz ME, Krischer JP, et al. Postoperative chemotherapy and delayed radiation in children less than three years of age with malignant brain tumors. N Engl J Med 1993; 328: 1725–31.

58 Grill J, Le Deley MC, Gambarelli D, et al. Postoperative chemotherapy without irradiation for ependymoma in children under 5 years of age: a multicenter trial of the French Society of Pediatric Oncology. J Clin Oncol 2001; 19: 1288–96.

59 Mason WP, Goldman S, Yates AJ, Boyett J, Li H, Finlay JL. Survival following intensive chemotherapy with bone marrow reconstitution for children with recurrent intracranial ependymoma – a report of the Children's Cancer Group. J Neurooncol 1998; 37: 135–43.

60 Zacharoulis S, Levy A, Chi SN, et al. Outcome for young children newly diagnosed with ependymoma, treated with intensive induction chemotherapy followed by myeloablative chemotherapy and autologous stem cell rescue. Pediatr Blood Cancer 2007; 49: 34–40.

61 Merchant TE, Haida T, Wang MH, Finlay JL, Leibel SA. Anaplastic ependymoma: treatment of pediatric patients with or without craniospinal radiation therapy. J Neurosurg 1997; 86: 943–9.

62 Paulino AC, Wen BC, Buatti JM, et al. Intracranial ependymomas: an analysis of prognostic factors and patterns of failure. Am J Clin Oncol 2002; 25: 117–22.

63 Jawahar A, Kondziolka D, Flickinger JC, Lunsford LD. Adjuvant stereotactic radiosurgery for anaplastic ependymoma. Stereotact Funct Neurosurg 1999; 73: 23–30.

64 Mansur DB, Drzymala RE, Rich KM, Klein EE, Simpson JR. The efficacy of stereotactic radiosurgery in the management of intracranial ependymoma. J Neurooncol 2004; 66: 187–90.

65 Merchant TE, Kiehna EN, Li C, Xiong X, Mulhern RK. Radiation dosimetry predicts IQ after conformal radiation therapy in pediatric patients with localized ependymoma. Int J Rad Oncol Biol Phys 2005; 63: 1546–54.

66 Vogel CL, Cobleigh MA, Tripathy D, et al. Efficacy and safety of trastuzumab as a single agent in first-line treatment of HER2-overexpressing metastatic breast cancer. J Clin Oncol 2002; 20: 719–26.

67 Lynch TJ, Bell DW, Sordella R, et al. Activating mutations in the epidermal growth factor receptor underlying responsiveness of non-small-cell lung cancer to gefitinib. N Engl J Med 2004; 350: 2129–39. Epub 004 Apr 29.

68 Paez JG, Janne PA, Lee JC, et al. EGFR mutations in lung cancer: correlation with clinical response to gefitinib therapy. Science 2004; 29: 29.

69 Druker BJ, Sawyers CL, Kantarjian H, et al. Activity of a specific inhibitor of the BCR-ABL tyrosine kinase in the blast crisis of chronic myeloid leukemia and acute lymphoblastic leukemia with the Philadelphia chromosome. N Engl J Med 2001; 344: 1038–42.

70 Romer JT, Kimura H, Magdaleno S, et al. Suppression of the Shh pathway using a small molecule inhibitor eliminates medulloblastoma in Ptc1(+/−)p53(−/−) mice. Cancer Cell 2004; 6: 229–40.

71 Gilbertson RJ, Rich JN. Making a tumor's bed: glioblastoma stem cells and the vascular niche. Nat Rev Cancer 2007; 7: 733–6.

72 Merchant TE, Li C, Xiong X, et al. Conformal radiotherapy after surgery for paediatric ependymoma: a prospective study. Lancet Oncol 2009 Mar; 10(3): 258–66. PubMed PMID: 19274783.

73 Merchant TE, Chitti RM, Li C, et al. Factors associated with neurological recovery of brainstem function following postoperative conformal radiation therapy for infratentorial ependymoma. Int J Radiat Oncol Biol Phys 2010 Feb 1; 76(2): 496–503. Epub 2009 May 21. PubMed PMID: 19464817.

74 Morris EB, Li C, Khan RB, et al. Evolution of neurological impairment in pediatric infratentorial ependymoma patients. J Neurooncol 2009 Sep; 94(3): 391–8. Epub 2009 Mar 29. PubMed PMID: 19330288; PubMed Central PMCID: PMC2731005.

75 Conklin HM, Li C, Xiong X et al. Predicting change in academic abilities after conformal radiation therapy for localized ependymoma. J Clin Oncol 2008 Aug 20; 26(24): 3965–70. PubMed PMID: 18711186; PubMed Central PMCID: PMC2654312.

76 Sanford RA, Merchant TE, Zwienenberg-Lee M, et al. Advances in surgical techniques for resection of childhood cerebellopontine angle ependymomas are key to survival. Childs Nerv Syst 2009 Oct; 25(10): 1229–40. Epub 2009 May 30. PubMed PMID: 19484252.

77 Di Pinto M, Conklin HM, Li C, et al. Investigating Verbal and Visual Auditory Learning After Conformal Radiation Therapy for Childhood Ependymoma. Int J Radiat Oncol Biol Phys 2009 Sep 22. [Epub ahead of print] PubMed PMID: 19783376.

4 Embryonal Tumors

Amar Gajjar[1] and Steven C. Clifford[2]

[1] Division of Neuro Oncology and Department of Oncology, St Jude Children's Research Hospital, Memphis, TN, USA and
[2] Northern Institute for Cancer Research, Newcastle University, The Medical School, Newcastle-upon-Tyne, UK

Introduction

Embryonal tumors are the most common type of malignant brain tumor to arise during the first and second decades of life [1, 2]. This group of tumors includes a range of different histologic disease types (Table 4.1). In this chapter we will focus on medulloblastoma, the most common childhood embryonal tumor, alongside providing a consideration of its rarer embryonal tumor counterparts; the supratentorial primitive neuroectodermal tumor (PNET) and the atypical teratoid rhaboid tumor (ATRT) (see Box 4.1 and Table 4.2).

Medulloblastoma

Histological classification of medulloblastoma

The latest (2007) World Health Organization (WHO) classification of tumors of the CNS lists the classic medulloblastoma and several variants: desmoplastic, anaplastic and large-cell medulloblastomas, and the medulloblastoma with extensive nodularity (MBEN) (Table 4.1 and Plate 4.1) [3].

Classic medulloblastoma

This is the most common histologic subtype accounting for around two-thirds of all tumors:
• Tumors are composed of small round or ellipsoid cells with a high nuclear:cytoplasmic ratio and round-to-oval or triangular hyperchromatic nuclei.
• Uniform cells with round nuclei, in which the chromatin is less condensed, are frequently intermingled with the hyperchromatic cells, and occasionally form the dominant population (Plate 4.1).
• Cell turnover in most medulloblastomas is high; indices of proliferation and apoptosis can be as great as in any other neuroepithelial tumor. However, these measures can be unexpectedly low in some classic tumors.

Pediatric Hematology and Oncology, 1st edition. Edited by Edward J. Estlin, Richard J. Gilbertson, and Robert F. Wynn. © 2010 Blackwell Publishing Ltd.

• Overall, the mitotic index for childhood medulloblastomas is usually in the range of 0.5 to 2% [5, 6]. The growth fraction, as assessed by Ki-67 immunolabeling, is generally greater than 20% [6, 7].

Anaplastic and large-cell medulloblastomas (Plate 4.1)
• Form a continuum; all large-cell medulloblastomas have regions of anaplasia.
• Large-cell and anaplastic tumors make up between 2 and 4%, and 10 and 22% of medulloblastomas, respectively [5–7].

Desmoplastic medulloblastomas
Desmoplastic medulloblastomas encompass the nodular/desmoplastic medulloblastoma and the MBEN which contribute approximately 7% and 3% of all medulloblastomas, respectively (Plate 4.1) [7, 8].
• Defined as having a biphasic architecture consisting of regions with dense intercellular reticulin and nodular reticulin-free zones, in which tumor cells show a neurocytic phenotype [8].
• Desmoplasia, a pericellular deposition of collagen in this context, and a nodular architecture may occur together or separately in medulloblastomas.
• Desmoplasia can be a reactive phenomenon when medulloblastoma cells invade the leptomeninges. The desmoplastic histopathological sub-type is common in infants (<3 years of age; ~50% of cases), but occurs less frequently in older children (≥3 years; ~5% of cases) [8].

Biology of medulloblastoma
Genetics and epigenetics
A series of key non-random molecular genetic and epigenetic abnormalities have been identified in medulloblastoma which: (i) have informed our understanding of the molecular mechanisms underlying its pathogenesis; (ii) identified key signaling pathways involved in medulloblastoma and; (iii) offer significant potential for improved treatment stratification and/or the identification of novel therapeutic targets.

Chromosomal aberrations in medulloblastoma
• Abnormalities of chromosome 17 are the most common chromosomal aberrations in medulloblastoma: isochromosome 17q (iso(17q)) is observed in approximately 40% of cases [9–13].

Table 4.1 World Health Organization 2007 pathological classification of childhood central nervous system (CNS) embryonal tumors[3].

Medulloblastoma
Desmoplastic/nodular medulloblastoma
Medulloblastoma with extensive nodularity (MBEN)
Anaplastic medulloblastoma
Large cell medulloblastoma

CNS primitive neuroectodermal tumor
CNS neuroblastoma
Medulloepithelioma
CNS ganglioneuroblastoma
Ependymoblastoma

Atypical teratoid rhabdoid tumor

Box 4.1 Key points regarding the epidemiology of embryonal tumors.

- Approximately 461 patients younger than 20 years of age are diagnosed with embryonal central nervous system tumors in the United States each year, the most common form being medulloblastoma.
- Peak incidence is between 4 and 9 years of age.
- Predominate in males (7.3 per million relative to 4.2 per million in females) and are more common in Caucasians as compared with African Americans.
- Arise most frequently in the posterior fossa.

- Isolated loss of 17p is observed in an additional ~20% of cases [10, 11, 13, 14].
- Gain of chromosome 7 occurs in ~40% of cases.
- Extensive non-random losses of chromosomes 8, 9, 10q, 11 and 16q are each observed in ~30% of cases [11, 13, 15].

Gene amplification
- *MYCN* (at 2p24) and *MYC* (at 8q24) are the most commonly amplified loci occurring in 5–15% of medulloblastomas, associated with the large-cell/anaplastic medulloblastoma variant [10, 16, 17].
- Additional rare gene amplifications have been documented including *OTX2, NOTCH2, hTERT, MYCL1, PDGFRA, KIT, MYB, PPM1D* and *CDK6* [18–21]. The incidence and biological and clinical significance of these events, require clarification.

Tumor predisposition syndromes
- Although only a small proportion of medulloblastomas (<5%) are associated with an inherited familial predisposition (Table 4.3), many of the genetic defects which cause these syndromes have subsequently been shown to play a more extensive role in sporadic medulloblastoma development.

Table 4.2 Medulloblastoma/primitive neuroectodermal tumor descriptive factors[4]. Percentages may not add to 100% due to rounding.

Age (years)	
0–3	244 (32%)
4–9	315 (41%)
10–14	140 (18%)
15–19	69 (9%)
All ages	768
Gender	
Male	487(63%)
Female	281(37%)
Ethnicity	
White	626(82%)
Black	70(9%)
Other	72(9%)
Anatomic location	
Supratentorial	53(7%)
Infratentorial	649(85%)
Mixed/overlapping	21(3%)
Brain (not otherwise specified)	45(6%)

- Mutations of *TP53, APC,* and *PTCH* in sporadic medulloblastoma have been uncovered through their causative roles in Li-Fraumeni, Turcot and nevoid basal cell carcinoma (NBCC) syndromes, respectively [22–26, 28, 29,36–42].
- Fanconi anemia subtype-D1 and subtype-N kindreds associated with *BRCA2* and *PALB2* mutations carry an increased risk of medulloblastoma [30, 31]. It is not known if these genes are mutated in sporadic medulloblastomas.

Epigenetic events in medulloblastoma
- Epigenetic alterations cause changes in gene expression which are not associated with changes in the nucleotide sequence, e.g. gene expression silencing caused by hypermethylation of promoter-associated CpG islands [43].
- Unlike genetic mechanisms of gene inactivation (e.g. gene mutation or deletion), gene silencing by DNA hypermethylation is reversible by DNA methyltransferase inhibitors or demethylating agents, and therefore may represent a potential therapeutic target [44].
- Multiple loci in medulloblastoma have been shown to be methylated [45–48], e.g. *RASSF1A* (in >90% of cases), *CASP8* (35–40%) and *HIC-1* (35–40%) [49–55].
- Epigenetic events may serve as prognostic biomarkers, e.g. methylation of *CASP8* has been associated with non-desmoplastic tumors and *S100A6* methylation is associated with the aggressive large cell/anaplastic disease sub-type. *HIC1* methylation levels in excess of those observed in the normal brain, and weak or low expression of the CASP8 protein, have both been reported as independent indicators of poor survival [48, 51, 53, 56].

Table 4.3 Medulloblastoma in hereditary cancer syndromes.

Syndrome	OMIM	Gene	Locus	Tumour susceptibilities	Risk	Reference
Brain tumor-polyposis syndrome 2/Turcot syndrome Type 2	175100	*APC*	5q21– q22	Medulloblastoma Multiple colorectal adenomas	79% 100%	[22, 23]
Nevoid basal cell carcinoma syndrome (NBCCS)/ Gorlin syndrome	109400	*PTCH*	9q22.3	Medulloblastoma Basal cell carcinoma	3–5% 100%	[24–27]
Li-Fraumeni syndrome	151623	*TP53*	17p13.1	Medulloblastoma Multiple primary neoplasms	~2% 3–25%	[28, 29]
Fanconi anemia (FA) subtype 'D1'	605724	*BRCA2*	13q12.3	Medulloblastoma Wilms' tumor Neuroblastoma	High	[30–32]
Fanconi anemia (FA) subtype 'N'	610832	*PALB2*	16p12.1	Hematological malignancies (pediatric kindred members) Breast cancer (adult kindred members)		
Rubenstein-Taybi syndrome	180849	*CREBBP*	16p13.3	Medulloblastoma Other nervous system tumors Neural crest tumors	Rare Rare Rare	[33]
Coffin-Siris syndrome	135900	–	–	Medulloblastoma	Rare	[34, 35]

Key cell signal pathways in medulloblastoma tumorigenesis

The discovery that genetic alterations target multiple members of the same signal pathways has identified these signaling systems as key regulators of medulloblastoma tumorigenesis.

Sonic hedgehog pathway

The sonic hedgehog (SHH) pathway plays a key role in normal cerebellar development. SHH is secreted by Purkinje neurons and promotes mitogenesis in external granule layer (EGL) progenitor cells during early development [57, 58]. Response to the SHH signal is controlled through two trans-membrane proteins, PTCH and its associated protein 'smoothened' (SMO) (Figure 4.1). In the absence of SHH ligand, PTCH suppresses SMO activity. Upon SHH stimulation, this inhibition is removed, leading to a SMO-induced transcriptional response, mediated by the activation and repression of target genes by the 'GLI' family of zinc-finger-containing transcription factors (GLI-1, GLI-2, GLI-3). In human cells, suppressor of fused (SUFU), co-operates with BTRCP, to inhibit GLI-1-mediated transcription. However, the mechanisms by which SMO activation is coupled to nuclear proteins in the mammalian SHH pathway are otherwise not well understood [57–59]. Key observations regarding SHH signaling in medulloblastoma include:

• Aberrant SHH pathway activation by genetic mutation occurs in at least 15% of medulloblastomas and include inactivating mutations in *PTCH* (~10% of cases), *SMO* activating mutations (~5% of cases), and inactivating mutations in *SUFU* (0–10% of cases) [37, 38, 41, 42, 60–62].

• Gene expression microarray studies indicate up to 25% of medulloblastomas display aberrant SHH signaling suggesting mechanisms in addition to mutation of *PTCH*, *SMO* and *SUFU* components operate in the disease [63].

• Mice in which the Shh pathway is aberrantly activated develop cerebellar tumors that mimic human medulloblastoma at both the histologic and gene expression level (e.g. *Ptch*$^{+/-}$ or *Ptch*$^{+/-}$, *Tp53*$^{-/-}$ mice; *Sufu*$^{+/-}$, *Tp53*$^{-/-}$ mice; *ND2:SmoA1* mice) [64–67].

• Aberrant SHH pathway activation appears to be associated with development of the nodular/desmoplastic medulloblastoma histological sub-type [11, 27, 37, 60]. However, the relationship between SHH defects and nodular/desmoplastic medulloblastomas is not absolute and pathway activation is also observed in classic and large cell/anaplastic tumors [41, 63].

The WNT/Wingless (WNT) pathway

APC is an essential component of the canonical WNT signaling pathway, which is necessary for normal development, including roles in the determination of neural cell fates [58, 68]. The canonical WNT pathway regulates intra-cellular localization of β-catenin, a key transcriptional activator (Figure 4.1). In the absence of pathway stimulation, β-catenin is phosphorylated and targeted for degradation by a complex that includes APC, GSK-3β and AXIN1 proteins. Stimulation of WNT signaling destabilizes the APC/GSK-3β/AXIN1 complex resulting in β-catenin accumulation and signaling [58, 69, 70]. Key observations regarding WNT signaling in medulloblastoma include:

• 10% of medulloblastomas contain oncogenic mutations in the *CTNNB1* gene (which encodes β-catenin). Mutations of alternative pathway components (*APC*, *AXIN1* and *AXIN2*) each affect a further ~2.5% of cases [39, 40, 71–74].

• Nuclear β-catenin protein stabilization provides a indication of WNT pathway activation in medulloblastoma, and affects 18–30% of cases overall [72, 75].

• WNT pathway activation defines a unique molecular subgroup of medulloblastomas, which display a distinct gene

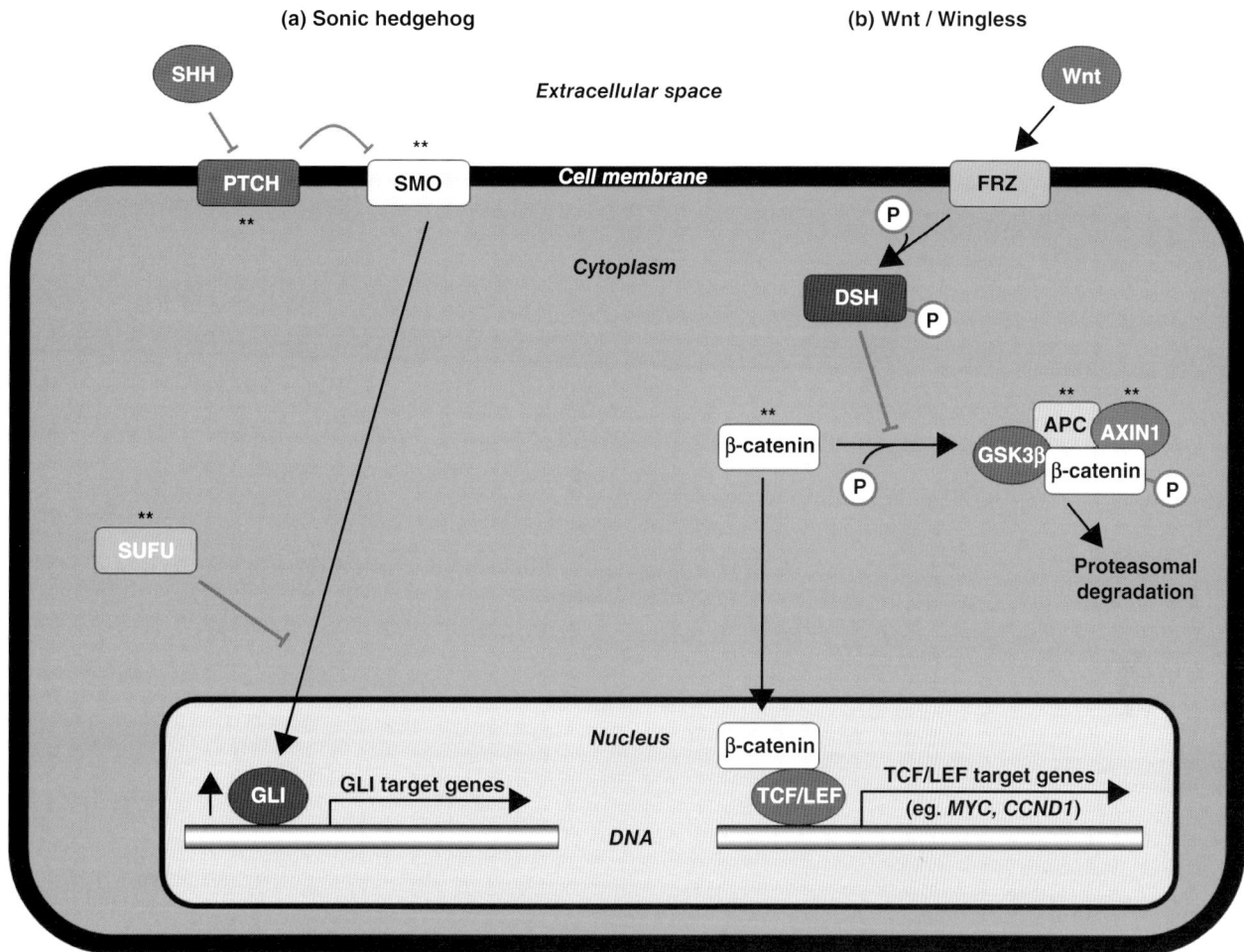

Figure 4.1 (a), The Sonic hedgehog and (b), Wnt/Wingless cell signaling pathways. Pointed arrows, stimulatory effect. Blunted arrows, inhibitory effect. P, phosphorylation. See text for detailed descriptions of each signaling cascade. Mutations in pathway components marked ** have been reported in medulloblastoma, associated with aberrant pathway activation. SHH, sonic hedgehog. PTCH, patched. SMO, smoothened. SUFU, suppressor of fused. GLI, GLI family of transcription factors. FRZ, frizzled. DSH, disheveled. GSK3β, glycogen synthase kinase 3 beta. APC, adenomatous polyposis coli protein. AXIN1, axis inhibition protein 1. TCF/LEF, TCF/LEF transcriptional complex. CCND1, cyclin D1.

expression profile and monsomy 6 and very favorable prognosis [63, 75–77].

TP53 and associated pathways

TP53 is a critical regulator of the cell cycle and apoptosis, and disruption of this gene occurs commonly in multiple cancer types. The TP53 pathway includes p14^{ARF}, a cell cycle inhibitor encoded by the *INK4A/ARF* locus. p14^{ARF} expression is induced in response to cellular stresses including oncogene activation. p14^{ARF} stabilizes TP53 by sequestering MDM2 (a negative regulator of TP53), thus diverting cells to either cell cycle arrest or apoptosis. Disruption of the TP53 pathway in cancer can occur by genetic events including mutation of *TP53*, p14^{ARF} inactivation (by hypermethylation, mutation, or deletion) or amplification of the *MDM2* oncogene [78, 79]. Key observations regarding *TP53* signaling in medulloblastoma include:

- *TP53* mutations have been found in around 10% of sporadic cases [36, 80–83]. A further 10% of medulloblastomas may contain mutually exclusive alterations in *ARF* (homozygous deletion or promoter hypermethylation); however, *MDM2* amplification is rarely observed [80, 83, 84].
- Elevated expression of the TP53 protein is observed in a significant proportion of cases and has been associated with a poor clinical outcome [82, 85, 86], and disruption of the TP53 pathway has been associated with the anaplastic histologic phenotype [80].

Additional aberrant cell signals in medulloblastoma

- Mutations in *PIK3CA*, a member of the family of the phosphatidylinositol 3′-kinase (PI3K) signaling pathway, have been reported in ~5% of medulloblastomas [87], and suggest that PI3K, its pathway components, and effectors may play a role in medulloblastoma tumorigenesis.

• Additional signaling networks, including those regulated through the neurotrophin, PDGFR, and ERBB2 receptor families, have been implicated by gene expression studies in human primary medulloblastomas. However, a genetic basis for their disruption has not yet been uncovered [88–92].

Clinical presentation

The typical presentation of a child with medulloblastoma includes:

• Morning headache relieved by projectile emesis.
• Irritability and lethargy.
• Infants whose fontanelles have not fused, often present with an enlarging head circumference.
• Ataxia, blurred vision, sixth nerve palsy, deterioration in handwriting at school, and on rare occasions back pain in patients with bulky spinal metastatic disease.
• Fundoscopy should be included in the examination of any child presenting with these symptoms. This will often reveal papilledema that is indicative of raised intracranial pressure and mandates further investigation.

Investigation and staging

Imaging

High-quality neuroimaging is required to stage accurately patients with medulloblastoma. For most patients, the initial modality used for imaging is computerized tomography (CT) of the head. The classic finding on CT scans is a mass in the fourth ventricle that is hyperdense on non-contrast imaging and enhances uniformly with contrast. Occasionally medulloblastomas only enhance centrally with contrast or present as hypodense non-enhancing masses [93].

All contemporary protocols stage patients according to the results of magnetic resonance imaging (MRI) [94]. MRI scans of the head are usually obtained with and without contrast pre-operatively and within 24–48 hours of surgical resection. Particular care should be taken to identify both the enhancing and non-enhancing portions of the tumor on the pre-operative MRI, so as to accurately determine the extent of tumor resection on the post-operative MRI. Care should also be taken to inspect all areas of the brain for metastasis, and especially the frontal horns of the lateral ventricles and folia of the cerebellum that are often overlooked (Figure 4.2a-c). Fluid attenuated inversion

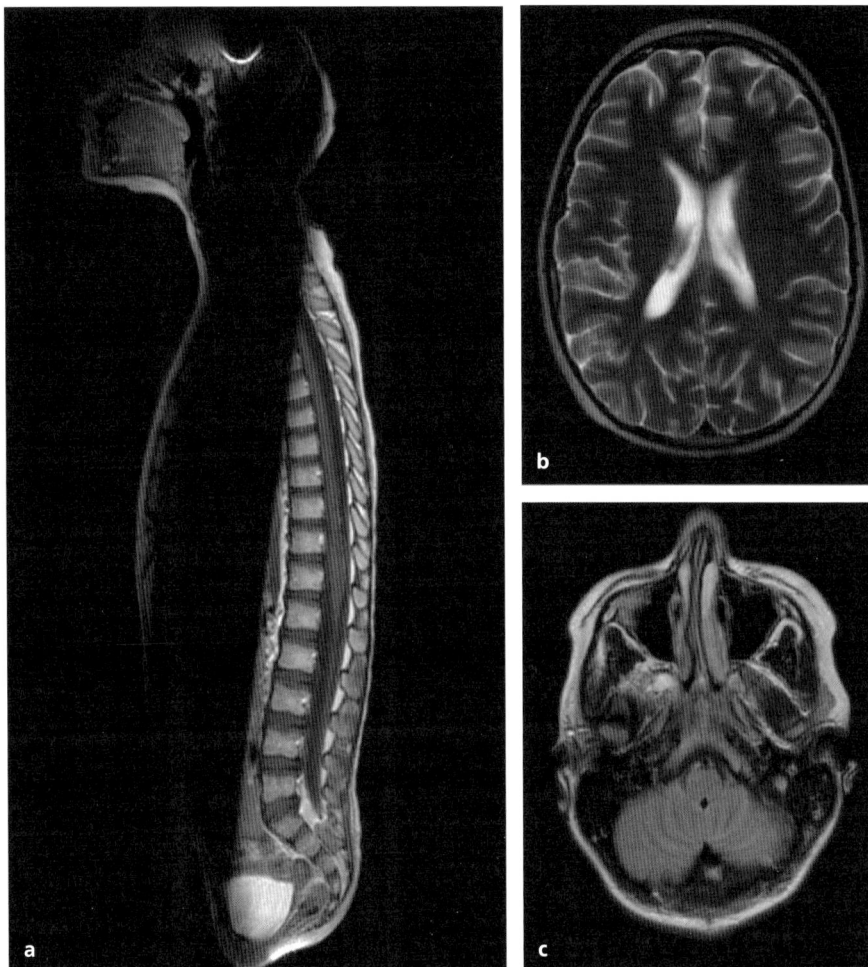

Figure 4.2 Medulloblastoma, showing (a), metastasis beyond the thecal sac, (b), metastasis in the anterior horn of the lateral ventricle, and (c), discrete enhancement in the folia of the cerebellum.

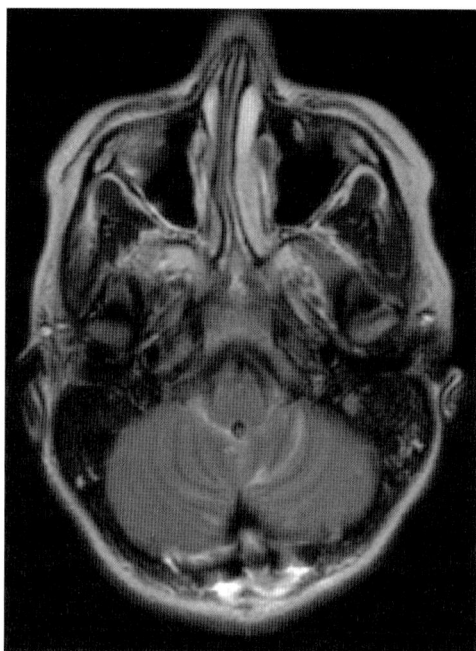

Figure 4.3 Fluid attenunated inversion recovery (FLAIR) sequences distinguish metastatic disease from non-specific enhancement.

Table 4.4 Risk-adapted classification for medulloblastoma (older children)[77].

	Standard risk	High risk
Extent of resection	Gross total resection or ≤ 1.5 cm^2 of residual disease	Residual disease ≥ 1.5 cm^2
Presence of metastatic disease	No metastatic disease	Presence of metastatic disease documented by lumbar cerebrospinal fluid cytology or gadolinium-enhanced magnetic resonance imaging scan of the head/spine

Table 4.5 Staging of metastatic disease[96].

M0	No metastatic disease
M1	Tumor cells present in the cerebrospinal fluid
M2	Presence of metastatic disease limited on the intracranial region only
M3	Presence of metastatic disease coating the spine
M4	Presence of metastatic disease outside the neuraxis

recovery (FLAIR) sequences can often assist in distinguishing subtle metastatic disease from non-specific enhancement (Figure 4.3).

MRI of the spine can be obtained either pre-operatively or 10–14 days post-operatively. Caution needs to be exercised when evaluating the spinal cord for metastatic disease. The entire length of the spinal cord needs to be imaged with sagittal T1 sequences both pre- and post-gadolinium enhancement. Note that metastatic deposits are often located at the tip of the conus or just caudal of this point and can be missed if the entire neuraxis is not imaged (Figure 4.2a). Any areas of concern within the spine should be reimaged with axial T1 sequences that can help to determine the presence of metastases. Since clinical outcome is correlated so closely with disease stage, it is recommended that all imaging studies of patients treated on prospective clinical trials undergo central review.

Imaging changes seen during the post-therapy period have been known to mimic recurrent disease; hence extreme caution needs to be exercised when interpreting scans during this period [95].

Risk stratification
The extent of tumor resection and presence of metastatic disease are the key factors that determine disease risk for newly diagnosed patients with medulloblastoma (Tables 4.4 and 4.5). The current system is based on the Chang staging system developed in the 1960s; however, improvements in surgical management have reduced the relevance of the tumor (T) stage component [96]. The presence of tumor cells in the cerebrospinal fluid (CSF) is

best confirmed on CSF that is obtained by lumbar puncture 2 weeks after surgical resection of the tumor [97]. Although the prognostic significance of several biologic factors have been evaluated, none of these factors are currently being used to assign disease risk [8, 85, 98, 99].

Staging of infants is similar to that of older children. Emerging data from several studies document that infants with desmoplastic medulloblastoma have an improved survival as compared to those infants with either classic or large cell/anaplastic histology [100]. The same principles of staging are utilized for staining PNET and ATRT patients. Similar to medulloblastoma patients, the extent of resection and presence of metastatic disease are important determinants of prognosis.

Treatment
Infants
Surgical resection, neuraxis radiation therapy, and chemotherapy are the three modalities that are used to successfully treat children diagnosed with medulloblastoma. Due to the devastating consequences of radiation therapy to the young brain, investigators have devised research protocols that seek to avoid or delay radiation therapy in children aged less than 3 years [101, 102] (Table 4.6). These studies demonstrated that radiation could be delayed or even omitted without compromising survival in a subset of medulloblastoma patients younger than 3 years of age at diagnosis.

Delayed radiation
The Pediatric Oncology Group (POG) and Children's Cancer Study Group (CCG) adopted a delayed radiotherapy approach

Table 4.6 Summary of outcome for infant studies.

Trial	n	5–year Event-free survival (±SE)*	5–year Overall survival (±SE)*	Reference
M0 no residual				
Baby POG	13		69%	[103, 104]
CCG 9921	38	41 ± 8%	54 ± 8%	[105]
Early studies that showed that these patients can be cured with chemotherapy and radiation therapy				
SFOP	47	29% (95% CI 18–44)	73% (95% CI 59–84)	[106]
HIT–SKK92	17	82 ± 9%	93 ± 6%	[100]
Head Start I + II (age > 3 year)	14	64 ± 13%	86 ± 9%	[107]
Next generation of studies that showed that >70% of infants can be cured with more aggressive chemotherapy or radiation therapy at the time of relapse				
M0 with residual				
CCG 9921	23	26 ± 9%	40 ± 11%	[105]
SFOP	17	6% (95% CI 1–27)	41% (95% CI 22–64)	[106]
HIT–SKK92	14	50 ± 13%	56 ± 14%	[100]
Head Start I + II (age > 3 year)	7	29 ± 17%	57 ± 19%	[107]
Infants with residual disease at the time of surgery had a lower event-free survival despite aggressive combined modality therapy				
Metastatic (M+)				
CCG 9921	31	25 ± 8%	31 ± 9%	[105]
SFOP	15	13% (95%CI 4–38)	13% (95%CI 4–38)	[106]
HIT–SKK92	12	33 ± 14%	38 ± 15%	[100]
Head Start II * (age < 6 year)	21	3-year EFS 49% (95%CI 27–72)	3-year OS 60% (95%CI 36–84)	[108]
Infants with metastatic disease have a dismal prognosis despite aggressive therapy.				

*The Head Start II protocol only included nine patients <3 years of age.

(POG 8633/34 [termed Baby POG-1] [103, 104] and CCG 921 trials [109]).

• Baby POG-1: children under the age of 3 years were treated with chemotherapy consisting of vincristine, cyclophosphamide, etoposide, and cisplatin. Neuraxis radiation was delivered after 1 or 2 years following diagnosis, but was successfully delayed in only 40% of patients. The 5-year progression-free survival (PFS) and overall survival (OS) for all medulloblastoma patients were 31.8 ± 8.3% and 39.7 ± 6.9% respectively. Patients with non-metastatic and gross totally resected tumors (M0R0) had much better outcomes, with 5-year OS of 69%.

• POG study 9233/34 (termed Baby POG-2) intensified the chemotherapy regimen. Patients were randomized between standard Baby POG-1 treatment or an intensified version of Baby POG-1 therapy in which the same drugs were administered at higher doses and more frequently. No difference in event-free survival (EFS) or OS was observed between patients receiving standard or intensified Baby POG therapy (unpublished data).

• CCG 921 [109] included children younger than 18 months of age. Patients were treated with the '8 in 1' chemotherapy regimen, followed by delayed neuraxis radiation or focal radiotherapy. Only 10% (nine of 91) of patients received the planned radiotherapy (RT) treatment. Patients with medulloblastoma had a

3-year PFS of 22%. The outcome for patients with M0R0 disease was marginally superior (5-year PFS 30%) [109].

• CCG 9921 [105] used a strategy of more intensive chemotherapy to improve outcome. Children younger than 3 years of age were randomly assigned to receive one of two five-cycle induction chemotherapy regimens, followed by a uniform regimen of maintenance chemotherapy for 56 weeks. Patients with residual or metastatic disease were to receive focal radiation or neuraxis radiotherapy at the end of maintenance or at 3 years of age, whichever came earlier. Only a minority (40%) of patients received RT treatment as planned. There was no difference in EFS or OS between chemotherapy arms.

Neuraxis radiation restricted to disease recurrence or progression

The Baby Brain Societe Française d'Oncologie Pediatrique (BBSFOP) trial treated patients younger than 4 years of age with conventional chemotherapy alone, reserving radiation (focal to the posterior fossa only) combined with high-dose chemotherapy and autologous stem cell rescue (ASCR), for patients whose tumors progressed or recurred [106]. The BBSFOP chemotherapy regimen resulted in a 5-year PFS of 29% (95% CI, 18–44) for M0R0 patients, revealing that this subset can achieve long-term survival with no radiation and relatively mild chemotherapy. Many patients were successfully salvaged with focal radiation and high-dose chemotherapy with ASCR, resulting in a 5-year OS for M0R0 patients of 73% (95% CI, 59 to 84) [106].

Strategies to avoid neuraxis radiation

• High-dose systemic and intensive intraventricular methotrexate combined with standard chemotherapy [100]. Using this approach, the HITSKK92 trial achieved the best results to date for children aged less than 3 years old with M0/M1R0 medulloblastoma (*n* = 17), with 5-year PFS and OS of 82 ± 9% and 93 ± 6% respectively. Outcomes for patients with residual disease (*n* = 14) were also somewhat better than in prior series, with 5-year PFS and OS of 50 ± 13% and 56 ± 14% respectively. Only patients with macroscopic metastasis (M2–M3) (*n* = 12) faired poorly, with 5-year PFS and OS of 33 ± 14% and 38 ± 15% respectively. This study reported no toxic deaths, but there was a very high frequency (19 of 23 [83%] evaluated patients) of asymptomatic leukoencephalopathy noted on MRI, most likely attributable to the intensive use of intrathecal methotrexate. This study revealed that the majority of young children without macroscopic metastasis and completely resected medulloblastoma can be cured with chemotherapy alone, but at a cost of methotrexate-induced neurotoxicity [100].

• Myeloablative chemotherapy with ASCR has also been investigated as an alternative to neuraxis irradiation. This approach was used by the Head Start II trial, which utilized five cycles of induction chemotherapy very similar to CCG 9921, but with the addition of high-dose intravenous methotrexate, followed by a single consolidation course of myeloablative therapy using carboplatin, thiotepa, and etoposide with ASCR. Using this strategy the Head Start II trial has achieved the best results to date for young children (defined as age less than 6 years in this trial) with metastatic medulloblastoma (M1–M3) (*n* = 21), with 3-year EFS and OS of 49% (95% CI, 27–72) and 60% (95% CI, 36–84), respectively [108]. Though promising, interpretation of these results is limited

by the small size of the study and inclusion of older children (only nine patients under age 3 years at diagnosis were enrolled). Children aged less than 3 years with M0 medulloblastoma treated on Head Start I and II trials were treated with identical therapy as patients with metastatic disease, except they did not receive high-dose methotrexate. For patients with M0R0 medulloblastoma (*n* = 14) the results of this trial are comparable with those of the German group, with 5-year EFS and OS of 64 ± 13% and 86 ± 9% respectively (unpublished data). This strategy appears to add no benefit for patients with non-metastatic residual disease (M0R1) (*n* = 7), since the 5-year EFS of 29 ± 17% for this group, is comparable to the CCG 9921 trial result of 26 ± 9%, which was achieved without the use of myeloablative chemotherapy with ASCR [105].

Older children with average-risk disease

Collectively, studies conducted among these patients have demonstrated that the addition of adjuvant chemotherapy has improved the cure rates for average-risk medulloblastoma (Table 4.7).

Reduced dose radiation

A series of initial studies demonstrated the efficacy of reduced-dose neuraxis radiation (23.4 Gy) with chemotherapy [110–112].

POG-CCG A9961. Patients were treated with neuraxis radiation (23.4 Gy) and with posterior fossa boost (55.8 Gy); vincristine was administered weekly during radiotherapy. After the completion of radiotherapy, patients were randomly assigned to groups that received either the standard regimen of lomustine, cisplatin, and vincristine or the alternative regimen of cyclophosphamide, cisplatin, and vincristine. The 5-year EFS for the 379 eligible patients enroled on the study was 81 ± 2% and there was no difference in the EFS of either arm of the study [113]. Based on this result, the current Children's Oncology Group (COG) is conducting a randomized study that is seeking to reduce further

Table 4.7 Results of prospective clinical trials for older children with standard-risk medulloblastoma. Large prospective studies demonstrating that approximately 80% of patients with standard-risk medulloblastoma can be cured with either standard dose (35 Gy) or lower dose (23.4 Gy) neuraxis radiation and adjuvant chemotherapy.

Trial	Treatment	Radiotherapy dose (Gy)	
		Neuraxis radiation	PF
Average risk (M0R0)			
CCG 9892 (1990–1994)	Reduced dose RT with weekly VCR followed by CHT (VCR, CDDP and CCNU)	23.4	55.8
SIOP-PNET3 (1992–2000)	Standard dose RT only vs Pre-RT CHT (VCR, VP-16, CBDA and Cyclo)	35	55
HIT-91 (1991–1997)	Pre-RT CHT (Ifos, ara-C, VP-16, HD-MTX, CDDP) vs Post-RT CHT (VCR, CDDP and CCNU)	35.2	55.2
A9961 (1996–2000)	Weekly VCR during RT then CCNU, CDDP, VCR. vs. Cyclo, CDDP, VCR	23.4	55.8
SJMB96 (1996–2003)	Reduced dose RT followed by four cycles of high-dose CHT with ASCR (VCR, CDDP and Cyclo)	23.4	55.8

EFS, event-free survival. Radiation, radiation therapy. CHT, chemotherapy. RD, residual disease. Neuraxis radiation, craniospinal irradiation. PF, posterior fossa. Cyclo, cyclophosphamide. CDDP, cisplatin. VCR, vincristine. CCNU, lomustine. VP-16- Etoposide, MTX, methotrexate; etoposide. 8-in-1, 8 chemotherapeutic agents administered in one day (consisting of VCR, methylprednisolone, CCNU, CDDP, hydroxyurea, procarbazine, ara-c and cyclo). *Unless otherwise stated.

the dose of neuraxis radiation to 18 Gy in patients ≥3–≤ 8 years of age while maintaining the same degree of disease control.

Timing of radiation

Studies by the International Society of Pediatric Oncology (SIOP) have attempted to answer the question of timing of chemotherapy in relation to radiation.

• SIOP II clearly demonstrated that use of prolonged pre-radiation chemotherapy negatively affects the EFS estimate for average-risk patients. The negative result could also be attributed to the choice of drugs given before radiation, because this chemotherapy regimen did not contain cisplatin, a drug that is particularly effective against medulloblastoma [114].

• SIOP III compared EFS estimates for patients treated with radiation alone with those for patients treated with vincristine, carboplatin, cyclophosphamide, and etoposide for four cycles and subsequent radiation. The dose of neuraxis radiation was 36 Gy, and the dose to the posterior fossa was 56 Gy. In contrast to United States studies that exclude M1 patients from average-risk protocols, patients with M0 and M1 disease were enroled on this study; therefore the comparison of these data with those from the United States is difficult. Of the 217 patients enrolled on the SIOP III study, 179 were eligible for analysis. The EFS probability at 5 years for the group that received chemotherapy and radiation was 74%, whereas that for the group that received only radiation was 60% (*P = 0.036*). This study confirms that post-operative standard-dose neuraxis radiation alone achieves 5-year EFS rates of between 60 and 65% and that this can be improved with the addition of platinum-based chemotherapy [115].

• HIT 91 compared the outcome of patients receiving pre- or post-radiation chemotherapy [116]. Two-hundred and eighty patients were enrolled on the study. Patients with M1 disease and residual tumor following surgery were included in the average-risk group. Included among the 234 average-risk patients were 69 patients with residual tumor and 49 patients with M1 disease. Once again, these disease risk criteria render any comparisons with US study data problematic. Post-radiation chemotherapy included eight cycles consisting of lomustine, cisplatin, and vincristine. Radiation for all patients consisted of neuraxis radiation (35.2 Gy) and irradiation of the posterior fossa (55.2 Gy). Pre-radiation chemotherapy included procarbazine, ifosfamide/etoposide, high-dose methotrexate, cisplatin, and Ara-C. Patients whose tumor responded poorly to the pre-radiation chemotherapy were given additional chemotherapy consisting of carboplatin, lomustine, and vincristine after radiation. The 5-year PFS estimate for patients in the post-radiation chemotherapy arm was 78% ± 6%, whereas that for patients in the pre-radiation chemotherapy group was 65% ± 5% (*P = 0.03*) [116]. The results for the post-radiation chemotherapy arm confirm those seen in United States studies in which a similar approach was used, albeit with a lower dose of neuraxis radiation and a more clearly defined group of average-risk patients.

Treatment of high-risk patients

Attempts to improve survival estimates for high-risk patients (≥1.5 cm² residual disease or presence of metastatic disease) have relied on a variety of chemotherapy regimens administered before or after radiation (Table 4.8). Historically, high-risk patients

Table 4.8 Prospective studies documenting poor survival for high-risk patients treated with neoadjuvant chemotherapy. The best results are documented in patients treated with high dose neuraxis radiation post-RT followed by moderately intense adjuvant chemotherapy.

Trial	Treatment	Radiotherapy dose (Gy) Neuraxis radiation	PF	5-year EFS (±SE)*
High risk (M1–M3 ± R1)				
HIT-91 (M2–M3) (1991–1997)	Pre-RT CHT (Ifos, ara-C, VP-16, HD-MTX, CDDP) vs Post-RT CHT (VCR, CDDP and CCNU) Separate results for the two treatment arms were not provided)	35.2	55.2	30 ± 15% (3 year EFS)
SIOP-PNET3 (M2–M3) (1992–2000)	Pre-RT CHT (VP-16 VCR, Cyclo and CBDA)	35	55	34.7%
CHOP (M1–M3)	Weekly VCR during RT then CCNU, CDDP, VCR	36	55.8	67 ± 15%
SJMB96 (M1–M3) (1996–2003)	Topotecan window pre-RT followed by four cycles of high dose CHT with ASCR (VCR, CDDP and Cyclo)	36 –39.6	55.8	70% (95%CI 55–85)

EFS, event-free survival. Radiation, radiation therapy. CHT, chemotherapy. Neuraxis radiation, craniospinal irradiation. PF, posterior fossa. Cyclo, cyclophosphamide. CDDP, cisplatin. VCR, vincristine. CCNU, lomustine. VP-16, Etoposide. MTX, methotrexate. * Unless otherwise stated.

treated with radiation alone have had 5-year PFS estimates of 25–40% [117]. In a trial conducted at five institutions and reported by Packer *et al.*, the 5-year PFS probability was 67% ± 15% for 15 patients with M+ disease treated with radiation with concurrent vincristine and adjuvant chemotherapy consisting of lomustine, cisplatin, and vincristine [118]. The impact of combined modality therapy on the PFS probability of high-risk patients has been confirmed in a recently reported POG study (POG 9031) [119]. Of the 224 patients enroled on the study, 94 patients had M+ disease. Patients were randomly assigned to groups that received three cycles of cisplatin and etoposide either before or immediately after RT; all patients subsequently received eight cycles of cyclophosphamide and vincristine. Patients with M1 disease received 35.2 Gy neuraxis radiation, and most patients with M2/M3 disease received 40 Gy neuraxis radiation with a boost of 4.8 Gy to gross sites of metastatic disease. The dose of irradiation to the posterior fossa ranged from 53.2 to 54.4 Gy. The 5-year EFS estimate for the patients with M+ disease was approximately 55%, a result that confirms the pilot experience of Packer *et al.*

Another large study in which pre-radiation and post-radiation arms were randomized was the CCG 921 study. This study enrolled 203 eligible patients with high-risk medulloblastoma; 188 patients were randomly assigned to two treatment groups. The experimental arm got two cycles of '8 in 1' chemotherapy pre-radiation and then received an additional six cycles of the same chemotherapy. In the standard arm, the chemotherapy was similar to the study by Packer *et al.* described above [118]. Patients received 36 Gy neuraxis radiation with a further radiation boost to the primary tumor site. The 5-year estimate of PFS for the entire cohort of patients was 54% ± 5%. Patients treated with the standard regimen of lomustine, vincristine, and prednisone had a 5-year PFS probability of 63% ± 5%. This estimate is similar to those noted from the Packer study and the POG study and superior to those achieved with the investigational '8-in-1' regimen [120].

For high-risk patients, the use of pre-radiation chemotherapy for a prolonged period of time yielded results that were clearly inferior to those obtained by the use of a shorter window (approximately 6–8 weeks of chemotherapy). Results from the PNET III trial and the HIT 91 trial that used pre-radiation chemotherapy did not demonstrate a survival advantage for patients despite the use of drugs that were active against medulloblastoma. The EFS for M2–M3 patients were 34.7% (*n* = 68) and 30% (*n* = 19) at 5 years and 3 years for the PNET III and HIT trials respectively [116, 121].

The best result for high-risk medulloblastoma to date has been published by a consortium of investigators led by St Jude Children's Research Hospital. Following maximal surgical resection of the tumor, therapy consisted of neuraxis radiation (36 Gy M0–M1; 39.6 Gy M2–M3) with an additional radiation boost to the primary tumor bed and a 2 cm margin delivered by a 3-dimensional conformal technique. Six weeks post-completion of radiation these investigators used four courses of cyclophosphamide-based dose intensive chemotherapy, with hematopoietic stem cell support, over 16 weeks. The 5-year EFS for 48 patients with high-risk medulloblastoma was 70% at 5 years [77]. This study suggests that chemotherapy does significantly improve the survival for patients with high-risk medulloblastoma, but the timing of chemotherapy in relation to radiation is critical to achieve good results. Despite using drugs with proven efficacy against medulloblastoma, neo-adjuvant chemotherapy used for a duration of greater than 6 weeks may have a detrimental impact on EFS in high-risk patients.

Prognostic factors

Only clinical variables are currently used in the therapeutic stratification of patients with medulloblastoma; molecular markers and histopathological subclassification do not currently influence therapeutic strategy. However, variability in outcome exists within current clinical risk groups. The accurate identification of disease risk thus remains a major goal, as a more robust stratification of disease-risk would facilitate the targeted use of adjuvant therapies; intensive regimens for aggressive tumors and reduced long-term side effects for patients with responsive tumors.

Assessment of the prognostic significance of molecular defects in medulloblastoma has frequently been limited by the retrospective analysis of individual markers in small, heterogenously treated cohorts. Nonetheless, a range of molecular markers with prognostic potential have now been identified in trial-based studies (Table 4.9).

• Markers associated with good prognosis: nuclear immunoreactivity of β-catenin [75, 77], expression of *TRKC* neurotrophin receptor [90]. The MBEN, which is a tumor of infancy, is associated with a good prognosis [122], and the wider desmoplastic variant (including MBENs) has consistently been associated with a more favorable outcome in trials-based studies in infants [8, 100].

• Markers associated with poor prognosis: amplification and or expression of the *MYC* and *MYCN* oncogenes [10, 98, 99], defects of chromosome 17 [10], and expression of the ERBB2 receptor tyrosine kinase [98]. Among the histopathological variants of medulloblastoma, an aggressive biological behavior has been established for the overlapping large-cell and anaplastic variants, which have been associated with a poor outcome in several clinical trial cohorts [6, 8, 77, 123, 124].

Treatment of other forms of embryonal tumors

Atypical teratoid rhabdoid tumors

Atypical teratoid/rhabdoid tumor (ATRT) has only recently been recognized as a distinct tumor entity from other CNS embryonal tumors [125, 126]. Key features are:

• Highly aggressive tumor.

• Occurs primarily in children younger than 2 years of age and frequently presents with metastatic disease at diagnosis [127, 128].

• Characterized by alterations in the *SMARCB1* (also known as *INI1/hSNF5*) gene on chromosome 22q11 [129].

Table 4.9 Molecular and histopathological markers of disease-risk in medulloblastoma, showing disease features which display consistent associations with prognosis in two or more clinical trials-based studies.

Disease feature	Method of detection	Prevalence	Survival (risk-group vs others)	Statistical analysis	Clinical trial	Cohort age range (years)	Reference
Favorable risk Wnt/Wg pathway activation-catenin nuclear((stabilization)	IHC	27/109 (25%)	92% vs 65% (5 year OS)	*P = 0.006*[m]	PNET3	3–16.8	[75]
		10/69 (14%)	100% vs 68% (5 year EFS)	*P = 0.03*[u]	SJMB96	3.1–20.2	[77]
Desmoplasia (in infants ≤3 years)	Histopathological assessment	20/43 (47%)	85% vs 34% (7 year PFS)	*P < 0.001*[m]	HIT-SKK'92	<3	[100]
		17/28 (61%)	53% vs 17% (5 year OS)	NR	CNS9204	<3	[8]
Adverse risk *MYC* gene amplification	FISH	5/84 (6%)	All dead at 5 years*	*P < 0.001*[m]	PNET3	>3	[10]
	qPCR	5/111 (4.5%)	40% vs 66% (7 year OS)	NS	HIT '91	3–18	[99]
Large-cell/anaplastic histology	Histopathological assessment	23/116 (20%)	57% vs ~80% (5 year EFS)	*P = 0.04*[u]	SJMB96	3.1–20.2	[77]
		52/315 (17%)	~55% vs ~75% (5 year OS)	*P = 0.024*[m]	PNET3	2.7–16.4	[8]

IHC, immunohistochemistry. FISH, fluorescence *in situ* hybridization. qPCR, quantitative polymerase chain reaction. OS, overall survival. EFS, event-free survival. PFS, progression-free survival. [m]multivariate analysis. [u]univariate analysis. NR, not reported. NS, not significant. COG, Children's Oncology Group. * Cases showing high-level gene amplification in >25% of tumor nuclei.

• The majority (85%) of ATRTs have inactivation of the *SMARCB1* gene, either through homozygous deletions or loss of one allele with concomitant mutation of the other copy.

• Older children with ATRT have been successfully treated with a combination of complete resection, neuraxis radiation, and high-dose chemotherapy with ASCR [130]. In contrast, possibly because of the omission of neuraxis radiation, outcomes for children younger than 3 years of age with a highly aggressive tumor are dismal. The 2-year EFS for 28 children less than 3 years old treated on the CCG 9921 trial was 14 ± 7% [105]. Likewise, in the St Jude experience reported by Tekautz *et al.* the 2-year EFS for the 22 children less than 3 years of age at diagnosis was 11 ± 6% [130]. Effective chemotherapy regimes for young children with ATRT remain elusive.

Supratentorial primitive neuroectodermal tumors including pineoblastoma

Supratentorial primitive neuroectodermal tumors (SPNET) in children are rare and represent less than 2.5% of childhood brain tumors [131]. Key features are:

1 SPNET are histologically similar to medulloblastomas [132].

2 SPNET are thought to be less curable than medulloblastoma (Table 4.10) [133, 134].

3 Higher doses of radiation therapy are used routinely to treat SPNET, regardless of the stage of the disease.

4 Pineal tumors have a better outcome as compared with non-pineal SPNET [133–137].

5 SPNET and medulloblastomas are molecularly distinct [138–141].

• SPNET display chromosomal losses affecting 1p12-22.1 and 9p, and gains at 19p, which are not commonly observed in medulloblastoma.

• SPNET show a reduced frequency of imbalances involving chromosome 17, the most common chromosome defect in medulloblastoma [142, 143].

6 Radiation therapy is an important component of the treatment of SPNET (Table 4.10).

• Timmerman *et al.* have recommended treating the entire neuraxis of patients with SPNET with at least 35 Gy and the primary tumor with at least 54 Gy [144].

• Massimino *et al.* treated children older than 4 years with SPNET with initial chemotherapy and then hyperfractionated craniospinal radiation therapy (31.2–39 Gy) and boost to the tumor site to a total dose of 59.7–60 Gy [145]. After the completion of hyperfractionated radiation therapy, these patients received either standard or high-dose chemotherapy followed by autologous stem-cell rescue. The 3-year EFS for all 15 patients was 34%.

• In the SIOP/UKCCSG experience by Pizer *et al.*, 68 patients were treated with radiation therapy that consisted of neuraxis radiation (35 Gy) with an additional 20 Gy boost to the primary tumor site [135]. Forty-four of these patients also received four cycles of chemotherapy before the start of radiation therapy, whereas the others received radiation therapy alone. The 5-year

Table 4.10 Results of prospective studies demonstrating that supratentorial primitive neuroectodermal tumors (PNET) have an inferior event-free S survival as compared with posteria fossa PNET despite aggressive therapy. Patients with pineoblastoma have a better prognosis in this age group.

Study	n	Radiation dose (neuraxis radiation)	Survival estimates	Pineal/non-pineal	Reference
CHOP/CNMC	22	34–40 Gy	5-year PFS, 37%	13/9	[137]
CCG	44	36–40 Gy	3-year PFS, 45%	17/27[a]	[133]
CCG	27	36 Gy for those older than 3 years	5-year PFS, 31%	0/27	[136]
		23.4 Gy for those 1.5–3 year ($n = 9$)			
HIT 88/89	63	35.2 Gy	3-year PFS, 39%	11/52[b]	[144]
CCG	17	36 Gy for those older than 3 years ($n = 15$)	3-year PFS, 61%	17/0	[134]
		23.4 Gy for those 1.5–3 years ($n = 2$)			
SIOP/UKCCSG	68	35 Gy	5-year EFS, 47%	14/54	[135]
Milan/Rome	15	31.2 Gy for those younger than 10 years	3-year EFS, 34%	3/12[c]	[145]
		39 Gy for those 10 years or older (6 patients)	3-year PFS, 54%		

Neuraxis radiation, craniospinal irradiation. PFS, progression-free survival. EFS, event-free survival. [a] PFS estimate for those with pineal tumors, 61%; PFS estimate for those with non-pineal tumors, 33%. [b] Disease in 46 patients was classified as M_0. [c] Ten patients received high-dose thiotepa and stem-cell rescue after the completion of neuraxis radiation (hyperfractionated). Second tumors developed in two patients. All patients received high dose chemotherapy prior to radiation. CHOP, Children's Hospital of Philadelphia. CNMC, Children's National Medical Center. CCG, Children's Cancer Group.

EFS was 40.7% for patients with non-pineal PNET and 71.4% for those with pineal PNET (14 patients). The overall 5-year EFS estimate was 47% for the entire group. The addition of pre-irradiation chemotherapy did not impact favorably on the EFS. This European experience demonstrates the relatively good outcome for pineal SPNET compared with non-pineal SPNET with all patients receiving at least 35 Gy to the craniospinal axis.

Treatment strategies for relapsed disease

Considerable debate remains as to the best therapeutic approach for patients who have recurrent disease. Infants who have not had irradiation as part of their original therapy and have a local relapse can clearly be salvaged by surgical resection and local radiation ± high dose chemotherapy (HDCT) [146]. For infants with metastatic relapse of medulloblastoma, HDCT alone is not effective and though neuraxis radiation can salvage a proportion of these patients the neurocognitive outcome is devastating [101, 102].

The outcome for patients with embryonal brain tumors who relapse following previous neuraxis radiation and who are retreated with 'conventional therapy' is abysmal. In this respect, HDCT has been widely investigated to improve the outcome of such patients. More than a decade ago, Finlay *et al.* published a landmark article in which they demonstrated that a subset of patients with recurrent brain tumors of diverse histological diagnosis could be salvaged with high-dose chemotherapy followed by ASCR [147]. Observations from this early series suggested that patients with minimal residual disease at the time of high-dose chemotherapy may be the appropriate candidates for this retrieval strategy. Patients with bulky, metastatic recurrent disease or

disease that did not respond to retrieval chemotherapy may not be the best candidates for this intervention. The toxicity of this approach was also a concern in this early series. Subsequently other investigators have further explored the role of high dose chemotherapy in patients with recurrent medulloblastoma [148, 149]. Recent data has demonstrated that high dose chemotherapy has failed to cure patients treated with radiation therapy and chemotherapy as part of their initial treatment [150].

The lack of randomized prospective studies that use HDCT vs standard dose chemotherapy for patients with recurrent disease make it difficult to compare the efficacy and short- and long-term toxicities between the two approaches.

Complications of treatment and important late-effects

Patients treated with multimodality therapy unfortunately do suffer from multiple early and late consequences of therapy. Early side effects include the expected side effects of therapy, many of which are reversible. Irreversible consequences of therapy are hearing loss [151, 152], endocrine deficiencies [153–158], neurocognitive decline [159–161], secondary malignancies [162], and sterility [163]. Age of the patient and dose of neuraxis radiation are key factors implicated in the degree of neurocognitive decline with the younger patients who are treated with higher dose irradiation suffering the worst decline [102, 164]. In addition to the decline in global IQ, these patients also demonstrate a decline in memory, attention, and processing speed [165–167]. Current attempts to reduce the dose of neuraxis radiation in standard-risk patients are seeking to reduce the degree of neuroendocrine and neurocognitive decline in this patient population while seeking to maintain a high cure rate [168, 169]. Current research initiates are focusing on introduction of intervention programs to compensate for the neurocognitive decline [170].

Novel therapeutic approaches

There has been a paucity of effective new traditional cytotoxic drugs which have shown efficacy against recurrent medulloblastoma [171–174]. In a phase II study in newly diagnosed patients with medulloblastoma/PNET, topotecan, a topoisomerase I inhibitor with good CSF penetration, showed efficacy in a third of the patients demonstrating response [175, 176]. However, this lack of newer effective chemotherapy agents has impeded the development of therapeutic strategies for medulloblastoma.

The application of novel small molecule inhibitors targeted against specific biological pathways offers promise for the improved therapy of embryonal brain tumors, with long-term potential for the development of therapies tailored to the biological profile of individual tumors, coupled with enhanced drug specificity and reduced toxicity/late-effects. Pre-clinical studies of compounds which target pathways constitutively activated by gene mutations in medulloblastoma pathogenesis are underway; small molecule inhibitors of the SHH pathway show significant pre-clinical activity against both xenograft models and tumors which arise spontaneously in transgenic ($ptch^{+/-}$; $p53^{-/-}$) models [177–179], while effective inhibitors of the canonical Wnt/Wg pathway are at much earlier stages in their development [180]. Additionally, inhibitors which target other pathways overexpressed in subsets of medulloblastomas (e.g. ERBB2, PDGFR and the RAS/MPK pathway) are at various stages of clinical development and merit investigation. The identification of specific biological pathways which could be targeted therapeutically in ATRT and SPNETs remains the focus of ongoing basic research investigations. Alongside the potential benefits offered by targeted therapies, careful consideration must be given to potential toxicities, associated with the delivery to young children of compounds which inhibit critical development pathways, in the planning of early clinical trials [181].

Summary and future directions for management

Therapeutic approaches to medulloblastoma have yielded very encouraging results over the last three decades; cure rates have gradually increased as a result of improvements in multimodality based therapy. Despite these successes, significant challenges remain, particularly in improving the long-term neurocognitive outcome for survivors and improving the cure rate for infants and high-risk presentations. Significant insights have been generated into the patho-biology of medulloblastoma using advanced molecular genetics. Future studies will seek to integrate this knowledge into front-line treatment protocols, through the development of risk-tailored stratification schemes, and therapies which target critical aspects of tumor biology [182]. International collaborations that increase the accrual to clinical protocols and tissue acquisition will be a cornerstone to making advances in curative strategies for this disease.

References

1 Cushing H. Experiences with the cerebellar medulloblastomas: a critical review. Acta Pathol Microbiol Scand 1930; 1: 1–86.

2 Park TS, Hoffman HJ, Hendrick EB, Humphreys RP, Becker LE. Medulloblastoma: clinical presentation and management. Experience at the Hospital For Sick Children, Toronto, 1950–1980. J Neurosurg 1983; 58: 543–52.

3 Louis DN, Ohgaki H, Wiestler OD, et al. The 2007 WHO classification of tumors of the central nervous system. Acta Neuropathol 2007; 114: 97–109.

4 McNeil DE, Cote TR, Clegg L, Rorke LB. Incidence and trends in pediatric malignancies medulloblastoma/primitive neuroectodermal tumor: a SEER update. Surveillance Epidemiology and End Results. Med Pediatr Oncol 2002; 39: 190–45.

5 Giangaspero F, Rigobello L, Badiali M, et al. Large-cell medulloblastomas. A distinct variant with highly aggressive behavior. Am J Surg Pathol 1992; 16: 687–93.

6 McManamy CS, Lamont JM, Taylor RE, et al. Morphophenotypic variation predicts clinical behavior in childhood non–desmoplastic medulloblastomas. J Neuropathol Exp Neurol 2003; 62: 627–32.

7 Ellison D. Classifying the medulloblastoma: insights from morphology and molecular genetics. Neuropathol Appl Neurobiol 2002; 28: 257–82.

8 McManamy CS, Pears J, Weston CL, et al. Nodule formation and desmoplasia in medulloblastomas – defining the nodular/desmoplastic variant and its biological behavior. Brain Pathol 2007; 17: 151–64.

9 Bigner SH, Mark J, Friedman HS, et al. Structural chromosomal abnormalities in human medulloblastoma. Cancer Genet Cytogenet 1988; 30: 91–101.

10 Lamont JM, McManamy CS, Pearson AD, Clifford SC, Ellison DW. Combined histopathological and molecular cytogenetic stratification of medulloblastoma patients. Clin Cancer Res 2004; 10: 5482–93.

11 Nicholson JC, Ross FM, Kohler JA, Ellison DW. Comparative genomic hybridization and histological variation in primitive neuroectodermal tumors. Br J Cancer 1999; 80: 1322–31.

12 Biegel JA, Rorke LB, Packer RJ, et al. Isochromosome 17q in primitive neuroectodermal tumors of the central nervous system. Genes Chromosomes Cancer 1989; 1: 139–47.

13 Reardon DA, Michalkiewicz E, Boyett JM, et al. Extensive genomic abnormalities in childhood medulloblastoma by comparative genomic hybridization. Cancer Res 1997; 57: 4042–7.

14 Gilbertson R, Wickramasinghe C, Hernan R, et al. Clinical and molecular stratification of disease risk in medulloblastoma. Br J Cancer 2001; 85: 705–12.

15 Avet–Loiseau H, Venuat AM, Terrier–Lacombe MJ, Lellouch–Tubiana A, Zerah M, Vassal G. Comparative genomic hybridization detects many recurrent imbalances in central nervous system primitive neuroectodermal tumors in children. Br J Cancer 1999; 79(11–12): 1843–7.

16 Eberhart CG, Kratz JE, Schuster A, et al. Comparative genomic hybridization detects an increased number of chromosomal alterations in large cell/anaplastic medulloblastomas. Brain Pathol 2002; 12: 36–44.

17 Aldosari N, Bigner SH, Burger PC, et al. MYCC and MYCN oncogene amplification in medulloblastoma. A fluorescence in situ hybridization study on paraffin sections from the Children's Oncology Group. Arch Pathol Lab Med 2002; 126: 540–4.

18 Boon K, Eberhart CG, Riggins GJ. Genomic amplification of orthodenticle homologue 2 in medulloblastomas. Cancer Res 2005; 65: 703–7.

19 Di C, Liao S, Adamson DC, et al. Identification of OTX2 as a medulloblastoma oncogene whose product can be targeted by all-trans retinoic acid. Cancer Res 2005; 65: 919–24.

20 Fan X, Mikolaenko I, Elhassan I, et al. Notch1 and notch2 have opposite effects on embryonal brain tumor growth. Cancer Res 2004; 64: 7787–93.

21 Fan X, Wang Y, Kratz J, et al. hTERT gene amplification and increased mRNA expression in central nervous system embryonal tumors. Am J Pathol 2003; 162: 1763–9.

22 Hamilton SR, Liu B, Parsons RE, et al. The molecular basis of Turcot's syndrome. N Engl J Med 1995; 332: 839–47.

23 Paraf F, Jothy S, Van Meir EG. Brain tumor-polyposis syndrome: two genetic diseases? J Clin Oncol 1997; 15: 2744–58.

24 Hahn H, Wicking C, Zaphiropoulous PG, et al. Mutations of the human homolog of Drosophila patched in the nevoid basal cell carcinoma syndrome. Cell 1996; 85: 841–51.

25 Johnson RL, Rothman AL, Xie J, et al. Human homolog of patched, a candidate gene for the basal cell nevus syndrome. Science 1996; 272: 1668–71.

26 Evans DG, Farndon PA, Burnell LD, Gattamaneni HR, Birch JM. The incidence of Gorlin syndrome in 173 consecutive cases of medulloblastoma. Br J Cancer 1991; 64: 959–61.

27 Schofield D, West DC, Anthony DC, Marshal R, Sklar J. Correlation of loss of heterozygosity at chromosome 9q with histological subtype in medulloblastomas. Am J Pathol 1995; 146: 472–80.

28 Malkin D, Li FP, Strong LC, et al. Germ line p53 mutations in a familial syndrome of breast cancer, sarcomas, and other neoplasms. Science 1990; 250: 1233–8.

29 Kleihues P, Schauble B, zur Hausen A, Esteve J, Ohgaki H. Tumors associated with p53 germline mutations: a synopsis of 91 families. Am J Pathol 1997; 150: 1–13.

30 Hirsch B, Shimamura A, Moreau L, et al. Association of biallelic BRCA2/FANCD1 mutations with spontaneous chromosomal instability and solid tumors of childhood. Blood 2004; 103: 2554–9.

31 Offit K, Levran O, Mullaney B, et al. Shared genetic susceptibility to breast cancer, brain tumors, and Fanconi anemia. J Natl Cancer Inst 2003; 95: 1548–51.

32 Reid S, Schindler D, Hanenberg H, et al. Biallelic mutations in PALB2 cause Fanconi anemia subtype FA-N and predispose to childhood cancer. Nat Genet 2007; 39: 162–4.

33 Taylor MD, Mainprize TG, Rutka JT, Becker L, Bayani J, Drake JM. Medulloblastoma in a child with rubenstein-taybi syndrome: case report and review of the literature. Pediatr Neurosurg 2001; 35: 235–8.

34 Fleck BJ, Pandya A, Vanner L, Kerkering K, Bodurtha J. Coffin-Siris syndrome: review and presentation of new cases from a questionnaire study. Am J Med Genet 2001; 99: 1–7.

35 Rogers L, Pattisapu J, Smith RR, Parker P. Medulloblastoma in association with the Coffin-Siris syndrome. Childs Nerv Syst 1988; 4: 41–4.

36 Cogen PH, Daneshvar L, Metzger AK, Duyk G, Edwards MS, Sheffield VC. Involvement of multiple chromosome 17p loci in medulloblastoma tumorigenesis. Am J Hum Genet 1992; 50: 584–9.

37 Pietsch T, Waha A, Koch A, et al. Medulloblastomas of the desmoplastic variant carry mutations of the human homologue of Drosophila patched. Cancer Res 1997; 57: 2085–8.

38 Raffel C, Jenkins RB, Frederick L, et al. Sporadic medulloblastomas contain PTCH mutations. Cancer Res 1997; 57: 842–5.

39 Huang H, Mahler-Araujo BM, Sankila A, et al. APC mutations in sporadic medulloblastomas. Am J Pathol 2000; 156: 433–7.

40 Koch A, Waha A, Tonn JC, et al. Somatic mutations of WNT/wingless signaling pathway components in primitive neuroectodermal tumors. Int J Cancer 2001; 93: 445–9.

41 Wolter M, Reifenberger J, Sommer C, Ruzicka T, Reifenberger G. Mutations in the human homologue of the Drosophila segment polarity gene patched (PTCH) in sporadic basal cell carcinomas of the skin and primitive neuroectodermal tumors of the central nervous system. Cancer Res 1997; 57: 2581–5.

42 Vorechovsky I, Tingby O, Hartman M, et al. Somatic mutations in the human homologue of Drosophila patched in primitive neuroectodermal tumors. Oncogene 1997; 15: 361–6.

43 Jones PA, Baylin SB. The fundamental role of epigenetic events in cancer. Nat Rev Genet 2002; 3: 415–28.

44 Egger G, Liang G, Aparicio A, Jones PA. Epigenetics in human disease and prospects for epigenetic therapy. Nature 2004; 429: 457–63.

45 Fruhwald MC, O'Dorisio MS, Dai Z, et al. Aberrant promoter methylation of previously unidentified target genes is a common abnormality in medulloblastomas – implications for tumor biology and potential clinical utility. Oncogene 2001; 20: 5033–42.

46 Vibhakar R, Foltz G, Yoon JG, et al. Dickkopf–1 is an epigenetically silenced candidate tumor suppressor gene in medulloblastoma. Neuro-oncology 2007; 9: 135–44.

47 Waha A, Koch A, Hartmann W, et al. SGNE1/7B2 is epigenetically altered and transcriptionally downregulated in human medulloblastomas. Oncogene 2007; 26: 5662–8.

48 Lindsey JC, Anderton JA, Lusher ME, Clifford SC. Epigenetic events in medulloblastoma development. Neurosurg Focus 2005; 19: E10.

49 Harada K, Toyooka S, Shivapurkar N, et al. Deregulation of caspase 8 and 10 expression in pediatric tumors and cell lines. Cancer Res 2002; 62: 5897–901.

50 Harada K, Toyooka S, Maitra A, et al. Aberrant promoter methylation and silencing of the RASSF1A gene in pediatric tumors and cell lines. Oncogene 2002; 21: 4345–9.

51 Lindsey JC, Lusher ME, Anderton JA, et al. Identification of tumor-specific epigenetic events in medulloblastoma development by hypermethylation profiling. Carcinogenesis 2004; 25: 661–8.

52 Lusher ME, Lindsey JC, Latif F, Pearson AD, Ellison DW, Clifford SC. Biallelic epigenetic inactivation of the RASSF1A tumor suppressor gene in medulloblastoma development. Cancer Res 2002; 62: 5906–11.

53 Rood BR, Zhang H, Weitman DM, Cogen PH. Hypermethylation of HIC–1 and 17p allelic loss in medulloblastoma. Cancer Res 2002; 62: 3794–7.

54 Zuzak TJ, Steinhoff DF, Sutton LN, Phillips PC, Eggert A, Grotzer MA. Loss of caspase–8 mRNA expression is common in childhood primitive neuroectodermal brain tumor/medulloblastoma. Eur J Cancer 2002; 38: 83–91.

55 Waha A, Koch A, Meyer-Puttlitz B, et al. Epigenetic silencing of the HIC-1 gene in human medulloblastomas. J Neuropathol Exp Neurol 2003; 62: 1192–201.

56 Pingoud-Meier C, Lang D, Janss AJ, et al. Loss of caspase-8 protein expression correlates with unfavorable survival outcome in childhood medulloblastoma. Clin Cancer Res 2003; 9: 6401–9.

57 Wechsler-Reya R, Scott MP. The developmental biology of brain tumors. Ann Rev Neurosci 2001; 24: 385–428.

58 Taipale J, Beachy PA. The Hedgehog and Wnt signalling pathways in cancer. Nature 2001; 411: 349–54.

59 Stone DM, Murone M, Luoh S, et al. Characterization of the human suppressor of fused, a negative regulator of the zinc-finger transcription factor Gli. J Cell Sci 1999; 112 (Pt 23): 4437–48.

60 Taylor MD, Liu L, Raffel C, et al. Mutations in SUFU predispose to medulloblastoma. Nat Genet 2002; 31: 306–10.

61 Koch A, Waha A, Hartmann W, et al. No evidence for mutations or altered expression of the Suppressor of Fused gene (SUFU) in primitive neuroectodermal tumors. Neuropathol Appl Neurobiol 2004; 30: 532–9.

62 Reifenberger J, Wolter M, Weber RG, et al. Missense mutations in SMOH in sporadic basal cell carcinomas of the skin and primitive neuroectodermal tumors of the central nervous system. Cancer Res 1998; 58: 1798–803.

63 Thompson MC, Fuller C, Hogg TL, et al. Genomics identifies medulloblastoma subgroups that are enriched for specific genetic alterations. J Clin Oncol 2006; 24: 1924–31.

64 Wetmore C, Eberhart DE, Curran T. The normal patched allele is expressed in medulloblastomas from mice with heterozygous germline mutation of patched. Cancer Res 2000; 60: 2239–46.

65 Goodrich LV, Milenkovic L, Higgins KM, Scott MP. Altered neural cell fates and medulloblastoma in mouse patched mutants. Science 1997; 277: 1109–13.

66 Lee Y, Kawagoe R, Sasai K, et al. Loss of suppressor-of-fused function promotes tumorigenesis. Oncogene 2007; 26: 6442–7.

67 Hallahan AR, Pritchard JI, Hansen S, et al. The SmoA1 mouse model reveals that notch signaling is critical for the growth and survival of sonic hedgehog-induced medulloblastomas. Cancer Res 2004; 64: 7794–800.

68 Marino S. Medulloblastoma: developmental mechanisms out of control. Trends Mol Med 2005; 11: 17–22.

69 Clevers H. Axin and hepatocellular carcinomas. Nat Genet 2000; 24: 206–8.

70 Morin PJ. Beta-catenin signaling and cancer. Bioessays 1999; 21: 1021–30.

71 Zurawel RH, Chiappa SA, Allen C, Raffel C. Sporadic medulloblastomas contain oncogenic beta-catenin mutations. Cancer Res 1998; 58: 896–9.

72 Eberhart CG, Tihan T, Burger PC. Nuclear localization and mutation of beta-catenin in medulloblastomas. J Neuropathol Exp Neurol 2000; 59: 333–7.

73 Dahmen RP, Koch A, Denkhaus D, et al. Deletions of AXIN1, a component of the WNT/wingless pathway, in sporadic medulloblastomas. Cancer Res 2001; 61: 7039–43.

74 Baeza N, Masuoka J, Kleihues P, Ohgaki H. AXIN1 mutations but not deletions in cerebellar medulloblastomas. Oncogene 2003; 22: 632–6.

75 Ellison DW, Onilude OE, Lindsey JC, et al. Beta–catenin status predicts a favorable outcome in childhood medulloblastoma: the United Kingdom Children's Cancer Study Group Brain Tumour Committee. J Clin Oncol 2005; 23: 7951–7.

76 Clifford SC, Lusher ME, Lindsey JC, et al. Wnt/Wingless pathway activation and chromosome 6 loss characterize a distinct molecular sub-group of medulloblastomas associated with a favorable prognosis. Cell cycle 2006; 5: 2666–70.

77 Gajjar A, Chintagumpala M, Ashley D, et al. Risk-adapted craniospinal radiotherapy followed by high–dose chemotherapy and stem–cell rescue in children with newly diagnosed medulloblastoma (St Jude Medulloblastoma-96): long-term results from a prospective, multicentre trial. Lancet Oncol 2006; 7: 813–20.

78 Sherr CJ. The INK4a/ARF network in tumor suppression. Nat Rev Mol Cell Biol 2001; 2: 731–7.

79 Sherr CJ, McCormick F. The RB and p53 pathways in cancer. Cancer Cell 2002; 2: 103–12.

80 Frank AJ, Hernan R, Hollander A, et al. The TP53-ARF tumor suppressor pathway is frequently disrupted in large/cell anaplastic medulloblastoma. Brain Res Mol Brain Res 2004; 121: 137–40.

81 Badiali M, Iolascon A, Loda M, et al. p53 gene mutations in medulloblastoma. Immunohistochemistry, gel shift analysis, and sequencing. Diag Mol Pathol 1993; 2: 23–8.

82 Burns AS, Jaros E, Cole M, Perry R, Pearson AJ, Lunec J. The molecular pathology of p53 in primitive neuroectodermal tumors of the central nervous system. Br J Cancer 2002; 86: 1117–23.

83 Adesina AM, Nalbantoglu J, Cavenee WK. p53 gene mutation and mdm2 gene amplification are uncommon in medulloblastoma. Cancer Res 1994; 54: 5649–51.

84 Batra SK, McLendon RE, Koo JS, et al. Prognostic implications of chromosome 17p deletions in human medulloblastomas. J Neurooncol 1995; 24: 39–45.

85 Ray A, Ho M, Ma J, et al. A clinicobiological model predicting survival in medulloblastoma. Clin Cancer Res 2004; 10: 7613–20.

86 Woodburn RT, Azzarelli B, Montebello JF, Goss IE. Intense p53 staining is a valuable prognostic indicator for poor prognosis in medulloblastoma/central nervous system primitive neuroectodermal tumors. J Neurooncol 2001; 52: 57–62.

87 Broderick DK, Di C, Parrett TJ, et al. Mutations of PIK3CA in anaplastic oligodendrogliomas, high-grade astrocytomas, and medulloblastomas. Cancer Res 2004; 64: 5048–50.

88 Gilbertson RJ, Clifford SC. PDGFRB is overexpressed in metastatic medulloblastoma. Nat Genet 2003; 35: 197–8.

89 Gilbertson RJ, Langdon JA, Hollander A, et al. Mutational analysis of PDGFR-RAS/MAPK pathway activation in childhood medulloblastoma. Eur J Cancer 2006; 42: 646–9.

90 Grotzer MA, Janss AJ, Fung K, et al. TrkC expression predicts good clinical outcome in primitive neuroectodermal brain tumors. J Clin Oncol 2000; 18: 1027–35.

91 Hernan R, Fasheh R, Calabrese C, et al. ERBB2 up-regulates S100A4 and several other prometastatic genes in medulloblastoma. Cancer Res 2003; 63: 140–8.

92 MacDonald TJ, Brown KM, LaFleur B, et al. Expression profiling of medulloblastoma: PDGFRA and the RAS/MAPK pathway as therapeutic targets for metastatic disease. Nat Genet 2001; 29: 143–52.

93 Tsuchida T, Tanaka R, Fukuda M, Takeda N, Ito J, Honda H. CT findings of medulloblastoma. Childs Brain 1984; 11: 60–8.

94 Buhring U, Strayle–Batra M, Freudenstein D, Scheel–Walter HG, Kuker W. MRI features of primary, secondary and metastatic medulloblastoma. Eur Radiol 2002; 12: 1342–8.

95 Fouladi M, Chintagumpala M, Laningham FH, et al. White matter lesions detected by magnetic resonance imaging after radiotherapy and high-dose chemotherapy in children with medulloblastoma or primitive neuroectodermal tumor. J Clin Oncol 2004; 22: 4551–60.

96 Chang CH, Housepian EM, Herbert C, Jr. An operative staging system and a megavoltage radiotherapeutic technic for cerebellar medulloblastomas. Radiology 1969; 93: 1351–9.

97 Gajjar A, Fouladi M, Walter AW, et al. Comparison of lumbar and shunt cerebrospinal fluid specimens for cytologic detection of leptomeningeal disease in pediatric patients with brain tumors. J Clin Oncol 1999; 17: 1825–8.

98 Gajjar A, Hernan R, Kocak M, et al. Clinical, histopathologic, and molecular markers of prognosis: toward a new disease risk stratification system for medulloblastoma. J Clin Oncol 2004; 22: 984–93.

99 Rutkowski S, von Bueren A, von Hoff K, et al. Prognostic relevance of clinical and biological risk factors in childhood medulloblastoma: results of patients treated in the prospective multicenter trial HIT'91. Clin Cancer Res 2007; 13: 2651–7.

100 Rutkowski S, Bode U, Deinlein F, et al. Treatment of early childhood medulloblastoma by postoperative chemotherapy alone. N Engl J Med 2005; 352: 978–86.

101 Gajjar A, Mulhern RK, Heideman RL, et al. Medulloblastoma in very young children: outcome of definitive craniospinal irradiation following incomplete response to chemotherapy. J Clin Oncol 1994; 12: 1212–6.

102 Walter AW, Mulhern RK, Gajjar A, et al. Survival and neurodevelopmental outcome of young children with medulloblastoma at St Jude Children's Research Hospital. J Clin Oncol 1999; 17: 3720–8.

103 Duffner PK, Horowitz ME, Krischer JP, et al. The treatment of malignant brain tumors in infants and very young children: an update of the Pediatric Oncology Group experience. Neurooncology 1999; 1: 152–61.

104 Duffner PK, Horowitz ME, Krischer JP, et al. Postoperative chemotherapy and delayed radiation in children less than three years of age with malignant brain tumors. N Engl J Med 1993; 328: 1725–31.

105 Geyer JR, Sposto R, Jennings M, et al. Multiagent chemotherapy and deferred radiotherapy in infants with malignant brain tumors: a report from the Children's Cancer Group. J Clin Oncol 2005; 23: 7621–31.

106 Grill J, Sainte-Rose C, Jouvet A, et al. Treatment of medulloblastoma with postoperative chemotherapy alone: an SFOP prospective trial in young children. Lancet Oncol 2005; 6: 573–80.

107 Finlay J, Sands S, Gardner I, Dunkel G, et al. Nondisseminated medulloblastoma in children less than three years of age: final report of the Head Start I and II protocols. Neuro-oncology 2006; 12th International Symposium on Pediatric Neuro-oncology (ISPNO): Abstract 107.

108 Chi SN, Gardner SL, Levy AS, et al. Feasibility and response to induction chemotherapy intensified with high-dose methotrexate for young children with newly diagnosed high-risk disseminated medulloblastoma. J Clin Oncol 2004; 22: 4881–7.

109 Geyer JR, Zeltzer PM, Boyett JM, et al. Survival of infants with primitive neuroectodermal tumors or malignant ependymomas of the CNS treated with eight drugs in 1 day: a report from the Childrens Cancer Group. J Clin Oncol 1994; 12: 1607–15.

110 Deutsch M, Thomas PR, Krischer J, et al. Results of a prospective randomized trial comparing standard dose neuraxis irradiation (3,600 cGy/20) with reduced neuraxis irradiation (2,340 cGy/13) in patients with low-stage medulloblastoma. A Combined Children's Cancer Group-Pediatric Oncology Group Study. Pediatr Neurosurg 1996; 24: 167–76; discussion 76–7.

111 Thomas PR, Deutsch M, Kepner JL, et al. Low-stage medulloblastoma: final analysis of trial comparing standard-dose with reduced-dose neuraxis irradiation. J Clin Oncol 2000; 18: 3004–11.

112 Packer RJ, Goldwein J, Nicholson HS, et al. Treatment of children with medulloblastomas with reduced-dose craniospinal radiation therapy and adjuvant chemotherapy: a Children's Cancer Group Study. J Clin Oncol 1999; 17: 2127–36.

113 Packer RJ, Gajjar A, Vezina G, et al. Phase III study of craniospinal radiation therapy followed by adjuvant chemotherapy for newly diagnosed average-risk medulloblastoma. J Clin Oncol 2006; 24: 4202–8.

114 Bailey CC, Gnekow A, Wellek S, et al. Prospective randomised trial of chemotherapy given before radiotherapy in childhood medulloblastoma. International Society of Paediatric Oncology (SIOP) and the (German) Society of Paediatric Oncology (GPO): SIOP II. Med Pediatr Oncol 1995; 25: 166–78.

115 Taylor RE, Bailey CC, Robinson K, et al. Results of a randomized study of preradiation chemotherapy versus radiotherapy alone for nonmetastatic medulloblastoma: the International Society of Paediatric Oncology/United Kingdom Children's Cancer Study Group PNET–3 Study. J Clin Oncol 2003; 21: 1581–91.

116 Kortmann RD, Kuhl J, Timmermann B, et al. Postoperative neoadjuvant chemotherapy before radiotherapy as compared to immediate radiotherapy followed by maintenance chemotherapy in the treatment of medulloblastoma in childhood: results of the German prospective randomized trial HIT '91. Int J Radiat Oncol Biol Phys 2000; 46: 269–79.

117 Hughes EN, Shillito J, Sallan SE, Loeffler JS, Cassady JR, Tarbell NJ. Medulloblastoma at the joint center for radiation therapy between 1968 and 1984. The influence of radiation dose on the patterns of failure and survival. Cancer 1988; 61: 1992–8.

118 Packer RJ, Sutton LN, Elterman R, et al. Outcome for children with medulloblastoma treated with radiation and cisplatin, CCNU, and vincristine chemotherapy. J Neurosurg 1994; 81: 690–8.

119 Miralbell R, Fitzgerald TJ, Laurie F, et al. Radiotherapy in pediatric medulloblastoma: quality assessment of Pediatric Oncology Group Trial 9031. Int J Radiat Oncol Biol Phys 2006; 64: 1325–30.

120 Zeltzer PM, Boyett JM, Finlay JL, et al. Metastasis stage, adjuvant treatment, and residual tumor are prognostic factors for medulloblastoma in children: conclusions from the Children's Cancer Group 921 randomized phase III study. J Clin Oncol 1999; 17: 832–45.

121 Taylor RE, Bailey CC, Robinson KJ, et al. Outcome for patients with metastatic (M2-3) medulloblastoma treated with SIOP/UKCCSG PNET-3 chemotherapy. Eur J Cancer 2005; 41: 727–34.

122 Giangaspero F, Perilongo G, Fondelli MP, et al. Medulloblastoma with extensive nodularity: a variant with favorable prognosis. J Neurosurg 1999; 91: 971–7.

123 Brown HG, Kepner JL, Perlman EJ, et al. 'Large cell/anaplastic' medulloblastomas: a Pediatric Oncology Group Study. J Neuropathol Exp Neurol 2000; 59: 857–65.

124 Eberhart CG, Kepner JL, Goldthwaite PT, et al. Histopathologic grading of medulloblastomas: a Pediatric Oncology Group study. Cancer 2002; 94: 552–60.

125 Packer RJ, Biegel JA, Blaney S, et al. Atypical teratoid/rhabdoid tumor of the central nervous system: report on workshop. J Pediatr Hematol Oncol 2002; 24: 337–42.

126 Kleihues P, Louis DN, Scheithauer BW, et al. The WHO classification of tumors of the nervous system. J Neuropathol Exp Neurol 2002; 61: 215–25; discussion 26–9.

127 Hilden JM, Meerbaum S, Burger P, et al. Central nervous system atypical teratoid/rhabdoid tumor: results of therapy in children enrolled in a registry. J Clin Oncol 2004; 22: 2877–84.

128 Reddy AT. Atypical teratoid/rhabdoid tumors of the central nervous system. J Neuro-oncol 2005; 75: 309–13.

129 Biegel JA, Kalpana G, Knudsen ES, et al. The role of INI1 and the SWI/SNF complex in the development of rhabdoid tumors: meeting summary from the workshop on childhood atypical teratoid/rhabdoid tumors. Cancer Res 2002; 62: 323–8.

130 Tekautz TM, Fuller CE, Blaney S, et al. Atypical teratoid/rhabdoid tumors (ATRT): improved survival in children 3 years of age and older with radiation therapy and high-dose alkylator-based chemotherapy. J Clin Oncol 2005; 23: 1491–9.

131 Gaffney CC, Sloane JP, Bradley NJ, Bloom HJ. Primitive neuroectodermal tumors of the cerebrum. Pathology and treatment. J Neuro-oncol 1985; 3: 23–33.

132 Rorke LB. The cerebellar medulloblastoma and its relationship to primitive neuroectodermal tumors. J Neuropathol Exp Neurol 1983; 42: 1–15.

133 Cohen BH, Zeltzer PM, Boyett JM, et al. Prognostic factors and treatment results for supratentorial primitive neuroectodermal tumors in children using radiation and chemotherapy: a Childrens Cancer Group randomized trial. J Clin Oncol 1995; 13: 1687–96.

134 Jakacki RI, Zeltzer PM, Boyett JM, et al. Survival and prognostic factors following radiation and/or chemotherapy for primitive neuroectodermal tumors of the pineal region in infants and children: a report of the Childrens Cancer Group. J Clin Oncol 1995; 13: 1377–83.

135 Pizer BL, Weston CL, Robinson KJ, et al. Analysis of patients with supratentorial primitive neuro-ectodermal tumors entered into the SIOP/UKCCSG PNET 3 study. Eur J Cancer 2006; 42: 1120–8.

136 Albright AL, Wisoff JH, Zeltzer P, et al. Prognostic factors in children with supratentorial (nonpineal) primitive neuroectodermal tumors. A neurosurgical perspective from the Children's Cancer Group. Pediatr Neurosurg 1995; 22: 1–7.

137 Reddy AT, Janss AJ, Phillips PC, Weiss HL, Packer RJ. Outcome for children with supratentorial primitive neuroectodermal tumors treated with surgery, radiation, and chemotherapy. Cancer 2000; 88: 2189–93.

138 Burnett ME, White EC, Sih S, von Haken MS, Cogen PH. Chromosome arm 17p deletion analysis reveals molecular genetic heterogeneity in supratentorial and infratentorial primitive neuroectodermal tumors of the central nervous system. Cancer Genet Cytogenet 1997; 97: 25–31.

139 Nicholson J, Wickramasinghe C, Ross F, Crolla J, Ellison D. Imbalances of chromosome 17 in medulloblastomas determined by comparative genomic hybridisation and fluorescence in situ hybridisation. Mol Pathol 2000; 53: 313–9.

140 Pomeroy SL, Tamayo P, Gaasenbeek M, et al. Prediction of central nervous system embryonal tumor outcome based on gene expression. Nature 2002; 415: 436–42.

141 Russo C, Pellarin M, Tingby O, et al. Comparative genomic hybridization in patients with supratentorial and infratentorial primitive neuroectodermal tumors. Cancer 1999; 86: 331–9.

142 Li MH, Bouffet E, Hawkins CE, Squire JA, Huang A. Molecular genetics of supratentorial primitive neuroectodermal tumors and pineoblastoma. Neurosurg Focus 2005; 19: E3.

143 Pfister S, Remke M, Toedt G, et al. Supratentorial primitive neuroectodermal tumors of the central nervous system frequently harbor deletions of the CDKN2A locus and other genomic aberrations distinct from medulloblastomas. Genes Chrom Cancer 2007; 46: 839–51.

144 Timmermann B, Kortmann RD, Kuhl J, et al. Role of radiotherapy in the treatment of supratentorial primitive neuroectodermal tumors in childhood: results of the prospective German brain tumor trials HIT 88/89 and 91. J Clin Oncol 2002; 20: 842–9.

145 Massimino M, Gandola L, Spreafico F, et al. Supratentorial primitive neuroectodermal tumors (S–PNET) in children: a prospective experience with adjuvant intensive chemotherapy and hyperfractionated accelerated radiotherapy. Int J Radiat Oncol Biol Phys 2006; 64: 1031–7.

146 Ridola V, Grill J, Doz F, et al. High-dose chemotherapy with autologous stem cell rescue followed by posterior fossa irradiation for local medulloblastoma recurrence or progression after conventional chemotherapy. Cancer 2007; 110: 156–63.

147 Finlay JL, Goldman S, Wong MC, et al. Pilot study of high-dose thiotepa and etoposide with autologous bone marrow rescue in children and young adults with recurrent CNS tumors. The Children's Cancer Group. J Clin Oncol 1996; 14: 2495–503.

148 Dunkel IJ, Boyett JM, Yates A, et al. High-dose carboplatin, thiotepa, and etoposide with autologous stem-cell rescue for patients with recurrent medulloblastoma. Children's Cancer Group. J Clin Oncol 1998; 16: 222–8.

149 Guruangan S, Dunkel IJ, Goldman S, et al. Myeloablative chemotherapy with autologous bone marrow rescue in young children with recurrent malignant brain tumors. J Clin Oncol 1998; 16: 2486–93.

150 Shih CS, Hale GA, Gronewold L, et al. High-dose chemotherapy with autologous stem cell rescue for children with recurrent malignant brain tumors. Cancer 2008; 112: 1345–53.

151 Bertolini P, Lassalle M, Mercier G, et al. Platinum compound-related ototoxicity in children: long-term follow-up reveals continuous worsening of hearing loss. J Pediatr Hematol Oncol 2004; 26: 649–55.

152 Knight KR, Kraemer DF, Neuwelt EA. Ototoxicity in children receiving platinum chemotherapy: underestimating a commonly occurring toxicity that may influence academic and social development. J Clin Oncol 2005; 23: 8588–96.

153 Chin D, Sklar C, Donahue B, et al. Thyroid dysfunction as a late effect in survivors of pediatric medulloblastoma/primitive neuroectodermal tumors: a comparison of hyperfractionated versus conventional radiotherapy. Cancer 1997; 80: 798–804.

154 Gurney JG, Kadan-Lottick NS, Packer RJ, et al. Endocrine and cardiovascular late effects among adult survivors of childhood brain tumors: Childhood Cancer Survivor Study. Cancer 2003; 97: 663–73.

155 Laughton SJ, Merchant TE, Sklar CA, et al. Endocrine outcomes for children with embryonal brain tumors after risk-adapted craniospinal and conformal primary-site irradiation and high-dose chemotherapy with stem-cell rescue on the SJMB-96 trial. J Clin Oncol 2008; 26: 1112–8.

156 Oberfield SE, Allen JC, Pollack J, New MI, Levine LS. Long-term endocrine sequelae after treatment of medulloblastoma: prospective study of growth and thyroid function. J Pediatr 1986; 108: 219–23.

157 Pasqualini T, Diez B, Domene H, et al. Long-term endocrine sequelae after surgery, radiotherapy, and chemotherapy in children with medulloblastoma. Cancer 1987; 59: 801–6.

158 Spoudeas HA, Charmandari E, Brook CG. Hypothalamo-pituitary-adrenal axis integrity after cranial irradiation for childhood posterior fossa tumors. Med Pediatr Oncol 2003; 40: 224–9.

159 Mulhern RK, Merchant TE, Gajjar A, Reddick WE, Kun LE. Late neurocognitive sequelae in survivors of brain tumors in childhood. Lancet Oncol 2004; 5: 399–408.

160 Mulhern RK, Palmer SL, Merchant TE, et al. Neurocognitive consequences of risk-adapted therapy for childhood medulloblastoma. J Clin Oncol 2005; 23: 5511–9.

161 Ris MD, Packer R, Goldwein J, Jones-Wallace D, Boyett JM. Intellectual outcome after reduced-dose radiation therapy plus adjuvant chemotherapy for medulloblastoma: a Children's Cancer Group study. J Clin Oncol 2001; 19: 3470–6.

162 Morris EB, Gajjar A, Okuma JO, et al. Survival and late mortality in long-term survivors of pediatric CNS tumors. J Clin Oncol 2007; 25: 1532–8.

163 Heikens J, Michiels EM, Behrendt H, Endert E, Bakker PJ, Fliers E. Long-term neuro-endocrine sequelae after treatment for childhood medulloblastoma. Eur J Cancer 1998; 34: 1592–7.

164 Mulhern RK, Horowitz ME, Kovnar EH, Langston J, Sanford RA, Kun LE. Neurodevelopmental status of infants and young children treated for brain tumors with preirradiation chemotherapy. J Clin Oncol 1989; 7: 1660–6.

165 Mabbott DJ, Penkman L, Witol A, Strother D, Bouffet E. Core neurocognitive functions in children treated for posterior fossa tumors. Neuropsychology 2008; 22: 159–68.

166 Nagel BJ, Delis DC, Palmer SL, Reeves C, Gajjar A, Mulhern RK. Early patterns of verbal memory impairment in children treated for medulloblastoma. Neuropsychology 2006; 20: 105–12.

167 Palmer SL, Goloubeva O, Reddick WE, et al. Patterns of intellectual development among survivors of pediatric medulloblastoma: a longitudinal analysis. J Clin Oncol 2001; 19: 2302–8.

168 Xu W, Janss A, Packer RJ, Phillips P, Goldwein J, Moshang T, Jr. Endocrine outcome in children with medulloblastoma treated with 18 Gy of craniospinal radiation therapy. Neuro-oncology 2004; 6: 113–8.

169 Jakacki RI, Feldman H, Jamison C, Boaz JC, Luerssen TG, Timmerman R. A pilot study of preirradiation chemotherapy and 1800 cGy craniospinal irradiation in young children with medulloblastoma. Int J Radiat Oncol Biol Phys 2004; 60: 531–6.

170 Thompson SJ, Leigh L, Christensen R, et al. Immediate neurocognitive effects of methylphenidate on learning-impaired survivors of childhood cancer. J Clin Oncol 2001; 19: 1802–8.

171 Fouladi M, Blaney SM, Poussaint TY, et al. Phase II study of oxaliplatin in children with recurrent or refractory medulloblastoma, supratentorial primitive neuroectodermal tumors, and atypical teratoid rhabdoid tumors: a pediatric brain tumor consortium study. Cancer 2006; 107: 2291–7.

172 Nicholson HS, Kretschmar CS, Krailo M, et al. Phase 2 study of temozolomide in children and adolescents with recurrent central nervous system tumors: a report from the Children's Oncology Group. Cancer 2007; 110: 1542–50.

173 Bomgaars LR, Bernstein M, Krailo M, et al. Phase II trial of irinotecan in children with refractory solid tumors: a Children's Oncology Group Study. J Clin Oncol 2007; 25: 4622–7.

174 Turner CD, Gururangan S, Eastwood J, et al. Phase II study of irinotecan (CPT–11) in children with high-risk malignant brain tumors: the Duke experience. Neuro-oncology 2002; 4: 102–8.

175 Stewart CF, Iacono LC, Chintagumpala M, et al. Results of a phase II upfront window of pharmacokinetically guided topotecan in high-risk medulloblastoma and supratentorial primitive neuroectodermal tumor. J Clin Oncol 2004; 22: 3357–65.

176 Zamboni WC, Gajjar AJ, Mandrell TD, et al. A four-hour topotecan infusion achieves cytotoxic exposure throughout the neuraxis in the nonhuman primate model: implications for treatment of children with metastatic medulloblastoma. Clin Cancer Res 1998; 4: 2537–44.

177 Berman DM, Karhadkar SS, Hallahan AR, et al. Medulloblastoma growth inhibition by hedgehog pathway blockade. Science 2002; 297: 1559–61.

178 Romer JT, Kimura H, Magdaleno S, et al. Suppression of the Shh pathway using a small molecule inhibitor eliminates medulloblastoma in Ptc1(+/–)p53(–/–) mice. Cancer Cell 2004; 6: 229–40.

179 Taipale J, Chen JK, Cooper MK, et al. Effects of oncogenic mutations in Smoothened and Patched can be reversed by cyclopamine. Nature 2000; 406: 1005–9.

180 van Es JH, Clevers H. Notch and Wnt inhibitors as potential new drugs for intestinal neoplastic disease. Trends Mol Med 2005; 11: 496–502.

181 Kimura H, Ng JM, Curran T. Transient inhibition of the Hedgehog pathway in young mice causes permanent defects in bone structure. Cancer Cell 2008; 13: 249–60.

182 Gilbertson RJ, Gajjar A. Molecular biology of medulloblastoma: will it ever make a difference to clinical management? J Neuro-oncol 2005; 75: 273–8.

5 Pediatric Spinal Cord Tumors

Annie Huang, Ute Bartels and Eric Bouffet

Pediatric Brain Tumor Program, Division of Hematology and Oncology, The Hospital for Sick Kids, Toronto, Ontario, Canada

General overview

Spinal cord tumors are between eight and 20 times less frequent than childhood brain tumors [1–3] and comprise 3–5% of all pediatric central nervous system (CNS) neoplasms [1]. Pediatric and adult tumors differ in location and histologies; 60% of intrinsic cord tumors in children are intramedullary compared with only 15–20% of adult tumors. Cervico-thoracic astrocytomas are most common in children; rare tumors include malignant astrocytoma, mixed gliomas, and primitive neuroectodermal tumors (PNET).

Intrinsic cord tumors include lesions of various histologies [4] that largely mirror the normal composition of the spine and associated coverings. Except for radiation exposure, no specific environmental factors are implicated; incidence of brain and spinal cord tumors are highest in Western, particularly European, countries [1], and reported to be lower in native and emigrant Asian populations, suggesting a strong genetic influence on tumor incidence. Although intramedullary tumors represent the majority of pediatric spinal neoplasms, their overall low incidence and varied histologies has significantly limited prospective evaluation. Existing literature report largely retrospective studies of adult and pediatric tumors collected over decades; thus extrapolation of these data to current practice is difficult. Nonetheless, management of intra-medullary pediatric tumors has evolved based on several observations.

Epidemiology and genetics
• Sixty to seventy percent present at >5 years of age.
• Neurofibromatosis (NF) types 1 and 2 predispose to spinal astrocytomas and ependymomas; one fifth of children with these tumor predisposition syndromes have intramedullary tumors [5], but only 7–10% of lesions are symptomatic [6, 7].

Malignant spinal tumors occur in the Li-Fraumeni syndrome, hereditary non-polyposis coli or Turcot, and rare uncharacterized familial glioma syndromes [8].

Pediatric Hematology and Oncology, 1st edition. Edited by Edward J. Estlin, Richard J. Gilbertson, and Robert F. Wynn. © 2010 Blackwell Publishing Ltd.

Histology and clinical presentation
• More than 85% of pediatric intra-medullary tumors are benign and compatible with long survival.
• Prodromes may span months to years.
• More than 70% present with back pain.
• Other signs at diagnosis include gait disturbances with sensory or motor deficits (>50%), spinal deformities (~30–40%), sphincter dysfunction (~20%) and hydrocephalus (~10%).
• Upper cervical tumors may cause torticollis, lower cranial nerve and brainstem dysfunction [9].
• Spinal tumors in children are associated with disease and treatment-related morbidities that are different to those observed in adults.

Diagnosis and clinical management (Table 5.1)
• Full sequence brain and spine magnetic resonance imaging (MRI) should be repeated within 24–48 hours post-surgery to provide an accurate assessment of tumor residuum, since non-specific changes that confuse image interpretation increase with time. Specific intra-spinal histology is not predicted reliably by MRI.
• Spine X-rays should be performed for associated scoliosis.
• Systemic investigations should be performed only as indicated by clinical history or exam.
• Aggressive measures, such as radical surgeries and radiation, do not always provide survival benefits and may compound treatment-related toxicity.
• Low dose chemotherapy is effective in a proportion of low grade astrocytomas, the most common pediatric intramedullary tumor.

Disease specific issues

Gliomas (Box 5.1)
Clinical presentation, investigations and staging
Spinal gliomas are characteristically large cervical tumors spanning five to seven vertebral segments and associated frequently with cysts or syrinx (40–50%); 5–10% are holocord [16]. Spinal deformities, seen in 40%, are associated with long histories, holocord, and lower grade tumors [14, 17].

Table 5.1 Differential diagnoses of pediatric spinal tumors.

Intradural – Intramedullary tumors
Astrocytoma
Ependymoma
Ganglioglioma
Hemangioblastoma

Intradural – extramedullary tumors
Myxopapillary ependymomas
Nerve sheath tumors (schwannoma, neurofibroma)
Meningioma
Dermoid/epidermoid
Teratoma
Lipoma
Primitive neuroectodermal tumor

Extradural tumors
Neuroblastoma
Sarcoma
Lymphoma
Metastatic tumors

Box 5.1 Glioma key facts.

- Ninety percent present by 10 years of age [10]; and <10% are seen in children <3 years old [11].
- Gliomas are the most common intramedullary spinal tumor [2, 6, 10] (Table 5.2).
- WHO grade 1 (juvenile pilocytic astrocytoma [JPA]) and grade II (fibrillary astrocytoma) tumors are the most common to arise in children.
- Pilomyxoid astrocytoma, a recently described aggressive intracranial pilocytic astrocytoma variant, arise occasionally in the spine [12].
- Less than 10% of spinal tumors are malignant astrocytomas. Higher proportions (30–50%) reported in multi-institutional studies [13,14] may reflect referral biases and differences in grading criteria. Approximately 70% of malignant spinal gliomas are grade III; grade IV tumors are more frequent in patients treated with prior radiotherapy [15].
- Malignant spinal gliomas are rare in very young children [11, 16].

Table 5.2 Epidemiological features of pediatric intraspinal tumors.

	Frequency	Median age range	M:F ratio	Associated genetic syndromes
Astrocytoma	>50%	5–7 years (3 months–18 years)	1–1.3:1	NF1, NF2, Li–Fraumeni Turcot
Ganglioglioma	<10%	7 years (7 months–18 years)	1:1	None known
Ependymoma	8–10%	11–12 years	1:1	NF2 >NF1 Chromosome 22 familial ependymoma
Myxopapillary ependymoma	5–10%	>8 years	2.2:1	Spinal dysraphism† Klinefelter's syndrome† MEN†

† Isolated cases.

Benign and malignant spinal gliomas manifest similar symptoms that differ in onset and severity. Low grade tumors may have minimal manifestations even with holocord involvement [17]; 50% of malignant tumors present with significant deficits. Prodromes in low grade tumors span a median of 9–12 months with 30–50% exceeding 1–2 years [17, 18]; median prodromes in malignant tumor is 5 weeks [19].

Shorter prodromes (median 5 months) are reported in children <3 years, without correlation to tumor grade, and probably reflects easier detection of motor delays which present in 50% of young children at diagnosis [11].

Intraspinal, leptomeningeal, or intracranial dissemination may be seen in both low (10–20%) and high grade (30–50%) spinal tumors [13, 19, 20]. Twenty to thirty percent of malignant spinal tumors present with hydrocephalus due to leptomeningeal disease.

Spinal gliomas enhance variably therefore diagnostic investigations should include MRI T2 or FLAIR sequences to delineate tumors completely. MRI spine is best for staging as cerebrospinal fluid (CSF) cytology is frequently negative in both benign and malignant tumors [13, 19]. Elevated CSF protein often accompanies leptomeningeal disease [9] and may be used to follow treatment response.

Treatment of low grade spinal astrocytoma
Surgery
Treatment guidelines for spinal cord gliomas are lacking. Since the first reported resection in the early 1900s [21], surgery

continues to be an important diagnostic and treatment modality for intrinsic spinal tumors. Tumor resectability is dependent on histology; circumscribed tumors like JPA are frequently completely respectable [22], radical removal of infiltrative grade II tumors is difficult with risk of additional neurological morbidity. Early studies advocated radical resection for all spinal tumors [17, 23]; however, longer follow-up studies indicate no significant benefit of radical resection on recurrence risk or overall survival for tumors with similar histology [14, 18, 23]. Therefore, maximal safe surgery to improve or preserve neurological function is most often undertaken.

Over 80% of children with grade 1 spinal gliomas survive >10 years even without radical surgery [14, 24]. Grade II spinal gliomas have variable outcomes and the role of adjuvant treatment for these tumors remains controversial. Multi-institutional studies have reported limited benefits of radiotherapy for improving long-term survival of primary and recurrent tumors [14, 25]. Therefore radiation is often deferred or avoided in pediatric low grade spinal gliomas to limit toxicity.

For progressive or recurrent tumors, repeat surgeries may be necessary to limit or reverse neurological symptoms, and may alone provide long-term control in a proportion of patients. Limited experiences suggest low grade spinal astrocytoma, like intracranial gliomas, may be chemoresponsive. Tumor reduction or stabilization, with neurological stabilization or recovery, has been reported in most progressive spinal tumors treated with various agents, including low dose carboplatin-based and more intensive regimens (Table 5.3). Treatment intensification appears to provide no additional benefits; the North American CCG 945 study, which used multi-agent chemotherapy and radiation in a small number of patients, reported 5 year progression free survival (PFS) (67%) and overall survival (OS) (83%) [26] comparable to more modest regimens [27, 28].

Chemotherapy

Similar to intracranial gliomas, response and duration of control with chemotherapy may be unpredictable for spinal tumors [26, 30]. Spinal gliomas are included in several prospective trials of vincristine and carboplatin in progressive low grade gliomas. These include the North American Children's Oncology Group CCG 9952, the German HIT and the European International Society for Paediatric Oncology (SIOP) glioma studies. Although formal results remain pending, vincristine–carboplatin is often used as first line treatment in recurrent spinal astrocytomas largely based on promising preliminary reports and published data on intracranial tumors. Monotherapy with temozolomide or vinblastine has also been used successfully in patients with inadequate response or poor tolerance of vincristine-carboplatin [27]. The relative efficacy of different drugs regimens in primary versus recurrent spinal astrocytoma remains unknown.

In addition to recurrent tumors, chemotherapy has been used in primary treatment of disseminated or inoperable spinal astrocytomas [30]. Although, a small study reported good neurological outcome and tumor control after conservative surgery and adjuvant chemotherapy in patients with focal spinal astrocytoma [33], the precise impact of chemotherapy on the unpredictable natural history of spinal astrocytomas remains to be studied in larger populations. In the absence of prospective data, our institutional approach for low grade spinal astrocytoma has been:
• Upfront chemotherapy only for patients with significant residual disease and/or persistent clinical signs/symptoms.
• Stable patients with small or no residual tumor are followed clinically and with surveillance MRI.
• Chemotherapy is considered if patients develop persistent clinical signs and symptoms not explained by reactive changes such as cysts or syrinx, and/or tumor progression on serial imaging, with or without change in clinical status. For symptomatic or

Table 5.3 Chemotherapy experience in treatment of low grade spinal tumors.

Study	No. of patients	Chemotherapy	Objective response or stable disease	Histology
Packer *et al.* (1993) [28]	1	Carboplatin/vincristine	1	LGA
Lowis *et al.* (1998) [29]	1	Carboplatin/vincristine	1	LGA
Doireau *et al.* (1999) [30]	6	BB SFOP	6	JPA, OA, A
Merchant *et al.* (2000) [31]	2	CDDP/VP16 Carboplatin	1	LGA
Hassall *et al.* (2001) [32]	2	Carboplatin	2	JPA
Fouladi *et al.* (2003) [26]		'8:1'chemotherapy	6	LGA
Townsend *et al.* (2004) [33]	4	Carboplatin/vincristine	3	LGA
Lafay-Cousin *et al.* (2005) [27]	1	Carboplatin/vincristine Vinblastine	1	LGA
Khaw *et al.* (2007) [34]	3	Temozolomide	3	LGA
Mora *et al.* (2007) [35]	2	Irinotecan/CDDP	2	LGA

LGA, low grade astrocytoma. OA, oligoastrocytoma. A, astrocytoma. JPA, juvenile pilocytic astrocytoma.

significant tumor re-growth, repeat surgery is considered prior to chemotherapy.

• Radiation is considered primarily for patients who have failed several lines of chemotherapy or earlier for patients with tenuous neurological function or deterioration on chemotherapy.

Clinical prognostic factors

Tumor grade is the strongest predictor of outcome [9, 14, 18, 25]. Bouffet *et al.* [14] reported progressive decline in 10 year OS of 83%, 69%, 40% and 0% respectively for grades 1–4 spinal astrocytoma. Not surprisingly, brief prodromes, increased neurological symptoms, and lower baseline function at diagnosis mirror aggressive pathology and correlate with decreased PFS and OS [14, 18, 33]. Interestingly, poor post-operative neurological status also correlates with worse median survival [24, 36], perhaps reflecting more aggressive surgical attempts at infiltrative tumors.

Spinal deformity at diagnosis, reflecting indolent tumor growth with gradual bony displacement [14, 33], predicts better outcome (Figure 5.1).

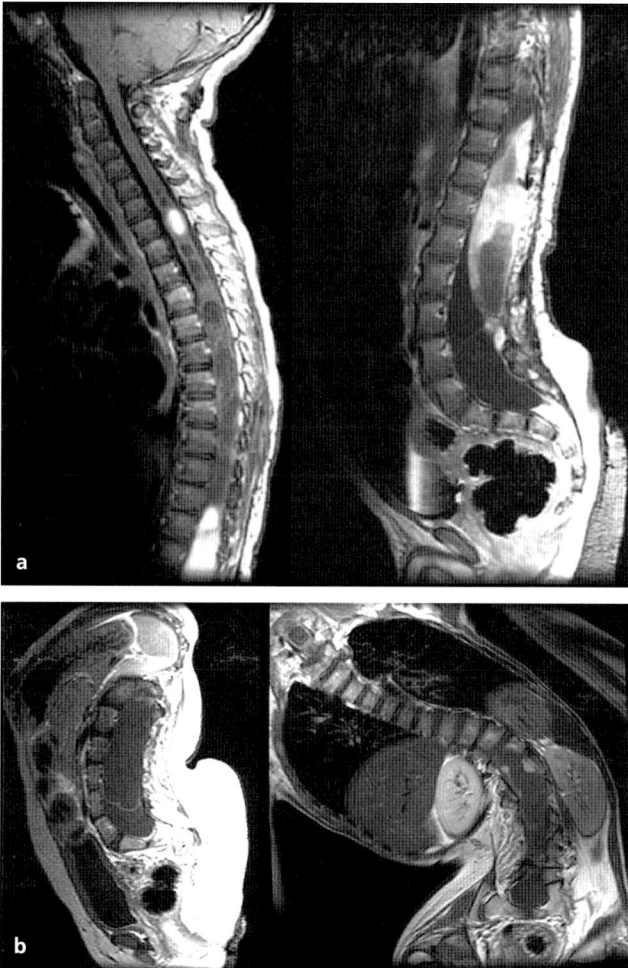

Figure 5.1 Progressive spinal deformity in a child with holocord low grade astrocytoma. (a), Images at diagnosis. (b), Images 9 years later, depict severe kyphoscoliosis due to progressive cysts and syrinxes.

Unlike in intracranial gliomas, younger patients are reported to fare as well or better than older children. A study of spinal astrocytoma in children <3 years old reported 3 and 5 year PFS (81 and 76%) [11] comparable to that in older children [11]. Similarly, better 10 year OS (76%) has been reported in children <7 years compared with those >7 years (38% 10 year OS) [14].

Factors inconsistently correlated with prognosis include tumor location, extent and patient gender [14, 23].

Treatment of high grade spinal astrocytoma

Malignant spinal gliomas have a 5–10 year OS of 20–30%. Factors associated with poorer outcome include prodrome (<2 months), grade IV histology, and dissemination [13, 19, 37]. Glioblastoma multiforme (GBM) with leptomeningeal dissemination have dismal outcomes with rapid death (<2 months) and no reported survivors. Extent of surgery trends with better outcome with shorter survival reported after incomplete surgery or biopsy [13].

With only limited survivors reported from heterogenous studies, optimal treatment strategies remain unclear. Despite upfront post-operative radiation most tumors exhibit distant and local progression within 10 months [15, 19]. Up to two-thirds of tumors disseminate at recurrence indicating a need for CNS prophylaxis. Best outcomes of 46% 5 year PFS and 54% OS were reported in a small cohort of tumors treated with a 'sandwich regimen' of post-operative '8 in 1' chemotherapy and involved field, spine, or craniospinal radiation in the North American CCG 945 study [13]. Although objective response to chemotherapy was reported in five of ten evaluable patients, the specific contribution of chemotherapy is unclear as most patients also received cranio-spinal irradiation.

For localized malignant spinal astrocytoma, the standard approach involves maximum safe surgery and focal radiation; whether specific chemotherapeutic agents, such as temozolomide, add survival benefits is unknown. The best approach to disseminated tumor is uncertain and may include high dose chemotherapy with or without craniospinal radiation.

Biological prognosticators and prospects for novel therapy of spinal cord glioma

Very few dedicated biological studies of spinal tumors have been published. Limited observations in the CCG945 study indicate an MIB-1 index >7% correlate with worse 5 year OS in low grade spinal astrocytoma [26]. Recent studies link telomere length [38], tumor vascularity [39], infiltrative histology and myelin basic protein expression with recurrence risk in intracranial low grade gliomas [40]. Similarities in clinical phenotypes of intracranial and spinal low grade astrocytoma suggest these factors are also likely to be relevant to spinal tumors.

For malignant spinal astrocytoma, increased mitotic indices, necrosis, and endothelial proliferation in grade III tumors are reported to correlate with worse outcome [24]. Whether genetic changes such as 1p/19q loss in mixed spinal tumors, and p53 gene mutations in grade III/IV spinal tumors have the same prognostic implications as intracranial tumors is unknown.

Chemotherapeutic approaches to spinal gliomas has largely been empirically extrapolated from intracranial tumors. Although direct comparative studies are pending, the similar clinical phenotypes of intracranial and spinal astrocytoma is suggestive of common molecular pathogenesis. Thus, emerging novel therapeutics in both low and high grade intracranial gliomas is likely to be relevant to treatment of spinal astrocytomas. Promising new agents include rapamycin and other inhibitors of mTOR – a direct NF1 target frequently upregulated in NF1-deficient astrocytomas [41]. Modulators of tumor angiogenesis and proliferation respectively by specific tyrosine kinase inhibitors and telomerase inhibition are also candidate novel therapies for spinal gliomas [42].

Spinal ependymomas (Box 5.2)
Epidemiology of intramedullary ependymomas
Only 8–10% of childhood spinal tumors are ependymomas [2, 3, 6] in contrast to adults where >50% of spinal tumors are ependymomas [43]. Incidence increases with age: <10% arise in children <5 years, and >50% are diagnosed in children >10 years old [2, 10].

Most tumors are sporadic, however, genetic associations are suggested in up to 20% of cases [44] (Table 5.2) with up to 15% reported in NF2 individuals [7]. Truncating NF2 mutations which is associated with earlier onset of NF2 predispose to intramedullary tumors [45, 46]. NF2 mutations are also frequent in sporadic tumors [47] and indicate an essential role for NF2 in the pathogenesis of spinal ependymoma.

Spinal and intracranial ependymomas have distinct genetic and biological features. Chr22q loss, NF2 mutations [47, 48] or decreased NF2 protein expression [49] seen in 30–70% of intramedullary ependymomas, are uncommon in intracranial tumors [50, 51]. Intracranial tumors also rarely exhibit chr 7 and 9 gains that is reported in most spinal ependymomas. Consistent with these observations, recent gene expression and genomic profiling studies [52, 53] indicate derivation of intracranial and spinal ependymomas from distinct precursor cell populations [53].

Histopathology and clinical presentation of intramedullary ependymomas
Intramedullary and intracranial ependymomas have similar histological spectra; World Health Organization (WHO) grade 2 tumors are most common, while grade 3 anaplastic tumors are rare. Grading criteria for ependymoma remains controversial, thus reported incidence of anaplastic spinal ependymoma is variable; although smaller pediatric series report incidence of <2–3% [23], a large series of 117 tumors reported no anaplastic spinal ependymoma [43]. Clinical presentation resembles that of low grade spinal astrocytoma. Some cases may present acutely with intra-tumoral hemorrhage after a trivial injury; a small proportion (<3%), have signs and symptoms of intracranial metastases at diagnosis.

Treatment, outcome and prognosis of intramedullary ependymomas
Pediatric intramedullary ependymomas have excellent outcomes. Lonjon *et al.* reported 5 and 10 year actuarial survival of 90%, and 5 and 10 year PFS of 93% and 70% respectively in the only exclusive study of 20 childhood spinal ependymomas [7]. Similar results have been reported from combined retrospective studies of adult and pediatric tumors [54]; in contrast intracranial ependymomas have a PFS of 30–50% [55].

Maximum surgery offers the best long-term outcome with 10 year OS of 86–100% achievable with surgery alone [7]. Most ependymomas are well circumscribed and >80% are completely respectable [10]; subtotal removal results in substantially decreased OS [10, 56] with ultimate progression in 20–50% of partially resected tumors. A multivariate study of 126 pediatric and adult spinal ependymomas, identified radiotherapy and extent of surgery as key predictors of survival. However, only surgical extent correlated with 15 year PFS [25], thus indicating survival advantages of radiation may not be independent of surgery. Sustained control of post-radiation relapse has been reported with repeat radical surgery [2, 7].

Adjuvant radiation has historically been advocated for partially resected tumors; however, in contrast to sustained remission in all patients with complete tumor resection [7], up to two-thirds of patients with irradiated incompletely resected tumors can recur, sometimes 6–7 years after radiotherapy.

Failures of spinal ependymomas are confined to the neuraxis, and in the majority of cases to the primary tumor location. Recurrent spinal ependymomas may have a higher incidence of intracranial metastases (6%) [57], thus full re-staging with MRI studies and CSF analysis are recommended for recurrent/progressive tumors.

Epidemiology of myxopapillary ependymoma
Less than 10% of childhood spinal tumors are myxopapillary ependymomas (MPE) [58] compared to 40% of adult spinal ependymomas are MPE [25].

Histopathology and clinical presentation of myxopapillary ependymoma
MPE is a distinct histopathological entity first described by Kernohan in 1931. These WHO grade 1 tumors typically arise in the conus and/or cauda equina and seldom at other CNS sites.

Box 5.2 Spinal ependymomas key facts.

- Commonly intramedullary cervico-thoracic tumors of cellular histology.
- Conal and cauda equina tumors are less common and characteristically of myxopapillary histology.
- Differ genetically from, and have superior outcomes compared with intracranial ependymomas.
- Grade I and II tumors are surgically curable.

Rare cases of subcutaneous MPE are proposed to originate from ependymal rests, or vestigial neural tube remnants. MPE are not linked to known genetic syndromes. However, rare cases are reported in sporadic [59] or syndrome-associated spinal dysraphism [60] . Unlike in intramedullary ependymomas, NF2 gene alterations are uncommon in MPE [48].

MPE are associated with a very favorable clinical outcome thus accurate histologic diagnosis is important. Histologically, MPE contain ependymal or perivascular rosettes, abundant perivascular myxoid deposits, low mitotic indices, rare nuclear pleomorphism, and frequent hemorrhage. MRI typically shows well-circumscribed, avidly enhancing, lumbar lesions with an enlarged filum, and multiple lumbar and sacral segments with associated cysts; tumors may extend to lower thoracic segments [61]. The indolent growth of MPE may result in bony displacement/deformity visible on X-rays.

Childhood MPE is typically localized. However, retrospective series indicate metastases in up to one-third of new or recurrent tumors [61–65]. Metastasis is usually confined to the neuraxis and may manifest as leptomeningeal infiltration, subarachnoid drop metastasis, or multifocal lesions; rare recurrent MPE involve extraneural sites [64]. Clinical presentation resembles that of other low grade spinal tumors with long non-specific prodrome (median 10.4 months; range 2–66 months). Almost all patients (>80%) present with back pain, lower extremity paresthesias, motor and gait abnormalities; one- to two-thirds have sphincter dysfunction [66]. Rare presentation of MPE include subarachnoid hemorrhage after minor trauma [67] and communicating hydrocephalus [68].

Treatment, outcome and prognosis of myxopapillary ependymoma

Only ~60 cases of pediatric MPE are reported to date; treatment approaches are extrapolated from adult data. Overall retrospective data indicate pediatric and adult MPE have a comparable excellent long-term outcome with 85–100% 5 year OS [61, 67].

Surgery is the primary treatment for MPE:
- Complete removal which can be safely achieved in 70–90% of tumors.
- Adjuvant treatment is unnecessary for completely resected MPE [58, 61, 67, 69].

MPE recurs in 15–30% of patients:
- Local recurrence is most common and can occur years after initial treatment.
- Incomplete surgery is more frequently associated with disease extension beyond the filum [61, 62, 67, 70, 71] and symptom durations <1 year [70] are associated with diminished 5 and 10 year PFS.

Due to favorable overall outcome of MPE, we generally advocate conservative management with surgery only. For children with new or recurrent unresectable tumors, histology and extent of tumor residual, time to progression, and risk of clinical deterioration are considered in deciding whether repeat surgery or radiation may be used.

Novel therapeutic approaches to spinal ependymomas

Therapeutic studies of pediatric spinal ependymomas are limited. The relatively good outcome of MPE and intramedullary ependymoma after surgery and radiation [72, 73] has precluded investigations of novel therapies in these rare tumors. Existing studies indicate that spinal and intracranial ependymomas are biologically distinct [52,53]. However, whether spinal tumors share the chemoresistant phenotypes of intracranial ependymoma is unknown. Promising responses has been reported in a few patients with recurrent spinal ependymomas or MPE using prolonged low dose etoposide with or without tamoxifen [74, 75], or Gleevec [76]. Cox-2 is overexpressed in up to 40% of spinal ependymomas [77], thus Cox-2 inhibitors which have demonstrated promising *in vitro* effects on intracranial ependymomas cell lines [78] represent additional novel agents. The role of other agents with activity against glial tumors [79], such as temozolomide, remains unexplored.

Rare intramedullary tumors
Gangliogliomas
- Gangliogliomas comprise 1–5% of pediatric cord tumors [31]; higher incidences (27–35%) reported in large single institutional series [18, 43] suggest referral bias.
- Most tumors are WHO grade I lesions with characteristic glioneuronal histology resembling cerebral gangliogliomas and present as cervico-thoracic or holocord lesions with clinical and radiologic features resembling low grade spinal gliomas; tumors may disseminate (Figure 5.2).
- Spinal gangliogliomas are reported at younger ages (mean age 7 years) than cerebral tumors.
- Data is limited to case reports [80, 81] and one large mixed pediatric and adult series [82]. Treatment approaches have been empiric and follow that of other low grade spinal tumors.
- Overall survival at 5 years and 10 years is excellent at 88–77% with surgery alone. However, spinal tumors have a three- to four fold higher recurrence risk [83] and inferior 10 year PFS (58%), indicating biological differences between cerebral and spinal gangliogliomas (Figure 5.2) [84].

Hemangioblastomas
- Hemangioblastomas are benign vascular lesions that may arise sporadically but are characteristically associated with Von-Hippel Lindau (VHL) disease.
- They comprise only 15% of all pediatric hemangioblastomas, most commonly present in the second decade [85].
- They are typically focal with associated syrinx/cysts and avid enhancement on MRI.
- Work-up for VHL disease is recommended for all children with CNS hemangioblastoma.
- VHL-associated hemangioblastomas may have unpredictable growth patterns [86]; therefore treatment is usually only undertaken with persistent and symptomatic tumor growth [86, 87]. Surgery, and more recently microsurgery, with or without embolization is the preferred treatment. SU5416, a VEGF receptor

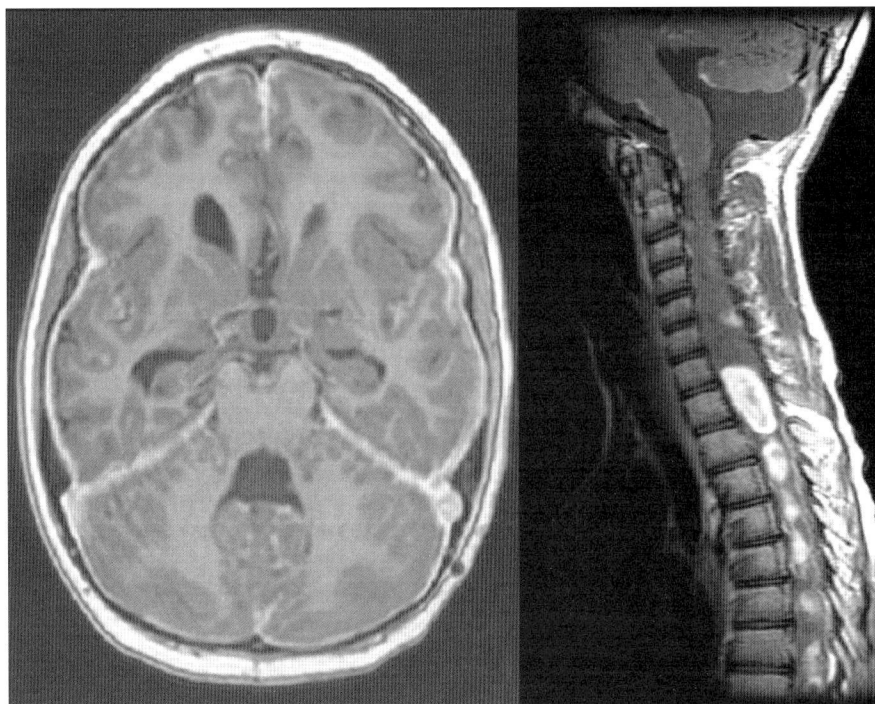

Figure 5.2 Intracranial and leptomeningeal dissemination of a spinal ganglioglioma.

inhibitor, has demonstrated promising results in retinal hemangioblastomas [88] and is currently on trial for surgically challenging CNS lesions [89]. It is exciting to anticipate future applications of such therapies for pre-symptomatic intervention in pre-disposed individuals.

Strategies for follow up and important late effects

Despite their benign nature, childhood spinal astrocytoma and ependymoma have significant risk of late recurrence or progression.
• We follow all patients with low grade spinal tumors with surveillance MRI for 3–5 years after completion of treatment. Initial MRI are scheduled every 3–4 months, and then weaned to an annual schedule over 2–3 years.
• Up to 50% of children have residual neurological and spinal deficits after treatment. In addition to sensory and motor deficits, bladder/bowel dysfunction may also persist [2, 18, 90, 91]. Worsening neurological symptoms may result from tumor associated cyst or syrinx, maturation of an old deficit (e.g spasticity), or progressive spinal deformities and may require neurosurgical, orthopedic, or plastic surgery intervention.
• Early post-operative rehabilitation is essential for minimizing morbidity, and maximizing functional recovery. Brief low dose steroid treatment to relieve cord edema may help early neurological recovery [92].

• Spinal deformity is the most significant and common late effect seen in almost all long-term survivors; up to 70% of children who received post-operative radiation required spondylodesis [3].
• Children often have progressive deficits that peak during periods of normal rapid growth. Uncorrected spinal deformities in extreme cases can result in cord compression and progressive myelopathy.
• All children require routine clinical monitoring for changes in neurological status, and imaging as clinically indicated.
• Children who receive spinal or cranio-spinal radiation should be followed for growth or thyroid hormone deficiencies, neurocognitive sequelae, malignant transformation of residual tumor, and second malignancies within the radiation field.
• Despite frequent and substantial physical morbidity, surprisingly, a small study reported psychosocial outcomes comparable to that of healthy controls in spinal tumor survivors [91].

Conclusions

As childhood intramedullary tumors are rare, establishment of treatment guidelines will continue to be challenging. Regardless of specific treatments, most children with intramedullary tumors will have long survival, often with substantial and progressive neurological deficits. Therefore, a multi-disciplinary approach is essential both in treatment planning and in follow up to maximize and preserve neurological function in this highly vulnerable population.

References

1 Stiller CA, Nectoux J. International incidence of childhood brain and spinal tumors. Int J Epidemiol 1994; 23: 458–64.

2 O'Sullivan C, Jenkin RD, Doherty MA, Hoffman HJ, Greenberg ML. Spinal cord tumors in children: long-term results of combined surgical and radiation treatment. J Neurosurg 1994; 81: 507–12.

3 Rickert CH, Paulus W. Epidemiology of central nervous system tumors in childhood and adolescence based on the new WHO classification. Childs Nerv Syst 2001; 17; 503–11.

4 Garg S, Dormans JP. Tumors and tumor-like conditions of the spine in children. J Am Acad Orthop Surg 2005; 13: 372–81.

5 Lee M, Rezai AR, Freed D, Epstein FJ. Intramedullary spinal cord tumors in neurofibromatosis. Neurosurgery 1996; 38: 32–7.

6 DeSousa AL, Kalsbeck JE, Mealey J, Jr, Campbell RL, Hockey A. Intraspinal tumors in children. A review of 81 cases. J Neurosurg 1979; 51: 437–45.

7 Lonjon M, Goh KY, Epstein FJ. Intramedullary spinal cord ependymomas in children: treatment, results and follow-up. Pediatr Neurosurg 1998; 29: 178–83.

8 Ohgaki H, Kleihues P. Epidemiology and etiology of gliomas. Acta Neuropathol 2005; 109: 93–108.

9 Reimer R, Onofrio BM. Astrocytomas of the spinal cord in children and adolescents. J Neurosurg 1985; 63: 669–75.

10 Innocenzi G, Raco A, Cantore G, Raimondi AJ. Intramedullary astrocytomas and ependymomas in the pediatric age group: a retrospective study. Childs Nerv Syst 1996; 12: 776–80.

11 Constantini S, Houten J, Miller DC, et al. Intramedullary spinal cord tumors in children under the age of 3 years. J Neurosurg 1996; 85: 1036–43.

12 Komotar RJ, Carson BS, Rao C, Chaffee S, Goldthwaite PT, Tihan T. Pilomyxoid astrocytoma of the spinal cord: report of three cases. Neurosurgery 2005; 56: 191.

13 Allen JC, et al. Treatment of high-grade spinal cord astrocytoma of childhood with '8-in-1' chemotherapy and radiotherapy: a pilot study of CCG-945. Children's Cancer Group. J Neurosurg 1998; 88: 215–20.

14 Bouffet E, Pierre-Kahn A, Marchal JC, et al. Prognostic factors in pediatric spinal cord astrocytoma. Cancer 1998; 83: 2391–9.

15 Cohen AR, Wisoff JH, Allen JC, Epstein F. Malignant astrocytomas of the spinal cord. J Neurosur 1989; 70: 50–4.

16 Przybylski GJ, Albright AL, Martinez AJ. Spinal cord astrocytomas: long-term results comparing treatments in children. Childs Nerv Syst 1997; 13: 375–82.

17 Epstein F, Epstein N. Surgical treatment of spinal cord astrocytomas of childhood. A series of 19 patients. J Neurosurg 1982; 57: 685–9.

18 Constantini S, Miller DC, Allen JC, Rorke LB, Freed D, Epstein FJ. Radical excision of intramedullary spinal cord tumors: surgical morbidity and long-term follow-up evaluation in 164 children and young adults. J Neurosurg 2000; 93: 183–93.

19 Merchant TE, Nguyen D, Thompson SJ, Reardon DA, Kun LE, Sanford RA. High-grade pediatric spinal cord tumors. Pediatr Neurosurg 1999; 30: 1–5.

20 Hukin J, Siffert J, Cohen H, Velasquez L, Zagzag D, Allen J. Leptomeningeal dissemination at diagnosis of pediatric low-grade neuroepithelial tumors. Neuro Oncol 2003; 5: 188–96.

21 Elsberg CA. Some aspects of the diagnosis and surgical treatment of tumors of the spinal cord: with a study of the end results in a series of 119 operations. Ann Surg 1925; 81: 1057–73.

22 Raco A, Esposito V, Lenzi J, Piccirilli M, Delfini R, Cantore G. Long-term follow-up of intramedullary spinal cord tumors: a series of 202 cases. Neurosurgery 2005; 56: 972–81; discussion 972–81.

23 Goh KY, Velasquez L, Epstein FJ. Pediatric intramedullary spinal cord tumors: is surgery alone enough? Pediatr Neurosurg 1997; 27, 34–9.

24 Innocenzi G, Salvati M, Cervoni L, Delfini R, Cantore G. Prognostic factors in intramedullary astrocytomas. Clin Neurol Neurosurg 1997; 99: 1–5.

25 Wahab SH, Simpson JR, Michalski JM, Mansur DB. Long term outcome with post-operative radiation therapy for spinal canal ependymoma. J Neurooncol 2007; 83: 85–9.

26 Fouladi M, Hunt DL, Pollack IF, et al. Outcome of children with centrally reviewed low-grade gliomas treated with chemotherapy with or without radiotherapy on Children's Cancer Group high-grade glioma study CCG-945. Cancer 2003; 98: 1243–52.

27 Lafay-Cousin L, Holm S, Qaddoumi I, et al. Weekly vinblastine in pediatric low-grade glioma patients with carboplatin allergic reaction. Cancer 2005; 103: 2636–42.

28 Packer RJ, Lange B, Ater J, et al. Carboplatin and vincristine for recurrent and newly diagnosed low-grade gliomas of childhood. J Clin Oncol 1993; 11: 850–6.

29 Lewis SP, Pizer BL, Coakham H, Nelson RJ, Bouffet E. Chemotherapy for spinal cord astrocytoma: can natural history be modified? Childs Nerv Syst 1998; 14: 317–21.

30 Doireau V, Grill J, Zerah M, et al. Chemotherapy for unresectable and recurrent intramedullary glial tumors in children. Brain Tumours Subcommittee of the French Society of Paediatric Oncology (SFOP). Br J Cancer 1999; 81: 835–40.

31 Merchant TE, Kiehna EN, Thompson SJ, Heideman R, Sanford RA, Kun LE. Pediatric low-grade and ependymal spinal cord tumors. Pediatr Neurosurg 2000; 32: 30–6.

32 Hassall TE, Mitchell AE, Ashley DM. Carboplatin chemotherapy for progressive intramedullary spinal cord low-grade gliomas in children: three case studies and a review of the literature. Neuro Oncol 2001; 3: 251–7.

33 Townsend N, Handler M, Fleitz J, Foreman N. Intramedullary spinal cord astrocytomas in children. Pediatr Blood Cancer 2004; 43: 629–32.

34 Khaw SL, Coleman LT, Downie PA, Heath JA, Ashley DM. Temozolomide in pediatric low-grade glioma. Pediatr Blood Cancer 2007; 49: 808–11.

35 Mora J, Cruz O, Gala S, Navarro R. Successful treatment of childhood intramedullary spinal cord astrocytomas with irinotecan and cisplatin. Neuro Oncol 2007; 9: 39–46.

36 Lee HK, Chang EL, Fuller GN, et al. The prognostic value of neurologic function in astrocytic spinal cord glioma. Neuro Oncol 2003; 5: 208–13.

37 Bouffet E, Amat D, Devaux Y, Desuzinges C. Chemotherapy for spinal cord astrocytoma. Med Pediatr Oncol 1997; 29: 560–2.

38 Tabori U, Vukovic B, Zielenska M, et al. The role of telomere maintenance in the spontaneous growth arrest of pediatric low-grade gliomas. Neoplasia 2006; 8: 136–42.

39 Bartels U, Hawkins C, Jing M, et al. Vascularity and angiogenesis as predictors of growth in optic pathway/hypothalamic gliomas. J Neurosurg 2006; 104: 314–20.

40 Wong KK, Chang YM, Tsang YT, et al. Expression analysis of juvenile pilocytic astrocytomas by oligonucleotide microarray reveals two potential subgroups. Cancer Res 65, 76–84.

41 Johannessen CM, Reczek EE, James MF, Brems H, Legius E, Cichowski K. The NF1 tumor suppressor critically regulates TSC2 and mTOR. Proc Natl Acad Sci USA 2005; 102: 8573–8.

42 Tabori U, Ma J, Carter M, et al. Human telomere reverse transcriptase expression predicts progression and survival in pediatric intracranial ependymoma. J Clin Oncol 2006; 24: 1522–8.

43 Miller DC. Surgical pathology of intramedullary spinal cord neoplasms. J Neurooncol 2000; 47: 189–94.

44 Garre ML, Capra V, Di Battista E, et al. Genetic abnormalities and CNS tumors: report of two cases of ependymoma associated with Klinefelter's Syndrome (KS). Childs Nerv Syst 2007; 23: 219–23.

45 Evans DG, Trueman L, Wallace A, Collins S, Strachan T. Genotype/phenotype correlations in type 2 neurofibromatosis (NF2): evidence for more severe disease associated with truncating mutations. J Med Genet 1998; 35: 450–5.

46 Patronas NJ, Courcoutsakis N, Bromley CM, Katzman GL, MacCollin M, Parry DM. Intramedullary and spinal canal tumors in patients with neurofibromatosis 2: MR imaging findings and correlation with genotype. Radiology 2001; 218: 434–42.

47 Birch BD, Johnson JP, Parsa A, et al. Frequent type 2 neurofibromatosis gene transcript mutations in sporadic intramedullary spinal cord ependymomas. Neurosurgery 1996; 39: 135–40.

48 Ebert C, von Haken M, Meyer-Puttlitz B, et al. Molecular genetic analysis of ependymal tumors. NF2 mutations and chromosome 22q loss occur preferentially in intramedullary spinal ependymomas. Am J Pathol 1999; 155: 627–32.

49 Rajaram V, Gutmann DH, Prasad SK, Mansur DB, Perry A. Alterations of protein 4.1 family members in ependymomas: a study of 84 cases. Mod Pathol 2005; 18: 991–7.

50 Hirose Y, Aldape K, Bollen A, et al. Chromosomal abnormalities subdivide ependymal tumors into clinically relevant groups. Am J Pathol 2001; 158: 1137–43.

51 Kramer DL, Parmiter AH, Rorke LB, Sutton LN, Biegel JA. Molecular cytogenetic studies of pediatric ependymomas. J Neurooncol 1998; 37: 25–33.

52 Korshunov A, Neben K, Wrobel G, et al. Gene expression patterns in ependymomas correlate with tumor location, grade, and patient age. Am J Pathol 2003; 163: 1721–7.

53 Taylor MD, Poppleton H, Fuller C, et al. Radial glia cells are candidate stem cells of ependymoma. Cancer Cell 2005; 8: 323–35.

54 McLaughlin MP, Laperriere NJ, Jaakkimainen L, et al. Ependymoma: results, prognostic factors and treatment recommendations. Int J Radiat Oncol Biol Phys 1998; 40: 845–50.

55 Massimino M, Giangaspero F, Garrè ML et al. Salvage treatment for childhood ependymoma after surgery only: pitfalls of omitting 'at once' adjuvant treatment. Int J Radiat Oncol Biol Phys 2006; 65: 1440–5.

56 Gomez DR, Missett BT, Wara WM, et al. High failure rate in spinal ependymomas with long-term follow-up. Neuro Oncol 2005; 7: 254–9.

57 Whitaker SJ, Bessell EM, Ashley SE, Bloom HJ, Bell BA, Brada M. Postoperative radiotherapy in the management of spinal cord ependymoma. J Neurosurg 1991; 74: 720–8.

58 Sonneland PR, Scheithauer BW, Onofrio BM. Myxopapillary ependymoma. A clinicopathologic and immunocytochemical study of 77 cases. Cancer 1985; 56: 883–93.

59 Kuo JS, Gonzalez-Gomez I, McComb JG. Unexpected myxopapillary ependymoma within a filum terminale tethering the spinal cord. Pediatr Neurosurg 2007; 43: 309–11.

60 Beschorner R, Wehrmann M, Ernemann U, et al. Extradural ependymal tumor with myxopapillary and ependymoblastic differentiation in a case of Schinzel-Giedion syndrome. Acta Neuropathol 2007; 113: 339–46.

61 Bagley CA, Kothbauer KF, Wilson S, et al. Resection of myxopapillary ependymomas in children. J Neurosurg 2007; 106: 261–7.

62 Akyurek S, Chang EL, Yu TK, et al. Spinal myxopapillary ependymoma outcomes in patients treated with surgery and radiotherapy at M.D. Anderson Cancer Center. J Neurooncol 2006; 80: 177–83.

63 Chinn DM, Donaldson SS, Dahl GV, et al. Management of children with metastatic spinal myxopapillary ependymoma using craniospinal irradiation. Med Pediatr Oncol 2000; 35: 443–5.

64 Mridha AR, Sharma MC, Sarkar C, et al. Myxopapillary ependymoma of lumbosacral region with metastasis to both cerebellopontine angles: report of a rare case. Childs Nerv Syst 2007; 23: 1209–13.

65 Fassett DR, Pingree J, Kestle JR. The high incidence of tumor dissemination in myxopapillary ependymoma in pediatric patients. Report of five cases and review of the literature. J Neurosurg 2005; 102: 59–64.

66 Nagib MG, O'Fallon MT. Myxopapillary ependymoma of the conus medullaris and filum terminale in the pediatric age group. Pediatr Neurosurg 1997; 26: 2–7.

67 Chan HS, Becker LE, Hoffman HJ, et al. Myxopapillary ependymoma of the filum terminale and cauda equina in childhood: report of seven cases and review of the literature. Neurosurgery 1984; 14: 204–10.

68 Tzekov C, Naydenov E, Kalev O. Ependymoma of the cauda equina starting with communicating hydrocephalus: a case report. Pediatr Neurosurg 2007; 43: 399–402.

69 Lin YH, Huang CI, Wong TT, et al. Treatment of spinal cord ependymomas by surgery with or without postoperative radiotherapy. J Neurooncol 2005; 71: 205–10.

70 Celli P, Cervoni L, Cantore G. Ependymoma of the filum terminale: treatment and prognostic factors in a series of 28 cases. Acta Neurochir (Wien) 1993; 124: 99–103.

71 Gagliardi FM, Cervoni L, Domenicucci M, Celli P, Salvati M. Ependymomas of the filum terminale in childhood: report of four cases and review of the literature. Childs Nerv Syst 1993; 9: 3–6.

72 Rezai AR, Woo HH, Lee M, Cohen H, Zagzag D, Epstein FJ. Disseminated ependymomas of the central nervous system. J Neurosurg 1996; 85: 618–24.

73 Combs SE, Thilmann C, Debus J, Schulz-Ertner D. Local radiotherapeutic management of ependymomas with fractionated stereotactic radiotherapy (FSRT). BMC Cancer 2006; 6: 222.

74 Chamberlain MC. Salvage chemotherapy for recurrent spinal cord ependymona. Cancer 2002; 95: 997–1002.

75 Madden JR, Fenton LZ, Weil M, Winston KR, Partington M, Foreman NK. Experience with tamoxifen/etoposide in the treatment of a child with myxopapillary ependymoma. Med Pediatr Oncol 2001; 37: 67–9.

76 Fakhrai N, Neophytou P, Dieckmann K, et al. Recurrent spinal ependymoma showing partial remission under Imatimib. Acta Neurochir (Wien) 2004; 146: 1255–8.

77 Naruse T, Matsuyama Y, Ishiguro N. Cyclooxygenase-2 expression in ependymoma of the spinal cord. J Neurosurg Spine 2007; 6: 240–6.

78 Kim SK, Lim SY, Wang KC, et al. Overexpression of cyclooxygenase-2 in childhood ependymomas: role of COX–2 inhibitor in growth and multi-drug resistance in vitro. Oncol Rep 2004; 12: 403–9.

79 Poppleton H, Gilbertson RJ. Stem cells of ependymoma. Br J Cancer 96, 6–10

80 Park CK, Chung CK, Choe GY, Wang KC, Cho BK, Kim HJ. Intramedullary spinal cord ganglioglioma: a report of five cases. Acta Neurochir (Wien) 2000; 142: 547–52.

81 Park SH, Chi JG, Cho BK, Wang KC. Spinal cord ganglioglioma in childhood. Pathol Res Pract 1993; 189: 189–96.

82 Jallo GI, Freed D, Epstein FJ. Spinal cord gangliogliomas: a review of 56 patients. J Neurooncol 2004; 68: 71–7.

83 Lang FF, Epstein FJ, Ransohoff J, et al. Central nervous system gangliogliomas. Part 2: Clinical outcome. J Neurosurg 1993; 79: 867–73.

84 Di Patre PL, Payer M, Brunea M, Delavelle J, De Tribolet N, Pizzolato G. Malignant transformation of a spinal cord ganglioglioma – case report and review of the literature. Clin Neuropathol 2004; 23: 298–303.

85 Vougioukas VI, Gläsker S, Hubbe U, et al. Surgical treatment of hemangioblastomas of the central nervous system in pediatric patients. Childs Nerv Syst 2006; 22: 1149–53.

86 Wanebo JE, Lonser RR, Glenn GM, Oldfield EH. The natural history of hemangioblastomas of the central nervous system in patients with von Hippel–Lindau disease. J Neurosurg 2003; 98: 82–94.

87 Lonser RR, Oldfield EH. Spinal cord hemangioblastomas. Neurosurg Clin N Am 2006; 17: 37–44.

88 Aiello LP, George DJ, Cahill MT, et al. Rapid and durable recovery of visual function in a patient with von hippel–lindau syndrome after systemic therapy with vascular endothelial growth factor receptor inhibitor su5416. Ophthalmology 2002; 109: 1745–51.

89 Harris AL. von Hippel–Lindau syndrome: target for anti-vascular endothelial growth factor (VEGF) receptor therapy. Oncologist 2000; 5 (Suppl 1): 32–6.

90 Poretti A, Zehnder D, Boltshauser E, Grotzer MA. Long-term complications and quality of life in children with intraspinal tumors. Pediatr Blood Cancer 2007.

91 Tobias ME, McGirt MJ, Chaichana KL, et al. Surgical management of long intramedullary spinal cord tumors. Childs Nerv Syst 2007.

92 McGirt MJ, Goldstein IM, Chaichana KL, Tobias ME, Kothbauer KF, Jallo GI. Neurological outcome after resection of intramedullary spinal cord tumors in children. Childs Nerv Syst 2008; 24; 93–7.

6 Pediatric Craniopharyngioma, Mixed Glioneuronal Tumors, and Atypical Teratoid/ Rhabdoid Tumor

Adrienne Weeks and Michael D. Taylor
Department of Neurosurgery, The Hospital for Sick Children, Toronto, Ontario, Canada

Introduction

Craniopharyngioma, mixed glioneuronal, and atypical teratoid/ rhabdoid tumors are among the rarest pediatric brain tumors. The treatment of these diseases remains controversial. The mixed glial neuronal tumors are a surgical success story with patients usually achieving a cure with a high quality of life after surgical resection alone. While craniopharyngioma can be cured also, this is often achieved at significant price to the child, and there is considerable debate within the medical community on how best to treat this disease. In contrast, atypical teratoid/rhabdoid tumor (ATRT) has a grave prognosis despite aggressive treatment.

Craniopharyngioma

Epidemiology
- Rare parasellar and sellar tumor accounting for approximately 1.8–4.4% of pediatric intracranial neoplasms [1, 2].
- No sex predilection.
- No known geographic distribution bias.
- Frequent juxtaposition to vital structures such as the optic apparatus, hypothalamus, cavernous sinus, cranial nerves, and the circle of Willis can result in high surgical morbidity.

Pathology and pathogenesis
Two subtypes of craniopharyngioma are recognized, the adamantinomatous and the papillary subtypes.

Adamantinomatous subtype
This occurs in childhood, is often highly calcified and cystic.
- Cysts contain fluid with a characteristic 'motor oil' consistency that is rich in cholesterol crystals [3].

Pediatric Hematology and Oncology, 1st edition. Edited by Edward J. Estlin, Richard J. Gilbertson, and Robert F. Wynn. © 2010 Blackwell Publishing Ltd.

- The cyst walls contain whorls and sheets of pallisading columnar cells arranged around stellate epithelial cells [3].
- Cysts can contain calcium or bone arising from desquamated cells of eosinophilic masses termed 'wet keratin'.

Histologically, these tumors resemble the embryonic tooth and therefore, the adamantinomatous subtype is thought to arise from epithelial cells derived from stomadeum in the remnants of the craniopharyngeal duct [4].

Papillary subtype
The papillary subtype occurs predominantly in adults.
- Typically solid.
- Usually not calcified.
- Well-differentiated squamous epithelium surrounding a fibrovascular core [4].
- Thought to arise as a result of metaplasia of the squamous epithelial rests in the craniopharyngeal duct remnants.

Clinical presentation and imaging characteristics
Symptoms at presentation depend on patient age and tumor location but often include one or more of three main problems [5, 6].
- Visual impairment: secondary to compression of the optic apparatus. The location of the lesion to some extent predicts visual changes, as impairment in acuity is higher in pre-chiasmatic lesions [7].
- Headache, nausea, and vomiting: secondary to hydrocephalus due to third ventricular compression.
- Endocrinopathies: secondary to compression of the hypothalamic-pituitary axis.

Initial CT imaging of craniopharyngioma shows an enhancing cystic sellar and/or suprasellar mass with calcification [8, 9] (Figure 6.1 and Box 6.1). The solid focus predominates in the sella with a suprasellar cystic extension [10].

Treatment
There is ongoing long-standing debate regarding the optimal treatment of craniopharyngioma.

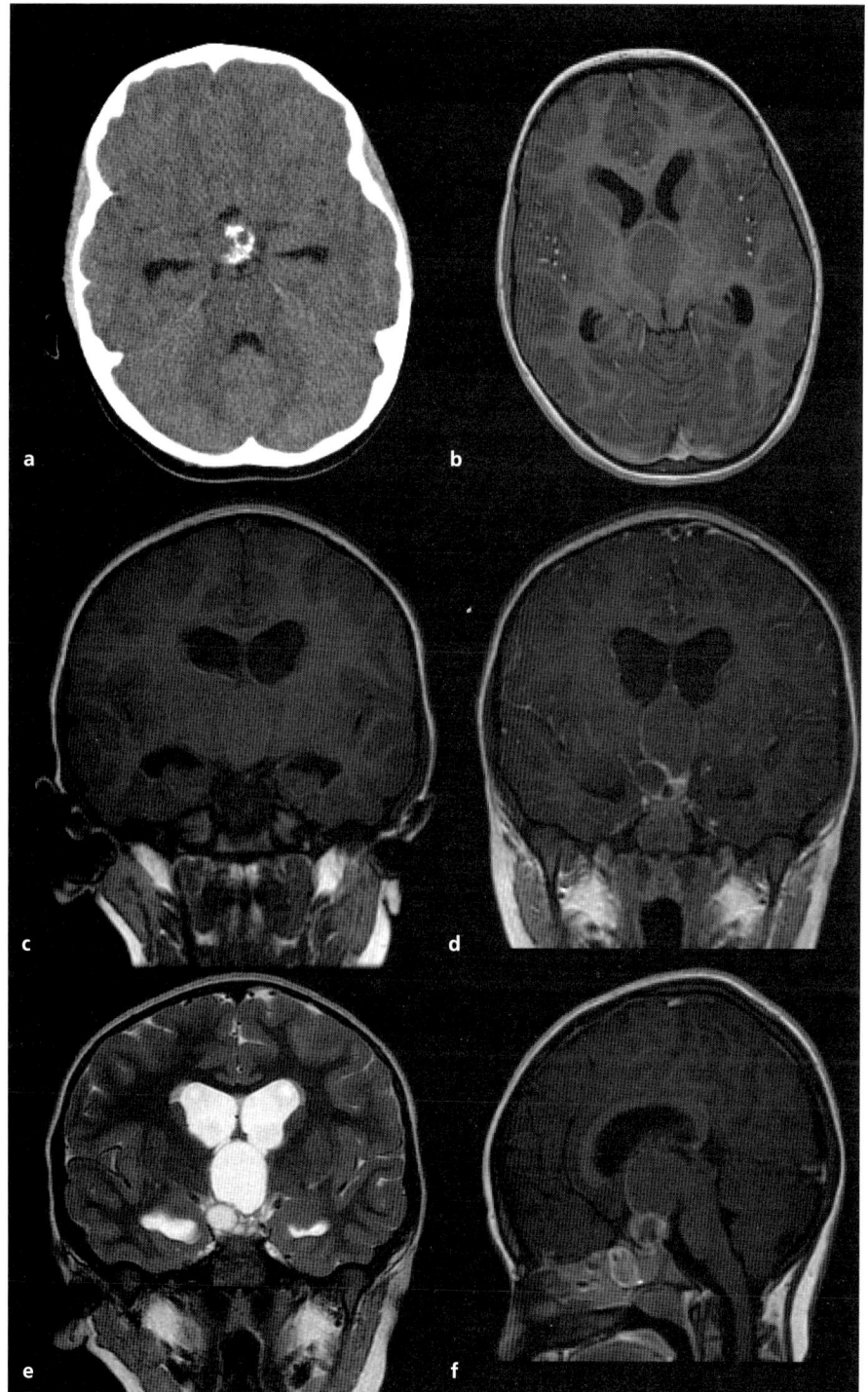

Figure 6.1 Radiographic appearance of craniopharyngioma. (a), Non-contrast CT showing suprasellar mass with calcification. (b), Axial T1 MRI showing suprasellar mass. (c, d), Coronal T1 MRI images with and without gadolinium showing suprasellar mass, compression of the Foramen of Monroe and associated hydrocephalus. (e), Coronal T2 images showing the cystic nature of suprasellar mass. f, Sagittal T1 MRI of suprasellar mass.

• Some clinicians advocate initial radical resection with the aim of achieving cure, improving visual function, and avoiding radiation treatment.

• Others advise a more conservative surgical approach followed by adjuvant radiation therapy in an effort to avoid the considerable risk of surgical morbidity that includes endocrine dysfunction, obesity, and neurocognitive decline.

• The longevity of the debate indicates that no single approach can be applied to all tumors, children, and families.

Surgical management

Surgical management has evolved dramatically since Harvey Cushing first attempted to reach the sellar/suprasellar region and remove a craniopharyngioma. The advent of the operating

Box 6.1 Key points regarding imaging of craniopharyngioma.

1 Can present a wide range of imaging characteristics:

T1 MRI sequences:

- Often isointense to hyperintense depending on the protein content of the cystic structure.
- Cholesterol clefts, fat, hemorrhage, and calcification can contribute to high T1 signal [11].

T2 MRI sequences:

- Heterogeneous solid component with a high signal in the cystic portion [9].

Gradient Echo images are useful to identify calcification.

Diffusion weighted imaging can be useful to exclude an epidermoid tumor [9].

2 Differential diagnosis of lesions in the sella include [9]:

- Pituitary adenoma.
- Hypothalamic/optic glioma.
- Rathke's pouch cyst.
- Epidermoid, thrombosed aneurysm.
- Simple arachnoid cyst.

microscope, advances in microsurgical technique, and the use of image-guided stereotactic surgery have allowed surgeons to access the sella/suprasellar regions and make gross total resection of craniopharyngioma possible. A variety of surgical approaches has been used to reach the sellar/suprasellar region, subfrontal, pterional, transcallosal, transtemporal, subtemporal, transfacial, transpheniodal, as well as combinations of the above [12].

Gross total resection

Proponents of radical resection suggest that in skilled hands with modern operating techniques, up front gross total resection should always be the goal. Key points relating to gross total resection of chraniopharyngioma include:

- Recurrence rates following gross total resection range from zero to 52.8% [13]. Van Effenterre and Boch reviewed their series of 122 adult and pediatric craniopharngiomas with 59% obtaining complete resection with an 11% total mortality rate, excellent functional outcome in 85% and an 18% recurrence rate [14].

  1 Other contemporary series suggest post-operative endocrine dysfunction is present in over 80% of patients, and approximately 15% of patients suffer from hypothalamic dysfunction [7, 14–18].

- Diabetes insipidus is almost unavoidable: 80% of cases require replacement of two or more hormones, and non-endocrine morbidity secondary to hypothalamic damage (obesity, cognitive impairment, and decreased sociability) are probably underestimated at 15% [15, 19].

2 The debilitating hypothalamic syndrome is unique to the pediatric population and may be underestimated in mixed adult and pediatric series [19].

3 Improved MRI image-based assessment of surgical resection suggest recurrence rates may be lower in cases of 'true' gross total resection.

- Zuccaro reported zero recurrence in the 69% of patients that had radiographic gross total resection (n=153) with a range of follow up from 1 to 16 years. Sixty-nine patients required combined surgical approaches [20]. Mortality rate was of 7%.
- Caldarelli et al. reported a recurrence rate of only 7.5% among 40 patients with radiographic evidence of gross total resection (five cases had multiple operations) [21]. Mortality rate was 3.5%.
- Morbidity was deemed acceptable in both studies, although endocrine dysfunction was present in over 80% of patients postoperatively in both series.

Conservative surgical approach

Other groups have taken a more conservative surgical approach, suggesting that pre-operative imaging characteristics such as hypothalamic involvement should guide decisions regarding gross total versus subtotal resection [15, 22].

1 Puget et al. reported a prospective study of children with craniopharyngioma plus hypothalamic involvement. Treatment included subtotal resection and radiation; none of the 22 children treated in this manner experienced hyperphagia, morbid obesity, or behavioral dysfunction [22].

2 A review by De Vile et al. suggested that the deleterious effects of radical surgery can be predicted pre-operatively by:

- Degree of hydrocephalus.
- Tumor size (classified by intracranial compartments involved).
- Age less than 5 years.
- Presence of hypothalamic dysfunction at presentation.

3 During surgery vascular complications and the degree of hypothalamic involvement may predict poor outcome [15, 23].

4 A more flexible approach that restricts radical surgical resection in those predictive of a good outcome may decrease surgical mortality, and improve cognitive status, but endocrine dysfunction and degree of hypothalamic dysfunction remain unchanged [15].

Radiation therapy

The serious morbidities associated with radical surgery, coupled with the variable rates of recurrence, has lead to the exploration of adjuvant treatments of craniopharyngioma [5, 7, 24–26]. The most common adjuvant treatment strategy is radiotherapy following subtotal resection.

1 The Royal Marsden Hospital reported the largest series of patients treated in this manner:

- 173 cases of craniopharyngioma, 148 having limited surgery plus radiation.
- 45% were pediatric patients.
- 10-year progression free and overall survival rates were 83% and 77% respectively [27].

• Younger age, and modern radiation therapy techniques were predictive of survival, but extent of surgical resection was not [27].

2 Boston's Children's Hospital series:
• 61 patients, 37 patients treated with radiation (mean dose of 54.6 Gy) and surgery.
• 10-year survival 91%.
• After 10 years of follow up there was statistical advantage in local control rates when radiation was employed [24].
• Diabetes insipidus and pituitary deficiency rates may be less than in aggressive surgical counterparts [24,27].

3 University of Pennsylvania:
• 10 year control rate was significantly lower (42% vs. 84%) among patients receiving surgery alone versus subtotal resection and radiation.
• Survival rates were similar for the two groups, and were attributed to the efficacy of salvage radiation [28].

4 Neurocognitive and neuropsychological sequelae from subtotal surgery and radiation may be less than that following radical surgery alone [29–31].

5 Radiation may be useful as a salvage strategy following recurrence after surgery [29].

Radiation therapy is not without serious complications. The proximity of the optic apparatus (tolerance of 54 Gy/30 fractions or 8–9 Gy in a single fraction), brainstem, hypothalamus, and pituitary present the same restrictions to radiation as they do to aggressive surgical treatment. The majority of these complications are dose related and must be balanced with the advantage of surgical sparing.

1 Optic neuropathy:
• Does not appear to occur in patients treated with 1.5 Gy fractions to total doses of 50 Gy [27], but may result when the total dose exceeds 60 Gy [32].

2 Neurocognition:
• Children less than 3 years are at particular risk.
• Surgical management, either radical resection or temporizing surgery, is indicated until such time as radiation is deemed safer.

3 Vasculopathy, and of moyamoya syndrome:
• Advances in stereotactic surgery, such as the gamma knife, may show some benefit. However, large and long-term studies are still pending and currently only small lesions <2.5 cm that are <3 mm away from the chiasm are amenable to radiosurgery [33–35].

4 Second malignancy:
• While rare, ependymomas, meningiomas, brainstem glioma, and glioblastoma multiforme have all been reported after radiation therapy for craniopharyngioma [28, 36–40].
• In the Royal Marsden series with a follow up of 12 years, no secondary malignancies have yet been reported [27].

Intracavitary treatments

Approximately 90% of craniopharyngiomas will present with cystic cavities as a portion of the tumor, either at initial diagnosis or at time of recurrence. These cyst cavities have been used as a means of delivering chemotherapy or radiotherapy to the lesion via catheters placed into the cyst [41,42]. Catheters are placed into the cyst using stereotactic, ultrasonic, or endoscopic guidance and attached to an Ommaya reservoir. Intracavity agents have included:

1 *Bleomycin:*
• Takeuchi first used the antitumoral antibiotic, bleomycin, in 1975 with favorable results [43].
• Standard dosing is 2–5 ml of bleomycin over a course of days to weeks [41].
• Bleomycin works on the walls of the cyst and is best used in patients harboring monocystic lesions with minimal solid components [44].
• The majority of studies show at least 50% reduction (from 50 to 100%) of the cystic component in a majority of patients undergoing this therapy for purely cystic craniopharyngiomas [45, 46].
• Toxicity has been reported with the use of intracavitary bleomycin. Death (rare) and hypothalamic injury secondary to bleomycin leakage outside the cyst walls, and acoustic nerve injury, optic neuritis, and vascular injury as a result of leakage into the subarachnoid space have been reported [47–50].
• Most authors support continual MRI evaluation during treatment to monitor for leakage and high-dose steroids to control bleomycin toxicity [41, 50].

2 Interferon alpha (IFN-α):
• Used in the treatment of cystic craniopharyngioma.
• Followed the use of systemic IFN-α that demonstrated moderate activity against craniopharyngioma [51].
• Cavalheiro *et al.* used IFN-α intralesionally via a catheter inserted subfrontally and attached to an Ommaya reservoir in 10 patients [52]. Patients had alternative days of IFN-α administration and cyst drainage with seven of the 10 having complete disappearance of the cyst in follow-up imaging [52]. This same group reported on these initial 10 patients plus 11 more in 2007, follow up ranging from 6 months to 4 years, 11 of 21 had a complete response, 7 of 21 had a partial response and three were non-responders [53]. It is unclear to what extent the reduction in lesional size can be attributed to IFN-α versus cyst decompression.

3 Intracavitary irradiation:
• Most commonly yttrium-90 and 32-phosphorus have been employed to treat cystic craniopharyngioma. Lack of cyst progression ranges from 55 to 100% [42, 54–60].
• Toxicity to intracavitary irradiation includes amarosis, chemical meningitis, moyamoya vessel changes, and death [24, 56, 58].

Conclusion

The optimal treatment of craniopharyngioma remains unclear. Arguably, the most strategic approach accounts for patient factors such as pre-operative endocrine and hypothalamic function, age, and imaging characteristics such as cystic size, and degree of hypothalamic involvement.

Mixed glioneuronal tumors

Overview

Mixed glial neuronal tumors present a rare, interesting, and diverse group of tumors (Box 6.2).

Ganglioglioma

Gangliogliomas (GG) represent 1% of all primary intracranial neoplasms and 4% of pediatric central nervous system (CNS) neoplasms. Of all tumors associated with epilepsy, 40% are identified pathologically as GG [62]. Histologically, GG are comprised of a dysplastic neuronal component and a variable glial component: pilocytic astrocytoma (93%), fibrillary astrocytoma (6%) [65]. The diagnosis may be aided by the identification of the marker CD34 in the neuronal component [61]. Malignant transformation of the glial (anaplastic or glioblastoma multiforme) constituent is rare, but occurs in approximately 2% of cases [65].

Clinically, the majority of GG present in patients with a history of epilepsy [66]. The most common location is the temporal lobe: temporal mesial (50%) and temporal lateral (29%) [65]. However, GGs can occur in the brainstem, spinal cord, mid-brain, as well as other cortical locations. On imaging they appear as circumscribed solid or cystic lesions, which are hypo- to iso-dense on non-contrast CT, with or without calcification, with approximately 50% showing enhancement [10]. On T1 MRI imaging the mass is hypo- to iso-intense to grey matter with possible associated areas of cortical dysplasia and broadening of the gyrus. T2 imaging shows a hyper-intense signal [67].

Complete surgical resection is curative, with only 3% of patients experiencing recurrent tumor and a 7.5 year survival rate of 97% [65]. Complete and sustained seizure relief after resection will be experienced by 60–84% of patients [65, 68]. Given the success of gross total resection there is little role for adjunctive chemotherapy or radiation in low-grade GG. Recurrences can usually be treated with re-operation [69]. The role of adjunctive therapy for completely resected high grade GG is limited given the rarity of the lesion, with some authors showing no difference between progression free survival rates regardless of grade in the setting of gross total resection [69]. However, adjunctive therapy is recommended in those instances where subtotal resection of a high-grade lesion has occurred [69].

Desmoplastic infantile ganglioglioma

Desmoplastic infantile ganglioglioma (DIG) is a very rare tumor that occurs predominantly in infants with a peak age of occurrence between 3 and 6 months [70]. Recent case reports have shown DIG can occur in older patients (eldest 25 years of age) [71–74]. The disease was first described in 1987 by VandenBerg *et al.* [75] as a tumor displaying:

- Divergent astrocytic and ganglionic differentiation.
- Prominent desmoplastic stroma.
- Voluminous size.
- Cystic component.
- Presentation within the first 18 months of life.
- Good prognosis.

The World Health Organization (WHO) classifies DIG as a grade I neoplasm. With the exception of one case in the literature, DIG occurs almost exclusively supratentorially [71]. Imaging reflects a solid superficial mass or plaque attached to the dura and associated with a large septated cystic component (Figure 6.2). The solid portion of the tumor is hyperdense on CT with marked contrast enhancement; on MRI the solid portion is hypointense on both T1 and T2 sequences [70]. The cystic portion does not enhance with contrast, and usually is large enough to cause ventricular compression [10].

Given the young age at presentation and the large size of DIG, patients present with a brief clinical history. Signs and symptoms of intracranial hypertension predominate, including a rapidly enlarging head circumference, bulging anterior fontanelle, cranial bulge at tumor location, lethargy, and vomiting [70].

The treatment of choice is gross total surgical resection resulting in an excellent prognosis [76]. However, gross total resection is attainable in less than 50% of cases [70, 76]. There are too few case studies to determine the effectiveness of adjunctive chemotherapy in these residual cases. Follow up of these residual tumors often shows no growth, or diminishing growth over time, and thus the majority of neuro-oncologists delay adjunctive chemotherapy until progression occurs [71].

Box 6.2 Key facts about mixed neuronal glial tumors.

1 Comprised of large dysplastic neurons mixed with a background of neoplastic glial cells. The World Health Organization (2007) recognizes six variants of mixed neuronal glial tumors:

- Ganglioglioma.
- Anaplastic ganglioglioma.
- Desmoplastic infantile ganglioglioma (DIG).
- Papillary glioneuronal tumor.
- Rosette forming glioneuronal tumor of the fourth ventricle.
- Benign biological behaviour and a low proliferative index [61, 62].

2 As a group they usually present with epilepsy in the pediatric population and are probably related to the focal cortical dysplasias [62].

3 Cortical dysplasia can often be found in the cortex adjacent to the glioneuronal tumor and it has been postulated that the focal cortical dysplasias and the glioneuronal tumors originate from the same precursor cells and/or the tumor arises from dysplastic cortical tissue [62–64].

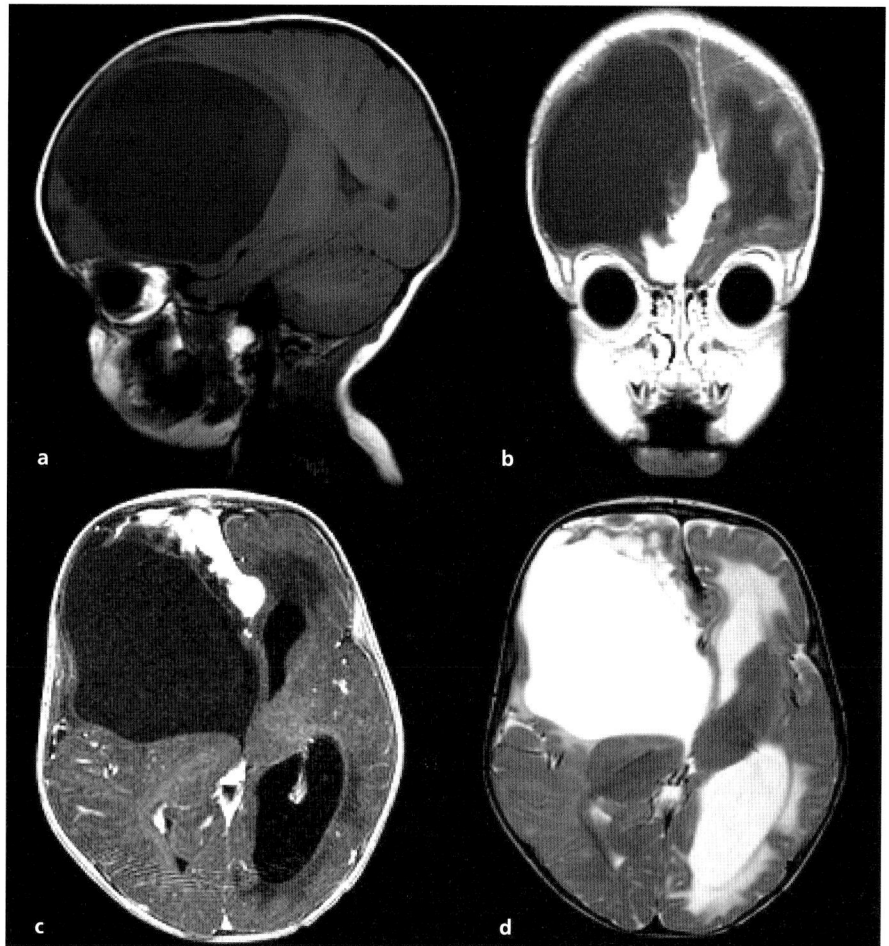

Figure 6.2 Radiographic appearance of desmoplastic infantile ganglioglioma. (a), Sagittal T1 MRI showing large cystic lesion. (b, c), Coronal and axial T1 MRI with gadolinium showing a large non-enhancing cystic lesion associated with an enhancing solid portion. There is a large mass effect and ventricular compression. (d), Axial T2 MRI showing the large cystic component of the tumor.

Dysembryoplastic neuroepithelial tumor

Daumas-Duport et al. first described dysembryoplastic neuroepithelial tumor (DNET) in 1988 as a tumor characterized by the following features:

• Indolent and highly epileptogeneic.
• Multiple nodules composed of astroyctoma, oligodendroglioma, and oligoastrocytoma intermixed with foci of dysplastic cortical organization arranged in columns perpendicular to the cortex [77, 78].

Focal cortical dysplasia is present in the surrounding cortex, suggesting this lesion is in the spectrum of a malformation. Reports of malignant transformation are rare and is usually from the glial component [79]. DNETs typically present as medically refractory seizures in children and young adults prior to the age of 20 [77].

The CT and MRI imaging are quite characteristic for DNET. DNETs are most commonly found in the temporal and frontal lobes. However, subcortical locations have been described [67] (Figure 6.3). DNETs are usually well circumscribed, wedge-shaped lesions involving a single expanded gyrus. They are typically described as 'bubbly' in appearance. There is often remodeling of the cranial vault overlying the lesion [80]. CT

imaging reveals a hypoattenuating cortical/subcortical lesion with possible calcification (20–36%) [10]. DNETs are usually non-enhancing. However, faint or patchy enhancement may be seen in up to 20% of cases and this may indicate a higher rate of recurrence [10]. A multinodular hypointense lesion on T1-weighted and hyperintense lesion on T2-weighted MRI sequences is characteristic. Again, faint contrast enhancement can be seen in approximately 20% of cases [10].

Treatment of DNET is surgical resection, either complete or partial with no adjunctive chemotherapy or radiotherapy required [81]. Clinically, DNET comprise 14% of epilepsy associated tumors [64]. Given the rarity of this lesion most series include DNET with other low grade gliomas in determining favorable seizure control rates after surgery (Engel class I rates of 50–90%) [64, 77, 81–86].

Atypical teratoid rhabdoid tumors

Malignant rhabdoid tumors were first described as a highly malignant subtype of Wilm's tumor [87]. It is now recognized

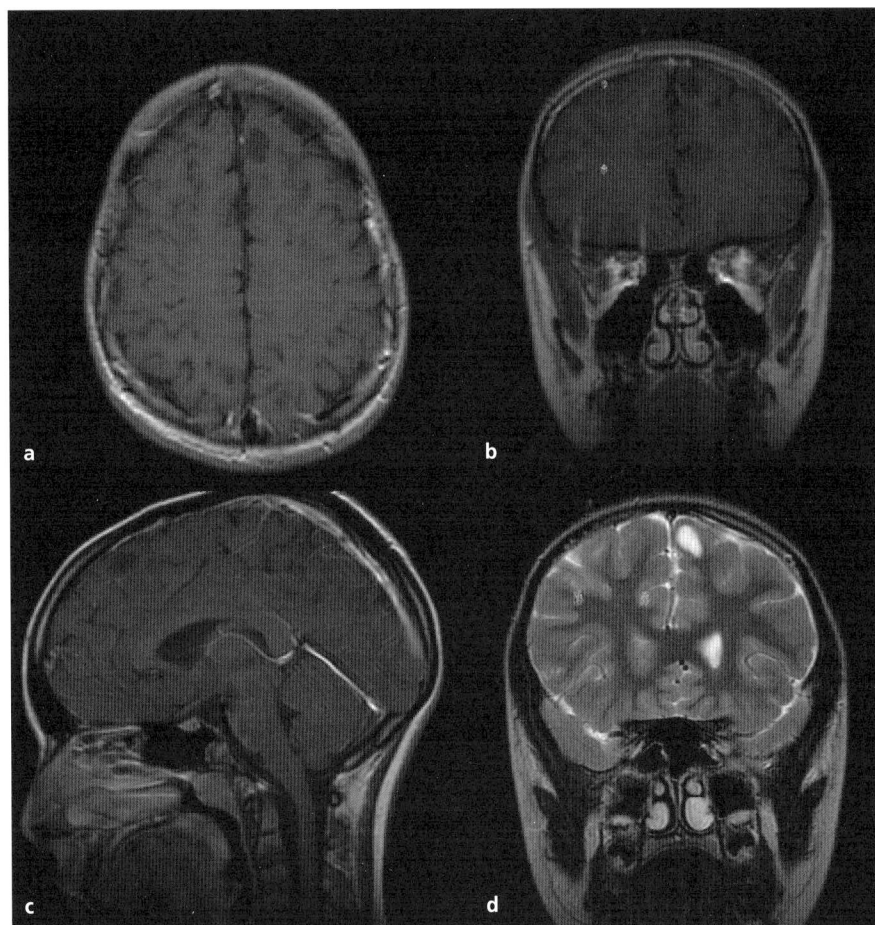

Figure 6.3 Radiographic appearance of dysembryoplastic neuroepithelial tumor. (a, c), Axial and sagittal T1 with gadolinium images showing a left frontal non-enhancing hypodense lesion expanding the gyrus. (b, d), Coronal T1 and T2 MRI images.

that rhabdoid tumors occur throughout the body. Biggs *et al.* first described the malignant intracranial rhabdoid tumor in 1987 [88]. These tumors were first termed atypical teratoid rhabdoid tumors (AT/RT) in a landmark paper in 1995 because of their histological constellation of neuroepithelial, peripheral epithelial, and mesenchymal elements [89]. The WHO first recognized AT/RT as a separate tumor entity in 2000.

Epidemiology

- AT/RT comprise 2–3% of all pediatric CNS tumors.
- AT/RT comprise 10–20% of primary intracranial malignancies in infants [89, 90].
- Median age of diagnosis is 20 months.
- Slight male predominance of 1.6:1 [89–91].
- Occur both supratentorially and infratentorially, notably in the cerebellopontine angle and cerebellum [90]. AT/RT have been reported to occur as intradural extramedullary/intramedullary lesions in the spine [92–96].
- At the time of presentation approximately 20% of patients will have disseminated disease [90]. Prior to the advent of intense multi-modal therapies, the vast majority children succumbed to their disease within a year [90].
- Two-year survival rate for AT/RT is around 15%.

Histology and molecular biology

AT/RT was diagnosed initially on the histological presence of rhabdoid cells (bland cells with eosinophilic cytoplasm) [97]. However, only a minority of AT/RT is composed entirely of nests or sheets of rhabdoid cells. Two-thirds of AT/RT contain rhabdoid cells intermixed with areas indistinguishable histologically from primitive neuroectodermal tumors (PNET) or medulloblastoma [89]. This variability underscores the importance of sampling error when biopsies for AT/RT are performed. AT/RT can less commonly resemble choroid plexus carcinoma, ependymoma, germ cell tumors, or glioblastoma [90, 91]. Improved understanding of the pathology and molecular biology of AT/RT has increased diagnostic accuracy considerably.

The majority of AT/RT stain positive for EMA (embryonal membrane antigen), vimentin, cytokeratin and SMA (smooth muscle actin), whereas PNET are histologically negative for these markers [91, 97]. AT/RT do not stain for germ cell markers such as alpha-fetoprotein, placental alkaline phosphatase, or human chorionic gonadotropin, allowing for differentiation from germ cell tumors [97].

Cytogenetic studies of AT/RT reveal minimal genetic alterations and lack of the classic isochromosome 17q typical of medulloblastoma [98].

Biegel *et al.* showed a high proportion of rhabdoid tumors have monosomy of chromosome 22 [98]. Further analysis revealed that a specific region of chromosome 22, 22q11.2 was deleted or translocated in AT/RT [95]. Using cloning strategies integrase interactor-1 (*INI-1*) was identified as the putative tumor suppressor in rhabdoid tumors [99].

INI-1 is part of the SWI/SNF complex:
• Remodels chromatin by disrupting the nucleosome and removing DNA from the histone octamer surface [100].
• Allows the SWI/SNF complex to transcriptionally activate or repress specific genes, although the signals for recruiting SWI/SNF to specific gene targets has yet to be elucidated [101].
• Truncating germline mutations of *INI-1* have been described by several groups with loss of the remaining wild type allele within the rhabdoid tumor [99, 101].
• Heritable truncating germline mutations of *INI-1* predisposing to rhabdoid tumors [102, 103]. Interestingly, in each case there was an asymptomatic adult carrier of the *INI-1* mutation.
• Deletion of *Ini-1* in mice is embryonically lethal; however, 5–10% of haploinsufficient mice (developmentally normal) develop rhabdoid tumors later in life [104, 105].
• The precise mechanism of *INI-1* tumor suppressor function has yet to be determined but current studies suggest it may play a role via the p16INK4a/cdk4/RB pathway [106].
• Two large series have been published that describe lack of INI1 nuclear staining as a marker for AT/RT:
  i Judkins *et al.* reviewed 53 pediatric CNS tumors. Twenty-five tumors had a microscopic diagnosis of AT/RT. Nineteen of the AT/RT had *INI-1* mutations, and one had lack of *INI-1* RNA expression. All of these tumors had lack of INI-1 nuclear staining. Five of the microscopic AT/RTs were re-classified as PNET due to a lack of *INI-1* mutation, and the presence of INI-1 nuclear positivity on immunohistochemistry [107]. Four of these five lacked the robust EMA staining typical of AT/RT. Of the 53 tumors, only two had negative nuclear staining for INI-1 without a diagnosis of AT/RT, one was a recurrent ependymoma (which on re-biopsy showed characteristic rhabdoid cells) and the other was an oligodendroglioma [107].
  ii Haberler *et al.* reviewed a larger series of 289 pediatric CNS tumors. All 17 tumors microscopically diagnosed as AT/RT lacked INI-1 nuclear staining. Six medulloblastomas and two PNET microscopically had negative INI-1 nuclear staining. These eight cases were re-reviewed and found to harbour no rhaboid cells. However, six of eight were positive for EMA [108]. In two of the eight post-mortem analysis of the tumor tissue found small focal areas of rhabdoid tumor cells, underscoring the importance of INI-1 nuclear staining in AT/RT diagnosis.

Clinical presentation

Signs and symptoms are dictated by both tumor location and age at presentation. Posterior fossa tumors often present with symptoms of hydrocephalus. Therefore vomiting, lethargy, irritability, headache, and macrocephaly (in infants) are common presenting features. Other signs and symptoms include cranial nerve palsies, ataxia, hemiplegia, reversal of motor milestones and head tilt. Supratentorial lesions may present with seizure, focal cortical neurological symptoms, and regression of previously attained milestones [90, 109]. Given the aggressive nature of AT/RT the duration of symptoms are relatively short prior to diagnosis.

Imaging characteristics

There are no distinguishing features on radiographic imaging that specifically distinguish AT/RT from other fourth ventricular tumors such as medulloblastoma (MB), ependymoma, choroid plexus carcinoma and cerebellar astrocytoma (Figure 6.4). Similarly to MB, the solid portions of AT/RT are predominantly hyperdense on CT, due to the tumor's high cellularity [109, 110]. The lesions commonly contain cysts, hemorrhagic foci (in contrast to MB), and flecks of calcium [94, 110–112]. There is heterogeneous contrast enhancement on CT. AT/RT are usually isointense on T1-W with foci of hyperintensity corresponding to areas of hemorrhage or cysts [110, 111, 113-117]. T2 images show heterogeneous areas within the tumor bed reflecting cystic and hemorrhagic areas. Administration of gadolinium results in heterogeneous enhancement and may reveal leptomeningeal spread, although a minority of AT/RT will homogenously enhance or not enhance at all [110]. In fact, 20–30% of imaging studies show leptomeningeal spread at initial imaging studies [90, 110, 117, 118]. Unlike AT/RT, cerebellar astrocytomas tend to have cystic lesions with an enhancing mural nodule with no evidence of leptomeningeal spread. In contrast to AT/RT, ependymomas can be seen to extend through fourth ventricular outlets (Magendie and Luschka). Unlike MB, supratentorial PNETs often show areas of hemorrhage and calcification making the differential diagnosis more difficult.

Treatment and outcome studies

Three major series have reported outcomes of AT/RT. Given the close similarity between AT/RT and other tumor types that can display very different prognoses, it is important to consider the diagnostic tools used when assessing the validity of studies of the clinical outcome of AT/RT.

The landmark paper defining AT/RT by Rorke *et al.* included 52 infants and children with microscopically diagnosed AT/RT.
1 Diagnosis:
  • Fluorescence *in-situ* hybridization (FISH) was performed on 15 cases, nine of which showed abnormalities of chromosome 22.
  • INI-1 nuclear staining was not yet described at the time of publication [90].
2 Chemotherapy:
  • Thirty-nine children received chemotherapy by a variety of protocols (baby POG, augment baby POG, high dose chemotherapy with stem cell rescue). Six had a documented 50% reduction in tumor mass. Ten children were treated with chemotherapy after relapse: none had an objective response to treatment.

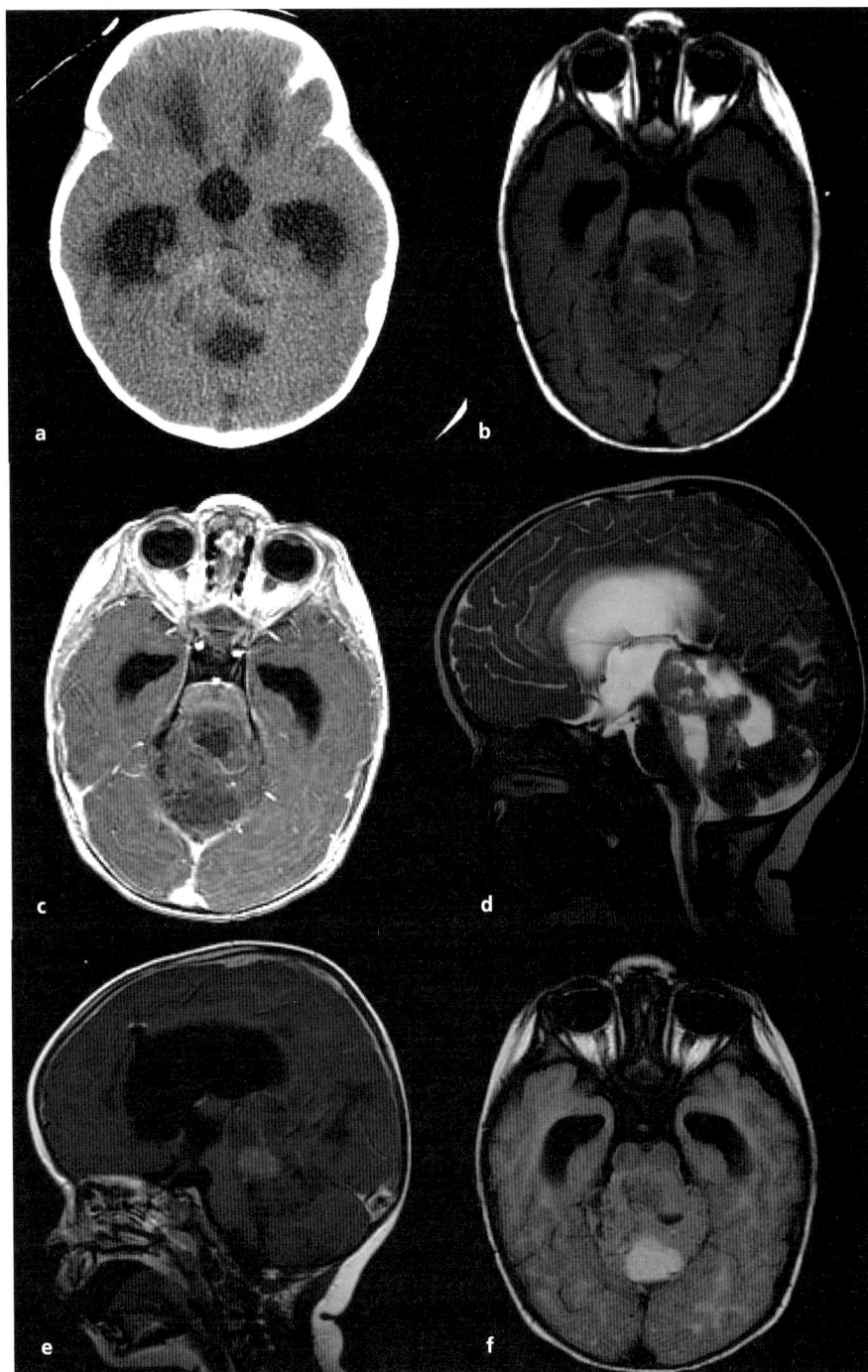

Figure 6.4 Radiographic appearance of atypical teratoid rhabdoid tumor. (a), Non–contrast CT showing fourth ventricular mass causing hydrocephalus. (b, c, e), Axial and sagittal T1 without and with gadolinium showing heterogenous mass with some enhancement invading the brainstem. (d), Sagittal T2 imaging showing the partially cystic nature of the lesion. f, FLAIR MRI sequence.

3 The median overall survival was 6 months.

The second case series was published in 2004 and presented 43 patients with AT/RT from a central registry in Cleveland [117].

1 Diagnosis:
  • Seventy-five percent of patients had a deletion of chromosome at 22q.

• Twenty-two tumors underwent gene sequence analysis: eight had no identifiable mutation. However, two of these patients harbored 22q deletions.
  • INI-1 staining was not performed.

2 Surgery:
  • Twenty patients had gross total resection. The median survival and event-free progression were 20 and 14 months

respectively. Of the 22 children receiving partial resection or biopsy, median survival and event-free progression was 15 months and 9.25 months, respectively. Ten of the 14 long-term survivors had gross total resection [117].

3 Chemotherapy:
• Forty-two patients received various chemotherapy regimes (in general combinations of cisplatin, etoposide, cyclophosphamide, and vincristine) including intrathecal chemotherapy (*n*=13) and high dose chemotherapy with stem cell rescue (*n*=16). Of the 22 patients assessable for response to chemotherapy (i.e. residual disease after surgery), 18 showed complete or partial response with a variety of protocols [117]. Of the 14 long-term survivors, six had surgery and chemotherapy alone without radiation [117]. Four of the six had high dose chemotherapy with stem cell rescue and one had intrathecal chemotherapy [117].

4 The median overall survival was 16.5 months [117].

The most recent case series was from St Jude Children's Research Hospital and includes 31 patients with AT/RT [118].

1 Diagnosis:
• Seventy-six percent of patients had deletion of chromosome 22q by FISH.
• Neither mutational analysis, nor INI-1 nuclear staining was performed.

2 Surgery:
• Extent of resection correlated positively with outcome.

3 Chemotherapy:
• Twenty-two children under 3 years of age were treated with various forms of intense chemotherapy (differing combinations of vincristine, cisplatin, cyclophosphamide, and carboplatin).
• Eighteen developed recurrent disease and succumbed to their disease despite.
• No change in median survival with rescue chemotherapy (3.6 months) or radiation (4.8 months) alone.
• Children receiving a salvage treatment of combined radiation and chemotherapy died with a median survival of 7.2 months.
• Of four survivors, one died of complications of surgery unrelated to disease, two are long-term survivors (both received radiation), and one received chemotherapy alone and was free of disease 10 months out [118].
• Of children >3 years of age (*n*=9), treated with the SJMB96 protocol including radiation (*n*=7), ICE only (*n*=1), and surgery only (*n*=1), four had relapse of disease [118]. Two of these relapses received no up-front radiation. Of the four relapses, three survived using a salvage treatment of chemotherapy and radiation.

4 Radiation:
• The addition of radiation therapy to AT/RT treatment regimes has probably done the most to increase long-term survivors.
• Of the 10 long-term survivors in the St Jude study (eight in the >3 years old group and two in <3 years old group) all but one received up-front radiation therapy [118].

5 Two-year overall survival was 78% for children >3 years old, and 11% for children aged <3 years [118].

Conclusion

AT/RT is an aggressive CNS tumor that presents a therapeutic challenge to clinicians. Long-term survivors are possible with a combination of surgery, intense chemotherapy and irradiation. However, the impact of treatment on quality of life is high.

References

1 Kaatsch P, Rickert CH, Kühl J, Schüz J, Michaelis J. Population-based epidemiologic data on brain tumors in German children. Cancer 2001; 92: 3155–64.
2 Rickert CH, Paulus W. Epidemiology of central nervous system tumors in childhood and adolescence based on the new WHO classification. Childs Nerv Syst 2001; 17: 503–11.
3 Miller DC. Pathology of craniopharyngiomas: clinical import of pathological findings. Pediatr Neurosurg 1994; 21(Suppl 1): 11–7.
4 Prabhu VC, Brown HG. The pathogenesis of craniopharyngiomas. Childs Nerv Syst 2005; 21: 622–7.
5 Sainte-Rose C, Puget S, Wray A, et al. Craniopharyngioma: the pendulum of surgical management. Childs Nerv Syst 2005; 21: 691–5.
6 Albright AL, Hadjipanayis CG, Lunsford LD, Kondziolka D, Pollack IF, Adelson PD. Individualized treatment of pediatric craniopharyngiomas. Childs Nerv Syst 2005; 21: 649–54.
7 Hoffman HJ, De Silva M, Humphreys RP, Drake JM, Smith ML, Blaser SI Aggressive surgical management of craniopharyngiomas in children. J Neurosurg 1992; 76: 47–52.
8 Fitz CR, Wortzman G, Harwood-Nash DC, Holgate RC, Barry JF, Boldt DW. Computed tomography in craniopharyngiomas. Radiology 1978; 127: 687–91.
9 Curran JG, O'Connor E. Imaging of craniopharyngioma. Childs Nerv Syst 2005; 21: 635–9.
10 Osborne A, Blaser S, Salzman K. Diagnostic Imaging: Brain. Osborne A (Ed.) AMIRSYS, 2004: 1050.
11 Ahmadi J, Destian S, Apuzzo ML, Segall HD, Zee CS. Cystic fluid in craniopharyngiomas: MR imaging and quantitative analysis. Radiology 1992; 182: 783–5.
12 Tsai EC, Santoreneos S, Rutka JT. Tumors of the skull base in children: review of tumor types and management strategies. Neurosurg Focus 2002; 12: e1.
13 Ohmori K, Collins J, Fukushima T. Craniopharyngiomas in children. Pediatr Neurosurg 2007; 43: 265–78.
14 Van Effenterre R, Boch AL. Craniopharyngioma in adults and children: a study of 122 surgical cases. J Neurosurg 2002; 97: 3–11.
15 Thompson D, Phipps K, Hayward R. Craniopharyngioma in childhood: our evidence-based approach to management. Childs Nerv Syst 2005; 21: 660–8.
16 de Vile CJ, Grant DB, Hayward RD, Kendall BE, Neville BG, Stanhope R. Obesity in childhood craniopharyngioma: relation to post-operative hypothalamic damage shown by magnetic resonance imaging. J Clin Endocrinol Metab 1996; 81: 2734–7.
17 Kang JK, Song JU. Results of the management of craniopharyngioma in children. An endocrinological approach to the treatment. Childs Nerv Syst 1988; 4: 135–8.

18 Sands SA, Milner JS, Goldberg J, et al. Quality of life and behavioral follow-up study of pediatric survivors of craniopharyngioma. J Neurosurg 2005; 103 (Suppl 4): 302–11.

19 Pierre-Kahn A, Recassens C, Pinto G, et al. Social and psycho-intellectual outcome following radical removal of craniopharyngiomas in childhood. A prospective series. Childs Nerv Syst 2005; 21: 817–24.

20 Zuccaro G. Radical resection of craniopharyngioma. Childs Nerv Syst 2005; 21: 679–90.

21 Caldarelli M, Massimi L, Tamburrini G, Cappa M, Di Rocco C. Long-term results of the surgical treatment of craniopharyngioma: the experience at the Policlinico Gemelli, Catholic University, Rome. Childs Nerv Syst 2005; 21: 747–57.

22 Puget S, Garnett M, Wray A, Grill J, et al. Pediatric craniopharyngiomas: classification and treatment according to the degree of hypothalamic involvement. J Neurosurg 2007; 106(Suppl 1): 3–12.

23 DeVile CJ, Grant DB, Hayward RD, Stanhope R Growth and endocrine sequelae of craniopharyngioma. Arch Dis Child 1996; 75: 108–14.

24 Hetelekidis S, Barnes PD, Tao ML, et al. 20-year experience in childhood craniopharyngioma. Int J Radiat Oncol Biol Phys 1993; 27: 189–95.

25 Villani RM, Tomei G, Bello L, et al. Long-term results of treatment for craniopharyngioma in children. Childs Nerv Syst 1997; 13: 397–405.

26 Yasargil MG, Curcic M, Kis M, Siegenthaler G, Teddy PJ, Roth P. Total removal of craniopharyngiomas. Approaches and long-term results in 144 patients. J Neurosurg 1990; 73: 3–11.

27 Rajan B, Ashley S, Gorman C, et al. Craniopharyngioma – a long-term results following limited surgery and radiotherapy. Radiother Oncol 1993; 26: 1–10.

28 Stripp DC, Maity A, Janss AJ, et al. Surgery with or without radiation therapy in the management of craniopharyngiomas in children and young adults. Int J Radiat Oncol Biol Phys 2004; 58: 714–20.

29 Kalapurakal JA. Radiation therapy in the management of pediatric craniopharyngiomas – a review. Childs Nerv Syst 2005; 21: 808–16.

30 Cavazzuti V, Fischer EG, Welch K, Belli JA, Winston KR. Neurological and psychophysiological sequelae following different treatments of craniopharyngioma in children. J Neurosurg 1983; 59: 409–17.

31 Merchant TE, Kiehna EN, Sanford RA, et al. Craniopharyngioma: the St Jude Children's Research Hospital experience 1984–2001. Int J Radiat Oncol Biol Phys 2002; 53: 533–42.

32 Flickinger JC, Lunsford LD, Singer J, Cano ER, Deutsch M. Megavoltage external beam irradiation of craniopharyngiomas: analysis of tumor control and morbidity. Int J Radiat Oncol Biol Phys 1990; 19: 117–22.

33 Chung WY, Pan DH, Shiau CY, Guo WY, Wang LW. Gamma knife radiosurgery for craniopharyngiomas. J Neurosurg 2000; 93 (Suppl 3): 47–56.

34 Chiou SM, Lunsford LD, Niranjan A, Kondziolka D, Flickinger JC. Stereotactic radiosurgery of residual or recurrent craniopharyngioma, after surgery, with or without radiation therapy. Neuro Oncol 2001; 3: 159–66.

35 Amendola BE, Wolf A, Coy SR, Amendola MA. Role of radiosurgery in craniopharyngiomas: a preliminary report. Med Pediatr Oncol 2003; 41: 123–7.

36 Habrand JL, Ganry O, Couanet D et al. The role of radiation therapy in the management of craniopharyngioma: a 25-year experience and review of the literature. Int J Radiat Oncol Biol Phys 1999; 44: 255–63.

37 Waga S, Handa H. Radiation-induced meningioma: with review of literature. Surg Neurol 1976; 5: 215–9.

38 Ushio Y, Arita N, Yoshimine T, Nagatani M, Mogami H. Glioblastoma after radiotherapy for craniopharyngioma: case report. Neurosurgery 1987; 21: 33–8.

39 Sogg RL, Donaldson SS, Yorke CH, Malignant astrocytoma following radiotherapy of a craniopharyngoima. Case report. J Neurosurg 1978; 48: 622–7.

40 Kitanaka C, Shitara N, Nakagomi T, et al. Postradiation astrocytoma. Report of two cases. J Neurosurg 1989; 70: 469–74.

41 Caceres A. Intracavitary therapeutic options in the management of cystic craniopharyngioma. Childs Nerv Syst 2005; 21: 705–18.

42 Schefter JK, Allen G, Cmelak AJ, et al. The utility of external beam radiation and intracystic 32P radiation in the treatment of craniopharyngiomas. J Neurooncol 2002; 56: 69–78.

43 Takeuchi K. A clinical trial of intravenous bleomycin in the treatment of brain tumors. Int J Clin Pharmacol Biopharm 1975; 12: 419–26.

44 Broggi G, Franzini A, Cajola L, Pluchino F. Cell kinetic investigations in craniopharyngioma: preliminary results and considerations. Pediatr Neurosurg 1994; 21(Suppl 1): 21–3.

45 Jiang R, Liu Z, Zhu C. Preliminary exploration of the clinical effect of bleomycin on craniopharyngiomas. Stereotact Funct Neurosurg 2002; 78: 84–94.

46 Mottolese C, Stan H, Hermier M, et al. Intracystic chemotherapy with bleomycin in the treatment of craniopharyngiomas. Childs Nerv Syst 2001; 17: 724–30.

47 Morantz RA, Kimler BF, Vats TS, Henderson SD. Bleomycin and brain tumors. A review. J Neurooncol 1983; 1: 249–55.

48 Haisa T, Ueki K, Yoshida S. Toxic effects of bleomycin on the hypothalamus following its administration into a cystic craniopharyngioma. Br J Neurosurg 1994; 8: 747–50.

49 Broggi G, Franzini A. Bleomycin for cystic craniopharyngioma. J Neurosurg 1996; 84: 1080–1.

50 Lafay-Cousin L, Bartels U, Raybaud C, et al. Neuroradiological findings of bleomycin leakage in cystic craniopharyngioma. Report of three cases. J Neurosurg 2007; 107(Suppl 4): 318–23.

51 Jakacki RI, Cohen BH, Jamison C, et al. Phase II evaluation of interferon-alpha-2a for progressive or recurrent craniopharyngiomas. J Neurosurg 2000; 92: 255–60.

52 Cavalheiro S, Dastoli PA, Silva NS, Toledo S, Lederman H, da Silva MC. Use of interferon alpha in intratumoral chemotherapy for cystic craniopharyngioma. Childs Nerv Syst 2005; 21: 719–24.

53 Ierardi DF, Fernandes MJ, Silva IR, et al. Apoptosis in alpha interferon (IFN-alpha) intratumoral chemotherapy for cystic craniopharyngiomas. Childs Nerv Syst 2007; 23: 1041–6.

54 Kobayashi T, Kageyama N, Ohara K. Internal irradiation for cystic craniopharyngioma. J Neurosurg 1981; 55: 896–903.

55 Strauss L, Sturm V, Georgi P, et al. Radioisotope therapy of cystic craniopharyngomas. Int J Radiat Oncol Biol Phys 1982; 8: 1581–5.

56 Julow J, Lányi F, Hajda M, et al. The radiotherapy of cystic craniopharyngioma with intracystic installation of 90Y silicate colloid. Acta Neurochir (Wien) 1985; 74: 94–9.

57 Guevara JA, Bunge HJ, Heinrich JJ, Weller G, Villasante A, Chinela AB. Cystic craniopharyngioma treated by 90-yttrium silicate colloid. Acta Neurochir Suppl (Wien) 1988; 42: 109–12.

58 Backlund EO. Colloidal radioisotopes as part of a multi-modality treatment of craniopharyngiomas. J Neurosurg Sci 1989; 33: 95–7.

59 Blackburn TP, Doughty D, Plowman PN. Stereotactic intracavitary therapy of recurrent cystic craniopharyngioma by instillation of 90-yttrium. Br J Neurosurg 1999; 13: 359–65.

60 Hasegawa T, Kondziolka D, Hadjipanayis CG, Lunsford LD. Management of cystic craniopharyngiomas with phosphorus-32 intracavitary irradiation. Neurosurgery 2004; 54: 813–20; discussion 820–2.

61 Blumcke I, Giencke K, Wardelmann E, et al. The CD34 epitope is expressed in neoplastic and malformative lesions associated with chronic, focal epilepsies. Acta Neuropathol 1999; 97: 481–90.

62 Blumcke I, Löbach M, Wolf HK, Wiestler OD. Evidence for developmental precursor lesions in epilepsy-associated glioneuronal tumors. Microsc Res Tech 1999; 46: 53–8.

63 Prayson RA, Estes ML Dysembryoplastic neuroepithelial tumor. Am J Clin Pathol 1992; 97: 398–401.

64 Prayson RA, Estes ML, Morris HH. Co-exsistence of neoplasia and cortical dysplasia in patients presenting with seizures. Epilepsia 1993; 34: 609–15.

65 Luyken C, Blümcke I, Fimmers R, Urbach H, Wiestler OD, Schramm J. Supratentorial gangliogliomas: histopathologic grading and tumor recurrence in 184 patients with a median follow-up of 8 years. Cancer 2004; 101: 146–55.

66 Luyken C, Blümcke I, Fimmers R, et al. The spectrum of long-term epilepsy-associated tumors: long-term seizure and tumor outcome and neurosurgical aspects. Epilepsia 2003; 44: 822–30.

67 Koeller KK, Henry JM. From the archives of the AFIP: superficial gliomas: radiologic-pathologic correlation. Armed Forces Institute of Pathology. Radiographics 2001; 21: 1533–56.

68 Morris HH, Matkovic Z, Estes ML, et al. Ganglioglioma and intractable epilepsy: clinical and neurophysiologic features and predictors of outcome after surgery. Epilepsia 1998; 39: 307–13.

69 Selch MT, Goy BW, Lee SP, et al. Gangliogliomas: experience with 34 patients and review of the literature. Am J Clin Oncol 1998; 21: 557–64.

70 Tamburrini G, Colosimo C Jr, Giangaspero F, Riccardi R, Di Rocco C. Desmoplastic infantile ganglioglioma. Childs Nerv Syst 2003; 19: 292–7.

71 Lonnrot K, Terho M, Kähärä V, Haapasalo H, Helén P. Desmoplastic infantile ganglioglioma: novel aspects in clinical presentation and genetics. Surg Neurol 2007; 68: 304–8; discussion 308.

72 Kuchelmeister K, Bergmann M, von Wild K, Hochreuther D, Busch G, Gullotta F. Desmoplastic ganglioglioma: report of two non-infantile cases. Acta Neuropathol 1993; 85: 199–204.

73 Onguru O, Celasun B, Gunhan O. Desmoplastic non-infantile ganglioglioma. Neuropathology 2005; 25: 150–2.

74 Marti A, Almostarchid B, Maher M, Saidi A. Desmoplastic non-infantile ganglioglioma. Case report. J Neurosurg Sci 2000; 44: 150–4.

75 VandenBerg SR, May EE, Rubinstein LJ, et al. Desmoplastic supratentorial neuroepithelial tumors of infancy with divergent differentiation potential ('desmoplastic infantile gangliogliomas'). Report on 11 cases of a distinctive embryonal tumor with favorable prognosis. J Neurosurg 1987; 66: 58–71.

76 Duffner PK, Burger PC, Cohen ME, et al. Desmoplastic infantile gangliogliomas: an approach to therapy. Neurosurgery 1994; 34: 583–9; discussion 589.

77 Daumas-Duport C, Scheithauer BW, Chodkiewicz JP, Laws ER Jr, Vedrenne C. Dysembryoplastic neuroepithelial tumor: a surgically curable tumor of young patients with intractable partial seizures. Report of thirty-nine cases. Neurosurgery 1988; 23: 545–56.

78 Raybaud C, Shroff M, Rutka JT, Chuang SH. Imaging surgical epilepsy in children. Childs Nerv Syst 2006; 22: 786–809.

79 Hammond RR, Duggal N, Woulfe JM, Girvin JP. Malignant transformation of a dysembryoplastic neuroepithelial tumor. Case report. J Neurosurg 2000; 92: 722–5.

80 Stanescu Cosson R, Varlet P, Beuvon F, et al. Dysembryoplastic neuroepithelial tumors: CT, MR findings and imaging follow-up: A study of 53 cases. J Neuroradiol 2001; 28: 230–40.

81 Chan CH, Bittar RG, Davis GA, Kalnins RM, Fabinyi GC. Long-term seizure outcome following surgery for dysembryoplastic neuroepithelial tumor. J Neurosurg 2006; 104: 62–9.

82 Fernandez C, Girard N, Paz Paredes A, Bouvier-Labit C, Lena G, Figarella-Branger D. The usefulness of MR imaging in the diagnosis of dysembryoplastic neuroepithelial tumor in children: a study of 14 cases. Am J Neuroradiol 2003; 24: 829–34.

83 Kirkpatrick PJ, Honavar M, Janota I, Polkey CE. Control of temporal lobe epilepsy following en bloc resection of low-grade tumors. J Neurosurg 1993; 78: 19–25.

84 Nolan MA, Sakuta R, Chuang N, et al. Dysembryoplastic neuroepithelial tumors in childhood: long-term outcome and prognostic features. Neurology 2004; 62: 2270–6.

85 Lee DY, Chung CK, Hwang YS, et al. Dysembryoplastic neuroepithelial tumor: radiological findings (including PET, SPECT, and MRS) and surgical strategy. J Neurooncol 2000; 47: 167–74.

86 Kameyama S, Fukuda M, Tomikawa M, et al. Surgical strategy and outcomes for epileptic patients with focal cortical dysplasia or dysembryoplastic neuroepithelial tumor. Epilepsia 2001; 42(Suppl 6): 37–41.

87 Beckwith JB, Palmer NF. Histopathology and prognosis of Wilms' tumors: results from the First National Wilms' Tumor Study. Cancer 1978; 41: 1937–48.

88 Biggs PJ, Garen PD, Powers JM, Garvin AJ. Malignant rhabdoid tumor of the central nervous system. Hum Pathol 1987; 18: 332–7.

89 Rorke LB, Packer R, Biegel J. Central nervous system atypical teratoid/rhabdoid tumors of infancy and childhood. J Neurooncol 1995; 24: 21–8.

90 Rorke LB, Packer RJ, Biegel JA. Central nervous system atypical teratoid/rhabdoid tumors of infancy and childhood: definition of an entity. J Neurosurg 1996; 85: 56–65.

91 Burger PC, Yu IT, Tihan T, et al. Atypical teratoid/rhabdoid tumor of the central nervous system: a highly malignant tumor of infancy and childhood frequently mistaken for medulloblastoma: a Pediatric Oncology Group study. Am J Surg Pathol 1998; 22: 1083–92.

92 Howlett DC, King AP, Jarosz JM, et al. Imaging and pathological features of primary malignant rhabdoid tumors of the brain and spine. Neuroradiology 1997; 39: 719–23.

93 Rosemberg S, Menezes Y, Sousa MR, Plese P, Ciquini O. Primary malignant rhabdoid tumor of the spinal dura. Clin Neuropathol 1994; 13: 221–4.

94 Bambakidis NC, Robinson S, Cohen M, Cohen AR. Atypical teratoid/rhabdoid tumors of the central nervous system: clinical, radiographic and pathologic features. Pediatr Neurosurg 2002; 37: 64–70.

95 Tamiya T, Nakashima H, Ono Y, et al. Spinal atypical teratoid/rhabdoid tumor in an infant. Pediatr Neurosurg 2000; 32: 145–9.

96 Cheng YC, Lirng JF, Chang FC, et al. Neuroradiological findings in atypical teratoid/rhabdoid tumor of the central nervous system. Acta Radiol 2005; 46: 89–96.

97 Rorke LB, Biegel JA. Atypical teratoid/rhabdoid tumor. In. Kleihues P, Cavenee WK (Eds), World Health Organization Classification of Tumors. Pathology and Genetics Tumors of the Nervous System. Lyon: IARC Press, 2000: 145–8.

98 Biegel JA, Rorke LB, Packer RJ, Emanuel BS. Monosomy 22 in rhabdoid or atypical tumors of the brain. J Neurosurg 1990; 73: 710–4.

99 Versteege I, Sévenet N, Lange J, et al. Truncating mutations of hSNF5/INI1 in aggressive paediatric cancer. Nature 1998; 394: 203–6.

100 Bazett-Jones DP, Côté J, Landel CC, Peterson CL, Workman JL. The SWI/SNF complex creates loop domains in DNA and polynucleosome arrays and can disrupt DNA–histone contacts within these domains. Mol Cell Biol 1999; 19: 1470–8.

101 Biegel JA. Molecular genetics of atypical teratoid/rhabdoid tumor. Neurosurgical Focus 2006; 20: E11.

102 Janson K, Nedzi LA, David O, et al. Predisposition to atypical teratoid/rhabdoid tumor due to an inherited INI1 mutation. Pediatr Blood Cancer 2006; 47: 279–84.

103 Taylor MD, Gokgoz N, Andrulis IL, Mainprize TG, Drake JM, Rutka JT. Familial posterior fossa brain tumors of infancy secondary to germline mutation of the hSNF5 gene. Am J Hum Genet 2000; 66: 1403–6.

104 Guidi CJ, Sands AT, Zambrowicz BP, et al. Disruption of Ini1 leads to peri-implantation lethality and tumorigenesis in mice. Mol Cell Biol 2001; 21: 3598–603.

105 Roberts CW, Leroux MM, Fleming MD, Orkin SH. Highly penetrant, rapid tumorigenesis through conditional inversion of the tumor suppressor gene Snf5. Cancer Cell 2002; 2: 415–25.

106 Imbalzano AN, Jones SN. Snf5 tumor suppressor couples chromatin remodeling, checkpoint control, and chromosomal stability. Cancer Cell 2005; 7: 294–5.

107 Judkins AR, Mauger J, Ht A, Rorke LB, Biegel JA. Immunohistochemical analysis of hSNF5/INI1 in pediatric CNS neoplasms. Am J Surg Pathol 2004; 28: 644–50.

108 Haberler C, Laggner U, Slavc I, et al. Immunohistochemical analysis of INI1 protein in malignant pediatric CNS tumors: lack of INI1 in atypical teratoid/rhabdoid tumors and in a fraction of primitive neuroectodermal tumors without rhabdoid phenotype. Am J Surg Pathol 2006; 30: 1462–8.

109 Parmar H, Hawkins C, Bouffet E, Rutka J, Shroff M. Imaging findings in primary intracranial atypical teratoid/rhabdoid tumors. Pediatr Radiol 2006; 36: 126–32.

110 Meyers SP, , Khademian ZP, Biegel JA, Chuang SH, Korones DN, Zimmerman RA. Primary intracranial atypical teratoid/rhabdoid tumors of infancy and childhood: MRI features and patient outcomes. Am J Neuroradiol 2006; 27: 962–71.

111 Arslanoglu A, Aygun N, Tekhtani D, et al. Imaging findings of CNS atypical teratoid/rhabdoid tumors. Am J Neuroradiol 2004; 25: 476–80.

112 Evans A, Ganatra R, Morris SJ. Imaging features of primary malignant rhabdoid tumor of the brain. Pediatr Radiol 2001; 31: 631–3.

113 Fenton LZ, Foreman NK. Atypical teratoid/rhabdoid tumor of the central nervous system in children: an atypical series and review. Pediatr Radiol 2003; 33: 554–8.

114 Martinez-Lage JF, Nieto A, Sola J, Domingo R, Costa TR, Poza M. Primary malignant rhabdoid tumor of the cerebellum. Childs Nerv Syst 1997; 13: 418–21.

115 Caldemeyer KS, Smith RR, Azzarelli B, Boaz JC. Primary central nervous system malignant rhabdoid tumor: CT and MR appearance simulates a primitive neuroectodermal tumor. Pediatr Neurosurg 1994; 21: 232–6.

116 Hanna SL, Langston JW, Parham DM, Douglass EC. Primary malignant rhabdoid tumor of the brain: clinical, imaging, and pathologic findings. Am J Neuroradiol 1993; 14: 107–15.

117 Hilden JM, Meerbaum S, Burger P, et al. Central nervous system atypical teratoid/rhabdoid tumor: results of therapy in children enrolled in a registry. J Clin Oncol 2004: 2877–84.

118 Tekautz TM, Fuller CE, Blaney S, et al. Atypical teratoid/rhabdoid tumors (ATRT): improved survival in children 3 years of age and older with radiation therapy and high-dose alkylator-based chemotherapy. J Clin Oncol 2005; 23: 1491–9.

II Hematological Disorders

7 Acute Lymphoblastic Leukemia

Robert F. Wynn

Blood and Bone Marrow Transplant Unit, Royal Manchester Children's Hospital, Manchester, UK

Introduction

Acute lymphoblastic leukemia (ALL) is the commonest leukemia of childhood. It accounts for 30% of new cases of childhood cancer in the USA and Western Europe and in absolute numbers about 2000 cases per annum in the USA and about 400 cases per annum in the UK or France.

The story of ALL is the story of childhood cancer. It is the story of improving treatment success through clinical trial. It is the story of childhood cancer epidemiology and pathogenesis. With increasing treatment success in ALL it is also the story of treatment refinement so that treatment intensity reflects disease risk. The numbers of patients with ALL have allowed focus on the costs of treatment success in terms of late effects to be set against the risk factors that can be identified for failure of treatment.

Our job as clinicians in the management of childhood cancer is this juggling of risk. Childhood ALL is a fatal disease without treatment. Our treatment also carries risk – both short-term morbidity and mortality during treatment and long-term morbidities. As clinicians we must neither inadequately treat the disease and risk treatment failure, nor over treat the disease and risk unnecessary toxicity. Understanding the disease through careful scientific study and well designed clinical trials over 40 years have allowed us to make these risk-based decisions and explain them, during treatment consent, to patients and their families.

In this chapter we will discuss first the pathology of ALL and its classification. Its epidemiology and pathogenesis will be reviewed before a discussion of the clinical features of ALL and its treatment, with a focus on risk-based therapy.

Epidemiology of acute lymphoblastic leukemia

Incidence

ALL is the commonest malignancy of childhood and accounts for 85% of childhood leukemias. Its incidence in the UK is 30 per

Pediatric Hematology and Oncology, 1st edition. Edited by Edward J. Estlin, Richard J. Gilbertson, and Robert F. Wynn. © 2010 Blackwell Publishing Ltd.

million children per year [1]. It has a peak incidence between the ages of 2 and 5 years and is commoner in white than black children. Its incidence is greater in developed than developing countries [2]. It is unclear whether it is becoming commoner with time as there are conflicting studies, but it is not thought that in developed countries there is much significant change [3–5].

Etiology

For any individual child the cause of leukemia is seldom apparent and is little more than an interesting question to family and clinician. For that child and his family this leukemia will represent a desperately unlucky chance and will not represent something that they as a family have done wrong or that is more likely to affect other children.

However the etiology of ALL is a research field in its own right and, on a population level, it is possible to make some statements about the origins of this leukemia.

Many cases of leukemia will have their clonal origin during fetal life. This is especially true of the ALL of early life, including the peak incidence leukemias of early childhood. This can be shown by:
• The increased concordance rate of leukemia in monozygotic as compared with dizygotic twins. It can be shown that this increased concordance rate is a consequence of twin to twin leukemia metastasis through a shared circulation [6].
• Backtracking leukemia specific genotypic change to a blood sample (usually the Guthrie card) taken in early life. Using the polymerase chain reaction (PCR) the leukemia-specific DNA (e.g. a leukemia specific translocation such as TEL-AML) can be found in this neonatal sample and long before the clinical presentation of leukemia [7].

The clinical relevance of this is that twins and especially monozygotic siblings of an index case diagnosed early in life should be regarded at high risk of leukemia and screened as such after discussion and consent.

Various possible causes of leukemia have been described.

Infection

In certain animal leukemias it is clear that there is a direct relationship between virus infection, usually with retrovirus, and leukemogenesis [8]. There is no such direct viral cause of leuke-mia in children. Epstein-Barr virus (EBV) is strongly associated with endemic Burkitt's lymphoma /leukemia but the molecular biology of this disease – c-myc translocation to the immunoglob-ulin gene – is the same as sporadic forms demonstrating that the virus has a facilitating effect rather than a causative effect [9].

However, the peak incidence of ALL strongly suggests an infectious etiology. This is not directly causal. Several other lines of evidence (international comparison, geographical clusters, inverse correlation with breast feeding, decreasing incidence with birth order) suggest that ALL is a rare response to a common infection and delayed exposure to the agent is critical to this aber-rant response. Population mixing may bring this agent into a susceptible community and some individuals are more prone genetically to such a response as shown by an association with HLA type [10, 11].

Genetic causes

Few cases of ALL have an association with a genetic syndrome. Down's syndrome (DS), Bloom syndrome, ataxia telangiectasia (AT) [12, 13] and neurofibromatosis (NF1)[14] all have an increased incidence of ALL compared with the general popula-tion [15]. In DS and NF1 the increased leukemia incidence is reduced for ALL compared with myeloid leukemia. A search for AT with genetics and measurement of serum alpha-fetoprotein should be undertaken in any individual with cerebellar ataxia and ALL, however mild the former might be. As discussed above there may be inherited differences that influence response to infection and that therein influence leukemia risk.

Physical causes

Undoubtedly, exposure to ionizing radiation is a cause of ALL. This will include pre-natal exposure during maternal X-rays [16] and there was an increase in the incidence of ALL following the nuclear bombs dropped in World War 2. However, there has been no detectable increase in ALL following the nuclear acci-dents and fallout at Chernobyl and Three Mile Island [17]. Similarly, there has been no increase in ALL close to nuclear plants that cannot be explained by other factors such as popula-tion mixing. It is unlikely that low energy electro-magnetic fields produced by electricity supply pylons will cause ALL as it does not damage DNA in the laboratory, although it has been a matter of considerable public debate [18].

Chemical and pesticide exposure

Exposure to certain chemicals and pesticides has been asso-ciated with leukemia but not usually ALL. The suggestion that parenteral vitamin K administration to neonates leads to an increased incidence of ALL has been disproved with further study [19].

Pathology of acute lymphoblastic leukemia

These are neoplasms of lymphoblasts committed to either B-cell lineage or T-cell lineage. Our understanding of leukemia is that it is a clonal disease and originates by mutation in a single cell and that the remainder of leukemia cells within the clone are derived from this one cell.

About 80–85% of ALL in childhood is of B-lineage. Several levels of classification are attempted as scientific techniques have advanced. Thus ALL can be classified according to clinical fea-tures, blast cell morphology, cytochemistry, immunophenotype, cytogenetics and molecular genetics.

In employing any classification system in ALL there are two questions to be answered:
• Am I certain that this is ALL and can treatment be instituted?
• Does this classification of ALL tell me anything about the risk that this leukemia poses the patient? This is the era of risk-based therapy and only at the beginning of therapy can a complete clas-sification of the clinical and biological features of the presenting leukemia be made (Table 7.1).

Table 7.1 Modalities of classification of acute lymphoblastic leukaemia (ALL).

Classification mode	Question	Aid definitive diagnosis?	Risk stratification?
Clinical	What are the presenting features of this leukemia?	No	Yes
Blast cell morphology	Do the blast cells appear as typical lymphoblasts using standard haematological stains? (FAB classification)	Yes	No
Cytochemistry	Do the blast cells lack cytochemical evidence of myeloid lineage commitment (MPO) and / or show the typical cytochemical properties of lymphoblasts (B or T-lineage) with PAS or AP stains.	Yes	No
Immunophenotype	Does the leukemia cell possess the membrane antigens that are present in normal precursor B and T-cells?	Yes	No
Cytogenetics	What are the chromosomal changes associated with the clone and are these recognized findings in ALL?	Yes	Yes
Molecular Genetics	Is there clonal immunoglobulin gene rearrangement (B-lineage ALL) or is there clonal T-cell receptor rearrangement (T-cell ALL)? Are there fusion genes that are described in ALL?	Yes	Yes

Morphology

For all our sophisticated immunophenotype tools and cellular and molecular genetics ALL is still diagnosed firstly by light microscopy of a bone marrow smear taken from a child with a suggestive history and abnormal peripheral blood cell counts. Diagnostic immunophenotyping should only be performed on a morphologically abnormal marrow or mistakes will be made.

The FAB classification is a morphological sub-classification of ALL. It describes three types of ALL – L1, L2 and L3 [20].
• In L1 disease the blast cells are small, uniform with a high nuclear/cytoplasmic (N/C) ratio, inconspicuous nucleoli and variable cytoplasmic vacuolation.
• In L2 disease there is pleomorphism with larger and more variable blasts, with variable cytoplasmic volume and vacuolation. Nucleoli may be multiple and prominent.
• In L3 ALL the blasts are large and uniform. There is moderate intensely basophilic cytoplasm with prominent vacuolation. There are multiple, prominent nucleoli.
Only the recognition of L3 leukemia has any modern relevance to diagnosis or relevance to therapy. As in acute promyelocytic leukemia (APML) a molecular change – in this case translocation of the c-myc oncogene to the transcriptionally active heavy or light chain regions of the immunoglobulin gene – defines a disease with typical clinical features, morphology, immunophenotype, cyto- and molecular genetics that responds poorly to standard leukemia therapy.

Otherwise morphology alone does not distinguish T- and B-lineage ALL and does not distinguish lymphoblastic leukemia from certain myeloid leukemias where there is little maturation of the abnormal clone (FAB AML M0 and M1).

Cytochemistry

The principle of cytochemistry is that an apparently primitive and microscopically bland blast cell will show lineage commitment in its enzymes. The principle importance in ALL is that ALL blasts do not have myeloperoxidase and are therefore Sudan Black negative and distinguishable from most cases of AML. ALL blasts of T- and B-lineage may be positive for periodic acid Schiff (PAS) stain, often in a characteristic block pattern and T-lineage leukemia may be positive in a characteristic polar pattern for acid phosphatase (AP) [20].

Immunophenotyping

Immunophenotyping is the cornerstone of modern leukemia diagnosis [21]. Just as cytochemistry assigns lineage commitment to an undifferentiated cell by its enzymatic capability, so immunophenotyping classifies leukemia by the membrane and cytoplasmic antigens it shares with cells of a certain lineage. In B-lineage leukemia there are therefore B-lineage antigens and in T-lineage leukemia there are T-lineage antigens. These antigens are specific to the lineage and not to the leukemia.

During normal B-cell or T-cell ontogeny or development there is serial and characteristic gain and loss of specified antigens. Thus the developmental stage of a B-lineage cell from uncommit-

ted stem cell to antibody producing plasma cell can be defined by its pattern of antigen expression. Leukemia may arise as a clonal disease from cells of different developmental stages and the antigen expression of the subsequent malignant clone reflects the antigen expression of the developmental stage at which malignancy arose.

Usually immunophenotypic analysis consists of two stages [22]:
• In the first instance a broad panel of antibodies is employed. Such a panel includes antibodies directed at common T-lineage, B-lineage and myeloid – including monocytic and erythroid – antigens. This will enable a broad immunophenotypic classification of leukemia to be made – in conjunction with morphology and cytochemistry.
• A second panel of more lineage specific antibodies will enable a more exact diagnosis and sub-classification of leukemia to be made. In the case of precursor B and precursor T lymphoblastic leukemias this second panel of antibodies will allow classification according to the normal cell ontogeny (Tables 7.2 and 7.3).
It should be noted that several different classifications of B-lineage ALL can be attempted. In the modern treatment era the importance of immunophenotyping is to make a certain diagnosis of precursor B-lineage leukemia and to make a certain diagnosis of B-cell leukemia as this has important treatment implications. The sub-classification of precursor B disease has little impact on prognosis compared with other criteria of risk stratification and little

Table 7.2 An immunophenotypic classification of acute lymphoblastic leukaemia (ALL).

Leukemia	Immunophenotype/ common antigens	Discriminatory antigens	Leukemia frequency
Early pre-B, CD10–	CD19, CD22, CD79a	TdT+, CD10–	8
Early Pre-B, CD10+	CD19, CD22, CD79a	TdT+, CD10+, Surface μ–	70
Late pre-B	CD19, CD22, CD79a	cytoplasmic μ+, SIgμ–, CD10+/–,	18
Mature B	CD19, CD22, CD79a	TdT–, CD10+/–, SIgμ+	4

Table 7.3 An immunophenotypic sub-classification of T-acute lymphoblastic leukaemia (ALL).

Leukemia	Immunophenotype/ common antigens	Discriminatory antigens
Pro-T	cyCD3, CD7	TdT+
Pre-T	cyCD3, CD7	TdT+, CD5+/–
Cortical T	cyCD3, CD7	TdT+, CD1a+, CD5+, CD4/8+/–
Mature T	cyCD3, CD7	TdT–, sCD3+, CD5+, CD4 or CD8+

sleep should be lost by the practising clinician in making such an exact diagnosis. Indeed the WHO classification of acute B-cell neoplasms is into precursor-B leukemia/lymphoma and Burkitt leukemia/lymphoma and further sub-grouping is based on cytogenetic abnormalities [21].

A similar sub-classification of T-cell ALL can be attempted where the leukemia immunophenotype reflects the stage of T-cell ontogeny in which malignant change has arisen. As in sub-classifications of B lineage ALL there is limited relevance to the treating clinician and the WHO classification does not attempt any classification beyond this, even with cytogenetics. The frequency of T-ALL is about 12% of all ALL.

Aberrant antigen expression is not uncommon in ALL and refers to the expression of antigens that are not associated with that leukemia's lineage. Aberrant antigens do not influence the diagnosis where there are immunological, cytogenetic and molecular features of a strong commitment to ALL. Over half of ALL cases will express some aberrant myeloid marker – usually CD13, 33 or 15. In these cases blasts are myeloperoxidase (MPO) negative and have the other typical immunophenotypic features of B-ALL (CD19, CD22 and CD79a positive) or T-ALL (CD7 and cyCD3). Such aberrant antigen expression does not appear to independently influence outcome after treatment. Myeloid antigen aberrant expression is common in infant ALL with the t(4;11) translocation which is associated itself with a poor prognosis.

Where there are co-expression of MPO and these typical ALL markers then this is a true bi-phenotypic leukemia. Mixed T-ALL and B-ALL leukemias are also described. Gene rearrangement and expression may help accurately classify these leukemias which pose otherwise a therapeutic difficulty for the clinician. Rarely there are two clear populations of blast cells expressing different antigens – this is termed bi-lineage leukemia.

Cytogenetics

Cytogenetics is the study of cellular chromosomal re-arrangements associated with leukemia and may find typical rearrangements that both confirm the diagnosis and aid prognosis and therefore therapy [23]. There are two techniques:
• Conventional cytogenetics. This remains the standard screening for karyotypic abnormalities in newly diagnosed leukemia. It will pick up abnormalities only in dividing cells (metaphase).
• 'Molecular cytogenetics'. In fluorescent *in situ* hybridization (FISH) a probe that is specific for normal (e.g. for a specific chromosome) or abnormal (e.g. for a particular translocation) part of the genome is applied to the cell that need not necessarily be dividing. It cannot be readily be used as a screen as it can only determine whether a particular probe binds or not, but it is useful for monitoring known abnormalities as in disease response monitoring.

Two patterns of cytogenetic alteration are described – alterations of chromosome number and structural abnormalities. Both can confer prognostic information.

Alterations of chromosome number
ALL can be classified into five types according to the number of chromosomes:

1 Hyperdiploidy (>50 chromosomes). This is a common finding and as many as 30% of ALL cases have a chromosome number between 51 and 68. Such hyperdiploidy, especially where the chromosome number is 51 to 55 chromosomes, is associated with other good risk features and an improved cure rate. Rarely there may be near tetraploid or, more rarely still near triploid karyotype. These do not appear in more recent analysis to have adverse outcome [24, 25]. The pattern of chromosome gain in hyperdiploidy is not random and the commonest chromosome gained is chromosome 21 and chromosomes 6, X and 14 are also commonly gained. Hyperdiploidy can also be detected by flow cytometry – expressed as DNA index, and this may sometimes be more sensitive than conventional cytogenetics [26].
2 Low hyperdiploidy (47–50 chromosomes). This does not confer such a good prognosis as higher hyperdiploidy but the prognosis is not adverse [27]. Where only chromosome 21 is gained then the prognosis is good [28] and where chromosome 8 is gained it is usually associated with T-cell disease and the prognostic significance is uncertain [29].
3 Pseudodiploidy. In this group, although there are 46 chromosomes, there are structural or numeric abnormalities. This is a heterogenous group therefore whose outcome with therapy will reflect the specific abnormality within the apparent normal chromosome number.
4 Diploidy. In this group there is apparent normal chromosome number and structure. About 10–15% of ALL are in this group. It may be commoner in T-cell ALL [30]. This group will contain children with cryptic translocations, e.g. t(12;21) in B-ALL and t(5;14) in T-ALL which will themselves confer prognostic significance.
5 Hypodiploidy and near haploidy. In this there are a reduced number of chromosomes. Where there is near haploid karyotype there is a poor prognosis even where there are relatively good presenting National Cancer Institute (NCI) features [23].

Structural chromosome changes
The commoner structural abnormalities in ALL , their lineage specificity and prognostic significance are given in Table 7.4 [23, 31].

Molecular genetics
Molecular genetics is the application of molecular biological techniques to determine the genes involved in ALL. Such techniques include analysis of the clonal origin of T and B leukemias and the acquired genetic origin of these illnesses [31].

B-cells and T-cells generate the antibody and T-cell receptor diversity necessary for an adaptive immune system by rearranging the germ line variable (V), diversity (D) and junctional (J) regions of the IG/TCR gene complexes. Each developing lymphocyte therefore obtains a specific VDJ combination and diversity is

Table 7.4 The commoner structural chromosome abnormalities in acute lymphoblastic leukemia (ALL).

Structural chromosome change	Lineage specificity	Genes	Frequency (%)	Prognostic significance
(1; 19)	B	E2A-PBX1	5	Adverse*
t(17; 19)	B	E2A-HLF	1	Adverse
t(4; 11)	B	MLL-AF4	5% (higher in infants)	Adverse
11q23 trans, inv, deletion	Usually B	Variable		Adverse, except deletion or inversion – these are neutral
t(9; 22)	B	BCR-ABL	<5	Adverse
t(12; 21)	B	TEL-AML	25	Good
Tan dup (21)	B	AML1 amplification	2	Adverse
Del (6q)	Non-specific	Unknown	10	Neutral
10q24, various partners	T	HOX11	0.5	Good
19p13, various partners	T	LYL1	1.5	Adverse
1p32	T	TAL1	6	Adverse
8q24	True B-cell	c-myc over expression	2	Good†

*This adverse treatment outcome can be overcome with intensive therapy. † Prognosis is good with short-term intensive chemotherapy.

further generated by nucleotide insertion and deletion during the VDJ coupling. As ALL is a clonal disorder arising from a developing lymphoid cell this unique DNA – specific to that developing cell – will act as a DNA 'fingerprint' for all its progeny. There are two implications in terms of leukemia diagnosis and risk stratification:

1 The presence of clonal TCR or IG gene rearrangement may aid diagnosis in difficult cases of leukemia such as biphenotypic or bilineage leukemias [32].

2 The unique DNA may be used as a target for monitoring the disappearance of the leukemia clone during therapy [33]. Thus primers for junctional regions are matched to either side of the junctions, generally within a distance of less than 500bp. Usually consensus primers will be used that recognize virtually all V or J gene segments – germ line DNA will not be amplified because of the long distance between these regions in unrecombined DNA. The PCR product – specific to the leukemia clone – can then be sequenced and patient specific (or allele specific) primers can be designed for the further monitoring of that leukemia clone during therapy. This is the basis of minimal residual disease (MRD) monitoring during ALL therapy and is strongly predictive of treatment outcome.

The structural chromosomal alterations usually disrupt genes that encode transcription factors. Leukemia specific translocations can activate transcription factors either by generating new fusion genes with oncogenic properties or by translocating those transcription factors to transcriptionally active portions of the genome – those coding for IG or the TCR. The importance to the clinician is twofold:

1 The chimeric gene is unique DNA and specific, within that patient, to the leukemic clone and can be monitored either by PCR or by FISH as analysis of MRD in the same way as the IG/TCR gene rearrangement [33].

2 The action of the fusion oncoprotein or the translocated transcription factor will enable us to better understand the molecular etiology of the leukemia and may in future allow the leukemia to be targeted more specifically [34]. In an analogous fashion the BCR-ABL fusion oncogene is specifically targeted in chronic myeloid leukemia (CML) and ALL by tyrosine kinase inhibitors such as imatinib [35].

Clinical presentation of acute lymphoblastic leukemia

Typical presentation and plan of investigation

In most cases the diagnosis of ALL is not difficult to make once there is sufficient clinical suspicion to merit investigation with blood tests. Leukemic blast infiltrate leads to marrow failure and the typical symptoms and signs of anemia, thrombocytopenia and leucopenia. There is frequently bone pain and fever. On physical examination there is frequently generalized lymphadenopathy and hepato-splenomegaly. The illness usually arises in a previously well child as there are few predisposing conditions (see Etiology).

In this typical case all institutions will have a standard series of investigations so that all information about the leukemia that might be conceivably useful can be gathered. Once therapy is initiated then the leukemia will soon be gone to sight and this opportunity will be lost. Most institutions will do these and any subsequent invasive bone marrows and lumbar punctures under general anesthetic or deep sedation. A comprehensive, clinical assessment of the fitness for such procedures should form part of the initial assessment of the child. Several points should be noted:
• In certain circumstances, e.g. large mediastinal mass (see below) causing respiratory compromise or superior vena cava

obstruction then it may not be possible to safely anesthetize or sedate. In these circumstances then as much as possible must be done without anesthetic. Where there are circulating blast cells then diagnosis may be made and samples taken for MRD and cytogenetic tests using the peripheral blood alone. Treatment may then be initiated and invasive procedures requiring anesthesia or sedation deferred until anesthetic or sedation is safe. The safety of the patient must not be compromised for the sake of the completeness of the diagnosis. This is sometimes a more critical issue in T-cell non-Hodgkin's lymphoma (NHL) where there is no circulating disease but a large mediastinal mass. Steroid therapy may be given in these circumstances to shrink the presenting tumor which is making anesthetic unsafe. Often over a matter of days this mass will shrink and the anesthetic will be perfectly safe. The child will require daily assessment by an experienced pediatric anesthetist to identify the window in which both anesthesia is safe and the tumor mass is not completely resolved.

• Tumor storage will require consent that is additional to the consent for the anesthesia and investigations.

• It is clearly appropriate to do as many investigations under the same anesthetic. It is our practice to give intrathecal chemotherapy at the time of first investigations where there are unequivocally circulating peripheral blood blasts. This saves the child returning for a second procedure (therapeutic lumbar puncture) once a diagnosis is made on a first marrow and means that intrathecal chemotherapy is always given with lumbar puncture and there is reduced risk of contamination of the CSF leading to later central nervous system (CNS) relapse through traumatic puncture (see CNS disease, below) [36].

Other presentations of acute lymphoblastic luekemia

Other organs might be involved. The commonest site of involvement is clearly the lymph nodes, liver, and spleen. Involvement of these organs may be in a patient with typical features as above or be the site of presenting symptoms and signs.

Central nervous system leukemia

Involvement of the CNS is more common in ALL than in other types of leukemia. It is more commonly a site of relapsed disease than presenting disease. It is commoner in T-cell disease, true B-cell leukemia and where the circulating white cell count is high. Its presentation may be on routine lumbar puncture or there may be symptoms and signs of disease including headache, vomiting, papilloedema or cranial nerve palsies and abnormal eye movements (cranial nerves III, IV or VI) or facial asymmetry (VII).

Diagnosis of CNS disease is on microscopic examination of a CSF cytospin in which the total white cell concentration has been counted. Three patterns of CSF are recognized:

1 CNS-1. No blast cells in the cytospin. There may be other cells present – often in considerable numbers either with infection or as a reaction to continuing intrathecal therapy. The frequent pres-

ence of other cells underlines the importance of experience in making this diagnosis of CNS involvement. Immunophenotyping of CSF can be helpful in difficult cases – where there is limited material the range of markers employed might be limited and will be guided by the immunophenotype of the patient's leukemia. TdT is useful in this circumstance in precursor B and T lymphoblastic leukemias.

2 CNS-2. There are unequivocally blasts in the CSF but their number is less than 5×106/litre.

3 CNS-3. There are unequivocally blasts and their number is greater than 5×106/litre.

Occasionally the pattern of disease is predominantly parenchymal. The presenting features are related to mass effect, neurological deficit, or seizures. Such pattern of involvement is more usually seen at relapse and parenchymal involvement is thought to be a later event in CNS invasion than meningeal involvement (which leads to CSF positivity). Epidural deposit of leukemia with spinal cord compression with a leukemic deposit is a rare presentation of ALL requiring urgent institution of appropriate therapy, including steroid therapy.

The management of CNS leukemias is separately discussed (below).

Hypoplastic presentation of acute lymphlastic leukemia

Rarely the diagnosis of ALL is preceded by an aplastic phase. This occurs in about 1–2% of these leukemias and the pathophysiology of this process is unclear. Characteristically there is fever with pancytopenia followed by restoration of normal counts and good health prior, within 6 months, to a diagnosis of overt leukemia. Uncommonly, there is no recovery of the peripheral blood counts but usually in these cases there might be marrow fibrosis and foci of blasts expressing TdT and (usually) CD10 [37].

Testicular disease

Testicular disease is rarely overtly present at diagnosis in boys, although it is commonly present at a sub-clinical level – as was demonstrated by studies of testicular biopsy at diagnosis of leukemia of boys without clinically apparent disease and is not associated with an adverse outlook [38]. Overt testicular disease was formerly a not uncommon site of relapse but the frequency of such relapse has diminished as protocol intensity has increased [39].

Mediastinal mass

This is usually a manifestation of T-cell leukemia although it is described to occur in precursor B disease rarely. It may be asymptomatic and simply noted on a posterior-anterior chest x-ray that is routinely done on all children presenting with leukemia at the time of initial investigations. It may present, however, as respiratory compromise or as a superior vena cava obstruction. In these circumstances, management of the presenting emergency is the physician's priority and investigations may be deferred whilst this is brought rapidly under control.

Bone and joint disease

Bone pain is common. In some children – usually with precursor B lymphoblastic disease, and often with a relatively normal blood count – bone pain may be the dominant finding leading to presentation to orthopedic or rheumatology teams and diagnostic difficulty and delay. In addition to these features there may be characteristic X-ray changes including transverse metaphyseal radiolucent lines, osteolytic lesions, diffuse osteoporosis and fracture [40]. No specific orthopedic intervention is necessary in these circumstances – simply management of the underlying leukemia.

Ocular disease

The incidence of eye involvement will depend on the intensity of the search [41]. Overt involvement is only commonly seen at relapse, and then more commonly in association with CNS disease. Like testicular disease contemporary treatment protocols have reduced the incidence of relapse in this site.

Treatment of acute lymphoblastic leukemia

Historical aspects

ALL treatment has proceeded from palliation to curative over the last 60 years. The majority of patients presenting with ALL can now expect to be cured of their disease [42]. The obstacles to successful treatment that have been progressively overcome have been:

• A lack of belief that anything other than transient responses and palliation of leukemia could be achieved with drug and radiation therapy.

• The lack of effective drugs capable of inducing response. Drugs that individually had some action in inducing response of the leukemia have been developed. The earliest drugs that had action were aminopterin (an early methotexate-like folate antagonist), corticosteroids, and the purine antagonists, 6MP and thioguanine.

• Primary and acquired resistance to applied anti-leukemia drug therapy. The use of multi-agent drug schedules that form the backbone of ALL therapy today were first employed in order to overcome such acquired resistance where children responded and achieved remission but later relapsed. Separate multi-agent schedules are employed in remission induction, consolidation and continuing therapy.

• CNS relapse leading to treatment failure even where there had been a medullary response. The development of strategies to prevent CNS relapse was initially achieved with prophylactic irradiation and subsequently with intrathecal administration of chemotherapy.

• The lack of a framework in which to test newer drugs and schedules. The concept of the randomized clinical trial in which new drugs, or different scheduling of the same drug, e.g. methotrexate or different combinations of drugs has allowed leukemia therapy to progressively and incrementally improve. These recent

incremental steps of the large cooperative oncology groups studying ALL therapy are discussed in more detail below.

Principles of treatment

ALL treatment is toxic and an important component of therapy is supportive care. Improvements in outcome are partly due to improvements in supportive care. Supportive care components are discussed separately in this book but any such care will require:

• Knowledge of the likely adverse effects of any applied therapy so that primary preventative therapy (prophylaxis) can be given.

• Early detection of problems so that therapy can be given early in the course of any complication.

• Effective drugs for the complications of the disease.

ALL treatment is risk directed. The risk of treatment failure in ALL is influenced by clinical factors and the National Cancer Institute has developed a uniform classification based on age at presentation and presenting white blood cell count [43]. Biological features of the leukemia including cytogenetics and molecular genetics will further inform this risk assessment and a treatment schedule will be selected. However, this risk assessment will be inaccurate and some children with apparently good disease by NCI criteria and disease biology will relapse during or after appropriate therapy. Conversely, some children with apparently poor risk disease by these criteria will apparently be cured with such treatment. One reason for the incomplete relation between applied therapy outcome and pre-treatment risk assessment is the individual response to drug treatment. Risk assessment can be improved by assessment of the disease response to therapy which will be influenced by pharmacodynamic and pharmacogenetic factors [44] – this response may be assessed crudely by morphological assessment of blast disappearance or using more sophisticated and quantitative measures of disease disappearance (flow cytometric or PCR molecular). This mode of disease assessment is summarized in Figure 7.1 and Box 7.1.

Results of cooperative studies in acute lymphoblastic leukemia treatment

There are several large collaborative consortia that have performed randomized trials in the therapy of childhood ALL. These trials have sometimes asked not dissimilar questions. Progress has been incremental, with each successive national trial testing the proposed improved treatment strategy against previous best (standard) therapy. The results of different national trial groups is summarized in Table 7.5 and in the succeeding section the accepted components of ALL therapy – remission induction, consolidation, re-induction and continuing therapy, and the drugs used in these components are discussed.

Components of acute lymphoblastic leukemia therapy

There is probably more randomized clinical trial information concerning the treatment of ALL in children than any other human malignancy. Therapy of ALL continues along the lines established in the early days of therapy:

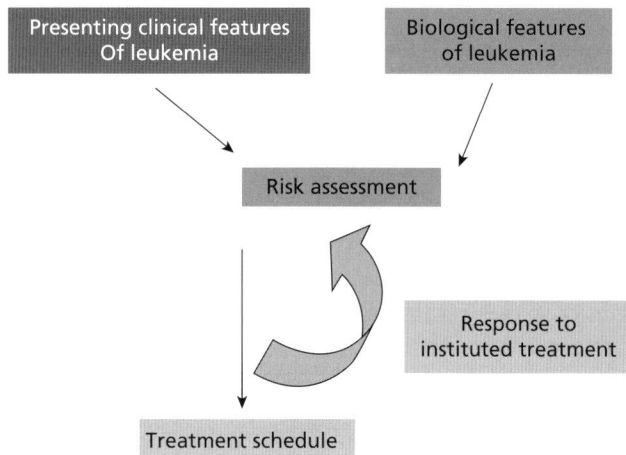

Figure 7.1 Determination of risk in acute lymphoblastic leukemia. Risk of treatment failure can be determined by clinical features of the patient and the leukemia, biological features of the leukemia, and the response of the disease to instituted therapy.

Box 7.1 Risk assessment in acute lymphoblastic leukemia (ALL) – what might change your treatment.

Consensus clinical criteria in ALL presenting outside infancy:

- High white blood cell count (>50)
- Age >10 years

Cytogenetics

- Philadelphia – some may be cured with chemotherapy alone but poor responders / with other risk criteria are usually transplanted
- MLL – some may be cured with chemotherpy alone, as Ph+ disease
- Near haploid karyotype – continuing dismal prognosis

Response to therapy

- Assessed by steroid response of peripheral blood blasts
- Assessed by repeat marrow aspirates during and at end of induction
- Assessed by MRD levels at end of induction chemotherapy and after consolidation therapy

---

- Remission induction therapy.
- Intensification/consolidation/re-induction therapy.
- CNS-directed therapy.
- Continuing/maintenance therapy.

Selected collaborative treatment group results are given in Table 7.5. This section will review these treatment phases and summarize the objectives of each phase, the consensus treatment and the evidence for that treatment.

Remission induction therapy
Definition and aim

This is the therapy that is given to a patient after a diagnosis is reached and once the patient's condition has been stabilized. Its aim is remission. Remission is defined as absence of detectable disease. The method of disease assessment needs to be defined in describing remission as different tools will have different sensitivities (Figure 7.2).

For any tool used, remission is defined as absence of detectable disease and residual disease is disease that remains present but undetected. This is a difficult concept for families. Leukemia cells are analogous to weeds in a flower bed and normal blood cells are the flowers in that flower bed. At presentation the gardener can only see weeds. After treatment there are only flowers to see but there might still be weeds within the flower bed that would grow back if treatment were stopped. The difference between cure and remission is that in cure there are no weeds left to grow back. MRD technology is a special test the gardener has developed for telling how many weeds are left behind even when he cannot see them.

The level of remission is not an academic issue. About 99% of children will be in remission at the end of remission induction therapy. Treatment failures will reflect a roughly equal mix of death due to toxicity and refractory disease. Patients with refractory disease have a dismal outcome with intensified therapy and transplant. With MRD, high level MRD (above 1%) have similarly dismal outcomes despite morphological remission [82].

MRD is currently estimated usually after induction (week 5) and after consolidation therapy (week 11). In current trials, high risk disease by MRD is defined as disease levels greater than 0.01% (10e-4) at week 5, and low risk disease as undetectable disease at week 11, having not been greater than 0.01% at week 5. Some disease is indeterminant by MRD, e.g. disease detectable but less than 0.01% at both time points. In the current UK trial the risk of subsequent relapse is about 5% in the high risk group and less than 0.5% in the low risk group. MRD is therefore a highly useful tool and it is hoped that treatment interventions based on MRD will improve overall survival – these interventions will usually be intensification of therapy in children with high risk disease and reduction of therapy in those with good risk disease as defined by MRD.

Drugs used

Remission induction therapy is a multiple drug regimen, following the earliest observation that multiple drug use has higher rates of remission induction that were translated into improved rates of overall survival. The leukemic clone is rapidly diminished so that drug resistant disease cannot emerge. Remission induction schedules in all current regimens will include both vincristine and steroids, and one or both of an anthracycline and L-asparaginase. In most cases, a three drug remission induction will be employed in standard risk disease. Four drugs will be reserved for those judged high risk by NCI criteria and for those with adverse geno-

Table 7.5 Key advances from collaborative group trials in the treatment of acute lymphoblastic anemia.

Study	Enrolment years	Event free survival	Lessons learned	References
AEIOP-91	1991–95	71	(1) Randomized exended Erwinia asparaginase did not improve response in intermediate risk ALL. (2) Multiple intensive blocks did not improve outcome in high risk ALL. (3) Intrathecal chemotherapy could replace cranial radiotherapy	[45–47]
AEIOP-95	1995–99	73	(1) Eight drug re-induction blocks (administered twice) improved outcome in high risk children (prednisolone poor response, t(9,22) or t(4; 11)) compared with the multiple intensive blocks of AEIOP-91. (2) Treatment reduction led to inferior results in good risk patients	[48–50]
BFM-90	1990–95	78	Continued improved outcome of ALL despite (1) reducing total anthracycline dose and (2) cranial radiotherapy dose	[51, 52]
BFM-95	1995–2000	79	(1) Vincristine and dexamethasone pulses do not add to therapy outcome in maintenance. (2) Increased relapse risk in CNS 2 (contaminated) LP	[53, 54]
MRC-UKALL XI	1990–1997	63	(1) No improvement in EFS and improved OS was due to better management of relapse. (2) Intensified treatment benefits all groups	[55–57]
MRC-ALL-97		81	(1) Benefit for dexamethasone as steroid in EFS and CNS relapse. (2) 6-MP is superior to 6-TG in maintenance therapy. (3) 6-TG in maintenance is associated with high incidence of liver disease	[58, 59]
POG	1986–1994	70.9 (B) and 51 (T)	(1) Intensive treatment blocks do not improve outcome in high risk ALL. (2) i.v. methotrexate is superior to oral in intensification. (3) i.v. mercaptopurine is not helpful to improving outcome. (4) NCI criteria did not predict outcome in T-cell disease which fared poorly	[60–63]
CCG-1800	1989–95	75	(1) Slow early responders have improved outcome with increased post-induction therapy. (2) Double delayed intensification improves outcome in intermediate risk ALL	[64–66]
CCG 1992	1993–1995	81	(1) Dexamethasone improves outcome in ALL and reduced CNS relapse in ALL. (2) ALL survival is not improved by i.v. 6-MP. (3) Triple intrathecal therapy does not improve outcome over IT methotrexate alone. (4) Any possible benefit in terms of disease control through use of 6-TG is offset by liver adverse effects	[67–69]
EORTC-58881	1989–98	71	(1) *E. Coli* asparaginase is superior (although more toxic) to Erwinia asparaginase. (2) Cytarabine added to methotrexate during continuing therapy does not improve outcome in ALL. (3) i.v. 6-MP is not helpful in improving EFS	[70–73]
NOPHO ALL92	1992–98	77	(1) High dose i.v. methotrexate can replace cranial irradiation. (2) 6-MP pharmacokinetics affects outcome including response and second malignancy	[74, 75]
SJCRH 13	1991–98	81	(1) i.v. 6-MP not helpful. (2) Additional early intrathecal therapy (triple) reduces CNS events	[44, 76–79]
TCCSG L92-13	1992–1995	63	Continuing therapy cannot be reduced despite earlier intensive therapy in standard risk but can be in high risk leukemia with good prednisolone response	[80, 81]

ALL, Acute lymphoblastic leukemia. LP, Lumbar puncture. EFS, Event free survival. OS, overall survival. CNS, Central nervous system. IV, Intravenous. NCI, National Cancer Institute. 6-MP, 6-mercaptopurine. 6-TG, 6-thioguanine.

type or who fail to respond appropriately to an instituted three drug regimen.

• Vincristine. This is administered on a weekly schedule. The usual dose is 1.5 mg/m^2/dose. Its toxicity is principally neuropathic. Excessive neurotoxicity is seen in hereditary sensorimotor neuropathies such as Charcot-Marie-Tooth disease, which might be revealed in family history and diagnosed genetically.

• Steroids. These are given by mouth. Several collaborative studies (Child's Cancer Group [CCG], Medical Research Council [MRC]) have addressed the question of which steroid should be used. There is evidence from these studies that use of dexametha-

sone has improved overall survival and reduced CNS relapse [58, 68]. It is unclear whether the dose of steroids is equipotent or whether the improved results seen with dexamethasone reflect simply higher glucocorticoid effect with the selected dose. There is increased toxicity with this dose of dexamethasone, which affects the bones with increased osteopenia, and causes behavioral disturbance, myopathy, and weight gain (both adding to the neuropathy of vincristine in reducing mobility of children during induction) [58].

• Asparaginase. Asparaginase cleaves asparagines into aspartic acid and ammonia. As asparagine is rate-limiting, it interrupts

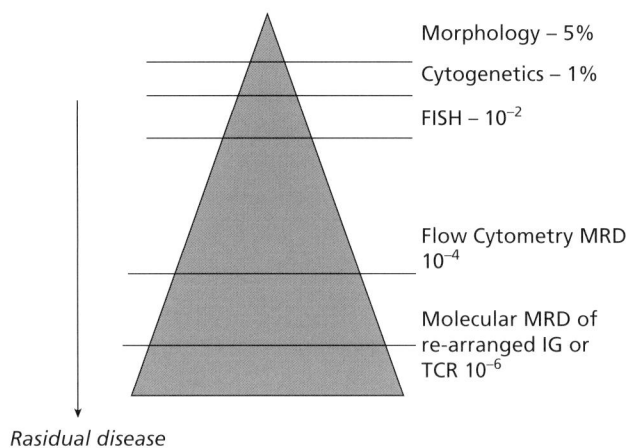

Morphology – 5%

Cytogenetics – 1%

FISH – 10^{-2}

Flow Cytometry MRD 10^{-4}

Molecular MRD of re-arranged IG or TCR 10^{-6}

Rasidual disease

Figure 7.2 The sensitivities of different methodologies in determining the level of residual disease in children with ALL.

protein synthesis. Asparaginase is an important drug in the treatment of ALL and children who are under-dosed for asparaginase have an inferior outcome to those that receive a more intensive treatment schedule. There are different preparations, with several products of different potency derived from *E. Coli* and a single commercial product of reduced potency derived from Erwinia. If the different half-lives (and there is a pegylated version of the Medac *E. Coli* asparaginase) and potencies of the different properties are taken into account in scheduling then comparable results will be achieved. Whilst its importance in ALL treatment is undoubted, the timing of administration in leukemia therapy is uncertain. It has considerable toxicity with thrombotic, infectious, and hepatic complications and these are especially evident in leukemia induction therapy. The Dana Faba cancer consortium has moved the administration of asparaginase into the post-induction period and demonstrated the importance of prolonged exposure whilst maintaining high remission induction rates [83, 84]. Therefore, the most appropriate timing of administration of the drug will remain the subject of further study.
• Anthracycline. The most extensively used anthracycline in ALL treatment has been daunorubicin. It is myelotoxic and significantly increases infection risk during induction therapy. It has a cumulative cardiac toxicity when doses above 400 mg/m² are used. It may not be necessary to use an intensive four drug remission induction therapy in standard risk cases where post-remission intensification therapy is being undertaken.

Intensification therapy
Definition and aim
In the early days of leukemia treatment, remission was maintained by prolonged continuing anti-metabolite (maintenance) therapy. Consolidation, intensification, and re-induction therapy is the therapy that follows achievement of morphological remission and that interrupts continuing therapy. The addition of such intensification blocks improves the outcome of all types of ALL, even those of lowest risk. The intensity should be sustained over

weeks rather than short blocks of chemotherapy, with a prolonged interruption in therapy thereafter as a consequence of bone marrow aplasia.

Drugs used
Different groups have evolved different schedules:
• Intensification therapy which is delivered following achievement of remission and is used principally in high risk leukemia. Usually cyclophosphamide, cytarabine and mercaptopurine are given which may be intensified further in those achieving remission more slowly by the addition of further agents including vincristine and asparaginase. This approach of augmented intensification has been shown in CCG trials to be beneficial in improving outcome in these high risk leukemias [64].
• Re-induction therapy in which the induction drugs are repeated 3 months after achieving remission and was pioneered by the Berlin-Frankfurt-Munster (BFM) group [39,51] or 'doubly' (repeated again at 32 weeks) which has been shown to improve outcome in higher risk disease [65].
• There are various other drugs used after induction that have been shown to be of benefit. The replacement of induction asparaginase with post-induction asparaginase was carried out by the Dana Faba group and shown to be beneficial [85] and asparaginase is an important component of the augmented delayed BFM consolidation therapy of CCG trials. Methotrexate after induction has been beneficial, especially in T-cell disease, where the blasts accumulate its active metabolites [51, 52].

Central nervous system prophylaxis
Definition and aim
This is therapy delivered specifically to the sanctuary site of the CNS. It is the story of leukemia therapy:
• CNS relapse was a huge problem in the early days, even where systemic leukemia control had been achieved, with as many as 50% of children suffering such relapse.
• Identification of a therapy that reduced such relapse – cranio-spinal irradiation.
• Identification of risk factors associated with CNS relapse (Box 7.2).
• Realization that radiation had long-term adverse sequelae on growth, neurocognitive function, and endocrine function.
• Gradual replacement of cranio-spinal irradiation with cranial irradiation and intrathecal therapy, then reduction of radiation

---

Box 7.2 Risk factors for central nervous system relapse.

High white blood cell count

T-cell immunophenotype

Traumatic lumbar puncture (LP) or CNS 2 LP at diagnosis

Adverse genotype – t(4; 11) or t(9; 22)

dose, and finally abolition of radiation with only intrathecal therapy and improved systemic therapy.

Drugs used

Effective prophylaxis of CNS relapse requires both effective systemic therapy and locally applied therapy. Local therapy is increasingly intrathecal therapy and there is equivalence of each treatment in meta-analysis of different trials [86]. Both St Jude's and MRC treatment protocols no longer give any CNS radiation therapy. Intrathecal therapy is either with single agent methotrexate or with triple agent therapy (methotrexate, hydrocortisone, and cytarabine). There is no proven benefit to triple therapy [67, 87].

Systemic therapy is better with dexamethasone, although this may reflect that those trials that have shown a beneficial dexamethasone effect did not select equivalent glucocorticoid efficacy in the prednisolone arm. Where a higher dose of prednisolone was used then no advantage of dexamethasone was demonstrated [88]. High dose methotrexate reduces systemic relapse rate but has little impact on CNS relapse. However, perhaps the effect is only at higher doses of methotrexate ($5 \, g/m^2$) [86].

Continuing (maintenance) therapy

Definition and aim

ALL is a unique malignancy in its requirement for a prolonged period of low dose but sustained and continuously delivered chemotherapy. Universally, it includes 6-mercaptopurine (6-MP) given daily and low dose methotrexate given weekly. This phase of treatment proceeds from achievement of completion of remission to completion of therapy but is interrupted for intensification or re-induction therapy. Children are relatively well during this phase of treatment and life can return to normal. However, children are significantly immune suppressed during this therapy and virus infection can be significant, even overwhelming. Particular problems are seen with parvovirus and prolonged red cell aplasia and transfusion may be needed.

Drugs used and duration

6-MP and methotrexate are the synergistic backbone of maintenance therapy. Methotrexate inhibits *de novo* purine synthesis and thereby enhances the conversion of mercaptopurine to its active metabolite thioguanine. In maintenance therapy:

• There is considerable variation in the individual patient's response to the administered drugs. In every day practice the dose of the drugs is adjusted so as to achieve myelosuppression, so that tolerant patients receive more of the drug. The effect on normal hematopoiesis is used as a surrogate for a presumed effect on malignant hematopoiesis. There is some evidence for the use of such a strategy, with children interrupting therapy for neutropenia faring better [89].

• Some children are deficient in the enzyme thiopurine-S-methyltransferase and these children show extreme sensitivity to 6-MP. Heterozygotes may show some sensitivity to the drug.

• The 6-MP is usually better given on an empty stomach and away from milk products. Methotrexate is as effective orally as parenterally [90].

• There is conflicting evidence about the benefit that the addition of pulses of vincristine and steroid beyond re-induction therapy brings and it is probably not very significant [91]. Such therapy brings continuing steroid toxicity.

• There is clear evidence that continuing therapy is necessary and despite the increased intensity of earlier therapy, and the evidence that such intensity is effective in improving cure rates, it has not been possible to reduce the duration of continuing therapy below 2 years. Some trials continue to offer increased therapy for boys (3 years), as opposed to 2 years for girls but there is little evidence for such a strategy and evidence that prolonging maintenance therapy beyond 3 years is not helpful [92, 93].

Treatment failure: predicting treatment failure and accounting for it

The factors associated with an increased risk of treatment failure are well described:

• Clinical factors encapsulated by the NCI consensus criteria.

• Disease-related factors, principally cytogenetic and molecular genetic factors.

There is considerable overlap between these assessment systems – thus genotypically favorable leukemias more typically have good clinical risk features. It is hoped that using gene expression profiles from an individual's leukemia might improve the sensitivity of risk determination by giving a molecular profile of the actual leukemia cells.

Some children with apparently good risk disease relapse and some children with apparently adverse leukemia are cured with standard chemotherapy. Assessment of leukemia disappearance using morphology or MRD is an attempt to take account of this variation in expected response. Some of this variation in response is due to inter-individual difference in drug metabolism. These pharmacogenomic differences mean that the drug dose delivered to leukemia cells is vastly different in some children than others and will explain why those drugs delivered in a formulaic fashion are sometimes more effective than expected and sometimes less so. Knowing these resistant mechanisms might mean that drug treatment can be more guided. Some of these differences are given in Table 7.6.

Special situations

Infant acute lymphoblastic leukemia

Features [110]

1 The cell from which ALL in infancy arises is a primitive cell in the early stage of commitment to the B lineage. As such:

• There is a high incidence of co-expressed myeloid antigens.

• It is frequently of a null phenotype with CD19+ and CD10–.

2 Eighty per cent of cases have MLL gene re-arrangement with the commonest translocation being t(4;11).

Table 7.6 Examples of inherited ('pharmacogenomic') differences in the handling of drugs used in the treatment of ALL that may be associated with differences in treatment outcome.

Drug	Metabolism	Pharmacogenomics
Methotrexate	(1) Entry into cell by folate carrier [94]. (2) Metabolism to methotrexate polyglutamates (MTXPG) by folylpolyglutamate synthetase (FPGS)[95]. (3) Hydrolysis and inactivation of MTXPG by gamma glutamyl hydrolase [96]	(1) Lower steady state concentrations during HD Mts infusion have increased risk of treatment failure [97, 98]. (2) Hyperdiploid blasts show higher levels of MTXPG [99]. (3) Increasing the dose of methotrexate overcomes this resistance in children whose blasts accumulate MTXPG less well [100]
Cytarabine	(1) Prodrug that is phosphorylated intracellularly into Ara-CTG [101, 102]. (2) Cellular uptake by membrane transporter (standard dose) or diffusion (high dose) [103, 104]	(1) Failure to retain intracellular AraCTP is commoner in relapsed compared with de novo ALL [105]. (2) Decreased activating enzyme as a means of resistance in ALL [106, 107]
6-MP	(1) Metabolized by HPRT to 6-TGNs. (2) Inactivated by TPMT [120]	(1) Accumulated intracellular TGN related to outcome [108, 109]. (2) Product of red cell MTXPG and TGN is predictive of outcome [109]. (3) Low TGN can discriminate compliance from pharmacological resistance

HPRT, hypoxanthine phosphoribosyl transferase. 6-TGN, 6-thioguanine nucleotides. TPMT, thiopurine methyl transferase.

3 Usually there are adverse clinical and genotypic risk factors and there is frequently a poor response to steroid induction chemotherapy.

4 Very young children do even worse.

Treatment

Because of the primitive nature of the leukemia, the co-expression of myeloid antigens, and because of the *in vitro* sensitivity to cytarabine, a recently reported protocol Interfant [99] attempted to improve treatment outcome with a protocol that included myeloid as well as lymphoid treatment elements, including cytarabine and high dose cytarabine [111]:

• This protocol reports an event-free survival (EFS) at 4 years of about 50%, which is an improvement on previous reports.

• MLL gene, high white blood cell count, younger than 6 months and poor steroid response were all independently associated with a poor outcome.

• CNS disease in infant leukemia is managed with intrathecal and systemic therapy only – radiotherapy is not employed in this age group.

Acute lymphoblastic leukemia in Down's syndrome

The incidence of ALL is increased in children with DS although the incidence of AML is increased even further, especially in young children. Usually there are no additional cytogenetic abnormalities in the ALL of DS, either favorable or adverse. Outcome is similar to children who do not have DS, in contrast to AML where a more favorable outcome is generally seen. Therefore, standard treatment protocols should be followed. Increased toxicity might be expected, especially with methotrexate administration [112].

Relapsed acute lymphoblastic leukemia

The salient features of relapsed ALL are summarized in the Box 7.3.

Many relapses will be predictable from adverse clinical or biological factors at diagnosis or from an observed slow response

---

Box 7.3 Relapsed acute lymphoblastic leukemia (ALL).

Affects about 15% of children in current leukemia protocols:

• May be systemic or extra-medullary

• CNS is commonest extra-medullary relapse

Prognosis depends on:

• Timing of relapse – earlier the worse

• Site of relapse – isolated CNS relapse of therapy will have prognosis as high as 70%

• Phenotype – T-cell will do worse

• Even extra-medullary relapse should be regarded as a manifestation of inadequately controlled systemic disease and requires systemic therapy as well as locally directed therapy

• The disease may show immunophenotypic, cytogenetic, or molecular clonal evolution compared with the original disease

---

to treatment. Relapse occurs most commonly in the first year after completing therapy and is uncommon, but not unheard of, 4 years after completing therapy. Relapse is managed as a systemic disease; even isolated extra-medullary disease is regarded as a failure of systemic therapy and a harbinger of systemic relapse [113].

Isolated, late CNS relapse has the best prognosis of relapse. As many as 70% of children will be cured with systemic therapy (including re-induction, consolidation and maintenance therapy for 24 months total therapy duration) and local radiotherapy [76].

For higher risk relapse (early, T-cell and where there has been a poor response to relapse therapy – as assessed molecularly), then allogeneic stem cell transplant will often form part of the relapse therapy. This is the major role for transplant in ALL although it may be offered to high risk leukemias in first remission. Usually transplant is applied in relapsed disease after remission re-induction therapy and consolidation therapy, and as continuing therapy would otherwise be starting. A chemotherapy approach alone may be adopted in lower risk cases – usually in non T-cell disease where there has been a prolonged first remission [114].

Transplant in acute lymphoblastic leukemia

Transplant is clearly effective in ALL and the following points can be made:

• It is a toxic therapy with appreciable short-term mortality risks and long-term morbidity risks (growth, infertility). Cases should be selected for transplant where it is unlikely that they will be cured by chemotherapy alone. Such cases may be in CR1, CR2 or >CR2. Different collaborative groups will have their own indications which are broadly similar – Children's Oncology Group (COG) indications are given (see Table 7.7).

• It should be a full intensity procedure with total tody irradiation (TBI) as part of the conditioning – usually with etoposide or cyclophosphamide.

• There is a clear relationship between burden of disease before transplant and relapse of disease after transplant. The higher the level of MRD then the greater the risk of relapse following transplant. Pre-transplant strategies should be directed therefore at monitoring and reducing the burden of disease prior to transplant.

• There is a reduced mortality risk for non-family donors, but this benefit is probably offset by increased transplant-related mortality.

Strategies for follow up and important late effects (Table 7.8)

Follow up, as in all pediatric oncology, has two purposes:

• To monitor disease response and detect relapse.
• To determine complications of applied treatment.

During therapy, patients are usually seen at least weekly during intensive phases of therapy and fortnightly during maintenance. Most children who will go on to relapse will do so in the first year of treatment. The remainder of relapses occurs usually by the end of the 4th year of treatment. During this period, marrow relapse can be detected by marrow examination, after abnormalities in the peripheral blood count have been detected. There is no need for serial bone marrow examinations. These may even be confusing as lymphoblasts (even CD10+ ones) may be seen in the marrow of normal children. CNS relapse will be diagnosed by examination of the CSF after suggestive symptoms are raised by the patient. Other extra-medullary relapses will be diagnosed on biopsy of the affected organ after suggestive history or findings on clinical examination.

With time, from completion of therapy, the focus of follow up will gradually change from detection of relapse to monitoring for adverse and long-term complications of therapy. A spectrum of complications will be seen in the long-term follow up clinic. The least complications will be in those treated on low intensity protocols and the most those that have received intensive therapy including allogeneic stem cell transplant and cranial or craniospinal radiation therapy.

Summary and future directions

The treatment of pediatric ALL is a success story and a story that the field of oncology is trying to replicate. It is not yet a finished story. Some children relapse. Children still die of ALL. Some children are cured but affected by the long-term consequences of

Table 7.7 Indications for stem cell transplant in acute lymphoblastic anemia.

Remission status	Indication
CR1	Alternative or sibling donors:
	• Ph+ patients requiring transplant
	• Extreme hypodiploidy (DNA index <0.81 or <44 chromosomes)
	• 11q23 (MLL) plus slow early response (>25% blasts at day 14 or MRD >0.1% at day 29)
	• Primary induction failure: overt disease at day 29 or <25% blasts or MRD >1% at day 29 who then fail consolidation with M2 or M3 marrow or MRD >1% at day 43
CR2	Matched sibling donor:
	• B-lineage after late bone marrow relapse (>36 months after diagnosis)
	• B-lineage ALL after early (<18 months from diagnosis) isolated extramedullary relapse
	Alternative or sibling donor:
	• B-lineage bone marrow relapse within 3 years of diagnosis
	• T-lineage bone relapse at any time
	• Ph+ positive marrow relapse at any time
	• T-lineage relapse isolated early extramedullary relapse)
CR3	Any lineage and at any time

MLL, Mixed Lineage Leukemia gene involvement. MRD, Minimal residual disease.

Table 7.8 Long-term effects of treatment of acute lymphoblastic leukemia.

Bone	(1) Reduced bone mineral density in survivors of childhood ALL, especially in those that have received cranial radiotherapy. It can occur but much less so in children treated with chemotherapy alone [115].
	(2) Avascular necrosis (AVN) can occur during therapy for ALL and is more common in older children, girls and those treated with dexamethasone. AVN may present after completion of therapy and will cause ongoing problems in many cases for the affected child [116].
CNS	Complicated field. Can see imaging abnormalities. Can see global (e.g. IQ) and specific change in performance. Might have impact on educational performance. Probably more common in children receiving radiation and therapy at an early age. Changes certainly seen with children receiving systemic therapy and intrathecal therapy only. Important is recognition assessment and support, including school support [117–119].
Cardiac	(1) The principle risk in chemotherapy protocols is related to anthracycline. The cumulative dose in non-relapse patients is $200–260\,mg/m^2$ and is below the threshold for risk of cardiac damage. However, some reduction in cardiac function is seen (especially young age at treatment, girls more than boys).
	(2) If there is reduction in cardiac function then this might be increased during pregnancy, with isometric exercise, and with cocaine/alcohol misuse.
	(3) Relapse treatment will give more anthracycline. TBI and cyclophosphamide will contribute to cardiac dysfunction after treatment.
Growth and pubertal development	(1) Cranial radiation is associated with significant effect on final height due to GH deficiency, abnormal including early puberty, hypothyroidism.
	(2) BMT with TBI causes significant effect on growth with irradiation of epiphyses of vertebral column and lower limbs and GH deficiency.
	(3) Probably little effect from chemotherapy only ALL schedules.
Pubertal development	(1) Cranial radiation for ALL causes early puberty. This is more marked in treated girls than boys.
	(2) Allogeneic transplant may cause ovarian failure and will be more marked with chemotherapy only conditioning (e.g. busulfan and cyclophosphamide). In girls who enter puberty after chemotherapy – TBI may subsequently experience premature menopause. Boys after TBI will retain hormonal function of testis.
	(3) Chemotherapy only schedules should not affect puberty.
Fertility	Will be markedly reduced or absent after stem cell transplant regardless of conditioning regimen. In children treated with chemotherapy fertility is preserved and there does not appear to be an effect on subsequent pregnancy or offspring.
Second malignancy	Second malignancy is NOT common – perhaps 5% at 10 years.
	CNS tumors, particularly meningiomas, are the commonest and cranial irradiation is the usual cause. Possible relation with genetic defects in thiopurine metabolism.
	Risk of AML is low unless etoposide used at regular scheduling and high dose.

ALL, Acute lymphoblastic leukemia. TBI, Total body irradiation. GH, Growth hormone. BMT, Bone marrow transplant. AML. Acute myeloid leukemia.

their treatment. Over the next 20 years of ALL therapy we would all wish to see fewer relapses and fewer long-term adverse consequences of therapy in cured children.

We contend that there are four areas where progress can be expected to take place in order to achieve these goals:

1 We need to be able to identify those children who are going to do well (better biological definitions of good risk with gene expression profiles, etc.) or who are doing well with therapy (MRD that has been shown to be reliable in allowing treatment reduction) so that good risk children receive even less treatment. No more children who are cured of their disease should die in delayed intensification blocks.

2 We need to be able to identify those who are going to do badly (better biological definitions of poor risk with gene expression profiles, etc.) or who are doing badly with therapy (MRD that has been shown to be reliable in predicting subsequent treatment failure) so that appropriate therapy can be offered in first response to children who will later fail that therapy.

3 We need to find better therapies for high risk disease including a better definition of the role and strategies of allogeneic stem cell transplant.

4 Basic scientific research into the mechanisms of leukemia needs to be translated into better and more specific drugs in the way that imatinib has transformed the therapy of CML. Rather the brown tablets taken twice a day than the intensive polychemotherapy and allogeneic stem cell transplant.

References

1 Gurney JG, Severson RK, Davis S, Robison LL. Incidence of cancer in children in the United States. Sex-, race-, and 1-year age-specific rates by histologic type. Cancer 1995; 75: 2186–95.

2 Ferlay J, Bray, F, Pisani, P, Parkin DM. GLOBOCAN 2000, Cancer Incidence, Mortality and Prevalence Worldwide. Lyon, France: IARC Press, 2001.

3 Linabery AM, Ross JA. Trends in childhood cancer incidence in the US (1992–2004). Cancer 2008; 112: 416–32.

4 Milne E, Laurvick CL, de Klerk N, Robertson L, Thompson JR, Bower C. Trends in childhood acute lymphoblastic leukemia in Western Australia, 1960–2006. Int J Cancer 2008; 122: 1130–4.

5 Svendsen AL, Feychting M, Klaeboe L, Langmark F, Schuz J. Time trends in the incidence of acute lymphoblastic leukemia among

children 1976–2002: a population-based Nordic study. J Pediatr 2007; 151: 548–50.

6 Greaves MF, Maia AT, Wiemels JL, Ford AM. Leukemia in twins: lessons in natural history. Blood 2003; 102: 2321–33.

7 Gale KB, Ford AM, Repp R, et al. Backtracking leukemia to birth: identification of clonotypic gene fusion sequences in neonatal blood spots. Proc Natl Acad Sci US A. 1997; 94: 13950–4.

8 Gross L. 'Spontaneous' leukemia developing in C3H mice following inoculation in infancy, with AK-leukemic extracts, or AK-embrvos. Proc Soc Exp Biol Med 1951; 76: 27–32.

9 Pagano JS. Epstein-Barr virus: the first human tumor virus and its role in cancer. Proc Ass Am Physicians 1999; 111: 573–80.

10 Bellec S, Baccaini B, Goubin A, et al. Childhood leukaemia and population movements in France, 1990–2003. Br J Cancer 2008; 98: 225–31.

11 Taylor GM, Dearden S, Payne N, et al. Evidence that an HLA-DQA1-DQB1 haplotype influences susceptibility to childhood common acute lymphoblastic leukaemia in boys provides further support for an infection-related aetiology . Br J Cancer 1998; 78: 561–5.

12 Loeb DM, Lederman HM, Winkelstein JA. Lymphoid malignancy as a presenting sign of ataxia-telangiectasia. J Pediatr Hematol Oncol 2000; 22: 464–7.

13 Taylor AM, Metcalfe JA, Thick J, Mak YF. Leukemia and lymphoma in ataxia telangiectasia. Blood 1996; 87: 423–38.

14 Korf BR. Malignancy in neurofibromatosis type 1. Oncologist 2000; 5: 477–85.

15 TaB JM. The hereditary basis of human leukemia. In: Henderson ES, Lister TA, Greaves M, (Eds), Leukemia. Philadelphia, PA: W.B.Saunders, 1996: 210–45.

16 Doll R, Wakeford R. Risk of childhood cancer from fetal irradiation. Br J Radiol 1997; 70: 130–9.

17 Cardis E. Current status and epidemiological research needs for achieving a better understanding of the consequences of the Chernobyl accident. Health Phys 2007; 93: 542–6.

18 Childhood cancer and residential proximity to power lines. UK Childhood Cancer Study Investigators. Br J Cancer 2000; 83: 1573–80.

19 Fear NT, Roman E, Ansell P, Simpson J, Day N, Eden OB. Vitamin K and childhood cancer: a report from the United Kingdom Childhood Cancer Study. Br J Cancer 2003; 89: 1228–31.

20 Loffler H, Gassmann W. Morphology and cytochemistry of acute lymphoblastic leukaemia. Baillieres Clin Haematol 1994; 7: 263–72.

21 Jaffe ES, Harris NL, Stein H, Vardiamn JW. World Health Organization Classification of Tumours. Pathology and Genetics of Tumours of Hematopoietic and Lymphoid Tissues. Lyon, France: IARC Press, 2001.

22 Bain BJ, Barnett D, Linch D, Matutes E, Reilly JT. Revised guideline on immunophenotyping in acute leukaemias and chronic lympho-proliferative disorders. Clin Lab Haematol 2002; 24: 1–13.

23 Harrison CJ, Foroni L. Cytogenetics and molecular genetics of acute lymphoblastic leukemia. Rev Clin Exp Hematol 2002; 6: 91–113; discussion 200–2.

24 Pui CH, Carroll AJ, Head D, et al. Near-triploid and near-tetraploid acute lymphoblastic leukemia of childhood. Blood 1990; 76: 590–6.

25 Raimondi SC, Zhou Y, Shurtleff SA, Rubnitz JE, Pui CH, Behm FG. Near-triploidy and near-tetraploidy in childhood acute lymphoblastic leukemia: association with B-lineage blast cells carrying the ETV6-RUNX1 fusion, T-lineage immunophenotype, and favorable outcome. Cancer Genet Cytogenet 2006; 169: 50–7.

26 Barlogie B, McLaughlin P, Alexanian R. Characterization of hematologic malignancies by flow cytometry. Anal Quant Cytol Histol 1987; 9: 147–55.

27 Williams DL, Tsiatis A, Brodeur GM, et al. Prognostic importance of chromosome number in 136 untreated children with acute lymphoblastic leukemia. Blood 1982; 60: 864–71.

28 Watson MS, Carroll AJ, Shuster JJ, et al. Trisomy 21 in childhood acute lymphoblastic leukemia: a Pediatric Oncology Group study (8602). Blood 1993; 82: 3098–102.

29 Raimondi SC, Roberson PK, Pui CH, Behm FG, Rivera GK. Hyperdiploid (47–50) acute lymphoblastic leukemia in children. Blood 1992; 79: 3245–52.

30 Raimondi SC, Behm FG, Roberson PK, et al. Cytogenetics of childhood T-cell leukemia. Blood 1988; 72: 1560–6.

31 Macintyre EA, Delabesse E. Molecular approaches to the diagnosis and evaluation of lymphoid malignancies. Semin Hematol 1999; 36: 373–89.

32 Felix CA, Poplack DG. Characterization of acute lymphoblastic leukemia of childhood by immunoglobulin and T-cell receptor gene patterns. Leukemia 1991; 5: 1015–25.

33 van der Velden VH, Boeckx N, van Wering ER, van Dongen JJ. Detection of minimal residual disease in acute leukemia. J Biol Regul Homeost Agents 2004; 18: 146–54.

34 Rubnitz JE, Pui CH. Recent advances in the treatment and understanding of childhood acute lymphoblastic leukaemia. Cancer Treat Rev 2003; 29: 31–44.

35 Hunter T. Treatment for chronic myelogenous leukemia: the long road to imatinib. J Clin Invest 2007; 117: 2036–43.

36 Gajjar A, Harrison PL, Sandlund JT, et al. Traumatic lumbar puncture at diagnosis adversely affects outcome in childhood acute lymphoblastic leukemia. Blood 2000; 96: 3381–4.

37 Breatnach F, Chessells JM, Greaves MF. The aplastic presentation of childhood leukaemia: a feature of common-ALL. Br J Haematol 1981; 49: 387–93.

38 Sirvent N, Suciu S, Bertrand Y, Uyttebroeck A, Lescoeur B, Otten J. Overt testicular disease (OTD) at diagnosis is not associated with a poor prognosis in childhood acute lymphoblastic leukemia: results of the EORTC CLG Study 58881. Pediatr Blood Cancer 2007; 49: 344–8.

39 Reiter A, Schrappe M, Ludwig WD, et al. Chemotherapy in 998 unselected childhood acute lymphoblastic leukemia patients. Results and conclusions of the multicenter trial ALL-BFM 86. Blood 1994; 84: 3122–33.

40 Kushner DC, Weinstein HJ, Kirkpatrick JA. The radiologic diagnosis of leukemia and lymphoma in children. Semin Roentgenol 1980; 15: 316–34.

41 Reddy SC, Menon BS. A prospective study of ocular manifestations in childhood acute leukaemia. Acta Ophthalmol Scand 1998; 76: 700–3.

42 Simone JV. History of the treatment of childhood ALL: a paradigm for cancer cure. Best Pract Res Clin Haematol 2006; 19: 353–9.

43 Smith M, Arthur D, Camitta B, et al. Uniform approach to risk classification and treatment assignment for children with acute lymphoblastic leukemia. J Clin Oncol 1996; 14: 18–24.

44 Pui CH, Campana D, Evans WE. Childhood acute lymphoblastic leukaemia – current status and future perspectives. Lancet Oncol 2001; 2: 597–607.

45 Conter V, Arico M, Valsecchi MG, et al. Extended intrathecal methotrexate may replace cranial irradiation for prevention of CNS relapse in children with intermediate-risk acute lymphoblastic leukemia treated with Berlin-Frankfurt-Munster-based intensive chemotherapy. The Associazione Italiana di Ematologia ed Oncologia Pediatrica. J Clin Oncol 1995; 13: 2497–502.

46 Rizzari C, Valsecchi MG, Arico M, et al. Effect of protracted high-dose L-asparaginase given as a second exposure in a Berlin-Frankfurt-Munster-based treatment: results of the randomized 9102 intermediate-risk childhood acute lymphoblastic leukemia study – a report from the Associazione Italiana Ematologia Oncologia Pediatrica. J Clin Oncol 2001; 19: 1297–303.

47 Conter V, Arico M, Valsecchi MG, et al. Long-term results of the Italian Association of Pediatric Hematology and Oncology (AIEOP) acute lymphoblastic leukemia studies, 1982–1995. Leukemia 2000; 14: 2196–204.

48 Arico M, Conter V, Valsecchi MG, et al. Treatment reduction in highly selected standard-risk childhood acute lymphoblastic leukemia. The AIEOP ALL-9501 study. Haematologica 2005; 90: 1186–91.

49 Arico M, Valsecchi MG, Conter V, et al. Improved outcome in high-risk childhood acute lymphoblastic leukemia defined by prednisone-poor response treated with double Berlin-Frankfurt-Muenster protocol II. Blood 2002; 100: 420–6.

50 Arico M, Valsecchi MG, Rizzari C, et al. Long-term results of the AIEOP-ALL-95 Trial for Childhood Acute Lymphoblastic Leukemia: insight on the prognostic value of DNA index in the framework of Berlin-Frankfurt-Muenster based chemotherapy. J Clin Oncol 2008; 26: 283–9.

51 Schrappe M, Reiter A, Zimmermann M, et al. Long-term results of four consecutive trials in childhood ALL performed by the ALL-BFM study group from 1981 to 1995. Berlin-Frankfurt-Munster. Leukemia 2000; 14: 2205–22.

52 Schrappe M, Reiter A, Ludwig WD, et al. Improved outcome in childhood acute lymphoblastic leukemia despite reduced use of anthracyclines and cranial radiotherapy: results of trial ALL-BFM 90. German-Austrian-Swiss ALL-BFM Study Group. Blood 2000; 95: 3310–22.

53 Conter V, Valsecchi MG, Silvestri D, et al. Pulses of vincristine and dexamethasone in addition to intensive chemotherapy for children with intermediate-risk acute lymphoblastic leukaemia: a multicentre randomised trial. Lancet 2007; 369: 123–31.

54 Burger B, Zimmermann M, Mann G, et al. Diagnostic cerebrospinal fluid examination in children with acute lymphoblastic leukaemia: significance of low leukocyte counts with blasts or traumatic lumbar puncture. J Clin Oncol 2003; 21: 184–8.

55 Eden OB, Harrison G, Richards S, et al. Long-term follow-up of the United Kingdom Medical Research Council protocols for childhood acute lymphoblastic leukaemia, 1980–1997. Medical Research Council Childhood Leukaemia Working Party. Leukemia 2000; 14: 2307–20.

56 Chessells JM, Harrison G, Richards SM, et al. Failure of a new protocol to improve treatment results in paediatric lymphoblastic leukaemia: lessons from the UK Medical Research Council trials UKALL X and UKALL XI. Br J Haematol 2002; 118: 445–55.

57 Hann I, Vora A, Richards S, et al. Benefit of intensified treatment for all children with acute lymphoblastic leukaemia: results from MRC UKALL XI and MRC ALL97 randomised trials. UK Medical Research Council's Working Party on Childhood Leukaemia. Leukaemia 2000; 14: 356–63.

58 Mitchell CD, Richards SM, Kinsey SE, Lilleyman J, Vora A, Eden TO. Benefit of dexamethasone compared with prednisolone for childhood acute lymphoblastic leukaemia: results of the UK Medical Research Council ALL97 randomized trial. Br J Haematol 2005; 129: 734–45.

59 Vora A, Mitchell CD, Lennard L, et al. Toxicity and efficacy of 6-thioguanine versus 6-mercaptopurine in childhood lymphoblastic leukaemia: a randomised trial. Lancet 2006; 368: 1339–48.

60 Maloney KW, Shuster JJ, Murphy S, Pullen J, Camitta BA. Long-term results of treatment studies for childhood acute lymphoblastic leukemia: Pediatric Oncology Group studies from 1986–1994. Leukemia 2000; 14: 2276–85.

61 Lauer SJ, Shuster JJ, Mahoney DH, Jr, et al. A comparison of early intensive methotrexate/mercaptopurine with early intensive alternating combination chemotherapy for high-risk B-precursor acute lymphoblastic leukemia: a Pediatric Oncology Group phase III randomized trial. Leukemia 2001; 15: 1038–45.

62 Mahoney DH, Jr, Shuster J, Nitschke R, et al. Intermediate-dose intravenous methotrexate with intravenous mercaptopurine is superior to repetitive low-dose oral methotrexate with intravenous mercaptopurine for children with lower-risk B-lineage acute lymphoblastic leukemia: a Pediatric Oncology Group phase III trial. J Clin Oncol 1998; 16: 246–54.

63 Mahoney DH, Jr, Shuster JJ, Nitschke R, Lauer S, Steuber CP, Camitta B. Intensification with intermediate-dose intravenous methotrexate is effective therapy for children with lower-risk B-precursor acute lymphoblastic leukemia: a Pediatric Oncology Group study. J Clin Oncol 2000; 18: 1285–94.

64 Nachman JB, Sather HN, Sensel MG, et al. Augmented post-induction therapy for children with high-risk acute lymphoblastic leukemia and a slow response to initial therapy. N Engl J Med 1998; 338: 1663–71.

65 Lange BJ, Bostrom BC, Cherlow JM, et al. Double-delayed intensification improves event-free survival for children with intermediate-risk acute lymphoblastic leukemia: a report from the Children's Cancer Group. Blood 2002; 99: 825–33.

66 Gaynon PS, Trigg ME, Heerema NA, et al. Children's Cancer Group trials in childhood acute lymphoblastic leukemia: 1983–1995. Leukemia 2000; 14: 2223–33.

67 Matloub Y, Lindemulder S, Gaynon PS, et al. Intrathecal triple therapy decreases central nervous system relapse but fails to improve event-free survival when compared with intrathecal methotrexate: results of the Children's Cancer Group (CCG) 1952 study for standard-risk acute lymphoblastic leukemia, reported by the Children's Oncology Group. Blood 2006; 108: 1165–73.

68 Bostrom BC, Sensel MR, Sather HN, et al. Dexamethasone versus prednisone and daily oral versus weekly intravenous mercaptopurine for patients with standard-risk acute lymphoblastic leukemia: a report from the Children's Cancer Group. Blood 2003; 101: 3809–17.

69 Jacobs SS, Stork LC, Bostrom BC, et al. Substitution of oral and intravenous thioguanine for mercaptopurine in a treatment regimen for children with standard risk acute lymphoblastic leukemia: a collaborative Children's Oncology Group/National Cancer Institute pilot trial (CCG-1942). Pediatr Blood Cancer 2007; 49: 250–5.

70 Vilmer E, Suciu S, Ferster A, et al. Long-term results of three randomized trials (58831, 58832, 58881) in childhood acute lymphoblastic leukemia: a CLCG-EORTC report. Children's Leukemia Cooperative Group. Leukemia 2000; 14: 2257–66.

71 van der Werff Ten Bosch J, Suciu S, Thyss A, et al. Value of intravenous 6-mercaptopurine during continuation treatment in childhood acute lymphoblastic leukemia and non-Hodgkin's lymphoma: final results of a randomized phase III trial (58881) of the EORTC CLG. Leukemia 2005; 19: 721–6.

72 Duval M, Suciu S, Ferster A, et al. Comparison of Escherichia coli-asparaginase with Erwinia-asparaginase in the treatment of childhood lymphoid malignancies: results of a randomized European Organisation for Research and Treatment of Cancer-Children's Leukemia Group phase 3 trial. Blood 2002; 99: 2734–9.

73 Millot F, Suciu S, Philippe N, et al. Value of high-dose cytarabine during interval therapy of a Berlin-Frankfurt-Munster-based protocol in increased-risk children with acute lymphoblastic leukemia and lymphoblastic lymphoma: results of the European Organization for Research and Treatment of Cancer 58881 randomized phase III trial. J Clin Oncol 2001; 19: 1935–42.

74 Gustafsson G, Schmiegelow K, Forestier E, et al. Improving outcome through two decades in childhood ALL in the Nordic countries: the impact of high-dose methotrexate in the reduction of CNS irradiation. Nordic Society of Pediatric Haematology and Oncology (NOPHO). Leukemia 2000; 14: 2267–75.

75 Schmiegelow K, Bjork O, Glomstein A, et al. Intensification of mercaptopurine/methotrexate maintenance chemotherapy may increase the risk of relapse for some children with acute lymphoblastic leukemia. J Clin Oncol 2003; 21: 1332–9.

76 Pui CH. Central nervous system disease in acute lymphoblastic leukemia: prophylaxis and treatment. Hematology Am Soc Hematol Educ Program 2006: 142–6.

77 Pui CH, Evans WE. Treatment of acute lymphoblastic leukemia. N Engl J Med 2006; 354: 166–78.

78 Pui CH, Schrappe M, Ribeiro RC, Niemeyer CM. Childhood and adolescent lymphoid and myeloid leukemia. Hematology Am Soc Hematol Educ Program. 2004: 118–45.

79 Pui CH, Boyett JM, Rivera GK, et al. Long-term results of Total Therapy studies 11, 12 and 13A for childhood acute lymphoblastic leukemia at St Jude Children's Research Hospital. Leukemia 2000; 14: 2286–94.

80 Tsuchida M, Ikuta K, Hanada R, et al. Long-term follow-up of childhood acute lymphoblastic leukemia in Tokyo Children's Cancer Study Group 1981–1995. Leukemia 2000; 14: 2295–306.

81 Toyoda Y, Manabe A, Tsuchida M, et al. Six months of maintenance chemotherapy after intensified treatment for acute lymphoblastic leukemia of childhood. J Clin Oncol 2000; 18: 1508–16.

82 Szczepanski T, Orfao A, van der Velden VH, San Miguel JF, van Dongen JJ. Minimal residual disease in leukaemia patients. Lancet Oncol 2001; 2: 409–17.

83 Silverman LB, Declerck L, Gelber RD, et al. Results of Dana-Farber Cancer Institute Consortium protocols for children with newly diagnosed acute lymphoblastic leukemia (1981–1995). Leukemia 2000; 14: 2247–56.

84 Silverman LB, Gelber RD, Dalton VK, et al. Improved outcome for children with acute lymphoblastic leukemia: results of Dana-Farber Consortium Protocol 91-01. Blood 2001; 97: 1211–18.

85 Goldberg JM, Silverman LB, Levy DE, et al. Childhood T-cell acute lymphoblastic leukemia: the Dana-Farber Cancer Institute acute lymphoblastic leukemia consortium experience. J Clin Oncol 2003; 21: 3616–22.

86 Clarke M, Gaynon P, Hann I, et al. CNS-directed therapy for childhood acute lymphoblastic leukemia: childhood ALL Collaborative Group overview of 43 randomized trials. J Clin Oncol 2003; 21: 1798–809.

87 Sullivan MP, Chen T, Dyment PG, Hvizdala E, Steuber CP. Equivalence of intrathecal chemotherapy and radiotherapy as central nervous system prophylaxis in children with acute lymphatic leukemia: a pediatric oncology group study. Blood 1982; 60: 948–58.

88 Igarashi S, Manabe A, Ohara A, et al. No advantage of dexamethasone over prednisolone for the outcome of standard- and intermediate-risk childhood acute lymphoblastic leukemia in the Tokyo Children's Cancer Study Group L95-14 protocol. J Clin Oncol 2005; 23: 6489–98.

89 Chessells JM, Harrison G, Lilleyman JS, Bailey CC, Richards SM. Continuing (maintenance) therapy in lymphoblastic leukaemia: lessons from MRC UKALL X. Medical Research Council Working Party in Childhood Leukaemia. Br J Haematol 1997; 98: 945–51.

90 Chessells JM, Leiper AD, Tiedemann K, Hardisty RM, Richards S. Oral methotrexate is as effective as intramuscular in maintenance therapy of acute lymphoblastic leukaemia. Arch Dis Child 1987; 62: 172–6.

91 Bleyer WA, Sather HN, Nickerson HJ, et al. Monthly pulses of vincristine and prednisone prevent bone marrow and testicular relapse in low-risk childhood acute lymphoblastic leukemia: a report of the CCG-161 study by the Childrens Cancer Study Group. J Clin Oncol 1991; 9: 1012–21.

92 Miller DR, Leikin SL, Albo VC, Sather H, Hammond GD. Three versus five years of maintenance therapy are equivalent in childhood acute lymphoblastic leukemia: a report from the Childrens Cancer Study Group. J Clin Oncol 1989; 7: 316–25.

93 Nesbit ME, Jr, Sather HN, Robison LL, Ortega JA, Hammond GD. Randomized study of 3 years versus 5 years of chemotherapy in childhood acute lymphoblastic leukemia. J Clin Oncol 1983; 1: 308–16.

94 Williams FM, Murray RC, Underhill TM, Flintoff WF. Isolation of a hamster cDNA clone coding for a function involved in methotrexate uptake. J Biol Chem 1994; 269: 5810–16.

95 Fabre I, Fabre G, Goldman ID. Polyglutamylation, an important element in methotrexate cytotoxicity and selectivity in tumor versus murine granulocytic progenitor cells in vitro. Cancer Res 1984; 44: 3190–5.

96 Li WW, Waltham M, Tong W, Schweitzer BI, Bertino JR. Increased activity of gamma-glutamyl hydrolase in human sarcoma cell lines: a novel mechanism of intrinsic resistance to methotrexate (MTX). Adv Exp Med Biol 1993; 338: 635–8.

97 Camitta B, Mahoney D, Leventhal B, et al. Intensive intravenous methotrexate and mercaptopurine treatment of higher-risk non-T, non-B acute lymphocytic leukemia: a Pediatric Oncology Group study. J Clin Oncol 1994; 12: 1383–9.

98 Evans WE, Crom WR, Abromowitch M, et al. Clinical pharmacodynamics of high-dose methotrexate in acute lymphocytic leukemia. Identification of a relation between concentration and effect. N Engl J Med 1986; 314: 471–7.

99 Whitehead VM, Vuchich MJ, Lauer SJ, et al. Accumulation of high levels of methotrexate polyglutamates in lymphoblasts from children with hyperdiploid (greater than 50 chromosomes) B-lineage acute lymphoblastic leukemia: a Pediatric Oncology Group study. Blood 1992; 80: 1316–23.

100 Whitehead VM, Shuster JJ, Vuchich MJ, et al. Accumulation of methotrexate and methotrexate polyglutamates in lymphoblasts and treatment outcome in children with B-progenitor-cell acute

lymphoblastic leukemia: a Pediatric Oncology Group study. Leukemia 2005; 19: 533–6.

101 Kufe DW, Major PP, Egan EM, Beardsley GP. Correlation of cytotoxicity with incorporation of ara-C into DNA. J Biol Chem 1980; 255: 8997–9000.

102 Momparler RL. Kinetic and template studies with 1–D-arabinofuranosylcytosine 5'-triphosphate and mammalian deoxyribonucleic acid polymerase. Mol Pharmacol 1972; 8: 362–70.

103 Muus P, Drenthe-Schonk A, Haanen C, Wessels H, Linssen P. In-vitro studies on phosphorylation and dephosphorylation of cytosine arabinoside in human leukemic cells. Leuk Res 1987; 11: 319–25.

104 Muus P, Haanen C, Raijmakers R, de Witte T, Salden M, Wessels J. Influence of dose and duration of exposure on the cytotoxic effect of cytarabine toward human hematopoietic clonogenic cells. Semin Oncol 1987; 14: 238–44.

105 Boos J, Hohenlochter B, Schulze-Westhoff P, et al. Intracellular retention of cytosine arabinoside triphosphate in blast cells from children with acute myelogenous and lymphoblastic leukemia. Med Pediatr Oncol 1996; 26: 397–404.

106 Kakihara T, Fukuda T, Tanaka A, et al. Expression of deoxycytidine kinase (dCK) gene in leukemic cells in childhood: decreased expression of dCK gene in relapsed leukemia. Leuk Lymphoma 1998; 31: 405–9.

107 Stammler G, Zintl F, Sauerbrey A, Volm M. Deoxycytidine kinase mRNA expression in childhood acute lymphoblastic leukemia. Anticancer Drugs 1997; 8: 517–21.

108 Lennard L, Lilleyman JS, Van Loon J, Weinshilboum RM. Genetic variation in response to 6-mercaptopurine for childhood acute lymphoblastic leukemia. Lancet. 1990; 336: 225–9.

109 Schmiegelow K, Schroder H, Gustafsson G, et al. Risk of relapse in childhood acute lymphoblastic leukemia is related to RBC methotrexate and mercaptopurine metabolites during maintenance chemotherapy. Nordic Society for Pediatric Hematology and Oncology. J Clin Oncol 1995; 13: 345–51.

110 Silverman LB. Acute lymphoblastic leukemia in infancy. Pediatr Blood Cancer 2007; 49: 1070–3.

111 Pieters R, Schrappe M, De Lorenzo P, et al. A treatment protocol for infants younger than 1 year with acute lymphoblastic leukemia (Interfant-99): an observational study and a multicentre randomised trial. Lancet 2007; 370: 240–50.

112 Whitlock JA. Down syndrome and acute lymphoblastic leukemia. Br J Haematol 2006; 135: 595–602.

113 Neale GA, Pui CH, Mahmoud HH, et al. Molecular evidence for minimal residual bone marrow disease in children with 'isolated' extra-medullary relapse of T-cell acute lymphoblastic leukemia. Leukemia 1994; 8: 768–75.

114 Gaynon PS. Childhood acute lymphoblastic leukemia and relapse. Br J Haematol 2005; 131: 579–87.

115 Arikoski P, Voutilainen R, Kroger H. Bone mineral density in long-term survivors of childhood cancer. J Pediatr Endocrinol Metab 2003; 16 (Suppl 2): 343–53.

116 Nachman JB. Adolescents with acute lymphoblastic leukemia: a 'new age'. Rev Clin Exp Hematol 2003; 7: 261–9.

117 Nathan PC, Patel SK, Dilley K, et al. Guidelines for identification of, advocacy for, and intervention in neurocognitive problems in survivors of childhood cancer: a report from the Children's Oncology Group. Arch Pediatr Adolesc Med 2007; 161: 798–806.

118 Krappmann P, Paulides M, Stohr W, et al. Almost normal cognitive function in patients during therapy for childhood acute lymphoblastic leukemia without cranial irradiation according to ALL-BFM 95 and COALL 06-97 protocols: results of an Austrian-German multicenter longitudinal study and implications for follow-up. Pediatr Hematol Oncol 2007; 24: 101–9.

119 Spiegler BJ, Kennedy K, Maze R, et al. Comparison of long-term neurocognitive outcomes in young children with acute lymphoblastic leukemia treated with cranial radiation or high-dose or very high-dose intravenous methotrexate. J Clin Oncol 2006; 24: 3858–64.

120 Krynetski EY, Krynetskaia NF, Yanishevski Y, Evans WE. Methylation of mercaptopurine, thioguanine, and their nucleotide metabolites by heterologously expressed human thiopurine S-methyltransferase. Mol Pharmacol 1995; 47: 1141–7.

8 Acute Myeloid Leukemia and Myelodysplastic Disorders

David K.H. Webb

Department of Haematology and Oncology, Great Ormond Street Hospital for Children NHS Trust, London, UK

Introduction

In this chapter three separate but closely related malignant myeloid disorders will be considered – acute myeloid leukemia (AML), myelodysplastic syndromes and myeloid disorders of Down's syndrome. The relevant features of epidemiology, pathogenesis, clinical presentation, investigation, and therapy of each will be considered in turn.

Acute myeloid leukemia

Epidemiology

AML comprises 5% of childhood cancer, with around 70 new cases in British children each year [1]. The age-specific incidence is highest in young children, and 20% of cases occur in the first 5 years of life, after which the incidence is essentially stable throughout childhood. The sex incidence is equal. The incidence shows geographical variation, and AML is more common in China, but less common in the Indian subcontinent. Environmental factors resulting in damage of DNA may be contributory. The diet of the mother in pregnancy (especially in regard to foods containing topoisomerase II inhibitors) may be influential, as a result of genetic polymorphisms. Exposure to petroleum products, benzene, heavy metals, or ionizing radiation are risk factors that are not generally implicated in most childhood cases.

Although the etiology of most cases is unknown, AML is more common in children with certain syndromes:
- Down's syndrome (considered separately, see page 104).
- Klinefelter syndrome.
- Bloom syndrome.
- Neurofibromatosis type I.
- Ataxia telangectasia.
- Congenital bone marrow failure disorders (Fanconi anemia, severe congenital neutropenia, Shwachman syndrome, Diamond-Blackfan anemia, thrombocytopenia-absent radius syndrome).

Classification

The first comprehensive classification used in AML was the French-American-British (FAB) type (Table 8.1) [2]. A diagnosis of AML required 30% leukemia cells (blasts) in the bone marrow. Patients with 5–30% had myelodysplasia (MDS, see below).

As immunophenotypic, cytogenetic, and molecular characteristics have been described, the usefulness of the FAB classification has proved limited, with the exception of acute promyelocytic leukemia (APL, FAB type M3) which is readily recognizable on light microscopy, and has critically important clinical features (see APL section). More recently, the World Health Organization (WHO) classification (Table 8.2) [3] has incorporated cytogenetic data, whilst lowering the percentage of blasts in the bone marrow necessary for the diagnosis of AML in adults to 20%.

Clinical presentation

AML presents with signs and symptoms attributable to bone marrow infiltration and bone marrow failure. Accordingly, pallor, bruising, fever, and bone pain are common. Organ infiltration results in hepatosplenomegaly. Gum infiltration, particularly in monocytic disease, and skin infiltrates may be observed. Some children present with an isolated, extramedullary mass of AML, termed a chloroma (as the cut surface is of greenish hue) or granulocytic sarcoma, and may have low percentages of leukemic blasts in the bone marrow, or no visible blasts at all. These masses commonly occur in and around the orbit, but may be paraspinal and cause cord compression. Where bone marrow disease is present, extramedullary masses are usually associated with FAB types M1 and M2 and cytogenetics most commonly show a t(8;21). Some cases, however, have a monocytic component, with FAB type M4 or M5.

Several groups of children with AML are at high risk of early life-threatening complications:

Pediatric Hematology and Oncology, 1st edition. Edited by Edward J. Estlin, Richard J. Gilbertson, and Robert F. Wynn. © 2010 Blackwell Publishing Ltd.

Table 8.1 French-American-British (FAB) classification of acute myeloid leukemia.

M0	Undifferentiated myeloblastic leukemia
M1	Myeloblastic leukemia without maturation
M2	Myeloblastic leukemia with maturation
M3	Acute promyelocytic leukemia
M4	Acute myelomonocytic leukemia
M5	Acute monoblastic leukemia
M6	Acute erythroblastic leukemia
M7	Acute megakaryoblastic leukemia

Table 8.2 World Health Organization classification of acute myeloid leukemia (AML).

AML with recurrent genetic abnormalities
AML with t(8;21)
AML with abnormal bone marrow eosinophils inversion 16 or t(16;16)
AML with t(15;17) and variants (Acute promyelocytic leukemia)
AML with 11q23 abnormalities

AML with multilineage dysplasia

AML and myelodysplasia, therapy related
AML not otherwise categorized
AML minimally differentiated
AML without maturation
AML with maturation
Acute myelomonocytic leukemia
Acute monoblastic leukemia
Acute erythroid leukemia
Acute megakaryoblastic leukemia
Acute basophilic leukemia
Acute panmyelosis with myelofibrosis
Myeloid sarcoma

AML of ambiguous lineage
Undifferentiated acute leukemia
Bilineal acute leukemia
Biphenotypic acute leukemia

• Patients with APL may have a severe coagulopathy, due to the release of cytoplasmic granules with procoagulant activity, with life-threatening bleeding or thrombosis.
• High count AML, especially monocytic disease, carries a risk of hyperviscosity syndrome, hemorrhage, and thrombosis in the CNS, and pulmonary infiltrates and respiratory insufficiency. Release of lysozyme from these monoblasts causes renal potassium loss, and hypokalemia may be profound. Monocytic AML is also associated with tumor lysis syndrome and coagulopathy. As a result, treatment is a medical emergency, and rapid white cell count reduction is important in symptomatic high count patients. Anthracyclines are the most useful drugs in this regard and should be given on day 1 of therapy.

Investigations

The complete diagnosis of AML will involve morphological, immunophenotypic, cytogenetic, and molecular aspects.
• The diagnosis of AML or MDS requires examination of a good quality blood film and bone marrow aspirate.
• Immunophenotyping is readily available in treatment centres and is able to ascribe lineage to most leukemia blast cell populations.
• Bone marrow cytogenetics should be obtained in every case, and G banding is now complemented by rapid assessment using fluorescent in-situ hybridization (FISH), and reverse transcriptase polymerase chain reaction (RT-PCR) for common fusion genes. In AML, favorable karyotypes comprise the t(15;17) characteristic of APL, t(8;21) and inversion of chromosome 16. Adverse karyotypes include monosomy 7, deletions of 5q, abnormal 3q, t(9;22), and complex karyotypes with three or more abnormalities. All remaining karyotypes are intermediate risk [4].
• Inversion 16 and t(8;21) involve genes encoding subunits of the core binding factor (CBF). The t(8;21) generates a novel fusion protein AML1/ETO, causing abnormal protein–protein signalling. The AML1/ETO interacts with CBF but recruits proteins involved in repression of transcription. Inversion 16 creates another fusion protein, CBF/MYHII, which also disrupts transcription via CBF by inhibiting binding of AML1. Accordingly the two karyotypic changes affect a common transcriptional pathway, leading to their description as CBF leukemias. The CBF pathway is under investigation for targets for new therapies. The match between FAB types and CBF leukemias is not exact, but most children with t(8;21) have FAB type M1 or M2, whilst most with inversion 16 have M4 with eosinophilia (M4Eo). The t(15;17) is tightly associated with APL, and is discussed in detail in the APL section of this chapter. In AML, abnormalities of 11q with a breakpoint at 11q23, the site of the MLL gene, are particularly but not exclusively associated with monocytic leukemia. These mutations disrupt the role of the MLL gene in transcriptional regulation. A large number of partner genes are observed, and it is possible that the different fusion genes have varying impact on prognosis – for example, several groups report a better outcome for children with the t(9;11). However, these findings are not consistent across studies, and require further elucidation, especially as the influence of prognostic factors may be protocol dependent [4].

Adverse karyotypes are associated with a reduced complete remission (CR) rate and increased relapse risk, with overall survival of less than 50%. Monosomy 7 carries a poor prognosis in AML and MDS, and occurs as a single abnormality, or as part of a more complex karyotype. Why monosomy 7 is adverse in AML and MDS is unknown, and this situation contrasts with several congenital bone marrow failure syndromes where monosomy 7 occurs as an opportunistic change which may disappear on follow up, without adverse influence on prognosis. Abnormalities of 5q, 3q and the t(9;22) are adverse risk factors in adults, but are very rare in children with AML. Complex karyotypes, varingly defined as more than three or more than five different changes are also adverse, and there is some evidence that the addition of abnormalities of 5q or 3q to monosomy 7 is especially high risk. Molecular characterization of AML has gained increasing importance, as a number of molecular markers may be used to refine the assessment of prognosis, and may be molecular targets (see section on new therapies).

Treatment

Emergency management of difficult clinical presentations – high white count, electrolyte disturbance, coagulopathy is discussed above. This section deals with chemotherapy treatment schedules, supportive care, role of stem cell transplant, management of relapsed disease, and important prognostic factors. Subsequent sections detail the management of APL and the summary experience of the major childhood cancer collaborative groups.

• Modern AML therapy is based on induction chemotherapy with an anthracycline combined with cytarabine, although schedules vary in choice of anthracycline (usually daunorubicin, idarubicin or mitozantrone), total doses, and methods of administration [5]. There is no convincing evidence for superiority of any anthracycline over daunorubicin. Most schedules include a third induction agent, although the superiority of additional agents compared with anthracycline and cytarabine alone has not been shown in a randomized study. With this combination 80–90% of children achieve CR after two courses. Induction death rates are in the region of 5%, with the remainder of induction failures due to resistant disease [6].

• Consolidation chemotherapy is necessary for cure, although the number of courses given varies between collaborative groups, and the optimum number within each regimen remains unknown. Consolidation courses usually contain high dose cytarabine, and it is unknown whether the addition of other drugs improves efficacy. This issue is being addressed in the current MRC AML 15 study.

• There is no evidence that extended maintenance therapy is beneficial in children treated with intensive induction and consolidation, although the Berlin-Frankfurt-Munster group protocols contain this element [7].

• Involvement of the central nervous system (CNS) at diagnosis occurs in 2% of children, and is associated with monocytic leukemia and AML in infants. The importance of CNS-directed therapy for the majority of children is unclear as CNS relapse is uncommon, and affects around 3% of children. A limited number of intrathecal injections with combinations of methotrexate, cytarabine and hydrocortisone are generally administered routinely to children who are CNS negative at diagnosis. There is no role for prophylactic cranial radiation, although this is included in BFM protocols because of a reduction in bone marrow relapse observed in a subgroup of patients in BFM 87 (see below).

AML chemotherapy is intensive, myelosuppressive, and associated with mucositis which may be severe. Treatment-related death rates of up to 20% have been described, but are now typically under 10%. Accordingly, supportive care needs are high, and therapy should only be administered in experienced units. It

is standard practice to keep children in hospital until bone marrow recovery occurs. Planned progressive therapy is required for febrile neutropenia, with early introduction of empiric antifungal drugs if fever persists. Since the early introduction of broad spectrum antibiotics for fever has become standard, Gram negative sepsis has been better controlled and most infection-related deaths are now fungal, although occasionally viral infections (cytomegalovirus, adenovirus, respiratory syncitial virus) have proved fatal.

Stem cell transplant (SCT) now has a very limited role in first line AML therapy, although this area remains contentious. There is no evidence that SCT improves outcome for children with adverse cytogenetics, and SCT is contraindicated in those with favorable cytogenetics due to the high cure rate with chemotherapy, and the toxicity associated with SCT (up to 20% of treatment-related deaths in most series). The situation is more complex in patients with intermediate karyotypes; although SCT may reduce relapse, the treatment-related death rate means that the overall survival benefit is small and European groups have generally discontinued SCT in first remission for these children. However, SCT continues to be considered in the United States for intermediate and poor risk cases.

Prognostic factors are to an extent protocol dependant but include [8]:
• Age (worse in adolescents and young adults).
• Presenting white cell count (worse with high counts).
• Presence of Down's syndrome (better prognosis).
• FAB type (M3 superior).
• Cytogenetics.
• Race (worse in African Americans treated in the United States).
• Response to therapy (patients with more than 15% blasts in the bone marrow on recovery from course 1 have an adverse prognosis).
• Performance score (worse with low score).
• Some molecular markers (see Table 8.11).

Of these prognostic factors, cytogenetics, M3 FAB type, response to therapy, Down's syndrome and internal tandem duplications of the fms-like tyrosine kinase (FLT3-ITD) are the most important on multivariate analyses.

Overall survival (OS) and event-free survival (EFS) range from 25 to 66% and 47 to 56% respectively in major collaborative studies (Table 8.3), with relapse rates of 30–50% the main cause of treatment failure. Although survival rates are broadly similar between leading collaborative groups, cumulative doses of anthracycline and cytarabine vary considerably (Table 8.4).

Salvage therapy cures around 25% of children who relapse, and the main prognostic factors at relapse are length of first remission and cytogenetics [9]. Children with favorable cytogenetics usually have long first remissions and the best outcome with retreatment, whilst those with adverse cytogenetics relapse early and are very difficult to cure. A wide range of standard AML chemotherapy regimens are satisfactory for reinduction of remission, achieving remission rates of 60–70% overall and with no clear differences in efficacy between them. In the United Kingdom high dose

Table 8.3 Key features of recent large (over 100 children registered) collaborative trials for the treatment of acute myeloid leukemia (AML) in children aged under 15 years.

Trial	n	CR rate (%)	Death in CR (%)	Relapse (%)	BMT (%)	EFS (%)	OS (%)
AML 12	564	92	6	35	15	56	66
BFM 93	427	83	4	28	7	51	58
NOPHO 93	223	92	2	39	25	49	66
AIEOP 92	160	89	7	32	29	54	60
CCG 2891	750	78	15	47	34	47	25
EORTC 58921	166	84	6	34	20	48	62
LAME 91	247	91	6	36	30	48	62
POG 8821	511	77	8	45	13	32	42

Children with Down's syndrome, secondary AML, and preceding myelodysplasia excluded. CR, complete remission. BMT, bone marrow transplant, EFS, event-free survival. OS, overall survival.

Table 8.4 Cumulative doses of anthracycline, cytarabine, and etoposide in major collaborative trials.

Trial	Anthracycline mg/m^2	Cytarabine g/m^2	Etoposide mg/m^2
AML 12	550	10.6	1500
BFM 93	300–400	41	950
NOPHO 93	300–375	49–61	1600
CCG 2891	180	14.6	1100
EORTC 58921	380	23–29	1350
LAME 91	460	9.8–13.4	400
POG 8821	360	55.7	2250

cytarabine and fludarabine (FLA) has been favored in recent years due to the high anthracycline dosage used in first line therapy.

Consolidation is usually by SCT, either from a matched donor or using autologous cells. The survival following SCT is around 40% with no significant differences between the source of stem cells – matched unrelated donor SCT has a lower rate of relapse but more treatment-related deaths than matched family donor SCT. Autologous SCT has the lowest treatment-related mortality but also the highest rate of relapse. Haploidentical SCT has been successfully used in the absence of a matched donor, but has the highest treatment-related mortality. Some children survive after chemotherapy alone in second remission, so this is an option if treatment toxicities preclude SCT.

Experience of major collaborative trial groups
Medical Research Council AML 10 and AML 12 trials [10, 11]
These two studies assessed different combinations of anthracycline and cytarabine-based induction chemotherapy (ADE versus DAT, AML 10), and found no difference in efficacy whether thioguanine or etoposide was used as the third drug. If mitozantrone was substituted for daunorubicin (MAE versus ADE, AML 12),

there was increased myelotoxicity with delayed recovery of the full blood count, but no difference in OS or EFS. The addition of either autologous or allogeneic SCT to four courses of chemotherapy reduced relapse in AML 10, but allogeneic SCT was associated with an increased treatment-related death rate which largely offset the reduction in relapse. As the reduction in relapse observed with SCT in AML 10 may have been due to a fifth course of treatment rather than SCT *per se*, AML 12 randomized children between four or five courses of treatment in all (fifth course of chemotherapy high dose cytarabine plus asparaginase). The addition of a fifth course was well tolerated but there was no improvement in OS or EFS. Analyses of AML 10 demonstrated that karyotype was a prime determinant of prognosis, with t(8;21), t(15;17) and inversion 16 favorable, whilst monosomy 7, abnormal 5q, abnormal 3q, t(9;22) or complex karyotypes were adverse. All other karyotypes were intermediate risk. This risk score was adapted to include response to the first course of chemotherapy (more than 15% blasts adverse) to define three risk groups for AML 12.

Berlin-Frankfurt-Munster (BFM) Group [12, 13]
BFM protocols have a backbone of induction, consolidation, and extended maintenance chemotherapy, currently to a total of 18 months treatment. Cranial radiation (CRT) is incorporated for all patients over 1 year of age, as children who did not receive CRT in BFM 87 had a higher relapse rate, both in bone marrow and the CNS. Accordingly, BFM therapy has major differences in design to most contemporary regimens. Children were divided between two risk groups; standard risk had FAB type M1 or M2 with Auer rods, M3, or M4Eo with <5% blasts in bone marrow at day 15, whereas all other children were high risk. In effect, FAB types were used as a surrogate for favorable cytogenetics as karyotypes were not uniformly available. BFM 93 was associated with improved survival compared with BFM 87, and randomized idarubicin and daunorubicin in induction for all patients, and high dose cytarabine with mitozantrone (HAM) in consolidation for

high-risk patients. HAM was given either before (early) or after (late) a standard BFM consolidation block. Results in high-risk patients improved compared with BFM 87, but not for the standard risk group. Although there was more rapid clearance of blasts as assessed on a day 15 bone marrow aspirate in children receiving idarubicin, there was no difference between idarubicin and daunorubicin in any measure of survival. There was some evidence that children given daunorubicin benefited from early rather than late HAM.

Children's Cancer Study Group (CCG) [14, 15]

Three studies were conducted between 1979 and 1995. The most recent study, CCG-2891, compared standard with intensified timing of induction chemotherapy using a five drug regimen (DCTER). In standard timing, hematologic recovery was allowed between courses unless there was evidence of resistant disease on a day 14 bone marrow, whereas with intensified induction therapy DCTER was timetabled for days 0–3 and 10–13. Remission rates were similar, but treatment-related deaths were more common, and relapse risk reduced in the intensive arm with a superior EFS. Children with Down's syndrome had better survival with standard intensity treatment, due to fewer therapy-related deaths. However, overall survival was disappointing and the current Children's Oncology study is based on the MRC AML 12 backbone.

Acute promyelocytic leukemia (APL) [16–19]

APL is uncommon, and comprises 8% of AML in children but has important biological and clinical characteristics. Around 95% of cases of APL are associated with a t(15;17) translocation, resulting in the PML/RAR fusion gene. In the remaining cases, RAR is fused to an alternative partner, in children most commonly the nucleophosmin gene (NPM1) in the t(5;17). Other subtypes include fusion with NuMA in the t(11;17), or the promyelocytic zinc finger (PLZF) gene. RAR is a member of the RA nuclear receptor family that acts as a ligand inducible transcription factor. PML controls p53 dependent induction of apoptosis, growth suppression, and is required for transcriptional repression by other tumor suppressors. The PML-RAR fusion protein functions as an aberrant retinoid receptor, and is resistant to physiologic concentrations of retinoic acid. The block is overcome, however, by therapeutic concentrations produced by all – transretinoic acid (ATRA), and arsenic trioxide (ATO) degrades the protein whilst also inducing apoptosis via induction of the proenzymes of caspase 2 and 3 and activation of caspases 1 and 3.

Besides the high risk of coagulopathy, APL has two unique features, namely a high sensitivity to anthracyclines, possibly due to low expression of P glycoprotein, and marked responsiveness to ATRA and ATO. ATRA as a single agent achieves a high CR rate, but relapse was common unless consolidation chemotherapy was administered. Several clinical trials demonstrated that ATRA administered prior to chemotherapy was associated with

improved survival compared with chemotherapy alone due to reduced relapse, but these results were subsequently improved by the simultaneous administration of ATRA with chemotherapy, until CR was achieved. Although anthracyclines are key components of therapy, questions remain as to whether any one anthracycline is superior to the others, and whether the addition of other agents, especially cytarabine, improves outcome.

Supportive care during induction therapy is of critical importance. ATRA usually leads to rapid resolution of DIC, but support of coagulation by transfusion of fresh frozen plasma, cryoprecipitate, and platelets must be used as necessary until the coagulopathy resolves. A standard approach is maintenance of fibrinogen above $1\,g/l$ and platelets above $50 \times 10^9/l$. A risk of both ATRA and ATO is the development of a differentiation syndrome characterized by fever, tachypnoea, hypoxia, pulmonary infiltrates, headaches, and confusion in around 10% of patients. This complication is more common with presenting white cell count above $10 \times 10^9/l$, and should be treated with dexamethasone $10\,mg/m^2$ twice daily. ATRA/ATO should be temporarily discontinued if the syndrome is severe, or fails to respond to dexamethasone. Up to 40% of children present with a white blood cell count over $10 \times 10^9/l$, associated with M3 variant morphology, FLT3-ITD, and a higher risk of treatment failure due to both increased induction deaths and relapse.

Evaluation of treatment response must be circumspect. Abnormal promyelocytes may persist for 40–50 days, and CR is achieved in virtually all patients. Molecular and cytogenetic tests at the end of induction have no prognostic value, and must not be misinterpreted as indicating resistant disease. Anthracycline-based consolidation therapy is associated with very high levels of molecular remission. The advantage of continued ATRA after remission has been achieved has not been proven in a randomized study. The role of cytarabine in consolidation is controversial. Variables confounding conclusions from the published series include differing combinations of anthracyclines, and total anthracycline doses. Cytarabine may be important in regimens with lower total anthracycline exposure.

The role of ATO is still under evaluation. Several studies have demonstrated high CR rates with ATO alone or especially when combined with ATRA. ATO has now been included in phase III studies for newly diagnosed disease in both children and adults, and as salvage therapy for molecular or hematologic relapse. The role of hemopoietic stem cell transplant (HSCT) is very limited. Children with persistent molecular disease (by end-stage polymerase chain reaction with low sensitivity of 10-3) at the end of consolidation, or following relapse, are considered for HSCT after salvage therapy with ATO and gemtuzamab. Autologous HSCT may be adequate in children who become molecularly negative, with allogeneic HSCT reserved for persistent molecular positivity. Molecular monitoring is important, as a better outcome has been shown for patients diagnosed and treated for molecular relapse rather than at hematological relapse.

Maintenance therapy with ATRA, mercaptopurine and methotrexate is of unproven benefit in APL. A study by the European

APL group indicated that maintenance was beneficial, especially for patients with a high white cell count at presentation, whereas a study by the GIMEMA group showed no benefit for maintenance (although the total dose of anthracycline was higher in this study). It is possible that efficacy is related to the intensity of initial therapy, that is maintenance is of benefit for patients receiving less intensive protocols with lower doses of anthracycline in induction and consolidation. Iin the future, the use of molecular monitoring may allow selection of patients for maintenance therapy.

Myelodysplastic syndromes

Classifications of myelodysplastic syndromes

Myelodysplastic and myeloproliferative disorders comprise under 5% of childhood leukemias. The myelodysplastic syndromes (MDS) were historically characterized by a cellular marrow with peripheral pancytopenia and were first described as smouldering leukemia or pre-leukemia; they were predominantly disorders of late adult life and have since been well classified in the extensive adult literature. Early reports of chronic leukemias in childhood made no distinction between chronic myeloid leukemia (CML) and what would now be deemed MDS and only in the last few years have any serious attempts been made to classify pediatric MDS [20], which differs in many important respects from the disease in adults [21–26].

The morphologic classification of MDS in adults was rationalized by the efforts of the FAB group (Table 8.5) [27], and terms such as pre-leukemia tended to be abandoned in favour of the appropriate FAB type of MDS. This FAB classification is unsatisfactory for childhood MDS for a number of reasons:

• Many children with MDS have a monocytosis which thus automatically classes them as having chronic myelomonocytic leukemia (CMML) which is clinically inappropriate [28].

• There are a number of patients, e.g. those with eosinophilia and dysplastic blood and bone marrows, for whom it is impossible to assign an FAB type.

• Both therapy-induced MDS and MDS occurring in association with congenital bone marrow disorders may defy classification by the scheme, the bone marrow showing hypoplasia and/or fibrosis in addition to dysplasia.

More recently, an international consensus has been developed, adapting the recent WHO classification (Table 8.6) [29], and subdividing MDS in children into a proliferative group comprising juvenile myelomonocytic leukemia, a group of adult-type MDS, and a number of very rare or secondary disorders [30]. MDS and AML of Down's Syndrome are dealt with separately.

Epidemiology and causes

There have been a number of recent estimates of the incidence of MDS in childhood. A population-based study in Denmark estimated that the incidence of MDS approximated that of AML at 4.0 new cases/million children/year, thus representing 9% of all hematologic malignancies, whereas in the northern region in England the estimated incidence was 0.53/million or 1% of malignancies [30]. A report from the national UK childhood MDS registry gave an annual incidence of 1.4/million over a 10-year period, with around 15 new cases each year [31]. These discrepancies could be due in part to the inclusion or exclusion of more aggressive forms (e.g. refractory anemia with excess of blasts in transformation) as either MDS or AML rather than any true variation in incidence. The diagnosis of MDS implies the finding of consistent hematologic abnormalities over a period of time, thus excluding patients with morphologic abnormalities in association with infection which may resolve spontaneously or patients whose abnormalities progress to frank AML within weeks. The

Table 8.5 French-American-British (FAB) classification of myelodysplastic syndromes.

Type	Blood film	Bone marrow
Refractory anemia (RA)	Blasts < 1%	Blasts < 5%
RA with ringed sideroblasts (RARS)	As in RA	As in RA but > 15% of erythroblasts as ringed sideroblasts
RA with excess of blasts (RAEB)	Blasts < 5%	Blasts 5–20%
RAEB in transformation (RAEBt)	Blasts > 5% Auer rods	As RAEB but 20–30% blasts Auer rods
Chronic myelomonocytic leukemia (CMML)	Monocytes > 1 × 10⁹/l Blasts < 5%*	Blasts < 20%

* CMML in children is often associated with a higher blast count in the blood, but marrow blasts should not exceed 20% and Auer rods should not be present.

Table 8.6 Pediatric modification of the World Health Organization classification of myelodysplastic disorders.

Proliferative
Juvenile myelomonocytic leukemia

Down's syndrome disease
Transient abnormal myelopoiesis
Myeloid leukemia of Down syndrome

Myelodysplastic syndrome
Refractory cytopenia
Refractory anemia with excess blasts
Refractory anemia with excess blasts in transformation
Refractory anemia with ring sideroblasts*

Myelodysplasia with eosinophilia

Other

* Extremely rare in children.

Table 8.7 Conditions associated with myelodysplasia in children.

Congenital
Down's syndrome
Neurofibromatosis type I
Noonan syndrome
Fanconi anemia
Diamond-Blackfan anemia
Shwachman-Diamond syndrome
Severe congenital neutropenia
Familial myelodysplasia

Acquired
Aplastic anemia
Prior cytotoxic or radiation therapy

distinction between refractory anemia with an excess of blasts with or without transformation and AML is an arbitrary one since patients may present with an abnormal count but a low percentage of blasts in the marrow and develop overt AML within weeks or even days. The diagnosis of true MDS implies a more indolent course demonstrating consistent hematologic abnormalities without evolution to AML over a 2-month period. The distinction is helped by careful review of morphology since patients with true MDS will exhibit multilineage dysplasia and also by the cytogenetic findings; t(8;21), t(15;17), t(9;11) and inv (16) all being associated with de novo AML (see section on investigations).

MDS arises more rarely in the previously well child than acute myeloid or lymphoid leukemias. Its causes and associations are given in Table 8.7 and discussed in greater detail here.

A characteristic feature of MDS in childhood is a strong association with congenital disorders and genetic syndromes. In recent non-population-based reports between one-quarter and one-half of patients have shown some phenotypic abnormality. There are a number of families described in the literature with no apparent congenital or genetic abnormality in whom more than one member has developed MDS or AML. MDS with monosomy 7 has been described in infant siblings, but in other families more than one member has developed AML or MDS in later childhood or adult life, sometimes in association with a familial platelet storage pool disorder. In several instances, the development of MDS has been associated with evolution of a cytogenetic abnormality in the bone marrow, most often monosomy 7 or 5.

Immunosuppressive therapy with antilymphocyte globulin and cyclosporin A has improved survival in patients with acquired aplastic anemia, particularly those without a histocompatible sibling donor. However, children treated by immunosuppression are at increased risk of MDS [32]. Secondary MDS with a predilection to development of AML was first described in patients treated for Hodgkin's disease, multiple myeloma, and ovarian cancer who had received alkylating agents, and more recently after high-dose chemoradiotherapy and infusion of autologous

bone marrow [33–37]. By contrast, secondary acute leukemia in patients who have been treated with topoisomerase II inhibitors usually occurs without any dysplastic prodrome.

Alkylating agent-induced MDS/AML tends to occur after 4–5 years, is associated with a preceding phase of MDS and is characterized by deletions from chromosomes 5 and 7. This disease is refractory to chemotherapy. The second, more recently described type of acute leukemia, is related to treatment with topoisomerase II inhibitors and is associated with a shorter induction period and presentation as acute leukemia without a preceding MDS. Alkylating agent-induced MDS does not always conform to the FAB subtypes. There is often a relatively low proportion of blasts at the time of diagnosis but this is accompanied by marked morphologic changes in all cell lines. There may be basophilia in both blood and bone marrow and cellularity is variable, with fibrosis in some cases producing a dilute aspirate. Clonal cytogenetic abnormalities are found in >90% of cases and the majority involves chromosomes 5 and 7. Topoisomerase inhibitor-related leukemia, which may be lymphoblastic or myeloblastic, has been more systematically studied in children because of its increased incidence in children with ALL receiving intensive epipodophyllotoxin treatment. This risk is protocol dependent. In one series, secondary AML was diagnosed in 21 of 734 patients treated for ALL [38]; the overall cumulative risk was 3.8% at 6 years, but in a subgroup of children receiving epipodophyllins weekly or twice weekly the risk was 12%. The scheduling of drug administration influenced the development of AML; the total dose, type of leukemia and radiotherapy had no influence on the risk of AML [39]. More detailed study showed that the majority of patients had myeloid or myelomonocytic leukemia and that chromosomal translocations predominantly involved the 11q23 region, most commonly as t(9;11) or t(11;19).

More recently, another group of therapy-related leukemias has been described in association with t(8;21), inv(16) and t(8;16) and t(15;17) after topoisomerase inhibitor therapy, alkylating agent therapy, or anthracycline therapy. These do not usually have a dysplastic prodrome and the risk factors have not been so precisely defined, but there is a similar correlation between the cytogenetic findings, morphology, and response to treatment, as in de novo AML, so that patients may respond to chemotherapy [40].

Clinical presentation

The symptoms and signs of MDS are more insidious than those of acute leukemia, and the diagnosis may even be made incidentally. Pallor is common, bacterial infections may be a consequence of neutropenia or defective neutrophil function and bruising may be due to thrombocytopenia or defective platelet function. Patients may also present with a prolonged history of repeated infections which is suggestive of congenital immune deficiency. Some children with juvenile myelomonocytic leukemia (JMML) develop weight loss and failure-to-thrive. Lymph node enlargement is unusual except in JMML. The liver and spleen may be enlarged or impalpable. A characteristic skin rash may occur on the face or trunk in JMML, and occasionally in infants with other types of MDS in association with monosomy 7.

JMML is an extremely heterogeneous disease which is more common in boys and in children aged less than 2 years. There is an association with neurofibromatosis, which may be found in 14% of patients, and Noonan syndrome. The clinical spectrum varies from a relatively benign disease in infants with hepatosplenomegaly and monocytosis to the classical disease usually in older children with bleeding, thrombocytopenia, enlarged lymph nodes and splenomegaly. Progression of the disease is accompanied by wasting, fever, infections, bleeding and pulmonary infiltrations. The typical skin rash, which may precede other symptoms by months, is classically of a butterfly distribution but may be more extensive, and on biopsy shows a non-specific infiltration with lymphocytes and histiocytes. The appearance of the blood film is more diagnostic than that of the bone marrow, and classically shows abnormal monocytes and blast cells with dysplasia in all cell lines.

The original detailed hematologic description of JMML has been complemented by a recent retrospective review of 110 cases strictly classified by the FAB criteria, except that >5% blasts were allowed in the blood. The median leukocyte count was $35 \times 10^9/l$ and exceeded $100 \times 10^9/l$ in only 7% of cases, eosinophilia was present in 8% of cases and basophilia in 28% while over half the patients had thrombocytopenia of $<50 \times 10^9/l$.

Investigations
General considerations
• Table 8.8 gives the diagnostic criteria for MDS and these criteria should be specifically sought for during investigation. It is important to consider differential diagnosis in this rare condition.

Table 8.8 Diagnostic criteria for myelodysplasia and juvenile monocytic leukemia in children.

At least two of the following
Blood cytopenia
Bilineage dysplasia
Excess of blasts in the bone marrow
Cytogenetic clone in bone marrow

Diagnostic criteria for juvenile myelomonocytic leukemia

Essential
Monocyte count $>1 \times 10^9/l$
<20% blasts in the bone marrow
Absence of t(9;22)

Plus two from
White blood count $>10 \times 10^9/l$
Myeloid precursors on blood film
Cytogenetic clone in bone marrow
Hypersensitivity to granulocyte-macrophage colony stimulating factor (GM-CSF)

• In the diagnosis of MDS (Table 8.8), it is essential to examine the blood film and bone marrow in tandem. The blood film is often more informative in reaching a diagnosis. A trephine biopsy of the bone marrow should be obtained in all cases and important observations include overall cellularity of the bone marrow, relative proportions, and morphology of the three cell lines, especially the megakaryocytes, presence of fibrosis and reticulin, and of abnormally-localized immature precursor cells (ALIP). These are aggregates of myeloblasts and promyelocytes in the intertrabecular region in the bone marrow biopsy.
• Other investigations, such as measurement of haemoglobin F (HbF), neutrophil function, and platelet function may serve to confirm abnormalities of development of the three cell lines. Measurement of the HbF before any transfusions of red cells is essential in JMML. Immunologic abnormalities may include low immunoglobulins, autoantibodies or even abnormalities of lymphocyte subsets. There may be antinuclear antibodies, anti-IgG antibodies, and autoimmune haemolysis and thrombocytopenia.
• It may be necessary to exclude congenital viral infections. The hematologic appearances of HIV infection in adults may mimic MDS but this presentation has not been described in children.

Investigation of juvenile myelomonocytic leukemia
A characteristic feature of JMML is an increase in the HbF level, which may increase progressively as the disease progresses, and a fetal pattern of alpha-globin chain synthesis. This is accompanied by a raised mean corpuscular volume (MCV), fetal pattern of 2,3-DPG and red cell enzyme production, red cell i/I antigen and carbonic anhydrase. While the diagnosis usually presents little difficulty, some patients with classic clinical features, including a grossly raised HbF, have a blood film with dominant normoblasts, almost suggestive of erythroleukemia, while in others the distinction from monocytic AML may be a fine one. Cytogenetic analysis in classical JMML with a grossly raised HbF is usually normal, but monosomy 7 may be found in some cases.

Investigation of refractory anemia
Refractory anemia must be distinguished from secondary changes due to systemic inflammatory disorders, congenital dyserythropoietic anemias and megaloblastic anemia and the presence of clonal cytogenetic abnormalities is helpful in confirming the diagnosis; without such abnormalities the diagnosis should be entertained with caution.

Refractory anemia with ringed sideroblasts (RARS) is exceptionally rare in pediatrics with only one case identified in the UK registry and can only be diagnosed with confidence in the presence of a cytogenetic abnormality. Several sideroblastic disorders must be excluded. Congenital sideroblastic anemia, due to abnormalities of heme synthesis, is usually associated with a dimorphic blood film; abnormalities of megakaryocytes and granulocytes are not seen. Sideroblastic anemia is also a feature of mitochondrial cytopathies, a group of disorders characterized by cortical neurologic impairment, metabolic acidosis and multiorgan involvement. The most typical of these is Pearson's syndrome of pancreatic insufficiency, neutropenia and a bone marrow showing vacuolated precursors and ringed sideroblasts. Hematologic abnormalities may be the dominant and indeed the only clinical feature of mitochondrial cytopathies at presentation and thus the distinction from MDS may be difficult. Mitochondrial cytopathies should be excluded in any patient with apparent sideroblastic anemia and it may be necessary to look for abnormal mitochondrial DNA on several occasions and to perform a muscle biopsy to confirm the diagnosis.

Reduced cellularity is a feature of around one-third of children with refractory cytopenia, and minor dysplastic changes are frequently observed in acquired aplastic anemia so on occasion there may be diagnostic uncertainty in distinguishing these disorders. The hypoplastic trephine appearances, absence of ALIP and absence of cytogenetic abnormalities in aplasia should help to make the distinction apparent.

The significance of cytogenetic abnormality

Cytogenetic abnormalities are found in about 50% of cases of primary MDS in both children and adults and in > 90% of patients with therapy-induced MDS. The results of cytogenetic analyses in children with JMML and MDS and included in the UK national registry are shown in Table 8.9. The most notable distinction between the cytogenetic findings in MDS and those in AML is the predominance of whole chromosome losses or partial deletions and the relative infrequency of translocations in MDS.

Monosomy 7 has a strongly adverse prognostic significance in refractory cytopenia and refractory anemia with excess blasts (RAEB), whilst age over 2 years, high HbF, and low platelet count are adverse in JMML.

Treatment of myelodysplastic syndromes

There is limited information about the role of chemotherapy in children with MDS as those data available are selected series, and differentiate poorly between the different FAB or WHO types. Generally it is possible to state:

Table 8.9 Cytogenetic findings in children with juvenile myelomonocytic leukaemia (JMML) and myelodysplasia (MDS) in the UK registry.

Abnormality	JMML (%)	MDS (%)
Normal karyotype	66	37
Monosomy 7	15	32
Other 7 abnormality	1.6	8
Trisomy 8	3.2	8
Complex	4.8	0
Others	9.6	13.6
Failed		1.3

- RAEB has responded more poorly to chemotherapy than *de novo* AML.
- Refractory anemia is unresponsive.
- JMML is not cured by chemotherapy, although temporary control of symptoms may be achieved.

In a series from the United Kingdom, children with RAEB in transformation had similar survival (63%) to those with *de novo* AML when treated with the same chemotherapy [41]. Although children with typical AML cytogenetic changes were excluded it was unclear whether all these children had stable MDS before treatment. Outcome for children with RAEB was significantly worse (28%). Monosomy 7 carried a strong adverse prognosis in both groups, and after allowance for adverse cytogenetics, which were more common in MDS, survival was similar to that for children with de novo AML.

High-dose chemotherapy and/or radiotherapy with SCT is the only curative treatment for most patients with MDS [42, 43]. The choice between chemotherapy alone for conditioning and regimens including TBI is in part dictated by consideration of the potential late effects of treatment, naturally an issue of extreme concern in the growing child (see late effects section). Currently, therefore, it seems appropriate to use chemotherapy alone as a preparative regimen, at least in standard transplants from an HLA-identical sibling. Reduced intensity conditioning may be appropriate for selected children with refractory cytopenia, for example children with normal cytogenetics or hypocellular bone marrows, or those with other organ system abnormalities and at increased risk of treatment toxicity.

There is a risk of relapse after SCT as after all other forms of treatment for MDS. This varies with the type and stage of MDS, and the type of donor and the results of treatment after relapse are unsatisfactory. Donor leukocyte infusions have shown some promise in the management of relapse in JMML, and should be considered as part of therapy in this setting [44].

Refractory anemia

An expectant approach is reasonable if the patient is well, not blood-product dependent, and has no evidence of disease progression, and is recommended particularly in the absence of any cytogenetic abnormality. Children who are transfusion dependent, with failure to thrive, infections or monosomy 7 should be considered for matched donor SCT.

Refractory anemia with excess of blasts and RAEB in transformation

In many national studies these patients are eligible for treatment with chemotherapy as if they had frank AML. In most centers these children are eligible for SCT, at least if they have a matched donor. However, the use of chemotherapy where SCT is planned is contentious, and many centres recommend elective SCT without prior AML chemotherapy in stable patients. If chemotherapy is used, and a CR obtained, it is reasonable to withhold SCT in children who do not have an adverse karyotype.

Juvenile monomyelocytic leukemia

Most children with JMML require SCT [43, 45]. In ill children, cytoreduction by chemotherapy and/or splenectomy are beneficial before SCT. A small proportion of children, especially those with Noonan syndrome, who clinically appear to have JMML have an indolent course, and gradually stabilize. Such individuals then remain well indefinitely. The molecular basis for this behaviour needs elucidation.

Myelodysplastic syndromes with eosinophilia

A raised eosinophil count is characteristic of chronic myeloproliferative disorders, CMML and the idiopathic hypereosinophilic syndrome, and may be secondary to infections or infestation. Rarely, children have eosinophilia and myelodysplasia, and this eosinophilic MDS is associated with translocations involving chromosome 5q [46, 47]. Other children have mutations of chromosome 4 at q12, with constitutive activation of a fusion tyrosine kinase gene formed between the platelet derived growth factor and the FIP-like-1 gene [48]. Recently, successful therapy with the tyrosine kinase inhibitor imatinib has been described in a number of these patients, and the mutation should be screened for in children with eosinophilic MDS.

Although both hydroxyurea and interferon therapy have been recommended in eosinophilic MDS, this has not been born out in clinical experience, and SCT would appear to be the most appropriate form of treatment provided that there is strong evidence of a clonal disorder.

Therapy-related myelodysplastic syndromes

There is relatively little reported pediatric experience in the management of secondary malignancies. It appears that the response to treatment can be predicted by the biology of the leukemia, but any remissions achieved tend to be short lived. Thus, secondary AML with chromosome 5 and 7 abnormalities is highly resistant to chemotherapy and while remissions can be achieved with combination chemotherapy in children with 11q23 leukemia, and even in half those receiving 2-chlorodeoxyadenosine as a single agent, the long-term survival rate is extremely poor. The only exception to this poor prognosis is the small group of patients with more favorable translocations such as t(8;21) or t(15;17), who tend to have a better response to treatment.

A recent study of intensive chemotherapy for secondary AML showed a 2-year disease-free survival of only 8% for patients with abnormal cytogenetics, thus confirming the dismal prognosis. It would appear that SCT affords the only chance of cure.

Down's syndrome and myeloid malignancy

Classification and pathogenesis

The association between Down's syndrome (DS) and leukemia was first described by Krivit and Good in 1957 [49]. The overall risk of leukemia is increased 10–20 fold, and is especially marked in the first 5 years of life, when it is 50 times that in normal children.

The spectrum of myeloid disease includes:
- A usually self-limiting myeloproliferative disorder of the newborn called transient abnormal myelopoiesis (TAM) or transient leukemia (TL) [50].
- MDS.
- AML [51].

MDS and AML in DS are closely linked with biological and clinical features distinct from the diseases in non-DS children, and are now recognized as a single specific entity. Myeloid leukemia of Down's syndrome (ML-DS) is the proposed WHO classification [52].

Although there are insufficient data to be precise regarding the incidence of TAM in DS, best estimates suggest 10–20% of all DS babies may be affected. The leukemic blasts in TAM and ML-DS are typically, but not exclusively, classified as FAB group M7. Recently, GATA-1 mutations have been described in DNA extracted from blast cells in DS children with TAM and ML-DS, and are already considered pathognomonic [53]. GATA-1 mutations have also been detected in Guthrie spot cards of several DS infants without TAM, although follow up was insufficient to exclude the later development of ML-DS in these infants. GATA-1 is a transcription factor necessary for the development of normal megakaryocytes, erythrocytes, eosinophils and mast cells, and in animal knockout models, absence of GATA-1 results in increased megakaryocyte proliferation with megakaryocyte dysplasia, differentiation arrest, and apoptosis in erythroid progenitors. As TAM is self-limiting, further unidentified genetic changes are considered necessary to produce the ML-DS phenotype.

Gene dosage or disomy of a leukemia predisposition gene or genes regulating haemopoiesis on chromosome 21 is a presumed mechanism of leukemogenesis in DS, although there is a lack of clear evidence to favor this hypothesis. The AML-1 gene (on chromosome 21 at q22.1-22.2), a partner in several leukemia translocations implicated in ALL, AML and MDS, is situated within the critical region for DS (21q22), and has a role in megakaryocyte differentiation, but has no proven role in ML-DS.

Clinical presentation and investigation

Transient abnormal myelopoiesis may affect the fetus, and is a cause of hydrops fetalis and intrauterine death. However, the majority of affected infants are asymptomatic, and TAM is detected with leucocytosis and circulating blasts on blood counts and blood films undertaken for other reasons. Some infants also have hepatosplenomegaly or skin infiltrates. In those most severely affected there may be ascites, pleural, or pericardial effusions, or liver dysfunction with obstructive jaundice from hepatic fibrosis, due to tissue infiltration and production of platelet-derived growth factor. In this group the disease may prove fatal, but TAM is usually self-limiting, with resolution of clinical and laboratory features over several months. Around 25% of children diagnosed with TAM subsequently develop ML-DS between 1 and 4 years of age. Rarely, ML-DS evolves directly from TAM with no intervening period of normality.

Table 8.10 Results of treatment of acute myeloid leukemia in Down's syndrome.

Study	Anthracycline cumulative dose (mg/m^2)	Cytarabine cumulative dose (g/m^2)	CR rate (%)	Resistant disease (%)	Relapse (%)	Treatment related deaths (%)	Event-free survival (%)
BFM 98	220–240	23–29	100	0	6	5	89
NOPHO 93	350	49	95	–	11	–	83
CCG 2861/2891 standard	350	31.5	95	2	8	9	74
CCG 2861/2891 intensive	350	31.5	64	4	8	32	52
MRC AML 12	550	9.6	94	0	3	12	85

BFM, Berlin Frankfurt Munster group. NOPHO, Nordic Organisation for Paediatric Haematology Oncology. CCG, Children's Cancer Study Group. MRC, Medical Research Council. CR, complete remission.

In children with TAM, haemoglobin and neutrophil numbers are most often normal, but wide variation in platelet counts is found, from severe thrombocytopenia to marked thrombocytosis. The white cell count is elevated, on occasion to very high levels, with blasts on the blood film. The blasts are deeply basophilic and may demonstrate characteristic cytoplasmic blebbing. Nucleated red cells and fragments of megakaryocyte cytoplasm are often present on the blood film. The bone marrow is hypercellular with an increase in blasts proportionate to the changes in the blood. Dysplastic changes are common in the erythroid series and megakaryocytes, which are increased in number. Immunophenotyping shows the blasts to be myeloid (CD33, CD34) with expression of megakaryocyte (CD41, CD61), and often erythroid markers (glycophorin A). Aberrant expression of CD7, a T lymphoid marker, is commonly found. Cytochemistry is negative for myeloperoxidase, Sudan black, chloracetate esterase and periodic acid-Schiff, but diffusely positive for acid phosphatase and non-specific esterase. Bone marrow cytogenetics invariably reveals trisomy for chromosome 21, even in recorded cases of TAM in phenotypically normal infants. Additional clonal cytogenetic abnormalities occur uncommonly, but include pentasomy 21, additional chromosomes 12 and 14, and polyploidy with 57 chromosomes.

Therapy of myeloid leukemia of Down's syndrome

A remarkable feature of ML-DS is the sensitivity of the leukemia to therapy, with disease resistance and relapse uncommon [54]. Conversely, DS children suffer high rates of treatment toxicity, with an increased risk of treatment-related death, primarily due to mucositis and infection [55]. TAM also shows marked sensitivity to treatment, and short courses of low dose cytarabine have proved effective in reducing white blood cell count in selected children. A number of genes have been identified on chromosome 21 where gene dosage could influence the effectiveness of chemotherapy. Most particularly in regard to therapy for AML, overexpression of cystathionine alpha synthase appears to confer increased sensitivity to cytarabine in the blasts of children with ML-DS. Assay of Ara-C triphosphate levels has shown a median

fivefold increase to non-DS blasts. *In vitro* studies using the MTT assay indicate a 12-fold increase in sensitivity to cytarabine for ML-DS blasts compared with non-DS blasts. This study also demonstrated increased sensitivity to anthracyclines (two- to sevenfold), mitoxantrone (ninefold), and etoposide (20-fold) in ML-DS [56].

Results of studies by several collaborative groups are shown in Table 8.10. Given the high potential for cure in ML-DS, but the risk of complications of therapy, the refinement of treatment to optimize cure rates whilst minimizing toxicity is the major focus of modern treatment protocols. As studies using reduced doses of anthracycline have proved very effective and limit mucositis and infective deaths, contemporary regimens for ML-DS include reduced doses of anthracycline compared with those for other children with AML.

Most children with TAM require observation alone, usually as outpatients, and the blood count normalizes within several months. Children with complications may benefit from therapy with low dose cytarabine [57], e.g. 20 mg/m^2/day for up to 7 days, and it is increasingly common to electively start treatment promptly in children with high white cell counts. Several collaborative groups (BFM group, Children's Oncology Group) have recently established clinical and laboratory studies of TAM, including treatment guidelines, to improve the epidemiology, understanding and therapy of the disorder.

Strategy for follow-up and important late effects

Most relapses of AML occur in the first 2–3 years from diagnosis, with 60% of relapses in the first year. It is customary to review children every 4–6 weeks in the first year off treatment, gradually extending the interval between visits as the relapse risk declines. Molecular monitoring, where it is applicable, will have an impact on this approach, and children treated for APL now have routine off treatment bone marrows for detection of RAR-PML transcripts because early detection and salvage therapy is beneficial in these cases.

Late effects of AML chemotherapy, unlike those of SCT, are limited, although there is considerable concern regarding the lifetime risk of cardiac failure due to anthracycline cardiomyopathy. The best cardioprotection strategy is reduced exposure, and so dose reduction is a prime issue in contemporary trials. The use of cardioprotectants remains limited, and the efficacy of liposomal daunorubicin is being studied by the BFM group. There is risk of otoxicity due to the routine use of aminoglycosides in the management of febrile neutropenia and this occurs in some children despite routine monitoring of serum levels of these drugs. Otoxicity is especially prevalent in rare children who carry the A1555G mitochondrial DNA mutation, a cause of familial deafness which confers exceptional sensitivity to aminoglycoside ototoxicity. This mutation should be screened for if there is a history of familial deafness [58].

Total body irradiation (TBI) used in SCT is associated with additional complications and younger children are most vulnerable. Children who have received TBI have growth failure which is in part due to spinal shortening and partly to hypothalamic-pituitary failure; this will be exacerbated if there is chronic GVHD. Delayed puberty and gonadal failure are common and there is a variable risk of hypothyroidism, cataracts, and learning problems. The combination of busulfan and cyclophosphamide has not been subjected to such rigorous long-term follow up studies as TBI and it may induce sterility, but it is unlikely to have such a significant effect on skeletal growth and neuropsychologic development.

Novel therapeutic approaches

Gemtuzamab is a new agent with considerable promise in AML, both as a single drug, and as part of combination chemotherapy. The drug comprises a recombinant, humanized anti-CD33 antibody conjugated to the anti-tumor antibiotic calicheamicin, a DNA damaging agent. CD33 is expressed by myeloid precursors in bone marrow and over 80% of cases of AML. The drug is myelotoxic, but in particular is hepatotoxic causing elevation of bilirubin and transaminases, and veno-occlusive disease of the liver in a minority of patients. Gemtuzamab shows good activity in relapsed AML, and has now been incorporated into phase III studies in *de novo* disease in adults and children [59].

A variety of molecular changes have been identified that are associated with prognosis (Table 8.11), and hold promise as a method of further refining prognosis or offering the prospect of targeted therapy. Internal tandem duplications of FLT3 are clearly a poor prognostic factor, particularly where the mutated to wild type allelic ratio is high, and FLT3 mutations have been shown as the strongest prognostic factor within cytogenetically normal AML. There is no clear evidence that treatment intensification improves prognosis, and inhibition of constitutively activated FLT3 is now the subject of phase III studies. Mutations of c-kit are found in up to 40% of patients with CBF leukemia, and specific tyrosine kinase (TK) inhibitors have activity against specific c-kit mutations. Accordingly, phase III studies considering TK inhibition are of interest in these patients [60].

Table 8.11 Genetic alterations affecting prognosis in patients with acute myeloid leukemia and normal karyotypes.

Genetic change	Effect
Fms-related tyrosine kinase (FLT3) gene internal tandem duplications	Adverse prognosis, especially when high FLT3 mutant to wild type allele ratio
Mixed lineage leukemia (MLL) gene partial tandem duplication	Adverse prognosis
Brain and acute leukemia (BAALC) gene overexpression	Adverse prognosis
v-ets erythroblastosis virus E26 (ERG) oncogene overexpression	Adverse prognosis
Nucleophosmin (NPM1) gene mutations	Favourable in absence of FLT3-ITD
CCAAT/enhancer binding protein (CEBPA) gene mutations	Favourable prognosis

Summary and future directions for management

The prognosis of AML has steadily improved through a combination of intensive chemotherapy and better supportive care. Prognostic groups have been identified, largely based on cytogenetics and response to therapy. The role of SCT has been restricted. It is likely further refinement is possible by the incorporation of molecular markers. However, further improvements to the control of disease by adjustments in conventional chemotherapy protocols are likely to be limited. This is especially true for children with poor risk disease. Increasingly, strategies will be developed for subgroups of children; this has already proved necessary in APL and Down's syndrome, and new targeted therapies, for example to FLT3-ITD or the CBF pathway, are needed or are under evaluation. Treatment strategies for MDS are mainly based on SCT. Progress in these diseases depends on improved knowledge of underlying biology to identify useful targets and treatment strategies.

References

1 Webb DK, Harrison G, Stevens RF, Gibson BG, Hann IM, Wheatley K. Relationships between age at diagnosis, clinical features, and outcome of therapy in children treated in the Medical Research Council AML 10 and 12 trials for acute myeloid leukaemia. MRC Childhood Leukaemia Working Party. Blood 2001; 98: 1714–20.

2 Bennett J, Catovsky D, Daniel MT, et al. Proposals for the classification of the acute leukaemias. French-American-British (FAB) co-operative group. Br J Haematol 1976; 33: 451–8.

3 Harris NL, Jaffe ES, Diebold J, et al. The World Health Organization classification of neoplastic diseases of the haematopoietic and lymphoid tissues: report of the Clinical Advisory Committee Meeting, Airlie House, Virginia, November 1997. Histopathology 2000; 36: 69–86.

4 Grimwade D, Walker H, Oliver F, et al. The importance of diagnostic cytogenetics on outcome in AML: analysis of 1612 patients entered into the MRC AML 10 trial. Blood 1998; 92: 2322–33.

5 Hann IM, Stevens RF, Goldstone AH, et al. Randomised comparison of DAT and ADE as induction chemotherapy in children and younger adults with acute myeloid leukaemia. Results of the Medical Research Council's 10th AML trial (MRC AML 10) Blood 1997; 89: 2311–18.

6 Lie SO, Jonmundsson G, Mellander L, Siimes MA, Yssing M, Gustafsson G. A population-based study of 272 children with acute myeloid leukaemia treated on two consecutive protocols with differ-ent intensity: best outcome in girls, infants, and children with Down's syndrome. Nordic Society of Paediatric Haematology and Oncology (NOPHO). Br J Haematol 1996; 94, 82–8.

7 Creutzig U, Zimmermann M, Ritter J, et al. Treatment strategies and long-term results in pediatric patients treated in four consecutive AML-BFM trials. Leukemia 2005; 19: 2030–42.

8 Wheatley K, Burnett AK, Goldstone AH, et al. A simple, robust, vali-dated and highly predictive index for the determination of risk-directed therapy in acute myeloid leukaemia derived from the MRC AML 10 trial. United Kingdom Medical Research Council's Adult and Childhood Leukaemia Working Parties. Br J Haematol 1999; 107: 69–79.

9 Webb DK, Wheatley K, Harrison G, Stevens RF, Hann I. Outcome for children with relapsed acute myeloid leukaemia following initial therapy in the Medical Research Council (MRC) AML 10 trial. MRC Childhood Leukaemia Working Party. Leukaemia 1999; 13: 25–31.

10 Hann IM, Webb DK, Gibson BE, Harrison CJ. MRC trials in child-hood acute myeloid leukaemia. Ann Hematol 2004; 83(suppl): S108–112.

11 Gibson BE, Wheatley K, Hann IM, et al. Treatment strategies and longterm results in pediatric patients treated in consecutive UK AML trials. Leukemia 2005; 19: 2130–8.

12 Creutzig U, Berthlod F, Boos J, et al. Improved treatment results in children with AML. Results of study AML-BFM 93. Klinik Padiatrik 2001; 213: 175–85.

13 Creutzig U, Zimmermann M, Reinhardt D, Dworzak M, Stary J, Lehrnbecher T. Early deaths and treatment-related mortality in chil-dren undergoing therapy for acute myeloid leukaemia: analysis of the multicenter clinical trials AML-BFM 93 and AML-BFM 98. J Clin Oncol 2004; 22: 4384–93.

14 Smith FO, Alonzo TA, Gerbing RB, Woods WG, Arceci RJ. Long-term results of children with acute myeloid leukaemia: a report of 3 consecutive Phase III trials by the Childrens Cancer Group : CCG 251, CCG 213 and CCG 2891. Leukaemia 2005; 19; 2054–62.

15 Lange BJ, Smith FO, Feusner J, et al. Outcomes in CCG-2961, a Childrens Oncology Group phase 3 trial for untreated pediatric acute myeloid leukaemia: a report from the childrens oncology group. Blood 2008; 111: 1044–53.

16 Avvisati G, Lo Coco F, Diverio D, et al. AIDA in newly diagnosed acute promyelocytic leukaemia: a GRUPPO Italiano Malattie Ematologiche Maligne dell'Adulto (GIMEMA) pilot study. Blood 1996; 88: 1390–8.

17 Testi AM, Biondi A, Lo Coco F, et al. GIMEMA-AIEOPAID. A pro-tocol for the treatment of newly diagnosed acute promyelocytic leu-kaemia (APL) in children. Blood 2005; 106: 447–53.

18 Sanz MA, Martin G, Gonzalez M, et al. Risk adapted treatment of acute promyelocytic leukaemia with all trans retinoic acid and anthra-cycline chemotherapy: a multicenter study by the PETHEMA group. Blood 2004; 103: 1237–43.

19 Ortega JJ, Madero L, Martin G, et al. Treatment with all-trans retinoic acid and anthracycline monochemotherapy for children with acute promyelocytic leukaemia: a multicenter study by the PETHEMA group. Blood 2005; 23: 7632–40.

20 Passmore SJ, Hann IM, Stiller CA, et al. Pediatric myelodysplasia: a study of 68 children and a new prognostic scoring system. Blood 1995; 85: 1742–50.

21 Hasle H. Myelodysplastic syndromes in childhood. Classification, epidemiology, and treatment. Leukemia Lymphoma 1994;13: 11–26.

22 Smith KL, Johnson W. Classification of chronic myelocytic leukemia in children. Cancer 1974; 34: 670–9.

23 Nix WL, Fernbach DJ. Myeloproliferative diseases in childhood. Am J Ped Hematol Oncol 1981; 3: 397–407.

24 Brandwein JM, Horsman DE, Eaves AC, et al. Childhood myelodys-plasia: suggested classification as myelodysplastic syndromes based on laboratory and clinical findings. Am J Ped Hematol Oncol 1990; 12: 63–70.

25 Hardisty RM, Speed DE, Till M. Granulocytic leukaemia in child-hood. Br J Haematol 1964; 10: 551–66.

26 Castro-Malaspina H, Schaison G, Passe S, et al. Subacute and chronic myelomonocytic leukemia in children (juvenile CML). Cancer 1984; 54: 675–86.

27 Bennett JM, Catovsky D, Daniel MT, et al. Proposals for the classifica-tion of the myelodysplastic syndromes. Br J Haematol 1982 ; 51: 189–99.

28 Niemeyer CM, Arico M, Basso A, et al. Chronic myelomonocytic leukemia in childhood: a retrospective analysis of 110 cases. Blood 1997; 89: 3534–43.

29 Hasle H, Niemeyer CM, Chessells JM, et al. A pediatric approach to the WHO classification of myelodysplasia and myeloproliferative dis-eases. Leukemia 2003; 17: 277–82.

30 Hasle H, Kerndrup G, Jacobsen BB. Childhood myelodysplastic syn-drome in Denmark: incidence and predisposing conditions. Leukemia 1995: 9: 1569–72.

31 Passmore SJ, Chessells JM, Kempski H, Hann IM, Brownbill PA, Stiller CA. Pediatric MDS and JMML in the UK: a population based study of incidence and survival. Br J Haematol 2003; 121: 758–67.

32 Fuhrer M, Burdach S, Ebell W, et al. Relapse and clonal disease in children with aplastic anemia after immunosuppressive therapy (IST): the SAA 94 experience. German/Austrian Pediatric Aplastic Anemia Working Group. Klinic Padiatrica 1998; 210: 173–9.

33 Stone RM, Neuberg D, Soiffer R, et al. Myelodysplastic syndrome as a late complication following autologous bone marrow transplanta-tion for non-Hodgkin's lymphoma. J Clin Oncol 1994; 12: 2535–42.

34 Darrington DL, Vose JM, Anderson JR, et al. Incidence and charac-terization of secondary myelodysplastic syndrome and acute myelog-enous leukemia following high-dose chemoradiotherapy and autologous stem-cell transplantation for lymphoid malignancies. J Clin Oncol 1994; 12: 2527–34.

35 Park DJ, Koeffler HP. Therapy-related myelodysplastic syndromes. Sem Hematol 1996; 33: 256–73.

36 Le Beau MM, Àlbain KS, Larson RA, et al. Clinical and cytogenetic correlations in 63 patients with therapy related myelodysplastic syn-dromes and acute non lymphocytic leukemias: further evidence for characteristic abnormalities of chromosome nos 5 and 7. J Clin Oncol 1986; 4: 325–45.

37 Rubin CM, Arthur DC, Woods WG, et al. Therapy-related myelod-ysplastic syndrome and acute myeloid leukemia in children:

correlation between chromosomal abnormalities and prior therapy. Blood 1991; 78: 2982–8.

38 Pui C, Ribeiro RC, Hancock MI, et al. Acute myeloid leukemia in children treated with epipodophyllotoxins for acute lymphoblastic leukemia. N Engl J Med 1991; 325: 1682–7.

39 Pui C, Relling MV, Rivera GK, et al. Epipodophyllotoxin-related acute myeloid leukemia: a study of 35 cases. Leukemia 1995; 9: 1990–6.

40 Quesnel B, Kantarjian H, Bjergaard JP, et al. Therapy-related acute myeloid leukemia with t(8;21), inv(16), and t(8;16): a report on 25 cases and review of the literature. J Clin Oncol 1993; 11: 2370–9.

41 Webb DK, Passmore SJ, Hann IM, Harrison G, Wheatley K, Chessells JM. Results of treatment of children with refractory anaemia with excess blasts (RAEB) and RAEB in transformation (RAEBt) in Great Britain 1990–1999. Br J Haematol 2002; 117: 33–9.

42 Locatelli F, Zecca M, Niemeyer C, et al. Role of allogeneic bone marrow transplantation for the treatment of myelodysplastic syndromes in childhood. The European Working Group on Childhood Myelodysplastic Syndrome (EWOG-MDS) and the Austria-Germany-Italy (AGI) Bone Marrow Transplantation Registry.

43 Locatelli F, Nollke P, Korthof E, et al. Hematopoietic stem cell transplantation in children with juvenile myelomonocytic leukaemia (JMML) results of the EWOG-MDS/EBMT trial. Blood 2005; 105: 410–19.

44 Worth A, Rao K, Webb DK, Chessells J, Passmore J, Veys P. Successful treatment of juvenile myelomonocytic leukaemia relapsing after stem cell transplant using donor lymphocyte infusion. Blood 2003; 101: 1713–14.

45 Niemeyer C, Kratz CP. Paediatric myelodysplastic syndromes and juvenile myelomonocytic leukaemia: molecular classification and treatment options. Br J Haematol 2008; 140: 610–24.

46 Peltier I, Le Mome PJ, Rialland X, et al. Myelodysplastic syndrome with t(5;12) (q31;p12-p13) and eosinophilia: a pediatric case with review of literature. J Pediatr Hematol Oncol 1996; 18: 285–8.

47 Jam K, Kempski HM, Reeves BR. A case of myelodysplasia with eosinophilia having a translocation t(5;12)(q31;q13) restricted to myeloid cells but not involving eosinophils. Br J Haematol 1994; 87: 57–60.

48 Gotlib J, Cools J, Malone JM, Scgrier SL, Gilliland G, Coutre SE. The FIP1L1-PDGFRα fusion tyrosine kinase in hypereosinophilic

syndrome and chronic eosinophilic leukaemia: implications for diagnosis, classification and management. Blood 2004; 103: 2879–91.

49 Krivit W, Good RA. The simultaneous occurrence of leukaemia and mongolism; report of four cases Am J Dis Child 1956; 91: 218–22.

50 Zipursky A, Poon A, Doyle J. Leukemia in Down syndrome: a review. J Ped Hematol Oncol 1992; 9: 139–49.

51 Zipursky A, Thorner P, De Harven E, Christensen H, Doyle J. Myelodysplasia and acute megakaryoblastic leukaemia in Down's syndrome. Leukemia Res 1994; 18: 163–71.

52 Lange B. The management of neoplastic disorders of haematopoiesis in children with Down's syndrome. Br J Haematol 2000; 110: 512–24.

53 Crispino JD. GATA-1 mutations in Down syndrome: implications for biology and diagnosis of children with transient myeloproliferative disorder and acute megakaryoblastic leukaemia. Pediatr Blood Cancer 2005; 44: 40–4.

54 Rao A, Hills RE, Stiller C, O'Marcaigh A, Hann IM, Webb DK. Treatment for myeloid leukaemia of Down syndrome: experience in the United Kingdom and results from the Medical Research Council AML 10 and AML 12 trials. Br J Haematol 2006; 132: 576–83.

55 Webb DK. Optimising therapy for myeloid disorders of Down Syndrome. Br J Haematol 2005; 131: 3–7.

56 Zwaan CM, Kaspers GJ, Pieters R, et al. Different drug sensitivity profiles of acute myeloid and acute lymphoblastic leukaemia and normal peripheral blood mononuclear cells in children with and without Down syndrome. Blood 2002; 99: 245–51.

57 Al Kasim F, Doyle JJ, Massey GV et al. Incidence and treatment of potentially lethal diseases in transient leukaemia of Down syndrome. Pediatric Oncology Group study. J Pediatr Hematol Oncol 2002; 24: 9–13.

58 Leisner RJ, Leiper AD, Hann IM, Chessells JM. Late effects of intensive treatment for acute myeloid leukemia and myelodysplasia in childhood. J Clin Oncol 1994; 12: 916–24.

59 Aplenc R, Alonzo TA, Gerbing RB, et al. Safety and efficacy of gemtuzumab ozogamicin in combination with chemotherapy for pediatric acute myeloid leukaemia: a report from the Children's Oncology Group. J Clin Oncol 2008; 26: 2390–5.

60 Kottaridis PD, Gale RE, Linch DC. Flt3 mutations and leukaemia. Br J Haematol 2003; 122: 523–38.

9 Non-Hodgkin's Lymphoma

Angelo Rosolen and Lara Mussolin

Clinica di Oncoematologia Pediatrica, Azienda Ospedaliera-Università di Padova, Padova, Italy

Introduction

Non-Hodgkin's lymphoma (NHL) represents a group of malignancies that combine features typical of the acute leukemias with a number of characteristics of solid tumors. As with most solid tumors, NHL form masses and can often be diagnosed due to signs and symptoms that such masses may cause. Nevertheless, they are usually generalized diseases from their very onset and have patterns of spread that mimic the physiological migration pattern of lymphoid cells.

NHL are among the pediatric malignancies that have benefited the most from recent advances in diagnosis, staging and treatment and, whilst once considered fatal diseases, at present they are among the most curable malignancies of childhood.

Combination chemotherapy introduced in the 1960s for acute leukemias has been adopted also for NHL. Histological diagnosis also improved from the pure morphological classification to a more complex definition of the different entities based on the identification of T- and B-cell lineage specific markers that gradually were associated with well defined immunophenotypic and clinical features. Table 9.1 summarizes landmarks in the management of these tumors.

The history of NHL may be considered to begin in the 1950s in Uganda, when the surgeon Denis Burkitt first described a disease, still identified by his name, that was originally believed to be a sarcoma [1]. At the same time it was recognized that a proportion of childhood lymphomas, defined then as lymphosarcomas, in Europe and in the United States were indistinguishable from Burkitt lymphoma as it was described in Africa, although the characteristic presenting features of a jaw tumor without bone marrow involvement were less frequent.

In the same period, early reports of limited, single institution series of children, described a low percentage of survivors with rather limited and differing treatments [2], indicating though that a high percentage of patients suffered a leukemic transformation of their disease. By the late 1960s, investigators suggested that chemotherapy combined with radiotherapy could achieve cure in localized lymphosarcoma patients, thus encouraging further developments of combination therapy for these diseases [3]. From those early observations, it was accepted that radiation and multi-agent chemotherapy should be the standard approach to pediatric NHL. This was, however, accompanied by severe and irreversible acute and long-term side effects.

It was only with the first randomized trial conducted at St Jude Hospital, Memphis, that Murphy and Hustu demonstrated that addition of involved field irradiation to combination chemotherapy was of no benefit in advanced stage NHL [4].

In addition to the St Jude efforts in improving the outcome of pediatric NHL, a combination chemotherapy derived from the leukemia regimen LSA2-L2 in conjunction with local radiation therapy on bulky disease was used by Wollner at Memorial Sloan Kettering Hospital. Results of the leukemia-derived therapy in the treatment of childhood NHL proved successful and demonstrated that intensive combination chemotherapy could significantly impact the poor prognosis of NHL [5].

More recently, a great deal of clinical knowledge has been gained that has allowed improvement in the diagnostic and therapeutic approach to pediatric NHL. This has been supplemented by an increase in the biological knowledge in the field of NHL and has led to the awareness that several distinct clinical, histological and biological subtypes of NHL exist and that they require specific management and therapy in order to reach satisfactory results. It is the consequence of the combined efforts of clinicians, pathologists, and biologists that NHL, with few exceptions, can be now considered among the pediatric malignancies with the best cure rates. A summary of the most significant early achievements in the field of pediatric NHL is reported in Table 9.1.

Epidemiology

NHL represent approximately 10–15% of all malignancies of childhood and constitutes the third most frequent group of

Pediatric Hematology and Oncology, 1st edition. Edited by Edward J. Estlin, Richard J. Gilbertson, and Robert F. Wynn. © 2010 Blackwell Publishing Ltd.

Table 9.1 Historical overview of early significant achievements in the field of pediatric non-Hodgkin's lymphoma (NHL).

Author/Group	Period	Findings	Reference
Denis Burkitt, Uganda	1958	First description of lymphoma (defined as a sarcoma of the jaw)	[1]
Memorial Hospital, New York	1958	Report of a series of 69 children with lymphosarcoma; 17% survivors with surgery, radiotherapy and single agent chemotherapy	[2]
St Jude Children Hospital, Memphis	1971	Effectiveness of multi-agent chemotherapy and radiotherapy	[3]
St Jude Children Hospital, Memphis	1975–78	First randomized clinical trial: no benefit of radiotherapy in addition to combination chemotherapy in advanced stage NHL	[4]
Memorial Hospital, New York	1976	Effectiveness of multi-agent chemotherapy used for acute lymphoblastic leukemia (LSA2-L2 regimen) in advanced stage NHL	[5]
Children's Cancer Study Group, USA	1977–79	Importance of stage and of histological subtype for treatment outcome; demonstration of differential efficacy of different chemotherapy regimen on lymphoblastic NHL	[7]
Pediatric Oncology Group, USA	1976–79	Efficacy of the leukaemia-like regimen LSA2-L2 in lymphoblastic lymphoma	[8]
Berlin-Frankfurt-Munster (BFM) Group, Germany	1975–81	Confirmed the prognostic relevance of stage, histology and immunophentotype in pediatric NHL	[9]
Societè Francaise de Oncologie Pediatrique (SFOP), France	1986	Efficacy of high-dose methotrexate and cytosine-arabinoside in B-cell NHL and B-cell acute leukemia	[10]
Berlin-Frankfurt-Munster (BFM) Group, Germany	1983–90	Optimization of outcome using stratification of therapy by biological subtype and stage	[11]

cancers in Europe and USA, after leukemias and central nervous system tumors. According to the National Cancer Institute (NCI) Surveillance, Epidemiology and End Results program (SEER), the annual incidence rate of NHL in the age group 0–19 years was 1.1 per 100 000 in the period 1999–2003 [6]. In the recent epidemiological reports for Western Countries, NHL constituted approximately 7% of all cancers in individuals below 20 years of age. Unlike Hodgkin's lymphoma that has a bimodal age distribution, NHL show a steady increase with age, although specific NHL categories have significant differences in age-distribution. Males are affected almost twice as frequently as females.

There is evidence that NHL incidence in childhood has increased during the last decades. During the period 1988–1997, the overall incidence of NHL was 9.4 per million in children under the age of 15 years with an increase in incidence rate of 0.9% per year on average. In adolescents aged 15–19 years, the age-specific incidence rate was 15.9 per million, increasing annually by 1.7% [12]. This increase in NHL prevalence was also observed in the USA.

It should also be considered that the incidence and relative frequency of NHL varies by geographic regions: within Europe, the South has the highest incidence rates for the individual diagnostic subgroups. The incidence of NHL is significantly higher in adults compared with children and this may reflect, at least in part, the different cellular composition of the immune system at different ages and, possibly, the different exposure to lymphomagenic stimuli, as environmental agents, that have been implicated in NHL pathogenesis.

In addition to the marked difference in incidence from region to region of the world, the relative frequency of the different types of NHL also varies greatly. In equatorial Africa, around 50% of all childhood cancers are NHL, and this is mostly the consequence of the high incidence of Burkitt lymphoma and the low incidence of acute leukemias, based on available information. In Europe and the USA 50–60% of NHL are mature B-cell NHL (Burkitt, Burkitt-like, large B-cell lymphomas), 30% are lymphoblastic lymphomas, 10–15% are anaplastic large cell NHL and less that 5% other rare histological subtypes.

It is especially important to distinguish the epidemiology of endemic (African) and sporadic Burkitt lymphoma. The incidence of Burkitt lymphoma in equatorial Africa is far higher than in Europe and USA, with an intermediate incidence in other regions of the world, from which, however, we lack reliable epidemiological data. African Burkitt lymphoma has distinct clinical features compared with the sporadic form (Table 9.2), and they include site of presentation, association with Epstein Barr virus (EBV) infection and characteristics of the chromosomal translocations involving the MYC oncogene. EBV genomes are found in more than 90% of the tumors in Africa, but only in 10–20% in sporadic Burkitt lymphoma. Also, a striking difference is that the vast majority of children have been EBV infected before the age of 3 years in Africa, whereas in the USA and Europe most individuals experience primary EBV infection during adolescence. Although the role of EBV is not fully understood yet, the expression of the EBV protein EBNA-1, that has some tumorigenic activity, is believed to play a role in the transformation process leading a normal B-lymphocyte to become a malignant cell in young individuals. This may have some relationships with the proliferation potential of lymphocytes in young children but is likely helped by the concomitance of other infections affecting individuals in the same region, such as malaria, that causes immunosuppression and has the same geographic distribution as Burkitt lymphoma in Africa.

Classification

NHL differ significantly in children compared with adults. In children, NHL are typically high grade, clinically aggressive, tumors whereas in adults the majority of NHL are low-grade lymphomas [4, 13, 14]. Contrary to adult lymphomas, NHL in childhood are diffuse cancers and follicular/nodular lymphomas are rare.

Immunophenotypically pediatric NHL are of T-cell phenotype in approximately 40% of the cases, whereas in adults T-cell NHL make up less than 10% of NHL.

A number of different classifications exist for NHL as they have developed based initially on morphology and cytochemical staining. They have evolved to classification systems incorporating immunophenotypic and molecular characteristics, thus giving more objective diagnostic elements to the pathologist. The most recent and used classification systems are the REAL [15] and the WHO (World Health Organization) [16] classification systems. However, in children there are four major categories of NHL, whose features are summarized in Table 9.3:

- B-cell NHL
- Lymphoblastic lymphomas
- Anaplastic large cell lyphoma
- Other subtypes, including peripheral T-cell lymphomas, follicular lymphomas and other rare entities that in total represent less than 3–5% of the cases.

Clinical presentation

Children with NHL usually present with clinical features that depend on histological subtype, localization, and stage of disease [17, 18]. In contrast to older patients who most often present with lymph node disease, children commonly have extranodal disease involving the abdomen (35–45% of cases), mediastinum (25–30%), or head and neck (25–30%) (Figure 9.1).

There is a close relationship between primary site of disease at presentation and Burkitt and lymphoblastic histologic subtypes. With very few exceptions, patients with Burkitt lymphoma present with primary involvement of the abdomen or head and neck region but not with mediastinum involvement, whereas children with lymphoblastic lymphoma usually have a mediastinal or head and neck presentation, but very rarely abdominal primary.

Often multiple sites are involved and dissemination to bone marrow (BM) and central nervous system (CNS) are not infrequent at diagnosis. This is a consequence of the characteristics of pediatric NHL as rapidly growing tumors, with a high cellular growth fraction, short doubling times ranging from 12 hours to a few days [19], and with a high predisposition to dissemination to distant sites via the blood stream.

Abdominal primary

In Europe and the USA, children with Burkitt and Burkitt-like lymphoma present with an abdominal mass in about 80% of the cases [20]. Although at physical examination the main finding is a palpable mass, often of large size, there are two types of abdominal primary.

- The first is a diffuse abdominal involvement of the mesentery and omentum with frequent involvement of the kidney, liver, and spleen and possible dissemination to the bone marrow and CNS. Patients often complain of abdominal pain or swelling, changes in bowel habits, nausea and vomiting with gastrointestinal bleeding and/or perforation possible, although infrequent before starting treatment.

Table 9.2 Characteristics of sporadic and endemic Burkitt lymphoma in children.

	Sporadic	Endemic
Average annual incidence	0.4 per 100 000	10 per 100 000
Sites involved	Abdomen, bone marrow, Waldeyer's ring	Jaw, abdomen, orbit, central nervous system, paraspinal
Association with Epstein Barr virus	15%	95%
MYC breakpoint in the t(8;14) chromosomal translocation	Within MYC gene	Upstream of the MYC gene

Table 9.3 Summary of World Health Organization categories, immunophenotype and major clinical features of childhood non-Hodgkin's lymphoma (NHL).

Histologic subtype	Immunophenotype	Cytogenetics	Primary site
Burkitt/Burkitt-like lymphoma, large B-cell lymphoma	B-cell	t(8;14), t(2;8), t(8;22)	Abdomen, head and neck
Lymphoblastic lymphoma	Precursor T-cell (80%), precursor B-cell (20%)	Many abnormalities	Medistinum, lymph-nodes
Anaplastic large cell lymphoma	T-cell or null	t(2;5)	Lymph-nodes, skin, mediastinum

Parotid 3 (0.9%)

Maxillary sinus 5 (1.5%)

Rhynopharynx 18 (5.6%)

Waldeyer ring 44 (13.6%)

Mediastinum 32 (10%)

Abdomen 160 (50%)

Testis/ovaries 1 (0.3%)

Lymph nodes 37 (11%)

Skin 2 (0.6%)

Bone 21 (6.5%)

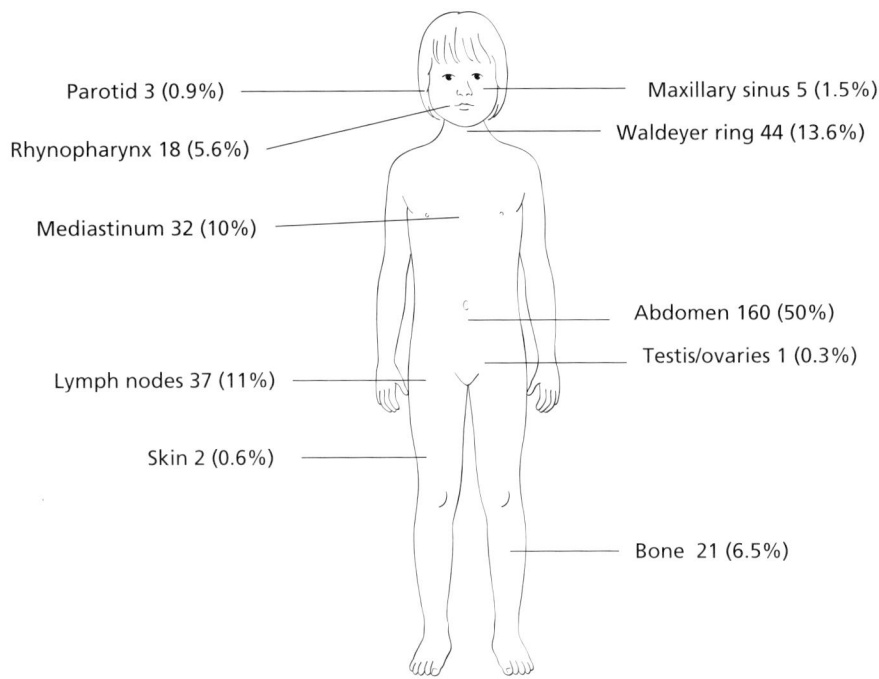

(a) B-cell LNH: total 323

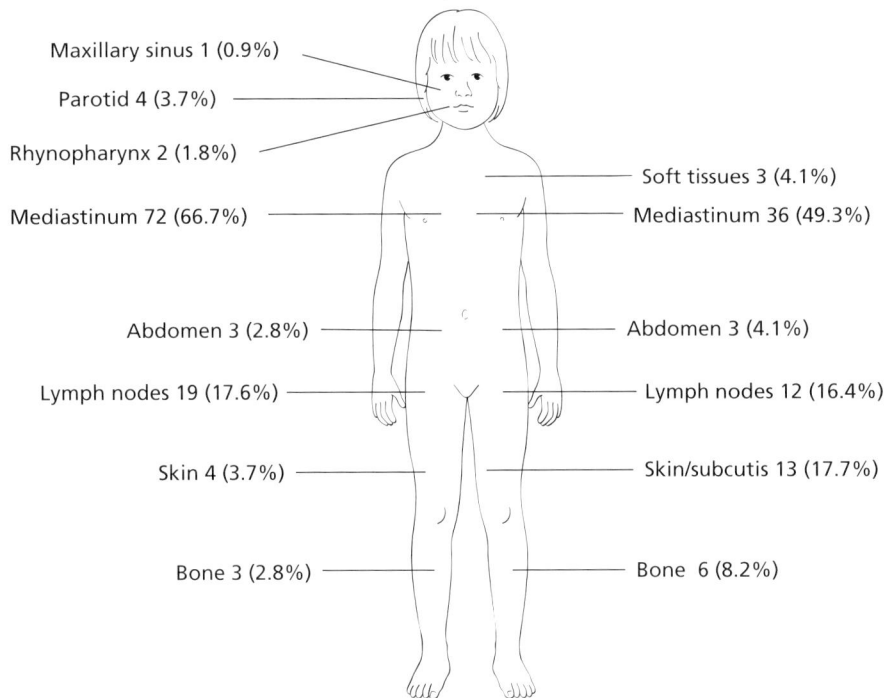

Maxillary sinus 1 (0.9%)

Parotid 4 (3.7%)

Rhynopharynx 2 (1.8%)

Soft tissues 3 (4.1%)

Mediastinum 72 (66.7%)

Mediastinum 36 (49.3%)

Abdomen 3 (2.8%)

Abdomen 3 (4.1%)

Lymph nodes 19 (17.6%)

Lymph nodes 12 (16.4%)

Skin 4 (3.7%)

Skin/subcutis 13 (17.7%)

Bone 3 (2.8%)

Bone 6 (8.2%)

(b) Lymphoblastic lymphoma: total 108

ALCL: total 73

Figure 9.1 Primary sites of disease in children affected by non-Hodgkin's lymphoma (NHL). Numbers indicate the prevalence (and percentage) of primary sites of patients enrolled in the Italian Association of Pediatric Hematology and Oncology protocols for NHL during the period 1998–2006. (a), B-cell NHL. (b), Lymphoblastic lymphomas (left) and anaplastic large cell lymphoma (ALCL) (right).

• The second type includes tumors localized to the bowel wall, most frequently involving the terminal ileum, believed to arise in Peyer's patches. This is a rarer presentation than the rapidly growing and diffuse abdominal form, and can be mistaken sometimes for acute appendicitis. A palpable right iliac fossa mass is frequently appreciated and intussusception can be the first sign of presentation of an ileum–cecal Burkitt lymphoma. Indeed, this is the most frequent cause of intestinal intussusception in children aged 5–10 years and may allow early diagnosis and therefore limit the subsequent treatment extent.

In both instances ascites and pleural effusion may occur and a number of other sites may be involved. Only occasionally do children present with jaw involvement, whereas in African Burkitt lymphoma, this localization accounts for up to 60% of primary site of disease, particularly in young children [21].

Mediastinal primary

Children with precursor T-cell lymphoblastic lymphoma usually have a mediastinal mass (50–70%) often with pleural effusion [14, 18] (Figure 9.2). Symptoms may include persistent slight cough, but more often severe respiratory distress resulting from airway compression or swelling of the neck, face, and upper limbs due to superior vena cava obstruction. Lymphadenopathy is usually supradiaphragmatic, involving neck, supraclavicular regions, and axillae. Abdominal nodes are rarely involved, with the exception of precursor B-cell lymphoblastic lymphoma that only occasionally can localize to the mediastinum. Hepatosplenomegaly is not uncommon and bone marrow and CNS involvement may occur. Lung involvement is very rare, except in the case of anaplastic large cell lymphoma (ALCL). Mediastinal localization represents a life-threatening condition if general anesthesia is to be performed for diagnostic purposes.

Localized disease

Localized NHL is not frequent in childhood. However, lymph-node swelling can be the only sign of presentation of a NHL, thus posing the need for differential diagnosis with other lymphadenopathies (Figure 9.3). Although enlarged lymph nodes can occur anywhere, most commonly they arise in the head and neck, sometimes concomitantly with Waldeyer's ring involvement. Pharyngeal masses are usually of B-cell origin. ALCL is the most frequent NHL that presents with isolated lymph-node involvement, particularly in the inguinal region. Other sites of NHL primaries include bone, skin, orbit, and kidney (mimicking Wilms' tumor). Testis can also be involved, usually by lymphoblastic lymphoma.

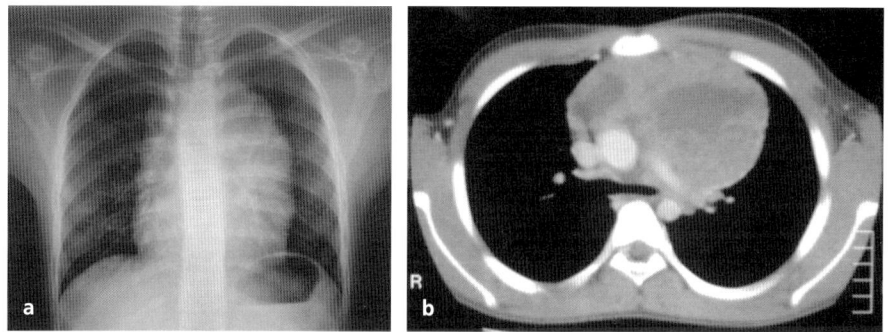

Figure 9.2 Typical clinical aspect of a T-cell lymphoblastic lymphoma at diagnosis. A 13-year-old boy underwent X-ray of the chest for cough and shortness of breath. The X-ray demonstrated an abnormally enlarged mediastinum. A subsequent CT scan of the chest confirmed the presence of a large mass of 13 × 12 × 9 cm in the anterior mediastinum.

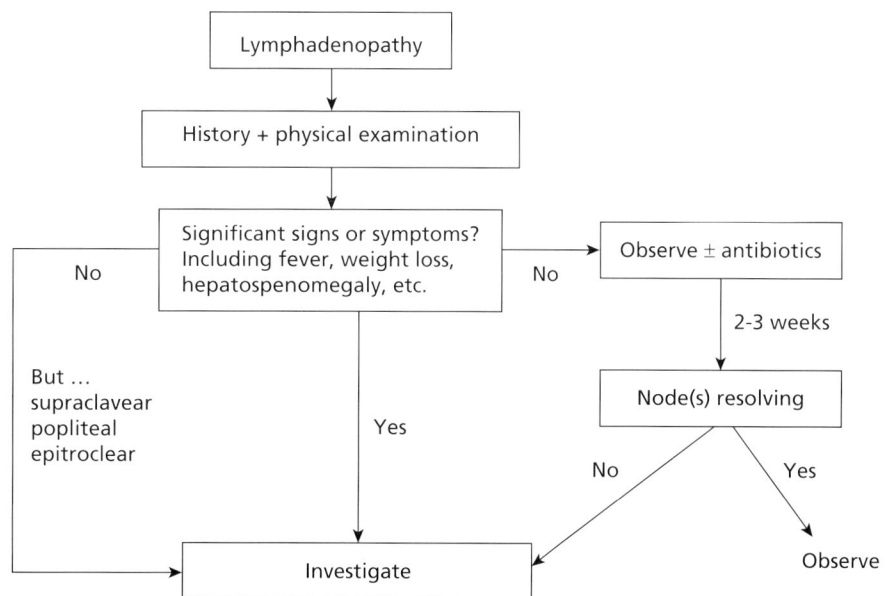

Figure 9.3 Initial management of a lymphadenopathy. An accurate clinical history must be collected in any individual with enlarged lymph nodes in order to evaluate the likelihood of an infectious lymph-node enlargement. In case no signs or symptoms suggestive of a malignant disease are present, a wait-and-see approach can be adopted with/without antibiotic treatment. In case the lymph nodes are in suspect areas (supraclavear, popliteal, etc.) or if lymphadenopathy persists after 2–3 weeks, further investigation, including biopsy, must be undertaken.

NHL localized to the bone can present as single lesion (requiring a differential diagnosis with other malignancies, particularly Ewing sarcoma/primitive neuroectodermal tumor (PNET)) or with multiple lesions, often painful, sometimes associated with hypercalcemia. Skin involvement may be found in T-cell lymphoblastic lymphoma, but is more common in ALCL, where it can be the only site of disease.

Bone marrow and central nervous system involvement

The BM is frequently involved in pediatric NHL and the prevalence of BM dissemination varies based on the sensitivity of the diagnostic approach used (morphology, molecular genetics, etc.). When more than 25% of cells in the BM are tumor cells, conventionally the disease is diagnosed as an acute leukemia. Depending on the infiltration degree, BM involvement may cause abnormalities of the peripheral blood cell counts in the same manner as a leukemic presentation.

Isolated CNS lymphoma is uncommon and can be found in immunodeficient children. More commonly the CNS is involved as part of the presentation of pediatric NHL, often in patients with BM dissemination of lymphoblastic or Burkitt lymphoma. Headache, vomiting, papilledema and cranial nerve palsy are the commonest signs of this disease localization.

Investigation and staging

Although the suspicion of NHL arises from clinical features that often relate to disease localization, diagnosis relies mostly on histology and immunohistochemistry. Immunophenotyping and molecular diagnostics have recently acquired a more relevant role in the diagnostic work-up.

Diagnosis should be made where possible on histological examination of an excised tumor mass that allows a complete histological, immunophenotypic and molecular characterization of the disease [13]. In patients presenting in extremis, such as with a large mediastinal mass, such an approach requiring general anesthesia may be contraindicated for patient safety. In this situation emergency control of the patient's symptoms takes priority and cytology may be helpful, for example of an aspirated pleural effusion. Every attempt should be made to obtain adequate tumor material once the patient's clinical condition has been stabilized.

Histology and immunophenotype

Morphology represents the keystone for the diagnosis of NHL, but immunohistochemical and flow-cytometric studies of tumor cells are required to achieve the exact diagnosis that is required before the institution of therapy. Specific features are associated with the major NHL subtypes.

Burkitt and large B-cell lymphoma

• Burkitt lymphoma cells have a high nuclear/cytoplasmic ratio, with multiple discernible nucleoli. Cytoplasm is scant and basophilic, due to the high RNA content and vacuoles are often present giving the typical L3 morphology (FAB classification) [22]. In the context of a tumor biopsy the characteristic, though not pathognomonic, pattern of 'starry sky' appearance is found as a result of the presence of macrophages interspersed among the tumor cells (Plate 9.1). While Burkitt lymphoma is composed of cells with rather regular shape and size, the Burkitt-like lymphoma is more pleomorphic, sometimes indistinguishable from large B-cell NHL.

• Nevertheless the diagnosis of Burkitt and Burkitt-like lymphoma can be made only when a very high proliferation rate, as evidenced by a high Ki-67 or MIB-1 positivity (>90%) is observed [23]. Burkitt lymphoma express surface immunoglobulin (SIg), being IgM, in more than 90% of the cases, associated with either kappa or lambda light chains. Other B-cell antigens are expressed, including CD19, CD20, CD22, CD79a and often CD10 [15, 23]. Terminal deoxynucleotidyl transferase (TdT) is negative. Large B-cell lymphoma express similar phenotype as Burkitt lymphoma, but CD10 may be negative and up to one-third of the cases are negative for SIg. SIg are generally absent from large B-cell lymphoma of the mediastinum that originates from a thymic B-cell.

Lymphoblastic lymphoma

• This entity is morphologically indistinguishable from acute lymphoblastic leukemia. Cells are usually of uniform appearance with a high nuclear–cytoplasm ratio and finely dispersed chromatin with small or inconspicuous nucleoli. Nuclei may show some indentations thus conferring a convoluted aspect [24].

• The most distinctive immunophenotypic feature of lymphoblastic lymphoma is the expression of TdT [25], an enzyme that participates in the generation of receptor diversity both in T- and B-cells during the process of T- or B-cell receptor gene rearrangements [26]. Only about 5% of cases are TdT negative [27]. Most tumors also express CD99/MIC2. Most lymphoblastic lymphomas originate from T-cell precursors and express T-cell markers corresponding to the stages of T-cell intra-thymic differentiation [28]: in different combination they include CD7, CD2, CD5, CD1, CD3, CD4 and CD8, as in T-cell acute leukemia [29, 30]. Approximately 10–15% of cases are of B lineage express precursor B-cell markers, including CD19, HLA-DR with CD10 but not SIg [31].

Anaplastic large cell lymphoma

• A relevant histological feature of this type of cancer is the propensity of the tumor cells to invade the lymph-node sinuses and the frequent partial involvement of the lymph node which is independent of the various morphological ALCL variants [32] (Plate 9.1). Specific difficulties may arise in the differentiation of ALCL from Hodgkin lymphoma, soft tissue sarcomas, lymphomatoid papulosis and reactive conditions affecting lymph nodes. Because marked hemohagocytosis can be present in the BM of ALCL patients, hemophagocytic syndromes should also be ruled out. Cells with abundant cytoplasm and horseshoe- or kidney-

Table 9.4 Immunophenotypic markers in use for anaplastic large cell lymphoma diagnosis. This table summarizes the antigens that should be studied by immunohistochemistry both as the minimal required panel (mandatory) or an extended panel of antibodies (mandatory plus optional antibodies) for the diagnosis of anaplastic large cell lymphoma (ALCL). Together with morphological features they allow the diagnosis of ALCL and the differentiation between ALCL and Hodgkin's lymphoma.

Mandatory antibodies	Optional antibodies
B-cell (CD79a, CD20)	T-cell (CD2, CD4, CD5, CD7, CD8)
T-cell (CD3, CD43)	Mib1 or Ki-67
CD30	perforin, TIA1, granzyme
ALK-1	Clusterin
EMA	BNH-9
CD15	
LMP-1 and/or EBER	

shaped nuclei, the so called hallmark cells, are frequently found in biopsies.

• Among the mandatory antibodies to be used in the histological diagnosis of ALCL are those recognizing CD30, EMA, CD15, T- and B-cell specific antigens and, most importantly, the Alk portion of the fusion protein originating from the reciprocal chromosomal translocation characteristic of ALCLs. Antibodies against NK cells, such as anti CD56, and those recognizing proteins associated with cytotoxic granules (perforin, granzyme) are useful (Table 9.4). A special group of CD30 positive lymphoproliferative lesions belonging to the ALCL are those localized to the skin. They include lymphomatoid papulosis that is characterized by a wax and wane behaviour, although it may precede a systemic ALCL. Both isolated cutaneous ALCL and lymphomatoid papulosis are usually Alk negative and this characteristic, along with morphology, is the basis for a correct diagnosis [33].

Cytogenetic and molecular features

Remarkable progress has been achieved in the last decade in the field of pediatric NHL biology. This is particularly relevant as it is hoped that through the understanding of the tumor biology we can identify new tumor markers, novel risk factors and ultimately devise new and more effective therapy approaches. Below is a summary of the most relevant findings in each of the three major NHL categories.

Burkitt and large B-cell lymphomas

Burkitt lymphoma (BL) often possess characteristic chromosomal translocations involving the MYC oncogene locus on chromosome 8q24 [34]. The most common translocation, t(8;14)(q24;q32), which involves the IgH gene locus, occurs in 80% of cases [35]. The consequence of MYC rearrangements in BL is deregulation of cMYC expression by juxtaposition to heterologous enhancers and by introduction of somatic point mutations in its 5' regulatory sequences as well as in exon 2. Because MYC

is a transcription factor that promotes cell cycle progression and cell transformation it is believed to be involved in tumorigenesis [36]. The most common translocation, t(8;14)(q24;q32), can be investigated by a long-distance polymerase chain reaction (LD-PCR) assay at the genomic level with a sensitivity of 10^{-4}. By this approach it is possible to analyze minimal BM infiltration at diagnosis and its response to chemotherapy [37].

Differently from BL, there are no specific or recurrent cytogenetic abnormalities associated with diffuse large B-cell lymphoma (DLBCL) in children and adolescents. Pasqualucci *et al.* [38] have suggested that the majority of BL and DLBCL are derived from lymph node germinal center (GC) regions where rapidly proliferating B-cell blasts (centroblasts) differentiate into centrocytes following hypermutation of the immunoglobulin variable region genes and transform into malignant BL and/or DLBCL by either activation of proto-oncogenes, disruption of tumor suppressor genes, and/or somatic hypermutation of proto-oncogenes.

BCL-6, located on chromosome 3q27, is a transcriptional repressor gene normally expressed within the GC of mature B cells. It has been proposed that repressor activity of BCL-6 is lost in DLBCL due to point mutations, thus contributing to lymphomagenesis in DLBCL [38]. Lossos *et al.* additionally demonstrated that low expression of BCL-6 mRNA in adult patients with DLBCL was associated with a poor prognosis [39]. It remains to be determined if similar genetic alterations are responsible for the pathogenesis of childhood DLBCL.

Lymphoblastic lymphoma

The vast majority of lymphoblastic lymphomas arise from immature T-cells corresponding to well-defined stages of thymocyte differentiation [40]. Fewer than 10% are of B-precursor cell origin.

Most immature B- and T-lymphoid cells express terminal deoxytidyl transferase (TdT), which can be detected by flow cytometric, immunohistochemical, or cytochemical methods and is an important marker of the disease. As a part of developing antigen recognition capabilities, T- and B-lymphocytes rearrange a series of V (variable), D (diversity), J (joining), and C (constant) genetic regions to produce unique antigen receptors. The antigen binding domains of T-cell receptors (TCR) and immunoglobulins (Ig) are unique and serve as clonal markers. Thus T- and B-cell receptor gene rearrangements can also help to distinguish the two subtypes. As a general rule, Ig gene rearrangements are observed in B-lineage lymphomas whereas TCR gene rearrangements are in T-cell disease. The recombinational events that lead to the diversity in antigen recognition may also leave TCR and Ig genes prone to recombination with oncogenes through chromosomal translocations. In contrast to other subtypes of NHL in which one or a few chromosomal rearrangements alter the function of a single gene locus (e.g. c-myc in BL and anaplastic lymphoma kinase (ALK) in ALCL), a number of translocations altering various proto-oncogenes (TAL1, TAL2, LMO1, LMO2, HOX11, HOX11L2, LYL1, c-myc, NOTCH1, LCK, FGFR1) occur in T-LL. A recent study demonstrated that pediatric lymphoblastic lymphoma had a high frequency of chromosome abnormalities, and these were most often structural, but also included numerical abnormalities [41].The variety of chromosomal abnormalities may contribute to different prognostic categories. Cytogenetic and molecular abnormalities in B-lineage disease are less well characterized. Classical chromosomal translocations which occur in B-precursor ALL, such as hyperdiploidy, t(12;21), t(1;19), and t(9;22) appear to occur less frequently in B-precursor lymphoblastic lymphoma. As expected, it usually shows monoclonal Ig gene rearrangements, but lacks evidence of somatic hypermutation [42].

Anaplastic large cell lymphoma

Systemic ALCLs are subdivided into two clinically significant subtypes based on expression of ALK, a tyrosine kinase that impacts many cellular responses including proliferation, growth, apoptosis, and cell transcription of specific genes(14). About 90–95% of pediatric ALCLs express ALK protein [43]. ALK is a novel receptor tyrosine kinase of the insulin receptor subfamily with homology to leukocyte tyrosine kinase. Its expression is highly tissue-specific and is normally restricted to cells of the nervous system where it is thought to play a role in neuronal development. ALK over-expression is linked to tumorigenesis in ALK-positive ALCL, as well as other tumors including inflammatory myofibroblastic tumors and some carcinomas [44]. In about 80% of tumors, ALK over-expression arises due to a t(2;5)(p23;q35) translocation that juxtaposes the ALK gene on chromosome 2p23 to the nucleophosmin (NPM) gene on 5q35. This fusion gene encodes a chimeric, constitutively activated tyrosine kinase, NPM-ALK, consisting of the N-terminal portion of the NPM fused to the catalytic domain of ALK.

The NPM-ALK fusion protein is detectable in more than 90% of cases by immunohistochemistry, and its transcript can be identified by reverse transcriptase polymerase chain reaction (RT-PCR), a highly sensitive and specific method for identification of ALK-rearrangements at RNA level.

Imaging

Although the diagnosis of NHL is based on histology, imaging studies are clearly involved in the investigation of a suspected NHL and in the subsequent staging of confirmed disease. An isolated anterior mediastinal mass would usually indicate, for example, a T-cell lymphoblastic lymphoma although only histological examination would exclude a large B-cell lymphoma of the mediastinum or even mediastinal ALCL. Conversely, a large abdominal mass would suggest a B-cell NHL and where the abdominal mass involves the bowel, the diagnosis of a Burkitt/Burkitt-like lymphoma is very likely. These assumptions should be considered with great caution but they form part of decision making and the formation of diagnostic hypothesis.

Independent of the NHL subtype, imaging procedures are similar for all patients with NHL.

• Chest X-ray is performed in any child and can detect a mediastinal mass or a pleural effusion.

• CT scan of the neck, thorax, and abdomen should also be performed. CT is the imaging approach of choice to study the mediastinum (and to define the volume of a mediastinal mass) and the lungs.

• The abdomen can be studied by ultrasonography, which is a fast and inexpensive approach to define liver, spleen, and kidney involvement. It may be less sensitive to define lymph-node involvement, mainly retroperitoneally. In our experience, however, it can complement CT scan findings: specific sites of disease can be more amenable to be studied by ultrasound and often it represents the method of choice for multiple consecutive evaluations of tumor response.

• A rather peculiar site of disease localization is the bone. Total skeletal scintigraphy with Tecnetium-99 is the approach used to assess possible bone localizations of NHL. Although it has been used systematically in the past, its current role in staging is less clear as accompanying bone localization apparently does not impact significantly on outcome of NHL [45]. Because scintigraphy may be positive in case of bone remodelling independently of any tumor involvement (i.e. post-traumatic bone lesions), all suspected lesions identified by this means should in any case be further studied by X-ray or MRI. In current clinical practice total skeletal or single bone imaging is considered mandatory only when there are symptoms of bone involvement such as pain.

• Brain MRI or CT scan is also indicated at diagnosis to exclude a CNS tumor. In case of symptoms or signs suggestive of CNS localization, which is a rare condition, MRI is the method of choice.

• Positron emission tomography (PET) is increasingly available for the investigation and follow up of lymphomas. PET is based on the uptake of 18-fluorodeoxyglucose (FDG) which is higher in malignant compared with normal cells. Indeed, incorporation of FDG is a characteristic of all actively proliferating cells, including inflammatory cells, and so caution must be exercised in the interpretation of positive PET findings. Abundant data are available in the literature for adult Hodgkin and non-Hodgkin lymphomas, whereas little experience is available in pediatric oncology [46]. PET has been evaluated in pre-treatment staging, monitoring during therapy and post-therapy surveillance in adults where it appears to be more sensitive than CT scan. The role of PET in pediatric lymphoma requires evaluation in large prospective trials although it is clearly a promising technique [47, 48]. In general, PET should be considered at present a useful tool for staging and response evaluation, but in the absence of a biopsy-proven result it is unwise to modify stage or therapy based on PET scans alone.

Staging

Staging classifications provide a means of describing the extent of disease and estimating prognosis. In NHL there is not infrequently widely disseminated disease at diagnosis. Staging reflects both the tumor volume as well as the degree of spread of disease. For this same reason, defining the 'primary site of disease' is difficult, except for the rare single site NHL, and consequently NHL

Table 9.5 St Jude staging system for pediatric non-Hodgkin's lymphoma.

Stage	Criteria for extent of disease
I	A single tumor (extranodal) or single anatomic area (nodal) with the exclusion of mediastinum or abdomen
II	A single tumor (extranodal) with regional node involvement
	Two or more nodal areas on the same side of the diaphragm
	Two single (extranodal) tumors with or without regional node involvement on the same side of the diaphragm
	A primary gastointestinal tumor usually in the ileocaeacal area with or without involvement of associated mesenteric nodes only, grossly completely resected
III	Two single tumors (extranodal) on opposite sides of the diaphragm
	Two or more nodal areas above and below the diaphragm
	All primary intra-thoracic tumors (mediastinal, pleural, thymic)
	All extensive primary intra-abdominal disease
	All paraspinal or epidural tumors regardless of other tumor site(s)
IV	Any of the above with initial central nervous system and/or bone marrow involvement

Table 9.6 Staging studies for non-Hodgkin's lymphoma.

Physical examination	
Blood cell count	
Clinical chemistry	Serum electrolytes; renal and liver tests; serum lactate dehyogrogenase, serum uric acid
Imaging studies	Chest X-ray; chest CT if X-ray suspiciously abnormal or abnormal; abdominal ultrasound examination; abdominal CT scan; FDP-glucose PET; MRI (CT) of the brain
Bone marrow aspirate, bilateral (±bone marrow biopsies)	
Cerebrospinal fluid examination (cytology)	
Bone scan	

FDP, fluoro-deoxy-glucose. PET, positron emission tomography.

are mostly divided into 'localized' versus 'extensive' disease to indicate the tumor burden.

Among localized diseases, stage I and stage II identify a single or multiple site NHL, respectively. Staging classifications for NHL have been influenced by staging systems used for Hodgkin lymphoma (Ann Arbor) [49], but this disease has a different pattern of initial localization from NHL and spread to extra-nodal localization has a prognostic impact. NHL in children as well as in adults are mostly extranodal and thus the considerations on which Hodgkin disease staging is based do not apply.

The stage of the disease in children with NHL is usually determined according to the St Jude staging system modified by Murphy [50] (Table 9.5) and relies on selected clinical, laboratory and imaging investigations aimed to determine disease burden and localization (Table 9.6).

In this staging classification, stage III (which accounts for 50–60% of all pediatric NHL) includes patients with primary intrathoracic (most often associated with lymphoblastic lymphoma, less frequently with primary mediastinal B-cell lymphoma (PBML) or extensive intra-abdominal tumor (most often a B-cell NHL) disease on both sides of the diaphragm, and paraspinal/epidural tumors. Definition of 'extensive' has changed with time as imaging techniques have evolved: this and other aspects may have to be taken into consideration for a possible update of the staging system.

Another condition that may be worth underlining, as pointed out by Murphy, is the artificial subdivision between stage IV disease due to less than 25% blast infiltration of the bone marrow and acute lymphoblastic leukemia (above 25%).

With time, additional specifications have been adopted to better define groups of patients with similar or different prognosis, based on additional parameters compared with those already included in the St Jude classification. Thus, the German Berlin-

Frankfurt-Munster (BFM) group defined as stage IV those children with multifocal bone disease and subdivided stage III B-cell lymphoma in two different groups: stage III with serum (lactate dehydrogenase) LDH between 5000 and 1000 IU/l and those with LDH above 1000 IU/ml [51]. In the French–American–British protocols, B-cell lymphomas are also subdivided based on stage and resectability, but serum LDH levels are not taken into account for the risk group definition [52].

Similarly, most protocols subdivide patients with lymphoblastic lymphoma based on disease extent and children with ALCL based on specific sites of disease that impact prognosis [53, 54] (Tables 9.7 and 9.8).

Within the pediatric NHLs 'stage' and 'risk group' refer to different categories: stage is more related to localization, distribution, and burden of the disease, whereas risk group is more related to treatment and is relevant for choosing the most appropriate therapy arm.

Treatment

Historical perspective

The modern era in the field of pediatric NHL therapy might be considered to have started in the early 1980s. From that time, with the advent of treatment protocols conducted by cooperative groups in the USA and in Europe, major advancements in remission and survival rates were made. There was increasing correlation of clinical and biological information that enabled physicians to adopt specific therapies for given subgroups of NHL.

In the late 1970s Wollner and co-workers had demonstrated that combination chemotherapy derived from the leukemia protocol LSA2-L2, in conjunction with irradiation of bulky disease, could achieve the cure of poor prognosis NHL [5]. The first randomized trial conducted by Murphy at St Jude Research

Table 9.7 Definition of therapy groups for B-cell non-Hodgkin's lymphoma.

BFM protocols*

Risk group 1	Stage I and II completely resected
Risk group 2	Stage I and II, not resected;
	Stage III and LDH < 500 U/l
Risk group 3	Stage III and LDH 500–999 U/l;
	Stage IV or B-cell leukemia and LDH < 1000 U/l, CNS negative
Risk group 4	Stage III and LDH ≥ 1000 U/l;
	Stage IV or B-cell leukemia and LDH ≥ 1000 U/l; CNS positive

FAB protocols†

Group A	Complete surgical resection stage I or abdominal stage II
Group B	All patients not eligible for group A or C
Group C	Any CNS involvement or bone marrow involvement ≥ 25%

* BFM, Berlin-Frankfurt-Munster protocols 95. † French-American-British protocols 96. LDH, lactate dehydrogenase. CNS, central nervous system.

Table 9.8 Current definition of therapy groups for lymphoblastic lymphoma and anaplastic large cell lymphoma within the European Intergroup for Childhood Non-Hodgkin's Lymphoma.

Lymphoblastic lymphoma

Localized disease	Stage I and II
Advanced stage disease	Stage III;
	Stage IV with bone marrow blasts ≤25% and CNS negative
Stage IV and CNS positivity	

ALCL

Isolated skin lesions	
Low risk	Stage I completely resected
Standard risk	No skin, mediastinal liver, spleen or lung involvement
High risk	Biopsy proven skin lesions (except isolated lesions or lesions overlying an involved node);
	Mediastinal, liver, spleen or lung involvement;
CNS involvement	

CNS, Central nervous system.

Hospital demonstrated that treatment results in advanced stage NHL were not improved by the addition of radiotherapy to systemic chemotherapy [4]. In the early 1980s a randomized trial conducted by the Children's Cancer Study Group compared the 10-drug based LSA2-L2 regimen with COMP (cyclophosphamide-vincristine-methotrexate-prednisone) regimen and demonstrated that, although both treatments were effective in curing most children with localized NHL, LSA2-L2 was significantly more effective than COMP in high-stage lymphoblastic lymphoma whereas the latter was more active in non-lymphoblastic lymphoma [7]. Concomitantly, the Pediatric Oncology Group confirmed the effectiveness of LSA2-L2 in children affected by NHL, excluding Burkitt lymphoma [8]. These trials not only demonstrated the efficacy of combination chemotherapy in the management of childhood NHL, but indicated that outcome greatly depends on the histological subtype.

In the same period in Europe, the French Society of Pediatric Oncology (SFOP) and the BFM groups designed the first trial for the diagnosis and treatment of NHL, and was conducted recently with very successful results. The BFM group developed treatments derived from the acute lymphoblastic leukemia protocols to treat NHL and confirmed the prognostic value of stage of disease, but also clearly indicated different prognosis based on immunophenotype [9] leading to further trials where B-cell derived NHL were treated differently from non-B cell NHL. Outcome of all NHL subtypes improved gradually to the current event free survival rates of 80% or above in subsequent trials [11] and results continue to improve. The French investigators, coordinated by Catherine Patte at the Institute Gustave-Roussy in Paris, designed a protocol to treat B-cell NHL and B-ALL, adding high-dose methotrexate and cytosine arabinosyde to a chemotherapy regimen already in use, thus initiating the successful series of LMB protocols, including LMB-89, that reached a failure-free survival of 91% [10]. Achievement of the LMB protocols encouraged an international collaboration among the French–American–British national groups who conducted a wide randomized clinical trial FAB/LMB-96 for B-cell NHL and ALL, the results of which have been published [55].

Description of major findings of most recent co-operative studies

Following the initial therapeutic protocols that showed the critical role of stage, histology, immunophenotype, and other clinical and biological risk factors, children with NHL were enrolled in specific disease-oriented clinical trials, designed to improve outcome and to optimize therapy intensity and duration. Three major disease groups were identified: (1) B-cell lymphoma, (2) lymphoblastic lymphoma and (3) ALCL, and the treatments of these is considered separately.

B-cell non-Hodgkin's lymphoma (Tables 9.9, 9.10 and 9.11)
Therapy for B-cell NHL has been developed based on clinical and biological characteristics of Burkitt lymphoma, but are effective also for DLBCL. Although the activity of cyclophosphamide (CP), vincristine (VCR) and methotrexate (MTX) were demonstrated from early studies in African Burkitt lymphoma [56], only in the context of more recent clinical trials developed in the USA (POG-Total B) and in Europe (French LMB and German–Austrian–Swiss BFM) have modern and more effective therapeutic approaches come into clinical practice. Burkitt lymphoma has

Table 9.9 Treatment characteristics and results of the most recent BFM and LMB/FAB trials for B-cell non-Hodgkin's lymphoma.

Therapy group	No. of patients	EFS	Chemotherapy cycles
BFM-95 (60)	**505**		
R1: Stage I, II, resected	10%	94% (3 y)	A-B
R2: Stage I, II, non-resected; III, LDH < 500 U/l	46%	94% (3 y)	P-A-B-A-B
R3: III-LDH > 500/< 999 U/l; BM+ and LDH < 1000 U/l	16%	85% (3 y)	P-AA-BB-CC-AA-BB
R4: LDH ≥ 1000 U/l and/or CNS+	28%	81% (3 y)	P-AA-BB-CC-AA-BB-CC
LMB/FAB-96 (55) (63)	**1134**		
A: stage I resected; II abdominal	12%	98% (3 y)	COPAD-COPAD
B: I-not resected; II non-abdominal; III; IV BM blasts ≤25% and CNS	67%	90% (4 y)	COP-COPADM1-*COPADM1/2-CYM-CYM ± M1
C: >25% BM blasts and/or CNS+	21%	79% (4Y)	COP-COPADM1-COPADM2-*CYVE1-CYVE2-M1-M2-M3-M4

P, cytoreductive pre-phase. BM, bone marrow. CNS, central nervous system.

In the BFM-95 trial MTX was administered randomly in 4 vs 24 hour i.v. infusion (1 g/m^2 in A and B; 5 g/m^2 in AA and BB): in R3 and R4 the 4-hour infusion showed lower efficacy that 24-hour. Equal efficacy in R1 and R2. *The LMB/FAB-96 trial, for Group B, was based on a factorial design to test, based on response after COP-COPADM1, COPADM2 (cyclophosphamide 3 g/m^2) vs COPADM1 (cyclophosphamide 1.5 g/m^2) and the role of adding cycle M1. Additionally, Group C was randomized to receive reduced intensity CYVE and omission of M2-M3-M4; CNS+ patients received additional HD-MTX at 8 g/m^2 instead of 3 g/m^2 and additional intrathecal therapy. Reduced intensity regimen showed inferior results in Group C.

a very high proliferation rate. In such a condition the use of high dose chemotherapy with four to five alternating drugs with different toxicity profiles allows the maintenance of effective anti-tumor concentrations of the individual chemotherapeutic agents while limiting toxicity. In addition, this will also permit the administration of subsequent cycles at relatively short time intervals. The recent protocols are designed based on the principles summarized in Box 9.1 and by using this approach, an event-free survival (EFS) up to 90% was achieved in most experienced cooperative groups [51, 55, 57–60, 63].

Another serious and possibly lethal complication is the massive tumor lysis syndrome (TLS) that, although with reduced incidence after the introduction of a low-dose chemotherapy (corticosteroids and CP) pre-phase and the availability of urate-oxidase, still remains a threatening clinical emergency to face at early therapy onset [62].

The progress observed in the treatment of B-cell NHL is strictly related to the aggressiveness of chemotherapy programs developed in the last two decades and tailored to well-defined prognostic groups: the success of such an approach depends on the availability of good supportive care. Consequently, treatment of B-cell NHL should be delivered in experienced hemato-oncology units by physicians who are familiar not only with the disease and with high-dose chemotherapy but also with all the preventive and supportive care measures to reduce the risk of lethal toxicity.

Lymphoblastic lymphoma (Table 9.11)

The initial management of a child with advanced stage lymphoblastic lymphoma might involve the potential oncologic emergen-

cies such as respiratory compromise from a mediastinal mass and metabolic abnormalities.

The immediate priority is to stabilize the patient, achieve a histological diagnosis and then to embark upon proven and effective chemotherapy. Drug therapy with steroids or low dose cyclophosphamide (100 mg/m^2/dose) might be needed to achieve clinical stability from a large tumor mass in order to allow surgical management. Decisions about investigating such a child should be made between oncologist, anesthetist, surgeon and pathologist.

The modern chemotherapy protocols originated from the early studies demonstrating that, except for limited stage disease, a leukaemia-like therapy is more efficacious than short chemotherapy regimens [7]. Thus, at present, most protocols for lymphoblastic lymphoma are modified versions of the 10-drug LSA2-L2 protocol or of the BFM group strategy: both were treatments designed for acute lymphoblastic leukemia.

The addition of high-dose MTX (3 g/m^2) to the LSA2-L2 protocol by the French Group gave a significant increase in survival bringing the EFS of stage III and IV to 79% and 72%, respectively [64]. Although in this study cranial radiation was limited to CNS positive patients only one of 77 CNS negative patients relapsed in the CNS. The advantage of increasing the dose of MTX (from 0.5 to 5 g/m^2 by 24 hour i.v. infusion) was also demonstrated by the BFM group that obtained a 5-year EFS of 73% compared with the previous 56% [65]. Although the therapeutic potentials of most single agents used in lymphoblastic lymphoma have not been elucidated, the role of L-asparaginase in T-cell lymphoblastic lymphoma has been demonstrated in the POG-8704 trial

Cycle	Daily dose	Administration	Days
Pre-phase			
Dexamethasone†	5–10 mg/m²/day	Orally or i.v. (in three fractions)	1–5
Cyclophosphamide	200 mg/m²/day	i.v. (1 h)	12
MTX+ARA-C+Pdn	12 mg‡ + 30 mg + 10 mg	i.t.	1
Cycle A			
Dexamethasone	10 mg/m²/day	Orally or i.v. (in three fractions)	1–5
MD-methotrexate	500 mg/m²/day	i.v. (1/10 in 30 min, 9/10 in 23,5 h)	1
Ifosfamide	800 mg/m²/day	i.v. (1 h)	1–5
Etoposide	100 mg/m²/day	i.v. (1 h)	45
Cytarabine	150 mg/m² every 12 h	i.v. (1 h)	45
MTX+ARA-C+Pdn	12 mg‡ + 30 mg + 10 mg	i.t.	1
Cycle B			
Dexamethasone	10 mg/m²/day	Orally or i.v. (in three fractions)	1–5
MD-methotrexate	500 mg/m²/day	i.v. (1/10 in 30 min, 9/10 in 23,5 h)	1
Cyclophosphamide	200 mg/m²/day	i.v. (1 h)	1–5
Adriamycin	25 mg/m²/day	i.v. (1 h)	45
MTX+ARA-C+Pdn	12 mg‡ + 30 mg + 10 mg	i.t.	1
Cycle AA			
Dexamethasone	10 mg/m²/day	Orally or i.v. (in three fractions)	1–5
HD-methotrexate	5 g/m²/da	i.v. (1/10 in 30 min, 9/10 in 23,5 h)	1
Ifosfamide	800 mg/m²/day	i.v. (1 h)	1–5
Etoposide	100 mg/m²/day	i.v. (1 h)	45
Cytarabine	150 mg/m² every 12 h	i.v. (1 h)	45
Vincristine	1.5 mg/m²/day (max 2 mg)	i.v.	1
MTX+ARA-C+Pdn	6 mg‡ +15 mg + 5 mg	i.t.	1
Cycle BB			
Dexamethasone	10 mg/m²/day	Orally or i.v. (in three fractions)	1–5
HD-methotrexate	5 g/m²/day	i.v. (1/10 in 30 min, 9/10 in 23,5 h)	1
Cyclophosphamide	200 mg/m²/day	i.v. (1 h)	1–5
Adriamycin	25 mg/m²/day	i.v. (1 h)	45
Vincristine	1.5 mg/m²/day (max 2 mg)	i.v.	1
MTX+ARA-C+Pdn	6 mg‡ +15 mg + 5 mg	i.t.	1
Cycle CC			
Dexamethasone	20 mg/m²/die	Orally or i.v. (in three fractions)	1–5
Etoposide	150 mg/m²/die	i.v. (1 h)	345
HD-cytarabine	2 g/m² every 12 h	i.v. (3 h)	12
Vindesine	3 mg/m²/die (max 5 mg)	i.v.	1
MTX+ARA-C+Pdn	12 mg‡ + 30 mg + 10 mg	i.t.	5

Table 9.10 Treatment schema of the BFM-95 protocol for B-cell non-Hodgkin's lymphoma*.

*The schema does not take into account the randomized schedule of HD-MTX used in the R3 and R4 patient groups. † Dexamethasone in the pre-phase was given at 5 mg/m²/day for the first 2 days and 10 mg/m²/day in the subsequent 3 days. ‡ Dose of intrathecal (i.t.) methotrexate (MTX, adjusted for children less than 3 years of age. Central nervous system positive patients were administered i.t. therapy daily intraventricularly on days 2 to 5 of each AA and BB cycles and on days 3 to 6 of CC cycles starting from the second cycle. Racemic folinic acid was administered at hours 42–48–54 from initiation of HD-MTX infusion and based on measured serum MTX levels thereafter. Pdn, prednisolone. MD, medium dose. HD, high dose. i.v., intravenously. H, hours.

Table 9.11 Recent cooperative group studies in pediatric non-Hodgkin's lymphoma (NHL).

Study	Period	No. of patients	Outcome (EFS)	Reference
B-cell NHL				
POG Total	1986–91	133	79% 4-year EFS for stage IV B-NHL; 65% for B-ALL	[59]
CCG-Orange	1991–93	42	77% 5-year EFS stage III–IV + B-ALL	[78]
LMB-89 SFOP	1989–96	561	91% 5-year EFS stage I–IV NHL+ B-ALL	[58]
BFM-90	1990–95	413	89% 6-year EFS stage I–IV + B-ALL	[51]
BFM-95*	1996–2001	505	89% 3-year EFS stage I–IV + B-ALL	[60]
FAB/LMB-96*	1996–2001	1109	89% 3-year stage I–IV + B-ALL	[55, 57]
Lymphoblastic NHL				
CCG-502*	1983–90	281	84% 5-year stage I–II; 67% stage III–IV	[79]
POG 8704*	1987–92	180	64–78% 4-year CCR†; stage III–IV	[66]
BFM-90	1990–95	105	90% 5-year EFS stage I–IV	[53]
BFM-95	1995–2001	198	82% 5-year EFS stage I–IV	[67]
LMT-96 SFOP	1997–2003	86	87%	[80]
ALCL				
HM89/91 SFOP	1988–97	82	66% 5-year EFS stage I–IV	[74]
BFM-90	1990–95	89	76% 5-year EFS stage I–IV	[73]
UKCCSG	1990–96	72	59% 5-year EFS stage I–IV	[75]
AIEOP	1993–97	34	65% 8-year EFS stage I–IV	[70]
POG-8704	1994–2000	86	72% 4-year EFS stage I–IV	[76]

EFS, event free survival. B-ALL, B-cell acute lymphoblastic leukemia (L3 ALL). ALCL, anaplastic large cell lymphoma.

* Randomized trials. † CCR, complete continuous remission: CCR for the two randomized arms.

Box 9.1 B-cell therapy

- 5 to 7-day cycles.
- Drug combinations from corticosteroids, VCR, CP or ifosfamide, HD-MTX, ARA-C, antracyclines, etoposide.
- The addition of intrathecal chemotherapy (usually MTX/ARA-C/corticosteroids) as CNS prophylaxis.
- Total treatment duration ranges from 1.5 to 5 months approximately, depending on the number of cycles administered, which is related to the prognostic group.
- The current treatments carry a high toxicity rate and even in the best clinical setting a 3–5% early toxic death rate may occur.
- Severe neutropenia and gastro-intestinal mucositis are the most frequent toxicities and they predispose to life-threatening infections that apparently cannot be prevented by the use of granulocyte colony-stimulating factor (G-CSF) [61].

where patients received or did not receive 20 weekly L-asparaginase administrations during the maintenance phase [66].

The BFM protocol for T-cell disease, stage III and IV, achieved a remarkable 90% EFS at 5 years in a cohort of 101 patients treated for 2 years. Patients were treated according to stage, but those who failed to achieve a reduction of the tumor mass of at least 70%, less that 5% blasts in the BM and a negative CSF, were shifted to a high-risk acute leukemia protocol [53]. Treatment consisted of a rather intensive chemotherapy lasting approximately 7 months and including three consecutive phases: induction of remission, consolidation, and reinduction of remission. Four doses of HD-MTX at $5 \, g/m^2$ in 24 hour i.v. infusion were administered at 2-week interval (consolidation) (Figure 9.4 and Table 9.12). The results were excellent and relapses occurred almost exclusively within the first year from diagnosis. All stage III and IV patients older than 2 years received cranial irradiation (1200 cGy in CNS negative children vs 2400 cGy in CNS positive patients). In the subsequent BFM95 trial, cranial irradiation was omitted for advanced stage CNS negative patients and CNS-free survival was not inferior to the previous BFM86 and BFM90 studies in which patients received prophylactic cranial radiotherapy [67], suggesting, together with the SFOP experience, that omitting radiotherapy may not influence the outcome significantly (Box 9.2).

Anaplastic large cell lymphoma (Table 9.11)

This specific histological subtype of pediatric NHL has been described rather recently and has been treated more heterogeneously that others. Because of its frequent T-cell phenotype, some

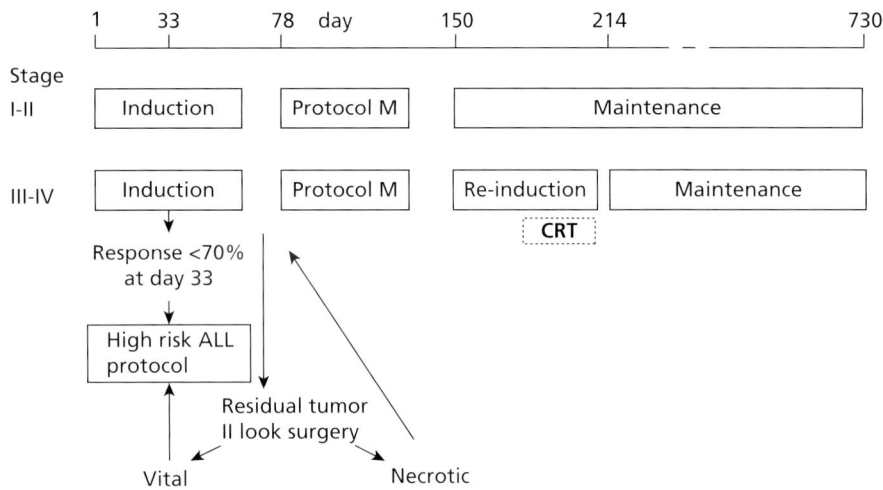

Figure 9.4 Schema of the BFM-90 protocol structure for the treatment of lymphoblastic lymphoma of childhood. All patients, independently of disease stage, received treatment based on induction, consolidation (Protocol M) and maintenance phases for a total duration of therapy of 24 months. Patients with stage III and IV disease according to the St Jude staging system received also a reinduction phase and prophylactic cranial irradiation. In case of a poor response at day 33 from start of treatment, patients were shifted to an intensified (high risk) chemotherapy protocol in use for acute lymphoblastic leukemia.

Table 9.12 BFM-90 protocol for T-cell lymphoblastic lymphoma.

Drug (dose)	Route of administration	Day of administration
Induction		
Prednisone (60 mg/m^2)	Oral	1–28 then tapering in 9 days
Vincristine (1.5 mg/m^2)	i.v.	8, 15, 22, 28
Daunorubicin (30 mg/m^2)	i.v. in 60 min	8, 15, 22, 28
L-Asparaginase (10000 IU/m^2)	i.v. in 60 min	12, 15, 18, 21, 14, 27, 30, 33
Cyclophosphamide (1 g/m^2) + Mesna	i.v. in 60 min	36, 64
Cytosine-arabinoside (75 mg/m^2)	i.v.	38–41, 45–48, 52–55, 59–62
6-mercaptopurine (60 mg/m^2)	Oral	36–63
Methotrexate (12 mg)*	i.t.	1, 15, 29, 45, 59
Protocol M		
6-mercaptopurine (25 mg/m^2)	Oral	1–56
Methotrexate (5 g/m^2)†	i.v. in 24 hours	8, 22, 36, 50
Methotrexate (12 mg)*	i.t.	8, 22, 36, 50
Re-induction		
Dexamethasone (10 mg/m^2)	Oral	1–21 then tapering in 9 days
Vincristine (1.5 mg/m^2)	i.v.	8, 15, 22, 29
Doxorubicin (30 mg/m^2)	i.v. in 60 min	8, 15, 22, 29
L-Asparaginase (10000 IU/m^2)		8, 11, 15, 18
Cyclophosphamide (1 g/m^2) + Mesna	i.v. in 60 min	36
Cytosine-arabinoside (75 mg/m^2)	i.v.	38–41, 45–48
6-thioguanine (60 mg/m^2)	Oral	36–49
Methotrexate (12 mg)*	i.t.	38, 45
Maintenance		
6-mercaptopurine (50 mg/m^2)	Oral	Daily
Methotrexate (20 mg/m^2)	Oral	Once a week

i.v., intravenously. i.t., intrathecal. * Doses according to age below age 3 years. † 10% of the dose in 30 minutes, the remaining in 23.5 hours, with leucovorin rescue: 30 mg/m^2 after 42 hours, 15 mg/m^2 after 48 and 54 hours from start of methotrexate infusion (increased doses if serum MTX levels above expected values). Cranial irradiation (CRT) was given to stage III and IV disease patients older than 1 year between Protocol-M and re-induction: 1200 cGy to CNS negative patients above 1 year; 1800 or 2400 cGy to CNS positive patients in the second year of life or older, respectively.

Box 9.2 The German Berlin-Frankfurt-Munster protocol for lymphoblastic non-Hodgkin's lymphoma.

- Steroid pre-phase (7 days)
- Four drug induction over 4 weeks – daunorubicin, vincristine, prednisolone, L-asparaginase (protocol IA)
- Three drug consolidation – cyclophosphamide, 6-mercaptopurine, cytarabine (protocol IB)
- Four doses of methotrexate ($5\,g/m^2$) with late folinic acid rescue
- Reinduction protocol – similar to IA (but with dexamethasone in place of prednisone) and IB (but only 50% of the dose of IB)
- Maintenance daily 6-MP and weekly oral methotrexate to complete 2 years treatment
- Intrathecal methotrexate in protocol IA,B, with HD methotrexate and in protocol IIB as CNS prophylaxis

---

groups, including the Italian group, treated these children with an ALL protocol derived from the LSA2-L2 [68–70], others with short, B-cell lymphoma like chemotherapy [71, 72]. This latter strategy is at present more widely used in Europe and in the USA – the total duration is significantly shorter than LSA2-L2 derived therapies being approximately 5 rather than 24 months.

In the study BFM-90, patients with ALCL were treated with a therapy derived from the B-cell NHL, based on 5-day courses of combination chemotherapy, given at 3-week intervals. By this approach an EFS of 76% at 9 years was achieved in the 89 patients enrolled into the study [73]. The EFS was 66% at 5 years in the French HM89/91 studies that used modified B-cell lymphoma protocols [74]. A similar approach was used in the UKCCSG study where advance stage disease patients were treated according to the French B-cell lymphoma protocols [75]. In all of these studies most relapses occurred within the first 20 months from diagnosis, but relapses as late as 5 years from diagnosis were observed.

A slightly different approach was employed by the POG study with the APO (doxorubicin, prednisone, vincristine) regimen. This treatment differed from the previous strategies in that it contained higher cumulative doses of anthracyclines and no alkylating agents and epipodophyllotoxins [76]. Therapy was stratified based mostly on stage of disease in the BFM and UKCCSG studies, whereas all children with ALCL received the same treatment in the French, Italian and POG studies. Indeed criteria for stratifying therapy in ALCL are not well established, but from a very recent European retrospective analysis, stage of disease may not be among the most relevant prognostic and more weight should be given to the presence of skin involvement, a mediastinal mass, or involvement of the lung, spleen, or liver [54].

Corticosteroids, vincristine, anthracyclines, and MTX were present in all of the studies reported above, although the total dose and fractionation differed significantly. Anthracyclines were given at a higher level in the APO and in the French HM91 regimens compared with the BFM, UKCCSG and AIEOP protocols. MTX was administered at a medium high dose in all of the studies, except for the APO regimen, that also did not include cyclophosphamide and epipodophyllotoxins. Thus, although one may speculate that anthracyclines, corticosteroids, and vincristine are the key component in the treatment of ALCL treatment, the role of other drugs is not clear. An interesting observation is the efficacy of vinblastine in the management of ALCL. The French group reported a high efficacy, even when used as single agent, in relapsed ALCL [77]. The role of vinblastine in front line therapy is one of the objectives of a large ongoing trial in Europe, but also within the American COG Group.

Limited stage disease

Independently from the histological subtype, stage I-II NHL have usually an excellent prognosis when treated with recent protocols. The 5-year EFS in localized disease is generally in the range of 85–95% in most NHL series and this has led to attempts to decrease intensity and/or duration of therapy with the aim of reducing the acute and long-term toxicity [81]. Among others, cardiac toxicity due to anthracyclines and sterility following alkylating agents are of major concern, although insufficient information on this specific issue is present in the literature. Based on the available results, it seems that the difference in outcome based on histology-oriented protocols (e.g. short-pulse chemotherapy for B-cell NHL vs leukemia-like treatments for lymphoblastic lymphoma) reported for advanced stage disease is not observed for localized NHL. In the case of B-cell NHL, the modern risk-oriented protocols that take into account other parameters besides stage, already have incorporated a reduced intensity and shorter duration of treatment, without a negative impact on survival [51, 57, 58, 60].

In contrast, in the case of lymphoblastic lymphoma most cooperative groups have continued to treat with relatively long therapies and a significant decrease in treatment duration may not be beneficial. Two previous studies from the POG group have demonstrated that omission of involved field radiation therapy and reduction of maintenance therapy do not impact negatively in B-cell and large cell NHL, but there was a benefit of maintenance therapy for lymphoblastic lymphoma [81–83]. Thus, although a prospective trial is warranted to determine whether treatment duration can be reduced in lymphoblastic lymphoma, T- and precursor B-lymphoblastic lymphoma behave differently. The current optimal approach to limited stage lymphoblastic lymphoma remains controversial and is one of the objectives of ongoing trials.

Rare subtypes (PMLBCL, peripheral T-cell)

In addition to the three main histological and immunological groups of pediatric NHL, there are other less frequent entities for which the treatment is still uncertain. Among the large B-cell NHL, the primitive mediastinal large B-cell lymphoma (PMLBCL) is one of those. Previously known as large B-cell lymphoma of the mediastinum with sclerosis, it affects mostly adolescents and young adults, with a higher incidence in females than males. Usually it presents with a large mediastinal mass, involving adjacent structures, and with vena caval obstruction.

Characteristically, PMLBCL is composed of B-cells expressing CD79a, CD19, CD20, CD22 but negative for Ig and CD21 expression, thus suggesting a thymic origin of the disease [84]. Only a few reports have been published on the epidemiology of this disease in childhood [85, 86].

Intensive multiagent chemotherapy with radiation therapy has proven to be efficacious in adults [87], but in children radiation therapy is used less frequently due to the burden of adverse late effects. The BFM experience suggests that high LDH value has a negative prognostic impact in patients treated with aggressive B-cell NHL-based therapy [84]. Whether other variables, including tumor volume, response kinetics and possibly any biological data may impact prognosis, is not known yet. Certainly the results obtained so far are inferior when compared with other B-cell NHL, suggesting therefore that modified therapies including a different use of standard chemotherapy or possibly the addition of anti-CD20 antibody may be of some relevance.

Other rare B-cell NHL in childhood is follicular lymphoma, which is the most frequent NHL in adults, and MALT (mucosa-associated lymphoma tissue) lymphoma. The former often presents as a localized disease, whereas the latter has frequently a nodal localization. Together they account for approximately 1% of all NHL of childhood. Optimal therapy for these very rare diseases is difficult to define, but generally, limited treatment may be used for localized and completely resected disease, whereas in other circumstances a B-cell based treatment may be indicated [88–90].

In the field of T-cell NHL, there is a wider heterogeneity of histological subtypes. Among rare types of NHL, we find the isolated CD30 positive cutaneous lesions, including lymphomatoid papulosis, the isolated cutaneous ALCL, the group of so called 'peripheral T-cell NHL', including panniculitis-like T-cell lymphoma and hepato-splenic T-cell lymphoma. Mycosis fungoides and Sezary syndrome are other rare entities. At present, all the CD30-positive lesions, which are usually localized to the skin, should not be considered among the peripheral T-cell lymphomas as they have distinct features. As pointed out by several authors, CD30 positive skin lesions, without involvement of lymph nodes or other sites, should be subject to an initial watch-and-wait approach as they may spontaneously regress [91]. This is most evident for lymphomatoid papulosis for which a wax-and-wane behaviour is part of the clinical definition of the disease [92]. Although spontaneous complete remission occurs in virtually all the cases, patients with lymphomatoid papulosis have an increased risk of developing a NHL, particularly an ALCL, or other malignancies.

Mycosis fungoides is a cutaneous lymphoma originating from epidermotropic T-cells and is the most common type of cutaneous T-cell lymphoma. It is a disease of adult patients, but can be occasionally diagnosed in childhood and adolescence. It may present with waxing and waning skin eruptions that may delay diagnosis. The outcome is excellent with a 5–10 year survival close to 95% [93]. Treatment of limited disease consists of topical steroids or retinoids. Ultraviolet A irradiation alone or combined with psoralen (PUVA) may be used in more extensive disease, whereas radiotherapy or systemic chemotherapy is rarely needed [94].

Sezary syndrome is exceptional in children and is the leukemic manifestation of mycosis fungoides that requires systemic therapy.

Panniculitis-like T-cell lymphoma and hepato-splenic T-cell lymphoma are rare in young individuals. They are often aggressive diseases that respond poorly to systemic therapy. Cure often depends on high-intensive treatment including bone marrow transplant [95, 96]. Other peripheral T-cell lymphoma not-otherwise specified (PTCL-NOS) have been described in children, but little is known about clinical behaviour and treatment.

Clinical emergencies in non-Hodgkin's lymphoma

Life-threatening conditions in childhood NHL may arise frequently due to the very high growth fractions of most of these tumors as exemplified by Burkitt lymphoma. Among others, mediastinal or superior vena cava syndrome, acute tumor lysis syndrome, complications due to intra-abdominal lymphoma and neurologic emergencies due to CNS involvement are the most relevant.

Mediastinal syndrome and superior vena cava syndrome

Mediastinal syndrome is the consequence of airways obstruction due to compression by a superior mediastinal mass whereas superior vena cava syndrome is caused by compression obstruction or thrombosis of the vena cava. Dyspnoea, cough, neck and face swelling and cyanosis are the most frequent symptoms in case of a large mediastinal mass. The most accurate method to assess the anatomical degree of compression is by CT scan. Severe airway obstruction is usually managed by initiating specific anti-lymphoma therapy, usually with corticosteroid treatment, with or without cyclophosphamide. Local radiation therapy has also been used in the past, but presently it is employed in cases where no symptomatic improvement has been achieved within a few days of initiation of chemotherapy. In cases of large mediastinal masses, bone marrow aspirate, biopsy of a peripheral lymph node or possibly examination of pleural fluid for tumor cells, performed under local anesthesia if needed, should be attempted to achieve a diagnosis. General anesthesia and sedation must be avoided as sudden death may occur in these conditions. If a diagnosis cannot be made by any other way then the resolution of the mass with instituted chemotherapy should be monitored. Diagnostic surgery should be undertaken when it is safe to do so and before the entire tumor has gone.

Because a large mediastinal mass may respond very rapidly to emergency treatment, tumor lysis prevention should be instituted during this early phase of therapy.

Acute tumor lysis syndrome (ATLS)

ATLS is frequent in NHL with a high growth fraction and high tumor burden that are highly sensitive to chemotherapy. These characteristics are more frequent in B-cell that in T-cell NHL [97, 98]. Tumor lysis syndrome may occur spontaneously in case of rapid tumor cell turnover, but is frequently initiated by acute and massive cell lysis induced by chemotherapy. Massive cytolysis results in increased purine metabolism leading to hyperuricemia and concomitant increase in plasma potassium and phosphate and decrease in calcium. Due to uric acid crystal formation and precipitation in the renal tubules, oliguric renal failure can develop that may cause death. ATLS is a life-threatening condition that needs to be prevented. Although specific therapy has to be initiated as soon as possible in NHL, in the presence of elevated uric acid plasma concentration and reduced urine output, the administration of chemotherapy would likely cause patient death due to acute metabolic abnormalities if appropriate preventive actions are not taken. Therefore biochemical abnormalities must be corrected before the initiation of specific therapy.

The first measure is to increase diuresis thus allowing a better elimination of the increased solute burden. Additionally, the administration of allopurinol, a xanthine oxidase inhibitor, prevents the formation of urate from xanthine, thus decreasing the probability of urate precipitation. Because allopurinol does not decrease the pre-existing urate, the use of urate oxidase has become current clinical practice and in some protocols has been introduced systematically at the early stage of therapy [62, 99, 100].

Because of the risk of sudden death from hyperkalemia that may occur soon after initiation of therapy, it is important to avoid additional potassium administration during the first days of chemotherapy. Hypocalcemia, a consequence of hyperphosphatemia, should be treated only if symptomatic and intravenous calcium chloride should be given with caution as it may favour extraosseous calcification in the presence of high serum phosphate levels. In critical metabolic conditions and/or renal failure, hemodialysis or hemofiltration should be used.

For all these reasons, protocols for the treatment of B-cell NHL start usually with a low-intensity chemotherapy (cyclophosphamide, vincristine, corticosteroids) to reduce the rate of response, thus reducing the risk of acute tumor lysis. Because of the quantity and quality of monitoring required, it is advisable to treat patients at high risk of ATLS in a critical care unit or in a unit with good experience in prevention of ATLS and with the possibility of rapid access to an intensive care unit.

Novel therapeutic approaches

Although remarkable progress has been achieved recently in the field of pediatric NHL a significant proportion of children with NHL still fail to be cured of their disease. The new techniques for the study of gene expression profiles and gene polymorphisms appear relevant to improve current diagnosis and to develop novel targeted therapies.

A better risk assessment will identify small subgroups of patients that need to be treated differently or more aggressively to be cured, but also those who could be treated with a less intensive therapy.

A form of NHL-directed therapy presently available is the use of monoclonal antibodies reacting with surface proteins such as CD20 and CD22. Anti-CD20 has entered clinical practice and has an established role in conjunction with chemotherapy such as the CHOP regimen in adult NHL of B-cell origin [101]. However, anti-CD20 has been used rarely in children, mostly to treat lymphoproliferative disease arising after organ transplant and only in a few cases of children with NHL in either first line or relapse settings [102]. Thus, although promising, whether this targeted therapy is beneficial in the treatment of pediatric B-cell NHL remains to be defined and is presently the object of ongoing clinical trials aiming to determine its activity. Less information is available on the use and potentials of other antibodies, including CD22.

Within the lymphoblastic lymphomas there is evidence that patients who fail first line chemotherapy have very little chance of being cured. The only patients who could be rescued after relapse are those undergoing allogeneic bone marrow transplant. This raises the question of whether some selected patients should undergo intensified therapy as front line therapy, but we do not have enough evidence that enables us to identify those children. New potential drugs to be used in lymphoblastic NHL, particularly of the T-cell subtype, as they have shown efficacy in acute lymphoblastic leukemia, are nucleoside analogs such as nelarabine [103], clofarabine [104] and forodesine [105]. Other novel drugs, among which is the proteasome inhibitor bortezomib which is undergoing preliminary clinical evaluation for its potential use in NHL [106], have distinct mechanisms of action that may increase standard chemotherapy efficacy, when used in combination.

In the field of ALCL, the anti-CD30 monoclonal antibody is undergoing phase II clinical studies, as it has shown anti-tumor activity and acceptable toxicity in preclinical and clinical studies when used as a naked antibody [107] or conjugated with toxins [108, 109]. Of great interest is the demonstration of anti-ALK circulating antibodies [110] and the presence of a T-cell antitumor response in patients with ALK-positive ALCL [111]. These observations suggest a potential role of naturally occurring immune-response to ALK-positive ALCL and open new possibilities of designing anti-tumor vaccines and tumor-specific cell therapies. They also give a strong rationale to consider allogeneic-BMT in high risk patients. Other studies are ongoing to design specific inhibitors of NPM-ALK kinase activity [112] that may be used against ALK-positive ALCL.

Not only are there new drugs that may be included in current therapeutic regimens, but also new formulations of drugs already in use, e.g. liposomal cytarabine that, due to its long half-life in the CSF, might be beneficial for the treatment of CNS disease [113].

Based on the present status of research in the field of pediatric NHL, in the immediate future a better risk-adaptation scheme in the context of specific subgroups of disease and specific treatments, together with new anti-lymphoma molecules that are now in the pipeline, may allow further improvements in the results of pediatric NHL treatment.

Summary and future directions for management

The field of pediatric NHL has witnessed significant progress in terms of knowledge and results in the last two decades. Most of the clinical improvements have originated from collaborative studies conducted at national and international levels in well-defined groups of diseases. Because pediatric NHL have a relatively low incidence and good to excellent prognosis with current therapies, large collaborative studies are needed to further improve results in selected subgroups of NHL that still show a rather unsatisfactory outcome. There are two remaining objectives for pediatric oncologists in this field:
• The identification of more effective treatments for children with aggressive and poor-responding NHL as salvage therapy for relapsed or refractory disease is rarely successful in B- cell and lymphoblastic lymphomas.
• Reduction of potential long-term toxicities of the current therapeutic strategies.
We hope that both of these objectives can be accomplished by increasing our knowledge of the biology of NHL and by designing better disease-targeted therapies that may integrate chemotherapy.

In considering NHL as a global pediatric health problem, one cannot ignore that the highly effective protocols in use in affluent countries are not feasible and affordable in limited resource countries. Thus, while applying increasingly highly technological approaches to diagnosis and treatment of NHL, consideration should be given to improve the existing facilities and treatments in developing countries. This will ultimately improve global survival rates of children with NHL and increase the knowledge of disease diversity and of the biological mechanisms of lymphomagenesis that are the basis for further progress.

References

1 Burkitt D. A sarcoma involving the jaws in African children. Br J Surg 1958; 46: 218–23.

2 Rosenberg SA, Diamond HD, Dargeon HW, Craver LF. Lymphosarcoma in childhood. N Engl J Med 1958; 259: 505–12.

3 Aur RJ, Hustu HO, Simone JV, Pratt CB, Pinkel D. Therapy of localized and regional lymphosarcoma of childhood. Cancer 1971; 27: 1328–31.

4 Murphy SB, Hustu HO. A randomized trial of combined modality therapy of childhood non-Hodgkin's lymphoma. Cancer 1980; 45: 630–7.

5 Wollner N, Burchenal JH, Lieberman PH, Exelby PR, D'Angio G, Murphy ML. Non-Hodgkin's lymphoma in children. A comparative study of two modalities of treatment. Cancer 1976; 37: 123–34.

6 SEER Cancer Statistics Review, 1975–2004. Bethesda: National Cancer Institute, 2007.

7 Anderson JR, Wilson JF, Jenkin DT, et al. Childhood non-Hodgkin's lymphoma. The results of a randomized therapeutic trial comparing a 4-drug regimen (COMP) with a 10-drug regimen (LSA2-L2). N Engl J Med 1983; 308: 559–65.

8 Sullivan MP, Boyett J, Pullen J, et al. Pediatric Oncology Group experience with modified LSA-L2 therapy in 107 children with non-Hodgkin's lymphoma (Burkitt's lymphoma excluded). Cancer 1985; 55: 323–36.

9 Muller-Weihrich S, Henze G, et al. BFM study 1975/81 for treatment of non-Hodgkin lymphoma of high malignancy in children and adolescents. Klin Padiatr 1982; 194: 219–25.

10 Patte C, Philip T, Rodary C, et al. Improved survival rate in children with stage III and IV B cell non-Hodgkin's lymphoma and leukemia using multi-agent chemotherapy: results of a study of 114 children from the French Pediatric Oncology Society. J Clin Oncol 1986; 4: 1219–26.

11 Reiter A, Schrappe M, Parwaresch R, et al. Non-Hodgkin's lymphomas of childhood and adolescence: results of a treatment stratified for biologic subtypes and stage–a report of the Berlin-Frankfurt-Munster Group. J Clin Oncol 1995; 13: 359–72.

12 Izarzuzaga MI, Steliarova-Foucher E, Martos MC, Zivkovic S. Non-Hodgkin's lymphoma incidence and survival in European children and adolescents (1978–1997): report from the Automated Childhood Cancer Information System project. Eur J Cancer 2006; 42: 2050–63.

13 Perkins SL. Work-up and diagnosis of pediatric non-Hodgkin's lymphomas. Pediatr Dev Pathol 2000; 3: 374–90.

14 Sandlund JT, Downing JR, Crist WM. Non-Hodgkin's lymphoma in childhood. N Engl J Med 1996; 334: 1238–48.

15 Harris NL, Jaffe ES, Stein H, et al. A revised European-American classification of lymphoid neoplasms: a proposal from the International Lymphoma Study Group. Blood. 1994; 84: 1361–92.

16 Jaffe ES, Harris NL, Stein H, Vardiman JW. World Health Organization Classification of Tumors. Pathology and Genetics of Tumors of Hematopoietic and Lymphoid Tissues. 2001.

17 Murphy SB. Management of pediatric lymphomas. Curr Opin Oncol 1989; 1: 42–6.

18 Magrath IT. Malignant non-Hodgkin's lymphomas in children. 4th edn. Philadelphia: Lippincott Williams & Wilkins, 2002.

19 Iversen U, Iversen OH, Bluming AZ, Ziegler JL, Kyalwasi S. Cell kinetics of African cases of Burkitt lymphoma. A preliminary report. Eur J Cancer 1972; 8: 305–8.

20 Shad A, Magrath I. Non-Hodgkin's lymphoma. Pediatr Clin North Am 1997; 44: 863–90.

21 Sariban E, Donahue A, Magrath IT. Jaw involvement in American Burkitt's Lymphoma. Cancer 1984; 53: 1777–82.

22 Bennett JM, Catovsky D, Daniel MT, et al. Proposals for the classification of the acute leukaemias. French-American-British (FAB) co-operative group. Br J Haematol 1976; 33: 451–8.

23 Harris NL, Jaffe ES, Diebold J, et al. World Health Organization classification of neoplastic diseases of the hematopoietic and lymphoid

tissues: report of the Clinical Advisory Committee meeting-Airlie House, Virginia, November 1997. J Clin Oncol 1999; 17: 3835–49.

24 Lukes RJ, Collins RD. New approaches to the classification of the lymphomata. Br J Cancer (Suppl.) 1975; 2: 1–28.

25 Braziel RM, Keneklis T, Donlon JA, et al. Terminal deoxynucleotidyl transferase in non-Hodgkin's lymphoma. Am J Clin Pathol 1983; 80: 655–9.

26 Desiderio SV, Yancopoulos GD, Paskind M, et al. Insertion of N regions into heavy-chain genes is correlated with expression of terminal deoxytransferase in B cells. Nature 1984; 311: 752–5.

27 Morabito F, Prasthofer EF, Pullen DJ, et al. Analysis of surface antigen profile, TdT expression, and T cell receptor gene rearrangement for maturational staging of leukemic T cells: a pediatric oncology group study. Leukemia 1987; 1: 514–7.

28 Killeen N, Irving BA, Pippig S, Zingler K. Signaling checkpoints during the development of T lymphocytes. Curr Opin Immunol 1998; 10: 360–7.

29 Bernard A, Boumsell L, Reinherz EL, et al. Cell surface characterization of malignant T cells from lymphoblastic lymphoma using monoclonal antibodies: evidence for phenotypic differences between malignant T cells from patients with acute lymphoblastic leukemia and lymphoblastic lymphoma. Blood 1981; 57: 1105–10.

30 Roper M, Crist WM, et al. Monoclonal antibody characterization of surface antigens in childhood T-cell lymphoid malignancies. Blood 1983; 61: 830–7.

31 Cossman J, Chused TM, Fisher RI, Magrath I, Bollum F, Jaffe ES. Diversity of immunological phenotypes of lymphoblastic lymphoma. Cancer Res 1983; 43: 4486–90.

32 Falini B. Anaplastic large cell lymphoma: pathological, molecular and clinical features. Br J Haematol 2001; 114: 741–60.

33 DeCoteau JF, Butmarc JR, Kinney MC, Kadin ME. The t(2;5) chromosomal translocation is not a common feature of primary cutaneous CD30+ lymphoproliferative disorders: comparison with anaplastic large-cell lymphoma of nodal origin. Blood 1996; 87: 3437–41.

34 Macpherson N, Lesack D, Klasa R, et al. Small noncleaved, non-Burkitt's (Burkit-Like) lymphoma: cytogenetics predict outcome and reflect clinical presentation. J Clin Oncol 1999; 17: 1558–67.

35 Dalla-Favera R, Martinotti S, Gallo RC, Erikson J, Croce CM. Translocation and rearrangements of the c-myc oncogene locus in human undifferentiated B-cell lymphomas. Science 1983; 219: 963–7.

36 Dang CV. c-Myc target genes involved in cell growth, apoptosis, and metabolism. Mol Cell Biol 1999; 19: 1–11.

37 Mussolin L, Basso K, Pillon M, et al. Prospective analysis of minimal bone marrow infiltration in pediatric Burkitt's lymphomas by long-distance polymerase chain reaction for t(8;14)(q24;q32). Leukemia 2003; 17: 585–9.

38 Pasqualucci L, Migliazza A, Basso K, Houldsworth J, Chaganti RS, Dalla-Favera R. Mutations of the BCL6 proto-oncogene disrupt its negative autoregulation in diffuse large B-cell lymphoma. Blood 2003; 101: 2914–23.

39 Lossos IS, Jones CD, Warnke R, et al. Expression of a single gene, BCL-6, strongly predicts survival in patients with diffuse large B-cell lymphoma. Blood 2001; 98: 945–51.

40 Crist WM, Shuster JJ, Falletta J, et al. Clinical features and outcome in childhood T-cell leukemia-lymphoma according to stage of thymocyte differentiation: a Pediatric Oncology Group Study. Blood 1988; 72: 1891–7.

41 Cairo MS, Raetz E, Lim MS, Davenport V, Perkins SL. Childhood and adolescent non-Hodgkin lymphoma: new insights in biology and critical challenges for the future. Pediatr Blood Cancer 2005; 45: 753–69.

42 Hojo H, Sasaki Y, Nakamura N, Abe M. Absence of somatic hypermutation of immunoglobulin heavy chain variable region genes in precursor B-lymphoblastic lymphoma: a study of four cases in childhood and adolescence. Am J Clin Pathol 2001; 116: 673–82.

43 Liang X, Meech SJ, Odom LF, et al. Assessment of t(2;5)(p23;q35) translocation and variants in pediatric ALK+ anaplastic large cell lymphoma. Am J Clin Pathol 2004; 121: 496–506.

44 Morris SW, Kirstein MN, Valentine MB, et al. Fusion of a kinase gene, ALK, to a nucleolar protein gene, NPM, in non-Hodgkin's lymphoma. Science 1994; 263: 1281–4.

45 Lones MA, Perkins SL, Sposto R, et al. Non-Hodgkin's lymphoma arising in bone in children and adolescents is associated with an excellent outcome: a Children's Cancer Group report. J Clin Oncol 2002; 20: 2293–301.

46 Mody RJ, Bui C, Hutchinson RJ, Frey KA, Shulkin BL. Comparison of (18)F Flurodeoxyglucose PET with Ga-67 scintigraphy and conventional imaging modalities in pediatric lymphoma. Leuk Lymphoma 2007; 48: 699–707.

47 Juweid ME, Stroobants S, Hoekstra OS, et al. Use of positron emission tomography for response assessment of lymphoma: consensus of the Imaging Subcommittee of International Harmonization Project in Lymphoma. J Clin Oncol 2007; 25: 571–8.

48 Seam P, Juweid ME, Cheson BD. The role of FDG-PET scans in patients with lymphoma. Blood 2007; 110: 3507–16.

49 Lister TA, Crowther SB, Sutcliffe SB, et al. Report of a committee convened to discuss the evaluation and staging of patients with Hodgkin's disease: Cotswolds meeting. J Clin Oncol 1989; 7: 1630–6.

50 Murphy SB. Classification, staging and end results of treatment of childhood non-Hodgkin's lymphomas: dissimilarities from lymphomas in adults. Semin Oncol 1980; 7: 332–9.

51 Reiter A, Schrappe M, Tiemann M, et al. Improved treatment results in childhood B-cell neoplasms with tailored intensification of therapy: a report of the Berlin-Frankfurt-Munster Group Trial NHL-BFM 90. Blood 1999; 94: 3294–306.

52 Patte C. Treatment of mature B-ALL and high grade B-NHL in children. Best Pract Res Clin Haematol 2002; 15: 695–711.

53 Reiter A, Schrappe M, Ludwig WD, et al. Intensive ALL-type therapy without local radiotherapy provides a 90% event-free survival for children with T-cell lymphoblastic lymphoma: a BFM group report. Blood 2000; 95: 416–21.

54 Le Deley MC, Reiter A, Williams D, et al. Prognostic factors in childhood anaplastic large cell lymphoma: results of a large European Intergroup Study. Blood 2008; 111: 1560–6.

55 Patte C, Auperin A, Gerrard M, et al. Results of the randomized international FAB/LMB96 trial for intermediate risk B-cell non-Hodgkin lymphoma in children and adolescents: it is possible to reduce treatment for the early responding patients. Blood 2007; 109: 2773–80.

56 Clifford P, Singh S, Stjernsward J, Klein G. Long-term survival of patients with Burkitt's lymphoma: an assessment of treatment and other factors which may relate to survival. Cancer Res 1967; 27: 2578–615.

57 Patte C, Gerrrard M, Auperin A, et al. Prognostic factors in childhood/adolescent B-cell lymphoma: results of the interantional FAB/LMB96 study. Ann Oncol 2005;16(Suppl. 5): v63.

58 Patte C, Auperin A, Michon J, et al. The Societe Francaise d'Oncologie Pediatrique LMB89 protocol: highly effective multiagent chemotherapy tailored to the tumor burden and initial response in 561 unselected children with B-cell lymphomas and L3 leukemia. Blood 2001; 97: 3370–9.

59 Bowman WP, Shuster JJ, Cook B, et al. Improved survival for children with B-cell acute lymphoblastic leukemia and stage IV small noncleaved-cell lymphoma: a pediatric oncology group study. J Clin Oncol 1996; 14: 1252–61.

60 Woessmann W, Seidemann K, Mann G, et al. The impact of the methotrexate administration schedule and dose in the treatment of children and adolescents with B-cell neoplasms: a report of the BFM Group Study NHL-BFM95. Blood 2005; 105: 948–58.

61 Patte C, Laplanche A, Bertozzi AI, et al. Granulocyte colony-stimulating factor in induction treatment of children with non-Hodgkin's lymphoma: a randomized study of the French Society of Pediatric Oncology. J Clin Oncol 2002; 20: 441–8.

62 Patte C, Sakiroglu C, Ansoborlo S, et al. Urate-oxidase in the prevention and treatment of metabolic complications in patients with B-cell lymphoma and leukemia, treated in the Societe Francaise d'Oncologie Pediatrique LMB89 protocol. Ann Oncol 2002; 13: 789–95.

63 Cairo MS, Gerrard M, Sposto R, et al. Results of a randomized international study of high-risk central nervous system B non-Hodgkin lymphoma and B acute lymphoblastic leukemia in children and adolescents. Blood 2007; 109: 2736–43.

64 Patte C, Kalifa C, Flamant F, et al. Results of the LMT81 protocol, a modified LSA2L2 protocol with high dose methotrexate, on 84 children with non-B-cell (lymphoblastic) lymphoma. Med Pediatr Oncol 1992; 20: 105–13.

65 Schrappe M, Tiemann M, Ludwig WD, et al. Risk-adapted therapy for lymphoblastic T-cell lymphoma: results from trials NHL-BFM86 and 90. Med Pediatr Oncol 1997; 29: 356–7.

66 Amylon MD, Shuster J, Pullen J, et al. Intensive high-dose asparaginase consolidation improves survival for pediatric patients with T cell acute lymphoblastic leukemia and advanced stage lymphoblastic lymphoma: a Pediatric Oncology Group study. Leukemia 1999; 13: 335–42.

67 Burkhardt B, Woessmann W, Zimmermann M, et al. Impact of cranial radiotherapy on central nervous system prophylaxis in children and adolescents with central nervous system-negative stage III or IV lymphoblastic lymphoma. J Clin Oncol 2006; 24: 491–9.

68 Vecchi V, Burnelli R, Pileri S, et al. Anaplastic large cell lymphoma (Ki-1+/CD30+) in childhood. Med Pediatr Oncol 1993; 21: 402–10.

69 Mora J, Filippa DA, Thaler HT, Polyak T, Cranor ML, Wollner N. Large cell non-Hodgkin lymphoma of childhood: analysis of 78 consecutive patients enrolled in 2 consecutive protocols at the Memorial Sloan-Kettering Cancer Center. Cancer 2000; 88: 186–97.

70 Rosolen A, Pillon M, Garaventa A, et al. Anaplastic large cell lymphoma treated with a leukemia-like therapy: report of the Italian Association of Pediatric Hematology and Oncology (AIEOP) LNH-92 protocol. Cancer 2005; 104: 2133–40.

71 Reiter A, Schrappe M, Tiemann M, et al. Successful treatment strategy for Ki-1 anaplastic large-cell lymphoma of childhood: a prospective analysis of 62 patients enrolled in three consecutive Berlin-Frankfurt-Munster group studies. J Clin Oncol 1994; 12: 899–908.

72 Massimino M, Gasparini M, Giardini R. Ki-1 (CD30) anaplastic large-cell lymphoma in children. Ann Oncol 1995; 6: 915–20.

73 Seidemann K, Tiemann M, Schrappe M, et al. Short-pulse B-non-Hodgkin lymphoma-type chemotherapy is efficacious treatment for pediatric anaplastic large cell lymphoma: a report of the Berlin-Frankfurt-Munster Group Trial NHL-BFM 90. Blood 2001; 97: 3699–706.

74 Brugieres L, Deley MC, Pacquement H, et al. CD30(+) anaplastic large-cell lymphoma in children: analysis of 82 patients enrolled in two consecutive studies of the French Society of Pediatric Oncology. Blood 1998; 92: 3591–8.

75 Williams DM, Hobson R, Imeson J, Gerrard M, McCarthy K, Pinkerton CR. Anaplastic large cell lymphoma in childhood: analysis of 72 patients treated on The United Kingdom Children's Cancer Study Group chemotherapy regimens. Br J Haematol 2002; 117: 812–20.

76 Laver JH, Kraveka JM, Hutchison RE, et al. Advanced-stage large-cell lymphoma in children and adolescents: results of a randomized trial incorporating intermediate-dose methotrexate and high-dose cytarabine in the maintenance phase of the APO regimen: a Pediatric Oncology Group phase III trial. J Clin Oncol 2005; 23: 541–7.

77 Brugieres L, Quartier P, Le Deley MC, et al. Relapses of childhood anaplastic large-cell lymphoma: treatment results in a series of 41 children – a report from the French Society of Pediatric Oncology. Ann Oncol 2000; 11: 53–8.

78 Cairo MS, Krailo MD, Morse M, et al. Long-term follow-up of short intensive multiagent chemotherapy without high-dose methotrexate ('Orange') in children with advanced non-lymphoblastic non-Hodgkin's lymphoma: a children's cancer group report. Leukemia 2002 ; 16: 594–600.

79 Tubergen DG, Krailo MD, Meadows AT, et al. Comparison of treatment regimens for pediatric lymphoblastic non-Hodgkin's lymphoma: a Childrens Cancer Group study. J Clin Oncol 1995; 13: 1368–76.

80 Bergeron C, Gomez F, Pacquement H, et al. Treatment of childhood T lymphoblastic lymphoma (TLL)-Results of the SFOP LMT96. Pediatr Blood Cancer 2006; 46: 967.

81 Link MP, Shuster JJ, Donaldson SS, Berard CW, Murphy SB. Treatment of children and young adults with early-stage non-Hodgkin's lymphoma. N Engl J Med 1997; 337: 1259–66.

82 Link MP, Donaldson SS, Berard CW, Shuster JJ, Murphy SB. Results of treatment of childhood localized non-Hodgkin's lymphoma with combination chemotherapy with or wiothout radiotherapy. N Engl J Med 1990; 322: 1169–74.

83 Neth O, Seidemann K, Jansen P, et al. Precursor B-cell lymphoblastic lymphoma in childhood and adolescence: clinical features, treatment, and results in trials NHL-BFM 86 and 90. Med Pediatr Oncol 2000; 35: 20–7.

84 Seidemann K, Tiemann M, Lauterbach I, et al. Primary mediastinal large B-cell lymphoma with sclerosis in pediatric and adolescent patients: treatment and results from three therapeutic studies of the Berlin-Frankfurt-Munster Group. J Clin Oncol 2003; 21: 1782–9.

85 Burkhardt B, Zimmermann M, Oschlies I, et al. The impact of age and gender on biology, clinical features and treatment outcome of non-Hodgkin lymphoma in childhood and adolescence. Br J Haematol 2005; 131: 39–49.

86 Piira T, Perkins SL, Anderson JR, et al. Primary mediastinal large cell lymphoma in children: a report from the Childrens Cancer Group. Pediatr Pathol Lab Med 1995; 15: 561–70.

87 Zinzani PL, Martelli M, Magagnoli M, et al. Treatment and clinical management of primary mediastinal large B-cell lymphoma with

sclerosis: MACOP-B regimen and mediastinal radiotherapy monitored by (67)Gallium scan in 50 patients. Blood 1999; 94: 3289–93.

88 Atra A, Meller ST, Stevens RS, et al. Conservative management of follicular non-Hodgkin's lymphoma in childhood. Br J Haematol 1998; 103: 220–3.

89 Lorsbach RB, Shay-Seymore D, Moore J, et al. Clinicopathologic analysis of follicular lymphoma occurring in children. Blood 2002; 99: 1959–64.

90 Claviez A, Meyer U, Dominick C, Beck JF, Rister M, Tiemann M. MALT lymphoma in children: a report from the NHL-BFM Study Group. Pediatr Blood Cancer 2006; 47: 210–4.

91 Bekkenk MW, Geelen FA, van Voorst Vader PC, et al. Primary and secondary cutaneous CD30(+) lymphoproliferative disorders: a report from the Dutch Cutaneous Lymphoma Group on the long-term follow-up data of 219 patients and guidelines for diagnosis and treatment. Blood 2000; 95: 3653–61.

92 Nijsten T, Curiel-Lewandrowski C, Kadin ME. Lymphomatoid papulosis in children: a retrospective cohort study of 35 cases. Arch Dermatol 2004; 140: 306–12.

93 Wain EM, Orchard GE, Whittaker SJ, Spittle MSMF, Russell-Jones R. Outcome in 34 patients with juvenile-onset mycosis fungoides: a clinical, immunophenotypic, and molecular study. Cancer 2003; 98: 2282–90.

94 Whittaker SJ, Marsden JR, Spittle M, Russell Jones R. Joint British Association of Dermatologists and UK Cutaneous Lymphoma Group guidelines for the management of primary cutaneous T-cell lymphomas. Br J Dermatol 2003; 149: 1095–107.

95 Santucci M, Pimpinelli N, Massi D, et al. Cytotoxic/natural killer cell cutaneous lymphomas. Report of EORTC Cutaneous Lymphoma Task Force Workshop. Cancer. 2003; 97: 610–27.

96 Belhadj K, Reyes F, Farcet JP, et al. Hepatosplenic gammadelta T-cell lymphoma is a rare clinicopathologic entity with poor outcome: report on a series of 21 patients. Blood 2003; 102: 4261–9.

97 Cohen LF, Balow JE, Magrath IT, Poplack DG, Ziegler JL. Acute tumor lysis syndrome. A review of 37 patients with Burkitt's lymphoma. Am J Med 1980; 68: 486–91.

98 Seidemann K, Meyer U, Jansen P, et al. Impaired renal function and tumor lysis syndrome in pediatric patients with non-Hodgkin's lymphoma and B-ALL. Observations from the BFM-trials. Klin Padiatr 1998; 210: 279–84.

99 Wossmann W, Schrappe M, Meyer U, Zimmermann M, Reiter A. Incidence of tumor lysis syndrome in children with advanced stage Burkitt's lymphoma/leukemia before and after introduction of prophylactic use of urate oxidase. Ann Hematol 2003; 82: 160–5.

100 Goldman SC, Holcenberg JS, Finklestein JZ, et al. A randomized comparison between rasburicase and allopurinol in children with lymphoma or leukemia at high risk for tumor lysis. Blood 2001; 97: 2998–3003.

101 Coiffier B. Rituximab in the treatment of diffuse large B-cell lymphomas. Semin Oncol 2002; 29(1 Suppl 2): 30–5.

102 de Vries MJ, Veerman AJ, Zwaan CM. Rituximab in three children with relapsed/refractory B-cell acute lymphoblastic leukaemia/Burkitt non-Hodgkin's lymphoma. Br J Haematol 2004; 125: 414–5.

103 Berg SL, Blaney SM, Devidas M, et al. Phase II study of nelarabine (compound 506U78) in children and young adults with refractory T-cell malignancies: a report from the Children's Oncology Group. J Clin Oncol 2005; 23: 3376–82.

104 Jeha S, Gaynon PS, Razzouk BI, et al. Phase II study of clofarabine in pediatric patients with refractory or relapsed acute lymphoblastic leukemia. J Clin Oncol 2006; 24: 1917–23.

105 Gandhi V, Balakrishnan K. Pharmacology and mechanism of action of forodesine, a T-cell targeted agent. Semin Oncol 2007; 34(6 Suppl 5): S8–12.

106 Houghton PJ, Morton CL, Kolb EA, et al. Initial testing (stage 1) of the proteasome inhibitor bortezomib by the pediatric preclinical testing program. Pediatr Blood Cancer 2008; 50: 37–45.

107 Bartlett NL, Younes A, Carabasi MH, et al. A phase 1 multidose study of SGN-30 immunotherapy in patients with refractory or recurrent CD30+ hematologic malignancies. Blood 2008; 111: 1848–54.

108 Pasqualucci L, Wasik M, Teicher BA, et al. Antitumor activity of anti-CD30 immunotoxin (Ber-H2/saporin) in vitro and in severe combined immunodeficiency disease mice xenografted with human CD30+ anaplastic large-cell lymphoma. Blood 1995; 85: 2139–46.

109 Schnell R, Staak O, Borchmann P, et al. A Phase I study with an anti-CD30 ricin A-chain immunotoxin (Ki-4.dgA) in patients with refractory CD30+ Hodgkin's and non-Hodgkin's lymphoma. Clin Cancer Res 2002; 8: 1779–86.

110 Pulford K, Falini B, Banham AH, et al. Immune response to the ALK oncogenic tyrosine kinase in patients with anaplastic large-cell lymphoma. Blood 2000; 96: 1605–7.

111 Ait-Tahar K, Barnardo MC, Pulford K. CD4 T-helper responses to the anaplastic lymphoma kinase (ALK) protein in patients with ALK-positive anaplastic large-cell lymphoma. Cancer Res 2007; 67: 1898–901.

112 Galkin AV, Melnick JS, Kim S, et al. Identification of NVP-TAE684, a potent, selective, and efficacious inhibitor of NPM-ALK. Proc Natl Acad Sci USA 2007; 104: 270–5.

113 Bomgaars L, Geyer JR, Franklin J, et al. Phase I trial of intrathecal liposomal cytarabine in children with neoplastic meningitis. J Clin Oncol 2004; 22: 3916–21.

10 Hodgkin's Lymphoma

Wolfgang Dörffel[1] and Dieter Körholz[2]

[1] Hospital for Children and Adolescents, HELIOS-Klinikum Berlin-Buch, Berlin, Germany and [2] Department of Pediatrics, Martin Luther University Halle/Wittenberg, Halle/Saale, Germany

Introduction

Hodgkin's lymphoma (HL, synonym: Hodgkin's disease, lymphogranuloma) is a malignant disease, histologically characterized by giant multinuclear Hodgkin's and Reed-Sternberg (H-RS) cells in the classical variant of HL (cHL), while lymphocytic and histiocytic (L & H) cells are characteristic of the nodular lymphocytic predominant HL (nLPHL or LPHL). These tumor cells usually account for less than 1% of cells in the tumor tissue and are embedded in a reactive infiltrate consisting of T-cells, histiocytes, eosinophils, plasma cells and others. The discussion about the origin of these cells and therefore of Hodgkin's disease (HD) itself has long been controversial and it has variably been considered an inflammatory or infectious disease, an unusual immunologic reaction, a true neoplasm, or a combination of these. Today there is clear evidence that the tumor cells in cHL and nLPHL differ in their immunophenotype and the mutational status of the immunoglobulin heavy chain gene and that the diseases they cause differ in clinical manifestations and course. Therefore, the World Health Organization (WHO) classification distinguishes these two different lymphomas as separate entities [1].

Prior to the middle of the last century HL was nearly always fatal. However, in the late 1960s, with the introduction of an effective treatment using high dose extended field radiotherapy (RT) for local disease and combination chemotherapy for advanced disease, the basis for the current high cure rates was laid. Such intensive treatment in children often caused severe side and late effects [2]. Therefore from the late 1970s onward cooperative study groups initiated trials for combined-modality therapy in pediatric HL [3–5] with the aim to further increase cure rates and to reduce the risk of potential late effects. Some trials in pediatric HD soon obtained cure rates of 90% and more. With risk and response adapted treatment strategies therapy of

HL is a paradigm of tailored therapies that extends beyond the field of pediatric oncology. Milestones in the history of HD, classification, and therapy are listed in Table 10.1.

Epidemiology and pathogenesis

In Germany incidence of HL is 0.7 children/100 000 children below the age of 15 years [14]. Distribution of HL regarding age and gender in children are illustrated by the proportions in the trial GPOH-HD 95 (Figure 10.1), but the number of adolescents older than 16 years is underestimated because many such patients were treated on adult treatment protocols.

The disease has two age peaks – at about 25 and later than 55 years. In developing countries the first peak appears earlier, suggesting that infections might play an important role in the pathogenesis of HL. In India the number of Epstein-Barr virus (EBV)-positive HL is much higher than in Europe. A study by Dinand et al. [15] showed that the prevalence of EBV was as high as 90% in children with HL in North India compared with about 30–50% in Western Countries. EBV positivity was significantly correlated with younger age and low socioeconomic status supporting the hypothesis that infections could contribute to the pathogenesis of HL in young patients.

The etiology of HL is so far unknown. Genetic factors might contribute, because monozygotic twins have a 50-fold increased risk of developing HL if one child is affected [16]. In addition, immunodeficiencies with DNA breakage syndromes seem to be associated with the development of HL. On the other hand, environmental factors might also contribute to the pathogenesis of the disease. Hjalgrim et al. [17] could demonstrate that infectious mononucleosis increases the risk for EBV-positive, but not EBV-negative HL about 3.2 fold. This risk was especially pronounced in the group of younger patients (below 44 years of age). HL occurred in these patients between 1.8 and 4.9 years after infectious mononucleosis.

Küppers et al. were the first to demonstrate that H-RS cells mainly derive from pre-apoptotic germ center B-cells with less

Pediatric Hematology and Oncology, 1st edition. Edited by Edward J. Estlin, Richard J. Gilbertson, and Robert F. Wynn. © 2010 Blackwell Publishing Ltd.

than 1% from T-cells [12, 18]. In many H-RS cells destructive mutations of the Ig genes were found, which normally lead to apoptotic cell death in physiological germinal center B-cells. However, in H-RS cells a constitutive overexpression of nuclear factor NF-kappa-B was found. This factor is able to inhibit apoptosis induction [19].

Although H-RS cells originate from germinal center B-cells, these cells mainly lack the B-cell gene expression profile of their normal counterpart [20]. Some of the key regulators of B-cell

Table 10.1 Milestones in recognition and treatment of Hodgkin's lymphoma.

1832	First description of the eponymous lymphomatoid disease by Thomas Hodgkin [6]
1898–1902	Description of the histological picture with characteristic cells by Carl Sternberg and by Dorothy Reed
1902	First X-ray irradiation of HD in a 4 year old boy (Pusey) [7]
1943	First chemotherapy of HD with nitrogen mustard (Goodman *et al.* 1946)
1964	Introduction of the combined chemotherapy MOPP (De Vita *et al.* 1970) [8]
1965	Rye-modification of the histologicical classification (Lukes *et al.* 1966) [9]
1966	Concept of the tumoricidal irradiation (Kaplan 1966) [10]
1970	Combined chemoradiotherapy for children (Donaldson and Link 1987) [3]
1971	Staging classification of Ann Arbor (Carbone *et al.*) [11]
1994	H-RS cells are clonally, mostly B-cell-derived malignant cells (Küppers) [12]
1997	WHO classification of lymphomas (Harris *et al.*1999) [13]

HD, Hodgkin's disease. MOPP, mechlorethamine + oncovin (vincristine) + prednisone + procarbazine. H-RS, Hodgkin's and Reed-Sternberg. WHO, World Health Organization.

specific gene expression such as E2A and EBF are retained but most of the down-stream target genes are not expressed [21, 22]. Recently, it was demonstrated that in HL-cells inhibitors of E2A-ID2 and ABF-1 are overexpressed. In normal B-cells overexpression of these proteins lead to inhibition of B-cell specific gene expression. On the other hand, inhibition of ABF-1 in H-RS-cells down-regulated aberrant T-cell specific genes expression, a phenomenon typical for H-RS cells. In addition to overexpression of ABF-1 or ID2, the expression of the transcription factor Notch-1 might explain the aberrant T-cell antigen expression which was observed in up to 5% of H-RS cells [23]. In conclusion, while a lot of facts are known about the potential molecular mechanisms of aberrant B-cell development in H-RS cells, the process inducing these aberrations is largely unknown.

The HL tumor mass consists mostly of less than 1% of classic HL cells, while 99% of the tumor mass is composed of infiltration lymphocytes and other cell types. Thus, not only the HL cells itself, but also the microenvironment and the interaction between HL cells and microenvironment might play important roles in the pathogenesis of this lymphoma. The HL cells produce several cytokines such as IL-13 which could stimulate an autocrine growth of HL-cells. Trieu *et al.* [24] report that inhibition of IL-13 could reduce proliferation of HL cells. In addition, HL cell growth was inhibited *in vivo* in mice by using an inhibitory soluble IL-13 receptor. Finally, production of Th-2 cytokines such as IL-13 by HL-cells could lead to infiltration of eosinophils, Th-2 and other regulatory cells as well as fibroblasts.

Other cytokines, such as IL-10, have been shown to be relevant for the development of systemic B-symptoms. In addition, Visco *et al.* [25] could show that IL-10 is an independent risk factor and that high IL-10 levels correlate with a poorer prognosis. This might be explained by the immunosuppressive effects of IL-10. Marshall *et al.* [26] found that HL infiltrating lymphocytes are

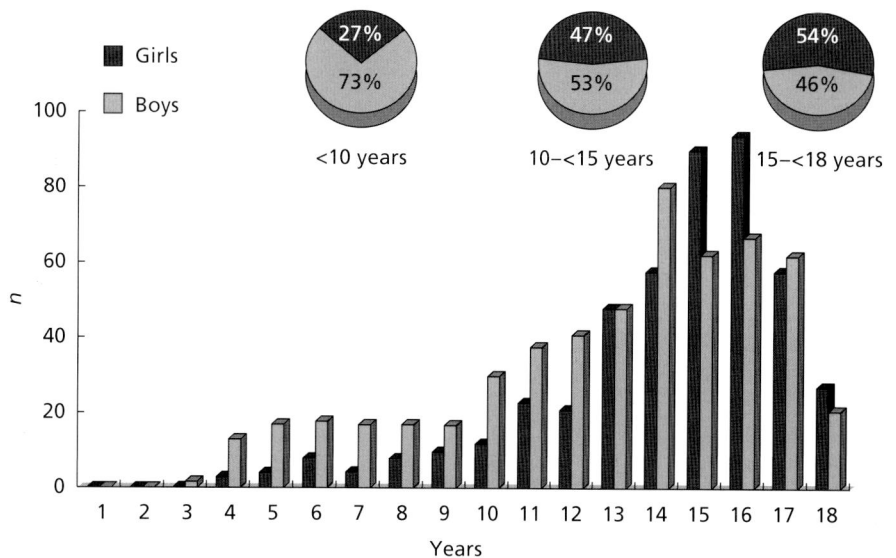

Figure 10.1 Age and gender in trial GPOH-HD 95. (Reproduced from Dörffel W [115], with permission from Springer Science and Business Media.)

mainly IL-10 secreting regulatory T-cells and that these cells are able to reduce function of regulatory T-cells.

Clinical presentation

The most common presenting sign in children and adolescents with HL is progressive, painless lymphadenopathy, most frequently in the neck. Figure 10.2(a) shows the incidence of lymph node involvement and Figure 10.2(b) extra nodal involvement in 1018 patients (GPOH-HD 95 trial).

About 80% of the patients present with mediastinal involvement, which can cause cough, shortness of breath or evidence of venous obstruction. Palpable enlargement of the liver and spleen or symptoms from osseous or pulmonary involvement are rare. About one-third of children present with systemic B-symptoms as defined by the Ann Arbor staging criteria (fever above 38°C, drenching night sweats, unexplained weight loss >10% within 6 months). Itching is a rare sign in children and without prognostic relevance.

The disease might present with paraneoplastic signs such as nephrotic syndrome, immunothrombocytopenia, or other syndromes. Children with HL can present with immunologic deficiencies and infection from an acquired cellular immune defect.

Anemia, leucocytosis or eosinophilia and, in advanced disease, lymphopenia might be observed. Marked pancytopenia should raise the suspicion of bone marrow involvement.

Investigation and staging

Accurate diagnosis of HL can only be made by histological examination of tissue from an excisional biopsy of enlarged lymph nodes or other involved sites. Needle-aspiration biopsy is insufficient for defining the histological pattern and for immunohistochemistry and molecular genetics. Identification of the characteristic H-RS cells, i.e. mono- (Hodgkin's cell) or multi-nucleated (Reed-Sternberg cells) giant cells with inclusion-like nucleoli can be made by cytological or histological examinations. However they are not pathognomonic for HL and can also be found in reactive processes including infectious mononucleosis and phenytoin-induced pseudolymphoma, and in non-Hodgkin's lymphoma.

The current classification of HL by the WHO [1], follows the Rye classification [9], but it describes two main entities: classic HL (cHL) with four subtypes (Table 10.2) and in addition nodular lymphocyte predominant HL (nLPHL).

Immunophenotyping of the H-RS cells (in cHL) and of lymphocytic and histiocytic (L & H) cells is essential in order to distinguish cHL and nLPHL.

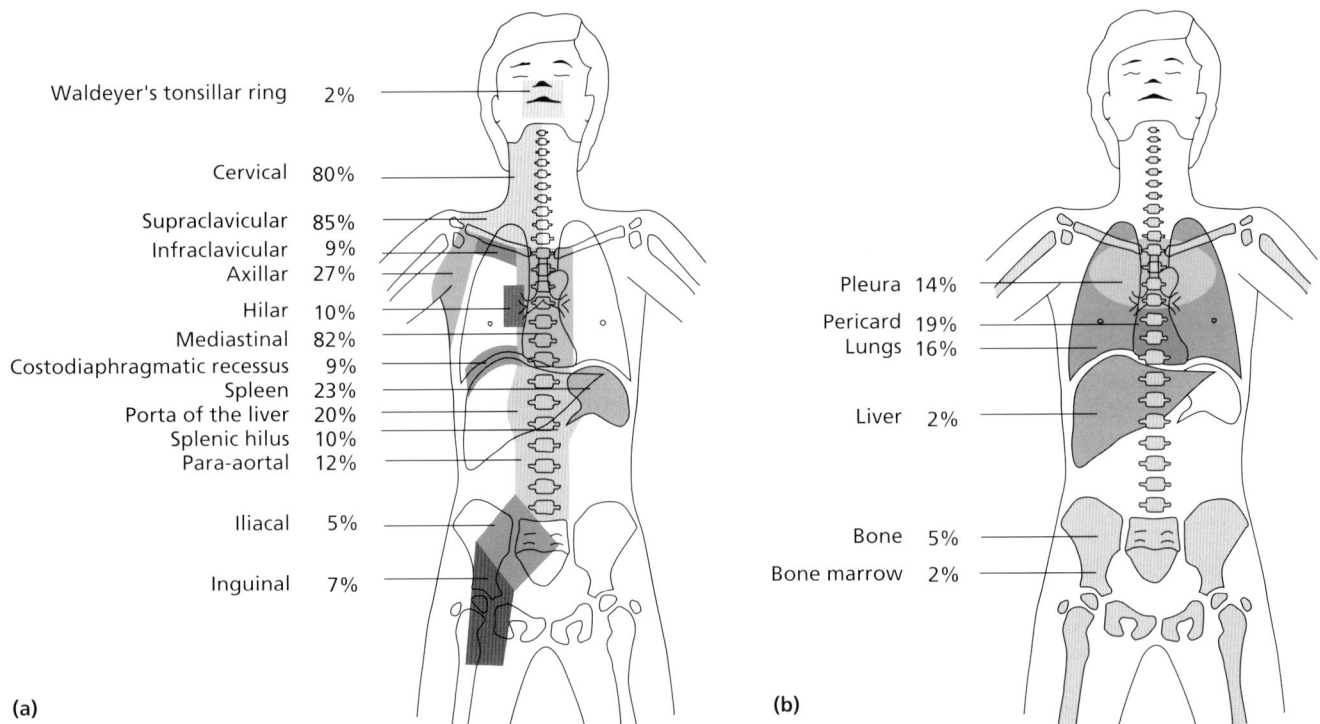

Figure 10.2 (a), Relevant nodal involvement, % in trial GPOH-HD 95 (*n* = 1018). Each independent lymph node region is one field (e.g. cervical and supraclavicular lymph node are together one field, but left and right are different independent fields). (b), Extranodal involvement, % in trial GPOH-HD 95 (*n* = 1018). (Modified from Dörffel W [115], with permission from Springer Science and Business Media.)

When a diagnosis of HL has been confirmed then staging procedures should be undertaken and carefully documented:
- The exact history of disease (e.g. systemic symptoms, paraneoplastic syndromes) should be recorded.
- Clinical examination of all palpable lymph nodes, palpation of spleen and liver, and examination of Waldeyer's tonsillar ring by an otolaryngologist should be performed.
- Laboratory tests are blood count, erythrocyte sedimentation rate, liver and renal function, serum protein and electrophoresis, immune status and serologic examinations for antibodies against relevant viral infection, and toxoplasmosis.
- Electrocardiogram and echocardiography are strongly recommended.
- The extent of diagnostic imaging depends on diverse factors including trial enrolment and socioeconomic conditions. Ultrasound, for example, is a reliable imaging procedure in the hands of experienced investigators for the detection of involved lymph nodes and the evaluation of abdominal organ enlargement, especially the spleen.

Table 10.2 WHO classification of Hodgkin's lymphoma and distribution (%) in trial GPOH-HD 95 (*n* = 1018).

	% of cases
Classic Hodgkin's lymphoma (cHL):	91
Lymphocyte rich classical HL (LRcHL)	1
Nodular sclerosis (NS)*	68
Mixed cellularity (MC)	21
Lymphocyte depletion (LD)	<1
Nodular lymphocyte predominant Hodgkin's lymphoma (nLPHL)	9

*According to Bennett *et al.*[27] we can perform a grading in type 1 and 2 (relation in GPOH-HD 95 pts like 3:), which may have prognostic relevance according to some trials.

- Chest radiograph is essential in all cases including measurement of mediastinal tumor size (ratio of maximum transverse tumor diameter to maximum intrathoracic diameter at T5/6 level). A ratio greater than or equal to one-third defines bulky mediastinal disease and is considered in many trials an indication of advanced disease, requiring intensified treatment. Thoracic computed tomography (CT) is the best method for the demonstration of lung involvement. Neck, abdomen, and pelvis can be investigated by CT or – without radiation exposure – with magnetic resonance imaging (MRI). Both imaging procedures can detect contiguous extranodal involvement of pleura, pericardium, or thoracic wall. Pleural effusions might also be secondary to lymphatic or venous obstruction within the mediastinum. For examination with regard to potential subdiaphragmatic involvement ultrasound, CT, or MRI have replaced diagnostic laparatomy and lymphangiography in the detection of subdiaphragmatic involvement. Splenectomy is obsolete and harmful in children with HL. Selective laparoscopy is indicated only in the rare case when subdiaphragmatic involvement cannot be excluded with other imaging methods. A surgical procedure might become necessary in females cases with subdiaphragmatic disease where the ovaries have to be omitted from the RT fields.
- Bone marrow biopsy remains mandatory in advanced cases (stage IIB–IV).
- Gallium scanning is a sensitive diagnostic procedure in HD and used in many countries, but it has limited accuracy in subdiaphragmatic sites. It will be replaced increasingly by fluor-deoxy-glucose-positron emission tomography (FDG-PET or PET).
- Bone scanning was mandatory in most trials but with the introduction of PET it can be limited to those cases with suspicious bone lesions.

FDG-PET is increasingly used in HL for initial staging and for response assessment after therapy (for overview see [29]). It can image the entire body and even detect foci in lung or bone. It can be used for differentiation between viable tumor and residual necrotic or fibrotic tissue and thus for evaluation of treatment response (Figure 10.3). Today PET–CT more and more

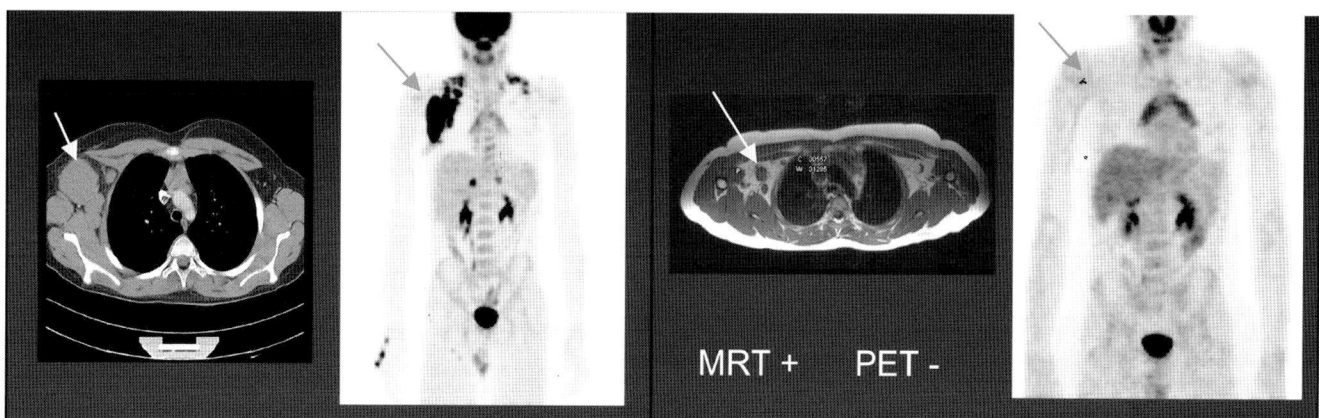

Figure 10.3 Imaging of a patient with axillary lymphadenopathy. Left panel: CT and PET prior to chemotherapy. Right panel: MRI and PET after chemotherapy. While the MRI shows residual lymph nodes, the PET is already negative. (Figures kindly provided by Prof. Dr R. Kluge, Leipzig.)

Table 10.3 Ann Arbor/Cotswold staging classification of Hodgkin's lymphoma (Lister *et al.* 1989 [28], modified phrase).

Stage	
I	Involvement of a single independent lymph node region (I) or lymphoid structure (e.g. spleen, thymus, Waldeyer's ring) or a single extralymphatic site (I$_E$)
II	Involvement of two or more lymph node regions on the same side of the diaphragm without (II) or with (II$_E$) involvement of extralymphatic organs or sites
III	Involvement of lymph node regions on both sides of the diaphragm without (III) or with (III$_E$) involvement of extralymphatic organs or sites
IV	Disseminated (multifocal) involvement of extra-nodal sites beyond 'E'-sites

Annotations to stage definitions:
A. No B symptoms
B. At least one of the following systemic symptoms
  1. Unexplained persisting or recurrent fever above 38°C
  2. Drenching night sweats
  3. Inexplicable weight loss of more than 10% during last 6 months
E. Extra-lymphatic structures or organs that are infiltrated per continuum out or proximal of a lymphatic mass are termed E-lesion (examples: lung, pleura, pericardium, bones) and do not automatically qualify for stage IV. Exceptions: liver or bone marrow involvement always implies stage IV.

substitutes for CT/MRI and PET. However, for correct staging it is absolutely necessary to have a CT scan with intravenous contrast to evaluate all lymph node regions correctly.

Clinical staging classification of HL uses the Cotswold revision of the Ann Arbor classification [28] (Table 10.3).

Most study groups use this staging system for treatment stratification and differentiate early (I, II and IIIA) from advanced (IIIB and IV) stages. Early stages can be further divided according to the presence of additional risk factors into 'early favorable' and 'early unfavorable or intermediate' stages. Generally B symptoms, extranodal involvement and advanced stages were considered risk factors for poor prognosis. Other factors like bulky disease (e.g. mediastinal bulky disease, or a defined number and size of involved lymph node regions), high erythrocyte sedimentation rate or anemia are more dependent on treatment regimen. With effective treatment strategies some of these factors have lost their impact on prognosis, such as tumor burden and histological subtype.

Treatment

With modern RT alone, cure rates in early stage HL are up to 80–90% in early stages and are about 50% in advanced stages. The recognition of the natural history with systematic spread of the disease from an initially involved node along known lymphatic pathways led to the development of the extended field (EF) RT technique; radiotherapy was not just applied to clinically

involved lymph nodes but also to the adjacent regions which often are subclinically infiltrated by HL [30].

The supradiaphragmatic lymph node regions and the mediastinum were encompassed in a so-called 'mantle field' and irradiated simultaneously, the lymph nodes below the diaphragm (para-aortic, iliac and inguinal) and the spleen were treated using the 'inverted Y-techniques', with the combination of both volumes resulting in 'total nodal irradiation' (TNI). In addition, it became obvious that a fractionated dose of about 40 Gy is needed for permanent local tumor control [10]. This wide field techniques and high dose RT can only be applied in a safe way with modern treatment equipment (megavolt linear accelerators, planning systems, customized blocks or leafs for the shielding of surrounding healthy tissue). However, despite using these modern techniques the very intensive RT can cause severe side and late effects, especially in children [2].

When effective chemotherapy became available it was recommended to reduce the dose [31] and volumes of RT [32] or both [4] in pediatric trials. Low-dose irradiation of involved regions only (IF-RT) in combination with chemotherapy ('combined modality therapy') became the standard [3, 33] for some time. A further reduction of the irradiation volumes to individualized or 'reduced involved' fields was performed in DAL trials (Figure 10.4) [34]. Nowadays efforts are directed towards response-adapted strategies with the avoidance of radiotherapy whenever it seems possible (see below).

During the past a variety of single antitumor agents were used for induction of and maintenance of remission in HD, e.g. with mechlorethamine, chlorambucil, vinca alkaloids, cyclophosphamide, procarbazine and others. But curative management of HD was not successful until the development of combination chemotherapy. De Vita *et al.* [8] tried to combine various single cytostatic agents with proven efficacy in HD but each agent had a different mode of action and a different toxicity profile. The most effective combination proved to be MOPP (mechlorethamine, oncovin [vincristin], prednisone and procarbazine).

When 188 patients with advanced HD were treated with MOPP the relapse-free survival (RFS) was 66% and the overall survival (OS) 48% at 20 years [8, 45]. In the following years several variants of MOPP with substitution of some agents were tried, such as COPP (substitution of M by cyclophosphamide, Table 10.4), LOPP (substitution of M by chlorambucil), ChlVPP (substitution of M by chlorambucil and of O by vinblastine) and others [46: overview]. Some of these combinations proved to be less toxic in comparison to MOPP but not more effective. The German-Austrian pediatric DAL group developed OPPA in which mechlorethamine was replaced by adriamycin, and the doses of prednisone and vincristine were increased. OPPA has a high efficacy and is considered the backbone of the DAL/GPOH trials. Another breakthrough was achieved with the development of ABVD (adriamycin, bleomycin, vinblastine and dacarbazine) by Bonadonna *et al.* [35]. ABVD proved equally efficacious in trials either alone or together with MOPP in alternative or hybrid regimens (e.g. COPP/ABV, Table 10.4) and superior to MOPP

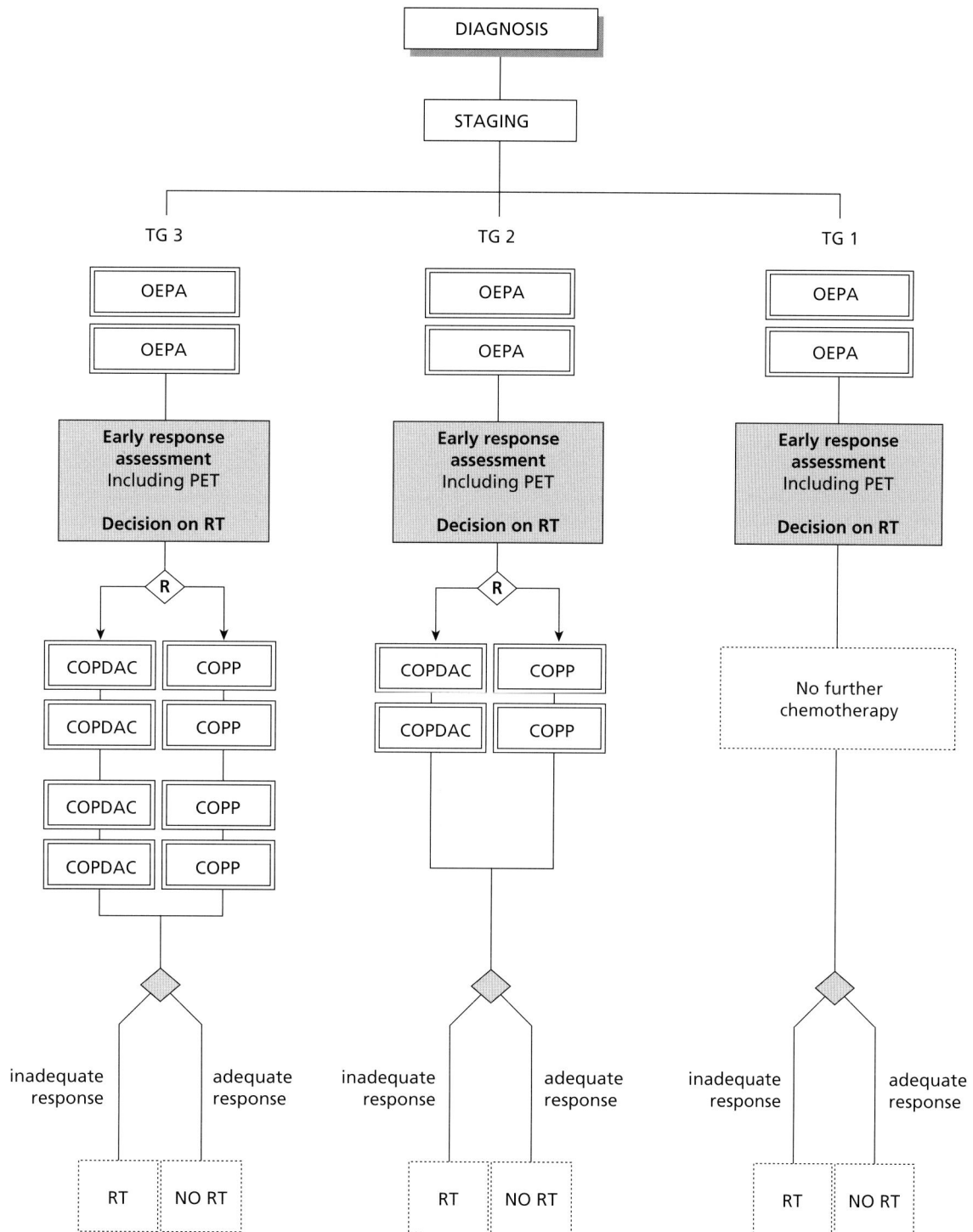

Figure 10.4 Radiation fields for total nodal irradiation, mantle field, involved field and individualized local field. (Reproduced from Dörffel W [115], with permission from Springer Science and Business Media.)

[47]. 'Stanford V' [40] and BEACOPP [39] are noteworthy examples of combination chemotherapy regimens, although largely employed in adult trials. Important regimens for children and adolescents are also VBVP, VAMP, OEPA and possibly COPDAC, which avoid some of the serious late effects of other combination chemotherapies.

There are many publications about chemotherapy alone in treatment of children with HL. They were reported either from

Table 10.4 Chemotherapeutic regimens in Hodgkin's lymphoma.

ABVD 28 d
Bonadonna *et al.* 1982 [35]

Adriamycin	25 mg/m^2	i.v.	d1+15
Dacarbacine	375 mg/m^2	i.v.	d1+15
Bleomycin	10 mg/m^2	i.v.	d1+15
Vinblastine	6 mg/m^2	i.v.	d1+15

COPP, 28 d, in brackets the modification used by the DAL/GPOH group
Morgenfeld 1972 [36]/ DAL: Breu 1982 [4]

Cyclophosphamide	650 (500) mg/m^2	i.v.	d1+8
Vincristine (O = oncovin)	1.4 (1.5) mg/m^2, max. 2 mg	i.v.	d1+8
Procarbazine	100 mg/m^2/d	p.o.	d1–14 (–15)
Prednison	40 mg/m^2/d	p.o.	d1–14 (–15)

COPP/ABV 28 d (regimen used by CCG)
Nachmann *et al.* 2002 [37]

Cyclophosphamide	600 mg/m^2	i.v.	d1
Vincristine	1.4 mg/m^2, max. 2 mg	i.v.	d1
Procarbazine	100 mg/m^2/d	p.o.	d1–7
Prednison	40 mg/m^2/d	p.o.	d1–14
Adriamycin	35 mg/m^2	i.v.	d8
Bleomycin	10 U/m^2	i.v.	d8
Vinblastine	6 mg/m^2	i.v.	d8

OPPA 28 d
Breu *et al.* 1982 [4]

Vincristine (O = oncovin)	1.5 mg/m^2, max. 2 mg	i.v.	d1+8+15
Procarbazine	100 mg/m^2/d	p.o.	d1–15
Prednison	60 mg/m^2/d	p.o.	d1–15
Adriamycin	40 mg/m^2	i.v.	d1+15

OEPA 28 d
Schellong *et al.* 1999 [34]
Schedule like OPPA, but Procarbazine substituted by:

Etoposide	125 mg/m^2	i.v.	d3–6
in the current version of the EuroNet –PHL-C1 trial	1	dose Etoposide more	d1–5

COPDAC 28 d
Körholz 2006 [38]

Cyclophosphamide	650 (500) mg/m^2	i.v.	d1+8
Vincristine (O = oncovin)	1.4 (1.5) mg/m^2, max. 2 mg	i.v.	d1+8
Dacarbazine	250 mg/m^2/d	i.v.	d1–3
Prednison	40 mg/m^2/d	p.o.	d1–15

BEACOPP-escalated, and in brackets: BEACOPP-basis 21 d
Diehl *et al.* 1997 [39]

Bleomycine	10 mg/m^2	i.v.	d8
Etoposide	200 (100) mg/m^2	i.v.	d1–3
Adriamycin 35	(25) mg/m^2	i.v.	d1
Cyclophosphamide	1250 (650) mg/m^2	i.v.	d1
Vincristine	1.4 mg/m^2, max. 2 mg	i.v.	d8
Procarbazine	100 mg/m^2	p.o.	d1–7
Prednisone	40 mg/m^2	p.o.	d1–14

Table 10.4 *Continued*

Stanford V 28 d
Bartlett *et al.* 1995 [40]

Adriamycin	25 mg/m²	i.v.	d1+15
Vinblastine	6 mg/m²	i.v.	d1+15
Mechlorethamine	6 mg/m²	i.v.	d1
Vincristine	1.4 mg/m², max. 2 mg	i.v.	d8+22
Bleomycin	5 U/m²	i.v.	d8+22
Etoposide	60 mg/m²	i.v.	d15+16
Prednisone	40 mg/m²	p.o.	alternating (each 2nd day)

VAMP 28 d
Donaldson *et al.* 2002 [41]

Vinblastine	6 mg/m²	i.v.	d1+15
Adriamycin	25 mg/m²	i.v.	d1+15
Methotrexate	20 mg/m²	i.v.	d1+15
Prednisone	40 mg/m²	p.o.	d1–14

VBVP 21 d
Landman-Parker 2000 [42]

Etoposide (V= VP 16)	100 mg/m²	i.v.	d1–5
Bleomycin	10 mg/m²	i.v.	d1
Vinblastine	6 mg/m²	i.v.	d1+8
Prednisone	40 mg/m²	p.o	d1–8

VEPA 28 d
Friedmann 2002 [43]

Vinblastine	6 mg/m²	i.v.	d1+15
Etoposide	200 mg/m²	i.v.	d1+15
Prednisone	40 mg/m²/d	p.o.	d1–14
Adriamycin	25 mg/m²	i.v.	d1+15

IEP 21 d
Schellong 2005 [44]

Ifosfamide	2000 mg/m²	in 24 h i.v.	d1–5
Etoposide	125 mg/m²	in 2 h i.v.	d1–5
Prednisone	100 mg/m²/d	p.o.	d1–5

countries with low resources and no availability of radiotherapy [e.g. 48–50] or from industrial countries, where pediatric oncologists have tried to avoid radiotherapy because of the unwanted late effects. But although some trials showed remarkably good outcome, they were not recognized, because most of these studies comprised only small numbers of additionally selected patients. Three large randomized US trials with and without RT as part of the treatment had good results in the chemotherapy only arm [37, 51, 52], but a superior outcome for patients treated with RT and therefore combined modality therapy remained standard treatment [53].

In the response adapted GPOH-HD 95 trial the omission of RT did not result in a poorer disease free survival (DFS) rate in 113 early stage patients who achieved a complete remission (CR) with chemotherapy and had no RT, in comparison with the DFS rate of 281 patients, who did not achieve a CR with chemotherapy

alone and therefore were irradiated (DFS after 5 years 97% versus 94%) [54].

Combined modality therapy is a strategy allowing the administration of less toxic, shorter chemotherapy and low-dose, limited-volume radiotherapy. In Table 10.5 pediatric treatment schedules for early stage HL are listed, reporting dose intensity and cumulative doses of different chemotherapeutics, RT dose and the resulting EFS values.

The rules for stratification differ in these study groups. Therefore different trials treat between 26% and 60% of all patients as early stage. But all trials achieved EFS values above 91%. The differences in chemotherapy regarding the dose intensity and cumulative dosage of the drugs are interesting. Dose intensity means the quantity of a single chemotherapeutic dose in mg/m² per week and determines, according to Hryniuk [57], the efficacy. The cumulative doses of the drugs on the other hand

Table 10.5 Pediatric treatment strategies and outcome in early stage Hodgkin's lymphoma. Chemotherapeutics with dose intensity in mg/m^2/week and cumulative doses in mg/m^2 (in brackets); applied radiotherapy and event-free survival (EFS). (Modified according to [114], with kind permission of Springer Science and Business Media.)

Trial	AIEOP-MH 89	France: MHD 90	USA: SSD	USA: CCG	GPOH-HD 95†
Publication	Vecchi et al. [55] 1997	Landman-P et al. [42] 2000	Donaldson et al. [56] 2007	Nachmann et al. [37] 2002	Dörffel et al. [54] 2003
Number of cycles	3 ABVD	4 VBVP*	4 VAMP	4 COPP/ABV	2 OPPA (f) or OEPA (m)
Treatment duration	12 weeks	12 weeks	16 weeks	16 weeks	8 weeks
Adriamycin	12.5 (150)		12.5 (200)	8.75 (140)	20 (160)
Bleomycin	5 (60)	3.3 (40)		2.5 (40)	
Cyclophosphamide				150 (2400)	
Dacarbazine	188 (2250)				
Etoposide		167 (2000)			m = 125 (1000)
Methotrexate			10 (160)		
Prednisone		93 (1120)	140 (2240)	140 (2240)	225 (1800)
Procarbazine				175 (2800)	f = 375 (3000)
Vinblastine	3 (36)	4 (48)	3 (48)	1.5 (24)	
Vincristine				0.35 (5.6)	1.1 (9)
IF-RT-dose	21 Gy	20 (–40) Gy and para-aortic field + spleen	15 (–25.5) Gy	21 Gy (36% of patients without RT)	20 (–35) Gy, 30% of patients without RT)
Patient (n=)	100	202	110	294	408
% of all HL-patients	39	60	34	26	40
EFS	91% (7 years)	91% (5 yearrs)	93% (5 years)	95% (3 years)	94% (5 years)

* In trial MHD 90 'poor responder' patients (tumor regression <70%, n= 27) received additionally 1–2 OPPA cycles. † In trial GPOH-HD 95 chemotherapy was different for girls (f) and boys (m).

are more relevant for toxic late effects. Therefore we favour schedules with high dose intensity and low cumulative doses. In addition there should be a low risk for organ dysfunction, infertility, and secondary malignant neoplasm, and for this reason the schedule should avoid radiotherapy, procarbazine, and high doses of adriamycin, bleomycin or alkylating agents. This strategy is currently applied in the EuroNet-Pediatric Hodgkin's Lymphoma Group trial 'EuroNet-PHL-C1' [38].

Comparing results in intermediate and advanced stages of HL is more difficult in view of the very different stratification of patients between different study groups. Stage IV disease has the most dismal outcome. For instance, the EFS of stage IV patients was only 49% in the UKCCSG study [58] and 62% in the first French pediatric study [59]. In the German-Austrian trial, DAL-HD 82, all 50 patients of stage IIIB and IV were treated with two cycles of OPPA, four cycles of COPP and involved field RT with 25 Gy (and boost doses up to 35 Gy for larger residual masses). The achieved EFS rate of 87% after 3.5 years was so encouraging that the Italian and French pediatric Hodgkin's groups participated in the SIOP-study HD-IV-87 for children with stage IV. The treatment was identical to the one employed for advanced stages in DAL-HD 82, but the IF-RT dose was

reduced to 20 Gy. Sixty-five children treated in this manner achieved an EFS of 77% and an OS of 93% after more than 7 years [60]. Nearly identical therapy was given in trial GPOH-HD 95, but boys received OEPA instead of OPPA and all patients who achieved a CR (defined as tumor volume regression >95% and maximal single lymphomas <2 ml) did not receive RT. The DFS for this cohort with advanced stages, mostly IIIB or IV, were 91% for 265 irradiated patients and 80% for 57 patients without RT after 5 years [54].

Similar results were obtained by the Children's Cancer Group trial CCG 5942. In this trial stage IV patients were treated with two cycles of high dose cytarabine and etoposide, two cycles COPP/ABV and two cycles of a combination chemotherapy with cyclophosphamide, adriamycin, vincristine, methylprednisolone and prednisone. Patients who achieved an initial CR (defined here as tumor volume regression of >70% and gallium negative) after chemotherapy were randomized to receive low-dose IF-RT or no further treatment. With an 'as treated' analysis, the 3-year EFS for the radiation cohort was 91% and 79% for patients without RT [37].

In the past, many study groups used treatment regimens with a higher burden of toxic chemotherapy and RT for patients with

Table 10.6 Pediatric treatment strategies and outcome in advanced stage Hodgkin's lymphoma.

Trial (published by)	Stage	Chemotherapy	RT	*n*	Outcome in % (years)
POG (Weiner 1991) [61]	III + IV	4 MOPP + 4 ABVD	21 Gy, TNI	80	80 (EFS 5), 87 (OS 5)
SFOP MDH 82 (Oberlin 1992) [59]	III	3 MOPP + 3 ABVD	20–40 Gy, EF	40	82 (DFS 6)
	IV			21	62 (DFS 6)
DAL-HD 82 [62] (Schellong 1992)	III B + IV	2 OPPA + 4 COPP	25 (–35) Gy, IF	50	86 (EFS 9)
St Jude (Hudson 1993) [63]	IV	5 COP + 4 ABVD	20 Gy, IF	27	85 (DFS 5), 86 (OS 5)
AIEOP-MH 1983 (Vecchi 1993) [64]	IIIB + IV	5 MOPP + 5 ABVD	25–40 Gy, EF or bulky d.	49	60,3 (FFP 7)
Stanford (Hunger 1994) [65]	IV	3 MOPP + 3 ABVD	15–25 Gy, IF	13	69 (EFS 10), 85 (OS 10)
SIOP HD-IV 87 [60] (Schellong 1996)	IV	2 OPPA + 4 COPP	20 (–35) Gy, IF	65	77 (EFS 7), 93 (OS 7)
CCG [52] (Hutchinson 1998)	III + IV	6 ABVD	21 Gy, IF, EF or TNI	54	87 (EFS 4), 90 (OS 4)
DAL-HD 90 [34] (Schellong 1999)	IIIB + IV	2 OPPA (m) or 2 OEPA (f) + 4 COPP	20 (–35) Gy, RIF	179	86 (EFS 5), 94 (OS 5)
UKCCSG HD 8201 + 9201 (Atra 2002) [58]	IV	6–8 ChlVPP	±20–35 Gy to bulky disease	67	49 (EFS 10), 77 (OS 10)
SSD [43] (Friedmann 2002)	III + IV	6 VEPA	15–25,5 Gy, IF	30	82 (EFS 5)
Toronto (Chow 2006) [66]	IV	6–8 MOPP/ABV	±15 Gy, EF	23	78 (EFS 10), 91 (OS 10)

EFS, event free survival. OS, overall survival. DFS, disease-free survival. FFP: freedom from progression. TNI, total nodal irradiation. EF, extended field. IF, involved field. RIF, reduced involved field. SSD, Stanford University Medical Centre, St Jude Children's Research Hospital and the Dana-Farber Cancer Institute.

advanced-stage disease. Some important trials in advanced-stage pediatric HL by different countries and groups are listed in Table 10.6.

In the current EuroNet-PHL-C1 trial, advanced-stage patients are treated with two cycles of OEPA and – in randomized fashion – with four cycles of COPP or COPDAC (see Table 10.4 and Figure 10.5). Response will be evaluated after two cycles for RT stratification. RT should be omitted in patients with adequate response, i.e. patients in CR or in partial remission (PR, defined as tumor volume regression equal or >50% or residual volume equal or <5 ml) measured with conventional imaging studies, and negative FDG-PET results. Patients with inadequate response will be irradiated, i.e. if at least one initially involved region is PET-positive or the residual masses are not at least in PR measured with conventional imaging procedures [38].

In trial HD9 of the German Hodgkin Study Group, 460 adult patients with unfavorable risk factor HL were treated with eight cycles of escalated BEACOPP (see Table 10.4) and RT for bulky tumors (30 Gy) and residual lymphomas after chemotherapy (40 Gy). They achieved a 'freedom from treatment failure' (FFTF) of 89% and OS of 91% after 3 years [67]. But this regimen contains high cumulative doses of adriamycin (280 mg/m²), bleomycin (80 mg/m²), cyclophosphamide (10 g/m²) and etoposide

(4800 mg/m²), and has potentially high risk for acute and late effects, and is particularly disadvantageous therefore for children and adolescents.

One-hundred and forty-two patients with unfavorable risk factors were treated with the 'Stanford V' regimen (Table 10.4) in combination with RT for initial bulky lymphomas, and they achieved an EFS of 89% and an OS of 96% after 5 years [68].

Data on treatment experiences in children with relapsed Hodgkin's lymphoma are very limited. A recent analysis of 174 patients with relapse/progression treated according to the DAL-HD-ST-86 treatment recommendations showed an estimated disease-free survival of 61% and an overall survival of 74% after 10 years [44].

For remission induction, relapsing patients received a combination of IEP (ifosfamide, etoposide and prednisone) alternating with ABVD, followed by radiotherapy. In patients with progressive disease, relapse induction treatment was mainly followed by autologous transplantation during recent years.

In a multivariant analysis, time of relapse was the only significant risk factor. The time of relapse was differentiated as progression (during front line therapy or until 3 months after the end of treatment), early relapse (>3 and <12 months after end of therapy) and late relapse (>12 months after end of front line therapy). DFS

EuroNet-PHL-C1 – second line treatment

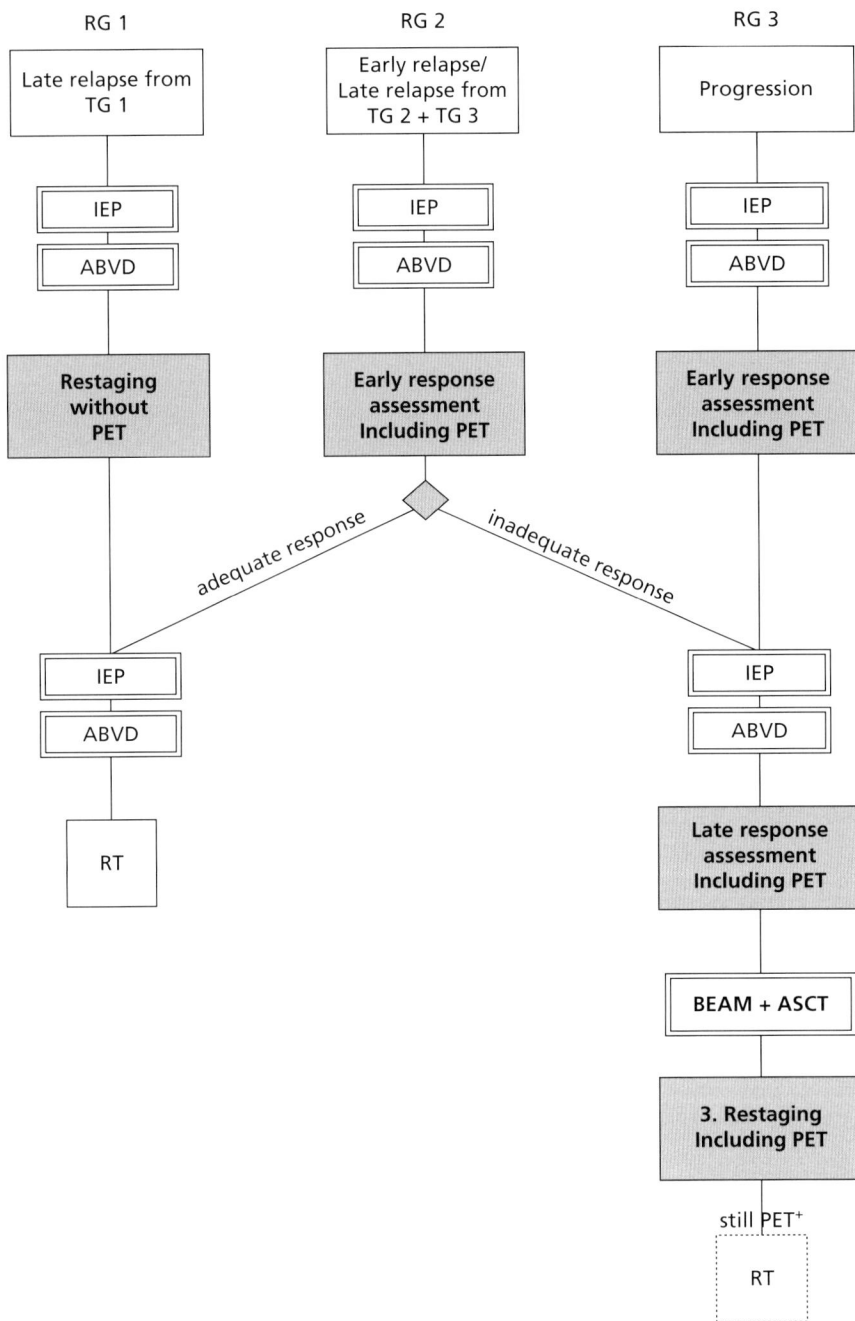

Figure 10.5 EuroNet-PHL-C1 schedule for front line therapy.

for patients with early and late relapse was 53% and 84% respectively. The best prognosis was obtained in patients with late relapse after initial diagnosis of an early stage (DFS of 96% after combined radio-chemotherapy). The initial stage of the disease seemed therefore to have some additional influence on the prognosis. These results are similar to those reported in adults [69].

Randomized studies comparing conventional chemotherapy versus mega-dose therapy followed by autologous stem cell trans-plantation showed an advantage of the more intensive treatment in adult patients with relapsed HL [70, 71]. In the study of Schmitz [71], patients with chemotherapy-sensitive early and late relapse (same definitions as above) benefited from the autologous transplantation. After 3 years', FFTF in patients with early relapse was 41% for those receiving high-dose treatment and 12% for those receiving conventional therapy. In those patients with late relapse, FFTF was 75% for those treated with high dose and 44%

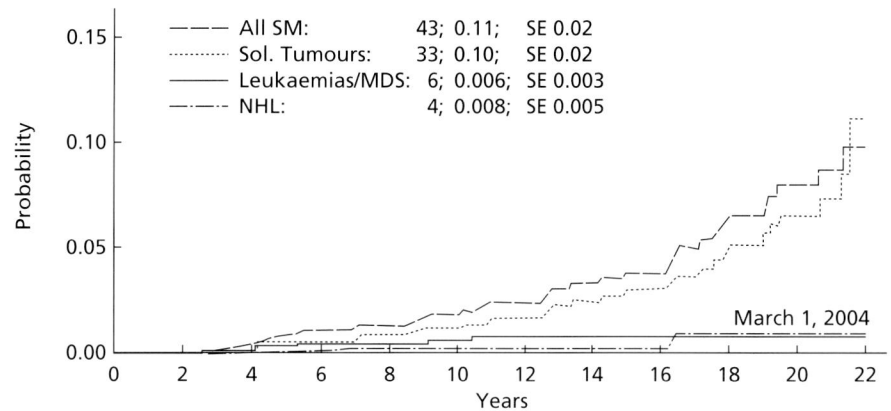

Figure 10.6 EuroNet-PHL-C1 schedule for treatment of progressive and recurrent HL.

for those treated with conventional therapy. Patients with multiple relapses did not benefit from peripheral blood stem cell therapy (SCT). The EFS at 4.8 years for 38 children treated with high dose chemotherapy plus autologous SCT is 42% [72]. A currently open transplant question is whether a positive FDG-PET result prior to autologous SCT is a negative predictor for outcome after transplantation. Becherer *et al.* [73] investigated the role of FDG-PET in 16 patients with NHL (*n*=10) or HL (*n*=6). Only one of eight patients with a negative or weakly positive PET scan before SCT relapsed, whereas seven of eight patients with moderate or strongly positive PET relapsed. Based on these experiences the strategy of the EuroNet-PHL-C1 protocol includes three relapse groups (Figure 10.6):

• RG1: Patients with late relapse after initial treatment for early stage disease.

• RG2: All patients with early relapse or patients with late relapse after initial diagnosis of an intermediate or advanced stage disease.

• RG3: All patients with progressive disease.

RG1 patients receive two double cycles of IEP-ABVD followed by radiotherapy of all regions involved at the time of relapse. Patients in RG3 receive two double cycles of IEP-ABVD followed by high-dose BEAM and autologous stem cell transplantation. Patients in RG2 with an adequate early response (definition similar to patients in front line therapy according to trial EuroNet-PHL-C1, see above) receive treatment according to RG1, whilst patients with an inadequate response receive treatment according to RG3.

Strategies for follow up and overview of important late effects

Follow up investigations after treatment of Hodgkin's lymphoma in children and adolescents have two aims – early detection of relapsing disease and recognition of late effects.

Recurrent disease occurs most frequently during the first three years, e.g. in DAL/GPOH studies about 90% of all recurrences occur after front line therapy. Therefore we recommend during the first 2 years regular clinical examinations every 6 weeks and investigations by laboratory and imaging procedures every 3

months, and for the third year the same procedures but 3 monthly clinical examinations and 6 monthly imaging. The details of imaging will depend on the primary involvement. Ultrasound is mandatory in all cases, but chest X-rays, MRI and CT investigations will vary according to site and FDG-PET only in case of suspected relapse. Regular investigations during later follow up should be restricted to clinical examinations at larger intervals because the first symptoms of late recurrent disease can be recognized earlier by the patient and relatives rather than by imaging studies [74].

Follow-up investigations for detecting late effects depend mainly on the kind of chemotherapy and radiotherapy, and one has to consider also the time interval after treatment (for overview see [75]). Some late effects do not appear until 15 or more years after treatment and our knowledge of these late effects is necessarily limited.

Cumulative mortality from reasons other than HL is already significant and will further increase over the following years in those patients treated during the 1970s and 1980s. An analysis of 387 children with HD treated at St Jude Children's Research Hospital between 1968 and 1990 showed that in this cohort the cumulative mortality due to other reasons than HD (i.e. secondary malignancy 4.3%, cardiac diseases 2.9%, infections 2.9%, accidents and suicides 2.1%) actually exceeded the mortality by HD (9.8%) after 20 years [76].

Table 10.7 shows an overview of the most relevant known late effects after treatment of HL in childhood and adolescents.

Overwhelming post-splenectomy infections are a relic of the previous era when exploratory laparotomy and splenectomy were obligatory staging measures. These procedures were reduced in a stepwise procedure and later completely abandoned during the course of DAL/GPOH studies. In the cohort of 1245 patients enrolled in the DAL studies HD-78 to HD-90 the OS rate after 24 years was 87% in the total group, 83% in 335 asplenic patients (with a fatal course in 11 of 18 overwhelming post-splenectomy infection events) and 93% in 910 non- or only partially splenectomized patients. In the large group of non-splenectomized patients only two non-fatal cases of septicaemia were observed and one event in a patient after irradiation of the spleen with

Table 10.7 Most relevant late effects after treatment of Hodgkin's lymphoma in childhood and adolescence.

Late effects	Radiotherapy	Chemotherapy
Septic infections (OPSI)	Spleen >20 Gy	
Local growth impairment	+	
Pulmonary dysfunction (fibrosis)	+	Bleomycin etc
Heart: cardiomyopathy	(+)	Anthracyclines a.o.
Heart: abnormalities of valves, coronaries, pericardium or conduction	++	(+)
Vascular disease: stroke a.o.	+	
Thyroid: hypothyroidism, nodules a.o.	++	
Ovarian dysfunction	+	Alkylating agents a.o.
Testicular dysfunction	(+)	Procarbazine a.o.
Secondary leukemia/ non-Hodgkin's lymphoma		++
Secondary solid tumors	+++	(+)

20 Gy [77]. Recommended measures for the prevention and treatment of infections in patients with an absent or dysfunctional spleen are well known [78].

Growth pattern and final height were sometimes affected following intensive radio- and chemotherapy in patients treated intensively in the past. More relevant now are the musculoskeletal effects that follow high-dose radiotherapy, especially when given in early childhood, in the region of the neck and upper thorax, with intraclavicular narrowing and shortening of the clavicles, and atrophy of the soft tissue in this region.

Lung dysfunction, mostly caused by pulmonary fibrosis, is a rather rare event today and relevant only for patients with higher dose and large volume radiation of the lungs and also for patients undergoing salvage therapy with lung toxic chemotherapy like bleomycin, nitrosureas and busulfan.

Cardiovascular late effects have been the most common nonmalignant sources of excess mortality among survivors of HD treated in the past, when the heart was completely irradiated with high doses and now obsolete radiation techniques [79]. These patients died from premature coronary artery disease with myocardial infarction, valvular dysfunctions, peri- or pancarditis, conducting system abnormalities or vascular diseases, including atherosclerosis, thrombosis, and stroke. Cardiomyopathies in survivors of HD can also result from chemotherapy, particularly with anthracyclines, but also from vinca alkaloids and alkylating agents in combination with radiotherapy. Because cardiac complications often do not occur until 20 or more years after completion of treatment, we do not know the exact risk of our currently used combined modality therapy. It is therefore imperative that we should monitor survivors by regular cardiac check ups. Special care should be taken with regard to cardiac function in pregnancy.

The risk for thyroid abnormalities after neck irradiation is increased for children and adolescents and it increases with higher radiation doses and with time after radiation. The most common abnormality is hypothyroidism, which might be overt or sub-clinical, but the spectrum of abnormality includes thyroid nodules, thyroid cancer, and other thyroid disorders. The risk for benign nodules and for thyroid cancer is different with increasing radiation dose. Whereas the risk for nodules rises continuously with increased dosage, and strongly over 25 Gy, the risk for thyroid cancer rises only with lower doses, but declines over doses of 30 Gy [80, 81].

Gonadal toxicity and infertility were relatively frequent events after treatment of HL in childhood and adolescents in the past. Damage by RT occurred more often in girls when the ovaries were not sufficiently protected. Infertility caused by chemotherapy, such as alkylating agents, was a more common problem until the current treatments were developed. A particularly toxic therapy in this regard for boys is procarbazine. For instance, two cycles of OPPA (1500 mg/m² procarbazine) led, in 28.9% of males, to an elevation of basal values of follicle stimulating hormone (FSH) which indicates a high suspicion for hypergonadotropic hypogonadism and azospermia. Boys who were treated with two cycles of OPA or OEPA without procarbazine showed FSH values within the normal range [82]. The agents in ABVD (see Table 10.4) do not usually cause permanent azospermia [83].

There is no data as to whether alkylating agents and procarbazine also damage the germ cells of girls and can induce premature menopause as in adult women. Younger women are very often fertile after HL therapy, as shown in former DAL studies, and there are already many healthy offspring from former DAL patients.

Secondary malignant neoplasias (SMN) occur more often after HL therapy in childhood and adolescence than after all other primary malignant neoplasias [84]. The cumulative incidence of SMN after pediatric HL increased in all different studies with time, but the absolute numbers are quite different. After 15 years they vary between 3.6% [85], 7% [86] and 12% [87], after 20 years between 7% [85, 88], 11% [89] and 19% [90] and after 30 years between 18% [85], 26% [89] and 31% [90]. Figure 10.7 shows the cumulative incidences after 22 years of follow-up for all SMN and individually for secondary non-Hodgkin's lymphoma (NHL), for leukemias/myelodysplastic syndromes, and for solid tumors.

Secondary leukemias and myelodysplastic syndromes manifest in the first 10–15 years after HL therapy only and are caused by different chemotherapy drugs. Drugs such as mechlorethamine and chlorambucil have a higher leukemogenic potential (2–6%) than cyclophosphamide. Therefore, only 0.6% of secondary leukemias were observed in DAL studies [91, 92].

The manifestation of NHL is also restricted to the first 10–15 years after HL therapy, but there is more speculation than evidence about the cause of these tumors. In DAL studies the cumulative incidence of secondary NHL is 0.8% [92].

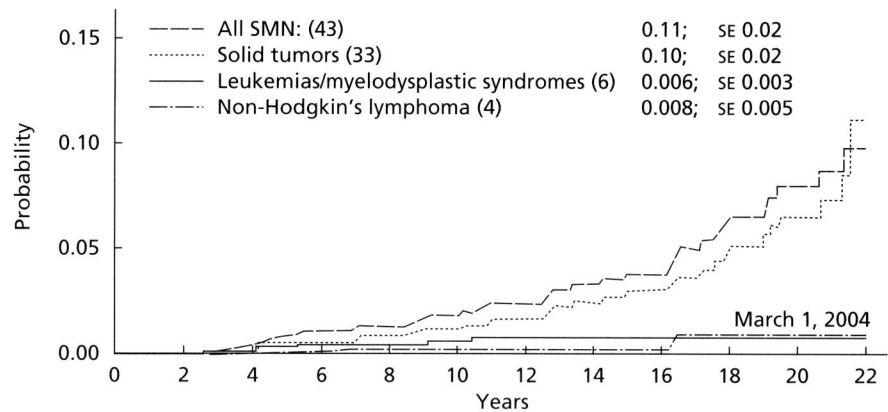

Figure 10.7 Cumulative incidences of secondary malignant neoplasms (SMN) in studies HD 78–HD 90. (Reproduced from Schellong G [77], with permission from Georg Thieme Verlag.)

In contrast to leukemias and NHL, secondary solid tumors most commonly appear 10, 15 or more years after treatment and the majority occur in the radiation fields or at their margins.

The commonest such tumors are thyroid, breast, and colorectal but others include skin tumors, tumors of the central nervous system, bone or soft tissue sarcomas and many others. According to some more recent publications the cumulative incidence of SMN rises linearly with RT – except for thyroid cancer, as discussed above – and so we can hope that the incidence will be markedly decreased in the recently treated HL patients who have received a lower dose and smaller volume radiation therapy.

We have some data about reduced quality of life, fatigue and other phenomena after treatment of HL in adults, but our knowledge of treated pediatric HL in this regard is limited.

Recommendations for follow-up investigations will be individualized according to the chemotherapy and/or radiotherapy that has been applied, and according to the anticipated late effects. Patients should be informed about late effects and the possibilities to reduce any risk including the practice of healthy behaviour.

Novel therapeutic approaches

Most of the patients with HL are cured after primary or secondary treatment. About 3% of the patients appear to have disease that is primarily refractory to conventional treatment. Recently in these patients, allogeneic transplantation with dose-reduced conditioning has successfully been applied. Peggs *et al.* [93] reported on 49 patients. Of the 49 patients, 44 received allogeneic transplantation for progression after autologous transplantation. Overall survival at 4 years was 55.7%. Sixteen patients received donor lymphocyte infusions (DLI) for relapse after allogeneic transplantation, and in eight of 16 patients a complete response was obtained, indicating a significant graft versus tumor (GvT) effect in HL patients. However, some patients presented with severe graft versus host disease III/IV and it is therefore necessary to determine the optimal strategy for such DLI. Therefore, Hart *et al.* [94] investigated the relevance of FDG-PET after allogeneic

stem cell transplantation. They showed that the FDG-PET results could influence the administration of donor lymphocytes in 9 of 15 patients with three patients receiving the DLI earlier or at a higher dose. In addition, monitoring with PET revealed a GvL effect in five patients.

In about 40% of HL patients tumor cells express EBV-specific membrane proteins (LMP1 an dLMP 2). Bollard *et al.* [95] used this antigen expression profile for specific immunotherapy using EBV-specific cytotoxic T-lymphocytes (CTL) in 14 patients. Gene marking revealed that after infusion these cells were further expanded *in vivo*. Five of 14 patients were in complete remission up to 40 months after cell therapy. In another patient Bollard [96] reported the use of donor-derived EBV-specific CTL after allogeneic transplantation. Immunotherapy induced a long-term remission in this patient with multiple relapses. Thus, allogeneic stem cell transplantation after dose-reduced conditioning in combination with specific immunotherapy might become an option for future treatment of refractory HL patients by increasing a GvT effect without severe GvHD.

Other strategies include the use of CD30 monoclonal antibodies. These antibodies are conjugated either to toxins or radioactive agents. Recently a CD30 antibody conjugated to Iodine-131 [97] was used in a phase I trial including 22 patients with refractory HL. One complete and five partial remissions were observed. In another trial this antibody was linked to the deglycosylated ricin A-chain [98]. However, the results of this trial were rather disappointing. Thus, monoclonal antibody strategies might be used as additional treatment option in refractory HL patients in future.

Nodular lymphocyte predominant Hodgkin's lymphoma

Lymphocyte-predominant HL (LPHL) is a rare CD-20 positive sub-type of HL which accounts for about 7% of all HL [99]. The malignant cells are composed of lymphocytic and histiocytic cell types which are frequently negative for CD15 and CD30, the typical markers of H-RS cells in cHL. Only a minority of these cells is EBV positive. However, the cells are positive for typical B-cell antigens such as CD20, CD79a or CD75 [100].

Gender distribution shows a male predominance. Patients present mainly with stage IA with cervical node involvement: In contrast to classic HL, mediastinal disease is exceptional. The prognosis seems to be favorable. Patients die from secondary malignancies such as aggressive B-cell lymphoma rather than from LPHL [101–103]. In up to 3% of patients LPHL transforms spontaneously into aggressive non-Hodgkin B-cell lymphoma.

In the past, treatment of LPHL was often related to classic HL protocols [104–106]. Since it was felt that most of these patients were overtreated, there are some approaches to reduce treatment intensity:
• In some institutions patients with limited stages have been treated with radiotherapy alone [107–109].
• Bone marrow biopsy remains mandatory in advanced cases (stage IIB–IV).
• For patients with stage IA, surgery alone might be a useful treatment. This approach could avoid severe long-term sequelae. Recently the EuroNet-PHL group reported the results of 58 patients treated with this strategy. About two-thirds of these patients experienced long-term remission. However, almost all patients with incomplete resection relapsed after surgery alone, but no relevant upstaging was observed [112].
In the upcoming EuroNet-PHL-LP-1 protocol patients with stage IA or IIA and incomplete resection will receive low intensity chemotherapy consisting of low dose cyclophosphamide (cumulative dose 1500 mg/m^2), prednisone (cumulative dose 840 mg/m^2) and vinblastine (cumulative dose 36 mg/m^2). Pilot data show that 17 of 18 patients with stage IA or IIA achieved complete remission after this chemotherapy. At a median follow up of 12 months (range 2–26 months) the overall survival is 100% and event free survival is 94% [113].

Summary and future directions for management

With the current treatment options, cure rate in children with HL is excellent. However, intensive treatment modalities could cause significant long-term sequelae such as infertility, early menopause, secondary malignancies, cardiac, and thyroid problems. Thus, clinical trials have to pursue furthermore two aims: keeping the high cure rates and minimizing late effects by controlled change and reduction of treatment. The aims of the current European protocols are prevention of infertility or early menopause as well as a significant reduction of the indication for radiotherapy, mostly to prevent the development of solid secondary tumors.

Early response assessment is used in several childhood and adult protocols. In the majority of these protocols FDG-PET is routinely used to evaluate response to chemotherapy. However, there are two problems using PET:
• Integration of FDG-PET into the staging results in the detection of more lesions could lead to unnecessary upstaging of patients.

But the aim is treatment reduction. Thus, upstaging due to PET should avoided in patients with a good prognosis, to avoid overtreatment.
• Response assessment using conventional imaging and PET is very complicated, so that incorrect treatment decisions are possible, especially at centres with few patients and little experience. Therefore, the EuroNet-PHL group established a real-time central review board, which reviews all clinical information as well as all imaging data sets. Based on these evaluations the reference stage of each individual patient is determined and response to chemotherapy and the decision for or against radiotherapy after chemotherapy is also centralized. As a result, each patient benefits from high expertise, independent of the experience of the local hospital with HL in children. The results of such a review panel have previously been published by Dieckmann *et al.* [114].

LPHL seems to be a special sub-entity which mostly is diagnosed at early stages. Although the prognosis is favorable, currently most patients receive the same intensive treatment as patients with cHL, which results in overtreatment in many patients. In the future, patients with stage IA disease should be treated with surgery alone if complete resection can be achieved. Using FDG-PET for a better identification of patients with incomplete resection should improve the results of this strategy. All patients without complete resection will receive low intensity chemotherapy. Taken together this concept should cure the majority of all LPHL-patients, avoiding treatment modalities leading to significant late effects.

Future protocols for patients with cHL or LPHL aim at avoiding and minimizing late effects. Thus prospective documentation and continuous evaluation of late effects within an international late effect registry will be necessary to develop suitable treatment strategies in future.

During the next years new treatment modalities, including allogeneic transplantation and tumor-specific immunotherapy, will be developed for patients with primary refractory disease. Using gene chip technology, it might become possible to identify these patients in the future before an insufficient treatment has been started. Thus, if these patients could ideally be identified at the time of initial diagnosis, the development of completely different protocols for these patients is possible.

References

1 Jaffe ES, Harris NL, Stein H, Vardiman JW (eds). World Health Organization Classification of Tumours. Pathology and Genetics of Tumours of Haematopoetic and Lymphoid Tissues. Lyon: IARS Press, 2001.
2 Donaldson SS, Kaplan H. Complications of treatment of Hodgkin's disease in children. Cancer Treatm Rep 1982; 66: 977–89.
3 Donaldson SS, Link MP. Combined modality treatment with low-dose radiation and MOPP chemotherapy for children with Hodgkin's disease. J Clin Oncol 1987; 5: 742–9.
4 Breu H, Schellong G, Grosch-Wörner I. Abgestufte Chemotherapie und reduzierte Strahlendosis beim Morbus Hodgkin im Kindesalter

– ein Bericht über 170 Patienten der kooperativen Therapiestudie HD 78. Klin Pädiat 1982; 194: 233–41.

5 Oberlin O, Boilletot A, Leverger G, et al. Clinical staging, primary chemotherapy and involved field radiotherapy in childhood Hodgkin's disease. Eur Paed Haematol Oncol 1985; 2: 65–70.

6 Hodgkin T. On some morbid appearances of the absorbent glands and spleen. Med-Chir Trans 1832; 17: 68–114.

7 Pusey W. Cases.of sarcoma and of Hodgkin's disease terated by exposures by X-rays: a preliminary report. JAMA 1902; 38: 166–9.

8 De Vita VT, Serpick AA, Carbone PP. Combination chemotherapy in the treatment of advanced Hodgkin's disease. Ann Intern Med 1970; 73: 891–5.

9 Lukes RJ, Craver LF, Hall TC, et al. Report of the Nomenclature Committee. Cancer Res 1966; 26: 1311.

10 Kaplan HS Evidence for a tumoricidal dose level in the radiotherapy of Hodgkin's disease. Cancer Res 1966; 26: 1221–4.

11 Carbone P, Kaplan HS, Musshoff K, et al. Report of the Comittee on Hodgkin's Disease Staging Classification. Cancer Res 1971; 31: 1860–1.

12 Küppers R, Rajewsky K, Zhao M, et al. Hodgkin's disease: Hodgkin and Reed–Sternberg cells picked from histological sections show clonal immunoglobulin gene rearrangements and appear to be derived from B cells at various stages of development. Proc Natl Acad Sci USA 1994; 91: 10962–6.

13 Harris NL, Jaffe ES, Diebold J, et al. World Health Organization Classification of Neoplastic Diseases of the Hematopoietic and Lymphoid Tissues: Report of the Clinical Advisory Committee Meeting – Airlie House, Virginia, November 1997. J Clin Oncol 1999; 17: 3835–49.

14 Kaatsch P, Spix C. Annual report 2004 from the German Childhood Cancer Registry, Mainz, 2004.

15 Dinand V, Dawar R, Arya LS, Unni R, Mohanty B, Singh R. Hodgkin's lymphoma in Indian children: prevalence and significance of Epstein-Barr virus detection in Hodgkin's and Reed-Sternberg cells. Eur J Cancer 2007; 43: 161–8.

16 Mack TM, Cozen W, Shibata DK, et al. Concordance for Hodgkin's disease in identical twins suggesting genetic susceptibility to the young-adult form of the disease. N Engl J Med 1995; 332: 413–8.

17 Hjalgrim H, Smedby KE, Rostgaard K, et al. Infectious mononucleosis, childhood social environment, and risk of Hodgkin lymphoma. Cancer Res 2007; 67: 2382–8.

18 Tzankov A, Bourgau C, Kaiser A, et al. Rare expression of T–cell markers in classical Hodgkin's lymphoma. Mod Pathol 2005; 18: 1542–9.

19 Bargou RC, Emmerich F, Krappmann D, et al. Constitutive nuclear factor-kappaB-RelA activation is required for proliferation and survival of Hodgkin's disease tumor cells. J Clin Invest 1997; 100: 2961–9.

20 Schwering I, Brauninger A, Distler V, et al. Profiling of Hodgkin's lymphoma cell line L1236 and germinal center B cells: identification of Hodgkin's lymphoma-specific genes. Mol Med 2003; 9: 85–95.

21 Mathas S, Janz M, Hummel F, et al. Intrinsic inhibition of transcription factor E2A by HLH proteins ABF-1 and Id2 mediates reprogramming of neoplastic B cells in Hodgkin lymphoma. Nat Immunol 2006; 7: 207–15.

22 Küppers R, Brauninger A. Reprogramming of the tumor B–cell phenotype in Hodgkin lymphoma. J Trends Immunol 2006; 27: 203–5.

23 Jundt F, Anagnostopoulos I, Forster R, Mathas S, Stein H, Dorken B. Activated Notch1 signaling promotes tumor cell proliferation and survival in Hodgkin and anaplastic large cell lymphoma. Blood 2002; 99: 3398–403.

24 Trieu Y, Wen XY, Skinnider BF, et al. Soluble interleukin-13Ralpha2 decoy receptor inhibits Hodgkin's lymphoma growth in vitro and in vivo. Cancer Res 2004; 64: 3271–5.

25 Visco C, Vassilakopoulos TP, Kliche KO, et al. Elevated serum levels of IL-10 are associated with inferior progression-free survival in patients with Hodgkin's disease treated with radiotherapy. Leuk Lymphoma 2004; 45: 2085–92.

26 Marshall NA, Christie LE, Munro LR, et al. Immunosuppressive regulatory T cells are abundant in the reactive lymphocytes of Hodgkin lymphoma. Blood 2004; 103: 1755–62.

27 Bennett MH, MacLennan KA, Easterling MJ, et al. The prognostic significance of cellular subtypes in nodular sclerosing Hodgkin's disease; an analysis of 271 non-laparotomised cases (BNLI report no. 22) Clin Radiol 1983; 34: 497–501.

28 Lister TA, Crowther D, Sutcliffe SB, et al. Report of a committee convened to discuss the evaluation and staging of patients with Hodgkin's disease: Cotswolds Meeting. J Clin Oncol 1989; 7: 1630–6.

29 Körholz D, Kluge R, Wickmann L, et al. Importance of F–18–fluorodeoxy–D–2–glucose positron emission tomography (FDG–PET) for staging and therapy of Hodgkin's lymphoma in childhood and adolescence – consequences for the GPOH – HD 2003 protocol. Onkologie 2003; 26: 489–93.

30 Gilbert R, Babaiantz I. Notre method de roentgentherapie de la lymphogranulomatose (Hodgkin): rcsultats eloignes. Acta Radiol 1931; 12: 523–9.

31 Donaldson SS. Pediatric Hodgkin's disease: focus on the future. In: Van Eys J, Sullivan MP (Eds), Status of the Curability of Childhood Cancers. New York: Raven Press, 1980: 235–49.

32 Oberlin O, Boilletot A, Leverger G, et al. Clinical staging, primary chemotherapy and involved field radiotherapy in childhood Hodgkin's disease. Eur Paed Haematol Oncol 1985; 2: 65–70.

33 Schellong G, Brämswig J, Ludwig R, et al. Kombinierte Behandlungsstrategie bei über 200 Kindern mit Morbus Hodgkin: Abgestufte Chemotherapie, Involved-Field-Bestrahlung mit erniedrigten Dosen und selektive Splenektomie. Ein Bericht der kooperativen Therapiestudie DAL–HD–82. Klin Pädiat 1986; 198: 137–46.

34 Schellong G, Pötter R, Brämswig J, et al. High cure rates and reduced long-term toxicity in pediatric Hodgkin's disease: the German-Austrian multicenter trial DA-HD-90. J Clin Oncol 1999; 17: 3736–44.

35 Bonadonna G, Santoro A. ABVD chemotherapy in the treatment of Hodgkin's disease. Cancer Treat Rev 1982; 9: 21–35.

36 Morgenfeld M. Treatment of malignant lymphoma with cyclophosphamide, vincristine, procarbazine and prednisone combination. XIV Internat Congr Hematolog Sao Paulo (abstract No 578), 1972.

37 Nachman JB, Sposto R, Herzog P, et al. Randomized comparison of low-dose involved-field radiotherapy and no radiotherapy for children with Hodgkin's disease who achieve a complete response to chemotherapy. J Clin Oncol 2002; 20: 3765–71.

38 Körholz D and steering committee. Protocol of the first International Inter-Group Study for Classical Hodgkin's Lymphoma in Children and Adolescents: EuroNet–PHL–C1. Halle 2006.

39 Diehl V, Sieber M, Rüffer U, et al. BEACOPP: an intensified chemotherapy regimen in advanced Hodgkin's disease. Ann Oncol 1997; 8: 143–8.

40 Bartlett NL, Rosenberg SA, Hoppe RT. Brief chemotherapy, Stanford V, and adjuvant radiotherapy for bulky or advanced-stage Hodgkin's disease: a preliminary report. J Clin Oncol 1995; 13: 1080–8.

41 Donaldson SS, Hudson MM, Lamborn KR, et al. VAMP and low-dose, involved-field radiation for children and adolescents with favorable, early–stage Hodgkin's disease: results of a prospective clinical trial. J Clin Oncol 2002; 20: 3081–7.

42 Landman–Parker J, Pacquement H, Leblanc T, et al. Localized childhood Hodgkin's disease: response-adapted chemotherapy with etoposide, bleomycin, vinblastine, and prednisone before low-dose radiation therapy – Results of the French Society of Pediatric Oncology Study MHD90. J Clin Oncol 2000; 18: 1500–7.

43 Friedmann AM, Hudson MM, Weinstein HJ, et al. Treatment of unfavourable childhood Hodgkin's disease with VEPA and low-dose, involved-field radiation. J Clin Oncol 2002; 20: 3088–94.

44 Schellong G, Dörffel W, Claviez A, et al. Salvage therapy of progressive and recurrent Hodgkin's disease: results from a multicenter study of the pediatric DAL/GPOH–HD Study Group. J Clin Oncol 2005; 23: 6181–9.

45 Longo DL, Young RC, Wesley M. 20 years of MOPP therapy for Hodgkin's disease. J Clin Oncol 1986; 4: 1295–306.

46 Hough RE, Hancock BW. Principles of chemotherapy in Hodgkin's disease. In: Mauch PM, Armitage JO, Diehl V, et al. (Eds), Hodgkin's Disease. Philadephia: Lippincott Williams & Wilkins, 1999: 377–94.

47 Canellos GP, Anderson JR, Propert KJ. Chemotherapy of advanced Hodgkin's disease with MOPP, ABVD or MOPP alternating with ABVD. N Engl J Med 1992; 327: 1478–84.

48 Olweny CLM, Katongole-Mbidde E, Kiire C, et al. Childhood Hodgkin's disease in Uganda. A ten year experience. Cancer 1978; 42: 787–92.

49 Jacobs P, King HS, Karabus C, et al. Hodgkin's disease in South Africa. Cancer 1984; 53: 210–13.

50 Baez F, Ocampo E, Conter V, et al. Treatment of childhood Hodgkin's disease with COPP or COPP–ABV (hybrid) without radiotherapy in Nicaragua. Ann Oncol 1997; 8: 247–50.

51 Weiner MA, Leventhal B, Brecher ML, et al. Randomized study of intensive MOPP–ABVD with or without low–dose total–nodal radiotherapy in the treatment of stages IIB, IIIA2, IIIB, and IV Hodgkin's disease in pediatric patients: a Pediatric Oncology Group study. J Clin Oncol 1997; 15: 2769–79.

52 Hutchinson RJ, Fryer CJH, Davis C. MOPP or radiation in addition to ABVD in the treatment of pathologically staged advanced Hodgkin's disease in children: results of the Children's Cancer Group phase III trial. J Clin Oncol 1998; 16: 897–906.

53 Donaldson SS. A discourse: The 2002 Wataru W. Sutow lecture Hodgkin disease in children – perspectives and progress. Med Pediatr Oncol 2003; 40: 73–80.

54 Dörffel W, Lüders H, Rühl U, et al. Preliminary results of the multicenter trial GPOH–HD 95 for the treatment of Hodgkin's disease in children and adolescents: analysis and outlook. Klin Pädiatr 2003; 215: 139–45.

55 Vecchi V, Burnelli R, Di Fabio F, et al. Childhood Hodgkin's disease: results of the Italian multicentric study AIEOP-MH'89-CNR. Med Paediat Oncol 1997; 29: 434.

56 Donaldson SS, Link MP, Weinstein HJ, et al. Final results of a prospective clinical trail with VAMP and low-dose involved-field radiation for children with low-risk Hodgkin's disease. J Clin Oncol 2007; 25: 332–7.

57 Hryniuk WM. The importance of dose intensity in the outcome of chemotherapy. Imp Adv Oncol 1988: 121–41.

58 Atra A, Higgs E., Capra M, et al. ChlVPP chemotherapy in children with stage IV Hodgkin's disease: results of the UKCCSG HD 8201 and HD 9201 studies. Br J Haematol 2002; 119: 647–51.

59 Oberlin O, Leverger G, Pacquement H, et al. Low-dose radiation therapy and reduced chemotherapy in childhood Hodgkin's disease: the experience of the French Society of Pediatric Oncology. J Clin Oncol 1992; 10: 1602–8.

60 Schellong G. The balance between cure and late effects in childhood Hodgkin's lymphoma: the experience of the German-Austrian Study-Group since 1978. Ann Oncol 1996; 7 (Suppl.4): 67–72.

61 Weiner MA, Leventhal BG, Marcus R, et al. Intensive chemotherapy and low-dose radiotherapy for the treatment of advanced-stage Hodgkin's disease in pediatric patients: a Pediatric Oncology Group study. J Clin Oncol 1991; 9: 1591–8.

62 Schellong G, Brämswig JH, Hörnig–Franz I. Treatment of children with Hodgkin's disease – results of the German Pediatric Oncology Group. Ann Oncol 1992; 3 (Suppl.4): 73–6.

63 Hudson MM, Greenwald C, Thompson E, et al. Efficacy and toxicity of multiagent chemotherapy and low-dose involved field radiotherapy in children and adolescents with Hodgkin's disease. J Clin Oncol 1993; 11: 100–8.

64 Vecchi V, Pileri S, Burnelli R, et al. Treatment of pediatric Hodgkin's disease tailored to stage, mediastinal mass, and age. An Italian (AIEOP) multicenter study on 215 patients. Cancer 1993; 72: 2049–57.

65 Hunger SP, Link MP, Donaldson SS, et al. ABVD/MOPP and low-dose involved-field radiotherapy in pediatric Hodgkin's disease: the Stanford experience. J Clin Oncol 1994; 12: 2160–6.

66 Chow ML, Nathan PC, Hodgson DC, et al. Survival and late effects in children with Hodgkin's lymphoma treated with MOPP/ABV and low-dose, extended-field irradiation. J Clin Oncol 2006; 24: 5735–41.

67 Diehl V, Franklin J, Paulus U, et al. BEACOPP chemotherapy improves survival, and dose escalation further improves tumor control in advanced-stage Hodgkin's disease: GHSG HD9 results. Leuk Lymphoma 2001; 42 (Suppl.2): 16–17.

68 Horning SJ, Hoppe RT, Breslin S, et al. Stanford V and radiotherapy for locally extensive and advanced Hodgkin's disease: mature results of a prospective clinical trial. J Clin Oncol 2002; 20: 630–7.

69 Josting A, Franklin J, May M, et al. New prognostic score based on treatment outcome of patients with relapsed Hodgkin's lymphoma registered in the database of the German Hodgkin's lymphoma study group. J Clin Oncol 2002; 1: 221–30.

70 Linch DC, Winfield D, Goldstone AH, et al. Dose intensification with autologous bone-marrow transplantation in relapsed and resistant Hodgkin's lymphoma: results of a BNLI randomised trial. Lancet 1993; 341: 1051–4.

71 Schmitz N, Pfistner B, Sextro M, et al. German Hodgkin's Lymphoma Study Group; Lymphoma Working Party of the European Group for Blood and Marrow Transplantation. Aggressive conventional chemotherapy compared with high-dose chemotherapy with autologous haemopoietic stem-cell transplantation for relapsed chemosensitive Hodgkin's lymphoma: a randomised trial. Lancet 2002; 359: 2065–71.

72 Zintl F, Suttorp M, Berthold F, Dörffel W. Autologe Stammzelltransplantation (ASZT) bei Kindern mit rezidivieren-

den oder therapierefraktären Hodgkin-Lymphomen (Abstract). Monatsschr Kinderheilkd 2002; 150: 555.

73 Becherer A, Mitterbauer M, Jaeger U, et al. Positron emission tomography with [18F]2-fluoro-D-2-deoxyglucose (FDG-PET) predicts relapse of malignant lymphoma after high-dose therapy with stem cell transplantation. Leukemia 2002; 16: 260–7.

74 Radford JA, Eardley A, Woodman C, et al. Follow up policy after treatment for Hodgkin's disease: too many clinic visits and routine tests? A review of hospital records. Br Med J 1997; 314: 343–6.

75 Donaldson SS, Hudson M, Oberlin O et al. Pediatric Hodgkin's disease. In: Mauch PM, Armitage JO, Diehl V et al. (Eds), Hodgkin's Disease. Philadelphia: Lippincott Williams & Wilkins, 1999: 531–62.

76 Hudson MM, Poquette CA, Lee J, et al. Increased mortality after successful treatment for Hodgkin's disease. J Clin Oncol 1998; 16: 3592–600.

77 Schellong G, Riepenhausen M. Late effects after therapy for Hodgkin's disease: update 2003/04 on overwhelming post-splenectomy infections and secondary malignancies. Klin Pädiatr 2004; 216: 364–9.

78 Waghorn DJ. Overwhelming infection in asplenic patients: current best practise preventing measures are not being followed. J Clin Path 2001; 54: 214–18.

79 Hancock SL. Cardiovascular late effects after treatment of Hodgkin's disease. In: Mauch PM, Armitage JO, Diehl V, et al. (Hrsg) Hodgkin's disease. Philadelphia: Lippincott Williams & Wilkins, 1999: 647–59.

80 Acharya S, Saratoglu K, LaQuaglia M, et al. Thyroid neoplasms after therapeutic radiation for malignancies during childhood and adolescence. Cancer 2003; 97: 2397–403.

81 Sigurdson AJ, Ronckers CM, Mertens AC, et al. Primary thyroid cancer after a first tumor in childhood (the Childhood Cancer Survivor Study): a nested case-control study. Lancet 2005; 365: 2014–23.

82 Gerres L, Brämswig JH, Schlegel W, et al. The effects of etoposide on testicular function in boys treated for Hodgkin's disease. Cancer 1998; 83: 2217–2222.

83 Kulkarni SS, Sastry PSRK, Saika TK, et al. Gonadal function following ABVD therapy for Hodgkin's disease. Am J Clin Oncol 1997; 20: 354–7.

84 Neglia JP, Friedmann DL, Yasui Y, et al. Second malignant neoplasms in five-year survivors of childhood cancer: Childhood Cancer Survivor Study. J Natl Cancer Inst 2001; 93: 618–29.

85 Sankila R, Garwicz S, Olsen JH, et al. Risk of subsequent malignant neoplasms among 1641 Hodgkin's disease patients diagnosed in childhood and adolescence: a population-based cohort study in the five Nordic countries. J Clin Oncol 1996; 14: 1442–6.

86 Bhatia S, Leslie MPH, Robison L, et al. Breast cancer and other second neoplasms after childhood Hodgkin's disease. N Engl J Med 1996; 334: 745–51.

87 Tarbell NJ, Gelber RD, Weinstein HJ, Mauch P. Sex differences in risk of second malignant tumors after Hodgkin's disease in childhood. Lancet 1993; 341: 1428–32.

88 Schellong G, Riepenhausen M. Spätfolgen nach Morbus Hodgkin bei Kindern und Jugendlichen. Ergebnisse der Studien DAL–HD–78 bis –HD–90. Projektbericht 2002. Eigenverlag, Münster, 2002.

89 Bhatia S, Yasui Y, Robinson LL. High risk of subsequent neoplasms continues with extended follow-up of childhood Hodgkin's disease: report from the Late Effects Study Group. J Clin Oncol 2003; 23: 4386–94.

90 Jenkin D, Greenberg M, Fitzgerald A. Second malignant tumors in childhood Hodgkin's Disease. Med Pediatr Oncol 1996; 26: 373–9.

91 Schellong G, Riepenhausen M, Creutzig U, et al. Low risk of secondary leukemias after chemotherapy without mechlorethamine in childhood Hodgkin's disease. J Clin Oncol 1997; 25: 2241–53.

92 Schellong G, Riepenhausen M. Late effects after therapy of Hodgkin's disease: update 2003/04 on overwhelming post-splenectomy infections and secondary malignancies. Klin Pädiatr 2004; 216: 364–9.

93 Peggs KS, Hunter A, Chopra R, et al. Clinical evidence of a graft-versus-Hodgkin's-lymphoma effect after reduced-intensity allogeneic transplantation. Lancet 2005; 365: 1934–41.

94 Hart DP, Avivi I, Thomson KJ, et al. Use of 18 FDG–PET following allogeneic transplantation to guide adoptive immunotherapy with donor lymphocyte infusions. Br J Haematol 2005; 128: 824–9.

95 Bollard CM, Aguilar L, Straathof KC, et al. Cytotoxic T lymphocyte therapy for EBV positive Hodgkin's disease. J Exp Med 2004; 200: 1623–33.

96 Bollard CM, Gottschalk S, Huls MH, et al. In vivo expansion of LMP1 and 2-specific T-cells in a patient who received donor-derived EBV specific T-cells after allogeneic stem cell transplantation. Leuk Lymphoma 2006; 47: 837–42.

97 Schnell R, Dietlein M, Staak JO, et al. Treatrment of refractory Hodgkin`s lymphoma patients with iodine-131 labeled murine anti-CD30 monoclonal antibody. J Clin Oncol 2005; 23: 4669–78.

98 Schnell R, Borchmann P, Staak JO, et al. Clinical evaluation of ricin A-chain immunotoxins in patients with Hodgkin's lymphoma. Ann Oncol 2003; 14: 729–36.

99 Harris NL, Jaffe ES, Diebold J, et al. World Health Organization classification of neoplastic diseases of the hematopoietic and lymphoid tissues: report of the Clinical Advisory Committee meeting, Airlie House, Virginia, November 1997. J Clin Oncol 1999;17: 3835–49.

100 Franklin J, Tesch H, Hansmann ML, et al. Lymphocyte predominant Hodgkin's disease: pathology and clinical implication. Ann Oncol 1998; 9 (Suppl 5): S39–44.

101 Regula DP Jr, Hoppe RT, Weiss LM. Nodular and diffuse types of lymphocyte predominance Hodgkin's disease. N Engl J Med 1988; 318: 214–9.

102 Borg–Grech A, Radford JA, Crowther D, Swindell R, Harris M. A comparative study of the nodular and diffuse variants of lymphocyte–predominant Hodgkin's disease. J Clin Oncol 1989; 7: 1303–9.

103 Pappa VI, Norton AJ, Gupta RK et al. Nodular type of lymphocyte predominant Hodgkin's disease. A clinical study of 50 cases. Ann Oncol 1995; 6: 559–65.

104 Nogova L, Reineke T, Josting A, et al. Lymphocyte–predominant and classical Hodgkin's lymphoma – comparison of outcomes. Eur J Haematol 2005: 75 (Suppl 66): 106–10.

105 Gobbi PG, Broglia C, Merli F, et al. Vinblastine, bleomycin, and methotrexate chemotherapy plus irradiation for patients with early-stage, favorable Hodgkin Lymphoma. Cancer 2003; 98: 2393–401.

106 Feugier P, Labourye E, Djeridane M, et al. Comparison of initial characteristics and long term outcome of Lymphocyte-predominant Hodgkin's lymphoma patients at clinical stage IA and IIA prospectively treated by brief anthracycline-based chemotherapies plus extended high dose irradiation. Blood 2004; 104: 2675–81.

107 Wirth A, Yuen K, Barton M, et al. Long-term outcome after radiotherapy alone for lymphocyte-predominant Hodgkin Lymphoma. Cancer 2005; 104: 1221–9.

108 Schlembach PJ, Wilder RB, Jones D, et al. Radiotherapy alone for lymphocyte-predominant Hodgkin's disease. Cancer 2002; 8: 377–83.

109 Wilder RB, Schlembach PJ, Jones D, et al. European Organization for Research and Treatment of Cancer and Groupe d'Etude des lymphomes de l'Adulte very favorable and favorable, lymphocyte-predominant Hodgkin disease. Cancer 2002; 94: 1731–8.

110 Ekstrand BC, Lucas JB, Horwitz SM, et al. Rituximab in lymphocyte–predominant Hodgkin disease: results of a phase 2 trial. Blood 2003; 101: 4285–9.

111 Rehwald U, Schulz H, Reiser M, et al.; German Hodgkin Lymphoma Study Group (GHSG). Treatment of relapsed CD20+ Hodgkin lymphoma with the monoclonal antibody rituximab is effective and well tolerated: results of a phase 2 trial of the German Hodgkin Lymphoma Study Group. Blood 2003; 101: 420–4.

112 Mauz–Koerholz C, Gorde–Grosjean S, Hasenlever D, et al. Resection Alone in 58 Children with Limited Stage Lymphocyte Predominant Hodgkin`s Lymphoma – Experience from the European Network Group on Paediatric Hodgkin's Lymphoma EuroNet–PHL Group. Cancer 2007; 110; 179–85.

113 Shankar A, Daw S, Gorde-Grosjean S, et al. Treatment of Children and Adolescents with early stage Nodular Lymphocyte Predominant Hodgkin's Lymphoma with a low intensity short duration chemotherapy regimen [CVP] – on behalf of the EuroNet-PHL Group ASH 2006 abstract No 2471).

114 Dieckmann K, Potter R, Wagner W, et al. Up-front centralized data review and individualized treatment proposals in a multicenter pediatric Hodgkin's lymphoma trial with 71 participating hospitals: the experience of the German-Austrian pediatric multicenter trial DAL–HD–90. Radiother Oncol 2002; 62: 191–200.

115 Dörffel W, Schellong G. Morbus Hodgkin. In: Gadner H, Gaedicke G, Niemeyer C, Ritter J (eds), Pädiatrische Hämatologie und Onkologie. Heidelberg: Springer Medizin Verlag, 2006: 752–69.

11 Histiocytic Disorders

Sheila Weitzman[1] and R. Maarten Egeler[2]

[1] Department of Pediatrics, University of Toronto, Toronto, Ontario, Canada and [2] Department of Pediatrics, Leiden University Medical Center, Leiden, The Netherlands

Introduction

The histiocytoses are defined as disorders that are due to abnormal accumulation of histiocytes, encompassing both increased proliferation and decreased apoptosis. The writing group of the Histiocyte Society has classified the histiocytoses into two major subtypes – disorders of variable biologic behavior and those disorders that are clearly malignant [1]. Malignant disorders are dealt with elsewhere in this book. The disorders of variable biologic behavior are further subdivided into disorders of the antigen presenting dendritic cells and disorders of the macrophage/monocyte (Table 11.1). This classification system provides a means of standardizing the nomenclature thereby making possible international cooperative studies of the two major histiocytic disorders, Langerhans cell histiocytosis and hemophagocytic lymphohistiocytosis (HLH).

Langerhans cell histiocytosis (LCH)

LCH is characterized by clonal proliferation and excess accumulation of pathologic Langerhans cells (LCs) at various sites. LCH has a wide spectrum of clinical presentation and prognosis and has been variously considered to be a neoplasm, a reactive disorder or an aberrant immune response [2].

Histopathology

The histopathology of LCH is that of a granulomatous lesion containing pathologic LCs and other cells such as eosinophils, macrophages, multinucleated giant cells, stromal cells and natural killer (NK) cells [3]. The diagnosis is clinico-pathologic, based on histology and immunohistochemistry within the correct clinical setting, to exclude reactive normal LCs in nodes in association with various diseases [4, 5].

Diagnosis requires demonstration by immunohistochemistry of either or both:

Pediatric Hematology and Oncology, 1st edition. Edited by Edward J. Estlin, Richard J. Gilbertson, and Robert F. Wynn. © 2010 Blackwell Publishing Ltd.

- CD1a
- Langerin and/or Birbeck granules (BG) which are typically rod- or racket-shaped cytoplasmic organelles seen on electron microscopy (EM).

Langerin (CD207) is a mannose-specific lectin involved with trafficking of exogenous antigens to the intracellular BG compartments [3]. Langerin positivity by immunohistochemistry is seen whenever BG are present, with 100% concordance [3, 6] and EM is therefore no longer needed for diagnosis. BG are usually absent from brain and liver LCH, even when these organs are clinically involved [7].

Pathogenesis

The lesional LCH-cell is most akin to the normal LC, but is clearly pathologic. Normal LCs, the sentinels of the immune system for foreign antigens, are strategically located at host/environmental interfaces such as epidermis, respiratory, and genital epithelia [3]. Put simply, LCs capture antigens, process them, express the antigenic peptides on their cell surface, migrate through lymphatics, and present antigen to peptide-specific naïve- and central memory-T cells in the T-cell areas of draining nodes and spleen [8,9]. These processes appear to be controlled by cytokines and chemokines produced by the keratinocytes, LCs, endothelial cells, and T-cells [10]. During normal maturation the LCs down-regulate CCR6, a receptor present on the cell surface, which keeps the LC in the epidermis and up-regulates CCR7 which responds to a chemokine within the lymph node allowing physiologic trafficking from skin to node. Lesional CD1a+ LCH cells fail to both down-regulate CCR6 and to up-regulate CCR7 preventing them from leaving their peripheral tissue sites where they accumulate and express other inflammatory chemokines, resulting in their own recruitment and retention, as well as that of other inflammatory cells, including eosinophils and T-cells. Ligation of CD40+LCH cells by the high number of lesional CD40L+ T-cells results in activation of both cells and erratic and uncontrolled production of various cytokines. The result is an amplification cascade, with cytokine upregulation in auto- and paracrine loops, creating the 'cytokine storm' [11, 12].

Many different cytokines have been demonstrated in LCH including IL-2, IL-4, IL-5, TNF-α, IL-1α, GM-CSF and IFN-γ,

Table 11.1 Classification of histiocytic disorder. Adapted from [1].

Disorders of varying biologic behavior
(a) Dendritic-cell related
Langerhans cell histiocytosis
Juvenile xanthogranulona and related disorders including:
- Erdheim Chester disease
- Solitary histiocytomas with JXG phenotype
Secondary dendritic cell disorders
(b) Macrophage-related
Hemophagocytic lymphohistiocytosis:
- Familial
- Secondary hemophagocytic syndromes
Sinus Histiocytosis with Massive Lymphadenopathy (Rosai-Dorfman disease

Malignant disorders
(a) Monocyte related
Leukemias:
- Monocytic leukemias M5A and B
- Acute myelomonocytic leukemia M4
- Chronic myelomonocytic leukemias
Extramedullary monocytic tumors or sarcoma (monocytic counterpart of granulocytic sarcoma)
Macrophage-related-histiocytic sarcoma (localized or disseminated)
(b) Dendritic-cell-related
Histiocytic sarcoma (localized or disseminated)

IL-3 and IL-7, contributing to the pathological sequelae including fibrosis, bone resorption, and necrosis.

Despite the plethora of studies and increasing knowledge the etiology of LCH remains unknown and there is continued debate as to whether LCH is a neoplastic or a reactive disease.

Genetic factors

Evidence of familial clustering of LCH, a higher concordance rate for monozygotic twins compared with dizygotic (87 vs 10%), as well as a younger median age at diagnosis (4 vs 32 months) and a higher prevalence of multisystem (MS) disease (87 vs 50%) in monozygotic twins, suggest a genetic predisposition for LCH [13]. Second malignancies, particularly T-cell acute lymphoblastic leukemia, a clonal malignancy of hematopoetic precursors, occur in LCH patients at a much higher than expected rate, giving further support for an underlying genetic abnormality in LCH cells [10]. Overall it appears that around 1% of children with LCH have an affected relative, and familial occurrence is not limited to the same generation [13].

Incidence, age, and gender

LCH can present at any age from the neonatal period until old age, with approximately 50–70% of cases being less than 15 years old. A recent Swedish study found an increased incidence in children of 8.9 per 10^6/y [14]. The increase was seen in MS and single site (SS) disease, suggesting that this was not solely due to improved recognition. These figures likely still underestimate the problem, as many patients with localized LCH are likely to go undiagnosed. Studies report a slight male preponderance overall, with an M:F ratio as high as 2:1 in MS patients.

The severity of disease tends to be age-related, with MS LCH seen mainly in children <2 years of age, multifocal SS disease in children between 2 and 5 years, while 50% of unifocal bone disease occurs in children over 5 [15, 16]. In adult patients, isolated pulmonary LCH (PLCH) is seen occurring most commonly in the 20–40-year-old age group. The vast majority of PLCH is seen in smokers, explaining why the incidence is increasing in young females, although there is still a male preponderance at the present time [17].

Clinical presentation

LCH in children is very diverse, with some patients presenting with localized disease that resolves spontaneously or with minimal therapy, while others develop a low grade chronic form of the disease with repeated reactivations and the risk of permanent long-term disabilities. At the other extreme, seen mainly in young infants, is the presentation with life-threatening disseminated LCH with rapid progression and death. The need for a uniform definition of extent of disease and 'risk-adjusted' therapy led to the definition of two categories of disease:
- single-system (SS-LCH)
- multisystem (MS-LCH)
  SS disease is further subdivided into:
- unifocal SS-LCH
- multifocal SS-LCH

MS disease is divided into 'risk' categories by the presence or absence of risk organ involvement. Approximately two-thirds of patients present with SS-LCH, most commonly in bone [10, 16]. SS disease may progress to become limited MS disease with involvement of the hypothalamo-pituitary axis and CNS. Young babies can also progress from SS-LCH (usually skin-only disease), to the disseminated, potentially fatal form of the disease, while conversely patients with risk organ MS-LCH who respond to therapy, can reactivate later in low risk organs (usually bone) and be at significant risk of long-term complications.

Bone Langerhans cell histiocytosis

Approximately 80% of pediatric LCH patients have bone disease:
- 80% have SS bone disease.
- 20% bone as part of MS-LCH.
- Unifocal bone (UFB) occurs in 78%.
- Multifocal bone (MFB) occurs in 22% [18].

The bone most commonly involved is the skull, followed by spine, lower extremity, pelvis, ribs, and upper extremity. Proximal long bones are more commonly involved than distal and the hands and feet are usually spared. In the long bones, the diaphysis and metaphysis are equally involved and the epiphysis is commonly spared, but epiphyseal location does not exclude LCH [19].

Presentation is with swelling and/or pain, present during activity and/or rest. Bone lesions may, however, be completely asymptomatic.

Additional symptoms depend on the area involved:
• Jaw LCH – jaw pain and loose teeth.
• Temporal bone LCH – chronic otitis media, with dermatitis of the auricular canal, mastoiditis and cholesteatoma – often in children less than 3 years of age [20, 21]. Radiologic changes may be out of proportion to clinical findings [22].
• Orbital LCH – proptosis, swelling and redness of eyelid, diplopia and/or ophthalmoplegia.
• Lower extremity lesions – limp or fracture.
• Vertebral body LCH – back pain and/or kyphoscoliosis or neurologic dysfunction including paraplegia.
LCH is the commonest cause of vertebra plana in children [23]. Other causes include osteomyelitis, infantile myofibromatosis [24], juvenile xanthogranuloma, aneurysmal bone cyst, osteogenesis inperfecta, leukemia, lymphoma, and malignant sarcomas [25].

Most patients with SS bone disease are afebrile, but fever should not exclude the diagnosis. Blood counts may show mild eosinophilia, but are otherwise normal, and the erythrocyte sedimentation rate (ESR) is often mildly elevated.

Because of the different outlook and therapy of UFB compared with MFB, every patient should have a complete work up at diagnosis, irrespective of presentation.

Radiologic investigation of bone Langerhans cell histiocytosis

Plain radiographs (skeletal survey) remains the first-line investigation and are more sensitive than Technetium-99 nuclear medicine scans for detection of LCH [26, 27] but both are recommended. Radiologic characteristics vary with site of involvement. The classic osteolytic lesion has sharply demarcated margins and little or no periosteal reaction (Figure 11.1) and may be associated with a soft tissue mass. Radiologically aggressive lesions resembling a malignant tumor may be seen particularly in the orbits, mastoid or other areas of the base of skull or even

in the long bones [26, 28].(Figure 11.2). With healing there is disappearance of the mass with development of a well- defined sclerotic rim. CT and MRI scans are useful in delineating uncertain lesions and the extent of soft tissue involvement but neither is useful in distinguishing LCH from malignancy in radiologically aggressive lesions [29]. The diagnosis should be proven by biopsy where possible. 18-FDG positive emission tomography (PET) is a sensitive technique for identifying active lesions and may differentiate active from healed lesions [30] and may prove helpful in follow up.

Natural history and therapy of bone Langerhans cell histiocytosis

Spontaneous healing of bone lesions is well known and healing at one site at the same time as, or followed by, progression in another is not uncommon.

In SS bone LCH, survival is almost universal but reactivations occur at a rate of:
• Unifocal bone – 3–12%
• Multifocal bone – 11–25%
• Bone in MS disease – 50–70% [16, 31].

The greater the reactivation rate, the higher the incidence of diabetes insipidus (DI) and other late complications.

'Risk' bones are those which give the highest risk of DI and include the facial bones and base of skull, particularly if associated with an intracranial soft tissue mass [32, 33].

Bone lesions are treated for two reasons:
• To treat symptoms such as pain or neurologic complications.
• To try to prevent reactivations and late effects.
Recommendations for therapy, therefore, vary for UFB compared with MFB and for 'risk' bone LCH compared with 'non-risk' bone LCH.
Patients who require therapy include those with:
• Intense pain.

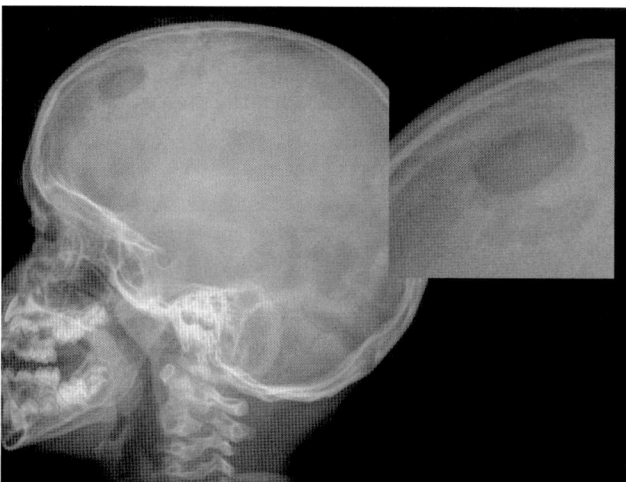

Figure 11.1 X-ray skull showing the typical punched out lesion of Langerhans cell histiocytosis.

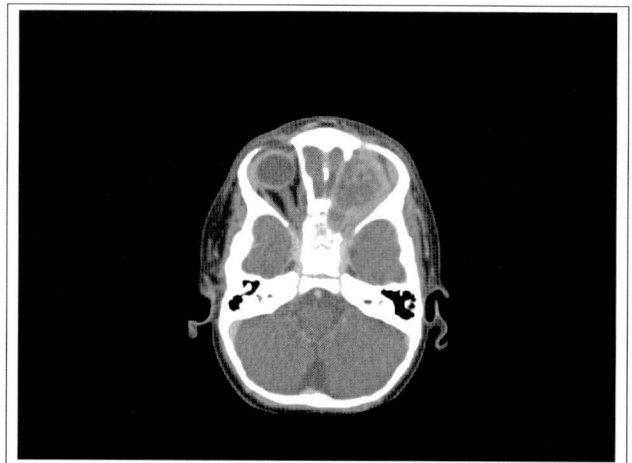

Figure 11.2 Computed tomography scan of an orbital Langerhans cell histiocytosis lesion showing the 'sarcomatous' appearance that may be found particularly in facial bones.

- Restriction of mobility.
- Unacceptable deformity.
- Involvement of a growth plate.
- Involvement of a bone likely to fracture [34].
  Treatment for bone LCH includes:
- Curettage to induce healing and provide tissue for diagnosis. This is often the only therapy required for UFB lesions at presentation.
- Intralesional corticosteroid under radiographic control. This is given only for a limited number of lesions and is effective and usually safe [34]. Around 10% require a repeat injection to achieve healing [35]. If a frozen section diagnosis is obtained, it can be given at the time of curettage or if there is local recurrence at the site of curettage (minority of patients).
- Surgery. Wide surgical resection is unnecessary, may lead to long term deformity, and is *contraindicated at any site*.
- Observation alone is limited to UFB in patients with a pathologic diagnosis.

UFB in 'risk' areas, particularly with a large intracranial soft tissue component, may require therapy to try to prevent progression to DI and other late effects.

Patients presenting with vertebra plana without a soft tissue mass or neurologic symptoms, can be observed without a firm diagnosis, but should be carefully followed.

- Low dose radiation therapy (6–10 Gy) is an effective therapeutic modality but is usually restricted to involvement of critical organs such as spinal cord or optic nerve [36]. At the suggested dose, long-term effects are unlikely and it is preferable to mutilating surgery.
- Indomethacin, a potent prostaglandin-E2 inhibitor, and other non-steroidal anti-inflammatory drugs (NSAIDS) have proved efficacious [37, 38].
- Bisphosphonate therapy [39–41]. Toxicity has been tolerable in most patients treated. The role of NSAIDS and bisphosphonates in preventing reactivations and late complications, however, is unclear and the long-term effects of bisphosphonates on growing bone, is unknown.
- Chemotherapy – MFB or bone LCH in MS disease. The commonest combination is vinblastine and steroid, although many drugs are effective. Chemotherapy is discussed in detail later

Natural history and therapy of skin Langerhans cell histiocytosis

Skin involvement in LCH occurs in 50% of patients and can occur at any age [42]. Isolated skin disease (skin-only LCH) is seen in 10% of cases, usually in the very young child, but does occur occasionally in older patients and adults [42, 43]. In MS LCH, skin-LCH may occur as part of limited disease together with bone and/or DI, or may be part of generalized disease. The commonest area involved is scalp followed by flexural creases, but any site may be involved including palms, soles, and nails. The commonest presentation is with a 'seborrhea-like' eruption on the scalp often misdiagnosed as 'cradle-cap', but papules, vesicles, crusted plaques, nodules, and purpuric nodules are all described [42].

LCH should be considered whenever seborrheic dermatitis or diaper dermatitis fails to respond to therapy or keeps recurring. The natural history is variable and patients with skin-only LCH may have:
- Spontaneous regression
- Regression and reactivation in skin.
- Progression, particularly in the infant, to disseminated and sometimes fatal disease.

Hashimoto and Pritzker [44] described a particular form of skin-LCH with spontaneous involution in all cases. The self-limited nature of the disease may be explained by the finding that the DCs are able to mature, eventually leading to their apoptosis. While a small percentage of babies with skin-only LCH fit this description, half of all babies with true skin-only LCH will progress to multisystem disease [45].

All young babies with skin-only LCH should be carefully followed [46, 47].

Therapy of cutaneous Langerhans cell histiocytosis

In view of the natural history and good prognosis of skin-only LCH, therapy should be restricted to severely symptomatic disease:
- Surgical excision – for small isolated lesions only, with no mutilating surgery.
- Local or systemic corticosteroids – first line therapy, but the effect is usually transient.
- Psoralen with ultraviolet therapy (PUVA) [48, 49].
- Topical nitrogen mustard [50, 51]. Despite the finding of no premalignant or malignant changes in the Mustine-treated skin of 20 children with median follow-up of 8.3 years [51], concerns with regard to late skin cancer persist.
- Topical tacrolimus (anecdotal reports). Like other topical therapy, the treatment may need to be repeated at intervals until the disease burns itself out. If a large surface area is treated, systemic tacrolimus levels should be followed.
- Thalidomide and interferon-α – experience tends to be limited to skin-LCH in adults[52, 53].
- Chlorambucil, prolonged, oral – reported in adults (Chu A).
- Etoposide, prolonged, oral, low dose [54].
- Multidrug chemotherapy – usually effective in skin-LCH – use usually limited to widespread symptomatic disease or skin as part of MS-LCH. This includes standard LCH chemotherapy as well as 2-CdA which is a good alternative for extensive skin disease.

Natural history and therapy of multisystem Langerhans cell histiocytosis

The clinical presentation depends on the organs involved:
- Limited MS-LCH usually refers to involvement of bone and/or skin and/or hypothalamo-pituitary axis of which DI is commonly the first manifestation.
- Disseminated MS-LCH usually occurring in children younger than 2 years of age. Almost all organs can be involved although kidney and gonadal disease is unusual.

The presentation is therefore with any or all of the following, fever, wasting, hepatosplenomegaly, abdominal distention, diarrhea, failure to thrive, lymphadenopathy, pancytopenia, edema, tachypnea, and respiratory distress. Skin and bone involvement are common in MS disease, and the manifestations described above in the relevant sections are also part of the clinical presentation of MS-LCH.

Liver and spleen.

Hepatosplenomegaly may indicate the presence of organ involvement by LCH, obstructive disease caused by enlarged nodes in the porta hepatis or indirectly from a cytokine effect [54]. Liver involvement is present in about one-third of patients and is considered to be a poor prognostic sign [55]. Documentation of liver dysfunction requires hypoalbuminemia, jaundice, or abnormal coagulation tests. Progression of cholestasis to sclerosing cholangitis, biliary cirrhosis, and liver failure may occur (see discussion later). Enlargement of the spleen may be an additional factor responsible for pancytopenia.

Lung

Pulmonary LCH (PLCH) predominantly affects young adults between 20 and 40 years of age and is seen almost exclusively in smokers who smoke more than 20 cigarettes per day. Ten to 20% progress to end-stage lung disease requiring lung transplant for cure [17]. Children with LCH who start smoking in adolescence or young adulthood have an increased incidence of PLCH compared with the normal population [56]. Symptoms may be minor or absent and dry cough, dyspnea or tachypnea with rib retraction may be the only clinical features. In the early stages the diagnosis is suggested by a diffuse micronodular pattern on chest radiographs which may progress to cyst formation and a 'honeycomb lung'. A characteristic CT appearance may be pathognomonic for LCH obviating the need for biopsy, and a high resolution CT is considered mandatory if PLCH is suspected. In later stages, large bullae may rupture causing spontaneous pneumothoraces. Emphysematous changes, along with increasing amounts of interstitial fibrosis, may occur in the final phase of PLCH. It has been suggested that more than 5% CD1a+ cells in bronchoalveolar fluid, where normally there should be <1% CD1a+ cells, is diagnostic of PLCH. Using the 5% cut off, the specificity is good but sensitivity is low [17] and lung biopsy is considered the gold standard for diagnosis and evaluation of disease activity in patients with radiologic findings suggestive of chronic disease. In children, PLCH is usually part of MS LCH and chemotherapy is the mainstay of treatment for active disease.

Hematopoetic system

Pancytopenia is a frequent manifestation of disseminated MS-LCH despite relative infrequency of morphologic infiltration of bone marrow, suggesting an effect of inhibitory cytokines on the marrow. In the LCH-I study 18% of MS patients had documented marrow infiltration but 36% had blood count abnormalities [20, 36]. Hematopoetic involvement is considered to be an important 'risk' factor and may be associated with secondary hemophagocytic syndrome (HLH) which requires therapy directed at the HLH component. Mortality is high if the patient does not respond quickly to therapy and salvage therapy with allogeneic transplant should be considered early in these young patients

Gastrointestinal tract

The commonest sign of GI disease is 'failure to thrive' due to malabsorption. Other symptoms include vomiting, diarrhea with or without blood, and protein-losing enteropathy. In most cases there is radiographic evidence of alternating dilated and stenotic segments in the small and large bowel. Endoscopic biopsy is needed for diagnosis. Several groups have suggested that GI involvement is a poor risk feature in MS LCH [12, 57].

Central nervous system (CNS)/endocrine

There is a well-described predilection of LCH for the hypothalamic–pituitary axis (HPA) and diabetes insipidus (DI) is the commonest manifestation of endocrine LCH. DI can occur prior to, concurrent with, or subsequent to the diagnosis of LCH [58], with the greatest risk being in patients with MS disease and those with lesions involving the facial bones and skull base [33]. Gadolinium-enhanced MRI scans demonstrate loss of the posterior pituitary 'bright spot', thickening of the pituitary stalk, a partial or completely empty sella, and sometimes a suprasellar mass [33, 58], but thread-like atrophy of the stalk may be seen. Differential diagnosis includes germinoma, hypophysitis and even lymphoma.

Anterior pituitary deficits are common complications of LCH [59] occurring usually in patients with preceding DI [60]. Growth hormone (GH) deficiency usually occurs first although growth failure in children with LCH is multifactorial with chronic illness, malabsorption and prolonged corticosteroid treatment [20]. Other HPA abnormalities include precocious or delayed puberty, amenorrhea in adult females, hyperprolactinemia, morbid obesity [60], sleeping disorders and disorders of thermoregulation [61]. Thyroid deficiency may occur as a result of TSH deficiency or thyroid gland infiltration [61–63].

Central nervous system–Non-Endocrine

The availability of MRI has revealed an increasing incidence of disease in other parts of the brain, notable even before clinical symptoms develop [33], usually occurring in patients with preceding DI. These include extraparenchymal lesions derived from meninges, choroid plexus or pineal gland, which may give focal neurologic symptoms and signs. Biopsy of these areas and the hypothalamo-pituitary lesions show active LCH, but CNS disease may progress to a chronic neurodegenerative stage in which only demyelination and gliosis is found, thought to be due to an autoimmune reaction to preceding LCH [33]. This end-stage disease is observed in about 3–5% of patients with LCH, but may occur in 10% or more of patients with DI. Areas affected are mainly cerebellum, pons, basal ganglia or cerebral grey or white matter. Clinical findings, including ataxia, dysarthia, nystagmus, tremor, dysdiadochokinesia, dysphagia, psychomotor retardation, and neuropsychologic problems, may develop years after the original diagnosis of LCH and may progress to produce severe disability and even death [33]. It is unclear whether all of the asymptomatic patients with abnormal MRI scans will progress to symptomatic neurodegenerative disease.

Like the late chronic disease in lung or liver described later, there is no known effective therapy for patients with neurodegenerative disease. At present, only DI with structural changes in the HPA, heralds involvement of other parts of the brain [33, 61]. Prevention of onset of DI is therefore likely to be very important. Attempts to detect partial DI before it becomes established have been largely unsuccessful.

Therapy of diabetes insipidus

Because of the significant neurologic consequences that appear to follow DI, and because of a few reports of reversibility of DI by early therapy [64], the current recommendation is to treat patients with recent onset of DI to try to prevent the uncommon but devastating late CNS disease [65]. Most DI will not reverse on therapy. The optimal therapy for recent-onset DI is unclear. Radiation therapy may be effective if given early before full ADH deficiency occurs, but there is no evidence that 'late' disease will respond to therapy [66] and the potential for late effects means that RT should be restricted to non-responsive growing masses. Standard LCH chemotherapy with vinblastine and prednisone will be effective for this extra-axial disease and it is unclear whether a drug such as cladribine (2-CdA), which crosses the blood–brain barrier (BBB), will be more effective in preventing progression from DI to other CNS/endocrine manifestations.

Therapy of central nervous system disease
Tumoral central nervous system Langerhans cell histiocytosis lesions

As these, like DI, have been shown pathologically to be due to active LCH, drugs that cross the BBB should be used for therapy. Cladribine (2-CdA) has been shown to be effective against active CNS LCH [64, 67, 68]. Other drugs which cross the BBB and have activity in LCH are cytosine arabinoside and methotrexate. As above, radiation therapy should be limited to non-responsive disease.

Late neurodegenerative disease

No therapy has to date been shown conclusively to affect the course of the neurodegeneration phase of CNS LCH. It has been suggested, but not proven, that multiple sclerosis type therapy with drugs such as tacrolimus may be effective (N. Grois, personal communication) and a low dose ara-C regimen appears to slow or stop progression and possibly to induce regression in a small number of patients [69], as has a regimen with cis-retinoic acid (J. Donadieu, personal communication). All these approaches need to be properly tested.

Therapy of multisystem Langerhans cell histiocytosis

Treatment of MS-LCH has dual aims:
- To improve survival.
- To prevent reactivations and late sequelae of the disease or therapy.

Most patients have been treated with systemic chemotherapeutic agents because of the progressive nature of generalized LCH. Results of the large non-randomized German/Austrian cooperative group DAL-HX studies, appears to support this approach. All patients with extensive disease were treated using vinblastine/prednisone/VP16 induction for 6 weeks, followed by maintenance with the same drugs plus 6-mercaptopurine (6-MP) for low risk patients, and 6-MP/MTX for those with organ dysfunction. Treatment duration was 12 months. Complete remission (CR) was obtained within 4 months in 89–91% of patients without organ involvement, and 67% of patients with organ involvement. Altogether 77% of patients have remained disease-free. No etoposide-induced second malignancies have been observed [70]. The rate of reactivation was low compared with previously reported studies as was the incidence of development of DI (estimated cumulative risk of 10% in patients without DI at presentation), suggesting that early therapy with relatively non-toxic chemotherapy could reduce the incidence of late complications. An important advance came with the creation of the Histiocyte Society and the instigation of international studies such as LCH-1, LCH-II and the open LCH-III study.

A different and conservative approach was suggested by McLelland who reported 44 children with extensive disease of whom 36 required systemic therapy. Of the 36, 17 responded to prednisolone alone, and 19 required the addition of vinblastine or etoposide. Overall survival was equivalent at 82%, but 60% of survivors had late effects and 36% developed DI [71], supporting the use of early chemotherapy for MS-LCH. The observation that the strongest predictor of survival was the early response to chemotherapy in the DAL-HX studies, the French study group trials as well as the LCH-1 and LCH-II studies also supports early chemotherapy in such patients [62, 72]. Comparison of the DAL-HX study and LCH-I and II studies, showed that the mortality for high risk patients with disseminated disease has not changed over the three studies. About 20% of young children with MS LCH did not respond to chemotherapy and most of the patients died. A recent study from the Japanese LCH study group (JLSG) suggests that the mortality from MS LCH can be reduced by increasing the early response rate using more intensive induction therapy and by prompt rescue of poor responders [73]. A pilot study from the French group suggests also that early switch to an effective salvage protocol will improve survival for the patients with refractory disease [74](see salvage therapy below).

For patients that respond to initial therapy, the problem is that of reactivation of disease and long-term consequences, rather than of survival. Both LCH-I and the succeeding LCH-II trial, showed that most reactivations in responding patients were in non-risk organs such as skin or bone, and were rarely fatal [70].

However, permanent disease-related disabilities occurred in more than 40% of patients.

Combining the results of the large multinational trials, therefore, allows the design of risk-tailored therapy. Patients with extensive disease, but without involvement of the risk organs (liver, spleen, lung, and hematopoetic system) have an excellent survival with minimal therapy. For this group, therapy should be given to prevent DI and other late complications. Whether this is best done by prolonged low-toxicity therapy as suggested by the DAL studies, or by using drugs such as 2-Cda which penetrate well into brain, or both, should be investigated.

Patients with extensive disease with risk organ involvement should be evaluated after induction therapy. Evaluation of response at 6 and 12 weeks, allows allocation to a group of 'responders' or 'non-responders'. The very high-risk group of non-responders (22% of 'risk' patients on LCH-II), should be moved early to a salvage protocol (see below), the aim of which is to improve survival. In this setting, toxicity and late-effects become secondary considerations.

Salvage therapies

The three groups of patients requiring salvage therapy are those with refractory MS disease, those with chronically relapsing disease associated with good survival but significant long-term complications, and patients with the late progressive involvement of liver, lung, and CNS

Salvage therapy for refractory MS disease includes chemotherapy, immunomodulatory approaches, and stem cell transplantation. A number of chemotherapy drugs and combinations have been tried in patients refractory to first line protocols. Cladribine (2-CdA), a nucleoside analog initially shown to be effective in adults with resistant LCH [75], proved to be effective in less than a third of refractory high-risk patients in a recently completed Histiocyte Society study [76]. *In vitro* and *in vivo*, the combination of 2-CdA and cytosine-arabinoside (ara-C) results in higher intracellular concentrations of the active metabolite ara-CTP [77]. A recent small series of 10 patients with progressive MS LCH, show encouraging results with 2-CdA/ara-C [74] and this combination is being tested in an open Histiocyte Society study.

A number of successful stem cell transplants (SCT) have been reported in refractory LCH patients. A review of the literature found 35 patients transplanted for refractory LCH [78]. A summary of 27 documented cases shows that 15/27(56%) were alive in complete continuous remission (CCR) from 12+ to 144+ (median 25+) months. The question of positive reporting bias remains but it seems that allogeneic, but not autologous transplant, is potentially curative in poor risk patients. The major cause of death is transplant-related toxicity and another Histiocyte Society study will evaluate reduced intensity SCT for patients refractory to salvage therapy.

Therapy of chronically reactivating disease
A number of drugs and drug combinations including vinblastine/prednisone, 2-CdA, a combination of low dose ara-C, vincristine,

and prednisolone[11] and even indomethacin [38], can successfully treat the acute reactivation, but do not appear to effectively prevent further reactivations. It has been suggested that low dose prolonged therapy for this low grade chronic form of the disease may be what is required. This can be achieved with the addition of a maintenance regimen of oral 6-MP daily and oral methotrexate weekly for 24 months to one of the induction regimens or possibly even the addition of prolonged indomethacin therapy. These hypotheses remain to be proven in prospective trials.

Late chronic Langerhans cell histiocytosis
Late progressive chronic LCH is seen in liver, lung (and CNS as described above), and appears to be due to late fibrosis (or gliosis). The initial lesions appear to be active LCH but at the late stage few LCH cells are found and it is felt that pro-and anti-inflammatory cytokines particularly TGF-β [79] play an important role in the development of this fibrosis [41, 80].
• Late chronic liver disease presents as sclerosing cholangitis (SC) and biliary cirrhosis progressing to liver failure. Patients may present with SC at diagnosis, or following active liver involvement as part of MS-LCH [81, 82].
• Late chronic lung fibrosis surrounds cystic spaces giving the classic honeycomb lung. Progression to pulmonary fibrosis and respiratory failure may result in death [17]. Clinically and radiologically, it is difficult to discriminate active LCH from end-stage fibrosis [83].

Therapy of chronic disease
In the early stages, therapy may control active LCH and stop progression of disease, but in the later stages no effective systemic therapy is known. Ursodeoxycholic acid may slow progress of liver fibrosis [84] but organ transplantation is the only proven effective therapy for end-stage lung and liver disease, and the results appear to be durable. A recent review of pediatric LCH patients transplanted for liver failure found that 78% of children were alive [85] and only two recurrences have been reported in the transplanted liver [86]. Similarly five of seven adult patients receiving a lung transplant for LCH are alive and well from 15 to 90 months post-transplant, and the two that recurred did so after resuming smoking [87]. An increased incidence of EBV-induced PTLD after liver transplant was found in one series and an increased incidence in severity and frequency of rejection in several series [88, 89].

Late effects of Langerhans cell histiocytosis
Results of the late effects study of the Histiocyte Society suggest that with a minimum of 3 years of follow up, at least 71% of MS and 24% of SS patients have at least one permanent consequence (PC) [90]. The most commonly reported PCs are:
• DI (24% overall and 40% of MS patients).
• Orthopedic problems (20%).
• Hearing loss (13%).
• Neurologic consequences (11%).
• Growth retardation (9%).

Other late effects include thyroid, gonadotrophin, and cortico-trophin deficiencies as well as other manifestations of the hypoth-alamic syndrome such as behavioral problems, abnormalities in temperature control, and morbid obesity.

LCH occurs in association with various malignancies at a higher frequency than would be expected by chance. The LCH-malignancy registry of the Histiocyte Society had 157 cases reported at the last update with solid tumors followed by acute myeloblastic leukemia (AML) being most commonly reported in the children [90]. Some of the associated malignancies arising after the LCH, appear to be therapy-related. Secondary AML may occur 3–8 years after long-standing chemotherapy for LCH, and solid tumors are sometimes seen within the radiation field of patients who received radiation therapy for their LCH, a practice that is significantly less common today. By contrast, LCH and acute lymphoblastic leukemia (ALL), particularly T-cell ALL, are frequently diagnosed close together, with the T-cell ALL as the primary diagnosis, or both diagnoses are made at the same time. This suggests a genetic defect as a causative factor in this association [10].

The late neurological problems may manifest many years after diagnosis, with a cumulative risk at 14 years of 20.4% in Haupt's study, confirming the findings of two large single institution studies which found incidences of PCs, particularly in MS patients, of 71 and 100% respectively, after longer follow up [91, 92]. From the point of view of therapeutic decision-making, most of the serious PC such as endocrine and CNS, occur in patients with MS disease and with lesions involving the facial bones and base of skull. Particular attention needs to be paid to these patients.

Hemophagocytic lymphohistiocytosis (HLH)

HLH is a life-threatening hyperinflammatory disorder resulting in infiltration of macrophages and activated T-cells into several organs, accompanied by significant hemophagocytosis. Without treatment, the uncontrolled inflammatory response may lead to death from multiorgan failure, cerebral dysfunction, or pro-longed neutropenia and associated bacterial or fungal infection

Pathogenesis
HLH is subdivided into primary and secondary forms with the majority of cases being due to secondary (acquired) disease, and an important minority due to familial (hereditary) HLH (FHLH). FHLH is a genetically heterogenous, autosomal recessive disor-der, with mutations described in:
• The perforin gene (FHLH-2)
• The hMunc 13.4 gene (FHLH-3)
• Syntaxin -11 (FHLH-4).
• hMunc 18.2 (FHLH-5) [93, 94].
• Unknown genetic cause. Except in the Turkish population, at least 50% of FHLH is due to as yet unknown mutations[95].
• HLH is also a predominant feature of a number of genetic syndromes such as the X-linked lymphoproliferative syndrome,

Chediak-Higashi, Griscelli type-2, and Hermansky-Pudlak type 2, the latter three having oculo-cutaneous albinism as part of their clinical picture.

All these conditions have in common genetic defects that lead to dysfunction of the perforin/granzyme cytolytic pathway resulting in infiltration of organs by activated lymphocytes and macro-phages and excess production of proinflammatory cytokines which together produce the clinical picture of HLH [96–98]. Failure of trafficking of melanosomes, as well as cytotoxic gran-ules, explains the association of immune dysfunction (HLH) and albinism in the three syndromes mentioned above.

The estimated incidence of FHLH is 1/50 000 live births, but this figure will almost certainly increase as more genetic defects are discovered. The male to female ratio is 1:1. The majority of patients present before the age of 1 year. However, with the descrip-tion of the gene mutations, it has become obvious that some FHLH may present at a much older age than previously suspected.

Congenital hemochromatosis may have a very similar clinical picture to FHLH including massive hyperferritinemia, and the two conditions, requiring very different therapy, may be difficult to distinguish without a liver biopsy.

Secondary HLH occurs as a result of macrophage activation by a known stimulus which can be infectious, malignant, autoim-mune, metabolic diseases, or the hyperlipidemia of total parenteral nutrition [99]. The commonest of the infection associated hemo-phagocytic syndrome (IAHS) is viral -associated(VAHS) due to Epstein-Barr virus (EBV) and other herpes viruses, but bacterial and other infectious causes are also described. At least in children, EBV-HLH appears to occur at a young age with more than 50% being less than 3 years old [99]. EBV and other infections may also trigger the familial form of the disease [100].

Clinical presentation and diagnosis
HLH usually presents with:
• fever which may be prolonged
• hepatosplenomegaly
• bi- or tri-lineage cytopenia
• lymphadenopathy
• neurologic symptoms (may be present)
• skin rash, jaundice and edema (may occur).
   Common laboratory findings include:
• hypertriglyceridemia, hyper- or hypocholesterolemia
• hypofibrinogenemia
• liver dysfunction including increased conjugated bilirubin (histiocytes have tropism for biliary tracts)
• hyperferritinemia which may reach extremely high levels
• increased soluble CD25 levels
• CSF pleocytosis [101].
Low NK cell activity is commonly found and persistence of this finding may suggest FHLH. Up to 20% of FHLH patients may have normal NK function, however, and normal function cannot be used to exclude HLH or a carrier status [102]. Activation of the coagulation and fibrinolytic pathways with resultant hem-orrhagic diathesis and high levels of D-dimers may occur.

Table 11.2 Diagnostic guidelines for hemophagocytic lymphohistocytosis (HLH). Adapted from [101].

---

(1) A molecular diagnosis consistent with HLH

(2) Diagnostic criteria for HLH fulfilled (five of eight criteria below):

Clinical criteria

- Fever
- Splenomegaly

Laboratory criteria

- Cytopenias (affecting ≥ two of three lineages). Hemoglobin <90 g/l. Platelets <100 × 10⁹/l. Neutrophils <1.0 × 10⁹/l. In infants <4 weeks: hemoglobin <100 g/l
- Hypertriglyceridemia and/or hypofibrinogenemia
- Low or absent natural killer-cell activity
- Ferritin ≥ 500 μm/l
- Soluble CD25 ≥ 2400 U/ml

Histopathologic criteria

- Hemophagocytosis in bone marrow or spleen or nodes

(3) On occasion the diagnosis may need to be made on strong suspicion even if not all the criteria are fulfilled!

Histopathologic findings:

• Accumulation of lymphocytes and macrophages.

• Hemophagocytosis may be seen especially in spleen, enlarged lymph nodes, bone marrow, and liver.

However, failure to find hemophagocytosis pathologically, particularly early in the disease, does not exclude HLH, nor does its presence make the diagnosis unless accompanied by other features. Hemophagocytosis is an epiphenomenon [54] and is neither sensitive nor specific for HLH!

The HLH study group of the Histiocyte Society have suggested revised diagnostic criteria for HLH (Table 11.2) [101].

Therapy

Diagnosis of HLH is often delayed and therapy compromised by failure to consider the syndrome. Once the diagnosis is made, a search for an underlying disease as well as evaluation of risk factors are critical.

Low-risk patients generally are older than 2 years of age with a negative family history, lack of severe neutropenia, no or mild disseminated intravascular coagulation (DIC), no CNS disease, absence of EBV and underlying malignancy, and a good response to initial therapy. In this group, therapy of underlying disease and prompt management of cytokine-induced symptoms by corticosteroids and intravenous immunoglobulin (IVIG) may be all that is necessary, but failure of response should result in early addition of other drugs.

For high-risk patients, which includes those with FHLH and severe secondary HLH, including most cases of EBV-HLH [99, 103], appropriate anti-HLH therapy and intensive supportive care should be started early, while the etiology is sought. If an underlying condition is found, specific therapy should be started promptly. However, even when an underlying condition is obvious at onset, specific therapy of the hemophagocytic component may be necessary to prevent a fatal outcome. For high-risk patients, a combination of etoposide, high dose corticosteroids and cyclosporin-A (CSA) with intrathecal therapy, form the basis of the most commonly used front-line protocol HLH-2004, an open study protocol of the Histiocyte Society [100, 101]. CSA has been shown to down-modulate the cytokine storm and appears to be an essential drug in high risk HLH with improved results if given early, particularly in neutropenic patients [98]. Despite concern about secondary leukemia, etoposide too has been shown to be an important drug in high-risk patients. Etoposide suppresses EBV nuclear antigen synthesis [104] and therapy of EBV-HLH should include early use of etoposide in children [98] and adults [100]. Therapy is given for 4–8 weeks except for FHLH patients and those with refractory disease. Intensive supportive care is required for these ill patients.

Experience has shown that patients failing to respond to a standard combination of dexamethasone and etoposide may respond to higher doses of the two drugs, as well as earlier use of CSA. If a patient fails to respond to adequate doses of standard therapy, salvage therapy with the anti-TNF antibody infliximab has been suggested [105]. Other salvage drugs include campath or antithrombin 3 [100]. A successful French protocol uses CSA, dexamethasone and anti-thymocyte globulin (ATG) in place of the etoposide [106], but ATG has not proved to be successful in non-responders to HLH-2004 therapy [107].

Stem cell transplant for hemophagocytic lymphohistiocytosis

It has become clear that despite initial response to therapy, all patients with FHLH will eventually relapse without an allogeneic stem cell transplant (SCT). SCT is therefore indicated for FHLH and XLP, but may also be necessary in refractory secondary HLH{94 287/id}. Experience with the HLH-94 protocol has shown that SCT results are better in patients who respond to initial therapy, and that SCT may be successful irrespective of the donor type[95]. Utilizing these principles, survival has improved from a 1 year survival close to 0% in 1983 to an estimated 3-year probability of survival of 55% at present [95] (Box 11.1).

Conclusion

Despite significant gains in knowledge with regard to the biology of histiocytes, as well as the dramatic improvement in survival in patients with HLH, much remains to be learnt. The high incidence of significant late effects found in patients with MS-LCH and those with chronically reactivating disease, has successfully demolished any tendency to complacency amongst treating physicians. Much work remains to be done and only international cooperation in clinical trials is likely to lead to the improvements required in the outcome of these patients.

Box 11.1 Hemophagocytic lymphohistocytosis (HLH).

- Familial HLH is a rare disease
- Secondary HLH is a syndrome at the severe end of the spectrum of hypercytokinemic responses to any severe underlying condition – it is not rare!
- Secondary HLH needs to be considered in any child presenting with multiorgan failure or acute liver necrosis
- The HLH component of severe secondary HLH needs to be treated separately from the therapy for the underlying disease or the patient may not survive long enough for the primary therapy to work
- HLH needs to be treated early, before irreversible damage occurs
- A high index of suspicion is needed!

References

1 Favara BE, Feller AC, Pauli M, et al. Contemporary classification of histiocytic disorders. The WHO Committee On Histiocytic/Reticulum Cell Proliferations. Reclassification Working Group of the Histiocyte Society. Med Pediatr Oncol 1997; 29: 157–66.

2 Bhatia S, Nesbit ME, Egeler RM, et al. Epidemiologic study of Langerhans cell histiocytosis in children. J Pediatr 1997; 130: 774–84.

3 Bechan GI, Egeler RM, Arceci RJ. Biology of Langerhans cells and Langerhans cell histiocytosis. Internat Review Cytol 2006; 254: 1–43.

4 Jaffe R. The histiocytoses. Clin Lab Med 1999; 19: 135–55.

5 Christie LJ, Evans AT, Bray SE, et al. Lesions resembling Langerhans cell histiocytosis in association with other lymphoproliferative disorders: a reactive or neoplastic phenomenon? Hum Pathol 2006; 37: 32–9.

6 Romani N, Holzmann S, Tripp CH, et al. Langerhans cells-dendritic cells of the epidermis. APMIS 2003; 111: 725–40.

7 Ladisch S, Jaffe ES. Histiocytoses. In Pizzo PA, Poplack DG (Eds), Principles and Practice of Pediatric Oncology. Philadelphia: Lippincott, 2002: 733–50.

8 Steinman RM, Pack M, Inaba K. Dendritic cells in the T-cell areas of lymphoid organs. Immunol Rev 1997; 156: 25–37.

9 Gunn MD, Tangemann K, Tam C, et al. A chemokine expressed in lymphoid high endothelial venules promotes the adhesion and chemotaxis of naïve T lymphocytes. Proc Natl Acad Sci 1998; 95: 258–63.

10 Beverley PC, Egeler RM, Arceci RJ, et al. The Nikolas Symposia and histiocytosis. Nat Rev Cancer 2005; 5: 488–94.

11 Egeler RM, de Kraker J, Voute PA. Cytosine-arabinoside, vincristine, and prednisolone in the treatment of children with disseminated Langerhans Cell Histiocytosis with organ dysfunction: experience at a single institution. Med Pediatr Oncol 1993; 21: 265–70.

12 Geissmann F, Lepelletier Y, Fraitag S et al Differentiation of Langerhans cells in Langerhans cell histiocytosis. Blood. 2001; 97: 1241–8.

13 Aricò M, Scappaticci S, Danesino C. The genetics of Langerhans cell histiocytosis. In Weitzman S, Egeler RM (Eds), Histiocytic Disorders of Infants and Children. Cambridge: Cambridge University Press, 2005: 83–94.

14 Karis J, Bernstrand C, Fadeel B, et al.. The incidence of Langerhans Cell Histiocytosis in children in Stockholm Count, Sweden 1992–2001. Proc of the XIX meeting of the Histiocyte Society, Philadelphia, 2003: 21.

15 Huang F, Arceci R. The histiocytoses of infancy. Semin Perinatol 1999; 23: 319–31.

16 Stuurman KE, Lau L, Doda W, et al. Evaluation of the natural history and long term complications of patients with Langerhans cell histiocytosis of bone. Proc of the XIX meeting of the Histiocyte Society, Philadelphia. 2003: 55.

17 Tazi A, Hiltermann TJN, Vassallo R. Adult lung histiocytosis. In Weitzman S, Egeler RM (Eds), Histiocytic Disorders of Infants and Children. Cambridge: Cambridge University Press, 2005: 187–207.

18 Titgemeyer C, Grois N, Minkov M, et al. Pattern and course of single-system disease in Langerhans cell histiocytosis. Data from the DAL-HX 83- and 90 study. Med Pediatr Oncol 2001; 37: 108–14.

19 Ghanem I, Tolo VT, D'Ambra P, et al. Langerhans cell histiocytosis of bone in children and adolescents. J Pediatr Orthop 2003; 23: 124–30.

20 Aricò M, Egeler RM. Clinical aspects of Langerhans Cell histiocytosis. Hematol/Oncol Clin N Am 1998; 12: 247–58.

21 Koch B. Langerhans cell histiocytosis of temporal bone: role of magnetic resonance imaging. Topics Magn Reson Imaging 2000; 11: 66–74.

22 Fernández-Latorre F, Menor-Serrano F, Alonso-Charterina S, et al. Langerhans' cell histiocytosis of the temporal bone in pediatric patients. Am J Roentg 2000; 174: 217–21.

23 Kamimura M, Kinoshita T, Itoh H, et al. Eosinophilic granuloma of the spine: early spontaneous disappearance of tumor detected on magnetic resonance imaging. J Neurosurg 2000; 932(suppl): 312–16.

24 Dautenheimer L, Blaser SI, Weitzman S, et al. Infantile myofibromatosis as a cause of vertebra plana. Am J Neuroradiol 1995; 164(Suppl): 828–30.

25 Yeom JS, Lee CK, Shin HY, et al. Langerhans cell histiocytosis of the spine. Analysis of 23 cases. Spine 1999; 24: 1740–9.

26 Ruppert D, Oria RA, Kumar R, et al. Radiologic features of eosinophilic granuloma of bone. Am J Roentgenol 1989; 153: 1021–6.

27 Meyer JS, Harty MP, Mabboubi S, et al. Langerhans cell histiocytosis: presentation and evolution of radiologic findings with clinical correlation. Radiographics 1995; 15: 1135–46.

28 Potepan P, Tesoro-Tess JD, Laffranchi A, et al. Langerhans cell histiocytosis mimicking malignancy: a radiologic appraisal. Tumori 1996; 82: 603–9.

29 Fisher AJ, Reinus WR, Friedland JA, et al. Quantitative analysis of the plain radiographic appearance of eosinophilic granuloma. Invest Radiol 1995; 8: 466–73.

30 Binkovitz LA, Olshefski RS, Adler BH. Coincidence FDG-PET in the evaluation of Langerhans cell histocytosis: preliminary findings. Pediatr Radiol 2003; 33: 598–602.

31 Howarth DM, Gilchrist GS, Mullan BP, et al. Langerhans cell histiocytosis. Diagnosis, natural history, management and outcome. Cancer 1999; 8: 2278–90.

32 Nanduri V, Titgemeyer C, Brock P. Long term outcome of orbital involvement in Langerhans cell histiocytosis. Proc of the XVII meeting of the Histiocyte Society, Stresa, 2001: 176.

33 Grois N, Prosch H, Lassmann H, et al. Central nervous system disease in Langerhans cell histiocytosis. In Weitzman S, Egeler RM (Eds), Histiocytic Disorders of Infants and Children. Cambridge: Cambridge University Press, 2005: 208–28.

34 Egeler RM, Thompson RC, Voûte PA, et al. Intralesional infiltration of corticosteroids in localized Langerhans cell histiocytosis. J Pediatr Orthop 1992; 12: 811–4.

35 Yasco AW, Fanning CV, Ayala AG, et al. Percutaneous techniques for the diagnosis and treatment of localized Langerhans cell histiocytosis (eosinophilic granuloma of bone). J Bone Joint Surg 1998; 80: 219–28.

36 Ladisch S, Gadner H, Aricó M, et al. A randomized trial of etoposide vs vinblastine in disseminated Langerhans cell histiocytosis. Med Pediatr Oncol 1994; 23: 107–10.

37 Arceci RJ, Brenner MK, Pritchard J. Controversies and new approaches to treatment of LCH. Hematol/Oncol Clin N Am 1998; 12: 339–57.

38 Munn SE, Olliver L, Broadbent V, et al. Use of indomethacin in Langerhans cell histiocytosis. Med Pediatr Oncol 1999; 32: 247–9.

39 Kamizono J, Okada Y, Shirahata A, Tanaka Y. Bisphosphonate induces remission of refractory osteolysis in Langerhans cell histiocytosis. J Bone Miner Res 2002; 17: 1926–8.

40 Farran RP, Zaretski E, Egeler RM Treatment of Langerhans cell histiocytosis with Pamidronate. J Pediatr Hematol/Oncol 2001; 23: 54–6.

41 Brown RE. Bisphosphonates as antialveolar macrophage therapy in pulmonary Langerhans cell histiocytosis. Med Pediatr Oncol 2001; 36: 641–3.

42 Munn S, Chu AC. Langerhans cell histiocytosis of the skin. Hematol/Oncol Clin N Am 1998; 12: 269–86.

43 Malpas JS. Langerhans cell histiocytosis in adults. Hematol/Oncol Clin N Am 1998; 12: 259–68.

44 Hashimoto K, Pritzker MS. Electronic study of retuiculo-histiocytoma: an unusual case of congential self healing reticulohistiocytosis. Arch Dermatol 1973; 107: 263–270.

45 Lau L, Krafchik B, Trebo M, et al. Cutaneous Langerhans cell histiocytosis in children under one year. Pediatr Blood Cancer 2006; 46: 66–71.

46 Esterly NB, Maurer HS, Gonzalez-Crussi F. Histiocytosis-X: a seven-year experience at a children's hospital. J Am Acad Dermatol 1985; 13: 481–96.

47 Longaker MA, Frieden IJ, Le Boit PT, et al. Congenital 'self-healing' Langerhans cell histiocytosis: the need for long term follow-up. J Am Acad Dermatol 1994; 31: 910–16.

48 Sakai H, Ibe M, Takahashi H, et al. Satisfactory remission achieved by PUVA therapy in Langerhans cell histiocytosis in an elderly patient. J Dermatol 1996; 23: 42–6.

49 Kwon OS, Cho KH, Song KY. Primary cutaneous Langerhans cell histiocytosis treated with photochemotherapy. J Dermatol 1997; 24: 54–6.

50 Gerlach B, Stein A, Fischer R, et al. Langerhans cell histiocytosis in the elderly. Hautarzt 1998; 49: 23–30.

51 Hoeger PH, Nanduri VR, Harper JL, et al. Long term follow up of topical mustine treatment for cutaneous langerhans cell histiocytosis. Arch Dis Child 2000; 82: 483–7.

52 Lair G, Marie I, Cailleux N, et al. Langerhans cell histiocytosis in adults: cutaneous and mucous lesion regression after treatment with thalidomiide. Rev Med Intern 1998; 19: 196–8.

53 Claudon A, Dietamann JL, Hamman De Compte A, et al. Interest in thalidomide in cutaneo-mucous and hypothalamo-hypophyseal involvement of Langerhans cell histiocytosis. Rev Med Interne 2002; 23: 651–6.

54 Helmbold P, Hegemann B, Holzhausen H-J, et al. Low dose oral etoposide monotherapy in adult Langerhans cell histiocytosis. Arch Dermatol 1998; 134: 1275–8.

55 Jaffe R The diagnostc histopathology of Langerhans cell histiocytosis. In Weitzman S, Egeler RM (Eds), Histiocytic Disorders of Infants and Children. Cambridge: Cambridge University Press, 2005: 14–39.

56 Bernstrand C, Cederlund K, Åhstrom L, et al. Smoking preceded pulmonary involvement in adults with Langerhans cell histiocytosis diagnosed in childhood. Acta Paediatr 2000; 89: 1389–92.

57 Choi SW, Bangaru BS, Wu CD, et al. Gastrointestinal involvement in disseminated Langerhans cell histiocytosis [LCH] with durable complete response to 2-chlorodeoxyadenosine and high-dose cytarabine. J Pediatr Hematol Oncol 2003; 25: 503–6.

58 Maghnie M, Cosi G, Genovese E, et al. Central Diabetes Insipidus in children and young adults. New Engl J Med 2000; 343: 998–1007.

59 Maghnie M, Bossi G, Klersy C, et al. Dynamic endocrine testing and magnetic resonance imaging in the long term follow-up of childhood Langerhans cell histiocytosis. J Clin Endocr Metab 1998; 83: 3089–94.

60 Municchi G, Marconcini S, D'Ambrosio A, et al. Central precocious puberty in multisytem Langerhans cell histiocytosis: a case report. Pediatr Hematol Oncol 2002; 19: 273–8.

61 Kaltsas GA, Powles TB, Fvanson J, et al. Hypothalamo-pituitary abnormalities in adult patients with Langerhans cell histiocytosis: clinical, endocrinological and radiological features and response to treatment. J Clin Endocr Metab 2000; 85: 1370–6.

62 Anon. A multicentre retrospective survey of LCH: 348 cases observed between 1983 and 1993. The French LCH Study Group. Arch Dis Child 1996; 75: 17–24.

63 Chong VF. Langerhans cell histiocytosis with thyroid involvement. Eur J Radiol 1996; 22: 155–7.

64 Ottaviano F, Finlay JL. Diabetes insipidus and Langerhans cell histiocytosis: a case report of reversibility with 2-Chlorodeoxyadenosine. J Pediatr Hematol/Oncol 2003; 25: 575–7.

65 Abla O, Weitzman S, Grois N, et al. Diabetes insipidus in Langerhans cell histiocytosis: when is treatment indicated? Pediatr Blood Cancer 2009; 52: 555–6.

66 Rosenzweig KE, Arceci R, Tarbell NJ. Diabetes insipidus secondary to Langerhans' cell histiocytosis: is radiation therapy indicated? Med Pediatr Oncol 1997; 29: 36–40.

67 Watts J, Files B. Langerhans cell histiocytosis: central nervous sytem involvement treated successfully with 2-chlorodeoxyadenosine. Pediatr Hematol Oncol 2001; 18: 199–204.

68 Giona F, Annino L, Bongarzoni V, et al. Unifocal Langerhans' cell histiocytosis involving the central nervous system successfully treated with 2-chlorodeoxyadenosine. Med Pediatr Oncol 2002; 38: 223.

69 Allen CE, Flores R, Rauch R, et al. Neurodegenerative central nervous system Langerhans cell histiocytosis and coincident hydrocephalus treated with vincristine/cytosine arabinoside. Pediatr Blood Cancer 2010; 54: 416–23.

70 Gadner H, Grois N, Arico M, et al. A randomized trial of treatment for multisystem Langerhans' cell histiocytosis. J Pediatr 2001; 138: 728–34.

71 McLelland J, Broadbent V, Yeomans E, et al. Langerhans cell histiocytosis: the case for conservative therapy. Arch Dis Child 1990; 65: 301–3.

72 Minkov M, Grois N, Heitger A, et al. Response to initial treatment of multisystem Langerhans cell histiocytosis: an important prognostic indicator. Med Pediatr Oncol 2002; 39: 581–5.

73 Morimoto A, Ikushima S, Kinugawa N, et al. Improved outcome in the treatment of pediatric multifocal Langerhans Cell Histiocytosis. results from the Japan Langerhans cell histiocytosis study group-96 protocol. Cancer 2006; 107: 613–19.

74 Bernard F, Thomas C, Bertrand Y, et al. Multicentre pilot study of 2-chlorodeoxyadenosine and cytosine-arabinoside combined chemotherapy in refractory Langerhans cell histiocytosis with haematological dysfunction. Eur J Cancer 2005; 41: 2682–9.

75 Saven A, Foon K, Piro L. 2-chlorodeoxyadenosine induced complete remissions in Langerhans cell histiocytosis. Ann Intern Med 1994; 21: 430–2.

76 Weitzman S, Arceci R, Braier J, et al. 2′;-Chlorodeoxyadenosine (2-CdA) as salvage therapy for Langerhans cell histiocytosis (LCH). Results of the LCH-S-98 protocol of the Histiocyte Society. Pediatr Blood Cancer 2009; 53: 1271–6.

77 Gandhi V, Estey E, Keating MJ, et al. Chlorodeoxyadenosine and arabinosylcytosine in patients with acute myelogenous leukemia: pharmacokinetic, pharmacodynamic and molecular interactions. Blood 1996; 87: 256–64.

78 Weitzman S, McClain K, Arceci R. Treatment of relapsed and/or refractory Langerhans cell histiocytosis. In Weitzman S, Egeler RM (Eds), Histiocytic Disorders of Infants and Children. Cambridge: Cambridge University Press, 2005: 254–71.

79 Kelly M, Kolb M, Bonniaud, et al. Re-evaluation of fibrogenic cytokines in lung fibrosis. Current Pharm Design 2003; 9: 39–49.

80 Egeler RM, Favara BE, van Meurs M, et al. Differential in situ cytokine profiles of Langerhans-like cells and T cells in Langerhans cell histiocytosis: abundant expression of cytokines relevant to disease and treament. Blood 1999; 94: 4195–201.

81 Braier J, Cioccca M, Latella A, et al. Cholestasis, sclerosing cholangitis, and liver transplantation in Langerhans cell histiocytosis. Med Pediatr Oncol 2002; 38: 178–82.

82 Marti L, Thomas C, Emilé JF, et al. Liver involvement in LCH. The French experience. Proc of the XIX meeting of the Histiocyte Society, Philadelphia, 2003: 20.

83 Sundar KM, Gosselin MV, Chung HL, et al. Pulmonary Langerhans cell histiocytosis. Emerging concepts in pathobiology, radiology, and clinical evolution of disease. Chest 2003; 123: 1673–83.

84 Debray D Sclerosing cholangitis in children: an overview. Proc of the XIX meeting of the Histiocyte Society, Philadelphia, 2003: 17.

85 Rajwal SR, Stringer MD, Davison SM, et al. Use of Basiliximab in pediatric liver transplantation for Langerhans cell histiocytosis. Pediatr Transplant 2003; 7: 247–51.

86 Hadzic N, Pritchard J, Webb D, et al. Recurrence of Langerhans cell histiocytosis in the graft after pediatric liver transplantation. Transplantation 2000; 15: 815–19.

87 Etienne B, Bertocchi M, Gamondes J-P, et al. Relapsing pulmonary Langerhans cell histiocytosis after lung transplantation. Am J Resp Crit Care Med 1998; 157: 288–91.

88 Stieber AC, Sever C, Starzl TE. Liver transplantation in patients with Langerhans' cell histiocytosis. Transplantation 1990; 50: 338–40.

89 Newell KA, Alonso EM, Kelly SM, et al. Association between liver transplantation for Langerhans cell histiocytosis, rejection and development of posttransplantation lymphoproliferative disease in children. J Pediatr 1997; 131: 98–104.

90 Haupt R, Nanduri V, Egeler RM Late effects of Langerhans cell histiocytosis and its association with malignancy. In Weitzman S, Egeler RM (Eds), Histiocytic Disorders of Infants and Children. Cambridge: Cambridge University Press, 2005: 272–92.

91 Willis B, Ablin A, Weinberg V, et al. Disease course and late sequelae of Langerhans' cell histiocytosis: a 25 year experience at the University of Southern California, San Francisco. J Clin Oncol 1996; 14: 2073–82.

92 Nanduri VR, Barelle P, Pritchard J, et al. Growth and endocrine disorders in multisystem Langerhans cell histiocytosis. Clin Endocrinol 2000; 53: 509–15.

93 zur Stadt U, Rohr J, Seifert W, et al. Familial hemophagocytic lymphohistiocytosis type 5 (FHL-5) is caused by mutations in Munc18-2 and impaired binding to syntaxin 11. Am J Human Genet 2009; 85: 482–92.

94 Côte M, Ménager MM, Burgess A, et al. Munc18-2 deficiency causes familial hemophagocytic lymphohistiocytosis type 5 and impairs cytotoxic granule exocytosis in patient NK cells J Clin Invest 2009 (Epub ahead of print).

95 Zur Stadt U, Beutel K, Kolberg S, et al. Mutation spectrum in children with primary hemophagocytic lymphohistiocytosis: molecular and functional analyses of PRF1, UNC13D, STX11, and RAB27A. Human Mutation 2006; 27: 62–8.

96 HenterJ-I, Andersson B, Elinder G, et al. Elevated circulating levels of interleukin-1 receptor antagonists but not IL-1 agonists in hemophagocytic lymphohistiocytosis. Med Pediatr Oncol 1996; 27: 21–5.

97 Osugi Y, Hara J, Tagawa S, et al. Cytokine production regulating Th-1 and Th-2 cytokines in hemophagocytic lymphohistiocytosis. Blood 1997; 89: 4100–3.

98 Imashuku S, Teramura T, Morimoto A, et al. Recent developments in the management of haemophagocytic lymphohistiocytosis. Expert Opin Pharmacother 2001b; 2: 1437–48.

99 Janke G, Imashuku S, Elinder G, et al. Infection- and malignancy-associated hemophagocytic syndromes: secondary hemophagocytic lymphohistiocytosis. Hematol/Oncol Clinics N Am 1998; 12: 435–44.

100 Imashuku S, Kuriyama K, Sakai R, et al. Treatment of Epstein-Barr Virus-associated hemophagocytic lymphohistiocytosis EBV-HLH in young adults: a report from the HLH-study center. Med Pediatr Oncol 2003; 41: 103–9.

101 Henter J-I, Horne AC, Aricó M, et al. HLH-2004: diagnostic and therapeutic guidelines for hemophagocytic lymphohistiocytosis. Pediatr Blood Cancer 2007; 48: 124–31.

102 Ueda I, Ishii E, Morimoto A, et al. correlation between phenotypic heterogeneity and gene mutational characteristics in familial hemophagocytic lymphohistiocytosis FHL. Pediatr Blood Cancer 2006; 46: 482–8.

103 Imashuku S, Kuriyama K, Teramura T, et al. Requirement for etoposide in the treatment of Epstein-Barr virus-associated hemophagocytic lymphohistiocytosis. J Clin Oncol 2001a; 19: 2665–73.

104 Kikuta H, Sakiyama Y. Etoposide VP16; inhibits Epstein-Barr virus determined nuclear antigen EBNA; synthesis. Br J Haematol 1995; 90: 971–3.

105 Henzan T, Nagafuji K, Tsukamoto H, et al. Success with infliximab in treating refractory hemophagocytic lymphohistiocytosis. Am J Hematol 2006; 81: 59–61.

106 Mahlaoui N, Ouachée-Chardin M, de Saint Basile G, et al. Immunotherapy of familial hemophagocytic lymphohistiocytosis with antithymocyte globulins: a single-center retrospective report of 38 patients. Pediatrics 2007; 120: e622–8.

107 Filipovich AH, Imashuku S, Henter JI, Sullivan KE. Healing hemophagocytosis. Clin Immunol 2005; 117: 121–4.

III   Solid Tumors of Childhood

12 Neuroblastoma

Sucheta J. Vaidya[1] and Andrew D. J. Pearson[2]

[1] Royal Marsden Hospital, Sutton, Surrey and [2] The Institute of Cancer Research & Royal Marsden Hospital, Sutton, Surrey, UK

Introduction

The neuroblastic tumors include neuroblastoma, ganglioneuroblastoma, and ganglioneuroma. These tumors are derived from the sympathetic nervous system and demonstrate a vast clinical spectrum from benign tumors, spontaneous regression, to extremely malignant behaviour. The German pathologist R.L.K. Virchow first described the histological appearance in 1864. J.H. Wright in 1910 used the term 'neuroblastoma'. He indicated that the migration of primitive nerve cells during embryogenesis explained the development of tumors of similar appearance in numerous sites within the body. The first patients of regressing disease were probably described in 1901 by W. Pepper as 'congenital sarcoma of the liver and suprarenal'. In 1907, R. Hutchison recorded older patients with 'sarcoma' of adrenal gland and metastases to the skull thereby describing the first patient with stage 4 disease. The three key features of neuroblastoma are:
- The capacity to undergo regression.
- The capacity to undergo maturation from undifferentiated neuroblastoma to ganglioneuroma mature.
- A superior prognosis for babies.

Epidemiology

- Neuroblastoma is the commonest extra-cranial solid tumor in children.
- Accounts for 8–10% of childhood cancers.
- Tumors arise from the sympathetic nervous tissue along the sympathetic chain or in other sympathetic ganglia.
- Annual incidence in UK is 9/million children under the age of 15 years [1] and incidence is fairly uniform throughout the developed world.
- Male: female ratio 1.2 : 1.
- Most common cancer of infancy.
- Median age of presentation is 18 months.

Pediatric Hematology and Oncology, 1st edition. Edited by Edward J. Estlin, Richard J. Gilbertson, and Robert F. Wynn. © 2010 Blackwell Publishing Ltd.

Clinical features

Symptoms
Symptoms from neuroblastoma may be non-specific and mimic many childhood illnesses. Symptoms may be attributed to:
- Site of primary tumor.
- Local infiltration.
- Sites of metastatic disease.
- Metabolic disturbances.

Sites of primary tumors and local infiltration
- Primary tumor is found in the abdomen in 60% cases (adrenal gland 32%), thorax (14%), pelvic region (6%), cervical (2%), and other areas in 18% patients [2].
- Tumors in the upper cervical and thoracic area can cause Horner's syndrome (unilateral ptosis, miosis, enophthalmos, and anhydrosis).
- Thoracic tumors can cause cough, dysphagia, breathlessness, thoracic inlet obstruction leading to superior vena caval syndrome.
- Abdominal tumors could present with abdominal pain, discomfort, fullness or rarely obstruction.
- Pelvic tumor could cause mechanical bladder or bowel obstruction.
- Some tumors have intra-spinal and extra-spinal components (dumb-bell tumors). Intra-spinal tumors can lead to cord compression causing flaccid paralysis and urinary and bowel disturbances.
- In 1% of patients, the primary tumor cannot be found, even with thorough investigations.

Metastatic tumors
- Common sites of metastases are lymph nodes, liver, skin, bone, and bone marrow. Brain involvement can be by direct extension of skull metastasis, but meningeal and parenchymal involvements are also seen. Lung metastasis is very rare [3].
- Infants may present with rapidly enlarging liver, sometimes accompanied with bluish, non-tender subcutaneous skin nodules and bone marrow involvement. Liver involvement can cause abdominal distension and respiratory compromise.

- Symptoms due to metastases in older children include bone pain, frequently manifesting as a limp and irritability. Signs and symptoms can sometimes mimic those of leukemia, consisting of anemia and mucosal or skin hemorrhage due to pancytopenia caused by bone marrow infiltration.
- Common sites of bone metastases include orbits, jaw, skull, and long bones.
- Metastases to orbit can produce unilateral or bilateral periorbital ecchymosis and proptosis (Racoon eye). This is due to retro bulbar and orbital infiltration by tumor.
- The pattern of metastases is changing with aggressive treatment strategies.

Paraneoplastic syndromes
- Opsoclonus–myoclonus syndrome or dancing eye syndrome consists of opsoclonus (rapid multi-directional conjugate eye movements), a movement disorder characterized by a jerky (sometimes myoclonic) ataxia and behavioural change consisting of irritability usually with sleep disturbance. This occurs in about 3% of patients with neuroblastoma.
- The high level of catecholamines and sometimes vasoactive intestinal peptides (VIP) produced by neuroblastoma cells can cause flushing, pallor, sweating, watery diarrhoea, and hypertension.
- Approximately 10% of patients with neuroblastoma present with hypertension [4]. This can result from either secretion of catecholamines or from effects on the renal artery and stimulation of the renin-angiotensin system.

Investigations

Plain radiographs
Plain radiographs may incidentally detect tumors in the chest or abdomen. The mass can have specks of calcification (Figure 12.1).

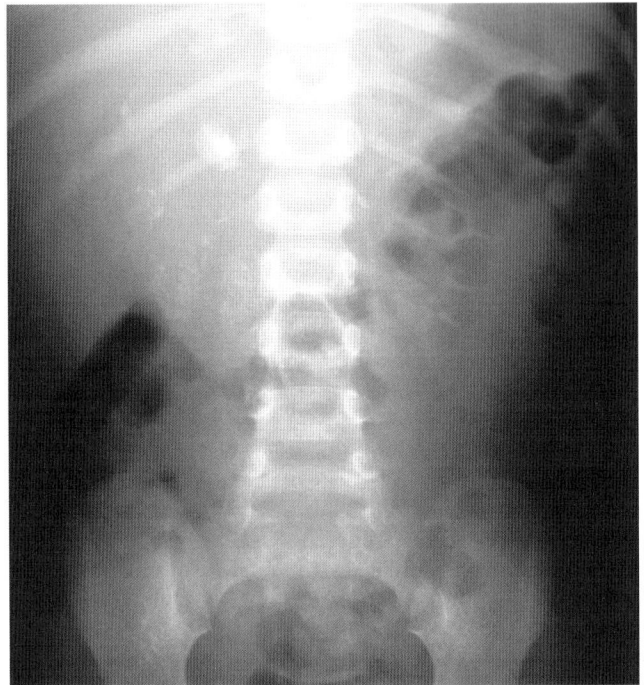

Figure 12.1 Plain X-ray showing a mass with calcification.

Eroded ribs and enlargement of intervertebral foramina can be found in cases of intra-spinal extensions.

Ultrasonography
Most tumors appear as a heterogeneous mass that may contain anechoic areas due to necrosis or hemorrhage. Direct invasion of the liver is suggested when there is a lack of movement between the tumor and liver during normal respiration.

Computerized tomography (CT) [5]
On CT, neuroblastoma often appears as a large, heterogeneous, lobulated mass that shows little or no contrast enhancement. Coarse, finely stippled, or curvilinear calcifications are seen in about 85% of tumors (Figure 12.2). Central, low-attenuation areas may be due to hemorrhage or necrosis. Encasing major blood vessels, including renal hilar vessels, the aorta, superior mesenteric artery, coeliac artery, and inferior vena cava, is a characteristic feature of neuroblastoma. The ipsilateral kidney is usually displaced by the primary tumor, and its identification helps in differentiation from Wilms' tumor. CT scan helps to confirm the site, size, extension, relation to internal organs and important vessels. It is often difficult to distinguish between primary tumor and contiguous lymphadenopathy by any imaging modality. Hepatic metastasis appear hypodense on CT and present classically as either diffuse involvement in regressing disease in infants or as focal, nodular deposits in metastatic disease in older patients. CT is the major imaging modality pre-

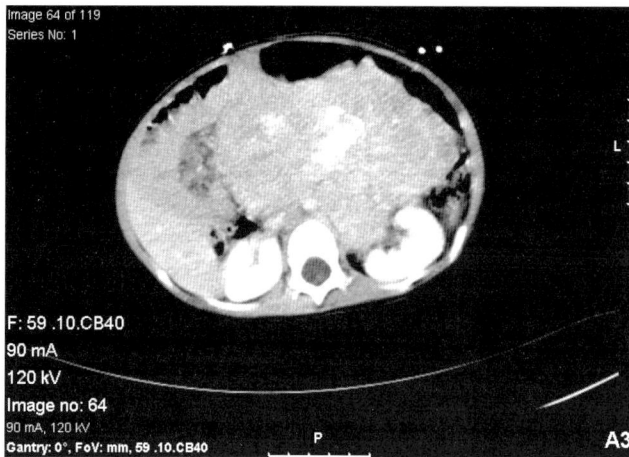

Figure 12.2 CT scan of abdomen showing a suprarenal mass with calcification.

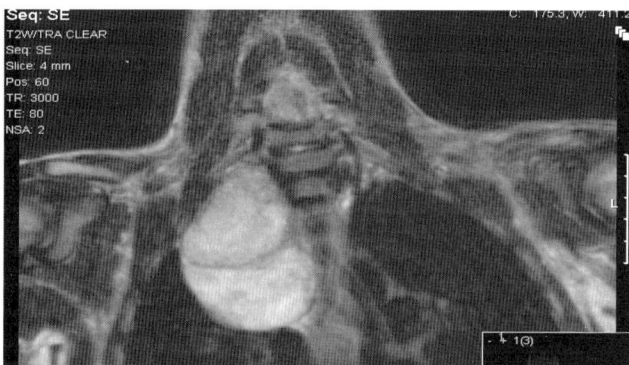

Figure 12.3 T2-weighted MRI scan showing a paravertebral ganglioneuroma.

surgery to demonstrate the relationship between tumor and blood vessels.

Magnetic resonance imaging (MRI)

On MRI, the primary and metastatic neuroblastoma show low T1- and high T2-weighted signal intensity, with little or no contrast enhancement. An MRI scan is extremely important to evaluate intraspinal extension of tumor (Figure 12.3). When this is suspected, detailed cranial and spinal MRI must be performed to assess for compression of the spinal cord and to exclude leptomeningeal spread. Bone marrow disease is seen either as diffuse infiltration or as focal disease with MRI signal characteristics similar to the primary tumor. Because lung metastases are rare, MRI has been proposed as superior to CT because it demonstrates bone and bone marrow abnormality, liver involvement, and intra-spinal tumor to a greater advantage. An important additional benefit of MRI is the lack of ionizing radiation and need for oral contrast. Whole-body MRI shows promise as an alternative to scintigraphy for the assessment of bone and bone marrow disease and is currently being investigated [6].

Nuclear magnetic investigations
Meta-iodo benzyl guanidine (MIBG) scan

MIBG can be labelled with ^{131}I or [123]I. This is specifically taken up by neural crest tumors by an active uptake mechanism at the cell membrane. Superior imaging quality and more positive lesions were observed with the ^{123}I when compared with[131]I [7]. Therefore ^{123}I is used for diagnostic purposes and is helpful in the diagnosis and staging. MIBG scan may help in identifying the primary when it is deemed to be occult by other standard radiological techniques. Other neural crest tumors such as pheochromocytoma, ganglioneuroma, paraganglioma, retinoblastoma and medullary thyroid carcinoma also take up MIBG. The sensitivity of MIBG scintigraphy is about 90% [8]. Once tumor MIBG avidity is documented, this is the preferred method for follow-up (Figures 12.4 and 12.5).

[99m]Technetium methylene diphosphonate bone scintigraphy (bone scan)

Approximately 10% of neuroblastomas fail to take up MIBG. Bone scan is important in these patients to assess cortical bone involvement. One major disadvantage of the use of the bone scan for assessing response to therapy is that abnormalities may persist (due to bone recovery) despite eradication of the tumor.

FDG-PET scan

The role of the PET scan has been evaluated in neuroblastoma. PET scan was equal or superior to MIBG scan in detecting soft tissue and extracranial disease. However the high FDG uptake by the brain failed to identify cranial vault lesions [9].

Tumor markers (Box 12.2)

Catecholamines

The first case of adrenaline-secreting neuroblastoma was described in 1957 [10]. It is now well documented that neuroblastoma cells secrete large amounts of one or more catecholamines (adrenaline, noradrenaline) or their metabolites (vanillylmandelic acid [VMA], homovanillic acid [HVA], dopamine). A random sample of urine is sufficient to detect these metabolites [11] and results are presented as ratios to creatinine. About 10% of patients do not secrete catecholamines. HVA and VMA are widely used for diagnosis, follow up, as well as for early detection in screening programmes. A recent study investigated the levels of urinary catecholamines in correlation to stages, biological features, and prognosis in 114 neuroblastoma patients. In 91% patients at least one of the three (VMA, HVA, dopamine) parameters was above normal. High VMA levels were associated with favourable biological features; high dopamine levels were predominantly found in biologically unfavourable disease. Patients with normal HVA levels had a significantly better outcome. The other parameters showed no significant association with prognosis. For

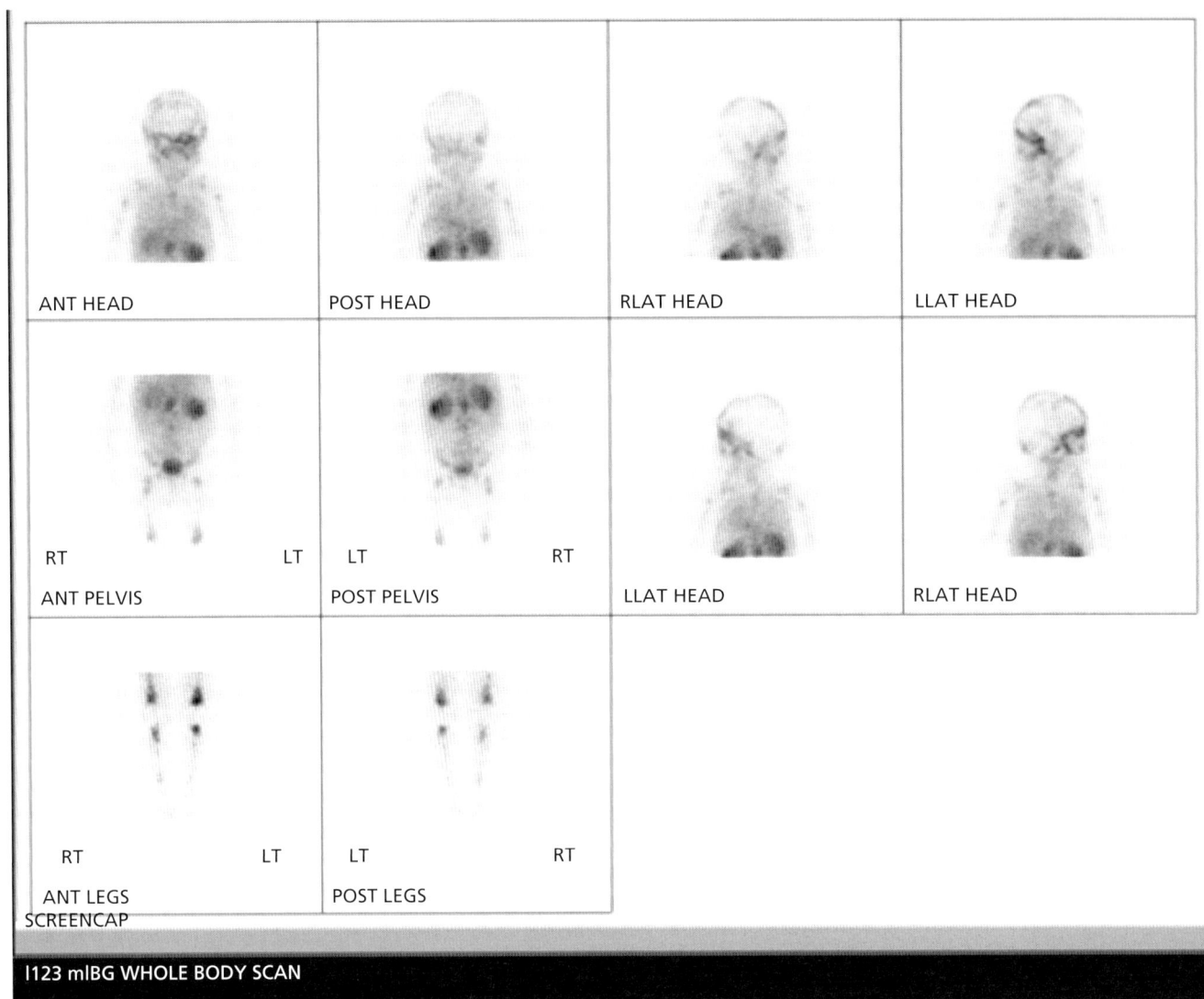

Figure 12.4 Whole body ^{123}I-MIBG planar imaging showing a MIBG-avid primary abdominal tumor mass, widespread metastatic skeletal uptake and also right orbital disease involvement, consistent with stage IV disease.

Box 12.2 Neuroblastoma key facts – tumor markers.

• Although tumor markers have prognostic value, none are currently included in risk group classification.
• The value of markers in monitoring response is minimal; the most useful is urinary catecholamine.
• Serum markers have no real value.

---

disseminated neuroblastoma of infancy, dopamine/VMA ratio proved to be helpful for the discrimination of stage 4 versus stage 4s, with the ratio being higher for patients with stage 4 disease [12].

Serum markers
Ferritin

Ferritin is a major tissue-binding protein. Raised ferritin in children with neuroblastoma results from direct secretion of ferritin by the tumor [13]. In a study, serum ferritin was studied in 241 patients with neuroblastoma. Serum ferritin was infrequently elevated in sera from patients with low stage disease but was elevated in the majority with high stage neuroblastoma. High levels of ferritin related to poor survival [14, 15]. In some recent studies, as patient survival has improved with more effective therapy, serum ferritin has lost its prognostic significance [16]. However, the International Neuroblastoma Risk Group (INRG) recently analysed the prognostic markers in 1483 stage 3 neuroblastoma patients. In patients over the age of 18 months, serum ferritin was an independent adverse prognostic factor on multi-

Common sites of metastases

Primary tumor sites

skull

lymph nodes

cervical 2%

thorax 14%

Liver

abdomen 60%

Bone marrow

adrenal 32%

pelvis 6%

Bones

Pediatric Oncology

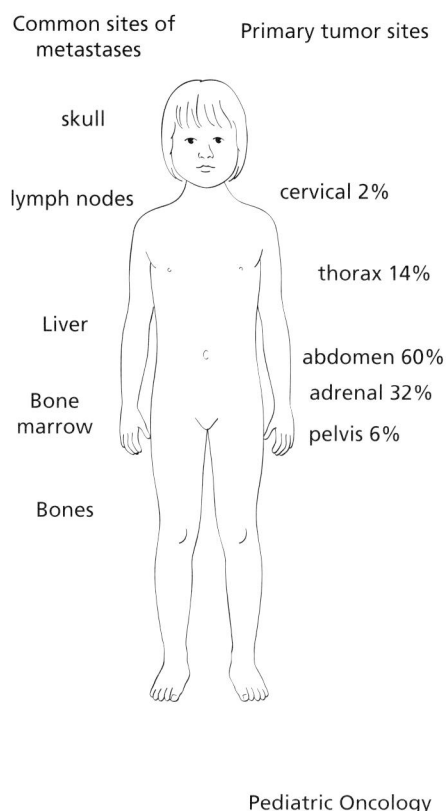

Figure 12.5 Sites of primary tumor and metastases.

variate analysis [17]. Also, in the cohort of patients ≥18 months with metastatic disease, serum ferritin (<vs ≥92 ng/ml) was shown to be prognostic by the event-free survival tree regression [18].

Lactic dehydrogenase (LDH)

LDH is an enzyme that catalyzes the reversible conversion of pyruvate to lactase. LDH was observed to be increased in 77–83% patients with newly diagnosed neuroblastoma [19, 20]. Absolute LDH levels correlate with prognosis with increased levels being more common in advanced disease as LDH levels correlate with rapid cell turn over. In 1992, in a large study, LDH was found to be an important prognostic marker [21].

Neuron specific enolase (NSE)

Enolases are glycolytic enzymes that convert 2-phosphoglycerate to phosphoenolpyruvate. There are three immunologically distinct subunits: alpha, beta, and gamma. Gamma enolase is found in neuron and called NSE. In children, although high serum NSE levels are suggestive of neuroblastoma, increased levels have been reported in other malignancies such as Wilms' tumor, Ewing's sarcoma, non-Hodgkin's lymphoma, acute leukemia and other diseases [22]. NSE is therefore not a specific marker and can also be raised following some non-malignant conditions, e.g. brain damage. Generally in stage 1 and stage 2 diseases, abnormal NSE levels are reported in less than 20% of cases. But in stage 3 and 4 diseases increased NSE levels are found in 80–95% cases [23]. In

general, a low level predicts a good prognosis and a high level a poor outcome, this being mainly due to the fact that children with advanced disease present with high serum NSE levels [24].

Gangliosides

Gangliosides are glycosphyngolipids, mainly present in the cell surface membrane. These membrane-bound glycolipids are released by a variety of cells, particularly tumor cells. Gangliosides are present in both tumors and the plasma of most children with neuroblastoma. In a study, the ganglioside composition of neuroblastoma samples from 53 patients was determined. Differences in ganglioside patterns were observed, with neuroblastoma from patients who were either disease positive or dead of disease tending to have more monosialogangliosides and fewer gangliotetraose gangliosides of the B series (GT1b) than tumors from patients who were disease-free. More specifically, six of the seven patients lacking GT1b died of disease, suggesting that the absence of GT1b is indicative of a poor prognosis [25]. Also, thoracic neuroblastoma patients who generally have good prognosis had higher levels of GT1b [26]. Circulating tumor-derived GD2 correlates inversely with prognosis. Randomized studies are evaluating the role of GD2 monoclonal antibodies on minimal residual disease.

Neuroblastoma staging

The first staging system for neuroblastoma was proposed by Evans et al. [27] in 1971 and used by the Children's Cancer Group (CCG) in the USA. The staging was based on involvement of lymph nodes and spread across the midline. Stage IV-S (special category) was described as a neuroblastoma which would be otherwise stage I or II but with remote disease confined to liver, skin, or bone marrow (minimal) without radiological evidence of bone metastases on skeletal survey. These tumors have a propensity for spontaneous regression [28] (Box 12.3).

In 1983, St Jude's proposed a surgico-pathological staging system based on extent of surgery and lymph node involvement [29]. In 1987, the TNM (tumor-node-metastasis) staging was proposed jointly by the American joint committee on staging and the Union Internationale Contre le Cancer (UICC) committee. In general, the different staging systems gave comparable results in distinguishing low-stage, good-prognosis patients from high-stage, poor-prognosis patients. However, some of the differences between the staging systems were substantial, particularly as applied to individual patients, so the results of one group could not be easily compared with another.

Points of disagreement included:
(1) Importance of resectability of the primary tumor;
(2) Prognostic significance of tumor 'crossing the midline';
(3) Prognostic importance of ipsilateral and/or contra-lateral lymph node involvement;
(4) Separation of patients (usually infants) with 'stage IV-S' from other children with disseminated disease.

Box 12.3 Neuroblastoma key facts – staging systems.

- 1971: First staging system by the Children's Cancer Group. Key points were concept of Stage IVS, lymph node involvement, and spread across the midline.
- 1983: St Jude's classification. Key points were extent of surgery and lymph node involvement.
- 1987: TNM (tumor node metastasis) classification.
- 1988: International Neuroblastoma staging system (INSS) and International Neuroblastoma Response Criteria (INRC).
- 1993: INSS modified. Post-surgical classification based on resection, lymph nodes. Pitfalls: not all patients are operated at diagnosis; staging depends on extent of surgical resection and thoroughness of surgery.
- 2009: INRGSS is a pre-treatment clinical staging system designed specifically for the INRG classification system. Localized tumors are classified depending on the presence of radiologically defined image-defined risk factors (IDRF).

In 1988, a proposal was made to establish an internationally accepted staging system for neuroblastoma – the International Neuroblastoma Staging System (INSS) – as well as consistent criteria for confirming the diagnosis and determine response to therapy – the International Neuroblastoma Response Criteria (INRC). Both have been universally adopted [30]. In 1993 these were modified [31].The INSS staging system is a post-surgical staging system and depends substantially on the assessment of resectability and surgical examination of lymph node involvement (Table 12.1).

Many countries around the world adopted the INSS. However, some difficulties have been encountered as the classification cannot be applied to every patient. As the INSS is a post-surgical classification, patients with localized disease who are observed because tumor regression is anticipated, cannot be properly staged using INSS criteria.

Since 1995, the European International Society of Paediatric Oncology Neuroblastoma Group (SIOPEN) has classified localized tumors as 'resectable' or 'unresectable' depending on the presence or absence of 'surgical risk factors' based on radiological characteristics of the tumors [32]. It was demonstrated that primary surgery in the presence of surgical risk factors was associated with both a lower complete excision rate and a greater risk of surgery-related complications [32].

The INRG classification system (see later) was developed to establish a consensus approach for *pre-treatment* risk stratification. As the INSS was based on post-surgical (post-therapy) assessment, it was not appropriate to be used in a pre-therapy setting. Also in the INSS the stage of locoregional tumors is based on the degree of surgical resection and the same tumor can be either stage 1 or 3 depending upon the extent of surgical excision,

Table 12.1 International Staging System for Neuroblastoma (INSS) [31].

Stage	Description
Stage 1	Localized tumor confined to the area of origin; complete gross excision, with or without microscopic residual disease. Representative ipsilateral and contralateral lymph nodes negative for tumor microscopically (nodes attached to and removed with the primary tumor may be positive)*.
Stage 2a	Localized tumor with incomplete gross excision; representative ipsilateral and non-adherent lymph nodes negative for tumor microscopically.
Stage 2b	Localized tumor with complete or incomplete gross excision; with ipsilateral non-adherent lymph nodes positive for tumor. Enlarged contralateral lymph nodes must be negative microscopically.
Stage 3	Unresectable unilateral tumor infiltrating across the midline[†] with or without regional lymph node involvement; or localized unilateral tumor with contralateral regional lymph node involvement or midline tumor with bilateral extension by infiltration (unresectable) or by lymph node involvement.
Stage 4	Any primary tumor with dissemination to distant lymph nodes, bone, bone marrow, liver, skin and/or other organs (except as defined in stage 4S).
Stage 4S	Localized primary tumor (as defined for stage 1, 2a or 2b) with dissemination limited to skin, liver and/or bone marrow[‡] (limited to infants less than one year old).

* Multifocal primary tumors (e.g. adrenal primary tumors) should be staged according to the greatest extent of the disease, as defined above, and followed by $_m$, e.g. 3_m. [†] The midline is defined as the vertebral column. Tumors originating on one side and 'crossing the midline' must infiltrate to or beyond the opposite side of the vertebral column. ‡ Marrow involvement of stage 4S should be minimal, i.e. fewer than 10% of total nucleated cells identified as malignant on bone marrow biopsy or on marrow aspirates. More extensive marrow involvement will be considered to be stage 4. The MIBG scan (if done) should be negative in marrow.

making direct comparison of clinical trials based on INSS stages difficult. Another limitation of the INSS is that assessment of lymph node involvement is necessary for proper staging. However, lymph node sampling is subject to the thoroughness of the individual surgeon and can be very variable; furthermore the assessment of extra-regional lymph node involvement is difficult to apply uniformly. Finally, the INSS depends on the midline which can be inconsistently defined.

Therefore based on the hypothesis that a staging system based on preoperative, diagnostic images would be more robust and reproducible than one based on operative findings and approach, the INRG Staging System (INRGSS) was developed [33] (Table 12.2). In the INRGSS, locoregional tumors are staged as L1 or L2 based on the absence or presence of one or more of 19 radiological 'Image Defined Risk Factors' (IDRFs) (Table 12.3). As digital radiographs can be reviewed centrally, the images can be evaluated

Table 12.2 The International Neuroblastoma Risk Group Staging System (INRGSS) [33].

Stage	Description
L1	Localized tumor not involving vital structures as defined by the list of image defined risk factors and confined to one body compartment.
L2	Locoregional tumor with presence of one or more image defined risk factors.
M	Distant metastatic disease (except Stage MS).
MS	Metastatic disease in children younger than 18 months with metastases confined to skin, liver and/or bone marrow.

Patients with multifocal primary tumors should be staged according to the greatest extent of disease as defined in the table.

uniformly. Metastatic tumors are defined as stage M, except for stage MS in which metastatic disease is confined to the skin, liver and/or bone marrow in children younger than 18 months of age.

Pathology

Neuroblastoma cells are described as 'small blue round cells'. The two important features of neuroblastoma are the degree of differentiation and the amount of Schwann cell (stroma) presence (Box 12.4). Historically neuroblastic tumors have been classified as neuroblastoma (NB), ganglioneuroblastoma (GNB), and ganglioneuroma (GN), the later being the most mature end of the spectrum. Systems for histological grading should take account of varying degrees of field to field differentiation within a tumor since the potential for metastasis is determined by the most undifferentiated component. Historically, the principal morphologic feature recognized to be of prognostic importance for neuroblastic tumors was the degree of neuroblastic maturation toward ganglion cells [34, 35]. In 1984, Shimada *et al.* took a new approach with their age-linked classification, which divided neuroblastic tumors into Schwannian stroma-rich and stroma-poor tumors [36]. The stroma-poor neuroblastoma and stroma-rich neuroblastoma were further divided into two prognostic categories: favourable histological features (FH) and unfavourable histological features (UH). The term mitosis-karyorrhexis index (MKI) was introduced for describing one of the prognostic indicators. Some modifications in this classification were published by Joshi *et al.* [37, 38] who suggested a high mitotic rate to be an unfavourable prognostic factor and tumor-associated calcification to be a favourable prognostic factor. The terms neuroblastoma and ganglioneuroblastoma were retained instead of stroma-poor NB and stroma-rich NB, recommended by Shimada *et al.* Undifferentiated neuroblastoma was considered a subtype separate from poorly differentiated neuroblastoma; and the term ganglioneuroblastoma was used only when there was a predominant ganglioneuromatous component admixed with the minor neuroblastomatous component.

Table 12.3 Image defined risk factors in neuroblastic tumors [33].

Ipsilateral tumor extension within two body compartments:
- Neck-chest, chest-abdomen, abdomen-pelvis

Neck:
- Tumor encasing carotid and/or vertebral artery and/or internal jugular vein
- Tumor extending to base of skull
- Tumor compressing the trachea

Cervico-thoracic junction:
- Tumor encasing brachial plexus roots
- Tumor encasing subclavian vessels and/or vertebral and/or carotid artery
- Tumor compressing the trachea

Thorax:
- Tumor encasing the aorta and/or major branches
- Tumor compressing the trachea and/or principal bronchi
- Lower mediastinal tumor, infiltrating the costo-vertebral junction between T9 and T12

Thoraco-abdominal:
- Tumor encasing the aorta and/or vena cava

Abdomen/pelvis:
- Tumor infiltrating the porta hepatis and/or the hepatoduodenal ligament
- Tumor encasing branches of the superior mesenteric artery at the mesenteric root
- Tumor encasing the origin of the coeliac axis, and/or of the superior mesenteric artery
- Tumor invading one or both renal pedicles
- Tumor encasing the aorta and/or vena cava
- Tumor encasing the iliac vessels
- Pelvic tumor crossing the sciatic notch

Intraspinal tumor extension whatever the location provided that:
- More than one third of the spinal canal in the axial plane is invaded and/or
- the perimedullary leptomeningeal spaces are not visible and/or
- the spinal cord signal is abnormal

Infiltration of adjacent organs/structures:
- Pericardium, diaphragm, kidney, liver, duodeno-pancreatic block, and mesentery

Multifocal primary tumors, intraspinal tumors (with or without symptoms of spinal cord compression), pleural effusion (with or without malignant cells) and ascites (with or without malignant cells) to be recorded, but not considered image defined risk factors.

The International Neuroblastoma Pathology Committee (INPC) was established in 1994. The goals and objectives of the INPC included standardization of terminology and morphologic criteria of neuroblastic tumors and establishment of a morphologic classification that was prognostically significant, biologically relevant, and reproducible [39]. Neuroblastic tumors were assigned to one of four basic morphologic categories:
- Neuroblastoma (Schwannian stroma-poor).
- Ganglioneuroblastoma, intermixed (Schwannian stroma-rich).

Box 12.4 Neuroblastoma key facts – pathology.

- Good prognosis tumors progress through undifferentiated neuroblastoma, poorly differentiated neuroblastoma, differentiating neuroblastoma, ganglioneuroblastoma-intermixed, ganglioneuroma maturing and ganglioneuroma mature with increasing patient age, i.e. undifferentiated tumors are not seen in older patients.

- In poor prognosis tumors this process of differentiation is arrested and undifferentiated neuroblastoma is seen in older patients.

- In ganglioneuroblastoma nodular tumors with undifferentiated or poorly differentiated nodules, the differentiation process does not occur in the nodules, possibly because a clone of cells are genetically distinct.

Table 12.4 International Neuroblastoma Pathology Classification [41, 42].

Favourable histology	Age <18 months	Neuroblastoma: poorly differentiated or differentiating and low or intermediate MKI
	Age ≥18 months–5 years	Differentiating neuroblastoma with low MKI. Neuroblastoma poorly differentiated with low MKI
	Any age	Ganglioneuroblastoma intermixed (GNB-I), ganglioneuroma
Unfavourable histology	Age ≥18 months	Poorly differentiated or intermediate MKI
	Any age	Neuroblastoma: undifferentiated or high MKI
	≥60 months	Differentiating neuroblastoma, neuroblastoma poorly differentiated with low MKI

MKI, mitosis-karyorrhexis index.

- Ganglioneuroma (Schwannian stroma-dominant).
- Ganglioneuroblastoma, nodular (composite Schwannian stroma-rich/stroma-dominant and stroma-poor).

(1) Neuroblastoma (Schwannian stroma poor) is a tumor composed of neuroblasts constituting the entire or predominant portion (at least 50% of the tumor mass) of the neuroblastic tumor. The neuroblasts are characteristically arranged in nests surrounded by fibro vascular septae. There are three subtypes of neuroblastoma:

- Undifferentiated neuroblastoma (virtually all tumor cells are undifferentiated) (Plate 12.1).
- Poorly differentiated neuroblastoma (less than 5% cells show a tendency towards differentiation).
- Differentiating neuroblastoma (at least 5% cells show a tendency towards differentiation toward ganglion cells) (Plate 12.2).

(2) Ganglioneuroblastoma contains predominantly a ganglioneuromatous component (more than 50% of the tumor mass) and a minor neuroblastomatous component showing variable differentiation and distribution. At present two distinct types of ganglioneuroblastoma are recognized:

- GNB nodular (composite Schwannian stroma-rich/stroma-dominant/stroma poor). Macroscopically, these are usually hemorrhagic nodules.
- GNB intermixed (Schwannian stroma rich). Neuroblastomatous component is present in the form of variably sized, fairly well-defined but unencapsulated nests of neuroblasts and neuropil intermixed with the predominant ganglioneuromatous component (Plate 12.3).

(3) Ganglioneuroma (Schwannian stroma dominant) has two subtypes:

- Ganglioneuroma maturing consisting of differentiating neuroblasts and mature ganglion cells.
- Ganglioneuroma mature consisting of mature Schwannian stroma and ganglion cells [38, 39] (Plate 12.4).

To test the prognostic effects of the International Classification, all neuroblastic tumors were classified into either a FH group or an UH group based on the age, MKI, and pathology. Regardless of the patient's age, tumors in the ganglioneuroblastoma, intermixed category and the ganglioneuroma category were classified into the FH group, whereas tumors in the ganglioneuroblastoma, nodular category were classified in the unfavourable group [40] However, in 2003 the international neuroblastoma pathology classification was revised to confirm favourable and unfavourable prognostic subsets in ganglioneuroblastoma, nodular tumors (GNB-N). GNB-N is a composite tumor with ganglioneuromatous and ganglioneuroblastomatous components and the prognostic grouping of the given tumor is determined by evaluating grade of neuroblastic differentiation and MKI of the neuroblastomatous nodules using the age dependent criteria [41]. Therefore it is only the GNB-N with unfavourable histology which is associated with a poor outcome and a tendency to be associated with metastatic disease. Analysis of 911 patients by these criteria substantiated the age-linked prognostic effects of the morphologic indicators (grade of neuroblastic differentiation and MKI) for patients with tumors in the neuroblastoma category, and supported the concept of an age-appropriate framework of maturation for patients with tumors. All these classifications are only applicable to tumors examined before any therapy. Previously treated primary tumors may have different appearances (Table 12.4).

In the INRG histological category (neuroblastoma, ganglioneuroblastoma- intermixed, ganglioneuroblastoma-nodular and ganglioneuroma maturing), grade of tumor differentiation (undifferentiated, poorly differentiated and differentiating), MKI, and age, were found to be of independent prognostic value. To prevent confounding of the effect of age, histological features (histological category, MKI, and grade of differentiation) were analyzed in lieu of the INPC.

The panel of immunohistochemical markers usually positive in neuroblastic tumors are: neuron specific enolase, chromogranin A, synaptophysin, tyrosine hydroxylase, protein gene product 9.5, GD2, NB84. Actin, desmin, low molecular weight cytokeratin, leukocyte common antigen, and vimentin are generally negative.

Neuroblastoma molecular pathology (Box 12.5)

Tumor cell ploidy

The prognostic implication of tumor cell ploidy in neuroblastoma has been accepted for over 30 years [43–45]. Locoregional tumors are commonly hyperdiploid, but diploidy is more common in advanced-stage tumors.

• Approximately 55% of the tumors have a hyperdiploid (near-triploid or penta-/hexaploid) DNA-content and about 45% of neuroblastic tumors are diploid.

• The prognostic significance of ploidy has been confirmed in infants and children up to 18 months of age with metastatic disease and without *MYCN* amplification. Children with hyperdiploidy without *MYCN* amplification had better event free survival (EFS) compared with diploid tumors without *MYCN* amplification [45–47].

The Children's Oncology Group has reported a retrospective study of clinical significance of ploidy and *MYCN* status in low stage disease and conclude that patients with hyperdiploidy and *MYCN* amplification have significantly higher overall survival (OS) as compared with patients with diploidy and *MYCN* amplification [48]. This needs to be confirmed in prospective studies.

MYCN amplification

The oncogene *MYCN* is located on chromosome 2p at 2p 23–24 [49]. Early reports suggested that amplification of *MYCN* was present in 25–50% patients with stage 3 and 4 disease and with amplification up to 300% [50, 51].

• The amplification of the gene most commonly occurred in double minutes in primary tumors, while amplification occurs in

---

Box 12.5 Neuroblastoma key facts – molecular pathology.

• *MYCN* amplification is an independent adverse prognostic factor for infants and localised disease.

• The presence of segmental alterations, with or without *MYCN* amplification, is the strongest predictor of relapse.

• Loss of 11q is prognostic for event free and overall survival especially in *MYCN* non-amplified tumors.

• Loss of 1p is prognostic for event free survival.

• Hyperdiploidy is associated with a superior prognosis in patients with metastatic disease under the age of 18 months.

---

cell lines in homogenous stained regions. Amplification in homogenous stained regions in tumors appears to have no clinical effect [52].

• *MYCN* amplification is an intrinsic biological property of a subset of neuroblastoma and if the amplification is going to occur, it is generally present at the time of initial diagnosis and this feature does not change with time [53].

• A relationship between higher tumor stage and rapid disease progression with *MYCN* copy number was first documented in 1985 [51].

Subsequently it was established that *MYCN* amplification is an independent prognostic factor [54]. However, amplification of *MYCN* does not have significance in stage 4 disease [55, 56].

It has been observed that frequently there is co amplification of genes in proximity to the *MYCN*. DEAD-box protein gene (DDX1) located at 2p24 is co amplified with *MYCN* in about two-thirds of patients [57]. Although there have been studies to suggest that co amplification of DDX1 and *MYCN* is associated with favourable outcome [58], this has been proven to be incorrect by others [59, 60]. The role of DDX1 and other genes such as NAG need to be further clarified.

In *MYCN* amplified tumors there is high level *MYCN* expression and this is associated with a poor outcome. However, high-level *MYCN* expression in neuroblastoma lacking *MYCN* amplification results in a benign phenotype. Thus, the high *MYCN* expression confers the opposite biological consequence in neuroblastoma, depending on whether or not *MYCN* is amplified [61].

Other non-random genetic abnormalities

In neuroblastoma, most structural chromosome aberrations are unbalanced, i.e. they are associated with physical losses or gains of parts of chromosomes. Balanced aberrations, i.e. reciprocal translocations without losses of genetic material, are relatively uncommon in neuroblastoma. The term 'structural' aberrations is used to refer to genomic amplifications together with gains or losses of parts of chromosomes and the term 'segmental' aberration is used when referring only to gains or losses of parts of chromosomes.

• In neuroblastoma, segmental chromosome aberrations represent unbalanced chromosome aberrations. Non-random genetic abnormalities in neuroblastoma can either be losses or gains of part of chromosomes (segmental aberrations) such as losses (1p36.3, 4p, 9p, 11q 23, 12p and 14q) or amplification/gains (*MYCN*, 17q) of genetic material.

• Genetic losses indicate the loss of function of some as yet unknown tumor suppressor genes. Of these, the better studied are 1p deletion, 11q deletions and *MYCN* gain and 17q gain. Multiplex ligation-dependent probe amplification (MLPA) is a novel technique which is currently being validated to simultaneously identify amplifications and whole and partial chromosomal gains and losses of a large number of chromosomal loci.

Chromosomal comparative genomic hybridization (CGH) is another method which has been well tested to assess whole or partial chromosome gains or losses. A recent study extensively analyzed 147 neuroblastoma samples at diagnosis, without *MYCN* amplification, by CGH. This showed gains or losses of entire chromosomes (type 1) in 71 cases, whereas partial chromosome gains or losses (type 2), including gain involving 17q, were observed in 68 cases. Atypical profiles were present in eight cases. A type 1 profile was observed more frequently in localized disease and in patients of less than 12 months at diagnosis. A type 2 genomic profile was associated with a higher risk of relapse in the overall population but also in the subgroup of patients with localized disease. In multivariate analysis, the genomic profile was the strongest independent prognostic factor. The study concluded that in patients without *MYCN* amplification, genomic alterations help predict the outcome [62]. It has been suggested that the analysis of the overall genomic pattern probably indicates genomic instability. These findings have been extended in a series of 493 *MYCN* amplified and non-amplified neuroblastomas. In tumors only with whole-chromosome copy number variations there were no disease-related deaths. In contrast the presence of segmental alterations with or without *MYCN* amplification was the strongest predictor of relapse [63].

1p deletion

Deletions of 1p were first detected in cytogenetic studies in 1977 [64]. Allelic loss of 1p occurs in about a third of neuroblastoma patients [65]. Loss of heterozygocity of distant chromosome is associated with *MYCN* amplification and implies an aggressive tumor [66, 67]. LOH of 1p was predictive of local recurrences in low stage disease [68] and associated with tumors with aggressive behaviours [69].

11q loss

11q aberrations are found in approximately 25% of patients. These are more associated with stage 4 disease and over the age of 2.5 years. These patients generally have a poor outcome. Common region of deletion is mapped at 11q23 [70]. In a large study, multivariate analysis confirmed that 11q status had prognostic significance for all patients with stage 1, 2, 3 and 4S disease in patients without *MYCN* amplification. 11q strongly correlated with increase incidence of relapse particularly metastatic relapses [71]. 11q aberrations are often not associated with *MYCN* amplification and are associated with reduced progression free survival, thereby strengthening its role as an independent prognostic factor [67].

17q gain

Gain in 17q is one of the commonest segmental aberration seen in patients with neuroblastoma [72]. Earlier studies showed that 17q gain is associated with adverse prognosis [73–76]. However this has not been universally confirmed [77].

Anaplastic lymphoma kinase (ALK)

ALK is an oncogene which was originally identified as a fusion kinase in anaplastic large cell lymphoma. It harbours mutations in the tyrosine kinase domain (TKD). It has recently been identified as a predisposition gene for familial neuroblastoma [78]. Somatic mutations are also found in about 12% of sporadic *high-risk* neuroblastoma tumors [78]. It is now also recognized as a frequent target of genetic alteration in advanced neuroblastoma [79]. This could be a potential future target for therapy.

Risk stratification

Risk assessment in neuroblastoma depends on several clinical and biological features. Different groups have used different criteria for risk stratification. For example, SIOPEN uses age, *MYCN* status, and surgical risk factors defined by imaging for assigning risk-group for locoregional tumors, whereas the COG uses age, *MYCN* status, stage, histology, and DNA ploidy [32, 80]. As an increasing number of genetic features have been included to guide therapy decisions [67, 73, 81], comparison of different trials is difficult (Box 12.6).

Efforts have been made in the last four years to develop a consensus approach that will allow comparison of results across the world. A Task Force representing the major paediatric cooperative groups globally was created in 2004 with the aim of developing INRG. From the major pediatric cooperative groups – COG (North American and Australia), GPOH (Gesellschaft für Pädiatrische Onkologie und Hämatologie, Germany), JINCS (Japan) and SIOPEN (Europe) – 8800 patients treated on studies between 1990 and 2002 were studied.

The prognostic significance of 13 potential risk factors was evaluated using survival tree regression using EFS as the primary endpoint. Cox proportional hazards regression models were used to identify the most highly statistically significant variable to create a given split or 'branch' in the survival tree [18].

Box 12.6 Neuroblastoma key facts – risk stratification.

- The INRG is an internationally agreed pre-therapy risk assessment system.

- Seven factors are employed – stage, age (<18 months versus ≥18 months), histological category (ganglioneuroma, ganglioneuroblastoma-intermixed), grade of tumor differentiation (differentiating versus undifferentiated or poorly differentiated), *MYCN* status, presence/absence of 11q aberration, and ploidy (≤1.0 versus >1.0).

- Sixteen statistically and/or clinically different pre-treatment groups, which are designated as very low, low, intermediate, or high pre-treatment risk subsets.

- The key is the assignment of patients in a given INRG row to a single treatment group without splitting that row in different treatment subgroups.

The analysis confirmed the previous results of London *et al.* [82] that the age cut-off of 18 months was prognostically significant. However, for patients with diploid, stage M, *MYCN* non-amplified tumor, the Task Force elected to use the more conservative age cut-off of 12 months (365 days).

Seven factors were identified that were highly statistically significant and also considered clinically relevant:
• Stage.
• Age (<18 months versus ≥18 months (547 days)).
• Histological category (ganglioneuroma, ganglioneuroblastoma – intermixed).
• Grade of tumor differentiation (differentiating versus undifferentiated or poorly differentiated).
• *MYCN* status.
• Presence/absence of 11q aberration.
• Ploidy (≤1.0 versus >1.0).
The INRGSS was used as a pre-therapy staging system for the INRG. A retrospective analysis supported the translation of INSS staging in the INRG Classification system [33]:
INSS 1 → INRGSS L1;
INSS 2, 3 → INRGSS L2;
INSS 4 → INRGSS M;
INSS 4S → INRGSS MS.

Sixteen statistically and/or clinically different pre-treatment groups of patients were identified and patients grouped using EFS cut points for 5-year. EFS of >85%, >75–≤85%, ≥50 ≤75% or <50%, were 28.2%, 26.8%, 9.0% and 36.1%, respectively. The categories were designated as very low, low, intermediate, or high pre-treatment risk subsets [18] (Table 12.5).

Screening and neuroblastoma (Box 12.7)

In Japan, a nationwide screening programme was commenced in 1985 as survival seemed to improve following pilot programmes. Prior to 1989, all infants aged 6 months were screened with qualitative spot tests for VMA in urine and subsequently by quantitative assay for VMA and HVA with high-performance liquid chromatography (HPLC). The total number of neuroblastoma cases diagnosed under the age of one year increased significantly. However, most patients were in favourable stages (stage 1, 2 or 4s), had a small primary mass and without unfavourable biological features. The survival rate for neuroblastoma diagnosed by screening was around 97% [83]. However, there was no decrease in the number of children diagnosed with neuroblastoma over 1 year of age. Also, mortality in children between 1 and 4 years of age from neuroblastoma did not decrease. It was therefore concluded that mass screening for neuroblastoma causes harm because of overdiagnosis, and it has little effect on decreasing the incidence or mortality from the disease at 1–4 years of age [84]. The Japanese government stopped the screening programme in 2004.

The Quebec screening programme screened infants at 3 weeks and 6 months of age and also concluded that screening for neuroblastoma markedly increases the incidence in infants without decreasing the incidence of unfavourable advanced stage disease in older children [85].

The German study investigated the role of screening at 1 year of age in 2.6 million children in six states while 2.1 million children in 10 states were not screened. There was significant overdiagnosis in the screened group and similar death rates, thereby confirming that screening was not useful [86]. Screening therefore results in overtreatment and psychological burden for families [87].

Treatment of neuroblastoma

Surgery
Surgery may be the only therapy necessary for localized (L1 without image- defined risk factors [IDRFs]) tumors with favourable histology and biology.

Initial approaches to localized neuroblastoma include:
• Immediate complete tumor excision with no need for subsequent therapy.
• Near-complete excision followed by adjuvant therapy in selected patients.
• No attempt at excision if the tumor has IDRFs. For these patients chemotherapy is generally administered to shrink the tumor and render it less vascular and friable to facilitate subsequent excision.
It is important that the surgical procedure is associated with no, or very low, morbidity (Box 12.8).

To develop guidelines for surgery for localized neuroblastoma, LNESG1 defined surgical risk factors (SRFs) based on imaging characteristics [88]:
• The adoption of SRFs as predictors of adverse surgical outcome was validated because their presence was associated with lower complete excision rate and greater risk of post surgical complications [32]. These are now called IDRFs. These were more recently tested with respect to the German NB97 trial and were useful in predicting risks and completeness of surgery [89].
• Most stage 3 tumors are deemed unresectable before or during operation. At presentation, usually only biopsy is possible, although there are some initial complete resections.
To stratify accurately patients with loco-regional tumors using the INRG classification system, adequate samples of tumor tissue are needed for genetic studies and for histological category determination. It is challenging to distinguish ganglioneuroblastoma-intermixed from ganglioneuroblastoma-nodular when the entire tumor is not resected. Surgical biopsy needs to be guided by the radiological appearances of the tumor, with any heterogeneous areas targeted. Adequate tissue samples are mandatory to evaluate histological grade in loco-regional neuroblastoma that lack *MYCN* amplification in children ≥18 months of age. In most cases, multiple image-guided core-needle biopsies 'true-cut' cores will yield sufficient tissue to determine tumor grade, but fine needle aspirates are not likely to provide adequate quantities

Table 12.5 The International Neuroblastoma Risk Group classification [18].

INRG stage	Age (months)	Histological category/grade of tumor differentiation	MYCN	11q aberration	Ploidy	Pre-treatment risk group
L1/L2		GN maturing GNB intermixed				A Very low
L1		Any, except GN maturing or GNB intermixed	NA			B Very low
			Amp			K High
L2	<18	Any, except GN maturing or GNB intermixed	NA	No		D Low
				Yes		G Intermediate
	≥18	GNB nodular, differentiating NB, differentiating	NA	No		E Low
				Yes		H Intermediate*
		GNB nodular, poorly differentiated or undifferentiated NB, poorly differentiated or undifferentiated	NA			H Intermediate*
			Amp			N High
M	<18		NA		Hyperdiploid	F Low
	<12		NA		Diploid	I Intermediate
	12–<18		NA		Diploid	J Intermediate
	<18		Amp			O High
	≥18					P High
MS	<18		NA	No		C Very Low
				Yes		Q High
			Amp			R High

GN, ganglioneuroma. GNB, ganglioneuroblastoma. NB, neuroblastoma. Amp, amplified. NA, not amplified.

* Pre-treatment risk group H has two entries. Tumor Stages: L1, localized tumor confined to one body compartment and with absence of image defined risk factors (IDRF); L2, locoregional tumor with presence of one or more IDRFs. M, distant metastatic disease (except Stage MS). MS, metastatic disease confined to skin, liver and/or bone marrow in children <18 months of age (definitions: 12 months = 365 days; 18 months = 547 days; Blank field = 'any'). Diploid (DNA index <1.0); hyperdiploid (DNA index >1.0 and includes near-triploid and near-tetraploid tumors). Very low-risk (5-year EFS >85%); low-risk (5-year EFS >75%-<85%); intermediate-risk (5-year EFS > 50%-<75%); High-risk (5-year EFS < 50%). EFS, event-free survival.

Box 12.7 Neuroblastoma key facts – screening for neuroblastoma.

Screening for neuroblastoma resulted in:

- Increased incidence of neuroblastoma in infants.
- Low stage and good biology tumors.
- Excellent cure rates for tumors detected by screening.
- Over treatment of patients and burden of therapy.
- Psychological distress to families.
- No reduction in the incidence of aggressive tumors in older children.
- No decrease in overall mortality from neuroblastoma.

Box 12.8 Neuroblastoma key facts – surgery

- Image-defined risk factors (IDRFs) are important to decide if attempts should be made for surgical resection of localized neuroblastoma tumors.
- For localized tumors (L1 and L2) there are three possible treatment options:
  (1) immediate complete tumor excision with no need for subsequent therapy (L1);
  (2) near-complete excision followed by adjuvant therapy in selected patients (this occurs very rarely);
  (3) No attempt at excision if the tumor has IDRFS (L2). These patients receive chemotherapy to attempt to shrink the tumor.
- For patients with stage M disease, surgery following clearance of metastatic deposits with chemotherapy is believed to help in local control.
- For patients with L2 with poor prognosis features surgery following chemotherapy is believed to help in local control.

of tissue for histological analysis and are not appropriate. In metastatic tumor, fine needle aspirates may provide adequate information for genetic analysis.

The conventional approach is delayed surgical resection following chemotherapy that causes tumor shrinkage. As the degree of resection is believed to be prognostic in poor prognosis tumors (see later) complete excision is the aim. Study by Kushner *et al.* in 1996 suggested that non-stage 4 patients without *MYCN* amplification can be spared cytotoxic therapy because residual post-surgical or recurrent biologically favourable (triploidy and non-amplified *MYCN*) neuroblastoma rarely evolves into lethal stage 4 disease [90].

For stage 4 neuroblastoma patients less than 18 months old, initial biopsy of the primary tumor is mandatory in view of the increasing importance of the molecular pathology. For infants with stage MS disease, excision of the primary tumor is not indicated [91, 92]. Biopsy is also recommended for patients over the age of 18 months. Biopsy should be associated with minimal morbidity and often done at the time of insertion of venous access. In stage 4 disease, the standard approach is to attempt surgical resection of the primary tumor after there has been a response to chemotherapy at the metastatic sites, particularly the bone marrow. Many studies have shown beneficial effects of surgery on survival in stage 4 disease [93–99]; and the aim should be complete resection. In one retrospective review the impact of complete resection in stage 4 diseases seemed less with the use of recent more aggressive chemotherapy. There remained, however, significant benefit for *MYCN* amplified tumors [100].

As a general principle, intensive local therapy, i.e. attempted total surgical resection and local radiotherapy, is utilized for high-risk disease. This is based on the data that in North America, with intensive local therapy, there is a local recurrence rate of less than 10%, compared with Europe where with historically, less aggressive surgery and no radiotherapy there is a local recurrence rate of 40%.

Role of chemotherapy in neuroblastoma (Box 12.9)

Induction therapy

The current practice is to use combination chemotherapy, as 'induction' therapy, for treatment of patients with unresectable localized disease with unfavourable histological or biologic features or those with stage 4 diseases.

There are significant challenges attempting to compare different induction regimens; there have been substantial changes in the techniques used and the thoroughness of application of these methodologies. Initially, bone marrow sampling procedures varied greatly and more recently MIBG scanning techniques and scoring vary. Furthermore, it is difficult to compare EFS and OS rates between different published induction regimens as the influence of myeloablative therapy, local treatment, and differentiation therapy have to be considered.

> **Box 12.9 Neuroblastoma key facts – chemotherapy.**
>
> - There are a number of induction regimens in current use – COJEC followed by TVD and cyclophosphamide and topotecan; cyclophosphamide, doxorubicin, and vincristine (CAV); cisplatin and etoposide (P/E). No randomized study has compared them.
> - Consolidation therapy with high dose therapy and stem cell rescue significantly improves outcome in patients with stage 4 neuroblastoma over 1 year.
> - Various conditioning regimens have been used: busulphan and melphalan, or carboplatin, etoposide and melphalan are the two most widely used. At present SIOPEN is conducting a randomized study comparing them.
> - A randomized trial has not shown any benefit of immunomagnetically purged stem cells as compared with non-purged stem cells.
> - Currently no role for allogeneic transplantation has been demonstrated.

Single agent phase II studies have demonstrated the effectiveness of various chemotherapy agents such as vincristine, cyclophosphamide, cisplatin, carboplatin, doxorubicin, etoposide, and melphalan in the treatment of neuroblastoma and these have become key agents in induction treatment of current protocols [101–103]. More recently topotecan, irinotecan, and temozolomide have been demonstrated to be active [104].

The initial chemotherapy combinations included vincristine, cyclophosphamide with doxorubicin or dacarbazine [105, 106]. However, long-term results were disappointing for children with aggressive disease over the age of one year.
- The introduction of cisplatin and epipodophyllotoxin-based regimens in the 1980s for the treatment of advanced neuroblastoma improved response rates and outcome [107].
- One of the first regimens to use these agents combined standard doses of vincristine, cisplatin, cyclophosphamide, and tenioposide [OPEC].
- Complete response rates in the bone marrow, by the standards then used, exceeded 80% and a number of patients achieved durable remission [108]. The French group used alternating sequence of non cross-resistant drugs cisplatin and tenioposide (PE) with cyclophosphamide, vincristine, and doxorubicin (CADO) and obtained an overall response rate of 96% (by 1987 criteria) [109].

The goal of induction therapy is to induce reduction in tumor bulk at both primary and metastatic sites. A retrospective study of 44 clinical trials over 25 year period suggested that maximum dose intensity of selective drugs over a short duration may improve outcome of poor risk neuroblastoma [110]. This was particularly relevant to platinum and epipodophyllotoxin compounds. However, a critical review of published data did not substantiate any effect of dose intensity on a number of patients who responded when bone marrow was used as a measure of metastatic disease [111]. A rapid schedule in which chemotherapy was administered every 10 days was developed [112].

ENSG5 compared the outcome and toxicity of increased dose intensity in induction chemotherapy in patients with stage 4 neuroblastoma in a randomized study. A rapid schedule administered over 10 days (COJEC, cisplatin, vincristine, carboplatin, etoposide, and cyclophosphamide) was compared with OPEC-OJEC (same five drugs) given every 21 days. Both EFS and OS were better with the rapid regimen compared with the standard regimen, but only the 5 year EFS reached statistical significance. In addition the rapid (COJEC) regimen achieved a higher overall complete response and very good partial response rate compared with the Standard regimen with less poor responders and progressions [113]. Earlier administration of myeloablative therapy might have also contributed to the improved outcome [114].

The Memorial Sloan Kettering Cancer Centre (MSKCC) protocols have used non-cross-resistant drug combinations: high dose cyclophosphamide (70 mg/kg/day $\times$ 2) plus doxorubicin and vincristine (CAV) with high doses of cisplatin (50 mg/m^2/d $\times$ 4) and etoposide (P/E) to achieve rapid cytoreduction in order to avert drug resistance. Reduction from seven courses to five courses still retained high response rate with lower toxicity [115].

Currently SIOPEN employs the COJEC regimen for induction therapy with topotecan, vincristine, and doxorubicin [116] for patients who fail to achieve adequate response following induction therapy. COG's previous induction therapy (A3973) was based on the MSKCC protocol with four courses of CAV and two courses of P/E [117]. COG's current induction protocol comprises two courses of cyclophosphamide and topotecan, two courses of CAV, and two courses of P/E. There have only been two randomized studies of induction therapy [113, 118] and there is a major need for mores such studies to determine the optimum induction therapy.

Consolidation therapy and role of high dose therapy (HDT) (myeloablative therapy), and hemopoietic stem cell rescue

The aim of consolidation therapy is to eliminate any residual tumor. Melphalan was the first drug chosen, as its main toxicity at conventional doses is myelosuppression and this could be overcome by autologous bone marrow transplantation (ABMT). The first published study on use of high dose melphalan with ABMT concluded that the median survival was longer than the historical compared group [119]. Subsequently, several single arm studies confirmed a trend towards improved survival in high-risk neuroblastoma patients [120, 121].

• Three randomized studies have evaluated the role of high dose chemotherapy as consolidation therapy in stage 4 neuroblastoma. In the ENSG 1 trial of the European Neuroblastoma Study Group conducted between 1982 and 1985, patients were randomized to receive high dose melphalan with ABMT or no further therapy.

For patients with stage 4 disease over the age of 1 year, the 5 year EFS was significantly better for the melphalan treated group (33% vs 17%) [122].

• In a multi-centre study conducted by the American Children's Study group, the role of HDT followed by purged ABMT was tested in a randomized fashion. The three year EFS was significantly better for patients assigned to receive ABMT compared with those who received continuation of chemotherapy [123]. A recent report has confirmed that the benefit of HDT is maintained with time and that HDT and hematopoietic cell rescue results in a significantly better five-year EFS and OS than non-myeloablative chemotherapy [124].

• A randomized study of 295 patients receiving ABMT with carboplatin, etoposide, melphalan (CEM) conditioning versus oral maintenance chemotherapy with cyclophosphamide showed better results for patients receiving megatherapy (3 year EFS 47% vs 31%) [125].

Various agents have been used as conditioning regimens prior to autologous bone marrow or peripheral stem cell transplantation. combination of melphalan and total body irradiation (TBI) was used by Pole et al. in 1991 [126]. A combination of vincristine, melphalan, and total body irradiation was used by Philip et al. [120]. A combination of carmustine (BCNU), tenioposide, and melphalan was used by Hartmann et al. [127]. Regimen have used vincristine, melphalan, etoposide, and carboplatin given over five days [128] or over a single day [129]. Busulphan and melphalan combination was used in Europe [130, 131].In a multivariate analysis of over 200 patients treated at one institution in Europe busulphan and melphalan was found to result in a superior EFS [131]. Therefore busulphan and melphalan has been adopted as 'the gold standard' European myeloablative regimen. In North America carboplatin, etoposide, and melphalan has been developed and refined in a number of studies and is the COG 'gold standard' [123, 132].

• The current SIOPEN high-risk neuroblastoma study (HR NB1) is testing the two approaches in a randomized study. The hypothesis is that busulphan and melphalan results in a superior 3 year EFS than CEM as myeloablative therapy.

• A retrospective multivariate analysis of 546 patients on the European bone marrow transplant (EBMT) registry from 1978 to 1992 was conducted to evaluate factors affecting EFS in stage 4 neuroblastoma patients over the age of 1 year who received myeloablative therapy. Two adverse prognostic factors were persistent bone marrow disease and persistent skeletal involvement (bone scan/MIBG san positive) [133].

• In a recent large report from the EBMT of 4098 patients, 'the quality of remission' was a significant prognostic factor. Also BMT with busulfan–melphalan conditioning in first remission achieved an OS of 48% compared with all other regimens [134].

The concept of repeating HDT with hemopoietic stem cell rescue on two occasions was first investigated by the LMCE group in France in the late 1980s [135]. More recently promising results have been observed in pilot studies with tandem cycles of HDT resulting in a 5 year EFS of 50% [136]. This approach is now being explored in a randomized study being planned by COG.

Purged versus non-purged marrow
The value of purging bone marrow for neuroblastoma cells has been debated for many years. However, a recently published randomized phase 2 trial of myeloablative autologous peripheral blood cell transplant for high-risk neuroblastoma using immunomagnetically purged versus unpurged peripheral blood stem cells (PBSC) in 489 patients did not impact on EFS or OS at 2 years [137].

Autologous versus allogeneic
In a non-randomized comparative study between allogeneic versus purged ABMT for high-risk neuroblastoma, there was no statistically significant difference in the survival (progression free survival 25% vs 49% at 4 years) [138].

Radiotherapy in neuroblastoma

Neuroblastoma is a radiosensitive tumor and this has been confirmed with both *in vitro* and *in vivo* studies [139–141]. Radiation therapy can be administered by:
• External beam radiotherapy: standard therapy or hyperfractionated therapy.
• Intra-operative radiotherapy.
• Targeted radiotherapy as MIBG therapy.
  The role of radiotherapy will be discussed in:
• Infants.
• Localized disease.
• Stage 4 disease.
• Radiotherapy as palliation.
• Radiotherapy as conditioning regimen for HDT.

External beam radiotherapy (EBRT)
This is the conventional method of administering radiotherapy. Most centres use standard once daily radiotherapy. There is general debate about optimum dose but the benefit of low doses (≤20 Gy) has been previously demonstrated [142]. The total dose has also been adapted to tumor burden by some groups and 36 Gy as intensified EBRT was used in a German study.

Hyperfractionated radiotherapy
In this method, radiotherapy is given over more that one dose per day. Studies have used pre-transplant hyperfractionated radiotherapy to local sites but generally radiotherapy is given after recovery from high dose chemotherapy [143]. This ensures better tolerance of the high dose chemotherapy. Hyperfractionated radiotherapy has also been suggested to be useful in children with stage 4 disease in combination with multimodality treatment [144]. No study has compared the role of standard versus hyperfractionated radiotherapy (RT) in a randomized method.

Intra-operative radiotherapy (IORT)
IORT has been found to achieve good local control after gross total resection of tumor in high-risk neuroblastoma patients, but as the sole radiotherapy to the primary it was inadequate for patients with extensive adenopathy or a sub-total resection of tumor [145].

In a recently published study, long-term outcomes and toxicities of intra-operative radiotherapy were studied in 31 high-risk neuroblastoma patients. The three-year local recurrence rate was 15%. Approximately 20% of patients developed vascular complications or hypertension [146].

Radiotherapy in infants
There is now general consensus that radiotherapy should be avoided in non high-risk infants with neuroblastoma. In a retrospective study in infants with neuroblastoma, locoregional control was excellent regardless of whether radiotherapy was used. Patients who received radiotherapy had significant long-term toxicity [147]. A Pediatric Oncology Groups (POG) study in infants also showed excellent results in infants with minimal chemotherapy and resection without radiotherapy [148]. Radiotherapy has in the past been used to control life-threatening symptoms in stage 4S disease, but chemotherapy, especially carboplatin and etoposide, are more effective and have less long-term side effects.

Localized neuroblastoma over the age of 1 year
For patients with Stage 1 and 2 neuroblastoma, irrespective of age, there is generally no role for RT [149]. In a POG randomized trial of children over the age of 1 year old with lymph node involvement (POG group C patients, i.e. completely or incompletely removed primary tumor with unattached nodes positive), RT to the primary tumor bed and regional nodes resulted in improved overall and disease free survival [150]. The significant difference in survival remained when adjusted for the Shimada classification.

For stage 3 disease with undifferentiated or poorly differentiated histology, the outcome is poor without radiotherapy, HDT, and 13-cis-retinoic acid (13-cis-RA). It has been suggested that radiotherapy, HDT, and 13-cis-RA improves outcome (5-year EFS 80%, 100% OS) [151]. SIOPEN is exploring if a good outcome can be achieved with localized EBRT and 13-cis-RA without HDT.

Role of radiotherapy in stage 4 disease
Studies have shown that patients over the age of 1 year with stage 4 disease benefit from intensive multimodality treatment [152]. In a CCG trial, the rate of local relapse after purged ABMT was not affected by the administration of local radiation (26% with radiation vs 31% without). However, only patients with gross residual disease were treated with radiation and the dose was only 10 Gy [153]. The role of EBRT on EFS and OS in stage 4 patients treated with the NB97 trial was retrospectively analyzed. Patients with residual disease were given intensified EBRT (36 Gy). EBRT

was found to be effective in highly intensive treatment of stage 4 patients [154]. The effect of local radiotherapy administered to primary disease sites in patients with high-risk neuroblastoma was studied in 539 patients enrolled on the CCG-3891 protocol. All patients were given 10 Gy of EBRT to gross residual disease following surgery and randomized to receive continuation chemotherapy or ABMT with TBI conditioning. Five year loco-regional relapse rate was significantly lower for patients who received TBI and HDT (51% vs 33%) [155].

Radiotherapy as palliation for control of pain and symptoms

Radiotherapy has been used in palliation of patients with soft tissue masses, bony masses, brain metastasis, and liver metastasis in patients with neuroblastoma [156]. Radiotherapy is highly effective in this setting especially in controlling pain and can be administered in one fraction.

Radiotherapy to relieve symptoms of spinal cord compression

Radiotherapy is effective in producing decompression in patients with spinal cord compression [157] and should be considered as an option.

Radiotherapy as a component of HDT

TBI has been a component of a number of HDT regimens. The benefit of including TBI has not been proven in randomized studies and the acute- and long-term morbidity and mortality associated with its use can be substantial [120, 158], and therefore it is no longer used.

Targeted radiotherapy

^{131}I-MIBG has a high tumor/non-tumor ratio and its relatively long intra-tumoral biological half-life is important for its therapeutic use. To offer MIBG treatment to patients, the patients have to be nursed in isolation facilities after adequate thyroid blockage with iodide. Although ^{131}I-MIBG has been shown to be an active therapeutic modality in neuroblastomas for over 20 years [159, 160] it has not found its role in frontline therapy of newly diagnosed patients. This is due to the technical difficulties in administering the agent and that only a few centres can undertake this therapy. There is a need for a randomized study to establish the role of MIBG therapy. However, this is hampered by logistic difficulties.

MIBG therapy can be used in three different ways:
- First-line therapy.
- Consolidation therapy.
- Recurrent disease.

As first line therapy

The role of ^{131}I-MIBG in the initial management of high-risk neuroblastoma was first explored in 1994 [161]. The objective of this approach was to reduce the tumor volume, enabling ade-

quate surgical resection of the tumor, and to avoid toxicity of combination chemotherapy at diagnosis prior to surgery in patients with advanced neuroblastoma. Thirty-one patients were treated and 70% had complete or >95% resection of primary tumor or did not require surgery. The toxicity was considerably less except for mild thrombocytopenia [162]. In a further expansion of the study on 44 patients, a 66% objective response rate was observed in children following two cycles of MIBG therapy as induction therapy [163]. MIBG therapy has also been combined with chemotherapeutic agents in the first line treatment of neuroblastoma [164]. It has been found to be well tolerated. However, treatment with MIBG needs detailed dosimetry and planning and is challenging at diagnosis.

As consolidation therapy

A retrospective analysis of the German 97 trial failed to show an independent benefit of MIBG therapy as consolidation treatment when HDT was used as well [165]. MIBG therapy has been incorporated in the conditioning regimen for high dose chemotherapy and ABMT and no clear benefit is evident as yet [166, 167].

A recent study has shown the feasibility and tolerability of two consecutive MIBG therapies at two week intervals with hematopoietic stem cell rescue. The recommended dose was 36 mCi/kg which could be taken forward into Phase III studies [168]. There is international interest in the use of ^{131}I-MIBG therapy as consolidation therapy for adolescent neuroblastoma.

Recurrent disease

MIBG therapy has been used for children with recurrent stage 4 neuroblastoma after previous treatment with chemotherapy and high dose chemotherapy. Of the 36 patients treated by the Amsterdam group, complete remission could be obtained and considerable prolongation of life was achieved but there were no long-term survivors after 4.5 years [169]. The palliative effect is considerable as there is no pain and minimal side effects. MIBG therapy has also been used following combination chemotherapy in relapsed or resistant neuroblastoma [164].

Differentiating therapy and neuroblastoma

When neuroblastoma cell lines are exposed to trans-retinoic acid or cis-retinoic acid *in vitro*, they exhibit decreased proliferation, decreased expression of the *MYCN* oncogene, and morphologic differentiation [170–172]. Cis-retinoic acid was chosen for clinical study in view of its lower toxicity and more favourable pharmacokinetics. Cis-retinoic acid has higher peak levels and much longer half-life when compared with Al-tran-retinoic acid and the levels are maintained consistently throughout course of treatment [173].

In the first clinical study, 13-cis retinoic acid was administered at 100 mg/m²/day in 28 patients with advanced refractory neuroblastoma patients. Only two patients demonstrated positive clinical response [174]. However, a phase I study of 13-cis-RA using an intermittent schedule, with two equally divided doses being given daily for 2 weeks followed by 2 weeks of rest period, reported responses in four out of 10 evaluable patients. This study also confirmed the maximum tolerated dose of 13-cis-RA to be 160 mg/m^2/day in two divided doses. The dose-limiting toxicities were hypercalcemia and a combination of skin, gastrointestinal, and hematological toxicities [175]. This study also confirmed that 13-cis-RA is well tolerated in children following HDT and has a possible role in a minimal residual setting.

In the ENSG study conducted from 1989 to 1997, patients with stage 3 and stage 4 neuroblastoma were randomized to receive either low dose daily cis-retinoic acid (0.75 mg/kg – approximately 22.5 mg/m^2) or placebo after completion of therapy. Maximum duration of retinoid therapy was 4 years or until relapse. This study did not show any significant benefit of cis-retinoic acid given in this schedule [176]. In the CCG study, 13-cis-RA was given intermittently for two out of every four weeks at a higher dose of 160 mg/m^2 in two divided doses.

• The EFS at three years was significantly better among the 130 patients who were assigned to receive 13-cis-RA compared with 128 patients assigned to receive no further therapy (46% vs 29%) [123] and the effect was maintained at 5 years [124].

• The main difference in the CCG and ENSG study was the dose and schedule used.

• Other differences, which may have influenced the outcome, include the later start of the 13-cis-RA in the European trial (median of 341 days from diagnosis), compared with an average of 290 days in the CCG study.

• Beginning 13-cis-RA relatively soon after cytotoxic therapy, before tumor cells can begin to grow, may be critical for this agent to be most effective. The greater efficacy of 13-cis-RA against minimal disease (compared with a larger tumor burden) is supported by the fact that the CCG study showed that the most significant effect of the 13-cis-RA was in children in apparent complete remission, with no significant difference seen when the analysis was restricted to those in partial remission [177].

Based on the CCG study 13-cis-RA is now considered standard therapy for high-risk neuroblastoma. However, there have been no randomized studies determining if six courses is the optimal duration of treatment. Furthermore, substantial interindividual variation in pharmacokinetics have been demonstrated and significantly lower plasma levels if the 13-cis-RA is administered after opening the capsules [178].

Neuroblastoma in infants

Although infants with neuroblastoma generally have a more benign clinical course, there are subsets of infants who can have aggressive disease and poor outcome. It is therefore of paramount importance to define risk groups and stratify treatment based on that. This would minimize therapy for patients with low risk tumors, improve therapy for patients with intermediate risk, and

---

Box 12.10 Key facts – neuroblastoma in infants.

• *MYCN* amplification is a major prognostic factor – 85% survival without amplification compared with 25% survival with *MYCN* amplification.

• The concept of stage 4S has been enlarged to include patients with an unresectable (stage 3), *MYCN* non-amplified primary tumor and metastases excluding those to the lung, central nervous system, and bone.

• Metastatic *MYCN* non-amplified infants require no chemotherapy or only a short course.

• Regression of unresectable *MYCN* non-amplified neuroblastoma has been documented in about 50% of patients.

• Infants with *MYCN*-amplified neuroblastoma should be treated as high-risk disease on the same protocol as children with stage M over 18 months of age.

• Pan genomic analysis on all infants with neuroblastoma may confirm the suggestion that those tumors with whole-chromosome copy number gains without segmental alterations require no therapy including surgery.

---

improve survival for patients with high-risk disease [179] (Box 12.10).

Incidence

The incidence of neuroblastoma in infants is higher than clinically apparent. Neuroblastoma (*in situ* neuroblastoma) were found incidentally in infants who died of unrelated causes at a much higher frequency than clinically evident tumors [180]. With the common use of ultrasound during pregnancy, there are more reported cases of perinatal neuroblastoma.

• These patients have low stage disease, *MYCN* non-amplified tumors and predominantly adrenal origin.

• A period of observation is important as they could regress spontaneously [181, 182].

• Analysis of an Italian neuroblastoma registry on antenatally detected neuroblastoma confirmed that most cases had good biology tumors and only those with unfavourable features should undergo surgical resection [183].

Screening for raised urinary catecholamines also resulted in a higher detection rate for infant neuroblastoma without decrease in number in the later years and in their natural course, these tumors would have spontaneously regressed [184].

Age cut-off

Previous studies have shown that infants under the age of 1 year have a more favourable prognosis than children over 1 year old [185]. Historically, the age of 1 year was considered for risk stratification and prognostication. However, two studies observed that children between the age of 12 and 18 months had comparable survival to those under the age of 1 year provided the tumor was not *MYCN* amplified [46, 186].

• Further analysis of the POG and CCG data on 3666 patients confirmed that patients less than 460 days old had a 4-year EFS of 82% compared with 42% for those over 460 days [82]. Graphical analysis revealed the continuous nature of prognostic contribution of age to outcome.

• Separate analysis of German data concurred with this [187]. Analysis of non-COG patients within the INRG cohort supports the optimal age cut-off to be between 15 and 19 months and for future stratification will be accepted as 18 months (547 days) [18].

However, for patients with diploid, stage M, *MYCN* non-amplified tumor, the Task Force have elected to use the more conservative age cut-off of 12 months (365 days).

Treatment

SIOPEN have recently enlarged the concept of stage 4S to include those patients less than 12 months with an unresectable (stage 3), *MYCN* non-amplified primary tumor and metastases excluding those to the lung, central nervous system, and bone [188].

For treatment purposes infants can be divided into 4 broad groups:

(1) Patients with localized MYCN non-amplified disease. Surgery may be the only treatment necessary for L1 tumors. There is an excellent prognosis for L2 tumors when treated with surgery and a short course of chemotherapy. The GPOH has followed 'a wait and watch strategy' after confirmation of histology and biology of the tumor. In almost 50% of patients observed with gross disease, spontaneous regression was observed [189]. This suggests that chemotherapy may not be needed in the majority of patients.

(2) Patients with Stage 4/4S tumors without MYCN amplification without lung, central nervous system or bone metastases. These metastatic patients, with no radiological bone abnormalities have an excellent survival (>95%) with no therapy or one or a few courses of carboplatin/etoposide to treat life- or organ-threatening symptoms [188].

(3) Patients with stage 4 disease without MYCN amplification with lung, central nervous system, or bone metastases. These patients have an excellent survival (OS>95%) with only four courses of chemotherapy (carboplatin /etoposide and cyclophosphamide/doxorubicin/vincristine) [188].

(4) Patients with MYCN amplification. In contrast, infants with MYCN-amplified neuroblastoma had a very poor prognosis (2 year EFS 29%) despite HDT but with relatively non-intensive induction therapy [190]. The consensus is that in the future this group should be treated on high-risk protocols, similar to children over the age of 1 year with stage 4 disease (chemotherapy, surgery, radiotherapy, high dose chemotherapy, differentiation therapy).

In the future, therapy for infants can be guided by additional genetic features. The presence of 11q aberration in MS patients may require therapy, even if there are no symptoms. The presence of hyperdiploidy in *MYCN* non-amplified metastatic patients between 12 and 18 months may indicate that HDT is not required for cure. Further developments and the ability to undertake pan genomic analysis on all infants with neuroblastoma may confirm the suggestion that those tumors with whole-chromosome copy number gains without segmental alterations require no therapy and this may include no surgery [63].

Neuroblastoma in adolescents

Neuroblastoma is rare beyond 5 years. Only 3% of neuroblastoma cases occur over the age of 10 years. Survival of patients under and over the age of 6 years was analyzed in a retrospective study from 1975 to 1992. Children over the age of 6 years tended to have *MYCN* non-amplified tumors. The patients also had an indolent course [191]. In another retrospective study, the presentation, biologic features, and outcome of adolescent and adult patients with neuroblastoma were compared to childhood neuroblastoma. Sixteen patients were identified over the age of 13 years (13–33 years). Less than 50% patients had raised urinary catecholamines and none of the six patients tested had *MYCN* amplification. Several of these patients had long courses from diagnosis to death, with multiple recurrences and/or chronic, persistent disease suggesting different biology and behaviour [192]. Similar conclusions of a slowly progressive disease have been demonstrated in other studies [193, 194] (Box 12.11).

It is envisaged that in the future the genetic profile of 'adolescent neuroblastoma' can be defined. A more recent study concluded that high-dose chemotherapy and surgery can achieve a minimal disease state in over 50% of older neuroblastoma patients. Local RT, and cis-retinoic acid, may improve the poor prognosis of these patients [195]. Myeloablative therapy probably has a role. Currently, proposals are in place to assess the role of

---

Box 12.11 Key facts neuroblastoma – adolescent neuroblastoma.

• Of patients with neuroblastoma 3% are above 10 years of age.

• Patients tend to have failure to achieve a complete response.

• Slow progression.

• Very poor survival.

• Poor survival for localized L2 unresectable disease.

• Histology – ganglioneuroblastoma – nodular, undifferentiated or poorly differentiated.

• Low frequency of *MYCN* amplification.

• High frequency 11q aberration.

• 'Adolescent' neuroblastoma probably occurs in younger children.

MIBG therapy in these patients as part of a COG–SIOPEN joint study.

Opsoclonus–myoclonus syndrome (OMS)/ dancing eye syndrome

OMS or dancing eye syndrome consists of opsoclonus (rapid multi-directional conjugate eye movements), a movement disorder characterized by a jerky (sometimes myoclonic) ataxia and behavioural change, consisting of irritability usually with sleep disturbance. There is great variability and not all features are necessarily present together [196].

• Patients with OMS and neuroblastoma generally have a low stage and low risk disease and have an excellent oncological prognosis.

• Many patients may not secrete catecholamines [197] and may not show MIBG uptake.

• There is predominance of paraspinal tumors [198].

• Over 90% of patients have favourable histology [199] and the majority have ganglioneuroblastoma intermixed histology with lymphoid infiltration, which possibly leads to favourable outcome [200].

• Unfavourable prognostic factors such as *MYCN* amplification have only rarely been found in patients with OMS [201].

However, many patients may experience significant amount of late neurological impairment and may have persistent issues with speech delay, cognitive deficits, motor delay, and behavioural problems [198, 202].

• Neurological outcome seems unrelated to the treatment of neuroblastoma [203].

• OMS is seen in 2–3% of patients with neuroblastoma typically between the ages of one and three years [202].

• Some studies suggest that in about 50% of patients with OMS, a neuroblastoma will be detected [204].

In the United Kingdom, a prospective study of 25% of cases of OMS had a detectable neuroblastoma tumor. There was considerable variation in the imaging protocols used to exclude neuroblastoma [205]. However, investigation using thin-cut CT of the thorax and abdomen detected a neuroblastoma tumor in over 80% of patients with OMS. One hypothesis is that very a large proportion of patients with OMS (possibly all) has at one stage had a neuroblastoma and the tumor has regressed in a substantial proportion. Studies have found that cerebrospinal fluid (CSF) B-cell expansion is characteristic of OMS [206]. It is thought that an immune-mediated mechanism is responsible for the symptoms of OMS, specifically that the T-cell dependent response to tumor-associated antigens leads to subsequent B-cell activation and antibody production [204].

Therapy should be directed separately for the neuroblastoma and OMS. Surgery is often the main stay of treatment for neuroblastoma for the majority of patients. Decision to give chemotherapy depends on the INRG group of the primary tumor. Occasional spontaneous resolution of symptoms in OMS may

occur, but therapy directed at immunosupression is usually needed. There are no large therapeutic studies in OMS. A number of therapeutic approaches may been described including the use of various steroids, including pulses [207], ACTH, immunoglobulins, azathioprine, rituximab [208], plasmapheresis [209], and cyclophosphamide, either given alone or in combination. Therapy with rituximab shows promise. However, there is no objective data demonstrating that these are effective in altering the outcome. Currently a COG study is in progress and one is in the final stages of planning by the Opsoclonus Myoclonus Collaboration Group (SIOPEN, GPOH and EPNS [European Paediatric Neurology Society]). In this, therapy is sequential. If there is not adequate response with dexamethasone, dexamethasone and cyclophosphamide is administered, and finally dexamethasone and rituximab is used if there is persistent lack of response. There is a major need for an international randomized study of OMS.

Late effects of treatment of neuroblastoma

Survivors of neuroblastoma fall into two broad groups:

(1) Patients treated with surgery alone or surgery with minimal chemotherapy.

In these patients, the late effects are minimal and are related to the site of the primary tumor and surgery. Study on long-term survivors of stage 4S neuroblastoma showed that the majority of patients had no clinically or radiologically significant sequelae but had some residual abnormalities from the tumor [210].

(2) High-risk patients treated with intensive chemotherapy including HDT, radiotherapy and surgery. For patients treated with intensive regimens, the late effects are related to effects of individual drugs and radiotherapy. Platinum compounds are used during induction and in some regimen as part of conditioning prior to high dose chemotherapy.

• A small study on 11 patients concluded that children receiving high-dose carboplatin as part of their conditioning regimen for ABMT have a high incidence of speech frequency hearing loss [211].

• A more recent study concluded that long-term neuroblastoma survivors, especially those with hearing loss, are at elevated risk for academic learning problems and psychosocial difficulties. The study also found strong concordance between parent-reported learning problems in the child and indications of distress in the child's self-reported quality of life [212].

As most neuroblastoma patients have an abdominal primary, children who receive radiation can demonstrate effects on fertility, chronic renal disease, and second neoplasms. Myelodysplasia/leukemia have been particularly reported with certain dose intense regimens [213]. From the Childhood Cancer Survivor Study, the cumulative incidence of second neoplasms at 20 years was 1.87%. There were 11 second neoplasms in 897 survivors [214]. Late relapses beyond 5 years have been reported [215].

Relapsed neuroblastoma

Neuroblastoma normally recurs in multiple sites after ABMT, particularly in areas of previous disease [153]. The commonest site for relapse after treatment for all stages of neuroblastoma is distant.

• After treatment of stage 4 neuroblastoma, a large Italian study confirmed that almost 60% of recurrences were at distant sites alone; 11% at primary sites and 30% had combined recurrences [216].

• For localized resectable patients, the incidence of local relapse alone was higher (31%), 43% at distant sites, and 25% of relapses were at local and distant sites [88].

• Intrinsic central nervous system (CNS) metastases (brain parenchyma or leptomeninges) are not uncommon and there is a trend towards increasing recognition in recent years. CNS metastases were documented in 16% of children in a retrospective study which assessed CT scans, MRI scans, CSF cytologies and autopsy records [217].

• A large retrospective study assessed the rate of CNS recurrence over a 15 year period (1985–2000). The risk of CNS recurrence was 8.0% at 3 years, with no significant change in risk over the 15-year period [218].

Treatment after relapsed neuroblastoma depends on stage of disease and previous treatment. For patients with low and intermediate risk and patients with local relapse, there are very good curative options using further therapies with surgery, chemotherapy, and radiotherapy. However, for patients with aggressively treated high-risk diseases, long-term disease control is very challenging.

New therapeutic approaches

The optimum development pathway is that agents are sequentially evaluated in Phase I then II studies, followed by inclusion in studies at first relapse or refractory setting, and progressing to evaluation in a randomized Phase III study. Between 1990 and 2007 there were only four new agents which entered the clinic: topotecan, irinotecan, temozolomide, and ^{131}I-MIBG. An exciting era is about to commence where there are potentially a number of very useful compounds which may become available, some of which target the underlying mechanisms that drive neuroblastoma.

Comparison of the results of different Phase II studies in neuroblastoma has been difficult due to inconstancies in the population of patients entered, endpoints, and response measurements. The INRG Task Force has created committee to establish international agreed criteria.

Topotecan–Irinotecan combinations

Topotecan and irinotecan [104, 219] have been shown to have single agent activity in neuroblastoma. Phase II studies have shown that combination therapies with topotecan–cyclophosphamide–etoposide and topotecan–etoposide have tolerable toxicity and encouraging responses [220, 221]. An Italian study found a 64% response rate with a combination of topotecan, vincristine and doxorubicin in relapsed and resistant neuroblastoma patients [116]. Temozolomide has shown activity in phase II study in relapsed and refractory neuroblastoma [222] and the irinotecan and temozolomide combination has shown tumor regression in 9/19 patients with refractory disease and 3/17 patients with relapsed disease [223]. A 10-day schedule of irinotecan–temozolomide has been studied [224]. However, a 5-day regime was found to have activity comparable with a 10-day irinotecan schedule in relapsed rhabdomyosarcoma [225]. Therefore, a 5-day temozolomide–irinotecan regimen, which has a number of practical advantages, is being taken forward. However, none of these combinations have been evaluated in randomized Phase II studies and the relative benefits in terms of activity and toxicity have not been determined.

Chemotherapy agents
ABT-751, an oral antimitotic agent that inhibits polymerization of microtubules, is being explored in neuroblastoma [226, 227].

Chemotherapy potentiating agents: bortezomib
Bortezomib is a selective and reversible inhibitor of the 26S proteasome that modulates cell-signalling molecules leading to apoptosis. It shows potent antitumor activity *in vitro* and *in vivo* against neuroblastoma cell lines. Furthermore there appears to be synergy with chemotherapeutic agents, including doxorubicin [228, 229].

Angiogenesis inhibitors
Angiogenesis is an attractive new target for neuroblastoma treatment [230]. Studies have shown that increased vascularity of tumors correlates with widely disseminated disease and poor survival [231, 232]. Also higher levels of pro-angiogenic factors such as VEGF-A, VEGF-B, bFGH, Ang-2 transforming growth factor alfa (TGF-alpha), and platelet-derived growth factor A (PDGF-A) were found in advanced stage disease compared with low stage diseases [233]. Therefore antiangiogenic therapy is a potential therapeutic option and preclinical studies have shown some promise [234].

PARP inhibitors
Recent evidence suggests that PARP inhibitors increase the efficacy of temozolomide and irinotecan [235].

Targeted delivery of radionucleotides
As discussed earlier, MIBG therapy has been previously shown to be effective in achieving short-term disease control in patients with relapsed neuroblastoma [169]. Myelosuppression was the main dose limiting toxicity when multiple MIBG doses were given [236, 237]. A phase I escalation study of MIBG therapy with myeloablative chemotherapy and autologous bone marrow

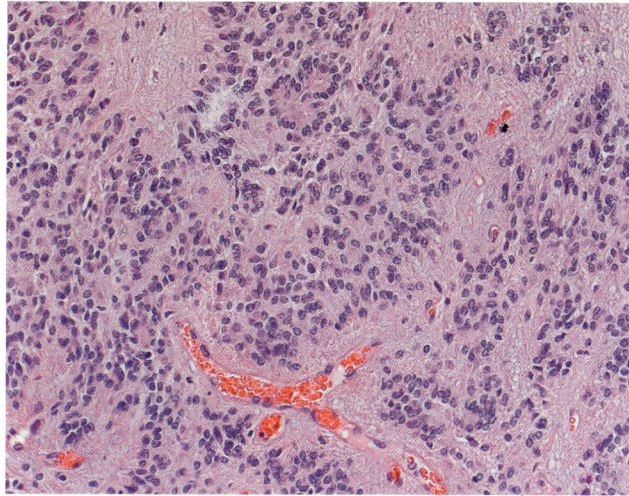

Plate 3.1 Pathology image demonstrating rosette formation.

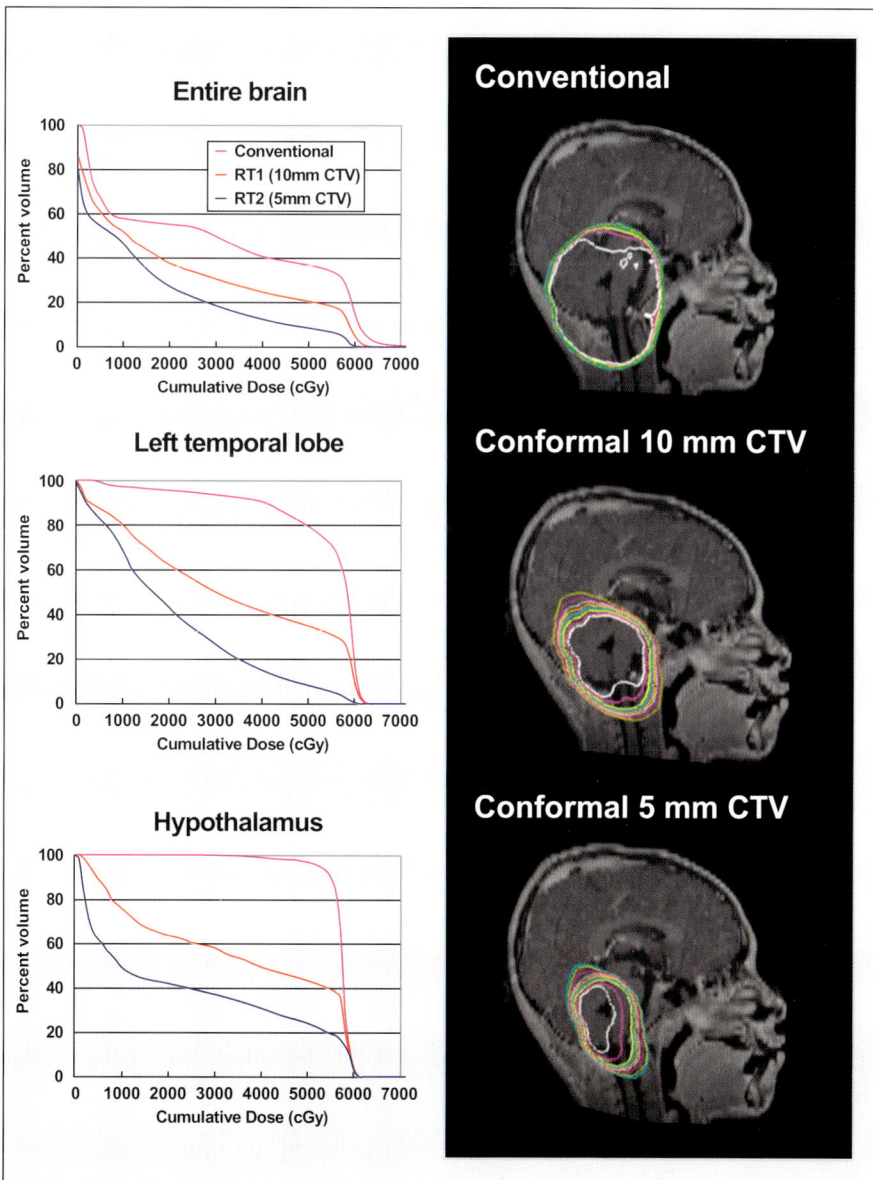

Plate 3.2 Dosimetry differences based on clinical target volume (CTV) margins.

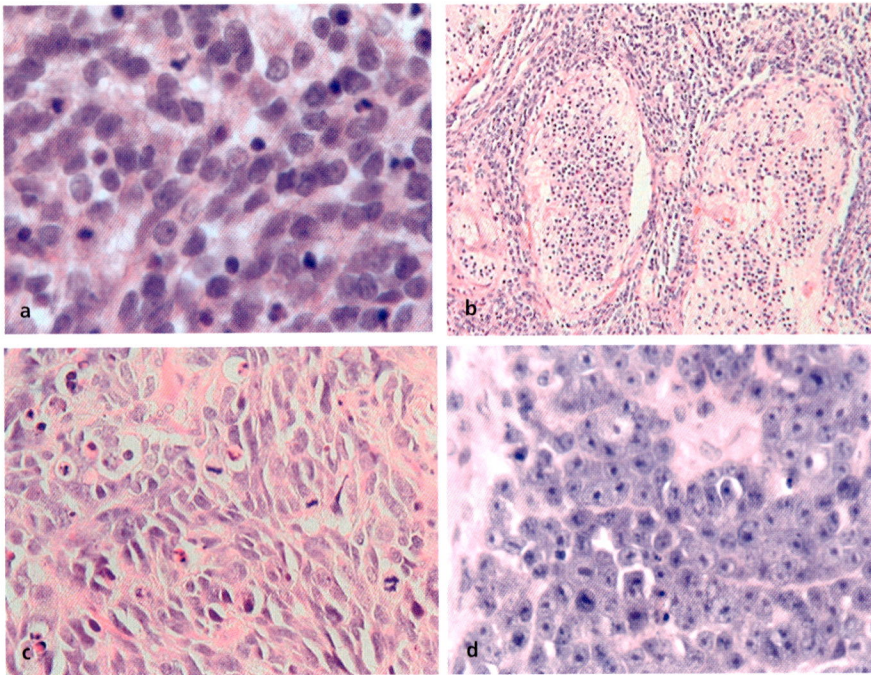

Plate 4.1 Medulloblastoma histopathological variants. a, The classic medulloblastoma consists of uniform densely packed cells with round nuclei (×400). b, The desmoplastic/nodular medulloblastoma contains nodules of neurocytic cells and internodular desmoplastic regions of more pleomorphic cells with polyhedral nuclei (×40). c, Pleomorphic nuclei molded to one another in a paving-stone pattern and abundant mitotic figures characterize the anaplastic variant (×120). d, Such cells are also seen in the large cell medulloblastoma, which also contain groups of large cells with a single nuceolus (×120). All hematoxylin & eosin. (Pictures courtesy of Dr David Ellison, MD, PhD.)

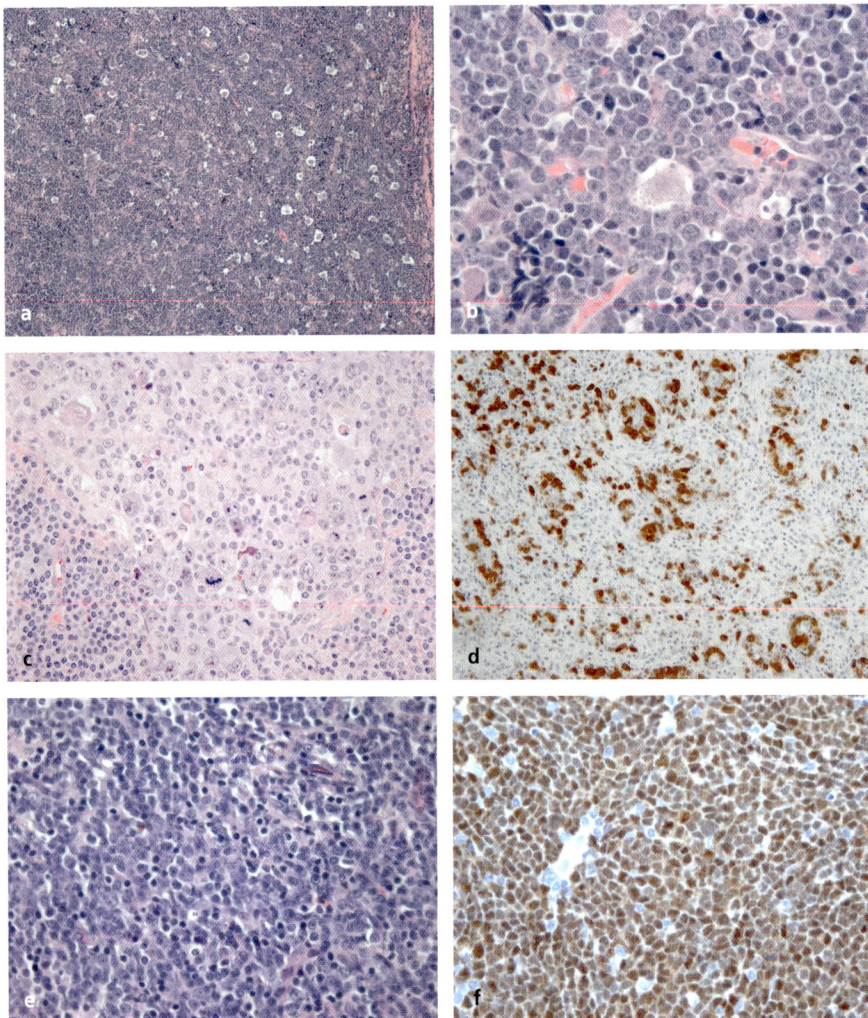

Plate 9.1 Histologic and immunophenotypical analysis of pediatric non-Hodgkin lymphoma. a, Burkitt's lymphoma: a low-power view of a lymph node involved by Burkitt's lymphoma demonstrating numerous tangible body macrophages conferring the 'starry sky appearance' (×50, hematoxylin & eosin stain). b, High-power view of the same specimen as (a). A vesicular chromatin and a relatively monomorphic pattern is evident. Burkitt lymphoma cells have a scant cytoplasm and prominent nucleoli (×600, hematoxylin & eosin stain). c, Anaplastic large cell lymphoma (ALCL): classic variant of anaplastic large-cell lymphoma with numerous large tumor cells including multinucleated and wreath-like forms (×400, hematoxylin & eosin stain). d, ALCL: classic pattern of anaplastic lymphoma kinase (ALK) staining of an ALCL with a t(2; 5) containing tumor with nuclear and cytoplasmic staining (×20, anti-ALK immunohostochemical stain). e, Precursor T-lymphoblastic lymphoma. Lymph node is completely infiltrated by blast cells with minimal cytoplasm, inconspicuous nucleoli and fine chromatin (×400, hematoxylin & eosin stain). f, Precursor T-lymphoblastic lymphoma. The panel shows diffuse effacement of lymph node architecture by an infiltrate of blast cells with minimal cytoplasm and typical intense staining with anti-TdT antibody (×400, anti-TdT immunohistochemical stain).

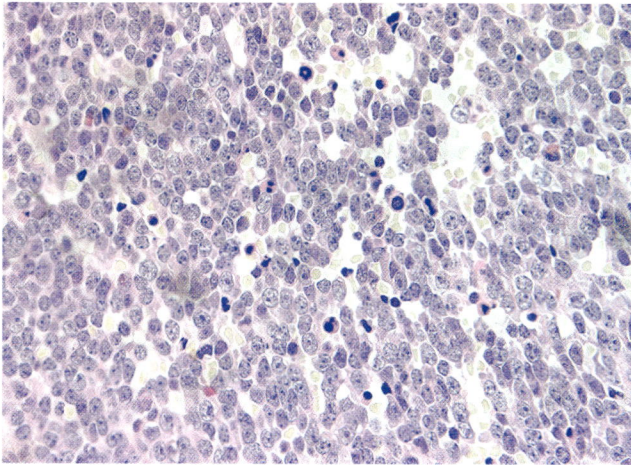

Plate 12.1 Undifferentiated neuroblastoma.

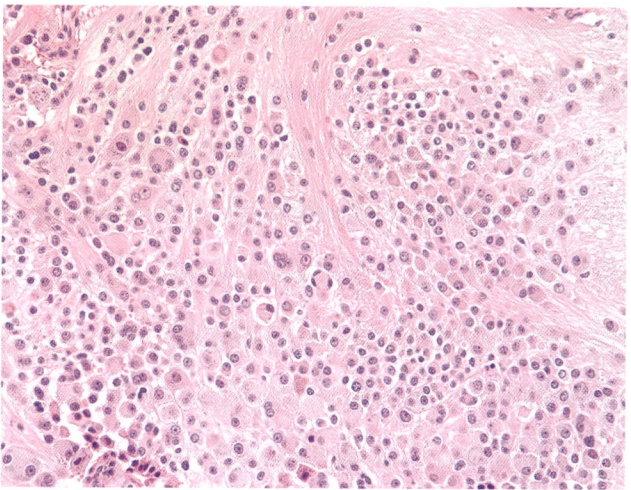

Plate 12.2 Differentiating neuroblastoma.

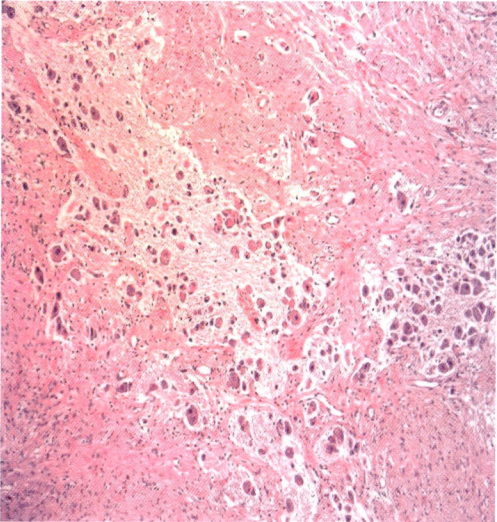

Plate 12.3 Ganglioneuroblastoma (intermixed).

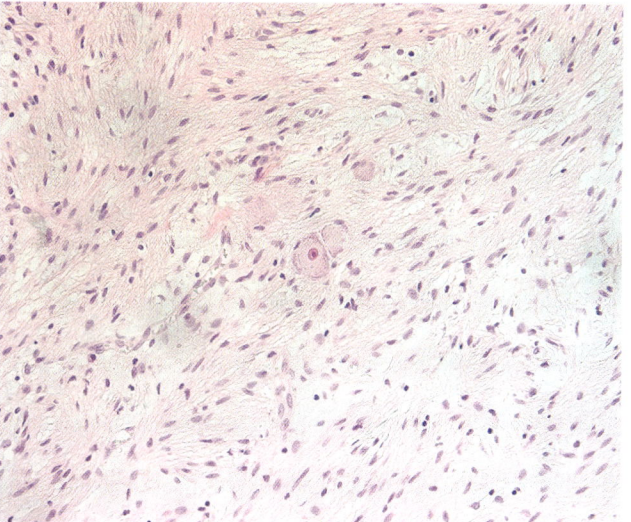

Plate 12.4 Ganglioneuroma.

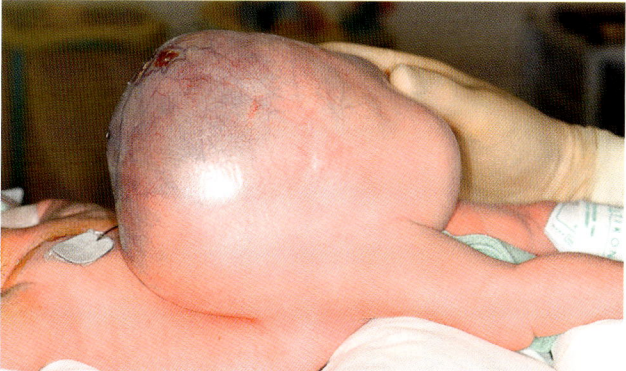

Plate 17.1 Neonatal sacrococcygeal teratoma (Altman Type I).

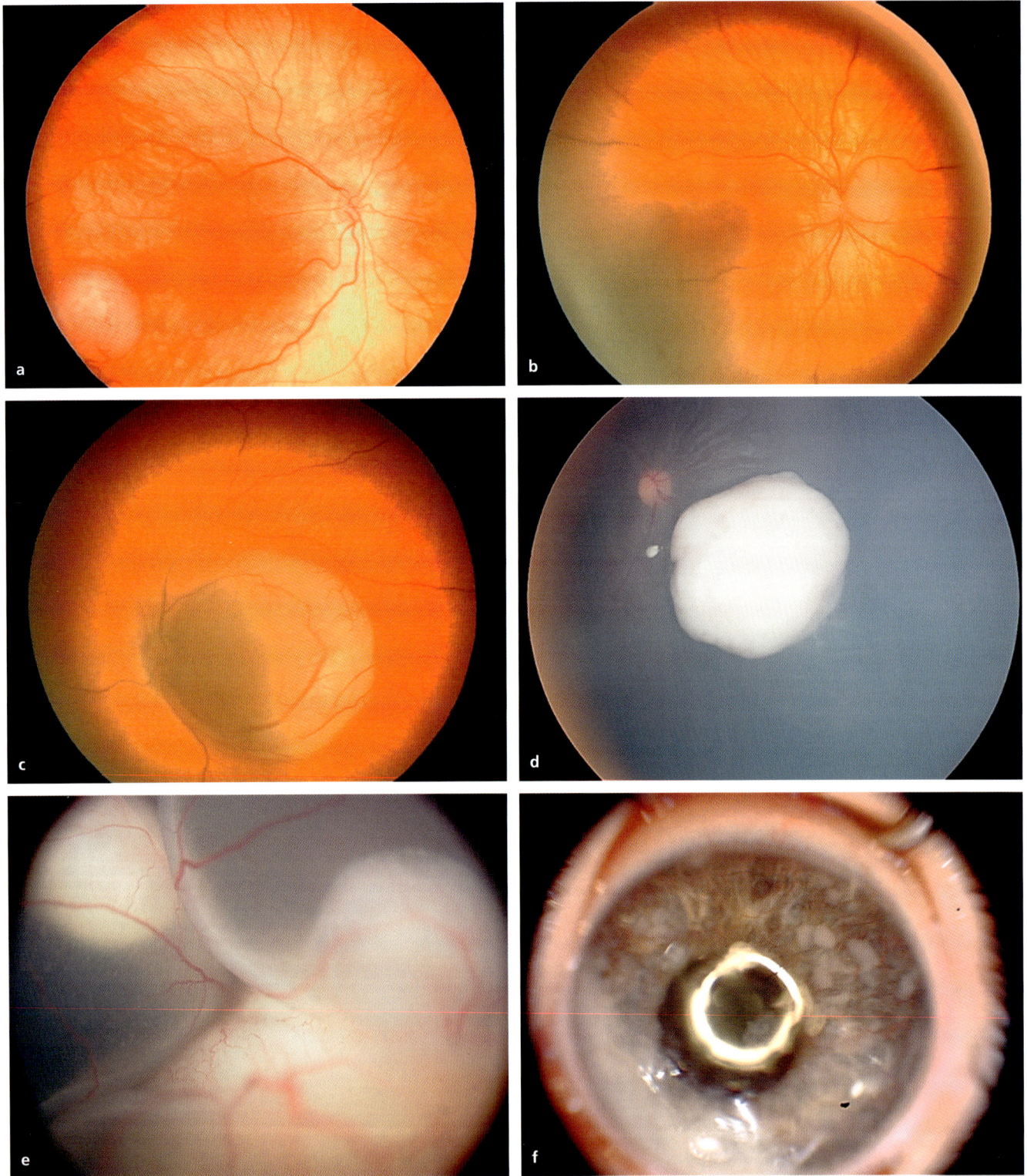

Plate 18.1 Retinoblastoma as visualized by retinography (a–e) and indirect ophthalmoscopy (f) as examples of the ABC Grouping System for retinoblastoma. The Figure designations denote the equivalent description from the ABD Grouping System.

rescue has shown this to be feasible, with a response rate of 31% and survival of 58% for resistant disease [238]. Current studies are exploring a combination of MIBG treatment with radiosensitizers such as topotecan and irinotecan. Combination of MIBG with topotecan has been found to have acceptable toxicity in an early European study [239]. In the future no carrier added MIBG may increase the therapeutic index [240].

Immunotherapy

GD2-targeted therapies using various monoclonal antibodies are currently being assessed in minimal residual disease in high-risk neuroblastoma [241].It has been shown that the chimeric human/murine anti-G(D2) monoclonal antibody (ch14.18) can induce lysis of neuroblastoma cells by antibody-dependent cellular cytotoxicity and complement-dependent cytotoxicity [242]. Most recent developments include the development of humanized antibodies linked to IL2 [243].

There is recent evidence from the Children's Oncology Group of North America clinical trial showing that chimeric anti-GD2 antibody ch14.18 combined with GMCSF and IL2 improves the EFS by 20% for high risk neuroblastoma patients when given in CR or VGPR after intensive induction and consolidation therapy [244]. This is the first time that immunotherapy has been shown to improve EFS in neuroblastoma. Previous single arm studies have led to very inconclusive results. Immunotherapy with 14.18 antibody IL2 and GMCSF is associated with significant toxicity; therefore further well designed studies are needed to improve efficacy and reduce toxicity of immunotherapy.

Retinoids

Fenretinide is a synthetic retinoid and induces apoptosis in neuroblastoma cell lines. A phase I study in children with neuroblastoma showed manageable toxicity and 41/53 patients had stable disease for a median period of 23 months [245, 246]. Pharmacokinetics support once a day oral administration [247].

Molecularly targeted agents

These target the underlying mechanisms that drive neuroblastoma and include lestaurtinib (tyrosine kinase inhibitor CEP-701), aurora kinase inhibitor, ALK kinase inhibitor, IGFR1, and PI3 kinase inhibitor. Phase I studies are being planned for these agents or have just commenced.

Summary

Neuroblastoma is a fascinating tumor with a wide disease spectrum from spontaneous regression, differentiation, to aggressive behaviour. Consequently the treatment options vary from observation to intensive multimodality treatment regimens. Better understanding of the disease and worldwide collaborative studies tailoring therapies for different risk groups have resulted in a significant improvement in outcome. Developing novel therapies

based on a new understanding of the disease would give an encouraging outlook for future patients.

References

1 Stiller CA, Kroll ME, Eatock EM. Incidence of Childhood cancer 1991–2000. In Stiller CA (Ed.), Oxford: Oxford University Press, 2007: 23–106.
2 Ninane J. Neuroblastoma. In Plowman PN, Pinkerton CR (Eds), Paediatric Oncology: Clinical Practice and Controversies. London: Chapman and Hall, 1992: 51–77.
3 DuBois SG, London WB, Zhang Y, et al. Lung metastases in neuroblastoma at initial diagnosis: a report from the International Neuroblastoma Risk Group (INRG) project. Pediatr Blood Cancer 2008.
4 Madre C, Orbach D, Baudouin V, et al. Hypertension in childhood cancer: a frequent complication of certain tumor sites. J Pediatr Hematol Oncol 2006; 28: 659–64.
5 Kaste SC, McCarville MB. Imaging pediatric abdominal tumors. Semin Roentgenol 2008; 43: 50–9.
6 Meyer JS, Siegel MJ, Farooqui SO, Jaramillo D, Fletcher BD, Hoffer FA. Which MRI sequence of the spine best reveals bone-marrow metastases of neuroblastoma? Pediatr Radiol 200; 35: 778–85.
7 Lynn MD, Shapiro B, Sisson JC, et al. Portrayal of pheochromocytoma and normal human adrenal medulla by m-[123I]iodobenzylguanidine: concise communication. J Nucl Med 1984; 25: 436–40.
8 Boubaker A, Bischof DA. Nuclear medicine procedures and neuroblastoma in childhood. Their value in the diagnosis, staging and assessment of response to therapy. Q J Nucl Med 2003; 47: 31–40.
9 Kushner BH, Yeung HWD, Larson SM, Kramer K, Cheung NK. Extending positron emission tomography scan utility to high-risk neuroblastoma: fluorine-18 fluorodeoxyglucose positron emission tomography as sole imaging modality in follow-up of patients. J Clin Oncol 2001; 19: 3397–405.
10 Mason GA, Hart-Mercer J, Millar EJ, Strang LB, Wynne NA. Adrenaline-secreting neuroblastoma in an infant. Lancet 1957: 17; 273(6990): 322–5.
11 Tuchman M, Morris CL, Ramnaraine ML, Bowers LD, Krivit W. Value of random urinary homovanillic acid and vanillylmandelic acid levels in the diagnosis and management of patients with neuroblastoma: comparison with 24-hour urine collections. Pediatrics 1985; 75: 324–8.
12 Strenger V, Kerbl R, Dornbusch HJ, et al. Diagnostic and prognostic impact of urinary catecholamines in neuroblastoma patients. Pediatr Blood Cancer 2007; 48: 504–9.
13 Hann HW, Stahlhut MW, Evans AE. Source of increased ferritin in neuroblastoma: studies with concanavalin A-sepharose binding. J Natl Cancer Inst 1986; 76: 1031–3.
14 Hann HW, Evans AE, Siegel SE, et al. Prognostic importance of serum ferritin in patients with Stages III and IV neuroblastoma: the Childrens Cancer Study Group experience. Cancer Res 1985; 45: 2843–8.
15 Evans AE, D'Angio GJ, Propert K, Anderson J, Hann HW. Prognostic factor in neuroblastoma. Cancer 1987; 59: 1853–9.
16 Mora J, Gerald WL, Cheung NK. Evolving significance of prognostic markers associated with new treatment strategies in neuroblastoma. Cancer Lett 2003; 197: 119–24.

17 Park JR, London WB, Maris JM, et al. Prognostic markers of stage 3 neuroblastoma (NB): a report from the International Neuroblastoma Risk Group (INRG) project. J Clin Oncol 2008; 26[15(S)]: 541.

18 Cohn SL, Pearson AD, London WB, et al. The International Neuroblastoma Risk Group (INRG) classification system: an INRG Task Force report. J Clin Oncol 2009; 27: 289–97.

19 Quinn JJ, Altman AJ, Frantz CN. Serum lactic dehydrogenase, an indicator of tumor activity in neuroblastoma. J Pediatr 1980; 97: 89–91.

20 Kinumaki H, Takeuchi H, Ohmi K. Serum lactate dehydrogenase isoenzyme pattern in neuroblastoma. Eur J Pediatr 1976; 123: 83–7.

21 Shuster JJ, McWilliams NB, Castleberry R, et al. Serum lactate dehydrogenase in childhood neuroblastoma. A Pediatric Oncology Group recursive partitioning study. Am J Clin Oncol 1992; 15: 295–303.

22 Cooper EH, Pritchard J, Bailey CC, Ninane J. Serum neuron-specific enolase in children's cancer. Br J Cancer 1987; 56: 65–7.

23 Hann HW, Bombardieri E. Serum markers and prognosis in neuroblastoma: Ferritin, LDH and NSE. In Brodeur GM, Sawada T, Tsuchida Y, Voute PA, (Eds), Neuroblastoma. Amsterdam: Elsevier, 2000: 371–82.

24 Zeltzer PM, Marangos PJ, Evans AE, Schneider SL. Serum neuron-specific enolase in children with neuroblastoma. Relationship to stage and disease course. Cancer 1986; 57: 1230–4.

25 Schengrund CL, Repman MA, Shochat SJ. Ganglioside composition of human neuroblastomas. Correlation with prognosis. A Pediatric Oncology Group Study. Cancer 1985; 56: 2640–6.

26 Shochat SJ, Corbelletta NL, Repman MA, Schengrund CL. A biochemical analysis of thoracic neuroblastomas: a Pediatric Oncology Group study. J Pediatr Surg 1987; 22: 660–4.

27 Evans AE, D'Angio GJ, Randolph J. A proposed staging for children with neuroblastoma. Children's cancer study group A. Cancer 1971; 27: 374–8.

28 D'Angio GJ, Evans AE, Koop CE. Special pattern of widespread neuroblastoma with a favourable prognosis. Lancet 1971; 1(7708): 1046–9.

29 Hayes FA, Green A, Hustu HO, Kumar M. Surgicopathologic staging of neuroblastoma: prognostic significance of regional lymph node metastases. J Pediatr 1983; 102: 59–62.

30 Brodeur GM, Seeger RC, Barrett A, et al. International criteria for diagnosis, staging, and response to treatment in patients with neuroblastoma. J Clin Oncol 1988; 6: 1874–81.

31 Brodeur GM, Pritchard J, Berthold F, et al. Revisions of the international criteria for neuroblastoma diagnosis, staging, and response to treatment. J Clin Oncol 1993; 11: 1466–77.

32 Cecchetto G, Mosseri V, De BB, et al. Surgical risk factors in primary surgery for localized neuroblastoma: the LNESG1 study of the European International Society of Pediatric Oncology Neuroblastoma Group. J Clin Oncol 2005; 23: 8483–9.

33 Monclair T, Brodeur GM, Ambros PF, et al. The International Neuroblastoma Risk Group (INRG) staging system: an INRG Task Force report. J Clin Oncol 2009; 27: 298–303.

34 Beckwith JB, Martin RF. Observations on the histopathology of neuroblastomas. J Pediatr Surg 1968; 3: 106–10.

35 Hughes M, Marsden HB, Palmer MK. Histologic patterns of neuroblastoma related to prognosis and clinical staging. Cancer 1974; 34: 1706–11.

36 Shimada H, Chatten J, Newton WA, Jr, et al. Histopathologic prognostic factors in neuroblastic tumors: definition of subtypes of ganglioneuroblastoma and an age-linked classification of neuroblastomas. J Natl Cancer Inst 1984; 73: 405–16.

37 Joshi VV, Cantor AB, Altshuler G, et al. Age-linked prognostic categorization based on a new histologic grading system of neuroblastomas. A clinicopathologic study of 211 cases from the Pediatric Oncology Group. Cancer 1992; 69: 2197–211.

38 Joshi VV, Cantor AB, Altshuler G, et al. Recommendations for modification of terminology of neuroblastic tumors and prognostic significance of Shimada classification. A clinicopathologic study of 213 cases from the Pediatric Oncology Group. Cancer 1992; 69: 2183–96.

39 Shimada H, Ambros IM, Dehner LP, Hata J, Joshi VV, Roald B. Terminology and morphologic criteria of neuroblastic tumors: recommendations by the International Neuroblastoma Pathology Committee 8. Cancer 1999; 86: 349–63.

40 Shimada H, Umehara S, Monobe Y, et al. International neuroblastoma pathology classification for prognostic evaluation of patients with peripheral neuroblastic tumors: a report from the Children's Cancer Group. Cancer 2001; 92: 2451–61.

41 Peuchmaur M, d'Amore ES, Joshi VV, et al. Revision of the International Neuroblastoma Pathology Classification: confirmation of favorable and unfavorable prognostic subsets in ganglioneuroblastoma, nodular. Cancer 2003; 8: 2274–81.

42 Sano H, Bonadio J, Gerbing RB, et al. International neuroblastoma pathology classification adds independent prognostic information beyond the prognostic contribution of age. Eur J Cancer 2006; 42: 1113–9.

43 Kaneko Y, Kanda N, Maseki N, et al. Different karyotypic patterns in early and advanced stage neuroblastomas. Cancer Res 1987; 47: 311–8.

44 Look AT, Hayes FA, Nitschke R, McWilliams NB, Green AA. Cellular DNA content as a predictor of response to chemotherapy in infants with unresectable neuroblastoma. N Engl J Med 1984; 311: 231–5.

45 Look AT, Hayes FA, Shuster JJ, et al. Clinical relevance of tumor cell ploidy and N-myc gene amplification in childhood neuroblastoma: a Pediatric Oncology Group study. J Clin Oncol 1991; 9: 581–91.

46 George RE, London WB, Cohn SL, et al. Hyperdiploidy plus non-amplified MYCN confers a favorable prognosis in children 12 to 18 months old with disseminated neuroblastoma: a Pediatric Oncology Group study. J Clin Oncol 2005; 23: 6466–73.

47 Ladenstein R, Ambros IM, Potschger U, et al. Prognostic significance of DNA di-tetraploidy in neuroblastoma. Med Pediatr Oncol 2001; 36: 83–92.

48 Schneiderman J, London WB, Brodeur GM, Castleberry RP, Look AT, Cohn SL. Clinical significance of MYCN amplification and ploidy in favorable-stage neuroblastoma: a report from the Children's Oncology Group. J Clin Oncol 2008; 26: 913–8.

49 Schwab M, Varmus HE, Bishop JM, et al. Chromosome localization in normal human cells and neuroblastomas of a gene related to c-myc. Nature 1984; 308: 288–91.

50 Brodeur GM, Seeger RC, Schwab M, Varmus HE, Bishop JM. Amplification of N-myc in untreated human neuroblastomas correlates with advanced disease stage. Science 1984; 224: 1121–4.

51 Seeger RC, Brodeur GM, Sather H, et al. Association of multiple copies of the N-myc oncogene with rapid progression of neuroblastomas. N Engl J Med 1985; 313: 1111–6.

52 Moreau LA, McGrady P, London WB, et al. Does MYCN amplification manifested as homogeneously staining regions at diagnosis predict a worse outcome in children with neuroblastoma? A Children's Oncology Group study. Clin Cancer Res 2006; 12: 5693–7.

53 Brodeur GM, Hayes FA, Green AA, et al. Consistent N-myc copy number in simultaneous or consecutive neuroblastoma samples from sixty individual patients. Cancer Res 1987; 47: 4248–53.

54 Matthay KK, Perez C, Seeger RC, et al. Successful treatment of stage III neuroblastoma based on prospective biologic staging: a Children's Cancer Group study. J Clin Oncol 1998; 16: 1256–64.

55 Combaret V, Gross N, Lasset C, et al. Clinical relevance of CD44 cell surface expression and MYCN gene amplification in neuroblastoma. Eur J Cancer 1997; 33: 2101–5.

56 George RE, Variend S, Cullinane C, et al. Relationship between histopathological features, MYCN amplification, and prognosis: a UKCCSG study. United Kingdom Children Cancer Study Group. Med Pediatr Oncol 2001; 36: 169–76.

57 Squire JA, Thorner PS, Weitzman S, et al. Co-amplification of MYCN and a DEAD box gene (DDX1) in primary neuroblastoma. Oncogene 1995; 10: 1417–22.

58 Weber A, Imisch P, Bergmann E, Christiansen H. Coamplification of DDX1 correlates with an improved survival probability in children with MYCN-amplified human neuroblastoma. J Clin Oncol 2004; 22: 2681–90.

59 De PK, Pattyn F, Berx G, et al. Combined subtractive cDNA cloning and array CGH: an efficient approach for identification of overexpressed genes in DNA amplicons. Genomics 2004; 5: 11.

60 De PK, Speleman F, Combaret V, Lunec J, Board J, Pearson A, et al. No evidence for correlation of DDX1 gene amplification with improved survival probability in patients with MYCN-amplified neuroblastomas. J Clin Oncol 2005; 23: 3167–8.

61 Tang XX, Zhao H, Kung B, et al. The MYCN enigma: significance of MYCN expression in neuroblastoma. Cancer Res 2006; 66: 2826–33.

62 Schleiermacher G, Michon J, Huon I, et al. Chromosomal CGH identifies patients with a higher risk of relapse in neuroblastoma without MYCN amplification. Br J Cancer 2007; 97: 238–46.

63 Janoueix-Lerosey I, Schleiermacher G, Michels E, et al. Overall genomic pattern is a predictor of outcome in neuroblastoma. J Clin Oncol 2009; 26: 1026–33.

64 Brodeur GM, Sekhon G, Goldstein MN. Chromosomal aberrations in human neuroblastomas. Cancer 1977; 40: 2256–63.

65 Caron H. Allelic loss of chromosome 1 and additional chromosome 17 material are both unfavourable prognostic markers in neuroblastoma. Med Pediatr Oncol 1995; 24: 215–21.

66 Fong CT, Dracopoli NC, White PS, et al. Loss of heterozygosity for the short arm of chromosome 1 in human neuroblastomas: correlation with N-myc amplification. Proc Natl Acad Sci USA 1989; 86: 3753–7.

67 Attiyeh EF, London WB, Mosse YP, et al. Chromosome 1p and 11q deletions and outcome in neuroblastoma. N Engl J Med 2005; 53: 2243–53.

68 Rubie H, Delattre O, Hartmann O, et al. Loss of chromosome 1p may have a prognostic value in localised neuroblastoma: results of the French NBL 90 Study. Neuroblastoma Study Group of the Societe Francaise d'Oncologie Pediatrique (SFOP). Eur J Cancer 1997; 33: 1917–22.

69 Spitz R, Hero B, Westermann F, Ernestus K, Schwab M, Berthold F. Fluorescence in situ hybridization analyses of chromosome band 1p36 in neuroblastoma detect two classes of alterations. Genes Chrom Cancer 2002; 34: 299–305.

70 Guo C, White PS, Weiss MJ, et al. Allelic deletion at 11q23 is common in MYCN single copy neuroblastomas. Oncogene 1999; 18: 4948–57.

71 Spitz R, Hero B, Simon T, Berthold F. Loss in chromosome 11q identifies tumors with increased risk for metastatic relapses in localized and 4S neuroblastoma. Clin Cancer Res 2006; 12: 3368–73.

72 Lastowska M, Nacheva E, McGuckin A, et al. Comparative genomic hybridization study of primary neuroblastoma tumors. United Kingdom Children's Cancer Study Group. Genes Chrom Cancer 1997; 18: 162–9.

73 Bown N, Cotterill S, Lastowska M, et al. Gain of chromosome arm 17q and adverse outcome in patients with neuroblastoma. N Engl J Med 1999; 340: 1954–61.

74 Bown N. Neuroblastoma tumor genetics: clinical and biological aspects. J Clin Pathol 2001; 54: 897–910.

75 Bown N, Lastowska M, Cotterill S, et al. 17q gain in neuroblastoma predicts adverse clinical outcome. UK Cancer Cytogenetics Group and the UK Children's Cancer Study Group. Med Pediatr Oncol 2001; 36: 14–9.

76 Lastowska M, Cotterill S, Pearson AD, et al. Gain of chromosome arm 17q predicts unfavourable outcome in neuroblastoma patients. UK Children's Cancer Study Group and the UK. Cancer Cytogenetics Group. Eur J Cancer 1997; 33: 1627–33.

77 Spitz R, Hero B, Ernestus K, Berthold F. Gain of distal chromosome arm 17q is not associated with poor prognosis in neuroblastoma. Clin Cancer Res 2003; 9: 4835–40.

78 Mosse YP, Laudenslager M, Longo L, et al. Identification of ALK as a major familial neuroblastoma predisposition gene. Nature 2008; 455: 930–5.

79 Chen Y, Takita J, Choi YL, et al. Oncogenic mutations of ALK kinase in neuroblastoma. Nature 2008; 455: 971–4.

80 Kushner BH, Cheung NK. Neuroblastoma–from genetic profiles to clinical challenge. N Engl J Med 2005; 353: 2215–7.

81 Caron H, van Sluis P, de Kraker J, et al. Allelic loss of chromosome 1p as a predictor of unfavorable outcome in patients with neuroblastoma. N Engl J Med 1996; 334: 225–30.

82 London WB, Castleberry RP, Matthay KK, et al. Evidence for an age cutoff greater than 365 days for neuroblastoma risk group stratification in the Children's Oncology Group. J Clin Oncol 2005; 23: 6459–65.

83 Sawada T. Past and future of neuroblastoma screening in Japan. Am J Pediatr Hematol Oncol 1992; 14: 320–6.

84 Ajiki W, Tsukuma H, Oshima A, Kawa K. Effects of mass screening for neuroblastoma on incidence, mortality, and survival rates in Osaka, Japan. Cancer Causes Control 1998; 9: 631–6.

85 Woods WG, Tuchman M, Robison LL, et al. Screening for neuroblastoma is ineffective in reducing the incidence of unfavourable advanced stage disease in older children. Eur J Cancer 1997; 33: 2106–12.

86 Schilling FH, Spix C, Berthold F, et al. Neuroblastoma screening at one year of age. N Engl J Med 2002; 346: 1047–53.

87 Dobrovoljski G, Kerbl R, Strobl C, Schwinger W, Dornbusch HJ, Lackner H. False-positive results in neuroblastoma screening: the parents' view. J Pediatr Hematol Oncol 2003; 5: 14–8.

88 De BB, Mosseri V, Rubie H, et al. Treatment of localised resectable neuroblastoma. Results of the LNESG1 study by the SIOP Europe Neuroblastoma Group. Br J Cancer 2008; 99: 1027–33.

89 Simon T, Hero B, Benz-Bohm G, von SD, Berthold F. Review of image defined risk factors in localized neuroblastoma patients: results of the GPOH NB97 trial. Pediatr Blood Cancer 2008; 50: 965–9.

90 Kushner BH, Cheung NK, LaQuaglia MP, et al. Survival from locally invasive or widespread neuroblastoma without cytotoxic therapy. J Clin Oncol 1996; 14: 373–81.

91 Nickerson HJ, Matthay KK, Seeger RC, et al. Favorable biology and outcome of stage IV-S neuroblastoma with supportive care or minimal therapy: a Children's Cancer Group study. J Clin Oncol 2000; 18: 477–86.

92 Guglielmi M, De BB, Rizzo A, Federici S, et al. Resection of primary tumor at diagnosis in stage IV-S neuroblastoma: does it affect the clinical course? J Clin Oncol 1996; 14: 1537–44.

93 Castel V, Tovar JA, Costa E, et al. The role of surgery in stage IV neuroblastoma. J Pediatr Surg 2002; 37: 1574–8.

94 Kaneko M, Ohakawa H, Iwakawa M. Is extensive surgery required for treatment of advanced neuroblastoma? J Pediatr Surg 1997; 32: 1616–9.

95 Adkins ES, Sawin R, Gerbing RB, London WB, Matthay KK, Haase GM. Efficacy of complete resection for high-risk neuroblastoma: a Children's Cancer Group study. J Pediatr Surg 2004; 9: 931–6.

96 Haase GM, O'Leary MC, Ramsay NK, et al. Aggressive surgery combined with intensive chemotherapy improves survival in poor-risk neuroblastoma. J Pediatr Surg 1991; 26: 1119–23.

97 La Quaglia MP, Kushner BH, Heller G, Bonilla MA, Lindsley KL, Cheung NK. Stage 4 neuroblastoma diagnosed at more than 1 year of age: gross total resection and clinical outcome. J Pediatr Surg 1994; 29: 1162–5.

98 La Quaglia MP, Kushner BH, Su W, et al. The impact of gross total resection on local control and survival in high-risk neuroblastoma. J Pediatr Surg 2004; 39: 412–7.

99 Kuroda T, Saeki M, Honna T, Masaki H, Tsunematsu Y. Clinical significance of intensive surgery with intraoperative radiation for advanced neuroblastoma: does it really make sense? J Pediatr Surg 2003; 38: 1735–8.

100 von SD, Hero B, Berthold F. The impact of surgical radicality on outcome in childhood neuroblastoma. Eur J Pediatr Surg 2002; 12: 402–9.

101 Carli M, Green AA, Hayes FA. Therapeutic efficacy of single drugs for childhood neuroblastoma: a review. In Raybaud E, Clement R, Lebreuil G, Bernard JL (Eds), Excerpta Medica, 1982: 141–50.

102 de Kraker J, Pritchard J, Hartmann O, Ninane J. Single-agent ifosfamide in patients with recurrent neuroblastoma (ENSG study 2). European Neuroblastoma Study Group. Pediatr Hematol Oncol 1987; 4: 101–4.

103 Pinkerton CR, Lewis IJ, Pearson AD, Stevens MC, Barnes J. Carboplatin or cisplatin? Lancet 1989; 2(8655): 161.

104 Vassal G, Giammarile F, Brooks M, et al. A phase II study of irinotecan in children with relapsed or refractory neuroblastoma: a European cooperation of the Societe Francaise d'Oncologie Pediatrique (SFOP) and the United Kingdom Children Cancer Study Group (UKCCSG). Eur J Cancer 2008; 44: 2453–60.

105 Ninane J, Pritchard J, Malpas JS. Chemotherapy of advanced neuroblastoma: does adriamycin contribute? Arch Dis Child 1981; 56: 544–8.

106 Finklestein JZ, Klemperer MR, Evans A, et al. Multiagent chemotherapy for children with metastatic neuroblastoma: a report from Childrens Cancer Study Group. Med Pediatr Oncol 1979; 6: 179–88.

107 Hayes FA, Green AA, Casper J, Cornet J, Evans WE. Clinical evaluation of sequentially scheduled cisplatin and VM26 in neuroblastoma: response and toxicity. Cancer 1981; 48: 1715–8.

108 Shafford EA, Rogers DW, Pritchard J. Advanced neuroblastoma: improved response rate using a multiagent regimen (OPEC) including sequential cisplatin and VM-26. J Clin Oncol 1984; 2: 742–7.

109 Bernard JL, Philip T, Zucker JM, et al. Sequential cisplatin/VM-26 and vincristine/cyclophosphamide/doxorubicin in metastatic neuroblastoma: an effective alternating non-cross-resistant regimen? J Clin Oncol 1987; 5: 1952–9.

110 Cheung NV, Heller G. Chemotherapy dose intensity correlates strongly with response, median survival, and median progression-free survival in metastatic neuroblastoma. J Clin Oncol 1991; 9: 1050–8.

111 Pinkerton CR, Blanc Vincent MP, Bergeron C, Fervers B, Philip T. Induction chemotherapy in metastatic neuroblastoma–does dose influence response? A critical review of published data standards, options and recommendations (SOR) project of the National Federation of French Cancer Centres (FNCLCC). Eur J Cancer 2000; 36: 1808–15.

112 Pearson AD, Craft AW, Pinkerton CR, Meller ST, Reid MM. High-dose rapid schedule chemotherapy for disseminated neuroblastoma. Eur J Cancer 1992; 28A: 1654–9.

113 Pearson AD, Pinkerton CR, Lewis IJ, Imeson J, Ellershaw C, Machin D. High-dose rapid and standard induction chemotherapy for patients aged over 1 year with stage 4 neuroblastoma: a randomised trial. Lancet Oncol 2008; 9: 247–56.

114 Matthay KK. Chemotherapy for neuroblastoma: does it hit the target? Lancet Oncol 2008; 9: 195–6.

115 Kushner BH, Kramer K, LaQuaglia MP, Modak S, Yataghene K, Cheung NK. Reduction from seven to five cycles of intensive induction chemotherapy in children with high-risk neuroblastoma. J Clin Oncol 2004; 22: 4888–92.

116 Garaventa A, Luksch R, Biasotti S, et al. A phase II study of topotecan with vincristine and doxorubicin in children with recurrent/refractory neuroblastoma. Cancer 2003; 98: 2488–94.

117 Kreissman SG, Villablanca JG, Diller L, et al. Response and toxicity to a dose-intensive multi-agent chemotherapy induction regimen for high risk neuroblastoma (HR-NB): a Children's Oncology Group (COG A3973) study. J Clin Oncol 2007; 25[18(S)]: 9505.

118 McWilliams NB, Hayes FA, Green AA, et al. Cyclophosphamide/doxorubicin vs. cisplatin/teniposide in the treatment of children older than 12 months of age with disseminated neuroblastoma: a Pediatric Oncology Group Randomized Phase II study. Med Pediatr Oncol 1995; 24: 176–80.

119 Pritchard J, McElwain TJ, Graham-Pole J. High-dose melphalan with autologous marrow for treatment of advanced neuroblastoma. Br J Cancer 1982; 45: 86–94.

120 Philip T, Zucker JM, Bernard JL, et al. Improved survival at 2 and 5 years in the LMCE1 unselected group of 72 children with stage IV neuroblastoma older than 1 year of age at diagnosis: is cure possible in a small subgroup? J Clin Oncol 1991; 9: 1037–44.

121 August CS, Serota FT, Koch PA, et al. Treatment of advanced neuroblastoma with supralethal chemotherapy, radiation, and allogeneic or autologous marrow reconstitution. J Clin Oncol 1984; 2: 609–16.

122 Pritchard J, Cotterill SJ, Germond SM, Imeson J, De KJ, Jones DR. High dose melphalan in the treatment of advanced neuroblastoma: results of a randomised trial (ENSG-1) by the European

Neuroblastoma Study Group. Pediatr Blood Cancer 2005; 44: 348–57.

123 Matthay KK, Villablanca JG, Seeger RC, et al. Treatment of high-risk neuroblastoma with intensive chemotherapy, radiotherapy, autologous bone marrow transplantation, and 13-cis-retinoic acid. Children's Cancer Group. N Engl J Med 1999; 341: 1165–73.

124 Matthay KK, Reynolds CP, Seeger RC, et al. Long-term results for children with high-risk neuroblastoma treated on a randomized trial of myeloablative therapy followed by 13-cis-retinoic acid: a Children's Oncology Group Study. J Clin Oncol 2009; 27: 1003–17.

125 Berthold F, Boos J, Burdach S, et al. Myeloablative megatherapy with autologous stem-cell rescue versus oral maintenance chemotherapy as consolidation treatment in patients with high-risk neuroblastoma: a randomised controlled trial. Lancet Oncol 2005; 6: 649–58.

126 Pole JG, Casper J, Elfenbein G, et al. High-dose chemoradiotherapy supported by marrow infusions for advanced neuroblastoma: a Pediatric Oncology Group study. J Clin Oncol 1991; 9: 152–8.

127 Hartmann O, Benhamou E, Beaujean F, et al. Repeated high-dose chemotherapy followed by purged autologous bone marrow transplantation as consolidation therapy in metastatic neuroblastoma. J Clin Oncol 1987; 5: 1205–11.

128 Corbett R, Pinkerton R, Pritchard J, et al. Pilot study of high-dose vincristine, etoposide, carboplatin and melphalan with autologous bone marrow rescue in advanced neuroblastoma. Eur J Cancer 1992; 28A(8–9): 1324–8.

129 Gordon SJ, Pearson AD, Reid MM, Craft AW. Toxicity of single-day high-dose vincristine, melphalan, etoposide and carboplatin consolidation with autologous bone marrow rescue in advanced neuroblastoma. Eur J Cancer 1992; 28A(8–9): 1319–23.

130 Valteau-Couanet D, Benhamou E, Vassal G, et al. Consolidation with a busulfan-containing regimen followed by stem cell transplantation in infants with poor prognosis stage 4 neuroblastoma. Bone Marrow Transplant 2000; 25: 937–42.

131 Hartmann O, Valteau-Couanet D, Vassal G, et al. Prognostic factors in metastatic neuroblastoma in patients over 1 year of age treated with high-dose chemotherapy and stem cell transplantation: a multivariate analysis in 218 patients treated in a single institution. Bone Marrow Transplant 1999; 23: 789–95.

132 Villablanca JG, Matthay KK, Ramsay NK. Carboplatin, etoposide, melphalan, and local irradiation (CEMLI) with autologous bone marrow transplantation (ABMT) for high risk neuroblastoma. Proc Am Soc Clin Oncol 1995; 14: 440.

133 Ladenstein R, Philip T, Lasset C, et al. Multivariate analysis of risk factors in stage 4 neuroblastoma patients over the age of one year treated with megatherapy and stem-cell transplantation: a report from the European Bone Marrow Transplantation Solid Tumor Registry. J Clin Oncol 1998; 6: 953–65.

134 Ladenstein R, Potschger U, Hartman O, et al. 28 years of high-dose therapy and SCT for neuroblastoma in Europe: lessons from more than 4000 procedures. Bone Marrow Transplant 2008; 41 (Suppl 2): S118–27.

135 Philip T, Ladenstein R, Zucker JM, et al. Double megatherapy and autologous bone marrow transplantation for advanced neuroblastoma: the LMCE2 study. Br J Cancer 1993; 67: 119–27.

136 George RE, Li S, Medeiros-Nancarrow C, et al. High-risk neuroblastoma treated with tandem autologous peripheral-blood stem cell-supported transplantation: long-term survival update. J Clin Oncol 2006; 24: 2891–6.

137 Kreissman SG, Villablanca JG, Seeger RC, et al. A randomized phase III trial of myeloablative autologous peripheral blood stem cell (PBSC) transplant (ASCT) for high-risk neuroblastoma (HR-NB) employing immunomagnetic purged (P) verus unpurged (UP) PBSC: a Children's Oncology Group Study. J Clin Oncol 2008; 26[15S]: 541.

138 Matthay KK, Seeger RC, Reynolds CP, et al. Allogeneic versus autologous purged bone marrow transplantation for neuroblastoma: a report from the Childrens Cancer Group. J Clin Oncol 1994; 12: 2382–9.

139 Deacon JM, Wilson P, Steel GG. Radiosensitivity of neuroblastoma. Prog Clin Biol Res 1985; 175: 525–31.

140 Deacon JM, Wilson PA, Peckham MJ. The radiobiology of human neuroblastoma. Radiother Oncol 1985; 3: 201–9.

141 Jacobson GM, Sause WT, O'Brien RT. Dose response analysis of pediatric neuroblastoma to megavoltage radiation. Am J Clin Oncol 1984; 7: 693–7.

142 Jacobson HM, Marcus RB, Jr, Thar TL, Million RR, Graham-Pole JR, Talbert JL. Pediatric neuroblastoma: postoperative radiation therapy using less than 2000 rad. Int J Radiat Oncol Biol Phys 1983; 9: 501–5.

143 Kushner BH, O'Reilly RJ, Mandell LR, Gulati SC, LaQuaglia M, Cheung NK. Myeloablative combination chemotherapy without total body irradiation for neuroblastoma. J Clin Oncol 1991; 9: 274–9.

144 Wolden SL, Gollamudi SV, Kushner BH, et al. Local control with multimodality therapy for stage 4 neuroblastoma. Int J Radiat Oncol Biol Phys 2000; 46: 969–74.

145 Haas-Kogan DA, Fisch BM, Wara WM, et al. Intraoperative radiation therapy for high-risk pediatric neuroblastoma. Int J Radiat Oncol Biol Phys 2000; 47: 985–92.

146 Gillis AM, Sutton E, Dewitt KD, et al. Long-term outcome and toxicities of intraoperative radiotherapy for high-risk neuroblastoma. Int J Radiat Oncol Biol Phys 2007; 69: 858–64.

147 Paulino AC, Mayr NA, Simon JH, Buatti JM. Locoregional control in infants with neuroblastoma: role of radiation therapy and late toxicity. Int J Radiat Oncol Biol Phys 2002; 52: 1025–31.

148 Castleberry RP, Shuster JJ, Altshuler G, et al. Infants with neuroblastoma and regional lymph node metastases have a favorable outlook after limited postoperative chemotherapy: a Pediatric Oncology Group study. J Clin Oncol 1992; 10: 1299–304.

149 Matthay KK, Sather HN, Seeger RC, Haase GM, Hammond GD. Excellent outcome of stage II neuroblastoma is independent of residual disease and radiation therapy. J Clin Oncol 1989; 7: 236–44.

150 Castleberry RP, Kun LE, Shuster JJ, et al. Radiotherapy improves the outlook for patients older than 1 year with Pediatric Oncology Group stage C neuroblastoma. J Clin Oncol 1991; 95: 789–95.

151 Park JR, Villablanca JG, London WB, et al. Outcome of high-risk stage 3 neuroblastoma with myeloablative therapy and 13-cis-retinoic acid: a report from the Children's Oncology Group. Pediatr Blood Cancer 2009; 52: 44–50.

152 Rosen EM, Cassady JR, Frantz CN, et al. Improved survival in neuroblastoma using multimodality therapy. Radiother Oncol 1984; 2: 189–200.

153 Matthay KK, Atkinson JB, Stram DO, Selch M, Reynolds CP, Seeger RC. Patterns of relapse after autologous purged bone marrow

transplantation for neuroblastoma: a Childrens Cancer Group pilot study. J Clin Oncol 1993; 11: 2226–33.

154 Simon T, Hero B, Bongartz R, Schmidt M, Muller RP, Berthold F. Intensified external-beam radiation therapy improves the outcome of stage 4 neuroblastoma in children >1 year with residual local disease. Strahlenther Onkol 2006; 182: 389–94.

155 Haas-Kogan DA, Swift PS, Selch M, et al. Impact of radiotherapy for high-risk neuroblastoma: a Children's Cancer Group study. Int J Radiat Oncol Biol Phys 2003; 56: 28–39.

156 Paulino AC. Palliative radiotherapy in children with neuroblastoma. Pediatr Hematol Oncol 2003; 20: 111–7.

157 Nguyen NP, Sallah S, Ludin A, et al. Neuroblastoma producing spinal cord compression: rapid relief with low dose of radiation. Anticancer Res 2000; 20(6C): 4687–90.

158 Flandin I, Hartmann O, Michon J, et al. Impact of TBI on late effects in children treated by megatherapy for Stage IV neuroblastoma. A study of the French Society of Pediatric oncology. Int J Radiat Oncol Biol Phys 2006; 64: 1424–31.

159 Treuner J, Klingebiel T, Feine U, et al. Clinical experiences in the treatment of neuroblastoma with 131I-metaiodobenzylguanidine. Pediatr Hematol Oncol 1986; 3: 205–16.

160 Lashford LS, Lewis IJ, Fielding SL, et al. Phase I/II study of iodine 131 metaiodobenzylguanidine in chemoresistant neuroblastoma: a United Kingdom Children's Cancer Study Group investigation. J Clin Oncol 1992; 10: 1889–96.

161 Hoefnagel CA, De KJ, Valdes Olmos RA, Voute PA. 131I-MIBG as a first-line treatment in high-risk neuroblastoma patients. Nucl Med Commun 1994; 15: 712–7.

162 Hoefnagel CA, De KJ, Valdes Olmos RA, Voute PA. [131I]MIBG as a first line treatment in advanced neuroblastoma. Q J Nucl Med 1995; 39(4 Suppl 1): 61–4.

163 De KJ, Hoefnagel KA, Verschuur AC, van EB, van Santen HM, Caron HN. Iodine-131-metaiodobenzylguanidine as initial induction therapy in stage 4 neuroblastoma patients over 1 year of age. Eur J Cancer 2008; 44: 551–6.

164 Mastrangelo S, Tornesello A, Diociaiuti L, et al. Treatment of advanced neuroblastoma: feasibility and therapeutic potential of a novel approach combining 131-I-MIBG and multiple drug chemotherapy. Br J Cancer 2001; 4: 460–4.

165 Schmidt M, Simon T, Hero B, et al. Is there a benefit of 131 I-MIBG therapy in the treatment of children with stage 4 neuroblastoma? A retrospective evaluation of The German Neuroblastoma Trial NB97 and implications for The German Neuroblastoma Trial NB2004. Nuklearmedizin 2006; 45: 145–51.

166 Miano M, Garaventa A, Pizzitola MR, et al. Megatherapy combining I(131) metaiodobenzylguanidine and high-dose chemotherapy with haematopoietic progenitor cell rescue for neuroblastoma. Bone Marrow Transplant 2001; 27: 571–4.

167 Corbett R, Pinkerton R, Tait D, Meller S. [131I]metaiodobenzylguanidine and high-dose chemotherapy with bone marrow rescue in advanced neuroblastoma. J Nucl Biol Med 1991; 35: 228–31.

168 Matthay KK, Quach A, Huberty J, et al. Iodine-131–Metaiodobenzylguanidine Double Infusion With Autologous Stem-Cell Rescue for Neuroblastoma: a New Approach to Neuroblastoma Therapy Phase I Study. J Clin Oncol 2009; 27: 1020–5.

169 Voute PA, Hoefnagel CA, De KJ, Valdes OR, Bakker DJ, van de Kleij AJ. Results of treatment with 131 I-metaiodobenzylguanidine (131 I-MIBG) in patients with neuroblastoma. Future prospects of zetotherapy. Prog Clin Biol Res 1991; 366: 439–45.

170 Reynolds CP, Kane DJ, Einhorn PA, et al. Response of neuroblastoma to retinoic acid in vitro and in vivo. Prog Clin Biol Res 1991; 366: 203–11.

171 Sidell N, Altman A, Haussler MR, Seeger RC. Effects of retinoic acid (RA) on the growth and phenotypic expression of several human neuroblastoma cell lines. Exp Cell Res 1983; 148: 21–30.

172 Thiele CJ, Reynolds CP, Israel MA. Decreased expression of N-myc precedes retinoic acid-induced morphological differentiation of human neuroblastoma. Nature 1985; 313: 404–6.

173 Reynolds CP, Schindler PF, Jones DM, Gentile JL, Proffitt RT, Einhorn PA. Comparison of 13-cis-retinoic acid to trans-retinoic acid using human neuroblastoma cell lines. Prog Clin Biol Res 1994; 385: 237–44.

174 Finklestein JZ, Krailo MD, Lenarsky C, et al. 13-cis-retinoic acid (NSC 122758) in the treatment of children with metastatic neuroblastoma unresponsive to conventional chemotherapy: report from the Childrens Cancer Study Group. Med Pediatr Oncol 1992; 20: 307–11.

175 Villablanca JG, Khan AA, Avramis VI, et al. Phase I trial of 13-cis-retinoic acid in children with neuroblastoma following bone marrow transplantation. J Clin Oncol 1995;13: 894–901.

176 Kohler JA, Imeson J, Ellershaw C, Lie SO. A randomized trial of 13-Cis retinoic acid in children with advanced neuroblastoma after high-dose therapy. Br J Cancer 2000; 83: 1124–7.

177 Matthay KK, Reynolds CP. Is there a role for retinoids to treat minimal residual disease in neuroblastoma? Br J Cancer 2000; 83: 1121–3.

178 Veal GJ, Cole M, Errington J, et al. Pharmacokinetics and metabolism of 13-cis-retinoic acid (isotretinoin) in children with high-risk neuroblastoma – a study of the United Kingdom Children's Cancer Study Group. Br J Cancer 2007; 96: 424–31.

179 Friedman GK, Castleberry RP. Changing trends of research and treatment in infant neuroblastoma. Pediatr Blood Cancer 2007; 49(7 Suppl): 1060–5.

180 Beckwith JB, Perrin EV. In situ neuroblastomas: a contribution to the natural history of neural crest tumors. Am J Pathol 1963; 43: 1089–104.

181 Sauvat F, Sarnacki S, Brisse H, et al. Outcome of suprarenal localized masses diagnosed during the perinatal period: a retrospective multicenter study. Cancer 2002; 94: 2474–80.

182 Acharya S, Jayabose S, Kogan SJ, et al. Prenatally diagnosed neuroblastoma. Cancer 1997; 80: 304–10.

183 Granata C, Fagnani AM, Gambini C, et al. Features and outcome of neuroblastoma detected before birth. J Pediatr Surg 2000; 35: 88–91.

184 Woods WG. Screening for neuroblastoma: the final chapters. J Pediatr Hematol Oncol 2003; 25: 3–4.

185 Cotterill SJ, Pearson AD, Pritchard J, et al. Clinical prognostic factors in 1277 patients with neuroblastoma: results of The European Neuroblastoma Study Group 'Survey' 1982–1992. Eur J Cancer 2000; 36: 901–8.

186 Schmidt ML, Lal A, Seeger RC, et al. Favorable prognosis for patients 12 to 18 months of age with stage 4 nonamplified MYCN neuroblastoma: a Children's Cancer Group Study. J Clin Oncol 2005; 23: 6474–80.

187 London WB, Boni L, Simon T, et al. The role of age in neuroblastoma risk stratification: the German, Italian, and children's oncology group perspectives. Cancer Lett 2005; 228: 257–66.

188 De BB, Gerrard M, Boni L, et al. Excellent outcome with reduced treatment for infants with disseminated neuroblastoma without MYCN gene amplification. J Clin Oncol 2009; 27: 1020–5.

189 Hero B, Simon T, Spitz R, et al. Localized infant neuroblastomas often show spontaneous regression: results of the prospective trials NB95-S and NB97. J Clin Oncol 2008; 26: 1504–10.

190 Canete A, Gerrard M, Rubie H, et al. Poor survival for infants with MYCN-amplified metastatic neuroblastoma despite intensified treatment: The International Society of Paediatric Oncology European Neuroblastoma Experience. J Clin Oncol 2009; 27: 1034–40.

191 Blatt J, Gula MJ, Orlando SJ, Finn LS, Misra DN, Dickman PS. Indolent course of advanced neuroblastoma in children older than 6 years at diagnosis. Cancer 1995; 76: 890–4.

192 Franks LM, Bollen A, Seeger RC, Stram DO, Matthay KK. Neuroblastoma in adults and adolescents: an indolent course with poor survival. Cancer 1997; 79: 2028–35.

193 Gaspar N, Hartmann O, Munzer C, et al. Neuroblastoma in adolescents. Cancer 2003; 98: 349–55.

194 Conte M, Parodi S, De BB, et al. Neuroblastoma in adolescents: the Italian experience. Cancer 2006; 106: 1409–17.

195 Kushner BH, Kramer K, LaQuaglia MP, Modak S, Cheung NK. Neuroblastoma in adolescents and adults: the Memorial Sloan-Kettering experience. Med Pediatr Oncol 2003; 41: 508–15.

196 Kinsbourne M. Myoclonic encephalopathy of infants. J Neurol Neurosurg Psych 1963; 25: 226.

197 Mitchell WG, Snodgrass SR. Opsoclonus-ataxia due to childhood neural crest tumors: a chronic neurologic syndrome. J Child Neurol 1990; 5: 153–8.

198 Russo C, Cohn SL, Petruzzi MJ, de Alarcon PA. Long-term neurologic outcome in children with opsoclonus-myoclonus associated with neuroblastoma: a report from the Pediatric Oncology Group. Med Pediatr Oncol 1997; 28: 284–8.

199 Cooper R, Khakoo Y, Matthay KK, et al. Opsoclonus-myoclonus-ataxia syndrome in neuroblastoma: histopathologic features – a report from the Children's Cancer Group. Med Pediatr Oncol 2001; 36: 623–9.

200 Gambini C, Conte M, Bernini G, et al. Neuroblastic tumors associated with opsoclonus-myoclonus syndrome: histological, immunohistochemical and molecular features of 15 Italian cases. Virchows Arch 2003; 442: 555–62.

201 Hiyama E, Yokoyama T, Ichikawa T, et al. Poor outcome in patients with advanced stage neuroblastoma and coincident opsomyoclonus syndrome. Cancer 1994; 74: 1821–6.

202 Rudnick E, Khakoo Y, Antunes NL, et al. Opsoclonus-myoclonus-ataxia syndrome in neuroblastoma: clinical outcome and antineuronal antibodies – a report from the Children's Cancer Group Study. Med Pediatr Oncol 2001; 36: 612–22.

203 Plantaz D, Michon J, Valteau-Couanet D, et al. [Opsoclonus-myoclonus syndrome associated with non-metastatic neuroblastoma. Long-term survival. Study of the French Society of Pediatric Oncologists]. Arch Pediatr 2000; 7: 621–8.

204 Matthay KK, Blaes F, Hero B, et al. Opsoclonus myoclonus syndrome in neuroblastoma a report from a workshop on the dancing eyes syndrome at the advances in neuroblastoma meeting in Genoa, Italy, 2004. Cancer Lett 2005; 228: 275–82.

205 Pang KK, Lange B, De Souza C, Pike MG. Prospective evaluation of Dancing Eye Syndrome (opsoclonus-myoclonus) management and outcome in UK paediatric neurology centres. Dev Med Child Neurol 2006; 48(Supp 104): 38.

206 Pranzatelli MR, Travelstead AL, Tate ED, Allison TJ, Verhulst SJ. CSF B-cell expansion in opsoclonus-myoclonus syndrome: a biomarker of disease activity Mov Disord 2004; 19: 770–7.

207 Ertle F, Behnisch W, Al Mulla NA, et al. Treatment of neuroblastoma-related opsoclonus-myoclonus-ataxia syndrome with high-dose dexamethasone pulses. Pediatr Blood Cancer 2008; 50: 683–7.

208 Pranzatelli MR, Tate ED, Travelstead AL, et al. Rituximab (anti-CD20) adjunctive therapy for opsoclonus-myoclonus syndrome. J Pediatr Hematol Oncol 2006; 28: 585–93.

209 Armstrong MB, Robertson PL, Castle VP. Delayed, recurrent opsoclonus-myoclonus syndrome responding to plasmapheresis. Pediatr Neurol 2005; 33: 365–7.

210 Levitt GA, Platt KA, De BR, Sebire N, Owens CM. 4S neuroblastoma: the long-term outcome. Pediatr Blood Cancer 2004; 43: 120–5.

211 Parsons SK, Neault MW, Lehmann LE, et al. Severe ototoxicity following carboplatin-containing conditioning regimen for autologous marrow transplantation for neuroblastoma. Bone Marrow Transplant 1998; 22: 669–74.

212 Gurney JG, Tersak JM, Ness KK, Landier W, Matthay KK, Schmidt ML. Hearing loss, quality of life, and academic problems in long-term neuroblastoma survivors: a report from the Children's Oncology Group. Pediatrics 2007; 120: e1229–36.

213 Kushner BH, Cheung NK, Kramer K, Heller G, Jhanwar SC. Neuroblastoma and treatment-related myelodysplasia/leukemia: the Memorial Sloan-Kettering experience and a literature review. J Clin Oncol 1998; 6: 3880–9.

214 Neglia JP, Friedman DL, Yasui Y, et al. Second malignant neoplasms in five-year survivors of childhood cancer: childhood cancer survivor study. J Natl Cancer Inst 2001; 93: 618–29.

215 Cotterill SJ, Pearson AD, Pritchard J, Kohler JA, Foot AB. Late relapse and prognosis for neuroblastoma patients surviving 5 years or more: a report from the European Neuroblastoma Study Group 'Survey'. Med Pediatr Oncol 2001; 36: 235–8.

216 De BB, Nicolas B, Boni L, et al. Disseminated neuroblastoma in children older than one year at diagnosis: comparable results with three consecutive high-dose protocols adopted by the Italian Co-Operative Group for Neuroblastoma. J Clin Oncol 2003; 21: 1592–601.

217 Blatt J, Fitz C, Mirro J, Jr. Recognition of central nervous system metastases in children with metastatic primary extracranial neuroblastoma. Pediatr Hematol Oncol 1997; 14: 233–41.

218 Matthay KK, Brisse H, Couanet D, et al. Central nervous system metastases in neuroblastoma: radiologic, clinical, and biologic features in 23 patients. Cancer 2003; 98: 155–65.

219 Bomgaars LR, Bernstein M, Krailo M, et al. Phase II trial of irinotecan in children with refractory solid tumors: a Children's Oncology Group Study. J Clin Oncol 2007; 25: 4622–7.

220 Simon T, Langler A, Harnischmacher U, et al. Topotecan, cyclophosphamide, and etoposide (TCE) in the treatment of high-risk neuroblastoma. Results of a phase-II trial. J Cancer Res Clin Oncol 2007; 133: 653–61.

221 Simon T, Langler A, Berthold F, Klingebiel T, Hero B. Topotecan and etoposide in the treatment of relapsed high-risk neuroblastoma: results of a phase 2 trial. J Pediatr Hematol Oncol 2007; 29: 101–6.

222 Rubie H, Chisholm J, Defachelles AS, et al. Phase II study of temozolomide in relapsed or refractory high-risk neuroblastoma: a joint Societe Francaise des Cancers de l'Enfant and United Kingdom Children Cancer Study Group – New Agents Group Study. J Clin Oncol 2006; 24: 5259–64.

223 Kushner BH, Kramer K, Modak S, Cheung NK. Irinotecan plus temozolomide for relapsed or refractory neuroblastoma. J Clin Oncol 2006; 24: 5271–6.

224 Wagner LM, Crews KR, Iacono LC, et al. Phase I trial of temozolomide and protracted irinotecan in pediatric patients with refractory solid tumors. Clin Cancer Res 2004; 10: 840–8.

225 Mascarenhas l, Lyden ER, Breitfeld PP, et al. Randomized phase II window study of two schedules of irinotecan (CPT-11) and vincristine (VCR) in rhabdomyosarcoma (RMS) at first relapse/disease progression. J Clin Oncol 2008: 26.

226 Fox E, Maris JM, Widemann BC, et al. A phase 1 study of ABT-751, an orally bioavailable tubulin inhibitor, administered daily for 7 days every 21 days in pediatric patients with solid tumors. Clin Cancer Res 2006; 12: 4882–7.

227 Fox E, Maris JM, Widemann BC, et al. A phase I study of ABT-751, an orally bioavailable tubulin inhibitor, administered daily for 21 days every 28 days in pediatric patients with solid tumors. Clin Cancer Res 2008; 14: 1111–5.

228 Brignole C, Marimpietri D, Pastorino F, et al. Effect of bortezomib on human neuroblastoma cell growth, apoptosis, and angiogenesis. J Natl Cancer Inst 2006; 98: 1142–57.

229 Combaret V, Boyault S, Iacono I, Brejon S, Rousseau R, Puisieux A. Effect of bortezomib on human neuroblastoma: analysis of molecular mechanisms involved in cytotoxicity. Mol Cancer 2008; 7: 50.

230 Armstrong MB, Schumacher KR, Mody R, Yanik GA, Opipari AW, Jr, Castle VP. Bortezomib as a therapeutic candidate for neuroblastoma. J Exp Ther Oncol 2008; 7: 135–45.

231 Rossler J, Taylor M, Geoerger B, et al. Angiogenesis as a target in neuroblastoma. Eur J Cancer 2008; 44: 1645–56.

232 Meitar D, Crawford SE, Rademaker AW, Cohn SL. Tumor angiogenesis correlates with metastatic disease, N-myc amplification, and poor outcome in human neuroblastoma. J Clin Oncol 1996; 14: 405–14.

233 Canete A, Navarro S, Bermudez J, Pellin A, Castel V, Llombart-Bosch A. Angiogenesis in neuroblastoma: relationship to survival and other prognostic factors in a cohort of neuroblastoma patients. J Clin Oncol 2000; 18: 27–34.

234 Eggert A, Ikegaki N, Kwiatkowski J, Zhao H, Brodeur GM, Himelstein BP. High-level expression of angiogenic factors is associated with advanced tumor stage in human neuroblastomas. Clin Cancer Res 2000; 6: 1900–8.

235 Katzenstein HM, Salwen HR, Nguyen NN, Meitar D, Cohn SL. Antiangiogenic therapy inhibits human neuroblastoma growth. Med Pediatr Oncol 2001; 36: 190–3.

236 Daniel RA, Rozanska AL, Thomas HD, et al. Inhibition of poly(ADP-ribose) polymerase-1 enhances temozolomide and topotecan activity against childhood neuroblastoma. Clin Cancer Res 2009; 15: 1241–9.

237 Howard JP, Maris JM, Kersun LS, et al. Tumor response and toxicity with multiple infusions of high dose 131I-MIBG for refractory neuroblastoma. Pediatr Blood Cancer 2005; 44: 232–9.

238 Matthay KK, Tan JC, Villablanca JG, et al. Phase I dose escalation of iodinc-131-metaiodobenzylguanidine with myeloablative chemotherapy and autologous stem-cell transplantation in refractory neuroblastoma: a new approach to Neuroblastoma Therapy Consortium Study. J Clin Oncol 2006; 24: 500–6.

239 Gaze MN, Flux GD, Mairs RJ, Becherer A, Staudenherz A. The early European experience of high activities of meta-iodobenzylguanidine and topotecan in neuroblastoma. Ped Blood Cancer 2008; 49(4): 554.

240 Mairs RJ, Cunningham SH, Russell J, et al. No-carrier-added iodine-131-MIBG: evaluation of a therapeutic preparation. J Nucl Med 1995; 36: 1088–95.

241 Kushner BH, Kramer K, Cheung NK. Phase II trial of the anti-G(D2) monoclonal antibody 3F8 and granulocyte-macrophage colony-stimulating factor for neuroblastoma. J Clin Oncol 2001; 19: 4189–94.

242 Ozkaynak MF, Sondel PM, Krailo MD, et al. Phase I study of chimeric human/murine anti-ganglioside G(D2) monoclonal antibody (ch14.18) with granulocyte-macrophage colony-stimulating factor in children with neuroblastoma immediately after hematopoietic stem-cell transplantation: a Children's Cancer Group Study. J Clin Oncol 2000; 18: 4077–85.

243 Osenga KL, Hank JA, Albertini MR, et al. A phase I clinical trial of the hu14.18-IL2 (EMD 273063) as a treatment for children with refractory or recurrent neuroblastoma and melanoma: a study of the Children's Oncology Group. Clin Cancer Res 2006;12: 1750–9.

244 Yu AL, Gilman AL, Ozkaynak M F, et al. A phase III randomized trial of the chimeric anti-GD2 antibody ch14.18 with GM-CSF and IL2 as immunotherapy following dose intensive chemotherapy for high-risk neuroblastoma: Children's Oncology Group (COG) study ANBL0032. J Clin Oncol 2009; 27: 15(suppl; abstr 10067z).

245 Garaventa A, Luksch R, Lo Piccolo MS, et al. Phase I trial and pharmacokinetics of fenretinide in children with neuroblastoma. Clin Cancer Res 2003; 9: 2032–9.

246 Villablanca JG, Krailo MD, Ames MM, Reid JM, Reaman GH, Reynolds CP. Phase I trial of oral fenretinide in children with high-risk solid tumors: a report from the Children's Oncology Group (CCG 09709). J Clin Oncol 2006; 24: 3423–30.

247 Formelli F, Cavadini E, Luksch R, et al. Pharmacokinetics of oral fenretinide in neuroblastoma patients: indications for optimal dose and dosing schedule also with respect to the active metabolite 4-oxo-fenretinide. Cancer Chemother Pharmacol 2008; 62: 655–65.

13 Renal Tumors

Edward J. Estlin[1] and Norbert Graf[2]

[1]Department of Pediatric Oncology, Royal Manchester Children's Hospital, Manchester, UK and [2]Department of Paediatric Haematology and Oncology, University Hospital of the Saarland, Homburg, Germany

Introduction

Renal tumors of childhood comprise one of the most common extracranial malignancies of childhood. A wide variety of oncological and non-oncological conditions can form tumors, and the range of diagnoses described when investigating renal tumors are presented in Table 13.1. This chapter will focus on the three most common and important conditions in relation to children with cancer of renal origin, namely Wilms' tumor or nephroblastoma, renal rhabdoid tumor and clear cell sarcoma of the kidney.

Wilms' tumor (nephroblastoma)

Prior to the introduction of systemic chemotherapy with vincristine and actinomycin-D in the early 1960s, Wilms' tumor carried a poor prognosis when treated by nephrectomy alone, or by nephrectomy plus local radiotherapy, with reported overall survival rates in the range of 11–40% [3, 4]. Table 13.2 outlines the early clinical studies of vincristine and actinomycin-D, and their role in establishing that these agents played a role in the palliation of advanced disease at diagnosis, and their prevention of the development of local and pulmonary relapse when administered alongside surgery and radiotherapy. In particular, early clinical studies of actinomycin D and vincristine demonstrated that (Table 13.2):
• Vincristine was as potent as radiotherapy in enhancing the operability of Wilms' tumor.
• Therapy with vincristine or actinomycin-D resulted in definite, but short-lived, tumor regressions for children with recurrent disease following surgery and radiotherapy.
• Early administration of these agents, in the adjuvant setting with surgery and local radiotherapy, markedly improved survival rates when compared with historical controls.

Pediatric Hematology and Oncology, 1st edition. Edited by Edward J. Estlin, Richard J. Gilbertson, and Robert F. Wynn. © 2010 Blackwell Publishing Ltd.

In the case of actinomycin-D, this improvement in survival was greater for children without evidence of metastases at diagnosis, and for children less than 3 years of age [5, 6].

In the setting of disease resistant to therapy with vincristine and actinomycin-D, doxorubicin was established in the early 1970s as an active agent, with a 50% response rate in the single agent setting [7]. Experience of doxorubicin in combination with vincristine during the late 1970s established this drug as part of the front-line therapy for Wilms' tumor [8]. The subsequent refinement of the role of this anthracycline is described below in the context of international collaborative studies.

Therefore, these early clinical studies underpinned the modern strategies for evaluation of combinations of chemotherapy in relation to Wilms' tumor, and in particular the early administration of chemotherapy, especially in the context of minimal residual disease, as evidenced by the lack of metastases at presentation, as an important means to improve the survival of children with Wilms' tumor.

Epidemiology

Malignant renal tumors comprise 6% of all childhood cancers, with Wilms' tumor being the most frequent type (90%) (Box 13.1). The epidemiology of Wilms' tumor is characterized by:
• An annual incidence of 9.1 per million children in Europe increasing by 0.7% per year [9], and 8.1 per million children in North America [10, 11].
• A male to female ratio of 0.9.
• Two peaks of incidence, occurring especially for females, at ages 1 and 3 years, respectively.
• A median age at diagnosis of 3 years for females compared with 2 years for males [9].
• A higher incidence in North America and Europe compared with Asia [12]. Epidemiological studies suggest that ethnicity affects the incidence rates more than geographical region of residence or other environmental factors [13–15].
• The majority of Wilms' tumors are solitary lesions, but approximately 12% of children develop multifocal tumors within a single kidney and almost 7% have bilateral involvement at diagnosis or later on [13, 14, 16].

Genetic predisposition to Wilms' tumor has long been recognized in patients with aniridia and the Wilms tumor, aniridia, genitourinary anomalies, and mental retardation syndrome (WAGR). Today we know that the genetic bases and molecular biology of Wilms' tumor is very heterogeneous and more complex than anticipated [17]. All underlying syndromes can be divided into overgrowth syndromes and others (Table 13.3). As well as gene mutations, loss of heterozygosity (LOH) and loss of imprinting (LOI) can be found in tumor cells. In the development of Wilms' tumor different genes and mutations are involved, making it difficult to explain pathogenesis by a simple 'two-hit' hypothesis. LOH affects most often the genes 1p, 7p, 11p, 16q and 22q [18]. Additional tumor suppressor or tumor-progressive genes may lie on chromosomes 16q and 1p as evidenced by LOH for these regions in 17% and 11% of Wilms' tumors, respectively. Patients classified by tumor-specific loss of these loci had significantly worse relapse-free and overall survival rates [19].

The genetics of the overgrowth syndromes are complex and carry a risk of Wilms' tumor in the order of 10%. As with the Beckwith-Wiedemann syndrome (BWS) they arise from mutations or abnormalities of imprinting in genes in the 11p15.5 region with different constitutional epigenotypes between BWS and hemi-hypertrophy [20]. If the analysis of the methylation status of several genes in this region will predict an individual risk of developing a Wilms' tumor, is an open question [21].

The WAGR syndrome is caused by a complete deletion of one copy of the Wilms' tumor gene, *WT1* and the adjacent aniridia gene, *PAX6* on chromosome 11p13 [22]. In patients with aniridia this information helps to identify those patients, who are at risk for developing Wilms' tumor, by screening them for the combined deletion of *WT1* and *PAX6*. *WT1* is also involved in the Denys-Drash syndrome (early onset nephrotic syndrome, Wilms' tumor, and ambiguous genitalia) [23] caused by a germ line point mutation. A similar constitutional WT1 mutation underlies the Frasier syndrome (nephropathy and gonadal tumors) [24]. It is of interest that in only 5% of Wilms' tumors a constitutional, and

Table 13.1 Differential diagnosis for renal tumors of childhood[1, 2].

Neuroblastoma	Benign teratoma
Mesoblastic nephroma	Adrenal haemorrhage
Renal cyst	Renal thrombosis
Renal cell carcinoma	Renal rhabdomyosarcoma
Polycystic kidney	Renal leiomyosarcoma
Multi-cystic kidney	Dysplastic kidney
Hydronephrosis	Extra-renal leiomyosarcoma
Hypernephroma	Multilocular cyst
Extra-renal fibrosarcoma	Lymphangiosarcoma
Renal carbuncle	

Box 13.1 Wilms' tumor key facts – epidemiology.

- 77% of cases are diagnosed prior to 5 years of age
- 15% of cases are diagnosed prior to 1 year of age
- 7% of cases have bilateral renal involvement, and present at a young age
- 1% of cases are familial
- 12% of cases have an underlying genetic cause/syndrome
- Association with abnormalities of 11p15 and overgrowth syndromes in 10% of cases
- Association with abnormalities of 11p13 LOH and WAGR/Denys-Drash in 4–5% of cases

---

Table 13.2 Major findings of early clinical trials for Wilms' tumor.

Study	Disease status	Chemotherapy	Clinical outcome	Reference
South West Cancer Study Group 13 children	Relapse following XRT and ACT-D	VCR	Short-lived response following vincristine for 8/13 children	[5]
South West Cancer Study Group 12 children	Metastatic disease at presentation	VCR	Complete regression of metastatic disease at presentation	[6]
South West Cancer Study Group 9 children	New diagnosis with localized disease	VCR	Vincristine improves operability rate for Wilms' tumor and 8/9 children remained disease free at 2 years of follow up	[6]
Howard (1965)	New diagnosis with localized disease	ACT-D	Improvement in survival from 11% for historical control to 62% with peri-operative ACT-D and delayed local XRT	[3]
Burgert & Glidewell (1967)	New diagnosis with localized disease	ACT-D	39% of 53 patients treated with surgery and XRT alive and free of disease at one year 59% of 49 patients who received adjuvant ACT-D alive and free of disease at one year.	[4]

XRT, radiotherapy.ACT-D, actinonmycin-D. VCR, vincristine.

Table 13.3 Syndromes and genetic loci that are associated with Wilms' tumor.

Syndrome	Characteristics	Gene	Risk	Link to OMIM*
Overgrowth syndromes				
	Hemihypertrophy	11p15 WT2	3–5%	http://www.ncbi.nlm.nih.gov/entrez/ dispomim.cgi?id=235000
Beckwith-Wiedemann EMG-Syndrome	**E**xomphalus **M**acroglossia **G**igantismus	11p15.5 WT2, IGF2, H19	10–20%	http://www.ncbi.nlm.nih.gov/entrez/ dispomim.cgi?id=130650
Soto's Syndrome	Rapid growth, acromegalic features Non-progressive cerebral disorder with mental retardation	5q35 NSD1		http://www.ncbi.nlm.nih.gov/entrez/ dispomim.cgi?id=117550
Simpson-Golabi-Behmel Syndrome	Post-natal overgrowth Coarse facies Congenital heart defects Other congenital abnormalities	Xq26 GPC3		http://www.ncbi.nlm.nih.gov/entrez/ dispomim.cgi?id=312870
Klippel-Trenaunay Syndrome	Cutaneous hemangiomata Hypertrophy of the related bones and soft tissues	5q13.3 VG5Q		http://www.ncbi.nlm.nih.gov/entrez/ dispomim.cgi?id=149000
Perlman	Renal hamartomas Nephroblastomatosis Fetal gigantism	?		http://www.ncbi.nlm.nih.gov/entrez/ dispomim.cgi?id=267000
Other syndromes				
	Aniridia	11p13 PAX6	30%	http://www.ncbi.nlm.nih.gov/entrez/ dispomim.cgi?id=106210
WAGR	**W**ilm's tumor **A**niridia **G**enitourinary anomalies Mental **R**etardation	11p13 WT1		http://www.ncbi.nlm.nih.gov/entrez/ dispomim.cgi?id=194072
Denys-Drash	Nephropathy Wilms' tumor Genital anomalies	11p13 WT1	30%	http://www.ncbi.nlm.nih.gov/entrez/ dispomim.cgi?id=194080
	Genitourinary malformations	11p13 GUD		http://www.ncbi.nlm.nih.gov/entrez/ dispomim.cgi?id=137357
Li-Fraumeni Syndrome	Inherited cancer syndrome	17p13 p53		http://www.ncbi.nlm.nih.gov/entrez/ dispomim.cgi?id=151623
Neurofibromatosis I Morbus Recklinghausen	Cafe-au-lait spots Fibromatous tumors of the skin	17q11.2 NF1		http://www.ncbi.nlm.nih.gov/entrez/ dispomim.cgi?id=162200

* Online Mendelian Inheritance in Man: http://www.ncbi.nlm.nih.gov/entrez/query.fcgi?db=OMIM

in further 10% a sporadic, *WT1* mutation can be found [25]. In those with germ line mutations bilateral Wilms' tumors are more frequent [26]. The WT1 protein functions as a transcription factor that is clearly critical for normal kidney development. There is a close correlation between *WT1* mutations and the histology of stromal predominant tumors with rhabdomyomatous features [27].

In familial Wilms' tumors, accounting for approximately 1% of patients, there is usually no associated congenital abnormality or predisposition to other tumor types. Genetic linkage studies in different families have localized one gene for familial Wilms' tumor, *FWT1*, to chromosome 17q [28] and another, *FWT2*, to 19q. Further *FWT* genes are waiting for identification, for there are other families known clearly unlinked to any currently identified Wilms' tumor locus [29].

Clinical presentation

The typical presentation of a child with a Wilms' tumor is an asymptomatic mass, and other complaints, signs, or symptoms are found in about 20% or less [30] (Table 13.4). In Germany, in about 10% of patients, an early diagnosis of Wilms' tumor is made during regular childhood routine examinations in an asymptomatic child [30]. In addition, Wilms' tumor is known to present with:

• Hypertension that is caused by an increase in renin activity and is sometimes difficult to control [31].

• Coagulopathy caused by an acquired von Willebrand syndrome [32]. In most cases an acquired coagulation disorder and the hypertension will resolve after tumor nephrectomy.

• Intra-tumoral hemorrhage may occur, resulting in an emergency situation with a rapid abdominal enlargement that requires urgent surgery.

• Extension of tumor and related thrombus may occur to involve the inferior vena cava and also the right atrium in 5% of cases [33]. This is rarely a cause of death due to massive cardiac insufficiency or can cause pulmonary emboli, but is usually successfully managed with initial chemotherapy and then surgery under cardiopulmonary bypass.

The pattern of presentation with metastatic Wilms' tumor, which is found for 13% of patients, is illustrated in Figure 13.1 [9].

Table 13.4 Symptoms in children with Wilms' tumor[30].

Symptom	Frequency (%)
Asymptomatic	10
Asymptomatic mass	56
Pain	25
Hematuria	18
Fever	10
Urinary tract infection	6
Weight loss	5
Constipation	6
Enteritis	4
Vomiting	6
Others	19

Investigation and staging
Imaging for Wilms' tumor
The imaging modalities of ultrasound, computerized X-ray tomography, and magnetic resonance imaging have all been evaluated in the context of the investigation and staging of Wilms' tumor, and the main features for this are as follows:
• Ultrasound provides a readily accessible imaging modality, which is of help in the initial diagnosis of Wilms' tumor and also the ongoing response to chemotherapy.
• Color flow Doppler ultrasound has an overall positive predictive value of almost 75% in assessing the patency and involvement of the inferior vena cava with tumor thrombus [34].
• With computed tomography (CT) and magnetic resonance imaging (MRI) scan evaluation, Wilms' tumor demonstrates a characteristic claw sign which is caused by the invasion of the kidney by tumor, with a rim of normal renal tissue appearing stretched around the adjacent tumor (Figure 13.2).
• On gadolinium-enhanced T1-weighted imaging, Wilms' tumors are hypo-intense in comparison with normal renal tissue and are iso-intense to normal renal cortex. The tumors demonstrate uptake of gadolinium, with an in-homogeneous signal intensity [35].
• All treatment modalities appear to have a poor correlation to histological staging [36].
Perhaps the main benefit of pre-surgical imaging is to help detect whether or not there is bilateral or Stage V Wilms' tumor at

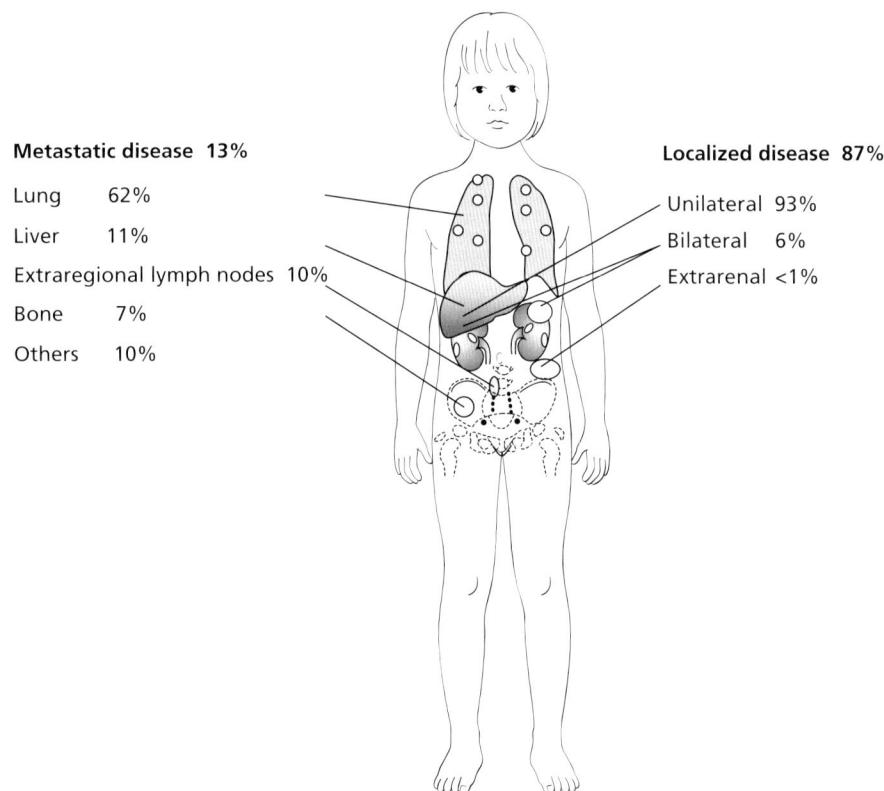

Metastatic disease 13%

Lung   62%

Liver   11%

Extraregional lymph nodes 10%

Bone   7%

Others   10%

Localized disease 87%

Unilateral 93%

Bilateral 6%

Extrarenal <1%

Figure 13.1 Sites of presentation for Wilms' tumor at diagnosis and relapse.

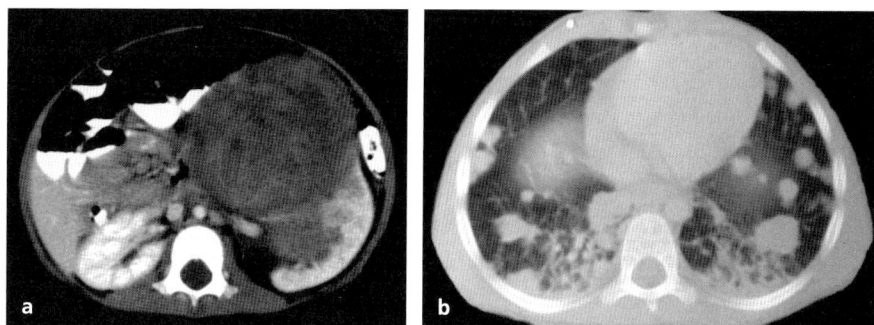

Figure 13.2 (a), Wilms' tumor of the left kidney demonstrating a characteristic claw sign. (b), Pulmonary metastases with Wilms' tumor.

diagnosis. However, the diagnosis of bilateral Wilms' was found to be missed in some 7% of patients on the National Wilms' Tumor Study Group-4 trial in comparison with operative findings. However, the majority of tumors that were missed, even by CT or MRI scan, tended to be less than 1 cm in greatest dimension [37]. Imaging by chest X-ray and thoracic CT scan is also required for the detection and diagnosis of pulmonary metastases and any of the imaging modalities can be expected to detect hepatic metastases arising from Wilms' tumor.

Histological classification

The histology of Wilms' tumor is characterized by a marked histological diversity and the tumor is thought to be derived from primitive metanephric blastema. In addition to expressing various cell types and aggregation patterns seen in the normally developing kidney, the neoplasms often contain tissues not found in the normal metanephros such as skeletal muscle, cartilage and squamous epithelial cells. The classical appearances of a nephroblastoma are made up of varying proportions of three cell types (blastemal, stromal, and epithelial), but these are not present in every case. For anaplastic Wilms' tumor, the characteristic anaplastic changes of gigantic polyploid nuclei may either be focal or diffuse.

The revised SIOP working classification of renal tumors of childhood [38] defines the appearance of tumors as ranked by their perceived risk for relapse (Table 13.5).

As well as the histological appearance of nephroblastoma, the intensity and duration of treatment for this malignancy treatment intensity and duration also depends on staging. For SIOP studies this is outlined as presented in Table 13.6. The effect of initial treatment modality on the relative frequency for the staging and occurrence of tumor rupture at laparotomy for Wilms' tumor is shown in Figure 13.3. The effect of initial treatment modality for diagnosis of the histological sub-types for Wilms' tumor is shown in Figure 13.4.

The staging criteria adopted by the North American Study Groups is essentially the same except for the recognition of chemotherapy induced changes at lymph nodes or resection margins due to the practice for achieving primary nephrectomy at diagnosis. The information gained by staging and histological subtype forms the basis for the current treatment modalities for Wilms' tumor as described in the following section, where other

Table 13.5 Risk-adapted classification for Wilms' tumor in relation to initial treatment modality.

Risk category	Primary nephrectomy	Pre-nephrectomy chemotherapy
Low	Mesoblastic nephroma Cystic partially differentiated nephroblastoma	Completely nephrotic nephroblastoma
Intermediate	Non-anaplastic nephroblastoma Nephroblastoma with focal anaplasia	Nephroblastoma: epithelial type stromal type mixed type regressive type Focal anaplasia
High	Nephroblastoma – diffuse anaplasia Clear cell sarcoma Rhabdoid tumors of the kidney	Nephroblastoma with diffusely anaplastic or blastemal type histology

factors such as tumor size and cytogenetic abnormalities are considered.

Treatment

Dramatic improvements in survival have occurred as the result of advances in anesthetic and surgical management, irradiation and chemotherapy. Contemporary treatments are based mainly on the findings of several multi-center trials and studies conducted by the International Society of Pediatric Oncology (SIOP) in Europe and the National Wilms' Tumor Study Group (NWTSG) (now incorporated into the Children's Oncology Group) in North America. Generally speaking, the differing investigational strategies adopted by the SIOP and NWTSG trials have helped inform contemporary therapies in different ways. For example, whereas the NWTSG studies established the importance of combination chemotherapy, the radiotherapy-sparing effect of doxorubicin for stage 3 disease, and the identification of subgroups where surgery alone might be possible, SIOP studies have sought to establish the role of pre-nephrectomy chemotherapy, and pursue response- and histology-directed reductions in treatment duration (Tables 13.7–9).

Table 13.6 SIOP criteria for Wilms' tumor staging.

Stage 1

(1) The tumor is limited to kidney or surrounded with a fibrous pseudocapsule if outside of the normal contours of the kidney. The renal capsule or pseudocapsule may be infiltrated with the tumor but it does not reach the outer surface, and it is completely resected (resection margins 'clear').

(2) The tumor may be protruding ('bulging') into the pelvic system and 'dipping' into the ureter (but is not infiltrating their walls).

(3) The vessels of the renal sinus are not involved.

(4) Intrarenal vessel involvement may be present.

Fine needle aspiration or percutaneous core needle biopsy ('tru-cut') does not upstage the tumor.

The presence of necrotic tumor or chemotherapy-induced change in the renal sinus and/or within the perirenal fat should not be regarded as a reason for upstaging tumor providing it is completely excised and does not reach the resection margins.

Stage II

(1) The tumor extends beyond kidney or penetrates through the renal capsule and/or fibrous pseudocapsule into perirenal fat but is completely resected (resection margins 'clear').

(2) Tumor infiltrates the renal sinus and/or invades blood and lymphatic vessels outside the renal parenchyma but it is completely resected.

(3) Tumor infiltrates adjacent organs or vena cava but is completely resected.

Stage III

(1) Incomplete excision of the tumor which extends beyond resection margins (gross or microscopical tumor remains post-operatively).

(2) Any abdominal lymph nodes are involved.

(3) Tumor rupture before or intra-operatively (irrespective of other criteria for staging).

(4) The tumor has penetrated through the peritoneal surface.

(5) Tumor implants are found on the peritoneal surface.

(6) The tumor thrombi present at resection margins of vessels or ureter, transsected or removed piecemeal by surgeon.

(7) The tumor has been surgically biopsied (wedge biopsy) prior to pre-operative chemotherapy or surgery.

The presence of necrotic tumor or chemotherapy-induced changes in a lymph node or at the resection margins is regarded as proof of previous tumor with microscopic residue and therefore the tumor is assigned stage III.

Stage IV

Hematogeneous metastases (lung, liver, bone, brain, etc.) or lymph node metastases outside the abdomino-pelvic region.

Stage V

Bilateral renal tumors at diagnosis. Each side should be substaged according to above classifications.

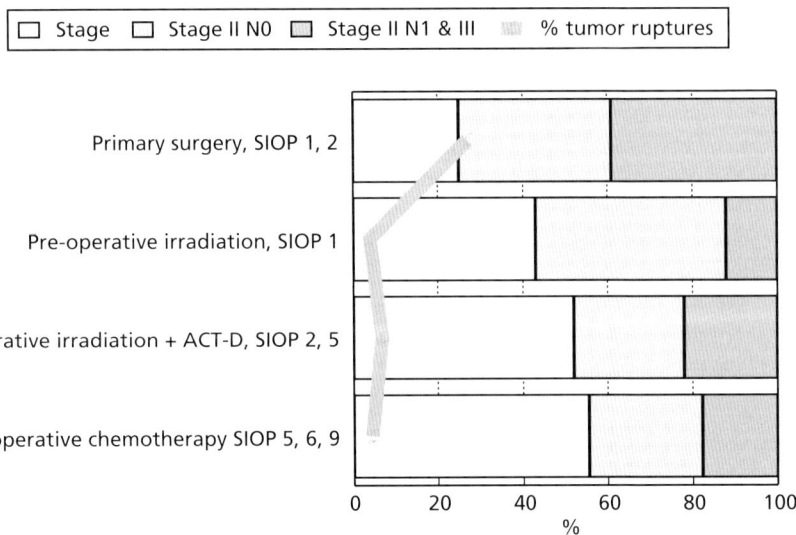

Figure 13.3 Stage distribution and tumor ruptures in the SIOP studies 1, 2, 5, 6 and 9.

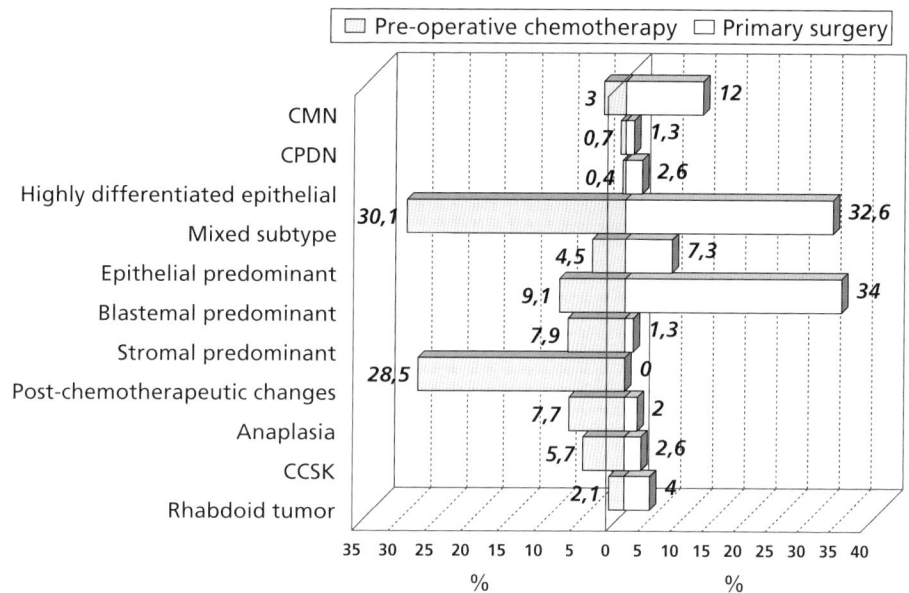

Figure 13.4 The influence of initial treatment modality on the frequency of histological sub-type. CMN, congenital mesoblastic nephroma. CPDN, cystic partially differentiated Wilms tumor. CCSK, clear cell sarcoma of the kidney.

Table 13.7 Major findings of successive NWTSG trials and studies.

Study	Stage	Chemotherapy	Irradiation	Reference
NWTS-1 1969–1973 606 patients	I	ACT-D	Unnecessary for children <2 years, when treated with chemotherapy	[52]
	II and III	Combination of VCR and ACT-D is better than each drug alone		
NWTS-2 1975–1978 775 patients	I	6 months of VCR and ACT-D sufficient	Unnecessary	[48]
	II, III, and IV	Addition of DOX increases relapse-free survival rate		
NWTS-3 1979–1985 2496 patients	I	11 weeks of VCR and ACT-D is sufficient (92.5% 16 year EFS, 97.6% OS)	Unnecessary	[48]
	II	DOX is unnecessary (89.6% 16 year EFS, 92.9% OS)	Unnecessary	
	III	DOX is necessary (80.4% 16 year EFS, 86.2% OS) DOX is unnecessary	10 Gy abdominal irradiation 20 Gy abdominal irradiation	
	IV	CYC is without benefit (76.5% 16 year EFS, 79.5% OS)		
NWTS-4 1986–1994 1687 patients	I-IV	'Pulse-intensive' chemotherapy as effective, less toxic, and less expensive (Stage I: 94.9% 2 year EFS, 98.7% OS) (Stage II: 83.6% 8 year EFS, 93.8% OS) (Stage III: 88.9% 8 year EFS, 93.0% OS) (Stage IV: 80.6% 2 year EFS, 89.5% OS)		[45, 46, 53]
	II, III, and IV	6 months of chemotherapy sufficient		
NWTS-5 1995–2002 2021 patients	I (age <24 m, tumor weight <550 g)	With surgery alone, 2 year OS rate remained 100% but relapse-free survival rate was 86% – arm closed		[19, 54]
	All stages	LOH at 1p and 16 q is an adverse prognostic indicator		

NWTSG, National Wilms'Tumor Study Group. ACT-D, actinomycin-D. VCR, vincristine. DOX, doxorubicin. EFS, event-free survival. OS, overall survival. LOH, Loss of heterozygosity. CYC, cyclophosphamide.

Table 13.8 Major findings of successive SIOP trials and studies.

Study	Stage	Chemotherapy	Irradiation	Reference
SIOP 1 1971–1974 398 patients	I–III	There is no evidence that prolonged ACT-D post-operatively contributes to a better disease free survival and/or survival	Pre-treatment reduces the number of ruptures and produces a more favourable stage distribution after surgery	[39, 55]
SIOP 2 1974–1976 138 patients	I–III	It is not necessary to give a two drug combination for more than 9 months post-operatively	Pre-operative XRT reduces tumor ruptures. Beware of the temptation to operate on small tumors	[55]
SIOP 5 1977–1979 433 patients	I–III	Chemotherapy is comparable to radiotherapy in efficacy for preparing the tumor for surgery. Due to fewer late effects, it is preferable to use chemotherapy rather than radiotherapy		[40, 55]
SIOP 6 1980–1987 1687 patients	I	After pre-operative chemotherapy and surgery, 17 weeks is as effective as 38 weeks post-operative chemotherapy with VCR and ACT-D (2 year DFS: 92% vs 88%, not significantly different.)		[41, 55]
	II N–	The stopping rule was activated due to an apparent increase in abdominal relapses in the non-irradiated group. No confirmation in the final analysis. (2 year DFS of 72% vs 78%, not significantly different.)		
	II N+, III	The DOX arm had a better 2 year DFS but equivalent 5 year OS (2 year DFS: 74% vs 49%) (5 year OS: 80% vs 77%, no significant difference.)		
SIOP 9 1987–1991 852 patients	I–III	Four weeks is equivalent to 8 weeks pre-operative chemotherapy for localized tumors in terms of proportion of stage I (64% vs 62%), intra-operative rupture rate (1% vs 3%), 2 year EFS (84% vs 83%) and 5 year overall survival (92% vs 87%)	According to the post-operative histology and local stage: Intermediate risk: II N+ and III: 15 Gy High risk: II and III: 30 Gy	[43, 55]
	IV	6 weeks of pre-operative VCR, ACT-D and DOX Post-operative CT depending on local stage and response to pre-operative CT	Local irradiation: as in patients without metastases Pulmonary irradiation: only in non-complete remission after pre-operative CT	
SIOP 93-01 1993–2000 410 patients	I	A reduction in duration of post-operative chemotherapy, from 18 to 4 weeks is safe in this group of patients	None	[44, 55]
	II–III	Same treatment as in SIOP 9 II N–: 92% 5 year EFS II N+, III: 82% 5 year EFS		
	IV	6 weeks of pre-operative VCR, ACT-D and DOX Post-operative CT depending on local stage and response to pre-operative CT	Local irradiation: as in patients without metastases Pulmonary irradiation: only in non-complete remission after pre-operative CT	
	All stages	Post-chemotherapy blastemal predominant subtype of Wilms' tumor has to be classified as high risk tumor (82% 5 year EFS) Local stage II N+ and III have the same outcome Focal anaplasia is doing better than diffuse		

SIOP, International Society of Pediatric Oncology. ACT-D, actinomycin-D.XRT, radiotherapy. VCR, vincristine. DFS, disease-free survival. DOX, doxorubicin. OS, overall survival. EFS, event-free survival. CT, computed tomography.

Table 13.9 Major findings of successive UK trials and studies.

Study	Stage	Chemotherapy	Irradiation	Reference
UKW 1 1980–1986 384 patients	I/FH	In FH single agent VCR ×26 weeks is efficient (89% 6 year EFS; 96% OS)	No	[56]
	II/FH	Two drugs VCR/ACT-D ×26 weeks is safe, an anthracycline can be omitted (85% 6 yr EFS, 93% OS)	Yes	
	III/FH	Sequential VCR/ACT-D + DOX × 1 year (82% 6 year EFS, 83% OS)	Yes	
	IV	VCR/Act-D + DOX + cyclophosphamide for one year (50% 6 year EFS, 65% OS)	Lung XRT only if no remission at week 12	
	UH	Same as stage IV/FH (50% OS)		
UKW 2 1986–1991 448 patients	I/FH	VCR, 10 weekly doses (87% 4 year EFS, 94% OS)	None	[57]
	II/FH	VCR + ACT-D, 6 months (82% 4 year EFS, 91% OS)	None	
	III/FH	VCR + ACT-D + DOX, 12 months (82% 4 year EFS, 84% OS)	XRT = 20 Gy, hemi-abdomen	
	IV	Intensive VCR + ACT-D + DOX, 6 months (70% 4 year EFS, 75% OS)	If local stage III 30 Gy to hemi-abdomen 12 Gy to whole lung	
	Unfavourable histology	Intensive VCR + ACT-D + DOX, 6 months (stage III: 12 months) (Anaplasia: 50% 4 year EFS, 36% OS)	Stage III, 30 Gy, hemi-abdomen	
UKW 3 1995–2002 205 patients	I-III	Randomization: immediate nephrectomy versus pre-operative chemotherapy. Significant improvement in stage distribution: Stage I: 65.2% vs 54.3% Stage II: 23.9% vs 14.9% Stage III: 9.8% vs 29.8% → 20% fewer children receiving radiotherapy and doxorubicin		[58]

FH, favourable histology. VCR, vincristine. EFS, event-free survival. OS, overall survival. ACT-D, actinomycin-D. DOX, doxorubicin. XRT, radiotherapy.

However, there is and remains a different approach in the treatment of nephroblastoma between SIOP and North America in that the Children's Oncology Group (COG) believes it is necessary to identify accurate tumor staging by immediate surgery, whereas the SIOP trials and studies largely focus on the issue of pre-operative therapy [39–47] (Box 13.2). The SIOP strategy of giving pre-operative chemotherapy is based on the premise that pre-operative therapy reduces the risk of tumor rupture during surgery, thereby reducing the likelihood of local and distant recurrence. However, there is a risk of up to 1.5% that chemotherapy will be administered to a benign tumor during the pre-operative phase [41, 43]. However, the main objectives of COG/NWTSG and SIOP trials are to treat patients according to well-defined risk groups in order to achieve highest cure rates, to decrease the frequency and intensity of acute and late toxicity, and to minimize the cost of therapy.

As an example of the COG strategy, the fourth NWTSG study investigated the efficacy, toxicity, and cost of different schedules of actinomycin-D and doxorubicin administration, finding that actinomycin-D could be given safely in 1 day rather than over 5 days and doxorubicin in 1 day rather than over 3 days [45, 46].

Box 13.2 Wilms' tumor key facts – international differences in treatment philosophies.

International Society of Pediatric Oncology (SIOP) strategy	Children's Oncology Group strategy
• Pre-nephrectomy chemotherapy with less tumor rupture	• Surgery at diagnosis to stage disease with more tumor rupture
• 60% stage 1	• 30% stage 1
• 50% receive anthracycline	• 35% receive anthracycline
• 17% receive radiotherapy	• 35% receive radiotherapy
• Small risk of inappropriate treatment for non-Wilms' tumor histology	• Correct histological diagnosis assured at presentation
• Response adapted approach for metastatic disease avoids pulmonary radiotherapy in 2/3 of patients with stage 4 disease	• Pulmonary irradiation mandated for involvement of lungs at presentation

These so-called pulse-intensive regimens were as effective as the standard courses but were accompanied by less severe hematological toxicity and fewer health-care encounters. As a consequence pulse-intensive therapy has become the standard of care for treatment of Wilms' tumor in North America [48–50].

In comparison, for the SIOP-93-01 trial, post-operative therapy was based on stage and pathological response to chemotherapy. From post-operative histology, tumors were classified as low, intermediate, or high risk according to the Stockholm working classification of renal tumors [51], and it could be shown by means of a prospective randomization that post-operative treatment for patients with stage I intermediate risk or anaplasia could be reduced to 4 weeks from the standard 18 weeks, while maintaining equivalent event-free survival [44]. Because about 60% of patients will have stage I disease after receiving pre-operative chemotherapy, most of the patients with unilateral disease can be cured after only 4 weeks of pre-operative chemotherapy, tumor nephrectomy and 4 weeks of post-operative chemotherapy with only two drugs (vincristine and actinomycin-D).

Post-operative treatment in both groups is mainly stratified according to the tumor stage and the histology after surgery. Through successive National Wilms' Tumor Study (NWTS), SIOP, and UK trials, the combination, length, and mode of administration of chemotherapy have been refined to optimize survival rates while minimizing acute and long-term toxicities. Radiation therapy, although still an important component of Wilms' tumor therapy, is restricted to treatment of stage III or IV disease. The conclusions drawn from each of these trials are summarized in Tables 13.7–9. Both approaches (SIOP and NWTS) result in similar tumor control rates but a different overall burden of treatment.

Although transatlantic differences in treatment philosophies with respect to pre-nephrectomy chemotherapy have underpinned nearly all of the SIOP and NWTSG/COG trails historically, the United Kingdom Children's Cancer Study Group (UKCCSG) sought to investigate the potential advantages for both of these approaches by means of a randomized clinical trial, UKW3 [58]. The main findings of this study, performed between 1991 and 2001 for children with non-metastatic Wilms' tumor, are summarized in Table 13.9 and by the following results:
• There was a significant improvement in the stage distribution for patients with Wilms' tumor receiving delayed surgery following 6 weeks of chemotherapy with vincristine and actinomycin, compared with those undergoing immediate nephrectomy.
• This improvement resulted in 20% fewer children receiving radiotherapy or doxorubicin.
• The event-free and overall survivals at 5 years were similar in the two groups.
The results suggest that all children with non-metastatic Wilms' tumor should receive chemotherapy prior to tumor resection. However, North American studies continue to advocate immediate tumor-nephrectomy, although the NWTSG has recommended pre-operative chemotherapy under certain circumstances [59], including:

• The occurrence of Wilms' tumor in a solitary kidney.
• Bilateral Wilms' tumor or tumor in a horseshoe kidney.
• Tumor thrombus in the inferior vena cava above the level of the hepatic veins.
• Respiratory distress resulting from the presence of extensive metastatic tumor.

The relationships between prognosis and clinical, tumor-related, and pharmacological factors

Prognosis following the diagnosis of Wilms' tumor has been found to relate to age and the features of any associated and predisposing syndrome, and also to tumor-related findings for histology, karyotype and for certain cellular determinants of chemosensitivity (Box 13.3). For an example of the influence of tumor predisposition, the diagnosis of WAGR carries with it a high risk of end stage renal disease as these patients approach adulthood, which has been shown to result in a fall off of survival from 95% at 4 years to just under 48% at 27 years when compared with only a modest reduction in survival for patients without this condition [60].

For those patient- and tumor-related factors that may influence prognosis, then both age and tumor size relate to outcome for Wilms' tumor. For example, nephrectomy without adjuvant therapy was suggested to be adequate treatment for a subset of patients with highly favorable clinical features in the 1970s. It was suggested by Green and Jaffe [61] because of the excellent survival of infants with small tumors on successive NWTS trials [62, 63]. Therefore, the NWTS-5 trial saw the prospective treatment of 75 children younger than 24 months with small (<550 g) stage I favorable histology tumors with nephrectomy only, but the study closed early according to predefined stopping rules because the risk of relapse at 2 years was 13.5%. However, all patients were successfully salvaged with standard therapy [64]. In light of the high overall survival (OS) rate achieved, the COG is re-evaluating the benefit of nephrectomy-only in this selected group of patients.

The definition of histological subtype, both at diagnosis and after initial chemotherapy is an important determinant of prognosis for Wilms' tumor as follows:

Box 13.3 Wilms' tumor key facts – determinants of prognosis.

• Associated tumor-predisposition syndrome
• Age
• Tumor size
• Histological subtype
• Complete necrosis in response to pre-nephrectomy chemotherapy
• Loss of heterozygosity for chromosome 1p and 16q
• Expression of MDR-1 by neovasculature of tumor
• Expression of MRP1 by blastemal/stromal elements of tumor

• The finding of diffuse anaplasia at diagnosis, especially in the context of higher stage disease, carries a poor prognosis [54].

• Children with the blastemal predominant tumors after pre-operative chemotherapy were found to have a poorer prognosis than other histological subtypes of the intermediate risk group [30].

• The extent of tumor necrosis following pre-nephrectomy chemotherapy is also a determinant of prognosis. For children receiving pre-nephrectomy chemotherapy, a statistically significant improvement in event free survival is found for those patients who have found to have a complete necrotic Wilms' tumor at delayed nephrectomy and this applies to patients with all stages of disease. In particular, children with stage IV disease were relatively over represented in the population of patients achieving complete tumor necrosis, and enjoyed an excellent prognosis [65].

The cytogenetic findings for Wilms' tumor, both at diagnosis and following chemotherapy, also relate to outcome. For children entering the NWTS-5 trial, loss of heterozygosity at chromosomes 1p and 16q has been found to be an adverse prognostic indicator [19]. Also, analysis of comparative genomic hybridization findings in primary Wilms' tumors of blastemal histology, has shown significant differences in the cytogenetic constitution between those tumors undergoing primary surgery and those receiving pre-operative chemotherapy. As a trend, tumors in the pre-nephrectomy chemotherapy group had fewer changes than those in the non-pre-nephrectomy chemotherapy group, and the frequencies of imbalances at 7p or +7q, respectively, were significantly lower. The results suggest that Wilms' tumor clones with +1q prevail after chemotherapy, while cytogenetically more complex clones with +7q and/or imbalances at 7p appear to be more responsive and are more likely to be eliminated by chemotherapeutic treatment [66]. This and the significantly higher reduction of tumor volume in intermediate risk than in high-risk tumors shows that response to pre-operative therapy is of prognostic value.

The major international treatment protocols for Wilms' tumor include vincristine and doxorubicin, which are both substrates for resistance mediated by the P-glycoprotein (MDR-1) and multi-drug resistance-associated protein-1 (MRP1) efflux mechanisms, and both of these cellular determinants of chemosensitivity relate to the prognosis for children with Wilms' tumor as follows:

• For children with nephroblastoma, increased microvascular density is predictive of relapse [67].

• Increased expression of P-glycoprotein/MDR-1 by the endothelial cells that line the newly formed capillaries in association with tumor growth is a determinant of poor prognosis rather than any association between P-glycoprotein expression by Wilms' tumor cells themselves [68].

• Furthermore, expression of MRP1 has been found to be heterogeneous and predominantly found in the blastemal and epithelial compartment compared with the stromal elements of nephroblastoma.

• A significant relationship between MRP1 expression and an adverse outcome has been demonstrated for patients with nephroblastoma [69], and MRP1 expression was found to relate to P53 levels, which is known to be associated with angiogenesis and clinically aggressive disease in favourable histology Wilms' tumor [70].

Therefore, mechanisms of drug resistance exist within Wilms' tumor as demonstrated by expression of MDR by the endothelial cells of the neovasculature associated with the tumor, and also a more complex interaction of MRP1 and P53 in the non-stromal elements of this tumor. This may be an important means by which cells may acquire or be intrinsically resistant to chemotherapy and at the molecular level the occurrence of WT1 gene mutations has been found to upregulate anti-apoptotic mechanisms such as the BCL-2 protein family [71]. This has been shown to be a determinant of chemo-resistance of vincristine and doxorubicin *in vitro*.

Age-related difference in the pharmacokinetic disposition of chemotherapy agents, or for the expression of cellular determinants of chemosensitivity such as MDR1 and MRP have not been explored in relation to outcome for Wilms' tumor, but may at least in part explain certain clinical observations for therapy and outcome for this disease. For example, age at presentation relates to outcome for children with favourable histology Wilms' tumor, as demonstrated by the findings of the UKW2 and UKW3 trials for the treatment of Wilms' tumor. For 242 children with stage I favourable histology disease who were treated with immediate nephrectomy followed by 10 weekly injections of vincristine, the 4-year event-free survival was 93.2% for children less than 2 years of age, which compared with a significantly lower event-free survival of 71.3% for children 4 years or older at diagnosis.

Similarly, and as discussed above, the pharmacodynamic response to chemotherapy in terms of the percentage of patients achieving complete necrosis induced by pre-operative chemotherapy has also been related to outcome for children with non-anaplastic Wilms' tumor. As with the observation of the apparent effect of age upon event-free survival for children receiving vincristine monotherapy, this observation may help to inform treatment intensity and prognosis following therapy, but has not yet been explained in integrated studies of clinical cellular pharmacology in relation to this condition.

Other treatment considerations – Stage IV and bilateral disease

Stage 4 disease (Box 13.4)

About 10% of patients are diagnosed with metastatic disease. The most common sites of metastases of Wilms' tumor are the lungs (Figure 13.2(b)), the regional nodes, and the liver (Figure 13.1). Of patients presenting with hematogenous metastases at diagnosis (stage 4 disease), the relative frequency of sites for metastases are [72]:

• The lungs are the only site in approximately 80% of cases.

• The liver, with or without lungs, is involved in 15% of cases.

• Bone and brain metastases are rare in Wilms' tumor, occurring in 0.5% of cases [73].

Box 13.4 Wilms' tumor key facts – Stage 4 and bilateral disease.

- 10% of cases present with metastatic disease
- The lungs are the predominant site for metastases
- The optimal strategy for the treatment of pulmonary metastases detected by computed tomograpy only is uncertain
- Synchronous bilateral tumors occur in 4–7% of cases
- Metachronous tumors occur in 1–2% of cases
- Nephrogenic rests predispose to Wilms' tumor in setting of bilateral disease
- Kidney-sparing surgery is advocated after initial chemotherapy
- Renal failure in the long-term may necessitate kidney transplantation

---

Although patients with stage disease are particularly challenging to treat, in comparison with other forms of childhood cancer such as neuroblastoma or rhabdomyosarcoma, the outlook for children diagnosed with stage 4 disease is good with 4-year relapse-free survival, in the context of favourable histology, of 72% reported for the NWTS-3 study. For children with lung metastases detected on the chest radiograph, whole lung irradiation continues to be administered in North America, whereas in Europe response to pre-operative chemotherapy is used for stratification of lung irradiation. In NWTS-3, the 4-year relapse-free survival was 71.9%, and the 4-year survival was 78.4% in children with favourable histology Wilms' tumor and lung metastases [74]. The outcome for patients treated under the auspices of the SIOP 93-01 study is not different to the NWTSG series with a 4-year relapse-free survival of 83% in patients achieving a complete remission after preoperative chemotherapy compared to 65% without a radiological remission at the same time point. The salient features for the treatment of stage 4 disease include:

- The optimal treatment strategy for children with pulmonary metastases that are detectable by CT scan but not by plain X-radiograph remains uncertain. However, SIOP investigators continue to avoid radiotherapy for patients with intermediate risk histology whose lung metastases disappear completely after 6 weeks of pre-nephrectomy chemotherapy with vincristine, actinomycin-D, and doxorubicin.
- Children with metastatic disease to lungs have a better prognosis than those with other metastatic sites.
- High malignancy and local stage III are bad prognostic features in stage IV patients (N. Graf, unpublished data of SIOP 93-01/ GPOH).
- Although there are genuine concerns about radiation toxicity, the poor outcome in children who relapse after initial treatment necessitates a critical assessment of the role of pulmonary irradiation in these patients [72].

Stage 5 and bilateral disease

Various reports record the incidence of synchronous bilateral Wilms' tumor as ranging from 4.4% to 7.0% and that of metachronous bilateral Wilms' tumor from 1.0% to 1.9% of Wilms' tumor patients. The existence of precursor lesions to Wilms' tumor, termed nephrogenic rests, has been recognized for many years. These nephrogenic rests are found in almost 1% of unselected pediatric autopsies, in 35% of kidneys with unilateral Wilms' tumor and in nearly 100% of kidneys with bilateral Wilms' tumor. The key characteristics for nephrogenic rests are [29]:

- Nephrogenic rests are composed of abnormally persistent embryonal nephroblastic tissue with small clusters of blastemal cells, tubules, or stromal cells, and are classified by their position within the kidney.
- Intralobar nephrogenic rests (ILNR) are randomly distributed, but tend to be situated deep within the renal lobe. These lesions are commonly stroma-rich and intermingle with the adjacent renal parenchyma.
- Perilobar nephrogenic rests (PLNR) are located at the periphery, and are usually sub-cortical, sharply demarcated, and contain predominantly blastema and tubules. These presumably reflect later developmental disturbances in nephrogenesis.

The term nephroblastomatosis is used to refer to the presence of multiple nephrogenic rests. Only a small number develop a clonal transformation into Wilms' tumor. When this happens, the Wilms' tumor is typically spherical and develops a pseudocapsule separating it from the nephrogenic rest.

About 6% of all children with Wilms' tumor present with simultaneous bilateral tumors (stage 5) at the time of diagnosis. Although more than 70% of such cases survive, these children are at high risk of renal failure [75]. This risk has led to the recommendation that such patients undergo preoperative chemotherapy to shrink the tumor and facilitate renal-sparing procedures. The key principles for the management of children with stage 5 Wilms tumor are:

- Primary excision of the tumor masses is not recommended. After 6–12 weeks of chemotherapy, the patient is reassessed and the feasibility of resection assessed. If there is no response to preoperative chemotherapy, further intensifying of treatment is seldom successful and surgical excision of the tumor should be performed [72].
- Post-operative treatment is recommended according to the criteria for unilateral disease, always based on the highest stage and worst histology of one side.
- The treatment for stage 5 disease in association with nephroblastomatosis has to be prolonged with vincristine and actinomycin-D.
- In the long follow up much attention has to be given to the renal function. An NWTSG review found that 9.1% of patients with synchronous bilateral Wilms' tumors and 18.8% of those with metachronous bilateral tumors have developed renal failure [75].
- The most common etiology for renal failure was the need for bilateral nephrectomy for persistent or recurrent tumor in the

remaining kidney after initial nephrectomy. Treatment-related injury (radiation-induced damage, surgical complications) to the remaining kidney was the second leading cause for renal insufficiency. Renal insufficiency secondary to hyperfiltration-induced injury (focal glomerulosclerosis) was rare [75]. Kidney transplantation has to be considered in these situations.

Kidney-sparing surgery

Partial nephrectomy as a primary tumor resection strategy remains controversial and is probably not indicated in routine treatment of Wilms' tumor. After successful inauguration of parenchymal-sparing surgery in children with bilateral Wilms' tumor [76, 77], recent reports emphasize conservative surgery for children with unilateral Wilms' tumor [78–80]. The salient features for the consideration of kidney sparing surgery include:
• For children presenting with non-metastatic, unilateral Wilms' tumors it was found that only 4.7% of patients would be eligible for partial nephrectomy [81, 82].
• Partial nephrectomy should only be attempted if the tumor involves one pole and less than one third of the kidney, if the affected kidney is functioning, if the collecting system or renal vein had no tumor involvement, and if clear margins existed between the tumor and surrounding structures.
• Because the rate of renal failure in patients with unilateral Wilms' tumor is less than 1% [75], kidney-sparing resection is not generally recommended and should be restricted to few experienced surgical centers.
• A recently published study [83] presented bench surgery with auto-transplantation as another new surgical technique for exploration in this area.

Treatment strategies for relapsed disease

Approximately 15% of patients with favorable-histology Wilms' tumor and 50% of patients with anaplastic Wilms' tumor experience relapse of their disease. Most recurrences occur within 2 years of diagnosis and mainly in the lungs, the tumor bed, and the liver. Less frequently bones, the brain, and distant lymph nodes are sides of relapses. Metachronous bilaterilization to the contralateral kidney likely represents second primary tumors rather than true relapses. Although surgical excision of pulmonary metastases does not improve outcome [84], surgical biopsy or excision of recurrence should nonetheless be performed to confirm histologically the presence of recurrent disease, and particularly in the case of intra-abdominal recurrence, to reduce the tumor burden prior to the initiation of radiation therapy and combination chemotherapy.

Children with relapsed Wilms' tumor have a variable prognosis. Outcome depends upon the initial stage, histology, site of relapse, time from initial diagnosis to relapse, and previous therapy. Favorable prognostic factors include [85, 86]:
• Favorable histology, no prior treatment with an anthracycline.
• Relapse more than 12 months after diagnosis.
• Sub-diaphragmatic relapse in a patient not previously given abdominal irradiation.

However, one-third of all relapses fulfil the above criteria. These patients have a good chance of achieving a second complete remission with a survival rate of more than 60% [85–87]. Two-thirds of patients have high risk relapses with a poor outcome of less than 40% survival rate [88–91].

Treatment regimens for recurrent Wilms' tumor are designed to include chemotherapy agents that were not used during primary therapy. Several highly effective chemotherapy combinations, including ifosfamide-carboplatin-etoposide (ICE), cyclophosphamide-etoposide, and carboplatin-etoposide, are considered first-line treatment for recurrent disease [88–91].

The effective use of high-dose therapy with stem cell rescue for the treatment of recurrent Wilms' tumor has been reported by several groups, and survival rates of 36–73% are described [88–91]. It has been suggested that high-dose chemotherapy with stem cell rescue should be employed in the management of patients with adverse prognostic factors at the time of relapse, although it remains unproved whether this approach is more efficacious and/or less toxic than conventional chemotherapy. In general, these children should be referred to centers that are conducting research into the treatment of children with recurrent solid tumors.

Short-term complications of presentation and treatment

The most frequent short-term complications of the treatment of Wilms' tumor include those that relate to the surgical procedures of laparotomy and biopsy, and medical complications that result from the use of cytotoxic chemotherapy agents. Surgical complications in relation to the treatment and diagnosis of Wilms' tumor include:
• Risk of tumor rupture and consequent upstaging of Wilms' tumor at laparotomy. In relation to the international differences in practice with respect to primary nephrectomy versus pre-nephrectomy chemotherapy, the incidence of intraoperative complications occurring with a rupture of tumor is lowered from approximately 25% to 8% following pre-operative chemotherapy in one institutional experience [92].
• Other surgical complications observed in the fourth National Wilms' Tumor Study (NWTS-4) following primary nephrectomy include bowel obstruction (5.1%), extensive hemorrhage and wound infection (1.9% each), extensive vascular injuries (1.4%), and injuries to other visceral organs (1%) [93]. Risk factors for surgical complications included intravascular extension into the inferior vena cava, the atrium, or both; a flank or paramedian surgical approach; and a tumor diameter greater than 10 cm. Interestingly, nephrectomy performed by a general surgeon carried a higher risk of complications than that performed by a pediatric surgeon or a pediatric urologist.
• Biopsy of tumor prior to pre-nephrectomy chemotherapy being administered is a relatively safe procedure, but is associated in a fall in hemoglobin and local cases and local pain in one-fifth of cases [58]. However, biopsy was associated with the requirement for emergency nephrectomy or death in less than 1% of cases, and in one case out of 241 biopsies a needle track recurrence occurred 8 months following the biopsy [94].

• The potential benefit of tumor volume reduction after pre-operative chemotherapy is also seen in a low total surgical complication rate of 8% in SIOP-9 patients [95]. The most frequent event was small-bowel occlusion, including intussusceptions (3.7%). This contrasts with the reported surgical complication rate in NWTS-3, in which small bowel obstruction was reported in 6.9% of the registered patients [96]. However, in other series this complication is not influenced by the initial modality of treatment [33].

• In the United Kingdom experience, 8% of children presenting with Wilms' tumor have evidence of intracaval extension which subsequently requires cavotomy and on rarer occasions cardiopulmonary bypass for intra-atrial extension with tumor [33].

In relation to the medical complications of therapy for Wilms' tumor, veno-occlusive disease has been characterized in relation to the treatment of Wilms' tumor, and different studies have highlighted the pharmacodynamic effects for the differing schedules of actinomycin-D administration that have been related to hepatotoxicity as follows [97]:

• The effect of actinomycin-D dose. For the NWTS-4, severe hepatotoxicity with veno-occlusive disease rates of 43% and 3.7% were observed for children receiving single, 3 weekly doses of $60\,\mu g/kg$ (equivalent to $1.8\,mg/m^2$) than for $45\,\mu g/kg$ (equivalent to $1.35\,mg/m^2$), respectively, and the risk of this complication also increases for children who received abdominal radiotherapy as part of their treatment.

• The effect of actinomycin-D schedule. For the SIOP-9 study, a veno-occlusive disease rate of 4.8% was found for children receiving standard fractionated actinomycin D at a dose intensity of 9.4–$22.5\,\mu g/kg/week$, but no such complications were experienced in children receiving single dose actinomycin D at a dose intensity of 3.75–$8\,\mu g/kg/week$ even in the face of abdominal radiotherapy [98].

Strategies for follow up and overview of important late effects

Children who survive more than three years from diagnosis of their Wilms' tumor are unlikely to suffer a recurrence, and the vast majority are at very low risk of developing second cancers related to their treatment. The aim of long-term follow up is therefore to monitor renal function. Survivors of renal malignancies should be examined regularly by a physician who is familiar with the natural history of this tumor, and the complications of therapy for this disease. Careful palpation of the abdomen will help detect local tumor recurrence, tumor growth in the liver, or contralateral tumor development. Suspicious findings on physical examination should be confirmed or clarified using abdominal ultrasound or CT. Lung irradiation may affect the thyroid gland, which therefore should be palpated yearly for life because of the known association between irradiation and thyroid neoplasms. In addition, these patients should have thyroid function tests performed at yearly intervals for 5 years to detect possible hypothyroidism (Table 13.10).

It is of interest that recent data from the NWTSG showed that children with Wilms' tumor and aniridia and also those with

Table 13.10 Checklist for the follow-up of patients with nephroblastoma.

	Year 1 and 2	Year 3 and 4	After 4 years
Regarding relapse			
Clinical examination, RR	3 monthly	6 monthly	1 yearly
Abdominal sonography	3 monthly	6 monthly	1 yearly
Lung X-ray or CT of lungs	3 monthly	6 monthly	1 yearly
MRI with and without contrast	In case of suspicious finding in sonography, ...		
Bone scintigraphy	CCSK, or in case of bone metastasis		
Regarding late effects			
Urine	3 monthly	6 monthly	1 yearly
Creatinine	3 monthly	6 monthly	1 yearly
Echocardiography	In case of treatment with anthracyclines		
Endocrinology	In case of irradiation (ovary, testis, thyroid)		
Audiology	In case of cisplatin or carboplatin treatment		
Lung function	In case of lung irradiation		
Neuropsychology	In case of mental retardation		
Second malignancies	About 1%		

RR, regarding relapse. CT, computed tomography. MRI, magnetic resonance imaging. CCSK, clear cell carcinoma of the kidney.

intra-lobar nephrogenic rests have a high incidence of renal failure with long-term follow up beyond 20 years [99]. It is therefore important that such information is imparted to their adult physicians or general practitioners.

Although no studies have been carried out to evaluate the most effective schedule of follow up, these proposed intervals are based on the fact that most recurrences (~90%) occur in the first 2 years after diagnosis and virtually the remainder in the next 2 years. Subsequent imaging studies should be obtained as clinically indicated.

For children with any of the Wilms' tumor-predisposing syndromes, or with nephrogenic rests in one or both kidneys, ultrasonography of the remaining kidney is performed for a longer period because the opposite kidney continues to be at risk for several years. This is particularly true for children younger than 12 months of age at diagnosis.

Because Wilms' tumor is usually a curable malignancy, it is essential to limit iatrogenic sequelae. Although the damage may be limited to the kidney (nephrectomy), additional treatment modalities may cause acute and chronic late effects to several organs such as the heart, lungs, liver, bones, and gonads. In addition, both chemotherapeutic agents and radiation therapy can induce second malignant neoplasms.

Current treatment strategies

The paradigm of maximizing cure while minimizing toxicity is being further evaluated in the ongoing SIOP-2001 protocol, in which post-operative chemotherapy is tailored according to histological features, as defined by the SIOP classification system [51]. In order to address concerns in relation to anthracycline-related cardiac toxicity, patients with stage II or III and histologically intermediate-risk disease are randomly assigned to receive a treatment with or without doxorubicin.

In relation to current COG strategies, having almost reached cure for most patients and knowing that better stratification parameters for treatment are only possible by finding prognostic molecular markers, the major aim of the closed non-randomized NWTS-5 trial therefore was to assess the prognostic value of loss of heterozygosity at chromosomes 1p and 16q and DNA ploidy. The results of NWTS-5 provide the framework for future Children's Oncology Group studies of Wilms' tumor. It could be shown that LOH at 1p and 16q is an adverse prognostic indicator [19]. For the first time molecular markers are now used as stratification parameters in the upcoming COG trials for nephroblastoma. On the basis of the lower than expected survival rate for patients with stage I anaplasia, the upcoming study will also augment therapy for this group of patients [53].

Novel therapeutic approaches

For children with high-risk Wilms' tumor, new approaches to therapy will be needed, and the pre-clinical evaluation of novel anticancer agents should include *in vivo* experience with tumor types thought to be of interest for clinical development. The potential importance of this principle can be found for early xenograft studies based on current modalities of treatment, whereby post-operative chemotherapy with vincristine, actinomycin and doxorubicin increased survival over surgery alone, an effect that was further enhanced by the addition of radiotherapy [100].

A Medline review of the involvement of Wilms' tumor xenografts in the pre-clinical evaluation of novel agents, or the publication of early clinical trials featuring children with Wilms' tumor in their populations, is presented Table 13.11. Broadly speaking, this activity relates to the exploration of:
- Early clinical trials with irinotecan and topotecan.
- The tubulin inhibitor ABT-751.
- The evolving field of angiogenesis inhibition.

In the setting of the biological study of Wilms' tumor, it is now being recognized that tumor proliferation and angiogenesis relates to epidermal growth factor [101] and ErbB2 [102], raising the possibility for therapy with novel receptor tyrosine kinase inhibitors that are potent inhibitors of these signaling pathways. However, perhaps the most extensively characterized interaction between novo-therapy and anti-tumor effect *in vivo* in the pre-clinical setting exists for the vascular endothelial growth factor (VEGF) and its receptors especially VEGFR-2. In the experimental setting, potent VEGF blockade as achieved by the decoy receptor VEGF-Trap trap exerts a potent effect on a Wilms' tumor xenograft [103]. VEGF expression has been found to relate to microvessel density as a measure of angiogenesis and outcome for children with Wilms' tumor [104]. As the recognition of acquired resistance to anti-angiogenesis agents evolves, *in vivo* studies employing VEGF-Trap continue to help to refine the optimal use of these novel agents such as titrating dosage to prevent vascular remodeling [102, 105]. These studies may serve as an important paradigm in the pre-clinical setting to help evolve treatment strategies involving VEGF inhibition that may find clinical application for children for whom an adverse outcome is expected with conventional therapies.

The cellular pharmacological determinants of chemo-sensitivity may prove to be an important determinant of outcome for children with Wilms' tumor and help develop rational therapies designed to overcome this phenomenon in children where adverse risk factors such as MDR and MRP expression indicate that chemotherapy with vincristine and doxorubicin may be of limited efficacy. However, the science of pharmacology has a relatively rare but important usage in the pharmacokinetically-guided dosing of carboplatin and etoposide during peritoneal dialysis and haemodialysis for children who are anephric following treatment of Wilms' tumor [106] and also for novel chemotherapy agents such as topotecan [107].

Summary and future directions for management

The treatment of Wilms' tumor will continue to be geared towards maximizing the chances of cure for children with this disease and also their quality of survival in the long term.

Table 13.11 Novel therapeutic approaches in relation to Wilms' tumor.

Context of study	New agent	Target	Reference
Preclinical			
Pre-clinical *in vivo*	Depsipeptide	Histone deacetylase	[108]
Pre-clinical *in vivo*	BMS247550	Microtubules	[109]
Pre-clinical *in vivo*	Blocking antibody	Epidermal growth Factor receptor	[110]
Clinical			
Phase I trial	Irinotecan	Topoisomerase I	[111]
Phase I trial	Topotecan-cyclophosphamide	Topoisomerase I	[112]
Phase I trial	ABT-751	Tubulin	[113]
Phase II trial	All trans retinoic acid and Interferon α2a	Multiple	[114]

Information that is now derived from the Automated Childhood Cancer Information System Project indicates that children with Wilms' tumor generally enjoy an excellent prognosis [9], but that survival rates for children who are older than 3 years of age at diagnosis and those with bilateral Wilms' tumor have a 10–15% poorer prognosis. However, this still relates to a survival rate of over 75% for children with favorable histology disease, and the impact of renal transplantation and renal-sparing surgery in relation to survivors of Denys-Drash syndrome related Wilms' tumor and other cases of bilateral disease [115], and ongoing evaluation of the cardiotoxicity of doxorubicin into the long term for survivors of Wilms' tumor [116], will continue to help inform health-related quality of life measures for children with Wilms' tumor. With this in mind, the recognition that important survivor-controlled differences for physical and psychosocial measures for survivors of Wilms' tumor indicate an ongoing need for studies to reduce treatment sequelae when this is possible in the maintenance of high cure rates [117].

Furthermore, novel effective agents are required for the therapy of advanced stage anaplastic or relapsed Wilms' tumors, for which the prognosis remains dismal. Understanding of the genesis of Wilms' tumor at the genetic level may allow an increased ability to identify individuals at highest risk for the development of the disease. Studies of gene expression profiles will hopefully shed light on the intracellular pathways of the Wilms' phenotype, allowing optimal prognostic factors to be discovered and ultimately to lead to novel therapeutic targets.

Renal rhabdoid tumors

Introduction

Rhabdoid tumors were first recognized as a separate pathological entity in the 1980s, and have now been reported widely at most anatomical sites in the body [118]. Rhabdoid tumor of the kidney is a rare, highly aggressive and frequently lethal tumor of childhood, and is characterized by the following features:
• These tumors occur mainly in children below the age of 2 years. After 5 years of age renal rhabdoid tumors are a rarity.
• Cytogenetic, fluorescence *in situ* hybridization (FISH), and LOH studies have revealed that malignant rhabdoid tumors frequently contain alterations at chromosome locus 22q11.1 [119, 120] (Box 13.5).

Because rhabdoid tumors demonstrate biallelic, inactivating mutations of *SMARCB1* (synonym: *INI1, hSNF5*), consistent with the 'two-hit' model of tumor formation, it is presumed that this gene functions as a classic tumor suppressor [121–23]. The observation that mice haplo insufficient for *SMARCB1* are predisposed to rhabdoid tumor supports this premise [124]. In most cases, the mutations are *de novo*, and not inherited from a parent. Germ line mosaicism has been suggested for several families with multiple affected siblings [125]. As a consequence for families with an affected child and the diagnosis of a *SMARCB1* mutation a genetic counselling is indicated. Only plexus carcinomas and

---

Box 13.5 Renal rhabdoid tumor key facts.

• Rare and highly aggressive
• Majority occur in children less than 2 years of age
• Characterized by genetic alterations at 22q11.1 and inactivating mutations of SMARCB1, which forms the basis for immunohistochemical diagnosis
• Approximate 40% survival for localized disease, but poor prognosis in setting of very young age and metastatic disease
• Current treatment strategies based on aggressive regimens based on the alkylating agents and etoposide

---

epitheloid sarcomas show also mutations of *SMARCB1*. At present, there is insufficient data to suggest an association between specific mutations and clinical outcome.

Investigations and staging

There are no typical clinical signs in children suffering from a renal rhabdoid tumor. The symptoms do not differ from children with other kidney tumors. However, the following features indicate the diagnosis of a renal rhabdoid tumor:
• Imaging studies are most important. In comparison with nephroblastoma, renal rhabdoid tumors are more lobulated, often showing peripheral subcapsular bleedings, more lymph node involvement and more often lung metastases [126, 127].
• In a small infant with a renal mass and metastasis to lung, renal rhabdoid tumor is the most likely tumor diagnosis.
• The diagnosis of renal rhabdoid tumor can only be done by histology, and detection of *SMARCB1* gene mutations is also possible by immunohistochemical techniques.

Nevertheless, in every case tumor material should be used for molecular genetic analysis to confirm the diagnosis of renal rhabdoid tumor and to perform gene array experiments for gaining further knowledge [128]. Tumor staging is the same as in nephroblastoma, but because of the coincidence of brain metastasis, cerebral MRI is always indicated.

Contemporary treatment philosophies

There have not been any prospective clinical trials published describing the management and treatment of renal rhabdoid tumor, but recently there have been reports of survivors, even when there has been metastatic disease, with the use of more intensive chemotherapy regimes including doxorubicin [129, 130].

In the United Kingdom (UK), patients with rhabdoid tumor of the kidney have historically been treated on two consecutive national Wilms' tumor protocols (UKW2 and UKW3) with a combination of vincristine, actinomycin D and doxorubicin. In a recent audit of 21 patients with renal rhabdoids treated on these protocols the overall survival was 35%, with all deaths within 13 months of diagnosis. The International Society of Pediatric Oncology (SIOP) reported similarly unfavorable outcomes [131].

In the United States, patients with rhabdoid tumor of the kidney historically have been treated on the National Wilms Tumor Study Group (NWTSG) trials with agents such as vincristine, actinomycin, and doxorubicin, with or without cyclophosphamide [132, 133]. The outcomes attained with these agents were poor [132–134]. In a review of 142 patients from NWTS 1-5, stage and age are significant prognostic factors. Patients with stage I and stage II disease had an OS rate of 42%; higher stage was associated with a 16% overall survival. Infants less than 6 months of age at diagnosis demonstrated a 4-year OS of 9%, whereas OS in patients aged 2 years and older was 41%. No survival differences were observed between males and females, between those treated with or without doxorubicin, or with or without radiotherapy [135].

Experience with other established or more novel cytotoxic agents is more limited, but several case reports have documented the successful treatment of advanced or metastatic renal rhabdoid tumor with the combination of:
- Ifosfamide/etoposide (IE) alternating with vincristine/doxorubicin/cyclophosphamide (VDCy) [129].
- Ifosfamide/carboplatin/etoposide (ICE) alternating with VDCy [2]. Gururangan *et al.* reported encouraging, transient responses to ICE chemotherapy in patients with advanced-stage renal and extrarenal rhabdoid tumor [136].
- Other promising drugs are topotecan and irinotecan against rhabdoid tumors as shown in xenograft models at the St Jude Children's Research Hospital (Jeff Dome, personal communication). Clinical data on the activity of irinotecan in patients with malignant rhabdoid tumor is limited. Blaney *et al.* reported that 1/2 patients with rhabdoid tumor had stable disease following treatment with irinotecan given on a daily ×5 regimen [137].

Future directions
The prognosis for renal rhabdoid tumor remains dismal, and treatment is not yet standardized. However, the COG in Northern America as well as SIOP in Europe are now initiating prospective multi-center trials for renal rhabdoid tumor, and it is of utmost importance that molecular biological investigations are conducted as part of this process in order to gain further insights into the biology of this rare tumor and thereby help to inform the rational development of novel treatment strategies.

Clear cell sarcoma of the kidney

Clear cell sarcoma of the kidney (CCSK) is a paediatric renal tumor that affects children primarily between the ages of 2 and 5, and accounts for 3–5% of all childhood renal tumors [138]. Kidd in 1970 [139] was first to recognize CCSK as an entity different from nephroblastoma, and in 1978 Morgan and Kidd [140], and Marsden and Lawler [141] simultaneously described the distinctive histopathological features of this tumor. Because of its propensity to metastasize to the bones, especially to the skull, Marsden defined it as a 'bone metastasizing renal tumor of

---

Box 13.6 Clear cell sarcoma of the kidney key facts.

- Rare tumor with similar presenting demography to that of nephroblastoma
- Lack of genetic characteristics, which necessitates a histological diagnosis which can be difficult
- Tendency to metastases to bone and brain
- Approximate 60% survival for more localized disease, but poorer prognosis in the setting of metastatic disease
- Current treatment strategies based on aggressive regimens based on the alkylating agents and etoposide

---

childhood' [141], and the other typical sites of metastasis are the lungs and the brain (Box 13.6).

Histologically, CCSK shows a tremendous morphologic diversity, which means that there can be difficulty in differentiating this from other renal tumors such as rhabdoid tumor of the kidney and mesoblastic nephroma [142]. Indeed, in studies up to 50% of all CCSK have initially been classified as an entity different from CCSK by local pathologists [142]. As with anaplastic Wilms' tumor and malignant rhabdoid tumors of the kidney, CCSK is classified as a tumor with unfavourable histology because of its metastatic potential to bones and tendency to recur, the latter sometimes happening many years after the original diagnosis [138].

Unlike Wilms' tumor, CCSK is not associated with any genetic syndrome and its molecular pathogenesis remains poorly understood.
- Biallelic IGF 2 expression, LOH (+19p, +1q, −10q, −19) and translocation t(10;17)(q20;p13) have been shown in CCSK, though a genetic alteration specific for CCSK has not been verified yet [143–145].
- Although Punnett *et al.* described a t(135;152) involving a breakpoint at the *p53* locus of chromosome 17p13 [146], the majority of CCSK cases to date have been shown to lack *p53* abnormalities, occurring only in tumors with anaplastic features.
- Reported cytogenetic abnormalities include deletion of chromosome 14q23 [147] t(145;152)(q157;p148) [148].
- Activation of the sonic hedgehog and Akt signalling pathways in CCSK with up-regulation of neural markers; the same study suggests that CD117 and epidermal growth factor receptor may be potential therapeutic targets in some cases of CCSK [149].

Together with the published literature, Brownlee *et al.* indicate that t(145;152) and interstitial deletions of chromosome 14q are recurring cytogenetic lesions in CCSK. The t(145;152) breakpoint and deletion of chromosome 14q24 suggest that other genes than p53 are involved in tumor pathogenesis [150].

Investigations and staging
The symptoms of children with CCSK do not differ from children with other kidney tumors, and most patients present with a median age that is not different from nephroblastoma.

- Most patients are diagnosed within the second and third year of life.
- Right- and left-sided tumors occur equally distributed.
- In comparison to nephroblastoma more boys are affected than girls.
- There is a 1.7:1 preponderance of male patients.

Diagnosis is made accordiong to thc gudelines described for Wilms' tumor, with imaging studies sharing similar characteristics. The diagnosis of CCSK can only be done by histology. Clear cell sarcoma of the kidney is typically centred in the medulla and is characterized grossly by a fleshy, tan, firm cut surface. Several histologic patterns are recognized, but nests and cords of cells typify the classic pattern, and are separated by fine, arborizing fibrovascular septa (so-called chicken-wire pattern), and collagenous material that is intermingled among the tumor cells. Nuclei are optically clear with fine chromatin, round to oval in shape, lack prominent nucleoli, and mitoses are generally infrequent. Anaplastic features may be seen in rare cases of CCSK [150]. In every case tumor material should be used for molecular genetic analysis to perform, for example, gene array experiments for gaining further knowledge. Tumor staging is the same as in nephroblastoma. Because of the coincidence of bone and brain metastasis a bone scan and a cerebral MRI is always indicated.

Treatment philosophies of contemporary therapies

Earlier reports, in which treatment was based on vincristine and actinomycin-D for CCSK, highlights the very poor prognosis for this disease, with survival rates in the region of 30% [142, 151]. However, the introduction of additional therapies has seen an improvement in outcome for this disease:

- The addition of anthracyclines (epirubicin or doxorubicin) saw an improvement in outcome, but survival rates remained below those found for nephroblastoma [152, 153].
- In the National Wilms' Tumor Study 3 cyclophosphamide in addition to these three agents did not improve the outcome [154].
- In the SIOP-9 study, patients with a CCSK received the triple drug regimen of vincristine, actinomycin-D and doxorubicin with additional ifosfamide. Five years after diagnosis the event-free survivial rate was below 60%, but OS was as good at 88% [155]. The OS in this study was remarkably better than the EFS. This suggests that salvage therapeutics used at the respective time such as etoposide, carboplatin, and cyclophosphamide could be more effective in the treatment of CCSK than classical nephroblastoma agents.

The results of recent trials support this observation [156]. In SIOP 93-01 and the ongoing SIOP 2001 trial and study, patients are treated with ifosfamide, doxorubicin, carboplatin, and etoposide, and only in localized stage I (which enjoys a more favourable prognosis) is treatment still based on the triple drug regimen alone. In the ongoing COG trial (AREN 0321), patients with localized stage I to III are treated according to regimen I consisting of vincristine, cyclophosphamide, doxorubicin, carboplatin, and etoposide. For stage IV patients, treatment is intensified as

for diffuse anaplastic nephroblastoma or rhabdoid tumor. Treatment duration is 24 weeks in localized disease. All patients will receive local irradiation in AREN 0321, whereas in SIOP only patients with a local stage higher than I are irradiated.

Preliminary results of 50 patients with CCSK treated within the SIOP 93-01/GPOH study confirm the benefit of these treatment regimens [156]. After a median observation period of 6.9 years the overall survival rate was 91%. Two of three patients with initial metastasis are in continuous complete remission. Only seven of the 50 patients relapsed, six of them had cerebral metastasis, four of which were fatal. No flank relapse occurred. Patients younger than 2 years of age at diagnosis had a lower event-free survival rate (74%) than older patients (93%). A local stage III was the only significant and independent risk factor in this study (event-free survival 97% versus 54%).

Future directions

With the introduction of carboplatin and etoposide to the treatment regimen prognosis of patients with CCSK has significantly improved. Even patients with initial metastatic disease can be cured today. Attention has to be given to the high intracerebral relapse rate. This clearly shows the importance of treating patients with this rare tumor in prospective multicenter trials. To achieve more insight into the pathogenesis of CCSK and to make further progress in the treatment of this entity, tumor material should always be stored for molecular genetic analysis.

References

1 D'Angio GJ, Evans AE, Breslow N, et al. The treatment of Wilm's tumor: results of the national Wilms' tumor study. Cancer 1976; 38: 633–46.
2 Lemerle J, Voute PA, Tournade MF, et al. Preoperative versus postoperative radiotherapy, single versus multiple courses of actinomycin D, in the treatment of Wilm's tumor. Preliminary results of a controlled clinical trial conducted by the International Society of Paediatric Oncology (SIOP). Cancer 1976; 38: 647–54.
3 Howard R. Actinomycin D in Wilm's tumor: treatment of lung metastases. Arch Dis Childh 1965; 40: 200.
4 Burgert EO, Jr, Glidewell O. Dactinomycin in Wilm's Tumor. JAMA 1967; 199: 464–8.
5 Sutow WW, Thurman WG, Windmiller J. Vincristine (Leurocristine) sulfate in the treatment of children with metastatic Wilm's tumor. Pediatrics 1963; 32: 800–87.
6 Sullivan MP. Vincristine (NSC-67574) Therapy for Wilm's Tumor. Cancer Chemother Rep 1968; 52: 481–4.
7 Ragab AH, Sutow WW, Komp DM, et al. Adriamycin in the treatment of childhood solid tumors. A Southwest Oncology Group study. Cancer 1975; 36: 1567–76.
8 Camitta B, Kun L, Glicklich M, et al. Doxorubicin-vincristine therapy for Wilm's tumor: a pilot study. Cancer Treat Rep 1982; 66: 1791–4.
9 Pastore G, Znaor A, Spreafico F, et al. Malignant renal tumors incidence and survival in European children (1978–1997): report from

the Automated Childhood Cancer Information System project. Eur J Cancer 2006; 42: 2103–14.

10 Gurney JG, Severson RK, Davis S, Robison LL. Incidence of cancer in children in the United States: sex-, race-, and 1-year age-specific rates by histologic type. Cancer 1995; 75: 2186–95.

11 Bernstein L, Linet M, Smith MA, et al. Renal tumor. In: Ries LAG, Smith MA, Gurney JG, et al. (Eds), Cancer incidence and survival among children and adolescents: United States SEER program. Bethesda: NIH Publication no 99–4649, 1999: 79–90.

12 Breslow N, Olsham A, Beckwith JB, Green DM. Epidemiology of Wilms tumor. Med Pediatr Oncol 1993; 21: 172–81.

13 Parkin DM, Kramárová E, Draper GJ, et al. (Eds). International Incidence of Childhood Cancer. International Agency for Research on Cancer, International Association of Cancer Registries, Vol. II. Lyon: IARC Scientific Publications No. 144, 1998.

14 Little J (Ed.). Epidemiology of Childhood Cancer. IARC scientific publications no. 149. Lyon: International Agency for Research on Cancer,1999.

15 Fukuzawa R, Breslow NE, Morison IA, et al. Epigenetic differences between Wilms' tumors in white and east-Asian children. Lancet 2004; 363: 446–51.

16 Green DM. Wilms' tumor. Eur J Cancer 1997; 33: 409–18.

17 Coppes MJ, Haber DA, Grundy PE. Genetic events in the development of Wilms' tumor. N Engl J Med 1994; 331: 586–90.

18 Klamt B, Schulze M, Thate C, et al. Allele loss in Wilms tumors of chromosome arms 11q, 16q, and 22q correlate with clinicopathological parameters. Genes Chrom Cancer 1998; 22: 287–94.

19 Grundy PE, Breslow NF, Li S et al. Loss of heterozygosity for chromosomes 1p and 16q is an adverse prognostic factor in favorable-histology Wilms tumor: a report from the National Wilms Tumor Study Group. J Clin Oncol 2005; 23: 7312–21.

20 Niemitz EL, Feinberg AP, Brandenburg SA, et al. Children with idiopathic hemihypertrophy and Beckwith-Wiedemann syndrome have different constitutional epigenotypes associated with Wilms tumor. Am J Hum Genet 2005; 77: 887–91.

21 Bliek J, Maas SM, Ruijter JM, et al. Increased tumor risk for BWS patients correlates with abherrant H19 and not KCNQ1OT1 methylation: occurrence of KCNQ10T1 hypomethylation in familial cases of BWS. Hum Mol Genet 2001; 10: 467–76.

22 Hastie ND. The genetics of Wilms' tumor; a case of disrupted development. Ann Rev Genet 1994; 28: 523–58.

23 Pelletier J, Bruening W, Kashtan CE, et al. Germline mutations in the Wilms' tumor suppressor gene are associated with abnormal urogential development in Denys-Drash syndrome. Cell 1991; 67: 437–47.

24 Koziell A, Charmandari E, Hindmarsh PC, et al. Frasier syndrome, part of the Denys Drash continuum or simply a WT1 gene associated disorder of intersex and nephropathy? Clin Endocrinol 2000; 52: 519–24.

25 Pritchard-Jones K. Molecular genetic pathways to Wilms' tumor. Crit Rev Oncog 1997; 8: 1–27.

26 Huff V. Wilms tumor genetics. Am J Med Genet 1998; 79: 260–7.

27 Schumacher V, Schneider S, Figg A, et al. Correlation of germ-line mutations and two-hit inactivation WT1 gene with Wilms' tumors of stromal-predominant histology. Proc Natl Acad Sci USA 1997; 94: 3972–7.

28 Rahman N, Arbour L, Tonin P, et al. Evidence for a familial Wilms' tumor gene (FWT1) on chromosome 17q12-q211. Nat Genet 1996; 13: 461–3.

29 Rapley EA, Barfoot R, Bonaiti-Pellie C, et al. Evidence for susceptibility genes to familial Wilms' tumor in addition to WT1, FWT1 and FWT2. Br J Cancer 2000; 83: 177–83.

30 Gutjahr P. Bundesweite Wilmstumor-Studie 1980 bis 1988. Dt Ärztebl 1990; 87: B2130–4.

31 Maas MH, Cransberg K, van Grotel M, et al. Renin-induced hypertension in Wilms tumor patients. Pediatr Blood Cancer 2007; 48: 500–3.

32 Leung RS, Liesner R, Brock P, et al. Coagulopathy as a presenting feature of Wilms tumor. Eur J Pediatr 2004; 163: 369–73.

33 Lall A, Pritchard-Jones K, Walker J, et al. Wilms' tumor with intracaval thrombus in the UK Children's Cancer Study Group UKW3 trial. J Pediatr Surg 2006; 41: 382–7.

34 Solwa Y, Sanyika C, Hadley GP, Corr P. Colour Doppler ultrasound assessment of the inferior vena cava in patients with Wilms' tumor. Clin Radiol 1999; 54: 811–4.

35 Gylys-Morin V, Hoffer FA, Kozakewich H, Shamberger RC. Wilms tumor and nephroblastomatosis: imaging characteristics at gadolinium-enhanced MR imaging. Radiology 1993; 188: 517–21.

36 Gow KW, Roberts IF, Jamieson DH, et al. Local staging of Wilms' tumor-computerized tomography correlation with histological findings. J Pediatr Surg 2000: 35: 677–9.

37 Ritchey ML, Green DM, Breslow NB, et al. Accuracy of current imaging modalities in the diagnosis of synchronous bilateral Wilms' tumor. A report from the National Wilms Tumor Study Group. Cancer 1995: 75: 600–4.

38 The revised SIOP working classification of renal tumors 2001.

39 Lemerle J, Voûte PA, Tournade MF, et al. Preoperative versus postoperative radiotherapy, single versus multiple courses of Actinomycin D, in the treatment of Wilms' tumor. Preliminary results of a controlled clinical trial conducted by the International Society of Pediatric Oncology (SIOP). Cancer 1976; 38: 647–54.

40 Lemerle J, Voûte PA, Tournade MF, et al. Effectiveness of preoperative chemotherapy in Wilms' tumor: results of an International Society of Paediatric Oncology (SIOP) Clinical Trial. J Clin Oncol 1983; 1: 604–9.

41 Tournade MF, Com-Nougué C, Voûte PA, et al. Results of the Sixth International Society of Pediatric Oncology Wilms' Tumor Trial and Study: a risk-adapted therapeutic approach in Wilms' Tumor. J Clin Oncol 1993; 11: 1014–23.

42 Voûte PA, Tournade MF, Lemerle J, et al. Results of studies conducted by the International Society of Paediatric Oncology (SIOP) from 1971–1978 concerning Wilms' tumor. Abstracts of the Tenth Meeting of the International Society of Paediatric Oncology (SIOP), Brussels, Belgium, September 1978: 3–5 (abstr 14).

43 Tournade MF, Com-Nougué C, de Kraker J, et al. Optimal duration of preoperative therapy in unilateral and nonmetastatic Wilms' tumor in children older than 6 months: results of the Ninth International Society of Pediatric Oncology Wilms' Tumour Trial and Study. J Clin Oncol 2001; 19: 488–500.

44 de Kraker J, Graf N, van Tinteren H, et al. Reduction of postoperative chemotherapy in children with stage I intermediate-risk and anaplastic Wilms' tumor (SIOP 93-01 trial): a randomised controlled trial. Lancet 2004; 364: 1229–35.

45 Green D, Breslow NE, Beckwith JB, et al. Effect of duration of treatment on treatment outcome and cost of treatment for Wilms' tumor: a report from the NWTSG. J Clin Oncol 1998; 16: 3744–51.

46 Green D, Breslow NE, Beckwith JB, et al. Comparison between single dose and divided dose administration of dactinomycin and doxorubicin for patients with Wilms' tumor: a report from the NWTSG. J Clin Oncol 1998; 16: 237–45.

47 Sutow WW, Breslow NE, Palmer NF, et al. Prognosis in children with Wilms' tumor metastases prior to or following primary treatment: results from the first National Wilms' Tumor Study (NWTS-1). Am J Clin Oncol 1982; 5: 339–47.

48 Green DM. The treatment of stages I-IV favorable histology Wilms' tumor. J Clin Oncol 2004; 22: 1366–72.

49 Kalapurakal JA, Dome JS, Perlman EJ, et al. Management of Wilms' tumor: current practice and future goals. Lancet Oncology 2004; 5: 37–46.

50 Metzger ML, Dome JS. Current Therapy for Wilms' Tumor. The Oncologist 2005; 10: 815–26.

51 Vujanic GM, Sandstedt B, Harms D, et al. Revised International Society of Paediatric Oncology (SIOP) working classification of renal tumors of childhood. Med Pediatr Oncol 2002; 38: 79–82.

52 Sutow WW, Breslow NE, Palmer NF, et al. Prognosis in children with Wilms' tumor metastases prior to or following primary treatment: results from the first National Wilms' Tumor Study (NWTS-1). Am J Clin Oncol 1982; 5: 339–47.

53 Breslow NE, Ou SS, Beckwith JB, et al. Doxorubicin for favorable histology, Stage II-III Wilms' tumor: results from the National Wilms' Tumor Studies. Cancer 2004; 101: 1072–80.

54 Dome JS, Cotton CA, Perlman EJ, et al. Treatment of anaplastic histology Wilms' tumor: results from the Fifth National Wilms' Tumor Study. J Clin Oncol 2006; 24: 2352–8.

55 Graf N, Tournade MF, de Kraker J. The role of preoperative chemotherapy in the management of Wilms' Tumor. The SIOP Studies. Urol Clin North Am 2000; 27: 443–54.

56 Pritchard J, Imeson J, Barnes J, et al. Results of the United Kingdom Children's Cancer Study Group (UKCCSG) first Wilms' tumor study (UKW-1). J Clin Oncol 1995; 13: 124–33.

57 Mitchell C, Morris JP, Kelsey A, et al. The treatment of Wilms tumor: results of the UKCCSG second Wilms tumor study. Br J Cancer 2000; 83: 602–8.

58 Mitchell C, Pritchard-Jones K, Shannon R et al. Immediate nephrectomy versus preoperative chemotherapy in the management of non-metastatic Wilms' tumor: Results of a randomised trial (UKW3) by the UK Children's Cancer Study Group. Eur J Cancer 2006; 42: 2554–62.

59 Shamberger RC. Pediatric renal tumors. Semin Surg Oncol 1999; 16: 105–20.

60 Breslow NE, Norris R, Norkool PA, et al. National Wilms Tumor Study Group. Characteristics and outcomes of children with the Wilms tumor- Anridia syndrome: a report from the National Wilms Tumor Study Group. J Clin Oncol 2003; 21: 4579–85.

61 Green DM, Jaffe N. The role of chemotherapy in the treatment of Wilms' tumor. Cancer 1979; 44: 52–7.

62 Larsen E, Perez-Atayde A, Green DM, et al. Surgery only for the treatment of patients with stage I (Cassady) Wilms' tumor. Cancer 1990; 66: 264–6.

63 Green DM, Breslow NE, Beckwith JB, et al. Treatment outcomes in patients less than 2 years of age with small, stage I, favourable histology Wilms' tumors: a report from the National Wilms' Tumor Study. J Clin Oncol 1993; 11: 91–5.

64 Green DM, Breslow NE, Beckwith JB, et al. Treatment with nephrectomy only for small, stage I/ favorable histology Wilms' tumor: a report from the National Wilms' Tumor Study Group. J Clin Oncol 2001; 19: 3719–24.

65 Boccon-Gibod L, Rey A, Sandstedt B, et al. Complete necrosis induced by preoperative chemotherapy in Wilms tumor as an indicator of low risk: report of the International Society of Pacdiatric Oncology (SIOP) Nephroblastoma Trial and Study 9. Medical and Pediatric Oncology 2000; 34: 183–90.

66 Schlomm T, Gunawan B, Schulten HJ, et al. Effects of chemotherapy on the cytogenetic constitution of Wilms tumor. Clin Cancer Res 2005; 11: 4382–7.

67 Abramson LP, Grundy PE, Rademaker AW, et al. Increased microvascular density predicts relapse in Wilms' tumor. J Pediatr Surg 2003; 38: 325–30.

68 Camassei FD, Arancia G, Cianfriglia M, et al. Nephroblastoma: mutlidrug-resistance P-glycoprotein expression in tumor cells and intramural capillary endothelial cells. Am J Clin Pathol 2002: 117: 484–90.

69 Efferth T, Thelen P, Schulten HG, et al. Differential expression of the multidrug resistance-related protein MRP1 in the histological compartments of nephroblastomas. Int J Oncol 2001; 19: 367–71.

70 Huang J, Soffer SZ, Kim ES, et al. p53 accumalation in favourable-histology Wilms tumor is associated with angiogenesis and clinically aggressive disease. J Pediatr Surg 2002: 37: 523–7.

71 Mayo MW, Wang CY, Drouin SS, et al. WT1 modulates apoptosis by transcriptionally upregulating the bcl-2 proto-oncogene. EMBO J 1999: 18: 3990–4003.

72 Kalapurakal JA, Dome JS, Perlman EJ, et al. Management of Wilms' tumor: current practice and future goals. Lancet Oncol 2004; 5: 37–46.

73 Lowis SP, Foot A, Gerrard MP, et al. Central nervous system metastases in Wilms tumor: a review of three consecutive United Kingdom trials. Cancer 1998; 83: 2023–9.

74 D'Angio GJ, Breslow N, Beckwith JB, et al. Treatment of Wilms' tumor: results of the Third National Wilms' Tumor Study. Cancer 1989; 64: 349–60.

75 Ritchey ML, Green DM, Thomas PR, et al. Renal failure in Wilms' tumor patients: a report from the National Wilms' Tumor Study Group. Med Pediatr Oncol 1996; 26: 75–80.

76 Horwitz JR, Ritchey ML, Moksness J, et al. Renal salvage procedures in patients with synchronous bilateral Wilms' tumors: a teport from the National Wilms' Tumor Study Group. J Pediatr Surg 1996; 31: 1020.

77 Kumar R, Fitzgerald R, Breatnach F. Conservative surgical management of bilateral Wilms tumor: results of the United Kingdom Children's Cancer study group. J Urol 1998; 160: 1450–3.

78 Moorman-Voestermans CGM, Aronson DC, Staalman CS, et al. Is partial nephrectomy appropriate treatment for unilateral Wilms' tumor? J Pediatr Surg 1998; 33: 165.

79 Cozzi F, Schiavetti A, Bonanni M, et al. Enucleative surgery for Stage I nephroblastoma with a normal contralateral kidney. J Urol 1996; 156: 1788.

80 Haecker FM, von Schweinitz D, Harms D, et al. Partial nephrectomy for unilateral Wilms tumor: results of study SIOP 93-01/GPOH. J Urol 2003; 170: 939–42.

81 Wilimas JA, Magill L, Parham DM, et al. Is renal salvage feasible in unilateral Wilms' tumor? Proposed computed tomographic criteria

and their relation to surgicopathologic findings. Am J Pediatr Hematol Oncol 1990; 12: 164–7.

82 Wilimas JA, Magill L, Parham DM, et al. The potential for renal salvage in nonmetastatic unilateral Wilms' tumor. Am J Pediatr Hematol Oncol 1991; 13: 342–4.

83 Desai D, Nicholls G, Duffy PG. Bench surgery with autotransplantation for bilateral synchronous Wilms' Tumor: a report of three cases. J Pediatr Surg 1999; 34: 632.

84 Green DM, Breslow N, Li Y, et al. The role of surgical excision in the management of relapsed Wilms' tumor patients with pulmonary metastases. J Pediatr Surg 1991; 26: 728–33.

85 Grundy P, Breslow NE, Green DM, et al. Prognostic factors of children with recurrent Wilms' tumor: results from the second and third National Wilms' Tumor Study. J Clin Oncol 1989; 7: 638–47.

86 Dome JS, Liu T, Krasin M, et al. Improved survival for patients with recurrent Wilms' tumor: the experience at St Jude Children's Research Hospital. J Pediatr Hematol Oncol 2002; 24: 192–8.

87 Wilimas JA, Champion J, Douglass EC, et al. Relapsed Wilms' tumor. Factors affecting survival and cure. Am J Clin Oncol 1985; 8: 324–8.

88 Garaventa A, Hartmann O, Bernard JL, et al. Autologous bone marrow transplantation for pediatric Wilms' tumor: the experience of the European Bone Marrow Transplantation Solid Tumor Registry. Med Pediatr Oncol 1994; 22: 11–14.

89 Pein F, Michon J, Valteau-Couanet D, et al. High-dose melphalan, etoposide, and carboplatin followed by autologous stem-cell rescue in pediatric high-risk recurrent Wilms' tumor: a French Society of Pediatric Oncology Study. J Clin Oncol 1998; 16: 3295–301.

90 Kremens B, Gruhn B, Klingebiel T, et al. High-dose chemotherapy with autologous stem cell rescue in children with nephroblastoma. Bone Marrow Trans 2002; 30: 893–8.

91 Campbell AD, Cohn SL, Reynolds M, et al. Treatment of relapsed Wilms' tumor with high-dose therapy and autologous hematopoietic stem-cell rescue: the experience at Children's Memorial Hospital. J Clin Oncol 2004; 22: 2885–90.

92 Stehr M, Deilmann K, Haas RJ, Dietz HG. Surgical complications in the treatment of Wilms' tumor. Eur J Pediatr Surg 2005; 15: 414–9.

93 Ritchey ML, Shamberger RC, Haase G, et al. Surgical complications after primary nephrectomy for Wilms' tumor: report from the National Wilms' Tumor Study Group. J Am Coll Surg 2001; 192: 63–8.

94 Vujanic GM, Kelsey A, Mitchell C, et al. The role of biopsy in the diagnosis of renal tumors of childhood: results of the UKCCSG Wilms tumor study 3. Med Pediatr Oncol 2003; 40: 18–22.

95 Godzinski J, Tournade MF, de Kraker J, et al. Rarity of surgical complications after postchemotherapy nephrectomy for nephroblastoma. Experience of the International Society of Paediatric Oncology – Trial and Study 'SIOP 9'. International Society of Paediatric Oncology Nephroblastoma Trial and Study Committee. Eur J Pediatr Surg 1998; 8: 83–6.

96 Ritchey ML, Kelalis PP, Etziono R, et al. Small bowel obstruction after nephrectomy for Wilms' tumor. A report of the National Wilms' Tumor Study – 3. Ann Surg 1993; 218: 654–9.

97 Estlin EJ, Veal GJ. Clinical and cellular pharmacology in relation to solid tumors of childhood. Cancer Treat Rev 2003; 29: 253–73.

98 Ludwig R, Weirich A, Abel U, et al. Hepatotoxity in patients treated according to the nephroblastoma trial and study SIOP-9/GPOH. Med Pediatr Oncol 1999; 33: 262–469.

99 Breslow NE, Takashima JR, Ritchey ML, et al. Renal failure in the Denys-Drash and Wilms' tumor-aniridia syndromes. Cancer Res 2000; 60: 4030–2.

100 Kedar A, McGarry M, Moore R, et al. Effect of postoperative chemotherapy and radiotherapy, on the survival of subcutaneously implanted Furth Wilms' tumor. Oncology 1981; 38: 65–8.

101 Yokoi A, McCrudden KW, Huang J, et al. Human epidermal growth factor receptor signalling contributes to tumor growth via angiogenesis in her2/meu-expressing experimental Wilms' tumor. J Pediatr Surg 2003: 38: 1569–73.

102 Pinthus JH, Fridman E, Dekel B, et al. ErbB2 is a tumor associated antigen and a suitable therapeutic target in Wilms tumor. J Urol 2004; 172: 1644–8.

103 Frischer JS, Huang J, Serur A, et al. Effects of potent VEGF blockade on experimental Wilms tumor and its persisting vasculature. Int J Oncol 2004; 25: 549–53.

104 Ghanem MA, van Steenbrugge GJ, Sudaryo MK, Mathoera RB, Nijman JM, van der Kwast TH. Expression and prognostic relevance of vascular endothelial growth factor (VEGF) and its receptor (FLT-1) in nephroblastoma. J Clin Pathol 2003; 56: 107–13.

105 Huang J, Soffer SZ, Kim ES, et al. Vascular remodelling marks tumors that recur during chronic suppression of angiogenesis. Mol Cancer Res 2004; 2: 36–42.

106 English MW, Lowis SP, Peng B, et al. Pharmacokinetically guided dosing of carboplatin and etoposide during peritoneal dialysis and haemodialysis. Br J Cancer 1996; 73: 776–80.

107 Iacano LC, Adams D, Homans AC, Guillot A, McCune JS, Stewart CF. Topotecan disposition in an anephric child. J Pediatr Hematol Oncol 2004; 26: 596–600.

108 Graham C, Tucker C, Creech J, et al. Evaluation of the antitumor efficacy, pharmacokinetics and pharmacodynmaics of the histone deacetylase inhibitor depsipeptide in childhood cancer models in vivo. Clin Cancer Res 2006; 12: 223–34.

109 Peterson JK, Tucker C, Favours E, et al. *In vivo* evaluation of ixabepilone (BMS247550), a novel epothilone B derivative, against pediatric cancer models. Clin Cancer Res 2005; 11: 6950–8.

110 Yokoi A, McCrudden KW, Huang J, et al. Human epidermal growth factor receptor signalling contributes to tumor growth via angiogenesis in her2/neu-expressing experimental Wilms' tumor. J Pediatr Surg 2003; 38: 1569–73.

111 Shitara T, Shimada A, Hanada R, et al. Irinotecan for children with relapsed solid tumors. Pediatr Hematol Oncol 2006; 23: 103–10.

112 Saylors RL, Stewart CF, Zamboni WC, et al. Phase I study of topotecan in combination with cyclophosphamide in pediatric patients with malignant solid tumors: a Pediatrc Oncology Group study. J Clin Oncol 1998; 16: 945–52.

113 Fox E, Maris JM, Widemann BC, et al. A phase I study of ABT-751, an orally bioavailable tubulin inhibitor, administered daily for 7 days every 21 days in pediatric patients with solid tumors. Clin Cancer Res 2006; 12: 4882–7.

114 Adamson PC, Matthay KK, O'Brien M, Reaman GH, Sato JK, Balis FM. A phase 2 trial of all-trans-retinoic acid in combination with interferon-alpha2a in children with recurrent neuroblastoma or Wilm's tumor: a Pediatric Oncology Branch, NCI and Childen's Oncology group study. Pediatr Blood Cancer 2007; 49: 661–5.

115 Kist-van Holthe JE, Ho PL, Stablein D, Harmon WE, Baum MA. Outcome of renal transplantation for Wilms' tumor and Denys-Drash syndrome: a report of the North American Pediatric Renal

Transplant Cooperative Study. Pediatr Transplant 2005; 9: 305–10.

116 Sorensen K, Levitt G, Sebag-Montefiore D, Bull C, Sullivan I. Cardiac function in Wilm's tumor survivors. J Clin Oncol 1995; 13: 1546–56.

117 Speechley KN, Barrera M, Shaw AK, Morrison HI, Maunsell E. Health-related quality of life among child and adolescent survivors of childhood cancer. J Clin Oncol 2006; 24: 2536–43.

118 Haas JE, Palmer NF, Weinberg AG. Ultrastructure of malignant rhabdoid tumor of the kidney: a distinctive renal tumor of children. Hum Pathol 1981; 12: 646.

119 Biegel JA, Rorke LB, Packer RJ, Emanuel BS. Monosomy 22 in rhabdoid or atypical tumors of the brain. J Neurosurg 1990; 73: 710–4.

120 Schofield DE, Beckwith JB, Sklar J. Loss of heterozygosity at chromosome regions 22q11-12 and 11p15.5 in renal rhabdoid tumors. Genes Chrom Cancer 1996; 15: 10–17.

121 Versteege I, Sevenet N, Lange J, et al. Truncating mutations of hSNF5/INI1 in aggressive paediatric cancer. Nature 1998; 394: 203–6.

122 Biegel JA, Zhou J-Y, Rorke LB, et al. Germ-line and acquired mutations of INI1 in atypical teratoid and rhabdoid tumors. Cancer Res 1999; 59: 74–9.

123 Rousseau-Merck M-F, Versteege I, Legrand I, et al. hSNF5/INI1 inactivation is mainly associated with homozygous deletions and mitotic recombinations in rhabdoid tumors. Cancer Res 1999; 59: 3152–6.

124 Roberts CWM, Galusha SA, McMenamin ME, et al. Haploinsufficiency of Snf5 (integrase interactor 1) predisposes to malignant rhabdoid tumors in mice. PNAS 2000; 97: 13796–800.

125 Sevenet N, Lellouch-Tubiana A, Schofield D, et al. Spectrum of hSNF5/INI1 somatic mutations in human cancer and genotype-phenotype correlations. Hum Mol Genet 1999; 8: 2359–68.

126 Schenk JP, Engelmann D, Rohrschneider W, et al. [Rhabdoid tumors of the kidney in childhood]. Rofo 2004; 176: 965–71.

127 Schenk JP, Engelmann D, Zieger B, et al. [Radiologic differentiation of rhabdoid tumor from Wilms' tumor and mesoblastic nephroma]. Urologe A 2005; 44; 155–61.

128 Huang CC, Cutcliffe C, Coffin C, et al. Classification of malignant pediatric renal tumors by gene expression. Pediatr Blood Cancer 2006; 46: 728–38.

129 Waldron PE, Rodgers BM, Kelly MD, Womer RB. Successful treatment of a patient with stage IV rhabdoid tumor of the kidney: case report and review. J Ped Hematol Oncol 1999; 21: 53–7.

130 Wagner L, Hill DA, Fuller C, et al. Treatment of metastatic rhabdoid tumor of the kidney. J Pediatr Hematol Oncol 2002; 24: 385–8.

131 Vujanic GM, Sandstedt B, Harms D, et al. Rhabdoid tumor of the kidney: a clinicopathological study of 22 patients from the International Society of Paediatric Oncology (SIOP) nephroblastoma file. Histopathology 1996; 28: 333–40.

132 D'Angio GJ, Breslow N, Beckwith JB, et al. Treatment of Wilms' tumor. Results of the Third National Wilms' Tumor Study. Cancer 1989; 64: 349–60.

133 Dome JS, Hill DA, McCarville, MB. Rhabdoid tumor of the kidney. eMedicine Journal 3, http://www.emedicine.com/ped/topic3012.htm, 2002. Boston Medical Publishing.

134 Weeks DA, Beckwith B, Mierau GW, Luckey DW. Rhabdoid tumor of kidney. Am J Surg Pathol 1989; 13: 439–58.

135 Tomlinson GE, Breslow NE, Dome J, et al. Rhabdoid tumor of the kidney in the National Wilms' Tumor Study: age at diagnosis as a prognostic factor. J Clin Oncol 2005; 23: 7641–5.

136 Gururangan S, Bowman LC, Parham DM, et al. Primary extracranial rhabdoid tumors. Cancer 1993; 71: 2653–9.

137 Blaney S, Berg SL, Pratt C, et al. A phase I study of irinotecan in pediatric patients: a pediatric oncology group study. Clin Cancer Res 2001; 7: 32–7.

138 Argani P, Perlman EJ, Breslow NE, et al. Clear cell sarcoma of the kidney: a review of 351 cases from the National Wilms Tumor Study Group Pathology Center. Am J Surg Pathol 2000; 24: 4–18.

139 Kidd JM. Exclusion of certain renal neoplasms from the category of Wilms' tumor. Am J Pathol 1970; 59: 16a.

140 Morgan E, Kidd JM. Undifferentiated sarcoma of the kidney: a tumor of childhood with histopathologic and clinical characteristics distinct from Wilms' tumor. Cancer 1978; 42: 1916–21.

141 Marsden HB, Lawler W, Kumar PM. Bone metastasizing renal tumor of childhood: morphological and clinical features, and differences from Wilms' tumor. Cancer 1978; 42: 1922–8.

142 Sandstedt BE, Delemarre JF, Harms D, et al. Sarcomatous Wilms' tumor with clear cells and hyalinization. A study of 38 tumors in children from the SIOP nephroblastoma file. Histopathology 1987; 11: 273–85.

143 Barnard M, Bayani J, Grant R, et al. Comparative genomic hybridization analysis of clear cell sarcoma of the kidney. Med Pediatr Oncol 2000; 34: 113–16.

144 Schuster AE, Schneider DT, Fritsch MK, et al. Genetic and genetic expression analyses of clear cell sarcoma of the kidney. Lab Invest 2003; 83: 1293–9.

145 Yun K. Clear cell sarcoma of the kidney expresses insulin like growth factor-II but not WT1 transcripts. Am J Pathol 1993; 142: 39–47.

146 Punnett HH, Halligan GE, Zaeri N, et al. Translocation 10;17 in clear cell sarcoma of the kidney. A first report. Cancer Genet Cytogenet 1989; 41: 123–8.

147 Douglass EC, Wilimas JA, Green AA, et al. Abnormalities of chromosomes 1 and 11 in Wilms tumor. Cancer Genet Cytogenet 1985; 14: 331–8.

148 Rakheja D, Weinberg AG, Tomlison GE, et al. Translocation (10;17) (q22; p13): a recurring translocation in clear cell sarcoma of the kidney. Cancer Genet Cytogenet 2004; 154: 175–9.

149 Cutcliffe C, Kersey D, Huang CC, et al. Clear cell sarcoma of the kidney: up-regulation of neural markers with activation of the sonic hedgehog and Akt pathways. Clin Cancer Res 2005; 11: 7986–94.

150 Brownlee NA, Perkins LA, Stewart W, et al. Recurring translocation (10;17) and deletion (14q) in clear cell sarcoma of the kidney. Arch Pathol Lab Med 2007; 131: 446–51.

151 Sotelo-Avila C, Gonzalez-Crussi F, Sadowinski S, et al. Clear cell sarcoma of the kidney: a clinicopathologic study of 21 patients with long-term follow-up evaluation. Hum Pathol 1985; 16: 1219–30.

152 Mitchell C, Jones PM, Kelsey A, et al. The treatment of Wilms' tumor: results of the United Kingdom Children's cancer study group (UKCCSG) second Wilms' tumor study. Br J Cancer 2000; 83: 602–8.

153 Green DM, Breslow NE, Beckwith JB, et al. Treatment of children with clear-cell sarcoma of the kidney: a report from the National Wilms' Tumor Study Group. J Clin Oncol 1994; 12: 2132–7.

154 Tournade MF, Com-Nougué C, de Kraker J, et al. Optimal duration of preoperative therapy in unilateral and nonmetastatic Wilms'

tumor in children older than 6 months: results of the Ninth International Society of Pediatric Oncology Wilms' Tumor Trial and Study. J Clin Oncol 2001; 19: 488–500.

155 Seibel NL, Li S, Breslow NE, et al. Effect of duration of treatment on treatment outcome for patients with clear-cell sarcoma of the

kidney: a report from the National Wilms' Tumor Study Group. J Clin Oncol 2004; 22: 468–73.

156 Furtwängler R, Reinhard H, Beier R, et al. Clear-cell sarcoma (CCSK) of the kidney – results of the SIOP 93-01/GPOH Trial. Pediatr Blood Cancer 2005; 45: 423: O155.

14 Soft Tissue Sarcoma

Gianni Bisogno[1] and John Anderson[2]

[1] Division of Hematology and Oncology, Department of Pediatrics, University Hospital of Padua, Padua, Italy and [2] Institute of Child Health and Great Ormond Street Hospital, London, UK

Introduction

The soft tissue sarcomas (STS) represent a diverse group of malignancies derived from mesenchymal cells. The different STS histotypes are identified according to the line of differentiation that may be recognized in the tumor cells. Thus rhabdomyosarcoma is composed of cells resembling normal fetal skeletal muscle, while fibrous structures are present in fibrosarcoma. In the pediatric population the histologies have been divided for reasons of convenience into rhabdomyosarcoma (RMS), which is by far the largest diagnostic group at approximately 50%, and the non-rhabdomyosarcoma soft tissue sarcomas (NRSTS) [1] This latter group comprises all the other STS seen in children and includes a variety of rare histotypes with the most common being synovial sarcoma, fibrosarcoma and malignant peripheral nerve sheath tumor.

- The incidence of soft tissue sarcoma in the 0–14 year age group is about 12 cases per million in North America [2].
- STS comprise approximately 8% of all pediatric malignancies.

Since its original description in 1854 by Weber, RMS has demonstrated to be a very aggressive tumor with less than one-third of children surviving in the 1960s after surgery and radiotherapy. In the 1970s, large cooperative national and international study groups started to adopt a systematic multidisciplinary approach including multidrug chemotherapy coordinated with surgery and radiotherapy. This led to a progressive increase of survival that is now above 70% [3, 4]. A less impressive improvement has been seen for children with NRSTS. Due to the rarity of the different histotypes it has been very difficult to build meaningful clinical trials, even on a multinational basis. Thus the management of NRSTS has been derived from the knowledge gathered with RMS and from adult experience [5] (Box 14.1).

Pediatric Hematology and Oncology, 1st edition. Edited by Edward J. Estlin, Richard J. Gilbertson, and Robert F. Wynn. © 2010 Blackwell Publishing Ltd.

Rhabdomyosarcoma

Epidemiology and genetics

RMS is the most common form of soft tissue sarcoma in children and young adults and accounts for approximately 4–5 % of all childhood malignancy.

- An annual incidence of 5.3 per million children under the age of 15 is recognized.
- RMS occurs more frequently in the first two decades of life and, in two-thirds of cases, arises before 6 years of age.
- A male predominance (1.4–1.7: 1) is generally reported.

Disease etiology is unclear. Genetic factors may play an important role as demonstrated by an association between RMS and a familial cancer syndrome (Li-Fraumeni), congenital anomalies (involving the genitourinary and central nervous system), and other genetic conditions, including neurofibromatosis type 1. The search for a relationship between environmental factors and RMS has no found substantial evidence.

Pathology and biology

RMS is broadly and functionally divided into embryonal and alveolar histological subtypes (Table 14.1). Within the embryonal grouping, botryoid, spindle cells and (more recently) pseudovascular sclerosing subtypes have been described [6–8]. A solid variant of alveolar has been shown to be functionally and biologically equivalent to classical alveolar [9]. All RMS show some immunohistochemical expression of:

- Myogenic transcription factors (MyoD, myogenin).
- Skeletal muscle specific proteins (desmin, myoglobin, muscle-specific actin).

However, ultrastructural features of striated muscle differentiation are often absent on light microscopic or electron microscopic appearance. It should be emphasized that there is no single or combination of ultrastructural or immunohistochemical features proven to distinguish the RMS subtypes, although recently the degree of nuclear staining of myogenin has been shown positively to correlate with alveolar subtype [10, 11].

As a result of careful analysis of reciprocal chromosomal trans-locations t(2;13)(q35;q14) and t(1;13)(p36:q14) characteristically occurring in alveolar RMS, the encoded fusion proteins PAX3-FOXO1A (formerly PAX3-FKHR) and PAX7-FOXO1A have been cloned and characterized.

Box 14.1 Comparison of presentation, epidemiology, and outcome for rhabdomyosarcoma (RMS) and non-rhabdomyosarcoma soft tissue sarcoma (NRSTS).

	RMS	NRSTS
Age at presentation	Mainly below age 6 years	Older child and adolescent
Sex	Male > female	Equal distribution
Sites of disease	Head and neck > GU and extremities	Mainly extremities
Localized at presentation	80%	80%
Metastatic at presentation	20% with lymph nodes, bone and lung	10%
Cytogenetics	t(2; 13), t(1;13)	No pattern
Molecular biology	Fusion proteins involving PAX	Not informative as yet
Survival for localised disease	60–70%	70–80%
Survival for metastatic disease	<25% depending on age and bony involvement	

- These fusion proteins function as transcription factors that activate transcription from the respective PAX binding sites but are 10 to 100 fold more potent than the wild type PAX3 and PAX7 proteins [12, 13].
- The fusion proteins themselves are also expressed at much higher levels in ARMS cells than the wild type proteins [14, 15] and it is hypothesized that the overexpression and increased transcriptional potency combine to cause high level expression of the normal PAX target genes, which in turn drive tumorigenesis through alterations in growth, differentiation, and apoptosis.

Microarray and transcriptional analysis of PAX3-FOXO1A target genes in tumor samples and cell lines respectively have to some degree validated this contention [16–18]. Recently it has been suggested that PAX3-FOXO1A has functions independent of transcription, for example through physical interaction with STAT3 and modulation of the tumor immune environment [19–21].

Although no recurrent chromosomal rearrangements have been described in embryonal RMS, allele loss at chromosome region 11p15.5 is reported to occur suggesting the presence of tumor suppressor gene/s in this region.

- Allele loss is most usually of maternally inherited copies in both rhabdomyosarcoma and other embryonal tumors such as Wilms' with allele loss at this locus.
- This suggests the involvement of imprinted genes, and the putative tumor suppressors H19 and p57/kip2 mapping to this region have both been shown to be paternally imprinted (maternally expressed).

It is therefore hypothesized that these, and other paternally imprinted genes in the region, are lost in embryonal RMS as a

---

Table 14.1 Histological subtypes of rhabdomyosarcoma.

Subtype	Clinical presentation	Histology	Prognostic significance	Biology
Classical embryonal	Any site; rarely limbs; age < 10	Strap-shaped cells with elongated nuclei; primitive to highly differentiated muscle cells	Intermediate	PAX-FOXO fusion proteins absent
Botryoid	Genitourinary; age < 10	Macroscopically resembles a bunch of grapes; cambial layer of tumor cells underlies intact epithelium	Favorable	PAX-FOXO fusion proteins absent
Spindle cell	Paratesticular	Spindle-shaped cells at low density	Favorable	PAX-FOXO fusion proteins absent
Pseudovascular sclerosing	Usually adults; can occur in childhood	Characterized by extensive hyaline fibrosis and pseudovascular growth patterns	Not known in children	PAX-FOXO fusion proteins absent
Classical alveolar	Often limbs; can occur elsewhere; usually >10 however PAX7-FOXO1A positive cases in a younger age group	Fibrovascular connective tissue septae lined by tumor cells	Unfavorable	PAX-FOXO fusion proteins present (in 80%)
Solid variant alveolar	Often limbs; can occur elsewhere ; age usually >10	Same cellular morphology as classical alveolar but without the alveolar growth pattern	Unfavorable	PAX-FOXO fusion proteins present (in 80%)

result of chromosome deletion of the maternal chromosome region resulting in a loss of tumor suppression. Whether genetic alteration of this region is also important in alveolar RMS is not clear; some studies have shown alterations of imprinting of the area in both histologies [22, 23], which might result in equivalent changes of protein expression by a different genetic mechanism.

Very significant genetic differences between alveolar and embryonal forms, however, are disclosed by analysis of gross chromosomal changes.

• Alveolar RMS is characterized by small amplifications and deletions but minimal changes in ploidy.

• Embryonal RMS typically shows whole chromosome gains and losses. Small-amplified regions (amplicons) are hypothesized to contain oncogenes, deregulated as a result of increased copy number of the whole gene and its regulatory sequences. For example, MDM2 and CDK4 are amplified in the 12q13-15 amplicon; MYCN is amplified at 2p24; and GPC5 from a 13q31 amplicon has been shown to be oncogenic in rhabdomyosarcoma [24].

• Similarly, a number of tumor suppressor genes are mutated or inactivated by other mechanisms in both histological types, such as for example, RB/CDKN2A pathway alterations and p53 inactivation, which can occur in sporadic RMA as well as families with inherited mutations of p53 (Li Fraumeni syndrome) [24].

More recently novel insights into the histogenesis of RMS have followed from murine transgenic or knock-in models in which putative genes involved in rhabdomyosarcoma development are de-regulated in the animal's somatic cells. Specifically, Ptch mutant mice, which are a model of Gorlin syndrome and which primarily develop medulloblastoma, show a high incidence of embryonal type RMS, as do HGF transgenic mice. It is important to note that the resemblance of these tumors to human RMS is not clearly defined. More convincing are tumors resembling alveolar RMS, arising in conditional knock-in mice in which PAX3-FOXO1A is switched on in late muscle differentiation. However, several other models of PAX3-FOXO1A expression in which the fusion protein expression is controlled by different genetic elements have either been non-viable or failed to develop tumors, indicating that the cellular environment is a critical determinant of PAX3-FOXO1A function [25].

Clinical presentation

RMS can develop in any anatomic location of the body where mesenchymal tissue other than bone is present. The most common primary sites are the head and neck (40%), genitourinary sites (20%) and extremities (20%). In 1986 European and US clinical investigators agreed an international definition of anatomical sites and identify six categories on the basis of frequency, treatment problem and different prognosis [26]:

1 Orbit (tumor confined into the orbital cavity without intracranial extension).

2 Parameningeal (all locations adjacent to the meninges, from whence the tumor can spread intracranially).

3 Head-neck non-parameningeal (includes scalp, parotid, check, oral cavity with oropharynx, larynx, thyroid area, and neck).

4 Genitourinary tract (includes two subcategories: (a) bladder and prostate; (b) non-bladder and prostate, i.e. vagina, vulva, uterus, paratesticular).

5 Extremities (up to the scapular area superiorly and the buttocks inferiorly).

6 Other sites: includes trunk wall, intrathoracic area, intra-abdominal, retroperitoneal, pelvic, perineal and paravertebral regions.

RMS tends to spread locally, invading the nearby organs, and disseminate along both lymphatic and hematogenous routes.

• At diagnosis, local lymph node involvement is evident in 0–25% of cases, being higher for pelvis-retroperitoneum or extremities RMS (23%) and virtually absent for orbital tumors.

• Distant metastases are discovered at diagnosis in approximately 20% of children, more frequently to lungs, bone marrow, bones, and distant lymph nodes. Less frequently other sites, such as abdominal organs, subcutaneous tissues or CNS, may be involved.

Symptoms are due to an enlarging mass and its effects on the surroundings organs. Therefore presentation is strongly influenced by site. Orbital tumors tend to present early with obvious displacement of the globe. In contrast, tumors arising in the head-neck region may result in a relatively long history of nonspecific symptoms with a final 'sudden' appearance of a progressive swelling.

Parameningeal RMS arises from head and neck locations adjacent to the meninges (including the nasopharynx, nasal cavity, middle ear/mastoid, paranasal sinus, pterygopalatine fossa, parapharyngeal space, and orbit with intracranial extension). These tumors have the potential to extend into the meninges and intracranially. The destruction of contiguous structure determines the symptoms: nasal discharge or obstruction from a mass in the nasopharynx, cranial nerve palsies or hypertension resulting from an intracranial mass lesion.

Bladder and prostate RMS may present with voiding difficulties or with symptoms mimicking cystitis. Paratesticular tumors present as a scrotal mass and are usually detected at an early stage in young children, whereas they might be hidden for a long time by adolescents. The presentation of abdominal or thoracic RMS is usually characterized by development of a mass not discovered until very large and invasive. Often the child is not unwell (for example in the case of extremity tumors) unless there is metastatic disease. In rare cases, the primary site is unknown but metastases are present and diagnosis is made through a bone marrow examination.

Investigation and staging

Diagnostic and staging investigations must aim to obtain a precise definition of the primary tumor with its locoregional extension, and an accurate assessment of the potential metastatic sites, prior to treatment planning. Imaging of the primary site should include tumor volume measurement and examination of regional lymph nodes, especially if not evaluable clinically, or if clinically suspicious. Pretreatment investigations may vary depending mainly on the anatomical sites affected but in general should include the following:

1 Biopsy or primary surgery. Adequate tissue must be obtained for morphological, histochemical and molecular/cytogenetic analysis following consultation with laboratories skilled in performing these techniques. Fresh tissue is required for optimal analysis which is often a requirement for accurate diagnosis. Storage of fresh material for research is extremely important. Fine needle aspiration biopsy is not recommended because the limited sample may cause problems to the pathologic and biological investigations. Endoscopic biopsies are often possible for bladder, prostate, or vaginal tumors. Primary surgery is indicated if there is no evidence of metastatic spread, and if clinical factors and imaging indicate a high likelihood of resection with clear margins.

2 Magnetic resonance imaging (MRI) or computed tomography (CT) scan of the primary site. The choice between MRI and CT often depends on local availability. MRI carries the potential advantage of more functional information. CT or MRI examination should be carried out with the use of contrast. MRI is preferable for most locations, other than the chest, including head and neck tumors with possible skull base invasion. MRI is mandatory for genito-urinary primaries and paraspinal tumors. CT is occasionally useful for assessing subtle bone destruction. The investigation may need to be performed again after surgical excision or biopsy if significant volume has been resected.

3 Chest CT scan: the presence of lung metastases must be evaluated in all patients at diagnosis by CT scan. Postero-anterior and lateral chest X-ray may be useful for follow up.

4 Abdomen-pelvic CT scan (during same acquisition as chest CT): for abdominal and pelvic primaries if MRI has not been performed and to assess the presence of liver metastasis and search for abdominal lymphadenopathy in case of paratesticular or lower limb primaries.

5 Radionuclide bone scan (with plain X-rays and/or MRI of any isolated abnormalsite). Mandatory in all patients at diagnosis.

6 Bone marrow aspiration and biopsy.

Other investigations may be appropriate according to the different the primary sites and include the following:

• Ultrasound of the primary tumor and possible metastatic site (liver, abdomen) is advisable in most cases to simplify the patient follow up.

• Cerebrospinal fluid (CSF) cytology in case of parameningeal tumors.

• Cystourethroscopy with biopsy for tumors arising in the bladder prostate site.

• Brain cross-sectional imaging should be considered in cases of extremity RMS as brain metastases seem to be more frequent in this setting.

• Spinal MRI is recommended in case of paraspinal tumors or the presence of neurological signs of medullary compression.

• Positron emission tomography (PET)-CT is an optional investigation according to local availability and local protocols. The diagnostic and prognostic meaning is not proven for pediatric

RMS although it is an important emerging field in adult soft tissue sarcoma [27, 28].

It is recommended that the same imaging procedure is used throughout the treatment for response evaluation. It is important to emphasize that clinical history and imaging are vital for staging and might strongly suggest a diagnosis of RMS, but diagnosis must be established histologically.

Staging

The most used classification of RMS is the one formulated by the Intergroup Rhabdomyosarcoma Study (IRS) in 1972 [29]. Patients were stratified into four groups according to the results of the initial surgery, and the spread of the tumor to local tissues and/or to the lymph nodes (Table 14.2). This system has been criticized because the clinical tumor characteristics (size, invasiveness) were not taken into account adequately and relied mainly on the ability and attitude of the surgeon.

European investigators taking part in the SIOP group chose to use a TNM (tumor, nodes and metastases) based classification relying on the clinical description of the disease, before and after initial surgery. Collaboration between groups has subsequently resulted in the incorporation of both clinical and surgical aspects

Table 14.2 IRS Clinical Grouping System.

Group I

Localized disease, completely resected. Regional nodes not involved.

(a) Confined to muscle or organ of origin.

(b) Continuous involvement: infiltration outside the muscle or organ of origin.

Group II

Total gross resection with evidence of regional spread.

(a) Grossly resected tumor with microscopic residual disease, no evidence of regional lymph node involvement (all visible tumor has been removed but the pathologist finds tumor at the margin of resection).

(b) Regional disease, completely resected with no microscopic residual but with involved nodes (both primary tumor and involved nodes are completely resected).

(c) Regional disease with involved nodes, grossly resected, but with evidence of microscopic residual disease.

Group III

Incomplete resection with gross residual disease.

(a) After biopsy only.

(b) After major resection (>50%) of the primary tumor.

Group IV

Distant metastases present at diagnosis.

• Be aware about node involvement: regional nodes infiltration place patients in the more favorable Group II or III, while distant node infiltration means evidence of metastatic disease (Group IV).

• Patients with positive cytology in the cerebrospinal fluid, pleural/effusion, ascites or pleural/peritoneal implants are usually treated as patients in Group IV.

Table 14.3 Risk stratification for EpSSG non-metastatic rhabomyosarcoma (RMS) study.

Risk group	Subgroups	Pathology	Post- surgical stage (IRS Group)	Site	Node stage	Size and age
Low risk	A	Favorable	I	Any	N0	Favorable
Standard Risk	B	Favorable	I	Any	N0	Unfavorable
	C	Favorable	II, III	Favorable	N0	Any
	D	Favorable	II, III	Unfavorable	N0	Favorable
High Risk	E	Favorable	II, III	Unfavorable	N0	Unfavorable
	F	Favorable	II, III	Any	N1	Any
	G	Unfavorable	I, II, III	Any	N0	Any
Very High Risk	H	Unfavorable	I, II, III	Any	N1	Any

(1) Pathology. Favourable, all embryonal, spindle cells, botryoid RMS. Unfavourable, all alveolar RMS (including the solid-alveolar variant). (2) Post surgical stage (according to the IRS grouping, see appendix A.2). Group I, primary complete resection (R0); Group II, microscopic residual (R1) or primary complete resection but N1; Group III, macroscopic residual (R2); (3) Site. Favorable: orbit, genitor-urinary non-bladder prostate (i.e. paratesticular and vagina/uterus) and non-parameningeal head & neck. Unfavourable: all other sites (parameningeal, extremities, GU bladder-prostate and 'other site'). (4) Node stage (according to the TNM classification, see appendix A1 and A5). N0, no clinical or pathological node involvement. N1, clinical or pathological nodal involvement. (5) Size and age. Favourable, tumor size (maximum dimension) ≤5 cm and age <10 years. Unfavourable, all others (i.e. size >5 cm or age ≥10 years).

into the contemporary staging systems for rhabdomyosarcoma. Unfortunately, this has led to more complicated classifications. As an example, the European Pediatric Soft Tissue Sarcoma Study Group (EpSSG) stratification (Table 14.3) takes into consideration six different prognostic factors leading to the identification of eight subgroups that will receive different treatments according to the resulting four risk groups.

Treatment

A multimodality approach involving surgery, chemotherapy, and radiotherapy is necessary in the treatment of children with RMS. The optimal timing and intensity of these three treatment modalities must be planned with regard to the prognostic factors, and consideration of the potential late sequelae of treatment.

Prognostic factors

Modern protocols determine treatment strategy according to disease extension (localized versus metastatic), histology, post-surgical status, tumor site and size, and patient age. The presence of metastatic disease at diagnosis represents the main prognostic factor that generally overshadows all the other factors in determining a dismal outcome. Therefore, more intensive or innovative treatments are required for this group of patients.

For non-metastatic RMS patients, the treatment is tailored on the balance of different prognostic characteristics. The most important are described in Table 14.4. It is important to note that these factors are often interdependent:
- Limb tumors are generally of the alveolar type whereas genito-urinary RMS are embryonal (or other favorable variants such as botryoid or spindle cell).
- Alveolar subtype shows a higher rate of metastasis and regional nodes involvement. Post-surgical status is strictly correlated with tumor site.

Table 14.4 Prognostic factors for localized rhabdomyosarcoma.

Histology	Favorable: embryonal, spindle cells, botryoid RMS Unfavorable: alveolar tumors (including the solid-alveolar variant)
Tumor site	Favorable: orbit, genito-urinary non-bladder prostate (i.e. paratesticular and vagina/uterus) and head and neck non-paramenigeal Unfavorable: parameningeal, extremities, genito-urinary bladder-prostate and 'other site'
Tumor size (maximum dimension)	Favorable: tumor size ≤5 cm Unfavorable: tumor size >5 cm
Lymph node involvement	According to the TNM classification: N0: no clinical or pathological node involvement N1: clinical or pathological nodal involvement
Initial surgery	This is defined according to the IRS Grouping
Patient age	Favorable: age <10 years (but infants age <1 year seem to have a worst prognosis) Unfavorable: age >10 years

- Complete resection is frequently possible for paratesticular RMS whereas is rare in cases of parameningeal location.

Biological prognostic factors are still lacking for RMS, but for the population with alveolar RMS the presence of t(2;13)(q35;q14) or t(1;13)(p36;q14) translocations seems to identify groups with different prognosis [30–32].

The combination of different prognostic factors broadly identifies distinct risk groups:

1 Low Risk Group: this represents a much-selected group of patients, accounting for 6–8% of the whole population of localized RMS, with an expected 90% event-free survival (EFS) at 5 years. Includes IRS Group I tumors with favorable histology and site. Most of these patients are represented by children with paratesticular RMS.

2 Intermediate Standard Risk Group: with 60–80% survival. Includes patients with favourable histology and site (i.e. embryonal RMS localized in orbit, head and neck site).
3 High Risk Group: survival below 60% (i.e. unfavourable site such as trunk, pelvis, extremities, and/or alveolar histology).
4 Very High Risk Group: this includes mainly metastatic RMS. In this group, survival is between 20 and 30%.

Surgery

The aim of surgery is to achieve tumor clearance with no, or minimal, long-term sequelae. The type and timing of surgery depends on the site and size of the primary tumor, the age of the patient and the response to initial chemotherapy. Surgical planning should include all reconstructive procedures with optimal timing of possible additional radiotherapy.

Tumor may be resected at diagnosis when an excision with adequate margins is anticipated without any danger or mutilation. This means that a layer of healthy tissue between tumor and resection margins should exist. The extent of this layer (2–5 cm) is not precisely defined in pediatric tumor surgery and could be very limited to avoid organ damage. A partial tumor resection (debulking) does not give any advantage in terms of survival, although recent data suggest this may not be true for all sites [33].

A primary re-excision (i.e. a second surgical resection before chemotherapy) should be considered when an initial operation results in positive margins.
• This applies particularly to trunk, limb, and paratesticular tumors, when it can be anticipated that clear margins of excision can be achieved without functional or cosmetic disadvantage [34].
• The interval between initial surgical approach and chemotherapy, including primary re-excision should be as short as possible (most protocols ask for less than 8 weeks). Extensive, 'mutilating' operations should never be considered at primary resection.

After chemotherapy a secondary operation should be considered in cases of residual mass or in doubtful cases. Marginal resections may also be acceptable, provided that they are followed by radiotherapy. Secondary operations should usually be conservative but 'mutilating' operations may sometimes be considered necessary after unsuccessful neo-adjuvant chemotherapy or radiotherapy.

Reconstructive procedures have to be included early enough in the planning of the resection. It is desirable to have the histological evaluation before reconstructive surgery. In cases, however, where reconstructive vascular surgery or microvascular surgery is involved, this is mostly not possible. Therefore in some cases resection and reconstructive surgery have to be performed at the same time without histological confirmation of the status of the resection.

Surgery should be also considered for lymph nodes and metastatic lesions. Clinically or radiologically suspicious regional lymph nodes should be sampled at diagnosis. Tru-cut biopsy may be useful to confirm nodal involvement but only if a conventional biopsy of the primary tumor has been obtained for diagnostic purposes. In extremity sites, systematic biopsy of regional nodes is recommended in the current EpSSG protocol even if nodes are not palpable or enlarged on imaging. New techniques of sentinel node mapping (with blue dye and/or radioactive tracer) are under investigation [35]. Radical lymph node dissections are generally not indicated and involved lymph nodes should be irradiated whether resected or not, if feasible. When the primary tumor control has been achieved, resection of all metastatic lesions should be considered if they are still evident after chemotherapy.

Radiotherapy

Radiotherapy is an essential treatment for most patients with rhabdomyosarcoma, but the awareness of the possible late effects, especially in young children, has led to attempts to identify categories of patients that can be cured without irradiation.
• The SIOP Group has adopted for many years the strategy to limit the use of radiotherapy to patients in whom clinical complete remission has not been achieved with chemotherapy [36]. This approach has been partially successful in the subsets of patients with orbital embryonal RMS where up to 40% of patients were cured without irradiation [37].
• These results have been criticized, however, because they are counterbalanced by a much higher rate of local relapse and the necessity for an aggressive second line approach to cure relapsed patients.

The only patients where radiotherapy can be safely withheld are those affected by embryonal RMS completely resected at diagnosis, or located in the vagina and in complete remission after chemotherapy [38, 39]. Data from different studies show that failure-free survival is significantly improved when radiotherapy is used in the other groups of patients (i.e. IRS I and unfavorable histology, IRS II and IRS III patients) [38]. However, reduction of late effects may also be achieved not only avoiding irradiation but also with better radiotherapy planning, reducing doses and investigation of new techniques such as intensity-modulated radiation therapy (IMRT).

As a consequence, radiotherapy should be performed only in centers with the most modern facilities and adequate pediatric experience. A 3-D-conformal radiotherapy planning is recommended when critical structures lie in or nearby the target volume. The target volume should be chosen according to the initial tumor volume plus adequate margins (1–2 cm), and should include scars of the initial or secondary surgery. In cases of large tumors, after the initial dose, a boost can be given to a more limited target field, i.e. including only the residual tumor plus a 1 or 2 cm margin.

Doses in excess of 50 Gy are not usually required when given by conventional (once a day) fractionation. However, there is also evidence that doses <40 Gy may be insufficient, particularly in patients with macroscopic residual disease. Current guidelines within the Children's Oncology Group (COG) and EpSSG protocols vary the prescribed dose from 40 to 55 Gy depending on site, size and histological subtype, as well as on the age of the child. Cooperative groups are also exploring the effectiveness of moderate radiation doses (32–36 Gy) for patients with favorable site and histology.

Different irradiation techniques are also under investigation. In the IRS IV trial, radiotherapy doses of 50.4 Gy in conventional fractionation were randomized against 59.4 Gy using hyperfractionation in patients with group III tumors [40]. Higher radiation doses did not improve the patients' outcome and the follow up is too short to assess a difference in late effects. Brachytherapy may be used in cases of incompletely resected tumors of vagina, perineum, bladder, prostate, and orbit, or as a boost technique before or after external beam irradiation.

Chemotherapy

Cyclophosphamide, ifosfamide, vincristine, actinomycin D, and doxorubicin have been employed in various combinations for the treatment of RMS, but only a limited amount of data concerning single agent responses is available. A review [41] of early phase II studies investigating single agent treatment of RMS indicated high tumor response rates with:

- Vincristine (50%).
- Cyclophosphamide (54%).
- Doxorubicin (31%).
- Actinomycin-D (24%).

For ifosfamide, response rates in the face of a total dose of 9g/m^2 fractionated over 5 days was associated with a response rate of 85% in the phase II setting [42], and this finding has encouraged the use of ifosfamide over cyclophosphamide in contemporary European as opposed to North American clinical trials [43].

Thus, chemotherapy is effective to reduce the primary tumor, and to control occult and evident metastasis. Despite its high activity against RMS, chemotherapy can rarely cure patients alone, but reduces the extent of subsequent surgery and radiotherapy. To improve its effect the most active drugs have been combined in different multidrug regimens and those most widely used are shown in Table 14.5.

In general, the North American investigators use vincristine and actinomycin-D (VA) for favorable tumors and vincristine, actinomycin-D, and cyclophosphamide (VAC) for intermediate and high-risk patients. The cyclophosphamide dose has varied in the different IRS protocols increasing up to 2.2g/m^2 in the IRS IV study [3]. This dose escalation was claimed as one of the reasons to explain the progressive improvement of results obtained in the successive IRS studies, but this observation has been recently questioned when further analysis showed no significant improvement in intermediate risk patients and a higher risk of veno-occlusive disease [44, 45].

Doxorubicin, as single drug, is very effective against RMS and other STS. Different randomized trials and historical comparisons performed by the IRS Group, however, did not show different results when patients with RMS are treated with VAC or VAC plus doxorubicin. Only a marginal improvement was noted in some subgroups, i.e. IRS group I/II alveolar histology and special pelvic sites [29, 46, 47]. Since the role of anthracyclines as part of

Table 14.5 Common chemotherapy combinations.

VA	Vincristine 1.5 mg/m² i.v. (max 2 mg) × 1 day
	Actinomycin-D 1.5 mg/ m² i.v. (max 2 mg) × 1 day
Pulse VAC	Vincristine 1.5 mg/ m² i.v. (max 2 mg)
	Actinomycin-D 0.015 mg/kg/day × 5 days or 1.5 mg/ m² i.v. (max 2 mg) × 1 day
	Cyclophosphamide 10 mg/kg/day × 3 days or 250 mg/ m²/day × 5–7 days
Intensive pulse VAC	Vincristine 1.5 mg/ m² i.v. (max 2 mg) × 1 day
	Actinomycin-D 0.015 mg/ m² (max 0.5 mg)/day i.v. × 5 days
	Cyclophosphamide 2.2 g/ m² × 1 day
IVA	Ifosfamide 3 g/m² i.v. × 2 or 3 days
	Vincristine 1.5 mg/ m² i.v. (max 2 mg) × 1 day
	Actinomycin-D 1.5 mg/ m² i.v. (max 2 mg) × 1 day
VAIA	It is composed of three cycles with IVA given as cycle 1 and 3 and IVAd as cycle 2.
	In IVAd actinomycin-D is replaced by adriamycin 40 mg/m² i.v. × 2 days
CEVAIE	It is composed of three cycles:
	(1) CEV: carboplatin 500 mg/m² i.v. × 1 day; epi-adriamycin 150 mg/m² i.v. × 1 day; vincristine 1.5 mg/m² (max 2 mg) i.v. × 1 day;
	(2) IVA as above
	(3) IVE as IVA but with etoposide 200 mg/ m²/day × 3 days replacing actinomycin-D
VTP	Vincristine 1.5 mg/ m² i.v. (max 2 mg) × 1 day
	Topotecan 0.75 mg/ m² × 5 days
	Endoxan 250 mg/ m² × 5 days
IVADo	IVA (as above) plus concomitant administration of Doxorubycin 30 mg/m² i.v. × 2 days

Most protocols recommend a 3 week interval between cycles and administer vincristine weekly for at least the initial 7–9 weeks.

a multi-drug regimen remains to be established, the E*p*SSG is testing a novel intensive combination doxorubicin-based (IVADo) in the initial part of the recently open RMS2005 protocol.

Since the replacement of cyclophosphamide by ifosfamide seemed to improve the response rate [48] the IVA or VAIA regimens were adopted in different European studies [49, 50]. More recently patients enrolled in the IRS IV study were randomized to receive chemotherapy with VAC or IVA or VIE (vincristine, ifosfamide, etoposide). No significant difference in outcome was noted and VAC was elected as gold standard by the American investigators due to the lower cost of cyclophosphamide and the possible nephrotoxicity of ifosfamide [3].

European groups have decided to keep therapy with IVA as a standard combination because there is only a small risk of significant renal toxicity at cumulative ifosfamide doses $<60 \text{g/m}^2$, and a higher risk of gonadal toxicity with cyclophosphamide. Further investigations aimed to test novel combinations or new drugs, namely CEVAIE, a six-drug regimen which includes all the most effective drugs against RMS, gave excellent response rates in metastatic patients [51], but has failed to translate to improvements in patient survival [52].

New drugs have recently been included in a randomized comparison in North American and European trials. Topotecan (VTP regimen) is under evaluation for intermediate risk patients in the ongoing COG D9803 study [4]. Vinorelbine in combination with low dose cyclophosphamide is included in one arm of the European trial RMS2005 [53]. Irinotecan, administered on a prolonged schedule, revealed an interesting response rate in patients with recurrent or metastatic RMS, especially when combined with vincristine. The low hematological toxicity profile of irinotecan suggests a possible use in association with more myelotoxic agents [54].

High and low dose chemotherapy

In the attempt to overcome tumor cell chemoresistance, different strategies of dose intensification have been tested. In particular, high dose chemotherapy (HDCT) followed by hematopoietic stem cell rescue (HSCR) has been explored in different trials.

• In the European MMT4 protocol the use of high-dose melphalan as consolidation therapy for children with metastatic disease in first complete remission resulted in an unsatisfactory 29% 3-year EFS.

• Similar poor results were achieved with other myeloablative regimens such as combination of melphalan, etoposide, and carboplatin (MEC regimen), thiothepa, cyclophosphamide and carboplatin, or melphalan and etoposide. The 2 or 3-year EFS in such studies ranged from 19 to 44% [55, 56].

An attempt to use repetitive courses of HDCT with HSRC earlier in the treatment pathway, has been evaluated recently by the SIOP and the Italian Groups without any advantage (unpublished).

In contrast, the German Group recently found a survival advantage for metastatic patients when low dose 'maintenance' chemotherapy (oral treatment with trofosfamide plus idarubicin) was administered instead of high dose chemotherapy (thiotepa, cyclophosphamide and melphalan, etoposide). The results in 62 patients are very promising with 3-year EFS above 50% for patients taking oral treatment (and EFS 20% after high dose). Since the comparison was not randomized, this result awaits confirmation.

Multimodality treatment according to site

Site is a major determinant for the application of the general principles of the multimodality approach. Indeed, whilst chemotherapy can be the same irrespective of the primary tumor location this is not the case for local treatment measures. Surgery has a limited role for orbital or parameningeal tumors so radiotherapy must be considered. On the contrary, surgery is a requirement for cure of children with paratesticular RMS, in combination with minimal chemotherapy and avoidance of radiotherapy. In other sites the administration of radiotherapy and surgery modalities must be carefully planned taking into account other variables

such as tumor response to chemotherapy and the patient's age. The different approaches according to tumor site are summarized in Table 14.6.

Results, survival, and outcome

The incremental increase in survival from 20% to above 70% clearly shows the improvement achieved from the initial protocols launched in the seventies to the most modern studies [3, 57] Remarkably, patients with localized RMS have benefited the most whilst prognosis has changed little for patients with metastatic disease where failure free survival remains between 20 and 30%. The 3-year overall and failure-free survival for patients with localized disease reported in the most recently published American study (IRS IV) were 77% and 86%, respectively, but did not significantly differ from the 5-year progression-free survival of 65% reported in IRS III.

These findings compare with the 57% and 71% 5-year EFS and overall survivals (OS) reported in SIOP MMT 89. The large difference between OS and EFS in the SIOP study reflects the strategy to limit the use of radiotherapy in localized disease. This has led to a higher relapse rate but also to an increased possibility to cure patients not receiving radiotherapy during first line treatment. The results achieved by the different cooperative Groups are presented according to site in Table 14.7.

When RMS recurs the event is typically within 3 years from diagnosis, and there is a very low rate of recurrence after 5 years [58].

• Treatment failure is mostly due to local or regional relapse (approximately 60% of failures), with metastatic relapse occurring in 30% of cases, and combined local and metastatic relapse in the remaining 10–20%.

• Local relapse is obviously associated with local treatment and it is higher when radiotherapy is not given. Distant relapse is more often associated with alveolar subtypes or primary tumor in the extremities.

Children suffering from tumor relapse are very difficult to cure and the estimated median survival after the first relapse is less than one year [59]. Recent studies showed that some favorable characteristics (embryonal histology, favorable primary site and the omission of radiotherapy during first line treatment), are associated with a second long-term complete remission. Children with alveolar histology or IRS group IV at diagnosis rarely survive after recurrence [60].

In the *in vitro* setting, the chemosensitivity of RMS cells related to the expression of MDR1 [61], where chemotherapy can up regulate the expression of multidrug-resistance associated proteins such as MRP and MDR1 in the xenograft setting [62]. These pre-clinical observations have not been widely investigated in clinical practice, but MDR1 expression has been found to relate to an adverse outcome for patients with orbital rhabdomyosarcoma [63]. However, whether or not MDR1 expression is an important determinant of disease outcome is uncertain, with conflicting reports of the relevance of MDR1 expression to the prognosis for RMS [64, 65].

Table 14.6 Multimodality treatment according to specific tumor.

	Initial surgery	Chemotherapy	Local treatment	Additional comments
Orbit (favorable)	Biopsy	VA or VAC or IVA	RT is preferred as complete resection is rarely possible	When a complete remission is achieved with chemotherapy 1/3 of the patients can be cured without RT Alveolar histotype needs more aggressive chemotherapy and higher RT doses In case of intracranial extension the tumor must be classified as PM
Paratesticular	Complete resection through an inguinal approach	IRS I: VA IRS II or III: VAC or IVA	No RT when IRS I In case of residual disease after initial CT, surgery is preferred and can avoid RT if complete	Retroperitoneal lymphadenectomy or node sampling at diagnosis is not recommended by European Groups but it is recommended by COG in children >10 years When the initial surgical approach has been through the scrotum hemiscrotectomy is usually recommended but recent data showed this may not be the case Alveolar histotype is very rare and may need a more aggressive CT (but no RT if in IRS I)
Vagina/uterus	Biopsy	IRS I: VA IRS II or III: VAC or IVA	No local treatment if in complete remission after CT	In case of residual tumor partial vaginectomy may be feasible, but brachytherapy is often preferable Alveolar histotype is very rare and may need a more aggressive approach including RT
Head and neck	Initial complete resection is rarely achieved so only a biopsy should be taken	IVA or VAC	Surgery and RT	In some circumstances a major tumor resection with reconstruction may be considered after neoadjuvant chemotherapy
Parameningeal (unfavorable)	Biopsy	VAC, IVA, VAIA, CEVAIE	RT is necessary. Surgery should be considered in case of post-RT residuals	In some circumstances a major tumor resection with reconstruction may be considered. Surgery should only be performed in centers with experience in this field More aggressive CT regimens are under study (IVADo, VTP)
Bladder Prostate	Biopsy possibly through a cystoscopy	VAC, IVA, VAIA, CEVAIE	RT is necessary in most cases	In some cases a post-CT conservative surgery may be considered (partial cystectomy and/or partial prostatectomy) in conjunction with brachytherapy Biopsy of suspicious residuals may be of help: specimens should be analyzed by expert pathologists to distinguish between residual neoplastic cells and rhabdomyoblasts More aggressive CT regimens are under study (IVADo, VTP)
Limbs	Complete tumor resection may be feasible (small non-invasive tumors) otherwise a biopsy is preferred. Regional lymph nodes biopsy is mandatory.	VAC, IVA, VAIA, CEVIE	Surgery and RT	Consider primary re-excision before starting chemotherapy in case of an initial resection with microscopic residuals At secondary operation, formal compartmental resection may be appropriate for some tumors but less 'anatomical' resections may be better providing an adequate margin of normal tissue Brachytherapy may be used in selected cases More aggressive CT regimens are under study (IVADo, VTP)
Other sites (trunk, abdomen, pelvis)	Tumor are usually very large so initial complete resection is rarely achieved and a biopsy should be taken	VAC, IVA, VAIA, CEVAIE	Surgery and radiotherapy	Some data suggest that debulking surgery may be of benefit at diagnosis Complete resection does not preclude the need for radiotherapy Consider whole abdominal irradiation in case of ascites with positive cytology More aggressive CT regimens are under study (IVADo, VTP)

Chemotherapy regimens are described in Table 14.5. RT, radiotherapy. CT, chemotherapy.

Table 14.7 Results by site.

Primary site	IRS IV		MMT 89		CWS 86		RMS 96	
	n	3-years FFS	*n*	5-years OS	*n*	5-years EFS	*n*	5-years OS
1Orbit	81	*94*	48	85	36	71	32	92
Head-neck	64	80	48	64	28	51	28	91
Parameningeal	222	72	135	64	55	60	56	69
GU bladder/prostate	90	79	62	80	30	70	27	74
GU non bladder-prostate	181	84	62	94	38	89	59	97
Extremity	113	68	51	46	25	56	30	86
Other	132	72	67	63	39	58	52	61

IRS-IV, Intergroup RMS Study IV. MMT-89, protocol of the International Society of Pediatric Oncology. CWS-86, protocol of the German Co-operative Soft Tissue Sarcoma Study. RMS 96 protocol of the Italian Soft Tissue Sarcoma Committee. FFS, failure free survival. OS, overall survival. EFS, event-free survival.

Late effects

As survival is improving the cost of the cure is becoming increasingly important. A correct patient stratification according to the risk of relapse is the main factor to avoid over-treatment in good prognosis patients. But aggressive therapy is necessary for most RMS patients and poor quality of life may be the long-term price.

The possible late effects must be anticipated during treatment and possibly avoided or corrected. Surgical sequelae are mainly due to mutilation, such as orbital exenteration, cystectomy, or amputation. New approaches are possible to avoid organ extirpation such as the use of partial cystectomy in conjunction with brachytherapy to avoid cystectomy [39]. If the bladder cannot be preserved, an orthotopic continent urinary diversion may be considered to allow patients to void spontaneously through the urethra [66]. Reconstructive surgery can give an acceptable function in case of amputation.

Radiotherapy is unavoidable in most RMS patients so cosmetic and organic problems are usually anticipated. The irradiated organs should be known to allow a tailored follow up:
• Periodical eye visit for orbital tumor and hormonal evaluation for patients with parameningeal RMS when the hypophyseal gland has been included in the irradiation field.
• Asymmetries due to bone irradiation must be searched for and reconstructive surgery can be proposed.

Chemotherapy is also associated with significant sequelae in some patients. Renal function (ifosfamide), fertility (cyclophosphamide), and heart function (doxorubicin) should be regularly checked. Finally the risk of second tumor seems to be relatively low in RMS patients but the systematic use of radiotherapy and alkylating agents warrants great attention.

New treatment approaches

The lack of improvements in survival in patients with metastatic disease despite intensive chemotherapy with or without bone marrow rescue or allogeneic transplantation has prompted the consideration of targeted pharmacological approaches, and investigation of entirely novel approaches such as immunotherapy.

• Novel agents that have shown antitumor activity in xenograft models of RMS include ixabepilone (BMS247550), one of a new class of microtubule-stabilizing antimitotic agents [67] and, in combination with irinotecan, irofulven, a derivative of a natural fungal toxin [68].
• In common with many other malignancies, RMS tumors express high levels of growth factors, such as insulin-like growth factors I and II (IGF-I/II), and their receptors, IGF-IR. The autocrine action of these growth factors appears to play an important role in the uncontrolled cellular proliferation within the tumor and such growth factors represent potentially important targets for therapy [69]. A monoclonal antibody directed against IGF-IR inhibits proliferation and survival of RMS cell lines *in vitro* [70] and insulin-like growth factor binding protein-6 (IGFBP-6), which avidly binds IGF-II, inhibits the proliferation of RMS cell lines *in vitro* and the growth of RMS xenografts in a nude mouse model [71].
• An alternative strategy has been the use of selective inhibitors for the IGF-IR kinase, such as NVP-AEW541 [72], although this agent appears to be more effective against Ewing's sarcoma cell lines than other forms of sarcoma including RMS [73].
• Alongside a possible role for growth factor inhibitors, there is growing interest in the use of cytokines, particularly tumor necrosis factor-related apoptosis-inducing ligand (TRAIL/Apo2 ligand), as anti-tumor agents. TRAIL induces cell death in a wide variety of tumor cell lines, but does not appear to be cytotoxic to normal cells. Experiments *in vitro* have demonstrated that TRAIL induces apoptosis in RMS cell lines when used as a single agent [74] or in combination with chemotherapy agents such as doxorubicin [75].
• Another potential treatment strategy involves the use of oncolytic viruses. For example, herpes simplex viruses, modified so as to restrict their ability to replicate to transformed target cells, have been shown to be effective against human rhabdomyosarcoma cell lines and xenografts [76, 77].

An area that is likely to become increasingly important is the development of immunotherapy techniques. One of the major

problems with conventional chemotherapy agents is their lack of specificity for malignant cells, such that their use in clinical practice is often limited by their systemic side effects. Novel agents targeting proteins expressed specifically by tumor cells hold out the prospect of a more directed approach.
• In ARMS, the PAX3-FOXO1A fusion protein represents one such potential target and preliminary experiments in mice have indicated that it is possible to generate cytotoxic T lymphocytes which specifically target tumor cells expressing this fusion protein [78]. Initial trials of such techniques in patients with recurrent RMS or Ewing's sarcoma (using fusion protein peptide vaccination) have not, however, demonstrated improved clinical outcomes [79].
• Recently *in vitro* studies of T-cell therapy successfully targeting the PAX3-FOXO1A fusion protein have been described [80].

An alternative promising technique is the use of adjuvants such as CpG oligodeoxynucleotides (ODNs) that contain CpG motifs characteristic of prokaryotic DNA and which are capable of stimulating a potent innate immune response. In a murine model of embryonal rhabdomyosarcoma administration of CpG ODNs, either in combination with conventional chemotherapy agents or following surgical resection of the tumor, resulted in suppression of tumor growth and improved survival [81]. Hence, in the search for novel therapeutic strategies, an important principle is tumor specificity, with agents designed to target epitopes, proteins or genetic pathways specific to the malignancy.

As with other pediatric cancers, the potential benefits of anti-angiogenesis therapies are being evaluated in the pre-clinical and clinical setting. For example, the vascular endothelial receptor (VEGF) inhibitors AZD2171 (a mall molecule inhibitor of the VEGF receptor tyrosine kinase) [82], VEGF-Trap (a soluble decoy receptor) [83], and the anti-vascular agent TNP-470 [84] have all shown activity in the xenograft setting for RMS. An understanding of the requirement to ensure blockade of both the host and tumor sources of VEGF in the xenograft setting [85], will be an important factor in the optimal introduction of specific anti-VEGF therapies into clinical practice for pediatric soft-tissue sarcoma.

Non-rhabdomyosarcoma soft tissue sarcomas

Excluding RMS, the rest of pediatric STS is composed of a group of rare and heterogeneous tumors of non-epithelial extraskeletal origin with different clinical, histological, and biological characteristics. Most histiotypes occur very rarely in children, being more common in older ages ('adult-type' STS). Finally, some entities are considered as intermediate-malignancy tumors because of their local aggressiveness but low potential of metastatic spread.

The relative frequencies of different histologic subtypes vary with age with infantile fibrosarcoma being more common in children less than 2 years old and synovial sarcoma (SS) and malignant peripheral nerve sheath tumor (MPNST) most commonly affecting adolescents. Other NRSTS include:

• Epithelioid sarcoma.
• Alveolar soft part sarcoma.
• Rhabdoid tumor.
• Vascular tumors (angiosarcoma, hemangiopericytoma).
• Desmoplastic small round cell tumor.
• Liposarcoma, malignant fibrous histiocytoma, leiomyosarcoma and undifferentiated sarcoma.

The incidence of the different NRSTS may vary according to the age limit adopted, the histologies considered and the Institutions involved: in fact adolescents with NRSRS may be treated in adult wards in some treatment centres. Figure 14.1 describes the relative frequencies of NRSTS registered in the Italian studies. The category of borderline tumors includes a large group of histiotypes with the fibroblastic and myofibroblastic lesions being the most frequent.

As for RMS, there is usually a painless growing mass that can occur anywhere in the body and causes symptoms when nearby organs are invaded. The most affected sites are the extremities, followed by the trunk wall and the retroperitoneum, while head and neck or genito-urinary sites are rarely involved. Compared with RMS, NRSTS have:
• A lower propensity to spread to the regional lymph nodes (10% of cases).
• A lower propensity to give rise to distant metastases (10–12%).
• In general high-grade NRSTS have a more invasive behaviour with high propensity to metastasize, in particular to the lungs.

Due to the rarity of these lesions histologic materials should be analyzed by an expert pathologist to confirm the diagnosis of NRSTS and to grade the tumor appropriately. Molecular biology is of increasing importance as a number of specific translocations have been identified. In general, the diagnostic work-up and the staging systems are the same as those adopted for RMS. The IRS grouping system and the TNM staging system are commonly used by pediatric oncologists to define the extension of surgery and the invasiveness and size of tumors. Different grading systems that take into account characteristics such as histology, amount of necrosis, number of mitoses, and cellular pleomorphism are in use in adult practice, but their prognostic value has not been established yet for pediatric NRSTS.

Pathology and biology

Although the cause of an individual's STS is usually unknown, host genetic factors are of importance in a minority of cases. For example, NF1 mutation in cases of malignant peripheral nerve sheath tumor and p53 mutation in sarcomas arising in patients within a Li Fraumeni family. A search for unifying genetic abnormalities underlying NRSTS through chromosome analysis has generally revealed a lack of consistent abnormalities. However, like RMS, consistent and characteristic chromosomal translocations have been identified for many adult and pediatric NRSTS and the resultant gene aberrations have been characterized. As for RMS, the presence of unique fusion transcripts and fusion genes within the tumors provides a molecular signature, which can be potentially exploited as a diagnostic marker. For example, reverse

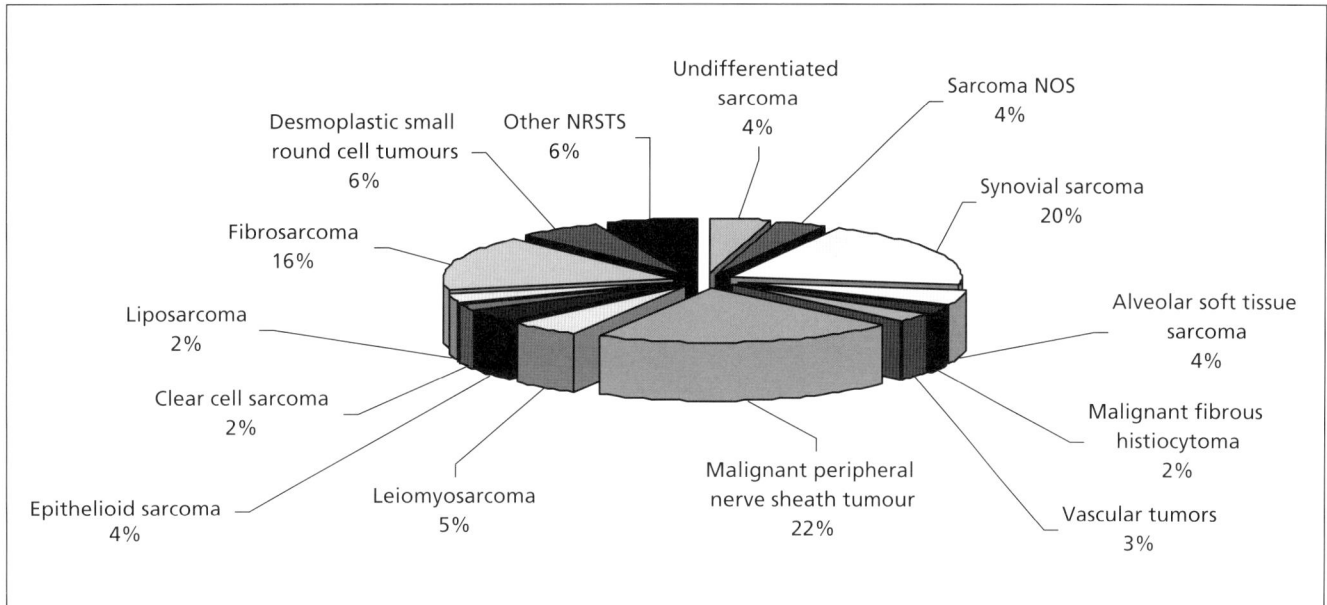

Figure 14.1 NRSTS distribution (334 patients registered into the Italian protocols from 1988 to 2006).

transcriptase/polymerase chain reaction (RT-PCR) or fluorescence *in situ* hybridization (FISH) can be performed on tumor-derived RNA and tumor section respectively, to identify the expression of the fusion gene or the presence of the fused/disrupted DNA respectively.

Treatment

Generally, the management of NRSTS has been derived from those adopted for RMS and from adult experience.
• A complete tumor resection with wide margins gives the best chance of cure and may be the only necessary treatment for some histotypes. Surgery tends to be more conservative in children, adopting limb sparing procedures and non-compartmental resections. It must be considered, however, that this approach may cause a higher relapse rate.
• Radiotherapy (40–50 Gy) is adopted when resection margins are uncertain, or to reduce the tumor mass before surgery.

The role of chemotherapy for NRSTS is controversial because response rates are usually low and few studies have reported an effect on survival. Recent reports have suggested that chemotherapy should probably be reserved for high risk tumors [5]. In fact data from larger series containing different histotypes or small series dedicated to single histotype have consistently identified several prognostic factors (see Table 14.8).
• In general patients with large invasive tumors of higher grade have an increased risk of local and especially metastatic relapse. Limited pediatric series have shown a lower metastatic relapse rate when chemotherapy was administered. This is confirmed by the comparison with adult sarcoma experience, where chemotherapy has been used less systematically, and the distant relapse rate is often the cause of treatment failure.

• Unfortunately, very few drugs demonstrate convincing activity against NRSTS and the doxorubicin-ifosfamide combination represents, as for adult sarcoma, the reference regimen with a response rate around 40% [86].

Overall, the survival rate for STS averages 60%, and exceeds 80% when the tumor is completely resected [5, 87]. Unresectable and/or metastatic tumor remains a challenge with survival below 50%. In these patients chemotherapy has been attempted to reduce tumor volume and obtain a delayed complete surgical resection. Although this has been possible for some patients, the impact of chemotherapy response on survival is not completely proven [5, 88].

Table 14.8 NRSTS prognostic factors.

Disease extension at diagnosis	Survival is poor when metastatic lesions are present
Surgery at diagnosis	Complete resection is necessary, and often enough, in most histotypes
Tumour size	Large lesions (>5 cm) have a higher risk of local and metastatic failure
Tumor invasiveness (according to the TNM system)	Often associated with tumor size, keep the same meaning
Histology	Histotypes may determine different biological behaviour and response to treatment
Grading	High grade lesions have a higher risk of local and metastatic failure
Age	Tumours in older children behave more like adult sarcomas and carry a worse prognosis

Synovial sarcoma

Synovial sarcoma is the most common NRSTS in pediatric practice, occurring most commonly in the extremities of adolescents and young adults, and demonstrate characteristic cytogenetic and molecular features.

• Fusion proteins SYT-SSX1 or SYT-SSX2, associated specifically with synovial sarcoma, were discovered following investigation of reciprocal chromosomal translocations t(X;18)(p11.2;q11.2) found within these tumor cells [89].

• More than 90% of synovial sarcomas express these proteins and their presence is effectively pathognomonic of the disease. Like PAX-FOXO1A fusions, synovial fusions are thought to act predominantly as transcription regulators. Monophasic synovial sarcomas can express either fusion subtype whereas biphasic histology is invariably associated with SYT-SSX1 [90].

• There is no difference between adult and pediatric SS in terms of these fusion proteins; however, it does not necessarily follow that the diseases in the two age groups are the same or that they should be treated equivalently.

The identification of optimal treatment for synovial sarcoma has been complicated by the lack of randomized clinical trials consequent on the relatively low incidence of the disease. There is evidence for significantly better event free survival in younger patients although this may be related to the more frequent use of adjuvant chemotherapy in pediatric practice [5]. Whereas there is limited evidence of chemoresponsiveness in low stage localized disease, larger tumors have favourable survival with adjuvant chemotherapy [91]. Current European risk-adapted therapy involves surgery only for completely resected tumors less than 5 cm in diameter, adjuvant chemotherapy (ifosfamide and doxorubicin) for completely resected greater than 5 cm tumors, and chemotherapy and involved field radiotherapy for microscopic and macroscopic incompletely resected tumors with doses determined by response (EpSSG NRSTS 2005 protocol).

Fibrosarcoma

Infantile fibrosarcoma and adult type fibrosarcoma occurring in children are different disease entities. Infantile fibrosarcoma occurs almost exclusively in infants and young children and can be congenital. The most common sites are the extremities and trunk.

• The tumors are characterized by the presence of a t(12;15)(p13;q25) translocation creating a ETV6-NTRK3 fusion, which is also seen in the cellular form of congenital mesoblastic nephroma, a renal tumor which shares a similar histological appearance (sheets of homogeneous spindle shaped cells with minimal collagen).

• Adult type fibrosarcoma in contrast does not have diagnostically or prognostically useful molecular genetic features.

As with the infantile form, immunohistochemistry is rather non-specific with positivity for vimentin and S100 being common. Metastatic spread is extremely rare and so the focus of treatment is achieving local control through good surgical clearance. Where complete resection is not possible without significant morbidity there is a role for adjuvant chemotherapy to induce tumor shrink-

age. First line agents for infantile fibrosarcoma are vincristine and actinomycin, although ifosfamide and doxorubicin are recommended as second line agents in the current EpSSG guidelines [92–94] and these latter drugs are considered first line adjuvant treatment for large adult type fibrosarcomas.

Malignant peripheral nerve sheath tumors

This disease represents one of the more frequent NRSTS in the pediatric age range. It is often observed in the context of neurofibromatosis type 1, arising within a pre-existing neurofibroma, although they can arise sporadically. The term 'MPNST' is preferred to 'malignant schwannoma' and to 'neurofibrosarcoma', because these tumors can show the appearance of any cell of the nerve sheath, including the Schwann cell, perineural fibroblast, or fibroblast.

The clinical presentation is characterized by an enlarging soft tissue mass of trunk, extremities or head and neck region, with or without pain and dysesthesia. Although nearly always localized at presentation, if relapse occurs it is frequently at distant metastatic sites, especially in the lungs [95]. There are no characteristic or diagnostic molecular genetic changes or rearrangements, and diagnosis is based on histological appearance.

MPNST behaves aggressively and surgical resection represents the mainstay of treatment, whereas the role of adjuvant treatment remains unclear. Recent reports support the use of post-operative radiotherapy in case of minimal residual tumor, whereas irradiation seems ineffective in controlling bulky disease. Response to chemotherapy up to 45% have been reported with a possible impact on survival that is around 80% when the tumor is resected at diagnosis, but is less than 50% in case of unresectable tumors [96]. Patients with NF1 rarely respond to chemotherapy and, in general, have a much worst outcome with survival reported less than 30% [97]. New approaches are under study targeting the epidermal growth factor receptor (EGFR), which is overexpressed in NF1 patients with high-grade MPNST and it is probably involved in their tumorigenesis [98].

Rhabdoid tumors

These are highly aggressive tumors usually occurring under the age of 5 years. Rhabdoid tumors arising in the brain are usually referred to atypical teratoid rhabdoid tumor (ATRT) but there is evidence that they are biologically equivalent to the extracranial disease which can arise within the kidney or in extra-renal sites. The feature in common between rhabdoid tumors in all these sites has recently been shown to be loss of expression of hSNF1/INI1, a component of the chromatin remodelling complex. The loss of protein expression can occur as a result of genetic deletion or mutation or by epigenetic mechanisms [99–101], and is a characteristic feature of the disease, having not been reported in other diagnoses. Interestingly, cases in which lesions arise in bilateral kidneys or in kidney and brain have been reported, suggesting a genetic predisposition syndrome and in rare cases, germline INI1 mutation has been described [102, 103]. Metastatic disease is usually fatal and current treatment approaches involve neoadjuvant multiagent chemotherapy to attempt tumor shrinkage prior to local therapy with radiotherapy and surgery. Recently age has been identified as an adverse prognostic factor with young children fairing particularly poorly [104].

Desmoplastic small round cell tumors

This rare but aggressive neoplasm, most commonly arising in the abdomen and with widespread metastatic deposits, is a predominantly pediatric condition, with a peak incidence in the second decade. A reciprocal chromosomal translocation t(11:22) (p12:q12) encoding the chimeric transcription factor EWS-WT1, is probably present in all cases of this tumor and can justifiably be thought of as pathognomonic since it has not been described in the context of any other histological diagnosis. Several treatment approaches have been described but survival rates are poor and cure has always been described in the context of multimodal therapy, incorporating intensive chemotherapy and surgery, typically with radiotherapy [105].

Fibroblastic and myofibroblastic lesions

These are fibrous tissue proliferations of intermediate malignancy, which typically present as localized lesions but with a locally invasive growth pattern and a tendency to localized recurrence. Several distinct pathological entities have been described, and they are grouped together here for reasons of similarity of clinical behaviour, not because of any known common features of histogenesis or biology. Aggressive fibromatosis (desmoid tumor) has several modes of presentation:
• In the context of familial adenomatous polyposis (Gardner syndrome) associated with inherited mutations in the APC gene. These lesions are typically abdominal and the development of lesions following surgery for polyposis has been described.
• Lesions that occur in aponeurotic structures, commonly on limbs.
• Lesions that arise in scars following previous surgery.

Fibromatosis is a surgical condition with likelihood of local relapse being related to achievement of clear margins. Repeat surgery following second or third local relapses can be curative if clear margins are achieved [106]. Medical treatment can be beneficial, especially if a degree of tumor shrinkage is desirable to achieve clear surgical margins whilst minimizing mutilating effects of surgery. The reported cytotoxic regimes generally involve fairly long courses of low dose agents such as vincristine, actinomycin, doxorubicin, vinorelbine, and methotrexate [107]. Anti-oestrogens (tamoxifen, teremofen) and, more recently, imatinib are anecdotally described as having useful activity, the latter resulting in clinical response in about 20% of cases and probably related to blockade of kit or platelet-derived growth factor receptor tryrosine kinases [108].

Myofibromatosis and its localized counterpart, myofibroma, are fibroblastic lesions with elements of myogenic differentiation. For localized lesions the treatment approach is the same as for aggressive fibromatosis although the usefulness of chemotherapy is less well established [109, 110] and in many cases good surgical

margins can be achieved without a requirement for trial of chemotherapy. In the rarer multicentric forms, especially those that involve viscera, prognosis is poor although cases responding to chemotherapy have been reported [109]. A recent report of over expression of PDGF and PDGF receptors in pediatric myofibromatosis suggests a trial of imatinib might be justified in unresectable cases [111].

A variant is the inflammatory myofibroblastic tumor (IMT) sometimes called inflammatory pseudotumor.
• These can occur at any site and are associated with fever, weight loss, and raised inflammatory markers, such that diagnoses such as chronic infections (e.g. tuberculosis) can form part of the differential. If possible, surgical resection with clear margins should be sought.
• There is little evidence for the value of chemotherapy and radiotherapy in these lesions. More recently there have been reports of responses following administration of non-steroidal anti-inflammatory drugs and a rational basis for their use in terms of high incidence of COX2 and VEGF staining [112].
• Medical treatment with cytotoxics and/or non-steroidals is advised in cases where complete surgical clearance is not deemed possible.

This diagnosis is most commonly made in the first two decades of life and often presents with fever and a mass lesion in the lung or abdomen. It is generally considered a low grade malignancy although both spontaneous regression and development of distant metastases has been described. The name results from the histological appearance of proliferating (myo)fibroblasts and inflammatory cells. A proportion of these tumors are characterized by translocations resulting in fusion with and consequent upregulation of the anaplastic lymphoma kinase (ALK). ALK1 immunopositivity is a useful diagnostic test in combination with vimentin although ALK1 staining is observed in a range of other STS. It is not established whether ALK1 staining is correlated with malignant potential or prognosis.

Dermatofibrosarcoma protuberans (DFSP) is of interest because of its characteristic chromosome translocation t(7:22) (q22:q13), which produces a novel gene fusion comprising the promoter of collagen 1A1 (COL1A1) gene, and the coding sequence of PDGF[113, 114]. The resultant over-expression of PDGFβ leads to continuous activation of the PDGFRβ protein tyrosine kinase that promotes DFSP tumor cell growth [115] and clinical responses to imatinib have been described [116].

References

1 Ries LAGMD, Krapcho M, Mariotto A, Feuer EJ. SEER Cancer Statistics Review 1975–2004.
2 Parkin DMKE, Draper GJ, Masuyer E, Michaelis J, Neglia J. International Incidence of Childhood Cancer. *Vol.* II. IARC Scientific Publication, No 144. 1998.
3 Crist WM, Anderson JR, Meza JL, et al. Intergroup rhabdomyosarcoma study-IV: results for patients with nonmetastatic disease. J Clin Oncol 2001; 19: 3091–102.

4 Breitfeld PP, Meyer WH. Rhabdomyosarcoma: new windows of opportunity. Oncologist 2005; 10: 518–27.

5 Ferrari A, Casanova M, Collini P, et al. Adult-type soft tissue sarcomas in pediatric-age patients: experience at the Istituto Nazionale Tumori in Milan. J Clin Oncol 2005; 23: 4021–30.

6 Newton WA, Jr, Gehan EA, Webber BL, et al. Classification of rhabdomyosarcomas and related sarcomas. Pathologic aspects and proposal for a new classification–an Intergroup Rhabdomyosarcoma Study. Cancer 1995; 76: 1073–85.

7 Kuhnen C, Herter P, Leuschner I, et al. Sclerosing pseudovascular rhabdomyosarcoma-immunohistochemical, ultrastructural, and genetic findings indicating a distinct subtype of rhabdomyosarcoma. Virchows Arch 2006; 449: 572–8.

8 Chiles MC, Parham DM, Qualman SJ, et al. Sclerosing rhabdomyosarcomas in children and adolescents: a clinicopathologic review of 13 cases from the Intergroup Rhabdomyosarcoma Study Group and Children's Oncology Group. Pediatr Dev Pathol 2005; 8: 141.

9 Tsokos M, Webber BL, Parham DM, et al. Rhabdomyosarcoma. A new classification scheme related to prognosis. Arch Pathol Lab Med 1992; 116: 847–55.

10 Morotti RA, Nicol KK, Parham DM, et al. An immunohistochemical algorithm to facilitate diagnosis and subtyping of rhabdomyosarcoma: the Children's Oncology Group experience. Am J Surg Pathol 2006; 30: 962–8.

11 Sebire NJ, Malone M. Myogenin and MyoD1 expression in paediatric rhabdomyosarcomas. J Clin Pathol 2003; 56: 412–16.

12 Bennicelli JL, Fredericks WJ, Wilson RB, Rauscher FJ, 3rd, Barr FG. Wild type PAX3 protein and the PAX3-FKHR fusion protein of alveolar rhabdomyosarcoma contain potent, structurally distinct transcriptional activation domains. Oncogene 1995; 11: 119–30.

13 Bennicelli JL, Edwards RH, Barr FG. Mechanism for transcriptional gain of function resulting from chromosomal translocation in alveolar rhabdomyosarcoma. Proc Natl Acad Sci USA 1996; 93: 5455–9.

14 Barr FG, Nauta LE, Davis RJ, Schafer BW, Nycum LM, Biegel JA. In vivo amplification of the PAX3-FKHR and PAX7-FKHR fusion genes in alveolar rhabdomyosarcoma. Hum Mol Genet 1996; 5: 15–21.

15 Davis RJ, Barr FG. Fusion genes resulting from alternative chromosomal translocations are overexpressed by gene-specific mechanisms in alveolar rhabdomyosarcoma. Proc Natl Acad Sci USA 1997; 94: 8047–51.

16 Davicioni E, Finckenstein FG, Shahbazian V, Buckley JD, Triche TJ, Anderson MJ. Identification of a PAX-FKHR gene expression signature that defines molecular classes and determines the prognosis of alveolar rhabdomyosarcomas. Cancer Res 2006; 66: 6936–46.

17 Khan J, Bittner ML, Saal LH, et al. cDNA microarrays detect activation of a myogenic transcription program by the PAX3-FKHR fusion oncogene. Proc Natl Acad Sci USA 1999; 96: 13264–9.

18 Margue CM, Bernasconi M, Barr FG, Schafer BW. Transcriptional modulation of the anti-apoptotic protein BCL-XL by the paired box transcription factors PAX3 and PAX3/FKHR. Oncogene 2000; 19: 2921–9.

19 Nabarro S, Himoudi N, Papanastasiou A, et al. Coordinated oncogenic transformation and inhibition of host immune responses by the PAX3-FKHR fusion oncoprotein. J Exp Med 2005; 202: 1399–410.

20 Anderson J, Himoudi N. PAX3-FKHR chimeric oncoprotein: hiding itself from immune detection? Cell Cycle 2006; 5: 563–4.

21 Lam PY, Sublett JE, Hollenbach AD, Roussel MF. The oncogenic potential of the Pax3-FKHR fusion protein requires the Pax3 homeodomain recognition helix but not the Pax3 paired-box DNA binding domain. Mol Cell Biol 1999; 19: 594–601.

22 Casola S, Pedone PV, Cavazzana AO, et al. Expression and parental imprinting of the H19 gene in human rhabdomyosarcoma. Oncogene 1997; 14: 1503–10.

23 Anderson J, Gordon A, McManus A, Shipley J, Pritchard-Jones K. Disruption of imprinted genes at chromosome region 11p15.5 in paediatric rhabdomyosarcoma. Neoplasia 1999; 1: 340–8.

24 Slater O, Shipley J. Clinical relevance of molecular genetics to paediatric sarcomas. J Clin Pathol 2007; 60: 1187–94.

25 Mercado GE, Barr FG. Fusions involving PASX and FOX genes in the molecular pathogenesis of alveolar rhabdomyosarcoma: recent advances. Curr Mol Med 2007; 7: 47–61.

26 Donaldson SS, Draper GJ, Flamant F, et al. Topography of childhood tumors: pediatric coding system. Pediatr Hematol Oncol 1986; 3: 249–58.

27 Schuetze SM, Rubin BP, Vernon C, et al. Use of positron emission tomography in localized extremity soft tissue sarcoma treated with neoadjuvant chemotherapy. Cancer 2005; 103: 339–48.

28 Ioannidis JP, Lau J. 18F-FDG PET for the diagnosis and grading of soft-tissue sarcoma: a meta-analysis. J Nucl Med 2003; 44: 717–24.

29 Maurer HM, Beltangady M, Gehan EA, et al. The Intergroup Rhabdomyosarcoma Study-I. A final report. Cancer 1988; 61: 209–20.

30 Sorensen PH, Lynch JC, Qualman SJ, et al. PAX3-FKHR and PAX7-FKHR gene fusions are prognostic indicators in alveolar rhabdomyosarcoma: a report from the children's oncology group. J Clin Oncol 2002; 20: 2672–9.

31 Anderson J, Gordon T, McManus A, et al. Detection of the PAX3-FKHR fusion gene in paediatric rhabdomyosarcoma: a reproducible predictor of outcome? Br J Cancer 2001; 85: 831–5.

32 Kelly KM, Womer RB, Sorensen PH, Xiong QB, Barr FG. Common and variant gene fusions predict distinct clinical phenotypes in rhabdomyosarcoma. J Clin Oncol 1997; 15: 1831–6.

33 Raney RB, Stoner JA, Walterhouse DO, et al. Results of treatment of fifty-six patients with localized retroperitoneal and pelvic rhabdomyosarcoma: a report from The Intergroup Rhabdomyosarcoma Study-IV, 1991–1997. Pediatr Blood Cancer 2004; 42: 618–25.

34 Cecchetto G, Guglielmi M, Inserra A, et al. Primary re-excision: the Italian experience in patients with localized soft-tissue sarcomas. Pediatr Surg Int 2001; 17: 532–4.

35 McMulkin HM, Yanchar NL, Fernandez CV, Giacomantonio C. Sentinel lymph node mapping and biopsy: a potentially valuable tool in the management of childhood extremity rhabdomyosarcoma. Pediatr Surg Int 2003; 19: 453–6.

36 Stevens MC. Treatment for childhood rhabdomyosarcoma: the cost of cure. Lancet Oncol 2005; 6: 77–84.

37 Oberlin O, Rey A, Anderson J, et al. Treatment of orbital rhabdomyosarcoma: survival and late effects of treatment–results of an international workshop. J Clin Oncol 2001; 19: 197–204.

38 Wolden SL, Anderson JR, Crist WM, et al. Indications for radiotherapy and chemotherapy after complete resection in rhabdomyosarcoma: a report from the Intergroup Rhabdomyosarcoma Studies I to III. J Clin Oncol 1999; 17: 3468–75.

39 Martelli H, Oberlin O, Rey A, et al. Conservative treatment for girls with nonmetastatic rhabdomyosarcoma of the genital tract: a report

from the Study Committee of the International Society of Pediatric Oncology. J Clin Oncol 1999; 17: 2117–22.

40 Donaldson SS, Meza J, Breneman JC, et al. Results from the IRS-IV randomized trial of hyperfractionated radiotherapy in children with rhabdomyosarcoma–a report from the IRSG. Int J Radiat Oncol Biol Phys 2001; 51: 718–28.

41 Pappo AS, Etcubanas E, Santana VM. A phase II trial of ifosfamide in previously untreated children and adolescents with unresectable rhabomyosarcoma. Cancer 1993; 71: 2119–25.

42 Treuner J, Burger D, Weinel P, et al. Comparison between the initial cytostatic response rate under a combination including cyclophospamide (VACA) and the same combination with ifosfamide (VAIA) in primary unresectable rhabomyosarcoma. Med Paed Oncol 1987; 15: 328.

43 Baker KS, Anderson JR, Link MP, et al. Benefit of intensified therapy with local and regional embroynal rhabdomyosarcoma: results from the Intergroup Rhabdomyosarcoma Study IV. J Clin Oncol 2000; 18: 2427–34.

44 Spunt SL, Smith LM, Ruymann FB, et al. Cyclophosphamide dose intensification during induction therapy for intermediate-risk pediatric rhabdomyosarcoma is feasible but does not improve outcome: a report from the soft tissue sarcoma committee of the children's oncology group. Clin Cancer Res 2004; 10: 6072–9.

45 Arndt C, Hawkins D, Anderson JR, Breitfeld P, Womer R, Meyer W. Age is a risk factor for chemotherapy-induced hepatopathy with vincristine, dactinomycin, and cyclophosphamide. J Clin Oncol 2004; 22: 1894–901.

46 Crist W, Gehan EA, Ragab AH, et al. The Third Intergroup Rhabdomyosarcoma Study. J Clin Oncol 1995; 13: 610–30.

47 Maurer HM, Gehan EA, Beltangady M, et al. The Intergroup Rhabdomyosarcoma Study-II. Cancer 1993; 71: 1904–22.

48 Treuner J, Koscielniak E, Keim M. Comparison of the rates of response to ifosfamide and cyclophosphamide in primary unresectable rhabdomyosarcomas. Cancer Chemother Pharmacol 1989; 24 (Suppl 1): S48–50.

49 Flamant F, Rodary C, Rey A, et al. Treatment of non-metastatic rhabdomyosarcomas in childhood and adolescence. Results of the second study of the International Society of Paediatric Oncology: MMT84. Eur J Cancer 1998; 34: 1050–62.

50 Koscielniak E, Jurgens H, Winkler K, et al. Treatment of soft tissue sarcoma in childhood and adolescence. A report of the German Cooperative Soft Tissue Sarcoma Study. Cancer 1992; 70: 2557–67.

51 Carli M, Koscielniak E, Bisogno G, et al. High-risk rhabdoyosarcoma. Early results of the Italian and German study ICS-CWSRMS96. Ped Blood Cancer 2005; 45: 415.

52 Carli M, Colombatti R, Oberlin O, et al. High-dose melphalan with autologous stem-cell rescue in metastatic rhabdomyosarcoma. J Clin Oncol 1999; 17: 2796–803.

53 Casanova M, Ferrari A, Bisogno G, et al. Vinorelbine and low-dose cyclophosphamide in the treatment of pediatric sarcomas: pilot study for the upcoming European Rhabdomyosarcoma Protocol. Cancer 2004; 101: 1664–71.

54 Pappo AS, Lyden E, Breitfeld P, et al. Two consecutive phase II window trials of irinotecan alone or in combination with vincristine for the treatment of metastatic rhabdomyosarcoma: the Children's Oncology Group. J Clin Oncol 2007; 25: 362–9.

55 Koscielniak E, Klingebiel TH, Peters C, et al. Do patients with metastatic and recurrent rhabdomyosarcoma benefit from high-dose therapy with hematopoietic rescue? Report of the German/Austrian Pediatric Bone Marrow Transplantation Group. Bone Marrow Trans 1997; 19: 227–31.

56 Walterhouse DO, Hoover ML, Marymont MA, Kletzel M. High-dose chemotherapy followed by peripheral blood stem cell rescue for metastatic rhabdomyosarcoma: the experience at Chicago Children's Memorial Hospital. Med Pediatr Oncol 1999; 32: 88–92.

57 Sutow WW, Vietti TJ, Lonsdale D, Talley RW. Daunomycin in the treatment of metastatic soft tissue sarcoma in children. Cancer 1972; 29: 1293–7.

58 Sung L, Anderson JR, Donaldson SS, Spunt SL, Crist WM, Pappo AS. Late events occurring five years or more after successful therapy for childhood rhabdomyosarcoma: a report from the Soft Tissue Sarcoma Committee of the Children's Oncology Group. Eur J Cancer 2004; 40: 1878–85.

59 Pappo AS, Anderson JR, Crist WM, et al. Survival after relapse in children and adolescents with rhabdomyosarcoma: a report from the Intergroup Rhabdomyosarcoma Study Group. J Clin Oncol 1999; 17: 3487–93.

60 Mazzoleni S, Bisogno G, Garaventa A, et al. Outcomes and prognostic factors after recurrence in children and adolescents with non-metastatic rhabdomyosarcoma. Cancer 2005; 104: 183–90.

61 Cocker HA, Pinkerton CR, Kelland LR. Characterization and modulation of drug resistance of human pediatric rhabdomyosarcoma cell lines. Br J Cancer 2000; 83: 338–45.

62 Seitz G, Warmann SW, Vokuhl CO, et al. Effects of standard chemotherapy on tumor growth and regulation of multidrug resistance genes and proteins in childhood rhabdomyosarcoma. Pediatr Surg Int 2007; 23: 431–9.

63 Staibano S, Franco R, Tranfa F, et al. Orbital rhabdomyosarcoma: relationship between DNA ploidy, p53, bcl-2, MDR-1 and Ki67 (MIB1) expression and clinical behavior. Anticancer Res 2004; 24: 249–57.

64 Chan HS, Thorner PS, Haddad G, Ling V. Immunohistochemical detection of P-glycoprotein: prognostic correlation in soft tissue sarcoma of childhood. J Clin Oncol 1990; 8: 689–704.

65 Gallego S, Llort A, Parareda A, Sanchez De Toledo J. Expression of multidrug resistance-1 and multidrug resistance-associated protein genes in pediatric rhabdomyosarcoma. Oncol Rep 2004; 11: 179–83.

66 Rigamonti W, Iafrate M, Milani C, et al. Orthotopic continent urinary diversion after radical cystectomy in pediatric patients with genitourinary rhabdomyosarcoma. J Urol 2006; 175: 1092–6; discussion 1096.

67 Peterson JK, Tucker C, Favours E, et al. In vivo evaluation of ixabepilone (BMS247550), a novel epothilone B derivative, against pediatric cancer models. Clin Cancer Res 2005; 11: 6950–8.

68 Woo MH, Peterson JK, Billups C, Liang H, Bjornsti MA, Houghton PJ. Enhanced antitumor activity of irofulven in combination with irinotecan in pediatric solid tumor xenograft models. Cancer Chemother Pharmacol 2005; 55: 411–19.

69 Dilling MB, Dias P, Shapiro DN, Germain GS, Johnson RK, Houghton PJ. Rapamycin selectively inhibits the growth of childhood rhabdomyosarcoma cells through inhibition of signaling via the type I insulin-like growth factor receptor. Cancer Res 1994; 54: 903–7.

70 Maloney EK, McLaughlin JL, Dagdigian NE, et al. An anti-insulin-like growth factor I receptor antibody that is a potent inhibitor of cancer cell proliferation. Cancer Res 2003; 63: 5073–83.

71 Gallicchio MA, van Sinderen M, Bach LA. Insulin-like growth factor binding protein-6 and CCI-779, an ester analogue of rapamycin, additively inhibit rhabdomyosarcoma growth. Horm Metab Res 2003; 35: 822–7.

72 Garcia-Echeverria C, Pearson MA, Marti A, et al. In vivo antitumor activity of NVP-AEW541-A novel, potent, and selective inhibitor of the IGF-IR kinase. Cancer Cell 2004; 5: 231–9.

73 Scotlandi K, Manara MC, Nicoletti G, et al. Antitumor activity of the insulin-like growth factor-I receptor kinase inhibitor NVP-AEW541 in musculoskeletal tumors. Cancer Res 2005; 65: 3868–76.

74 Petak I, Douglas L, Tillman DM, Vernes R, Houghton JA. Pediatric rhabdomyosarcoma cell lines are resistant to Fas-induced apoptosis and highly sensitive to TRAIL-induced apoptosis. Clin Cancer Res 2000; 6: 4119–27.

75 Tomek S, Koestler W, Horak P, et al. Trail-induced apoptosis and interaction with cytotoxic agents in soft tissue sarcoma cell lines. Eur J Cancer 2003; 39: 1318–29.

76 Cinatl J, Jr., Michaelis M, Driever PH, et al. Multimutated herpes simplex virus g207 is a potent inhibitor of angiogenesis. Neoplasia 2004; 6: 725–35.

77 Currier MA, Adams LC, Mahller YY, Cripe TP. Widespread intra-tumoral virus distribution with fractionated injection enables local control of large human rhabdomyosarcoma xenografts by oncolytic herpes simplex viruses. Cancer Gene Ther 2005; 12: 407–16.

78 Mackall C, Berzofsky J, Helman LJ. Targeting tumor specific trans-locations in sarcomas in pediatric patients for immunotherapy. Clin Orthop Relat Res 2000: 373; 25–31.

79 Dagher R, Long LM, Read EJ, et al. Pilot trial of tumor-specific peptide vaccination and continuous infusion interleukin-2 in patients with recurrent Ewing sarcoma and alveolar rhabdomyosarcoma: an inter-institute NIH study. Med Pediatr Oncol 2002; 38: 158–64.

80 Himoudi N, Nabarro S, Yan M, Gilmour K, Thrasher AJ, Anderson J. Development of anti-PAX3 immune responses; a target for cancer immunotherapy. Cancer Immunol Immunother 2007; 56: 1381–95.

81 Weigel BJ, Rodeberg DA, Krieg AM, Blazar BR. CpG oligodeoxynucleotides potentiate the antitumor effects of chemotherapy or tumor resection in an orthotopic murine model of rhabdomyosarcoma. Clin Cancer Res 2003; 9: 3105–14.

82 Maris JM, Courtright J, Houghton PJ, et al. Initial testing of the VEGFR inhibitor AZD2171 by the pediatric preclinical testing program. Pediatr Blood Cancer 2008; 50: 581–7.

83 Holash J, Davis S, Papadopoulos N, et al. VEGF-Trap: a VEGF blocker with potent antitumor effects. Proc Natl Acad Sci USA 2002; 99: 11393–8.

84 Landuyt W, Theys J, Nuyts S, et al. Effect of TNP-470 (AGM-1470) on the growth of rat rhabomyosarcoma tumors of different sizes. Cancer Invest 2001; 19: 35–40.

85 Gerber HP, Kowalski J, Sherman D, Eberhard DA, Ferrara N. Complete inhibition of rhabomyosarcoma xenograft growth and neovascularization requires blockade of both tumor and host vascular endothelial growth factor. Cancer Res 2000; 60: 6253–8.

86 Pappo AS, Devidas M, Jenkins J, et al. Phase II trial of neoadjuvant vincristine, ifosfamide, and doxorubicin with granulocyte colony-stimulating factor support in children and adolescents with advanced-stage nonrhabdomyosarcomatous soft tissue sarcomas: a Pediatric Oncology Group Study. J Clin Oncol 2005; 23: 4031–8.

87 Spunt SL, Poquette CA, Hurt YS, et al. Prognostic factors for children and adolescents with surgically resected nonrhabdomyosarcoma soft tissue sarcoma: an analysis of 121 patients treated at St Jude Children's Research Hospital. J Clin Oncol 1999; 17: 3697–705.

88 Spunt SL, Hill DA, Motosue AM, et al. Clinical features and outcome of initially unresected nonmetastatic pediatric nonrhabdomyosarcoma soft tissue sarcoma. J Clin Oncol 2002; 20: 3225–35.

89 Clark J, Rocques PJ, Crew AJ, et al. Identification of novel genes, SYT and SSX, involved in the t(X;18)(p11.2;q11.2) translocation found in human synovial sarcoma. Nat Genet 1994; 7: 502–8.

90 Ladanyi M, Antonescu CR, Leung DH, et al. Impact of SYT-SSX fusion type on the clinical behavior of synovial sarcoma: a multi-institutional retrospective study of 243 patients. Cancer Res 2002; 62: 135–40.

91 Okcu MF, Munsell M, Treuner J, et al. Synovial sarcoma of childhood and adolescence: a multicenter, multivariate analysis of outcome. J Clin Oncol 2003; 21: 1602–11.

92 Shetty AK, Yu LC, Gardner RV, Warrier RP. Role of chemotherapy in the treatment of infantile fibrosarcoma. Med Pediatr Oncol 1999; 33: 425–7.

93 Loh ML, Ahn P, Perez-Atayde AR, Gebhardt MC, Shamberger RC, Grier HE. Treatment of infantile fibrosarcoma with chemotherapy and surgery: results from the Dana-Farber Cancer Institute and Children's Hospital, Boston. J Pediatr Hematol Oncol 2002; 24: 722–6.

94 Cecchetto G, Alaggio R, Dall'Igna P, et al. Localized unresectable non-rhabdo soft tissue sarcomas of the extremities in pediatric age: results from the Italian studies. Cancer 2005; 104: 2006–12.

95 Wong WW, Hirose T, Scheithauer BW, Schild SE, Gunderson LL. Malignant peripheral nerve sheath tumor: analysis of treatment outcome. Int J Radiat Oncol Biol Phys 1998; 42: 351–60.

96 Carli M, Ferrari A, Zanetti I, et al. Pediatric malignant peripheral nerve sheath tumor: the Italian and German soft tissue sarcoma cooperative group. J Clin Oncol 2005; 23: 8422–30.

97 Ferrari A, Bisogno G, Macaluso A, et al. Soft tissue sarcomas in children and adolescents with neurofibromatosis type 1. Cancer 2007; 109: 1406–12.

98 Ling BC, Wu J, Miller SJ. Role for epidermal growth factor receptor in neurofibromatosis-related peripheral nerve tumorigenesis. Cancer Cell 2005; 7: 65–75.

99 Versteege I, Sevenet N, Lange J, et al. Truncating mutations of hSNF5/INI1 in aggressive paediatric cancer. Nature 1998; 394: 203–6.

100 Sevenet N, Lellouch-Tubiana A, Schofield D, et al. Spectrum of hSNF5/INI1 somatic mutations in human cancer and genotype-phenotype correlations. Hum Mol Genet 1999; 8: 2359–68.

101 Rousseau-Merck MF, Versteege I, Legrand I, et al. hSNF5/INI1 inactivation is mainly associated with homozygous deletions and mitotic recombinations in rhabdoid tumors. Cancer Res 1999; 59: 3152–6.

102 Janson K, Nedzi LA, David O, et al. Predisposition to atypical teratoid/rhabdoid tumor due to an inherited INI1 mutation. Pediatr Blood Cancer 2006; 47: 279–84.

103 Sevenet N, Sheridan E, Amram D, Schneider P, Handgretinger R, Delattre O. Constitutional mutations of the hSNF5/INI1 gene predispose to a variety of cancers. Am J Hum Genet 1999; 65: 1342–8.

104 Tomlinson GE, Breslow NE, Dome J, et al. Rhabdoid tumor of the kidney in the National Wilms' Tumor Study: age at diagnosis as a prognostic factor. J Clin Oncol 2005; 23: 7641–5.

105 Kushner BH, LaQuaglia MP, Wollner N, et al. Desmoplastic small round-cell tumor: prolonged progression-free survival with aggressive multimodality therapy. J Clin Oncol 1996; 14: 1526–31.

106 Faulkner LB, Hajdu SI, Kher U, et al. Pediatric desmoid tumor: retrospective analysis of 63 cases. J Clin Oncol 1995; 13: 2813–18.

107 Skapek SX, Ferguson WS, Granowetter L et al. Vinblastine and methotrexate for dsmoid fibromatosis in children: results of a Pediatric Oncology Group Phase II trial. J Clin Oncol 2007; 25: 501–6.

108 Heinrich MC, McArthur GA, Demetri GD, et al. Clinical and molecular studies of the effect of imatinib on advanced aggressive fibromatosis (desmoid tumor). J Clin Oncol 2006; 24: 1195–203.

109 Gandhi MM, Nathan PC, Weitzman S, Levitt GA. Successful treatment of life-threatening generalized infantile myofibromatosis using low-dose chemotherapy. J Pediatr Hematol Oncol 2003; 25: 750–4.

110 Williams W, Craver RD, Correa H, Velez M, Gardner RV. Use of 2-chlorodeoxyadenosine to treat infantile myofibromatosis. J Pediatr Hematol Oncol 2002; 24: 59–63.

111 Gibson S, Sebire N, Anderson J. Platelet derived growth factor receptors and ligands are upregulated in paediatric fibromatoses. Histopathology 2007; 51: 752–7.

112 Applebaum H, Kieran MW, Cripe TP, et al. The rationale for non-steroidal anti-inflammatory drug therapy for inflammatory myofibroblastic tumors: a Children's Oncology Group study. J Pediatr Surg 2005; 40: 999–1003; discussion 1003.

113 Sirvent N, Maire G, Pedeutour F. Genetics of dermatofibrosarcoma protuberans family of tumors: from ring chromosomes to tyrosine kinase inhibitor treatment. Genes Chrom Cancer 2003; 37: 1–19.

114 Simon MP, Navarro M, Roux D, Pouyssegur J. Structural and functional analysis of a chimeric protein COL1A1-PDGFB generated by the translocation t(17;22)(q22;q13.1) in Dermatofibrosarcoma protuberans (DP). Oncogene 2001; 20: 2965–75.

115 Shimizu A, O'Brien KP, Sjoblom T, et al. The dermatofibrosarcoma protuberans-associated collagen type Ialpha1/platelet-derived growth factor (PDGF) B-chain fusion gene generates a transforming protein that is processed to functional PDGF-BB. Cancer Res 1999; 59: 3719–23.

116 McArthur GA, Demetri GD, van Oosterom A, et al. Molecular and clinical analysis of locally advanced dermatofibrosarcoma protuberans treated with imatinib: Imatinib Target Exploration Consortium Study B2225. J Clin Oncol 2005; 23: 866–73.

15 Bone Tumors

Richard Gorlick[1], Martha Perisoglou[2] and Jeremy Whelan[2]

[1]Department of Pediatrics, The Children's Hospital at Montefiore, New York, USA and [2]Department of Oncology, University College Hospital, London, UK

Introduction

Bone tumors refer to a group of tumors that arise in a particular anatomic site rather than a specific histological entity. Tumors that involve the bone include (Table 15.1):
• Metastases from cancers in other organs.
• Malignancies arising from the hematopoietic system secondarily involving the bone.
• A variety of benign bone neoplasms.
• Several primary malignant bone neoplasms.
Given the markedly higher incidence of a variety of cancers which have a tendency to metastasize to bone and hematological malignancies, these lesions are much more common than primary bone tumors. This is particularly true in adults, in which the prevalent cancers involving the lungs, breast, prostate, and kidney among others, appear as bone metastases at a much higher incidence than primary bone lesions. In children, as in adults, metastatic bone lesions are more common than primary tumors, but the predominant histologic types are neuroblastoma, lymphoma, and rhabdomyosarcoma [1]. The treatment of hematopoietic cancers and metastatic bone lesions, although potentially different from the management of localized disease, generally follows the principles for management of the primary malignancy and therefore is beyond the scope of this chapter. A variety of benign neoplasms arise in bone. In general, these lesions are successfully managed with surgery as the sole therapy and therefore less focus will be placed on these entities.

The most common primary malignant bone tumors are chondrosarcoma, osteosarcoma, and the Ewing's Sarcoma Family of Tumors (ESFT) [1]. The focus of this chapter is children and young people and therefore chondrosarcoma will not be discussed, as it is a relatively rare entity in individuals less than 21. Other rare primary malignant bone neoplasms exist such as adamantinomas, but these also will be beyond the scope of this chapter. This chapter will therefore concentrate on the two distinct and commoner primary bone malignancies, osteosarcoma and ESFT (Table 15.1). Although primary bone tumors overall are rare, they are the sixth most common malignant neoplasm in children [2], and are characterized by the following epidemiological features:
• For adolescents and young adults, they are the third most frequent neoplasm, with only leukemias and lymphomas being more common.
• Malignant bone tumors occur in the United States at an annual rate of approximately 8.7 cases per million children and adolescents younger than 20 years [2]. In England and Wales, the crude rate per million is 6.6 per million under 20 years. Within this there is some variation, both by gender (boys: 7.6 cases per million, girls 5.6 cases per million) and age (e.g. 18.3 cases per million boys aged 15 to 19 compared with 1.4 per million boys aged 1 to 4 years) (Personal Communication, National Cancer Intelligence Centre, Office of National Statistics).
• Of the bone tumors occurring in childhood, osteosarcoma is the most frequent [3, 4], accounting for approximately 35% of all primary sarcomas of bone considering all age groups [5]. If one only considers those between 0 and 20 years it is over 50%. ESFT, the second most frequent primary bone cancer, is more common than osteosarcoma in children younger than 10 years.

Although presented in a single chapter since they arise in a common site, osteosarcoma and ESFT are linked as much by their differences as by their similarities. In fact, contrasting the features of these two entities is frequently used as a didactic tool (Table 15.2). Similarly, the recognition of these conditions as clinical entities is quite disparate. Evidence of the existence of osteosarcoma can be found in mummified remains dating from over 5000 years ago in ancient Egyptians with amputation a documented form of surgical intervention [5]. In contrast, ESFT, which are histologically difficult to distinguish from other small round blue cell tumors, was only described as a clinical entity by James Ewing in 1921 [6].

Benign bone tumors

Benign bone tumors can be classified into:
• Lesions that produce osteoid, e.g. osteoid osteoma, osteoblastoma.

Pediatric Hematology and Oncology, 1st edition. Edited by Edward J. Estlin, Richard J. Gilbertson, and Robert F. Wynn. © 2010 Blackwell Publishing Ltd.

- Collagen lesions, e.g. non-ossifying fibroma, fibrous dysplasia.
- Cartilage producing lesions, e.g. osteochondroma, enchondroma, chondroblastoma.
- Vascular or of unknown histogenesis, e.g. aneurysmal bone cysts, giant cell tumors and eosinophilic granulomas [1, 4].

Many of these conditions appear in the differential diagnosis of malignant tumors and can mimic their presentation, radiographic, or histologic appearance. As two examples of the category of benign bone tumors, osteoid osteoma and aneurysmal bone cyst will be presented in additional detail.

Osteoid osteoma

Osteoid osteoma is a benign bone neoplasm clinically characterized by pain and swelling. The tumors peak incidence is in the second decade of life [4]. The most common sites are the femur and tibia, although osteoid osteoma can occur anywhere in the skeleton. The radiographic appearance is typically a sclerotic lesion in the long bones with a lucent nidus [7]. The usual clinical history involves the abrupt onset of pain which awakens the patient at night. In 75% the pain is relieved by non-steroidal anti-inflammatory medications. Surgery is recommended for patients whose pain is not relieved by this medication. The only part of an osteoid osteoma that needs to be dealt with surgically is the nidus which is the neoplastic portion of the tumor with the remainder of the lesion being reactive bone. Increasingly, less invasive techniques such as radiofrequency thermoablation are replacing surgery.

Aneurysmal bone cyst

Aneurysmal bone cyst is a rare, benign bone lesion characterized by dilated vascular spaces [8]. The lesion usually occurs in the metaphyses of long bones, but it can also affect the bones of the axial skeleton. The radiographic appearance characteristically is a well-demarcated expansile lesion that thins the cortex and produces a 'bubble' appearance [4]. As their location and radiographic appearance mimic telangiectatic osteosarcoma it is important to keep this differential consideration in mind [8]. Aneurysmal bone cysts typically produce painless swelling of the affected area but pathologic fracture can occur. Aneurysmal bone cysts are primarily treated by thorough curettage and in some institutions cryosurgery. Occasionally they recur, and additional treatment measures are necessary [8].

Osteosarcoma

Osteosarcoma, the most common primary malignant bone tumor, is a highly aggressive disease in which dramatic progress has been made in treatment and outcome over the past several decades. Its overall features are summarized in Box 15.1.

Table 15.1 Bone tumors.

Malignant	Hematopoietic	Benign
Osteosarcoma*	Multiple myeloma	Osteoid osteoma
Ewing's sarcoma family tumors*	Lymphoma	Aneurysmal bone cyst
Chondrosarcoma	Granulocytic sarcoma	Osteoblastoma
Metastatic cancers		Non-ossifying fibroma
Adamantinoma		Giant cell tumors
Giant cell tumors		Fibrous dysplasia
Malignant fibrous histiocytoma (of bone)		Enchondroma
Malignant mesenchymoma (of bone)		Chondroblastoma
		Eosinophilic granuloma
		Osteochondroma
		Chondromyxoid Fibroma
		Chordoma

*The most common malignant primary bone tumors in children and adolescents.

Table 15.2 Comparison of clinical features of Ewing's sarcoma family tumors and osteosarcoma.

	Ewing's sarcoma family tumors	Osteosarcoma
Peak incidence/epidemiology	Peak incidence in second decade Rare after age 30 No known causal factor	Peak incidence in second decade Occurs in adults particularly in Paget's, radiation exposure or genetically predisposed
Racial predilection	Uncommon in Blacks or Asians	None
Genetics	A consistent chromosomal translocation is observed Simple karyotype	Frequent genetic abnormalities at the p53 and retinoblastoma gene loci Complex chromosomal derangements
Pathology	Small round blue cell tumor	Spindle cell sarcoma with osteoid
Skeletal location	Diaphyses	Metaphyses
Radiographic	'Onion skin'	'Sunburst'
Appearance	Codman's Triangle	Codman's Triangle
Common sites of metastases	Lungs, bone, bone marrow	Lungs, bone
Treatment modalities	Surgery, radiation, chemotherapy	Surgery, chemotherapy

---

Box 15.1 Treatment and prognosis for osteosarcoma.

- For localized disease the survival is 60–70%
- Complete resection of primary tumor essential for cure
- Induction chemotherapy is currently based on cisplatin, doxorubicin, and methotrexate
- Tumour necrosis in response to induction therapy allows stratification of the nature and intensity of post-surgical treatment, with the inclusion of ifosfamide and etoposide
- For metastatic disease at presentation, the survival is less good (<25% overall) depending on nature and extent of disease burden, with patients presenting with bony involvement faring worse than those with pulmonary disease alone
- Long-term morbidities include cardiac and nephrological sequelae
- Novel therapies being explored in clinical and pre-clinical setting

---

Epidemiology and pathogenesis

Several features characterize the epidemiology of osteosarcoma and provide some clues to its pathogenesis.

- A bimodal age distribution with the first peak in the second decade of life and the second among older adults.
- The approximate incidence of osteosarcoma is 4.8 per million children younger than 20 years of age [2]. This is as low as 0.3 per million in children under the age of 5 years, 2.8 per million at the age of 5–9 years, 8.3 per million at the age of 10–14 years and 9.4 per million at the age of 15–19 years [2].
- There are approximately 400 new cases in those under 20 each year in the United States and 60 cases in England and Wales.
- The male to female ratio is approximately 1.3:1 in this age range.
- It is slightly commoner in black children than in white children.

The etiology of osteosarcoma remains uncertain. The peak age of incidence coincides with a period of rapid bone growth in young people, suggesting a correlation between rapid bone growth and the evolution of osteosarcoma. Other evidence supporting this relationship includes the higher incidence of osteosarcoma in large dog breeds as compared with small breeds [9], and the earlier peak age in girls as compared with boys, corresponding to the earlier age of their growth spurt [10]. At the same time, it must be recognized that osteosarcoma arises in many patients both well before and long after the adolescent growth spurt. Radiation exposure is a well-documented etiological factor [11–13], but as the interval between irradiation and the appearance of osteosarcoma is typically long, this is not relevant to most pediatric patients [4, 14, 15].

The occurrence of osteosarcoma also relates to syndromes that predispose to malignancy as follows:

- The incidence of osteosarcoma is dramatically increased among survivors of retinoblastoma [1], where the majority of second malignancies are sarcomas, and of these almost 50% are osteosarcomas [16]. In the hereditary form of retinoblastoma, germ line mutations of the retinoblastoma gene are common. This is the probable basis for the increased frequency of secondary cancers in this population, since the rate in survivors of unilateral sporadic retinoblastoma is much less [17].
- Germ line mutations in the p53 gene can lead to a high risk of developing malignancies including osteosarcoma which has been described as the Li-Fraumeni syndrome [18]. Loss of function of the p53 and retinoblastoma tumor suppressor genes is believed to have an important role in tumorigenesis in osteosarcoma [18, 19].
- The p53 gene product in normal cells increases in response to DNA damage and directs the cell to either stop progression through the cell cycle or to undergo apoptosis [20, 21]. The retinoblastoma gene product likewise regulates cell-cycle progression [22]. Although germ line mutations of p53 and the retinoblastoma gene are rare, these genes are altered in the majority of osteosarcoma tumor samples [23, 24].
- Numerous oncogenes and tumor suppressor genes are altered in osteosarcoma tumor cells. Although it is clear that alterations in tumor suppressor genes and oncogenes are necessary to produce osteosarcomas, it is not clear which of these events occurs first and why or how it occurs.

A viral etiology has been suggested based on evidence that bone sarcomas can be induced in select animals by viruses, in hamsters by the injection of cell-free extracts of human osteosarcoma, and the presence of SV40-like sequences in some human osteosarcomas [25]. However, no convincing data have emerged that viruses are a major etiological factor. Finally, trauma has often been associated with the diagnosis of osteosarcoma, but little evidence exists to support a causal relationship [1].

Presentation

The most common features in the clinical presentation of osteosarcoma are:

- Pain from the involved region, either with or without an associated soft tissue mass. Pain is often attributed to trauma or vigorous physical exercise, both of which are common in the patient population.
- Symptoms are usually present for several months before the diagnosis is made [1, 4].
- Occasionally patients can present more dramatically with a pathologic fracture.
- The most common site is the metaphysis of a long bone but osteosarcoma can occur in any bone of the body.
- Approximately half of all osteosarcomas originate in the region around the knee. The anatomic distribution of osteosarcoma is shown in Figure 15.1 [4].
- Approximately 20% of patients with osteosarcoma present with metastatic disease which can be detected radiographically. Eighty-percent of patients present with localized disease but the vast

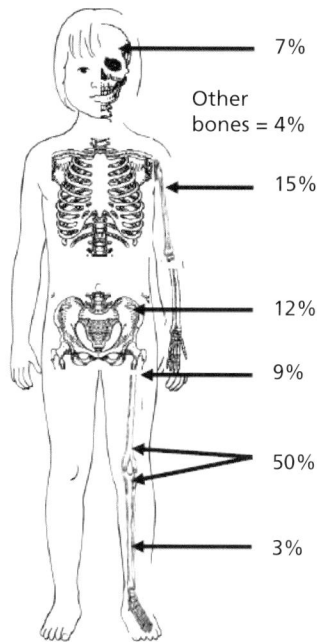

Figure 15.1 Site of primary tumor in patients with osteosarcoma.

majority of this group are known to have subclinical, microscopic metastases [3].
• The most frequent site of metastases is the lung. Much less frequently, metastases at initial diagnosis can occur in other bones. Death from osteosarcoma is almost always the result of progressive pulmonary metastasis. Bone lesions, although extremely painful, are usually not life threatening [1, 4]. Pain at multiple sites does not rule out the possibility of osteosarcoma as this can be from metastatic disease. Metastases in the lungs only produce respiratory symptoms when there is extensive involvement. When osteosarcoma is widely metastatic, which happens more frequently at recurrence than at the time of initial diagnosis, it can spread to the central nervous system or gastrointestinal tract [1, 4].
• Systemic symptoms, such as fever and weight loss, occur rarely [3].

Investigation and staging

The evaluation of suspected osteosarcoma begins with history, physical examination, laboratory evaluations, and plain radiographs. History may be significant only for pain. Physical examination is typically remarkable only for a soft tissue mass at the primary site which is not always present. Laboratory evaluation is seldom revealing. Elevation of the serum alkaline phosphatase and lactate dehydrogenase are observed in a large proportion of patients but are not sensitive or specific. The differential diagnosis for pain at a bone site in this age group includes the malignant bone tumors, osteosarcoma and ESFT, along with the benign bone tumors listed previously and a variety of non-neoplastic conditions with osteomyelitis among the more common. In a patient

with a suspected bone tumor obtaining a plain radiograph of the site is most critical for the proper recognition of the entity [1, 4].

The diagnosis of osteosarcoma is typically suspected by its radiographic appearance, with the following characteristics:
• Osteosarcoma can present as a lytic, sclerotic or as a mixed lytic-sclerotic lesion. As with other malignant tumors in bone, plain films reveal bone destruction with poorly defined zones of transition.
• Ossification in the soft tissue in a 'sunburst' pattern is classic for osteosarcoma but is not a sensitive or specific feature.
• Periosteal new bone formation with lifting of the cortex leads to the appearance of a Codman's triangle. Features such as its location in the metaphysis and the bone involved as well as patient age help to distinguish osteosarcoma and ESFT [1, 4].

The diagnosis of osteosarcoma can be predicted accurately in two-thirds of cases based on radiographic location and appearance, but should never be made from images alone. It is mandatory to obtain a biopsy for pathological confirmation of the diagnosis. The biopsy must be performed by someone experienced in performing these procedures as a poorly placed biopsy can necessitate a subsequent amputation or have other morbidities. The diagnosis of osteosarcoma is made by histologic examination of the biopsy.

The diagnosis of osteosarcoma is based on certain histopathological criteria, and also depends on the presence of malignant spindle cells associated with the production of tumor osteoid. Great variability exists in the histologic patterns seen in this tumor and in the degree of osteoid production, so that extensive review of the pathologic material may be required to demonstrate tumor osteoid.
• As osteosarcomas arise from mesenchymal tissue capable of differentiating toward fibrous tissue, cartilage, or bone, osteosarcoma can have chondroblastic, fibroblastic, and osteoblastic components [1, 4].
• Chondrosarcomas and fibrosarcomas are distinguished from osteosarcoma, with which they can be histologically confused, by their lack of production of osteoid.

The World Health Organization classifies osteosarcomas into central (medullary) and surface (peripheral) tumors and recognizes a number of subtypes within each group (Table 15.3) [26].
• Conventional high-grade central osteosarcoma accounts for 80–90% of all osteosarcomas and it is the predominant form in children and adolescents. The cancer is a primary intramedullary high-grade malignant tumor in which the neoplastic cells produce osteoid, even if only in small amounts. Based on the predominant differentiation of the tumor cells, the most frequent subtypes of conventional osteosarcoma are osteoblastic (50%), chondroblastic (25%) and fibroblastic (25%).
• In osteoblastic osteosarcoma, the tumor appears to be a mixture of large, atypical, spindle-shaped cells that are cytologically highly malignant, with large irregular nuclei and abnormal mitotic figures [3, 4]. Interspersed are areas of osteoid production and calcification in close proximity to the malignant cells. The value of these sub-classifications (osteoblastic, chondroblastic,

Table 15.3 The World Health Organization's histologic classification of osteosarcomas.

Central (medullary)	Surface (peripheral)
• Conventional high-grade central	• Parosteal (juxtacortical) well- differentiated (low-grade)
• Telangiectatic	
• Intraosseous well-differentiated (low-grade)	• Periosteal osteosarcoma, low- to intermediate-grade
• Small-cell osteosarcoma	• High-grade surface

fibroblastic) is unclear as they are very dependent on sampling with mixed histology frequent in a given tumor. Moreover, no difference in clinical behaviour or outcome based on subtype has been discerned.

Conventional high-grade osteosarcomas may develop on the surface of bone and are similar to conventional osteosarcoma both histologically and clinically. Therefore, they should be managed in the same way.

• Telangiectatic osteosarcoma [1, 3, 4] is an unusual subtype that is notable because it appears to be a purely lytic lesion on plain radiographs, leading to diagnostic confusion with aneurysmal bone cyst [27] and giant cell tumor. These tumors are grossly cystic and histologically demonstrate dilated blood-filled spaces with viable tumor cells confined to the periphery of the lesion. Although they have been reported to be associated with an unfavorable outcome [28], other studies treating them as a typical high-grade osteosarcoma fail to demonstrate any difference in prognosis [29].

• Small cell osteosarcoma [30] is a subtype notable because it can be easily confused histologically with Ewing's sarcoma. Immunocytochemical studies or molecular pathology studies may be necessary to make the distinction [31].

Other rarer subtypes and clinical variants of osteosarcoma are also reported and include entities which occur primarily in older patients, and as with low-grade lesions, will not be discussed further [32].

• The malignant fibrous histiocytoma subtype of osteosarcoma.

• Osteosarcoma of the jaw.

• Giant cell rich osteosarcoma.

• Extraosseous and juxtacortical (parosteal) osteosarcoma.

To determine the local and distant extent of disease at presentation various radiographic studies are indicated as part of the diagnostic evaluation. The extent of osteosarcoma in both bone and soft tissue is best appreciated with cross-sectional imaging techniques that have increasingly been based on magnetic resonance imaging (MRI) [1, 4, 5]. A radionuclide bone scan, such as methylene diphosphonate labelled with technetium-99m, defines the extent of the primary tumor and is useful in the detection of 'skip lesions' within the same bone, as well as in detecting distant bone metastases [33].

An unusual presentation of osteosarcoma is multifocal osteosarcoma, a rare entity in which multiple synchronous skeletal tumors are present at diagnosis with each lesion resembling the primary tumor radiographically, suggesting a multi-centric origin. It is unclear whether such sarcomas arise in multiple sites or if one of the lesions is the true primary which has metastasized rapidly to other skeletal sites in the absence of lung metastases. Routine postero-anterior and lateral radiographs of the chest allow detection of metastases in the majority of cases. Computed tomography (CT) of the chest is more sensitive in detecting pulmonary metastases and has become the imaging procedure of choice. However, there are false- positive results, particularly with smaller lesions [1, 4].

Successful treatment of high grade osteosarcoma requires the use of systemic chemotherapy. Many of the agents have both acute and long-term toxicity; therefore, it is essential to obtain baseline studies prior to the initiation of chemotherapy so that these toxicities can be monitored. Baseline evaluations of renal function, cardiac function, and hearing are usually performed. All young men past the age of puberty typically are offered the opportunity to carry out sperm banking [1]. Newer techniques for maintaining fertility of women have been developed but their indications have not completely been established.

The most widely utilized staging system for bone tumors including osteosarcoma is the system developed by Wolf and Enneking [34]. This system categorizes localized malignant bone tumors by grade (low grade – stage I; high grade – stage II) and by the local anatomic extent (intracompartmental – A; extracompartmental – B), and has the following features [1, 4, 5].

• The compartmental status is determined by whether or not the tumor extends through the cortex of the bone.

• Patients with distant metastases are stage III. There are very few high-grade intramedullary lesions (i.e. stage IIA), because most high-grade osteosarcomas break through the cortex early in their natural history.

• In the younger age group, the vast majority of osteosarcomas are high-grade lesions; hence, virtually all patients are stage IIB or III distinguished by the presence or absence of detectable metastatic disease.

General principles of treatment

Almost all patients with high-grade osteosarcoma have at least microscopic metastatic disease. This necessitates the use of systemic chemotherapy in all patients. Despite the effectiveness of chemotherapy against microscopic disease it cannot control clinically detectable disease. Tumors at the primary site as well as at all sites of radiographically visible metastatic disease require local control. Osteosarcoma is considered resistant to radiation therapy, and therefore local control is usually surgery. Advances made in surgery have significantly improved the clinical practice and options available.

Surgery

Complete surgical resection of primary and metastatic disease is the cornerstone for successful treatment [35]. Surgical procedures employed worldwide include amputation, limb salvage techniques and rotation-plasty. All three approaches should incorporate the basic principle of *en bloc* excision of the tumor and biopsy site through normal tissue planes.

• The type and extent of surgery depends on the position and size of the tumor, the anatomy of the affected site as well as the patient's age and skeletal development.

• The ultimate aim is to achieve radical excision or at least excision with wide margins while maintaining adequate function and satisfactory cosmetic result.

• Marginal or intra-marginal margins are associated with increased risk of local recurrence and poor outcome [36] and those patients warrant revision surgery.

At present, most patients are managed with limb-salvage techniques. Carefully selected patients treated by experienced surgeons with limb-preserving operations do not appear to have a survival disadvantage [37–43]. However, amputation may be the most suitable option in patients with adverse tumor features.

Radiotherapy

Osteosarcomas are not responsive to conventional-dose radiotherapy which is only reserved where complete surgery cannot be achieved. It is recommended for inoperable sites or those that could only be operated with inadequate margins.

Chemotherapy – the evolution of current treatment templates

Despite the use of radical surgery, the outcome of patients with osteosarcoma was in the past very poor. Approximately 85–90% of patients presenting with apparently localized disease who underwent radical surgery rendering them grossly free of disease subsequently had recurrences [1, 44]. This high probability demonstrates that the great majority of patients with localized disease at presentation actually harbour sub-clinical metastases. In the 1970s several investigators reported that chemotherapy had activity against relapsed or metastatic osteosarcoma. The agents that were reported to demonstrate activity included doxorubicin, cisplatin, high-dose methotrexate with folinic acid rescue, and ifosfamide [1, 45–48]. When these agents were administered to patients with relapsed or metastatic osteosarcoma, tumor responses were observed, but it must be noted that compared with other pediatric malignancies, the list of drugs shown to be effective was relatively short. Subsequent studies have then underpinned the importance of adjuvant chemotherapy for osteosarcoma as summarized below.

• With this rationale, several investigators embarked on trials of adjuvant chemotherapy for the treatment of osteosarcoma, especially in the setting of disease that was not clinically detectable following initial surgery. In the 1970s and early 1980s, all of these trials were single arm, non-randomized treatments employing adjuvant chemotherapy, comparing results against historical controls. Every reported trial of adjuvant chemotherapy for osteosarcoma demonstrated a disease-free survival superior to the historical rate of 20% [1, 49, 50].

• Not all investigators were convinced that chemotherapy was appropriate for all patients with osteosarcoma as the use of historical comparisons can be flawed [1, 4]. For example, it was postulated the improved survival might be the result of identification of a cohort of patients with an intrinsically better outcome. Earlier diagnosis or improved surgical technique could have also contributed to improved outcome [51], and this was supported by a Mayo clinic trial performed in the early 1980s where chemotherapy was randomized with no apparent improvement to the overall 40% survival rates achieved [52, 53].

• To clarify the issues surrounding the value of adjuvant chemotherapy, the Multi-Institution Osteosarcoma Study (MIOS) was initiated in the early 1980s [54]. Patients were eligible for study entry after amputation or tumor resection if they did not have clinically detectable metastatic disease. The intent of the study was to randomize patients between observation and adjuvant multi-agent chemotherapy. Results were analyzed for both the randomized patients and the larger group who were not randomized with both having identical results. Patients who did not receive chemotherapy after surgery had a probability of disease-free survival (DFS) of 11% as compared with 66% for those who received chemotherapy. This study unequivocally demonstrated that the natural history of osteosarcoma had not changed and adjuvant chemotherapy was of clear benefit [52–54]. With longer follow up, an OS advantage with adjuvant chemotherapy became apparent in accordance with the DFS rates observed earlier, and the majority of patients surviving 3 years without evidence of recurrence were likely to be cured.

• In the same era, Rosen *et al.* introduced the concept of giving chemotherapy before carrying out definitive surgery on the primary tumor [55, 56]. This treatment has been referred to as pre-operative or neoadjuvant chemotherapy, or more recently induction chemotherapy [1]. The concept of induction chemotherapy arose from the need for time to make the custom endo-prostheses required for a limb salvage procedure, creating an interval during which chemotherapy could be administered. In addition, theoretical advantages of induction chemotherapy included early treatment of micro-metastatic disease and facilitation of the eventual surgical procedure, because of tumor shrinkage and decreased vascularity. It also became possible to examine the histologic response of the tumor to induction chemotherapy to assess the effectiveness of therapy.

A strong correlation between the degree of necrosis (Huvos grade) and the probability of subsequent DFS was observed [55], and this has been confirmed in multiple clinical trials since [42, 55, 57].

• A theoretical concern with this approach is that the delay in removal of the bulk tumor could lead to the emergence of chemotherapy resistance.

• A prospective trial by the Pediatric Oncology Group addressed this concern by randomizing patients to immediate definitive surgery or to receive induction chemotherapy followed by definitive surgery with the total chemotherapy given in both arms identical. Reports from this study indicate that there was no advantage to immediate surgery [58].

Given the advantages in facilitating limb salvage procedures and in assessing chemotherapeutic efficacy, the use of induction chemotherapy has become the standard treatment approach for osteosarcoma.

Soon after the identification of the prognostic value of the degree of necrosis following induction chemotherapy it was suggested that chemotherapy be modified for the patients with less necrosis which is currently referred to as:

• Either standard or poor responders, and variably defined as <90 or <98% tumor necrosis.

• Or the persistence of more than rare viable tumor cells, with more than very rare viable tumor clumps.

This may allow the development of response-directed treatment stratification in order to increase their probability of DFS. Modifying therapy to achieve a better outcome in patients with a poor histologic response was initially reported as showing benefit in an influential publication describing the results of the T10 protocol at The Memorial Sloan-Kettering Cancer Center [43, 55, 59]. Longer follow up of this patient population, however, showed no benefit to the therapy intensification [60].

Numerous cooperative groups and institutions, including the Children's Cancer Group, the Cooperative Osteosarcoma Study Group (COSS), and Istituto Rizzoli among others have undertaken studies using a similar strategy, delivering a variety of intensified regimens to patients with standard response in an attempt to improve their outcome. The vast majority of studies have demonstrated that:

• Intensified therapy cannot change the outcome of a patient who has had a standard response [42, 57, 61].

• Intensification of therapy in the induction period to increase the proportion of patients with greater amounts of necrosis (currently referred to as favorable responders), likewise did not change the outcome [62].

Several trials have been conducted to clarify the role of the various chemotherapeutic agents in the treatment of osteosarcoma as well as their method of delivery. The combination of bleomycin, cyclophosphamide, and actinomycin-D was once commonly utilized for osteosarcoma treatment but subsequent studies demonstrated the combination was not effective [63] and it is no longer recommended.

Studies of pre-surgical chemotherapy administered via the intra-arterial route have been performed. Most commonly doxorubicin and cisplatin were administered directly into the arterial supply of extremity tumors with the theoretical advantage that the drug delivery to the tumor vasculature and tumor would be maximized [42, 64]. High local drug concentrations were documented by pharmacokinetic studies [65], and dramatic responses in primary tumors were observed. Reviewing studies of intra-arterial chemotherapy in general demonstrate that if improvements occur in local control, which is controversial, it may be at the expense of treating systemic disease. An update of studies from the M.D. Anderson Hospital where intra-arterial chemo-

therapy was pioneered [66] indicates that the overall DFS for patients treated with intra-arterial cisplatin, definitive surgery, and post-operative adjuvant chemotherapy is 60%, a disappointing result for a single institutional trial. Therefore, the use of intra-arterial chemotherapy has declined in recent years.

Contemporary international experiences for the treatment of osteosarcoma

More recent group collaborative efforts has seen the investigation of strategies such as increasing overall dose-intensity, the introduction of other chemotherapy agents such as interferon, and the intensification of chemotherapy based on histological response, with a particular emphasis on the role of ifosfamide and etoposide.

For example, the last North American-based randomized Phase III pediatric cooperative group study (INT-0133) jointly administered by the Children's Cancer Group and the Pediatric Oncology Group addressed two study questions [1].

• The study tested whether the addition of ifosfamide and/or muramyl tripeptide – phosphatidyl ethanolamine (MTP–PE) to the three other agents used in the standard treatment of osteosarcoma (doxorubicin, cisplatin, high dose methotrexate) would improve the probability of disease-free survival. Muramyl tripeptide is a component of the bacillus Calmette-Guerin (BCG) cell wall. It is conjugated to phosphatidyl ethanolamine and liposome encapsulated to improve delivery to the reticuloendothelial system [67].

• The primary rationale supporting the use of this relatively non-specific immune adjuvant were the encouraging results obtained in a prospective randomized trial of this compound in canines [68]. The results of this trial did not demonstrate a benefit for the patients who were treated with the addition of ifosfamide or muramyl tripeptide–phosphatidyl ethanolamine alone [69]. Further analysis of the results has been undertaken producing some discrepant findings.

The Scandinavian Sarcoma Group (SSG) has performed four non-randomized clinical trials for high-grade osteosarcoma localized to the extremities.

• The first study (SSG-II: 1982–1989) was based on the MSKCC T10 regimen, and contained the BCD combination (bleomycin, cyclophosphamide, and actinomycin-D). The OS (OS) and event-free survival (EFS) rates were inferior to the MSKCC results [70]. However, the latter were from a single institution, and might therefore be expected to be better than those achievable in a multi-institutional setting.

• The subsequent SSG osteosarcoma trial (SSG-VIII: 1990–1997) used a three-drug combination of methotrexate, doxorubicin, and cisplatin (MAP) pre-operatively. Good responders were given three further cycles of MAP whilst poor responders received five cycles of etoposide and ifosfamide. The 5-year projected OS was 74%, which represented an improvement of 9% compared with the SSG-II [71]. However, the relatively low dose of ifosfamide ($4.5\,g/m^2$) failed to improve the outcome in poor histological responders, and therefore poor response to pre-operative chemotherapy does not justify discontinuation of the drugs used upfront.

• The following study, a joint Italian/Scandinavian study (ISG/SSG I: 1997–2000), explored the benefit of adding high-dose ifosfamide ($15\,g/m^2$) to induction therapy, which did not improve outcome compared with previous trials [72].

• In the next SSG osteosarcoma study, SSG XIV, all patients received two MAP cycles pre-operatively and three further cycles post-operatively. Poor responders also received ifosfamide (10–$14\,g/m^2$). The results of this study have yet to be published.

As the SSG trials were being conducted, the German-Austrian-Swiss Cooperative Osteosarcoma Study Group (COSS) performed a series of studies using multi-agent regimens.

• COSS 80 (1979–1982) compared the effect of cisplatin with that of the BCD combination, within the context of sequential multi-drug chemotherapy with doxorubicin and high-dose methotrexate. After surgery patients were further randomized to receive or not to receive fibroblast interferon in addition to chemotherapy. There was no difference in DFS rates in the patients receiving BCD versus cisplatin or receiving interferon versus no interferon [56].

• COSS 82 tried to spare some patients from the chronic toxicity of doxorubicin and cisplatin by using these only in poor response to a less aggressive pre-operative regimen. However, poor responders were not salvaged by post-operative intensification suggesting that osteosarcoma chemotherapy should be as aggressive as possible from initiation [61].

• In the subsequent study, COSS 86, patients were stratified into a high- and a low-risk stratum, based on tumor length, initial tumor histology and radiological response to chemotherapy. Low risk patients received MAP, whereas high-risk patients received MAP and ifosfamide. Actuarial overall and EFS rates at 10 years were 72% and 66%, respectively [73]. In Italy, the Rizzoli Institute, using a five-drug regimen (MAP with ifosfamide and etoposide for poor responders to pre-operative chemotherapy) achieved a 5-year EFS of 63% [74].

The European Osteosarcoma Intergroup (EOI) collaboration used an alternative approach to the prolonged multi-drug regimens used by the American, German, and Italian groups. EOI used shorter dose-intense regimens in a series of large prospective randomized controlled studies.

• An initial study demonstrated no benefit to the addition of methotrexate to doxorubicin and cisplatin, the two-drug combination producing a 5-year DFS of 57% [75].

• A second study made the important comparison of doxorubicin and cisplatin with a multi-agent combination very similar to the T10 regimen [76]. This reported no benefit from the longer multi-agent protocol, although the overall 5-year event survival for the whole study group, at 43.7%, was inferior to the results of the previous EOI study. Nevertheless, the doxorubicin and cisplatin combination was adopted as standard treatment.

• The subsequent study, BO06, determined whether it was possible to improve results by increasing dose intensity by use of colony stimulating factors [77]. Results showed that while the

proportion of good responders (achieving ≥90% necrosis in the resection specimen) was increased in the more dose-intense arm, this did not translate into improved overall or EFS rates. Moreover, survival in EOI studies remained inferior to that achieved in Germany, Italy and the USA.

Thus, the COSS, EOI, and SSG experiences have confirmed that MAP-based chemotherapy is effective in the treatment of osteosarcoma, but that the addition of drugs such as ifosfamide and etoposide do not necessarily improve survival rates, even in the context of increased tumor necrosis rates at the time of definitive surgery. These studies are summarized in Table 15.4 and Table 15.5 [78].

The EURAMOS 1 clinical trial, launched in 2005, epitomizes the current management of osteosarcoma. EURAMOS 1 is the culmination of collaboration between the North American Children's Oncology Group (COG), the German-Austrian-Swiss Cooperative Osteosarcoma Study Group (COSS), the European Osteosarcoma Intergroup (EOI) and the Scandinavian Sarcoma Group (SSG). The aim of the study is to evaluate whether it is possible to improve the outcome of both poor and good responders to pre-operative chemotherapy by modification of post-operative chemotherapy. All patients receive pre-operative methotrexate, doxorubicin and cisplatin (MAP) as given in the control arm of the INT-0133 study. Poor responders are randomized to receive MAP with or without ifosfamide and etoposide. Good responders will continue on MAP chemotherapy, and are randomized to maintenance pegylated interferon-α or observation. In contrast with previous studies, EURAMOS 1 includes axial as well as extremity tumors, and patients with metastatic as well as non-metastatic disease (www.euramos.org).

Treatment of metastatic disease

The standard management of patients with metastatic disease follows the same general principles as those who present with localized disease, and the overall 5-year survival of approximately 50% is influenced by the nature and burden of the metastatic spread of disease [1, 79]. For example, patients with more than eight pulmonary nodules, bilateral lung involvement and lymph node or bone involvement have fared poorly with survival of 25–35%, in comparison with the much better survival of patients with less extensive metastases, where survival rates are comparable with those patients with apparently localized disease at presentation [79]. Therefore, patients undergo surgery wherever possible to remove all evidence of bulk disease. Several chemotherapy and surgical timing approaches have been reported for the treatment of these patients. Survival has clearly been enhanced by aggressive treatment designed with a curative intent [79].

Recurrent disease

Recurrent disease still occurs in approximately 30–40% of osteosarcoma patients despite a complete surgical removal and intensive chemotherapy treatment. The overall outcome for those patients is poor [60, 80], and apart from surgery, there is currently no universally accepted standard of multimodal treatment.

Table 15.4 Studies of neoadjuvant chemotherapy in non-metastatic extremity osteosarcoma [78]. (From Whelan J *et al.*[78], with permission from Current Medicine Group, LLC.)

Study	Type	Patients (*n*)	Chemotherapy	Good responders	Modify post-op chemotherapy by histologic response?	Outcome	Outcome better for poor responders by changing chemotherapy?
MSKCC T7 [59, 60]	Single centre	75	Pre-op and post-op: BCD, MTX, V, D	65%	No	12-year DFS 72%	NA
MSKCC T10 [59, 60]	Single centre	153	Pre-op: MTX, V Post-op: D, P, BCD (poor) *or* D, MTX, BCD (good)	34%	Yes	5-year DFS 72%	No
SSG-1 (T10) [70]	Multicentre	97	Pre-op: MTX, V Post-op D, P, BCD (poor) *or* D, MTX, BCD (good)	17%	Yes	5-year DFS 54% 5-year OS 64%	No
CCSG-782 (T10) [57]	Multicentre	268	Pre-op: MTX, BCD Post-op: D, P, BCD (poor) *or* D, MTX, BCD (good)	28%	Yes	8-year DFS 53% 8-year OS 60%	No
COSS-80 [56]	RCT	158	Pre-op: MTX, D; BCD *or* P Post-op: MTX, D; BCD *or* P ± IFN	Not reported	No	2.5-year DFS 68%	NA
COSS-82 [61]	RCT	125	Pre-op: MTX, BCD *or* MTX, D, P Post-op: modified on response	MTX, BCD 28% MTX, D, P 60%	Yes	4–year MFS 58%	No
COSS-86 [73]	Multicentre	171	Pre-op and post-op: MTX, D, P; I (high risk patients)	76%	No	10-year EFS 66% 10-year OS 72%	NA
Rizzoli study 1 [42]	Single centre	127	Pre-op: MTX, P Post-op: MTX, D, P (good) or D, BCD (poor)	52%	Yes	5-year DFS 49%	No
Rizzoli study 2 [74]	Single centre	164	Pre-op: MTX, D, P Post-op: MTX, D, P (good) or MTX, D, P, I, E (poor)	71%	Yes	5-year DFS 63%	Yes
EOI study 1 [75]	RCT	198	Pre-op and post-op: P, D ± MTX	30%	No	D, P: 5-year DFS 57%, 5–year OS 64% D, P, MTX: 5-year DFS 57%, 5-year OS 64%	NA
EOI study 2 [76]	RCT	391	Pre-op: D, P or MTX, D, V Post-op: D, P or MTX, D, V, BCD	D,P 30% multidrug 29%	No	5-year PFS 44% 5-year OS 55%	NA
EOI study 3 [77]	RCT	504	Pre-op and post-op: D, P ± GCSF	D, P 36% D, P, GCSF 51%	No	D, P: 5-year DFS 37%, 5-year OS 54% D, P, GCSF: 5-year DFS 40%, 5-year OS 56%	NA
INT-0133 [69]	RCT	507	Pre-op and post-op: MTX, D, P ± I, ±MTP-PE	Not reported	No	3-year EFS: D, P, MTX 71%; D, P, MTX, MTP-PE 69%; D, P, MTX, I 60%; D, P, MTX, I, MTP-PE 78%	NA

BCD, bleomycin, cyclophosphamide, actinomycin-D. COSS, Cooperative Osteosarcoma Study. D, doxorubicin. DFS, DFS. E, etoposide. EFS, EFS. EOI, European Osteosarcoma Intergroup. GCSF, granulocyte colony stimulating factor. I, ifosfamide. IFN, interferon. MFS, metastasis free survival. MSKCC, Memorial Sloan-Kettering Cancer Centre. MTP-PE, muramyl tripeptide phosphatidyl ethanolamine. MTX, methotrexate. NA, not applicable. OS, overall survival. P, cisplatin. PFS, progression-free survival. Post-op, post-operative. Pre-op, pre-operative. RCT, randomized controlled trial. SSG, Scandinavian Sarcoma Group. V, vincristine.

Table 15.5 Studies of non-metastatic extremity osteosarcoma in which pre-operative chemotherapy has been intensified aiming to increase the proportion of patients with a good histological response to pre-operative chemotherapy. (From Whelan J *et al.*[78], with permission from Current Medicine Group, LLC.)

Study	Type	n	Chemotherapy	% good responses	Outcome	Intensification judged beneficial?
COSS 86 [73]	Multi-centre	171	Methotrexate, doxorubicin, cisplatin, ± ifosfamide (in high risk patients)		10-year EFS 66% 10-year OS 72%	No
MSKCC T12 [62]	RCT	73	Methotrexate, BCD, ± cisplatin, doxorubicin	Standard arm 37% Intensified 44%	5-year EFS 73% 5-year OS 78%	No
INT–0133 [69]	RCT	507	Methotrexate, doxorubicin, cisplatin ± ifosfamide and/or MTP-PE	Not reported	3-year EFS: Standard 71% Ifosfamide, MTP-PE 78%	Yes
ISG/SSG [78]	Multi-centre	181	Methotrexate, doxorubicin, cisplatin, ifosfamide	60%	3-year EFS 68% 3-year OS 86%	No

BCD, bleomycin, cyclophosphamide, actinomycin-D. COSS, Cooperative Osteosarcoma Study. EFS, event-free survival. ISG, Italian Study Group. MSKCC, Memorial Sloan-Kettering Cancer Centre. MTP, PE-muramyl tripeptide phosphatidyl ethanolamine. OS, overall survival. RCT, randomized controlled trial. SSG, Scandinavian Sarcoma Group.

Ferrari *et al.* reported a projected 5-year post-relapse survival rate of 28% in patients with recurrent osteosarcoma of the extremity [81] while Bielack *et al.* described an actuarial 5-year survival rate of 23% in patients with recurrent osteosarcoma of any site [35]. Prognosis appears to relate to:

• Complete surgery seems to be a prerequisite for cure [80, 82]. Patients with recurrence in unresectable locations have very little probability of survival.

• A long interval between first diagnosis and relapse and a small number of involved sites are favorable prognostic indicators [80].

• Treatment with chemotherapy, especially with agents not used during front-line treatment, may benefit in some cases, and patients who don't achieve second complete surgical remission and received chemotherapy survived significantly longer than those who did not. However, the role of chemotherapy in relapsed patients who achieved second complete surgical remission is equivocal [80, 81].

Prognostic factors

The outcome of osteosarcoma patients depends on several factors that include clinical, histological, and pharmacological factors.

• The most consistent prognostic factor at diagnosis is the presence of clinically detectable metastatic disease, which confers a unfavorable prognosis [1, 79, 83]. With currently available regimens, approximately 60–70% of patients with non-metastatic osteosarcoma of the extremity will survive without evidence of recurrence.

• In most large reported studies, only 10–20% of patients who presented with clinically detectable metastatic disease were continuously free of disease 5 years from diagnosis [1, 79, 82, 83].

• In some series the outcome of patients presenting with metastatic disease has been reported to be as high as 50% but these studies typically included patients with isolated pulmonary nodules which were not histologically confirmed [79].

• The site of the primary tumor has some prognostic significance, with axial lesions prognostically inferior to tumors of the appendicular skeleton.

• Both serum lactate dehydrogenase and the alkaline phosphatase correlate with outcome; higher levels of either enzyme predict an inferior prognosis [1, 84–86]. These factors most likely influence outcome by reflecting the size of the tumor or its resectability.

• The histological response to induction chemotherapy is a consistent prognostic factor but cannot be assessed at diagnosis [2].

• In patients with disease metastatic at diagnosis, the number of pulmonary nodules as well as their laterality are of prognostic significance [79, 82, 86].

The received dose-intensity of chemotherapy has been studied in the setting of osteosarcoma, where a higher dose-intensity has been found to relate to the extent of tumor necrosis [87], where there was a lower overall- and progression-free survival for patients with a received dose-intensity (RDI) of 0.6 or less. However, these differences were not statistically significant at 5-year follow up for patients with non-metastatic disease treated with cisplatin and doxorubicin [88], even in the setting of the known improvement in pre-operative histological response [87]. Similarly, the dose-intensity of drug achieved by day 200 for a regimen containing cisplatin, doxorubicin, high-dose methotrexate (HDMTX), and ifosfamide in this clinical setting was not found to relate to prognosis [89].

The outcome for osteosarcoma has also been related to pharmacokinetic and cellular pharmacological determinants of chemosensitivity for HDMTX in particular. Considerable inter-patient pharmacokinetic variability has been described for HDMTX. For example, HDMTX infusions of $5\,g/m^2$ administered over 24 hours achieve steady-state plasma concentrations of $25–100\,\mu M$

[90]. The importance of steady-state MTX concentrations achieved during HDMTX-based therapy for childhood acute lymphoblastic leukaemia (ALL) and osteosarcoma have been reported in relation to prognosis. For childhood ALL, median plasma MTX concentrations achieved during a 24-hour infusion of >16 µM optimize the metabolism of MTX to more potent moieties and are protective against bone marrow relapse. Furthermore, pharmacologically-guided HDMTX consolidation therapy, designed to achieve above median systemic exposure when compared with conventional surface area dosing has improved survival in a randomized trial [91].

• For osteosarcoma, dose intensity [92] and pharmacokinetic variability have been related to outcome.

• For example, DFS has been related to MTX systemic exposure [93], and a better prognosis has been found for patients who achieve high steady-state MTX concentrations following a HDMTX infusion of 12 g/m².

• In the latter studies, plasma MTX concentrations of >700 µM at the end of a 6 hour infusion [94], or >1000 µM at the end of a 4 hour HDMTX infusion were significantly related to DFS [95].

• A further suggestion of the importance of MTX pharmacology comes from the improvement in 5-year DFS found for patients who undergo MTX dose escalation to achieve higher systemic exposures and dose intensities, albeit in a non-randomized study [96].

However, the importance of end-infusion MTX concentrations has not been found for all studies involving patients with osteosarcoma [97]. Moreover, a recent study brings an element of caution to the assumption that high levels of MTX are always protective, and this group have found a negative impact for very high steady-state plasma concentrations (>1500 µM) and systemic exposure following HDMTX [98].

The cellular pharmacology of MTX has been less well studied for osteosarcoma in comparison with childhood ALL.

• However, xenografts of osteosarcoma cells have been found to form predominantly short-chain (and less pharmacologically potent) MTX polyglutamates [99].

• Moreover, a study from the Memorial Sloan-Kettering group has described the occurrence of relatively low-levels of reduced folate carrier (RFC) mRNA expression for 65% of osteosarcoma samples studied at diagnosis, a factor that is known to limit MTX uptake into cells. This patient group formed two-thirds of the patients who responded poorly on histological grounds to initial chemotherapy [100].

• Although occurring in two-thirds of patients at relapse, relatively high tumoral levels of the target enzyme dihydrofolate reductase were only found for 10% of patients at diagnosis [100]. The findings of the Memorial Sloan-Kettering group have been supported by the findings of Ifergan *et al.* (1993) [101], where lower RFC protein levels also relate to poor histological response.

Therefore, based on this profile of the potential cellular determinants of sensitivity to MTX for osteosarcoma, short-term exposures to methotrexate may not be optimal for all patients, especially for those tumors with low RFC expression and a low potential for MTX polyglutamation. This will be especially true for extracellular MTX concentrations at which the RFC is a limiting factor for drug uptake, an occurrence that is found very soon after the end of a HDMTX infusion for many patients.

The main cellular determinants for chemosensitivity of doxorubicin and cisplatin, namely cellular MDR-1 phenotype and glutathione or glutathione-transferase levels, respectively, have not been studied extensively in relation to received dose-intensity or the pharmacokinetic variables of the drugs currently employed in the treatment of osteosarcoma. Studies of MDR1 mRNA expression and outcome have shown either a negative [102] or neutral [103] impact upon outcome, and although the expression of glutathione-s-transferase relates to cisplatin and doxorubicin resistance *in vitro* [104], this finding has not yet been explored in the clinical setting.

Follow up and late effects

After treatment completion, careful follow up is required to monitor for signs of recurrence and treatment-related complications. Either surgery or/and chemotherapy may be associated with long-term disability of some degree. Both limb salvage surgery and amputation may have functional and cosmetic/psychological consequences. Revision surgery may be required in case of prosthesis-related infection, loosening or breakage. Furthermore, skeletally immature children will require sequential lengthening of their prosthesis.

Doxorubicin can cause acute and late cardiac toxicity which may become manifest clinically as congestive heart failure or malignant arrhythmias. The risk of cardiac toxicity is related to both dose intensity and total cumulative dose. Lifelong follow up with serial echocardiograms is essential.

The North American-based pediatric cooperative group, the Children's Oncology Group, has completed a series of pilot feasibility studies assessing increased dose doxorubicin with dexrazoxane cardioprotection in combination with the other standard agents, increased dose ifosfamide and etoposide in combination with the other standard agents or standard dose ifosfamide in combination with increased dose doxorubicin with dexrazoxane cardioprotection in patients with a standard chemotherapy response. The results of this study have not been published as of yet but the treatments were generally tolerable.

Cisplatin is responsible for high frequency hearing loss, reported as in as high as 11% of the patients [69]. However, only a few patients who survive their osteosarcoma require hearing aids.

Treatment with cisplatin or ifosfamide may result in chronic renal failure. Moreover, gonadal damage may be evident in survivors of osteosarcoma (males more so than females). In addition, secondary malignancies (such as leukemia, breast, lung, kidney, central nervous system, and colon cancer) have been observed in 2–3% of patients at a median of 7.6 years (1–25 years) after primary osteosarcoma treatment [105].

Novel therapeutics and future directions for management

Intensive efforts in recent years have been made to increase the understanding of the basic biology of osteosarcoma. As intensification of therapy after an inferior histologic response has generally failed to improve outcome and prognostic factors at diagnosis are limited, efforts have been directed towards identifying biological factors which predict outcome. Examples of this include studies of P-glycoprotein expression, DNA ploidy, human epidermal growth factor receptor-2 overexpression, cDNA expression profiling, and comparative genomic hybridization. Many molecular markers are currently under study, but sufficient data have not yet been accrued to allow any to be recommended as prognostic factors [1, 106–109].

Another area of active research has been the use of radiographic studies as predictors of the degree of necrosis at the time of definitive surgery. Several techniques have been proposed for this purpose but none thus far has been proven to be sufficiently sensitive or reliable. Assessment of disease by conventional radiographs, computed tomography, and MRI show definite changes in response to pre-surgical chemotherapy, but the changes do not correlate reliably with histologic response. Studies suggest three phase bone scans and thallium scintigraphy may predict the histologic tumor response [110]. Dynamic MRI and positron emission spectroscopy are also promising [111]. Ultimately, if radiographic studies are effective at determining the degree of necrosis at definitive surgery, earlier or repeated evaluation of tumor response could be performed. These radiographic studies would serve as a prognostic factor or an earlier determinant of the effectiveness of therapy.

New therapies are clearly needed for the treatment of osteosarcoma patients. Patients who present with metastatic disease or develop recurrent disease have a poor prognosis and are appropriate for consideration for clinical trials of novel agents.
- Monoclonal antibodies against osteosarcoma may prove useful as treatments or for delivering drugs or radiopharmaceuticals directly to the tumor. Therapies such as trastuzumab, which targets the epidermal growth factor receptor type-2, are being tested in osteosarcoma [1]. Newly developed antibodies targeting insulin-like growth factor receptor are of potential interest and clinical trials are rapidly being developed.
- Other biologic approaches such as the use of inhaled granulocyte macrophage colony stimulating factor and interferon are being tested.
- Bone-seeking isotopes such as samarium may allow the delivery of extremely high dose local radiation therapy, perhaps providing an appropriate treatment approach for sites of mineralized disease [112].
- Adenoviral gene therapy approaches using selective promoters, such as the promoter driving osteocalcin expression, controlling a suicide gene (thymidine kinase), is being developed [113]. Studies of new drugs such as pemetrexed are also being developed.

The study of vascular endothelial growth factor (VEGF)-related biology in relation to osteosarcoma may also lead to novel approaches to the therapy of this disease. Plasma VEGF levels have been found to relate both to the degree of tumoral angiogenesis and risk of developing pulmonary metastases [114], and tumoral VEGF expression both at diagnosis [115] and following pre-operative chemotherapy [116] negatively impact upon DFS and OS. Thus, the ongoing evaluation of specific VEGF inhibitors in the pediatric setting [117] may result in specific strategies being developed in the setting of osteosarcoma. Thus, the eventual incorporation of the agents of proven activity and these newer agents into front-line chemotherapy protocols will hopefully further improve the outcome of all osteosarcoma patients.

Ewing's sarcoma family tumors (ESFT)

The ESFT are comprised of two major entities, Ewing's sarcoma and primitive neuroectodermal tumors, which although initially considered to be distinct are now believed to be a spectrum of the same entity [1]. In the early 1980s it was discovered that Ewing's sarcoma and primitive neuroectodermal tumor have the same reciprocal translocation between chromosomes 11 and 22, t(11;22)(q24;q12) [118]. The combination of the shared translocation, and the similar clinical behaviour led these two tumors, along with Askin's tumor (a similar tumor specifically of the chest wall), to be described subsequently as the ESFT [119]. Its overall features are summarized in Box 15.2.

Epidemiology and pathogenesis

Based upon SEER (Surveillance Epidemiology and End Results) data, the incidence of ESFT in children and adolescents is 2.9/1 000 000 per year [2], and has the following epidemiological features.

Box 15.2 Treatment and prognosis for Ewing's sarcoma family tumors.

- For localized disease the survival is 60–70%
- Local control measures include surgery and radiotherapy and are important for cure
- Induction chemotherapy is intensive and is currently based on vincristine, ifosfamide, doxorubicin and etoposide
- Tumour necrosis in response to induction therapy may allow stratification of the nature and intensity of treatment post-surgery/radiotherapy for local control, but the role of high-dose chemotherapy treatment uncertain, with the inclusion of ifosfamide and etoposide
- Limb-sparing surgery is possible for most patients
- For metastatic disease at presentation, the survival is less good (25–35%) depending on nature and extent of disease burden
- Long-term morbidities include cardiac and otological sequelae
- Novel therapies being explored in clinical and pre-clinical setting

---

- There is a slight male predominance.
- Its incidence peaks in the latter half of the second decade.
- The age distribution of ESFT shows 27% occur in the first decade, 64% in the second decade, and 9% in the third decade [120].
- It has an unusual and unexplained race distribution. The incidence in whites is at least ninefold higher than in blacks. This is in contrast to osteosarcoma, which has a relatively equal race distribution. This racial predilection is not related to geography [2].

There is no known cause of ESFT, and all cases are thought to be sporadic. However, family members of ESFT patients have an increased incidence of neuroectodermal and stomach malignancies [121]. Growth parameters such as height and weight have not been linked to developing an ESFT [122]. ESFT rarely occurs as a second neoplasm [123]. ESFT are thought to derive from cells of neuroectodermal origin, possibly post-ganglionic cholinergic neurons [124], although the exact cell of origin of ESFT has yet to be identified.

- The translocation t(11;22)(q24;q12), or another in a series of related translocations occurs in greater than 95% of ESFT. Some researchers argue that such a translocation is pathognomonic and sufficient for a diagnosis of ESFT [125].
- The classic t(11;22)(q24;q12) translocation joins the EWS gene (Ewing's Sarcoma) located on chromosome 22 to an ETS family gene, FLI-1 (Friend Leukemia Insertion) located on chromosome 11.

The EWS/FLI1 fusion transcript encodes a 68 kD protein with two primary domains. The EWS domain is a potent transcriptional activator, while the FLI1 domain contains a highly conserved ETS DNA binding domain.

- The EWS/FLI1 fusion protein thus acts as an aberrant transcription factor. EWS/FLI-1 transforms mouse fibroblasts.
- To effect this transformation, both the EWS and FLI-1 functional domains must be intact [126].
- The insulin-like growth factor type 1 receptor (IGF-IR) is required for EWS/FLI-1 to transform fibroblasts [127].

Thus, the EWS/FLI-1 fusion protein is implicated in the pathogenesis of ESFT. However, there are no data as to the underlying etiology of the translocation. Early investigations of EWS/FLI-1 induced transformation of mouse fibroblasts demonstrated that not all fibroblasts could be equally transformed. The fibroblasts that were transformable were immortalized and were found to lack some component of the G1 checkpoint, most often p16(INK4a) [128]. Over half of all ESFT from patients have been shown to lack some component of the G1 checkpoint, either p16, p15, p14, p53, or p21 [128]. The exact role of these additional alterations in the pathogenesis and their clinical significance in ESFT remains unclear.

Presentation

ESFT patients usually present with pain and a palpable mass. As compared with osteosarcoma there is a greater propensity to develop in the axial skeleton, although appendicular sites remain the most common site of presentation.

- Long bone lesions can present with a pathologic fracture.
- Back pain may indicate tumors in a paraspinal, retroperitoneal, or deep pelvic location and must be considered in the differential diagnosis of this symptom [1, 4].
- Systemic symptoms of fever and weight loss can occur and often indicates the presence of metastatic disease.
- ESFT can occur in virtually any location, even remote from bones rarely, so that careful examination of painful sites by inspection and palpation is critical.
- Since ESFT can present in close juxtaposition to vertebrae, tumors can result in neuropathic pain mimicking sciatica or producing nerve dysfunction. Thus, a comprehensive neurological exam is critical to evaluate asymmetric weakness or numbness.
- Patients with lung metastases may present with asymmetric breath sounds, pleural signs, or rales.
- Unlike osteosarcoma, ESFT metastasizes to the bone marrow and patients with significant disease in this site can present with petechiae or purpura from thrombocytopenia [1, 4].

The most frequent primary sites for ESFT include the pelvis, femur, ribs, and spine (8%) (Figure 15.2). Approximately 25% of patients will present with metastatic disease at diagnosis [129]. Less than 40% of the patients that present with metastatic disease at diagnosis will have it confined to lung or pleura. The majority of patients with metastatic disease will have bone and/or bone marrow metastases either alone or in addition to pulmonary/pleural disease, which again contrasts with osteosarcoma [129]. A pelvic location of the tumor, high levels of lactate dehydrogenase, fever, age older than 12 years and an interval between onset

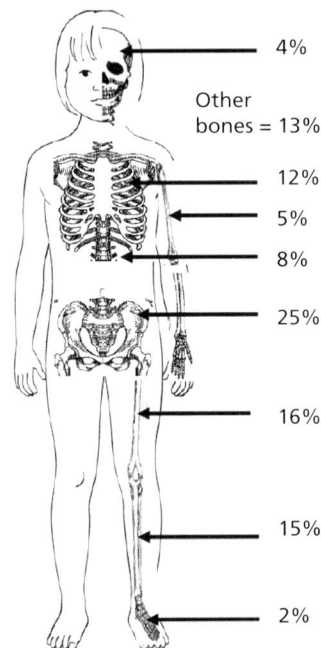

Figure 15.2 Site of primary tumor in patients with Ewing sarcoma family tumors of the bone.

of symptoms and diagnosis of less than 3 months, tends to associate with having clinically evident metastatic disease at diagnosis [130].

Investigation and staging

The evaluation of suspected ESFT begins with history, physical examination, laboratory evaluations, and plain radiographs. History and physical examination are as described previously. There are no blood tests with which to diagnose ESFT. Serum lactate dehydrogenase level, if elevated, suggests malignancy but is neither sensitive nor specific. Anemia, neutropenia, and thrombocytopenia can suggest bone marrow infiltration but are also not specific for ESFT [1, 4].

ESFT should be included in the differential diagnosis of any bone or soft tissue mass in patients from age three through to the third decade of life. The differential diagnosis of a bone lesion should include other neoplasms both malignant and benign including osteosarcoma and other non-neoplastic entities such as osteomyelitis. If a mass is palpated or if persistent bone pain is reported, plain radiographs are indicated [1, 4, 131].

The classic radiological description of an ESFT is a lamellar (onion skin) lesion on plain film which if it involves a long bone is typically in the diaphysis. Additional radiographic findings may include bone sclerosis, elevation of the periosteum with periosteal reaction (Codman's triangle) and radial streaks of bone beyond the cortical walls.

Once a bone tumor is suspected from a radiograph, the suspected primary lesion should be imaged for biopsy planning purposes among other reasons [1, 4, 131]. An MRI of the region can help to identify extent of disease, and is generally more precise than CT scan. The CT scan, however, delineates bone involvement better.

Tumors that are adjacent to critical neurological structures require rapid MRI scanning and consideration of emergency therapy to prevent neurological deterioration. The radiological evaluation for metastases must include a chest CT scan and radio-isotope bone scans. Bone marrow aspiration and biopsy are required, to exclude malignant infiltration, as this is a potential site of metastases [1, 4, 131].

ESFT are typically staged based on the radiographic findings and grade of the tumor (which is always high grade) using the Enneking staging system described previously. Pre-chemotherapy treatment evaluations should be performed as described for osteosarcoma. A biopsy is always required to confirm the diagnosis. The biopsy needs to be evaluated by routine staining as well as by immunohistochemistry to exclude other small round blue cell tumors such as rhabdomyosarcoma and lymphoma. The diagnosis should be confirmed using cytogenetics, reverse transcriptase-polymerase chain reaction (RT-PCR), and fluorescent *in situ* hybridization (FISH) to identify the t(11;22) or a related translocation.

ESFT range from completely undifferentiated (Ewing's sarcoma) to differentiated (peripheral primitive neuroectodermal tumor). Immunohistochemical markers include:

• Membranous staining of CD99 (MIC2), present on greater than 90% of ESFT, and are well preserved using standard tissue fixation [132].
• Muscle, lymphoid, and adrenergic markers should be negative.
• Immature tumors lack most immunohistochemical markers, but do contain abundant glycogen.
• More differentiated tumors express membrane and cytoplasmic markers including neuron specific enolase, S-100, neurofilaments, CD57, CD45, and synaptophysin.

Differentiating tumors often contain pseudo-rosettes and sometimes contain classical rosette formation. Tumor differentiation markers can help with diagnosis of ESFT but despite reports that differentiation might be prognostic [133], this has not been confirmed in large series [120, 133]. Identifying an ESFT-specific translocation is pathognomonic for the diagnosis.

• This includes chromosomal breakpoints t(11;22), t(21;22) and t(7;22).
• These breakpoints are often seen by standard cytogenetic karyotyping. Standard cytogenetics and FISH can also reveal additional karyotypic abnormalities including trisomies 8 and 12, and chromosomes 1 and 16 abnormalities (see section on prognostic factors) [134].
• Some of the t(21;22) remain cryptic by standard cytogenetic techniques and require RT-PCR or FISH. Ideally every small round blue cell tumor should be evaluated by a multiplex RT-PCR assay that will identify any of the known translocations and identify translocations of histologically similar small round blue cell tumors such as rhabdomyosarcoma [124, 135].

Treatment

Survival of patients with ESFT prior to the use of chemotherapy was poor; studies reported a 5-year survival of 10% [131]. The first chemotherapeutic agents with efficacy in ESFT were cyclophosphamide (C), actinomycin-D (A), and vincristine (V). Patients with ESFT began to be treated with these agents individually in the early 1960s and in combination by the late 1960s. Evaluation of survival curves from ESFT studies is generally unstable for a minimum of 5 years from diagnosis.

The most consistent stratification factor is the presence or absence of metastatic disease at diagnosis, and this is currently used to stratify patients. Alkylating agents (cyclophosphamide, ifosfamide, melphalan, and busulfan) and doxorubicin are the most active single agents in ESFT, while the combination of ifosfamide plus etoposide showed significant activity in a classic phase II setting [131, 136]. Platinum derivatives have not shown significant efficacy in ESFT [131]. The European experience and historical perspectives for the therapy of ESFT highlights the development of those principles that underpin contemporary treatment approaches such as:

• The importance of the combined modalities of surgery and radiotherapy for local control.
• The early consideration of local control in the treatment pathway.
• The dose intensity of alkylating agents such as ifosfamide.

- The continued challenge to improve the survival of high risk/metastatic patients.

European clinical trials

The SSG has conducted two clinical trials for Ewing's sarcoma, the SSG IV and SSG IX. Following those, as part of the Scandinavian/Italian (Italian Sarcoma Group, ISG) cooperation two further trials have taken place, the ISGSSG-III and ISGSSG-IV, for localized and metastatic disease, respectively.

- In SSG IV (1984–1990, $n = 52$), patients with localized and metastatic disease received five blocks of a 12-week cycle of chemotherapy with vincristine, methotrexate, doxorubicin, cyclophosphamide, bleomycin, and dactinomycin. After two blocks of chemotherapy, surgery (if possible) was performed and radiotherapy as daily fractions of 2 Gy to a total dose of 40–60 Gy. Metastasis-free and sarcoma-related survival at 5 years were 43% and 46% respectively with a high local recurrence rate of 19% [137].

- In SSG IX (1990–1999, $n = 88$, localized or metastatic disease), chemotherapy consisted of four cycles of a VAI (vincristine, adriamycin, ifosfamide)/PAI (cisplatin, adriamycin, ifosfamide) combination. Local treatment with surgery and hyperfractionated/accelerated radiotherapy was performed earlier, at week 9. Metastasis-free and sarcoma-related survival rates at 5 years for patients with localized disease were 58% and 70% respectively, with local recurrence rate of 10% [138].

In the ISGSSG-III and ISGSSG-IV trials (1999-ongoing), multi-agent chemotherapy includes vincristine, adriamycin, actinoycin-D, cyclophosphamide in combination with etoposide and ifosfamide. Local treatment follows the principles from the SSG IX trial. Poor responders to neoadjuvant therapy in ISGSSG-III and all ISGSSG-IV patients are salvaged with high-dose chemotherapy (melphalan-busulfan) and stem cell support. Preliminary results seem promising but caution should be taken with the short follow up [139].

In Italy, prior to the previously described SSG-ISG cooperation, the Rizzoli Institute conducted the REN-3 clinical trial for patients with non-metastatic Ewing's sarcoma (1991–1997, $n = 157$).

- Induction chemotherapy consisted of two cycles of VAC (vincristine, adriamycin, cyclophosphamide) alternated with one cycle of VIAc (vincristine, ifosfamide, actinomycin). After local treatment, patients received three more cycles of VAC, two of VIAc, three cycles of ifosfamide and etoposide and two cycles of vincristine, cyclophosphamide, and actinomycin.

- The 5-year EFS and OS rates were 71% and 76.5% respectively. These results were significantly better than the ones achieved in the previous Italian studies, in which a three-drug VAC regimen (REA-1), a four-drug VACAc regimen (REA-2 and REN-1) was used, and in REN-2, which was based on a six-drug regimen as in REN-3, but where ifosfamide and actinomycin were used only after local treatment [140].

The French Society of Pediatric Oncology (SFOP) conducted the EW-88 study (1988–1991, $n = 141$) for patients with localized ESFTs. Therapy included induction chemotherapy consisting of vincristine and cyclophosphamide, followed by surgery (where possible), followed by radiotherapy (0–60 Gy, depending on the quality of resection and the histological response to induction chemotherapy) and maintenance chemotherapy with vincristine, cyclophosphamide, actinomycin, and doxorubicin. The projected 5-year DFS and OS rates were 58% and 66% respectively [141].

ET-1 (1978–1986, $n = 142$) was the first study conducted by the United Kingdom Children's Cancer Study Group (UKCCSG), for patients with localized and metastatic Ewing's sarcoma. Induction chemotherapy (vincristine, adriamycin, and cyclophosphamide) was followed by surgery (where possible), followed by radiotherapy combined with vincristine and cyclophosphamide, followed by maintenance chemothearapy with VACA (vincristine, cyclophosphamide, and adriamycin alternating with actinomycin-D). The 5-year DFS and OS rates were 38% and 44% respectively for patients with localized disease and 9% and 14% respectively for metastatic patients [142].

In the second UKCCSG study ET-2 (1987–1993, $n = 243$), patients with localized and metastatic Ewing's sarcoma received four cycles of induction chemotherapy with ifosfamide, vincristine, adriamycin followed by surgery (where possible), followed by radiotherapy combined with vincristine and cyclophosphamide, followed by maintenance chemothearapy with three cycles of ifosfamide, vincristine, adriamycin, and 10 cycles of ifosfamide, vincristine, and actinomycin-D.

- The 5-year DFS and OS rates were 56% and 62% respectively. For those with localized disease at diagnosis the DFS rate was 62% and for those with metastases, 23% [143].

- The improved survival rates, compared with those achieved in ET-1, were attributed to the use of higher doses of ifosfamide compared with relatively low doses of cyclophosphamide in ET-1.

The German Society of Pediatric Oncology initiated the Cooperative Ewing's Sarcoma Study CESS-81 (1981–1985, $n = 93$) using a four-drug combination with VACA, prior to definitive local control with surgery and/or radiotherapy. The estimated 3-year DFS rate was 60%. For patients with small tumors (<100 ml) the estimated 3-year DFS was 80% and for those with large tumors (>100 ml), 31% [144]. The following study, CESS-86 (1986–1991, $n = 301$) aimed at improving EFS in patients with high-risk localized Ewing's tumor of bone. Tumors of volume >100 ml and/or central axis sites qualified patients for 'high risk' (HR), and small extremity lesions for 'standard risk' (SR). SR patients received 12 courses of VACA; HR patients received ifosfamide instead of cyclophosphamide (VAIA). The 10-year EFS rate was 52% and did not differ between SR and HR patients. HR patients seem to have benefited from the intensified treatment that incorporated ifosfamide [145].

The EICESS-92 study (1992–1999, $n = 1062$) was the product of cooperation between the German/Dutch/Austrian Cooperative Ewing's Sarcoma Group (GPOH) and UKCCSG. SR patients (localized, <100 ml) received four courses of VAIA induction therapy and were then randomized to eight courses of either

VAIA or VACA. HR patients (≥100 ml) were randomized to receive 14 courses of either VAIA or EVAIA (VAIA plus etoposide). Superiority of any randomized treatment strategy was not shown. The 5-year EFS for SR patients was 63.4% and 67% for SR-VAIA and SR-VACA respectively ($P = 0.9437$). The 5-year EFS for HR patients was 43.1% and 52.1% for HR-VAIA and HR-EVAIA respectively ($P = 0.1220$) [146].

In late 1999, the European Ewing Tumor Working Initiative of National Groups (Euro-EWING), the product of collaboration of several European study groups (GPOH, UKCCSG, SFOP, SIAK [Schweizerisches Institut für Angewandte Krebsforschung] and EORTC-STBSG [European Organisation for Research and Treatment of Cancer – Soft Tissue and Bone Sarcoma Group]), has initiated the EURO-EWING-99 study. All patients receive induction with six courses of vincristine, ifosfamide, doxorubicin, and etoposide (VIDE), followed by consolidation therapy stratified and randomized according to the initial tumor volume (<200 ml or >200 ml), presence and site of metastatic disease at diagnosis and histologic response to induction therapy. Standard risk patients with good histologic response to VIDE are randomized to receive vincristine, actinomycin-D and ifosfamide (VAI) or vincristine, actinomycin-D and cyclophosfamide (VAC). High risk patients with poor response to VIDE are randomized to receive VAI or high-dose treatment with busulphan and melphalan and autologous stem cell support. In high-risk patients with initial lung metastases, VAI plus lung irradiation is compared with high-dose treatment. The study is ongoing. The main endpoints are to determine EFS, OS, and toxicity, to evaluate the role of high-dose therapy in high-risk patients and to evaluate the prognostic value of EWS-FLI1 transcript type and the prognostic significance of minimal disease in bone marrow and peripheral blood progenitor cell (PBPC) harvest as determined by the presence or absence of EWS-FLI1 transcript type.

US trials

• In 1973, the first Intergroup Ewing Sarcoma Study (IESS-1) evaluated the efficacy of VAC compared with VAC plus lung radiation therapy (RT) or VAC plus doxorubicin (D) in patients with localized disease. IESS-1 showed that for patients with localized disease, VAC alone provided a 24% 5-year DFS, VAC plus lung RT a 44% DFS, and VAC plus D provided a 60% DFS [147]. Besides the dramatic improvement in OS. IESS-1 identified large primary, and in particular, patients with pelvic tumors as having poorer survival.

• The follow-up study, IESS-2 was begun in 1978. Patients with pelvic tumors were treated in a separate stratum with VAC plus a higher dose of D. Localized, non-pelvic, patients in IESS-2 were randomized to a doxorubicin dose that was moderate and continuous versus high dose and intermittent. Survival for those patients with large pelvic tumors was higher than in IESS-2 compared with IESS-1; other studies have reproduced the success of these early studies [146, 148].

• A further improvement in survival was reported by the addition of ifosfamide and etoposide to the three drug VDC regimen (vincristine/doxorubicin-dactinomycin /cyclophospamide) [149].

• Subsequently, the IESS compared a 30-week dose intensive regimen of alkylators to the previous 48-week regimen and showed no difference between therapeutic arms with results that have been presented but not published. The question asked in the most recently completed COG study is whether compression of the time between chemotherapy cycles to 2 weeks will improve DFS. Several of these studies are summarized in Table 15.6.

Table 15.6 ESFT localized disease clinical trials.

Study	Type	n	Chemotherapy	F/U time (years)	EFS (%)	OS (%)	Intervention beneficial
IESS [149]	Multi	398	VACD vs VACD/IE	5	54 69	61 72	Yes
IESS [180]	Multi	483	30 week VDC/IE vs 48 week VDC/IE	5	70 72	80 78	No
Instituto Rizzoli [180]	Single	44	VACD/IE	5	54	63	N/A
SFOP [141]	Multi	141	Induction: C(150 mg/m²)/D Maintenance: V/A plus C/D	5	58	66	N/A
CESS-86 [146]	Multi	SR: 52 HR: 241	SR: VACD HR: VAID	10	52 51		No
Instituto Rizzoli [181]	Single	140	Induction: 2 × VDC, 1 × VAI. Maintenance: 5 × (3 × VDC, 2 × VAI); then 5 × (3 × EI, 2 × VAC)	3	78	84	N/A
UKCCSG [182]	Multi	191	IVAD	5 10	67	69	N/A

F/U, follow up. EFS, event-free survival. OS, overall survival. SR, standard risk. HR, high risk. V, vincristine. A, actinomycin-D. C, cyclophosphamide. E, etoposide. D, doxorubicin. I, ifosfamide.

ESFT with metastases at presentation

ESFT patients with disease metastatic at initial diagnosis have been identified as having a poor outcome since early multiagent trials [150].

• Patients with multiple sites of metastatic disease have the lowest survival rate [1, 131].

• Patients with metastases confined to the lungs may represent a group of patients with better prognosis than patients with bone or bone marrow metastases.

• Studies conducted of patients with metastatic disease are summarized in Table 15.7.

Early chemotherapy regimens included low dose regimens, such as oral cyclophosphamide 150 mg/m^2 for 7 days followed by doxorubicin alternating with vincristine, dactinomycin, and BCNU [151, 52]. To improve survival, high dose regimens consisting of vincristine/doxorubicin/cyclophosphamide and ifosfamide/etoposide induction followed by total body irradiation/melphalan or thiotepa/carboplatin have been employed [153]. These studies have assured the feasibility of high dose regimens requiring stem cell support but also demonstrated significant toxicity. They were driven by the hypothesis that the dose response to alkylator therapy for ESFT cells is very steep, and that, therefore, increasing the dose intensity of these agents would kill adequate ESFT cells to ensure patient survival. This is particularly true for melphalan and busulfan, where therapeutic dosing requires stem cell support. However, despite dose intensification to megadose therapy followed by stem cell rescue, survival has not improved [146, 153, 154]. It is equally unclear that addition of ifosfamide/etoposide is successful at curing more patients with metastatic disease than standard regimen with doxorubicin/vincristine/cyclophosphamide/dactinomycin [151, 153].

More recently, poor prognosis patients were treated with melphalan, busulfan, and thiotepa with or without total marrow irradiation in a pilot study using a tandem autologous stem cell rescue. This study, which included patients with recurrent disease who have historically had dismal survival, showed encouraging results, with a 36% 2-year EFS [152]. One possible mechanism for disease recurrence in the patients who have undergone autologous transplant could be the presence of tumor cells in the stem cell preparation [153]. The actual incidence of ESFT tumor cells in pheresed stem cell preparations is likely based upon many factors including chemotherapy prior to harvest, method of stem cell mobilization, and possibly stem cell handling. Some studies report a low incidence of contaminating tumor [155]. A quantitative method to estimate tumor cell contamination in stem cell preparations has the potential to clarify the role of contaminating cells in recurrent disease as well as for use in tumor cell purging strategies [156].

As suggested in earlier studies [153], the role of megatherapy with stem cell support for ESFT is best evaluated in the context of controlled clinical trials. As discussed previously, there is presently a randomized study, EURO-EWING 99, in which patients with pulmonary only metastases or bulky or unresectable primary tumors are randomized to chemotherapy versus megatherapy with stem cell support.

Prognostic factors

ESFT survival is highly dependent on the initial presentation and therefore potentially the biologic properties of the disease.

• OS in patients with ESFT is 60%. However, for patients with localized disease it approaches 70%, while patients with metastatic disease have less than a 25% likelihood of long-term survival.

• Metastatic disease at diagnosis has been reproducibly the most significant adverse prognostic factor in the treatment of patients with ESFT despite aggressive chemotherapy [120].

• Patients who present with metastatic disease are now stratified to different therapy from the time of diagnosis.

The prognostic factors which have been repeatedly evaluated in many clinical trials include age at diagnosis, sex, serum lactate dehydrogenase levels (LDH), size of tumor, location of tumor, and neural differentiation. Response to therapy as measured by amount of viable tumor present after induction chemotherapy cycles has been shown to be a predictor of outcome, however, not technically a prognostic factor [141, 157]. More recently, and as discussed below, a number of biologic features of the tumors have begun to be evaluated as prognostic factors.

• In early ESFT studies, the most reproducible prognostic factors in patients who present with localized disease include the tumor volume. In general, larger tumors (often axial) had a poorer prognosis and correlated with other poor prognostic factors. Aggressive, multi-agent chemotherapy as well as effective local management has somewhat reduced the prognostic value of such indices.

Table 15.7 ESFT metastatic disease clinical trials, non-megatherapy.

Study	Type	n	Chemotherapy	Follow up time (years)	EFS (%)	OS (%)
IESS [178]	Multi	121	VAC(1.2 g/m^2)D vs VAC(1.2 g/m^2)D/I(9 g/m^2)E	4	19	38
IESS [179]	Multi	60	VAC(2.2 g/m^2)D/I(14 g/m^2)E	2	26	35
UKCCSG [166]	Multi	42	IVAD	5	23	
EICESS [144]	Multi	171	IVAD+/−E (36 patients received 'megatherapy')	4	27	

EFS, event-free survival. OS, overall survival. V, vincristine. A, actinomycin-D. C, cyclophosphamide. E, etoposide. D, doxorubicin. I, ifosfamide.

• LDH has been reported as a prognostic factor. In particular, high LDH identifies patients with a higher likelihood of metastases [158], and later in therapy is useful as a predictor of recurrent disease [159]. More recent studies evaluating LDH level have reported mixed findings with regard to prognostic significance [141].

• Most studies show a trend to improved survival in those patients who present at a younger age (less than 10 or 15 years), but not all are in agreement here[141, 146].

Many molecular markers have begun to be evaluated as prognostic indicators in patients with ESFT. Among these include t(11;22) breakpoint regions, other chromosomal abnormalities, cell cycle/checkpoint genes and p-glycoprotein expression.

• The t(11;22) in any individual patient fuses one of many observed combinations of exons together from EWS and FLI1 to form the fusion message.

• The most common combination is the EWS exon 7 fused to FLI1 exon 6 (type 1 translocation), which occurs in approximately 50–64% of ESFT.

• Retrospective analyses have shown that patients who have localized tumors with the 7/6 fusion have a 70% 4-year survival while patients with the other variants had a 20% 4-year survival [148, 160, 161].

• Prospective studies are currently in progress to validate these findings and to determine whether they could be used for stratification.

Cell cycle and checkpoint genes have been evaluated as prognostic markers in ESFT. While any specific checkpoint gene has been found mutated or deleted in small numbers of tumors, as a group these abnormalities are found in over 50% of ESFT (discussed previously). In patients with ESFT, 80% of p16INK4a mutations or deletions were found in patients with metastatic disease in one study [162, 163], while another study showed no difference in p16INK4a based upon extent of disease at presentation [164]. Both studies showed that patients with p16INK4a abnormalities had a poor prognosis. The role of p16INK4a requires a prospective study to clarify whether this is a true independent prognostic marker.

TP53 mutations are often identified by overexpression as measured by increased immunoreactivity in tissues. There is reasonable correlation between overexpression and true mutations of tp53. Overexpression of tp53 occurs in approximately 10% of patient ESFT samples [165]. The presence of tp53 overexpression has been shown to independently identify patients with a poor prognosis in retrospective studies [162, 165]. Like p16INK4a, prospective evaluation is required to determine if overexpression of tp53 can serve to stratify patients who will have a poor outcome with existing chemotherapeutic regimens.

As with osteosarcoma, pharmacological variables have been related to outcome for ESFT. Although an earlier study reported by Delephine *et al.* [166] suggested a significant relationship between received drug intensity for vincristine and actinomycin--D and both histological response and outcome for patients with Ewing's sarcoma, increasing the dose-intensity *per se* of chemo-

therapy increases toxicity but without improvement in outcome [167]. MDR1 expression occurs in the context of ESFT, but the paucity of studies performed does not allow a clear relationship between MDR1 expression and response to be related to outcome [168].

Follow up and late effects

Toxicity is an important consideration in the therapy of ESFT since the doses of effective agents are pushed to the maximum tolerated dose.

• Cumulative cardiotoxicity from doxorubicin may complicate therapy. In one small study, sarcoma patients randomized to receive the cardioprotectant dexrazoxane (ICRF-187) tolerated higher doses of doxorubicin with less cardiotoxicity and no effect on disease outcome [169].

• High dose intensity of alkylating agents can result in Fanconi's syndrome of renal electrolyte wasting [170], and at the extreme may result in hypophosphataemic rickets [171].

• Other side effects will occur based upon the toxicity profiles of the individual cytotoxic agents.

Patients treated for ESFT are at risk for the development of a second malignancy. The majority of second malignancies are acute myeloid leukemia, myelodysplastic syndrome, and sarcomas in the radiation field [149, 172, 173]. The overall likelihood of developing a second malignancy is approximately 2%, with most leukemias occurring within 3 years from diagnosis but can be as high as 11% [149, 172, 173].

Patients who have been successfully treated for ESFT over the past 15 years have received high doses of alkylator therapy, epipodophyllotoxins, and anthracyclines; however, none of these has been dosage linked to second malignancy [149, 172, 173]. The IESS trial that compared VDC with VDCIE showed no difference in second malignancies between therapeutic arms, suggesting that, in the dose and schedule employed, the addition of etoposide did not independently increase the risk of second malignancy [149, 170]. On the other hand, it is notable that arm C of the Children's Cancer Group/Pediatric Oncology Group intergroup study (POG 8850), designed for patients with disease metastatic at diagnosis, in which very high cumulative dosages of ifosfamide and cyclophosphamide were prescribed, also demonstrated a very high rate of induced leukemia [173]. There may be a threshold or stepwise effect, with a low rate of induced leukemia with conventional dosage treatment, but a much higher rate at the high cumulative dosages prescribed in arm C. Radiation dosage is important to the rate of development of secondary cancers, with the vast majority of induced tumors being osteosarcomas [149, 172, 173].

Because of these studies, recommendations for radiation usage and dosage are being evaluated and modified [172, 173]. Patients who have received radiation therapy should be evaluated for sarcoma development in the radiation field if symptoms arise since these second malignancies continue to occur more than 15 years from diagnosis. In addition, since the risk of osteosarcoma was shown to rise after as little as 10 Gy, evaluation should not be limited to the irradiated bone [172, 173].

Novel therapeutics and future directions for management

New agents are needed to improve the survival of ESFT patients. A phase II trial of cyclophosphamide ($250\,mg/m^2$)/topotecan ($0.75\,mg/m^2$) administered daily for 5 days induced complete or partial responses in six of 17 patients and stable disease in six additional patients with recurrent disease [174]. In an up-front window study of newly diagnosed patients with ESFT metastatic at initial diagnosis, topotecan/cyclophosphamide showed 56% PR [175].

The tumor necrosis factor-related apoptosis-inducing ligand (TRAIL) can activate tumor necrosis factor modulated apoptotic pathways in ESFT [176, 177]. TRAIL activated apoptosis occurs through caspase-8 in ESFT and most ESFT cell lines express caspase-8. Thus, TRAIL may represent a biologic approach to inducing apoptotic cell death in ESFT.

As with osteosarcoma, higher tumoral VEGF expression relates to a poorer progression-free and overall survival for patients with Ewing's sarcoma, and the promising results obtained with specific VEGF-receptor blockade in the pre-clinical xenograft setting [178] is underpinning current early clinical studies with avastin in this disease setting. Moreover, clinical strategies that incorporate fenretinide, an agent that causes cell death via involvement of the reactive oxygen species-dependent pathway, especially in the setting of EWS-Fli-1 activation, are in development [179].

Thus, as with osteosarcoma, it is hoped that incorporation of the agents of proven activity and these newer agents into front-line chemotherapy protocols will hopefully further improve the outcome of all ESFT patients.

References

1 Gorlick R, Bernstein ML, Toretsky JA, et al. Bone tumors. In: Holland J, Frei E (Eds), Cancer Medicine, 7th edn. Hamilton, Ontario, BC Decker, 2006: 2019–27.

2 Gurney JG, Swensen AR, Bulterys M. Malignant bone tumors. In: LAG Ries, MA Smith, JG Gurney, et al. (Eds), Cancer Incidence and Survival among Children and Adolescents: United States SEER Program 1975–1995. National Cancer Institute, SEER Program. NIH Pub. No. 99-4649. Bethesda, MD, 1999: 99–110.

3 Dahlin DC, Unni KK. Bone Tumors: General Aspects and Data on 8542 Cases, 4th edn. Springfield, IL, Charles C. Thomas, 1986.

4 Huvos A. Bone Tumors: Diagnosis, Treatment and Prognosis, 2nd edn. Philadelphia, WB Saunders, 1991.

5 Capasso LL. Antiquity of cancer. Int J Cancer 2005: 113: 2–13.

6 Ewing J. Diffuse endothelioma of bone. Proc NY Path Soc 1921; 21: 17.

7 Freiberger R, Loitman B, Helpern M, Thompson T. Osteoid osteoma – a report of 80 cases. Am J Roentgenol 1959; 82: 194.

8 Dabska M, Buraczewski J. Aneurysmal bone cyst. Cancer 1968; 23: 371–84.

9 Tjalma RA. Canine bone sarcoma: estimation of relative risk as a function of body size. J Natl Cancer Inst 1966; 36: 1137–50.

10 Price C. Primary bone-forming tumors and their relationship to skeletal growth. J Bone Joint Surg [Br] 1958; 40: 574–93.

11 Varela-Duran J, Dehner L. Post-irradiation osteosarcoma in childhood: a clinicopathologic study of three cases and review of the literature. Am J Pediatr Hematol Oncol 1980; 2: 263–71.

12 Freeman C, Gledhill R, Chevalier L, et al. Osteogenic sarcoma following treatment with megavoltage radiation and chemotherapy for bone tumors in children. Med Pediatr Oncol 1980; 8: 375–82.

13 Haselow R, Nesbit M, Dehner L, et al. Second neoplasms following megavoltage radiation in a pediatric population. Cancer 1978; 42: 185–91.

14 Sim F, Cupps R, Dahlin D, Ivins J. Postradiation sarcoma of bone. J Bone Joint Surg [Am] 1972; 54: 1479–89.

15 Newton WA, Meadows AT, Shimada H, et al. Bone sarcomas as second malignant neoplasms following childhood cancer. Cancer 1991; 67: 193–201.

16 Abramson D, Ellsworth R, Kitchin F, Tung G. Second nonocular tumors in retinoblastoma survivors. Are they radiation induced? Ophthalmology 1984; 91: 1351–5.

17 Knudson A. Mutation and cancer: statistical study of retinoblastoma. Proc Natl Acad Sci USA 1971; 68: 820–3.

18 Malkin D, Li FP, Fraumeni JF, et al. Germ line p53 mutations in familial syndrome of breast cancer, sarcomas and other neoplasms. Science 1990; 250; 1233–8.

19 Friend S, Bernards R, Rogelj S, et al. A human DNA segment with properties of the gene that predisposes to retinoblastoma and osteosarcoma. Nature 1986; 323: 643–6.

20 Lane DP. P53, guardian of the genome. Nature 1992; 358: 15–16.

21 Diller L, Kassel J, Nelson CE, et al. p53 functions as a cell cycle control protein in osteosarcomas. Mol Cell Biol 1990; 10: 6772–5781.

22 Huang H-JS, Yee J-K, Shew J-Y, et al. Suppression of the neoplastic phenotype by replacement of the RB gene in human cancer cells. Science 1988; 242: 1563–6.

23 Miller CW, Aslo A, Tsay C, et al. Frequency and structure of p53 rearrangements in human osteosarcoma. Cancer Res 1990; 50: 7950–4.

24 Wadayama B, Toguchida J, Shimizu T, et al. Mutation spectrum of the retinoblastoma gene in osteosarcomas. Cancer Res 1994; 54: 3042–8.

25 Finkel M, Biskis B, Jinkins P. Virus induction of osteosarcoma in mice. Science 1966; 151: 698–701.

26 Fletcher CDM, Unni KK, Mertens F (Eds). World Health Organization Classification of Tumours. Pathology and Genetics of Tumours of Soft Tissue and Bone. IARC Press: Lyon, 2002.

27 Vergel De Dios AM, Bond JR, Shives TC, McLeod RA, Unni KK. Aneurysmal bone cyst. A clinicopathologic study of 238 cases. Cancer 1992; 69: 2921–31.

28 Dahlin D, Unni K. Osteosarcoma of bone and its important recognizable varieties. Am J Surg Pathol 1977; 1: 61–72.

29 Huvos A, Rosen G, Bretsky S, Butler A. Telengiectatic osteogenic sarcoma: a clinicopathologic study of 124 patients. Cancer 1982; 49: 1679–89.

30 Sim FH, Unni KK, Beabout JW, Dahlin DC. Osteosarcoma with small cells simulating Ewing's tumor. J Bone Joint Surg [AM] 1979; 61: 207–15.

31 Perlman EJ, Dickman PS, Askin FB, et al. Ewing's sarcoma – routine diagnostic utilization of MIC – 2 analysis: a Pediatric Oncology Group/Children's Cancer Group intergroup study. Human Pathol 1994; 25: 304–7.

32 Ballance WA, Mendelsohn G, Carter JR, et al. Osteogenic sarcoma. Malignant fibrous histiocytoma subtype. Cancer 1988; 62: 763–71.

33 McKillop J, Etcubanas E, Goris M. The indications for and limitations of bone scintigraphy in osteogenic sarcoma. A review of 55 patients. Cancer 1981; 48: 1133–8.

34 Wolf RE, Enneking WF. The staging and surgery of musculoskeletal neoplasms. Orthop Clin North Am 1996; 27: 473–81.

35 Bielack S, Kempf-Bielack B, Günter D, et al. Prognostic factors in high-grade osteosarcoma of the extremities or trunk: an analysis of 1792 patients treated on neoadjuvant Cooperative Osteosarcoma Study Group protocols. J Clin Oncol 2002; 20: 776–90.

36 Picci P, Sangiorgi L, Rongraff BT, et al. The relationship of chemotherapy-induced necrosis and surgical margins to local recurrence in osteosarcoma. J Clin Oncol 1994; 18: 4016–27.

37 Grimer RJ, Taminiau AM, Cannon SR. Surgical outcomes in osteosarcoma. J Bone Joint Surg Br 2002; 84-B: 395–400.

38 Rougraff BT, Simon MA, Kneisl JS, et al. Limb salvage compared with amputation for osteosarcoma of the distal end of the femur. A long-term oncological, functional, and quality-of-life study. J Bone Joint Surg Am 1994; 76: 649–56.

39 Simon MA. Limb salvage for osteosarcoma. J Bone Joint Surg Am 1988; 70: 307–10.

40 Lindner NJ, Ramm O, Hillmann A, et al. Limb salvage and outcome of osteosarcoma. The University of Muenster experience. Clin Orthop Relat Res 1999; 358: 83–9.

41 Gherlinzoni F, Picci P, Bacci G, et al. Limb sparing versus amputation in osteosarcoma. Correlation between local control, surgical margins and tumor necrosis: Instituto Rizzoli experience. Ann Oncol 1992; 3 (Suppl 2): S23–7.

42 Bacci G, Picci P, Ruggieri P, et al. Primary chemotherapy and delayed surgery (neoadjuvant chemotherapy) for osteosarcoma of the extremities. The Instituto Rizzoli experience in 127 patients treated postoperatively with intravenous methotrexate (high versus moderate doses) and intraarterial cisplatin. Cancer 1990; 65: 2539–53.

43 Rosen G, Murphy ML, Huvos AG, et al. Chemotherapy, en block resection, and prosthetic bone replacement in the treatment of osteogenic sarcoma. Cancer 1976; 37: 1–11.

44 Marcove RC, Mike V, Hajek JV, et al. Osteogenic sarcoma under the age of twenty- one. A review of 145 operative cases. J Bone Joint Surg [Am] 1970; 52: 411–23.

45 Cortes EP, Holland JF, Wang JJ, Sinks LF. Doxorubicin in disseminated osteosarcoma. JAMA 1972; 221: 1132–8.

46 Baum ES, Gaynon P, Greenberg L, et al. Phase II study of cis-dichlorodiammineplatinum (II) in childhood osteosarcoma: Children's Cancer Study Group Report. Cancer Treat Rep 1979; 63: 1621–7.

47 Marti C, Kroner T, Remagen W, et al. High-dose ifosfamide in advanced osteosarcoma. Cancer Treat Rep 1985; 69: 115–17.

48 Jaffe N, Frei E, Traggis D, Bishop Y. Adjuvant methotrexate and citrovorum-factor treatment of osteogenic sarcoma. N Engl J Med 1974; 291: 994–7.

49 Goorin A, Delorey M, Gelber R, et al. The Dana-Farber Cancer Institute/The Children's Hospital adjuvant chemotherapy trials for osteosarcoma: three sequential studies. Cancer Treat Rep 1986; 3: 155–9.

50 Sutow WW, Sullivan MP, Fernbach DJ, et al. Adjuvant chemotherapy in primary treatment of osteogenic sarcoma. A Southwest Oncology Group Study. Cancer 1975; 36: 1598–602.

51 Carter SK. Adjuvant chemotherapy in osteogenic sarcoma: the triumph that isn't? J Clin Oncol 1984; 2: 147–8.

52 Link MP, Goorin AM, Miser AW, et al. The effect of adjuvant chemotherapy on relapse-free survival in patients with osteosarcoma of the extremity. N Engl J Med 1986; 314: 1600–6.

53 Eilber F, Giuliano A, Eckardt J, et al. Adjuvant chemotherapy for osteosarcoma: a randomized prospective trial. J Clin Oncol 1987; 5: 21–6.

54 Link MP, Goorin AM, Horowitz M, et al. Adjuvant chemotherapy of high grade osteosarcoma of the extremity: updated results of the Multi-Institutional Osteosarcoma Study. Clin Orthop 1991; 270: 8–14.

55 Rosen G, Marcove RC, Caparros B, et al. Primary osteogenic sarcoma. The rationale for preoperative chemotherapy and delayed surgery. Cancer 1979; 43: 2163–77.

56 Winkler K, Beron G, Kotz R, et al. Neoadjuvant chemotherapy for osteogenic sarcoma: results of a Cooperative German/Austrian Study. J Clin Oncol 1984; 2: 617–24.

57 Provisor AJ, Ettinger LJ, Nachman JB, et al. Treatment of nonmetastatic osteosarcoma of the extremity with preoperative and postoperative chemotherapy: a report from the Children's Cancer Group. J Clin Oncol 1997; 15: 76–84.

58 Goorin AM, Schwartzentruber DJ, Devidas M, et al. Presurgical chemotherapy compared with immediate surgery and adjuvant chemotherapy for nonmetastatic osteosarcoma: Pediatric Oncology Group Study POG–8651. J Clin Oncol 2003; 21: 1574–80.

59 Rosen G, Caparros B, Huvos AG, et al. Preoperative chemotherapy for osteogenic sarcoma: selection of postoperative adjuvant chemotherapy based on the response of the primary tumor to preoperative chemotherapy. Cancer 1982; 49: 1221–30.

60 Meyers PA, Heller G, Healey J, et al. Chemotherapy for non-metastatic osteogenic sarcoma: The Memorial Sloan-Kettering experience. J Clin Oncol 1992; 10: 5–15.

61 Winkler K, Beron G, Delling G, et al. Neoadjuvant chemotherapy of osteosarcoma: results of a randomized cooperative trial (COSS-82) with salvage chemotherapy based on histological tumor response. J Clin Oncol 1988; 6: 329–37.

62 Meyers PA, Gorlick R, Heller G, et al. Intensification of preoperative chemotherapy for osteogenic sarcoma: results of the Memorial Sloan-Kettering (T12) protocol. J Clin Oncol 1998; 16: 2452–8.

63 Pratt CB, Epelman S, Jaffe N. Bleomycin, cyclophosphamide, and dactinomycin in metastatic osteosarcoma: lack of tumor regression in previously treated patients. Cancer Treat Rep 1987; 71: 421–3.

64 Jaffe N, Prudich J, Knapp J, et al. Treatment of primary osteosarcoma with intra – arterial and intravenous high-dose methotrexate. J Clin Oncol 1983; 1: 428–31.

65 Jaffe N, Knapp J, Chuang VP, et al. Osteosarcoma: intra-arterial treatment of the primary tumor with cis-diamminedichloroplatinum II (CDP). Angiographic, pathologic and pharmacologic studies. Cancer 1983; 51: 402–7.

66 Hudson M, Jaffe MR, Jaffe N, et al. Pediatric osteosarcoma: therapeutic strategies, results and prognostic factors derived from a 10-year experience. J Clin Oncol 1990; 8: 1988–97.

67 Kleinerman ES, Jia S-F, Griffin J, Seibel NL, Benjamin RS, Jaffe N. Phase II study of liposomal muramyl tripeptide in osteosarcoma: the cytokine cascade and monocyte activation following administration. J Clin Oncol 1992; 10: 1310–6.

68 MacEwen EG, Kurzman ID, Rosenthal RC, et al. Therapy for osteosarcoma in dogs with intravenous injection of liposome-

encapsulated muramyl tripeptide. J Natl Cancer Inst 1989; 81: 935–8.

69 Meyers PA, Schwartz CL, Krailo M, et al. Osteosarcoma: a randomized, prospective trial of the addition of ifosfamide and/or muramyl tripeptide to cisplatin, doxorubicin, and high-dose methotrexate. J Clin Oncol 2005; 23: 2004–11.

70 Saeter G, Alvegard TA, Elomaa I, et al. Treatment of osteosarcoma of the extremities with the T – 10 protocol, with emphasis on the effects of preoperative chemotherapy with single-agent high-dose methotrexate: a Scandinavian Sarcoma Group study. J Clin Oncol 1991; 9: 1766–75.

71 Smeland S, Müller C, Alvegard TA, et al. Scandinavian Sarcoma Group Osteosarcoma Study SSG VIII: prognostic factors for outcome and the role of replacement salvage chemotherapy for poor histological responders. Eur J Cancer 2003; 39: 488–94.

72 Ferrari S, Smeland S, Mercuri M, et al. Neoadjuvant chemotherapy with high-dose ifosfamide, high-dose methotrexate, cisplatin, and doxorubicin for patients with localized osteosarcoma of the extremity: a joint study by the Italian and Scandinavian Sarcoma Groups. J Clin Oncol 2005; 23: 8845–52.

73 Fuchs N, Bielack SS, Epler D, et al. Long-term results of the co-operative German-Austrian-Swiss osteosarcoma study group's protocol COSS-86 of intensive multidrug chemotherapy and surgery for osteosarcoma of the limbs. Ann Oncol 1998; 9: 893–9.

74 Bacci G, Picci P, Ferrari S, et al. Primary chemotherapy and delayed surgery for nonmetastatic osteosarcoma of the extremities. Results in 164 patients preoperatively treated with high doses of methotrexate followed by cisplatin and doxorubicin. Cancer 1993; 72: 3227–8.

75 Bramwell VH, Burgers M, Sneath R, et al. A comparison of two short intensive adjuvant chemotherapy regimens in operable osteosarcoma of limbs in children and young adults: the first study of the European Osteosarcoma Intergroup. J Clin Oncol 1992; 10: 1579–91.

76 Souhami RL, Craft AW, Van der Eijken JW, et al. Randomised trial of two regimens of chemotherapy in operable osteosarcoma: a study of the European Osteosarcoma Intergroup. Lancet 1997; 350: 911–17.

77 Lewis IJ, Nooij MA, Whelan J, et al. Improvement in histologic response but not survival in osteosarcoma patients treated with intensified chemotherapy: a randomized phase III trial of the European Osteosarcoma Intergroup. J Natl Cancer Inst 2007; 99: 112–28.

78 Whelan J, Seddon B, Perisoglou M. Management of osteosarcoma. Curr Treat Options Oncol 2006; 7: 444–55.

79 Harris MB, Gieser P, Goorin AM, et al. Treatment of metastatic osteosarcoma at diagnosis: a Pediatric Oncology Group study. J Clin Oncol 1998; 16: 3641–48.

80 Kempf-Bielack B, Bielack S, Jürgens H, et al. Osteosarcoma relapse after combined modality therapy: an analysis of unselected patients in the Cooperative Osteosarcoma Study Group (COSS). J Clin Oncol 2005; 23: 559–68.

81 Ferrari S, Briccoli A, Mercuri M, et al. Postrelapse survival in osteosarcoma of the extremities: prognostic factors for long-term survival. J Clin Oncol 2003; 21: 710–15.

82 Goorin A, Delorey M, Lack E, et al. Prognostic significance of complete surgical resection of pulmonary metastases in patients with osteogenic sarcoma: analysis of 32 patients. J Clin Oncol 1984; 2: 425–31.

83 Putnam JB, Roth J, Wesley M, et al. Survival following aggressive resection of pulmonary metastases from osteogenic sarcoma: analysis of prognostic factors. Ann Thorac Surg 1983; 36: 516–23.

84 Lockshin M, Higgins I. Prognosis in osteogenic sarcoma. Clin Orthop 1968; 58: 85–101.

85 Simon R. Clinical prognostic factors in osteosarcoma. Cancer Treat Rep 1978; 62: 193–7.

86 Levine A, Rosenberg S. Alkaline phosphatase levels in osteosarcoma tissue are related to prognosis. Cancer 1979; 44: 2291–3.

87 Lewis IJ, Nooji MA, Whelan J et al. Improvement in histological response but not survival in osteosarcoma patients treated with intensified chemotherapy: a randomized phase II trial of the European Osteosarcoma Intergroup. J Natl Cancer Inst 2007; 99: 112–28.

88 Lewis IJ, Weeden S, Machin D, Stark D, Craft AW. Received dose and dose-intensity of chemotherapy outcome in nonmetastatic extremity osteosarcoma. European Osteosarcoma Intergroup. J Clin Oncol 2000; 18: 4828–37.

89 Esselgrim M, Grunert H, Kuhne T, et al. Dose intensity of chemotherapy for osteosarcoma and outcome in the Cooperative Osteosarcoma Study group (COSS) trials. Pediatr Blood Cancer 2006; 47: 42–50.

90 Borsi JD, Moe PJ. A comparative study of the pharmacokinetics of methotrexate in the dose range 0.6 g to 33.6 g in children with acute lymphoblastic leukaemia. Cancer 1987; 60: 5–13.

91 Estlin EJ, Burke GAA, Ronghe M, Lowis SP. Optimising antimetabolite-based chemotherapy for the treatment of childhood acute lymphoblastic leukaemia. Br J Haematol 2000; 110: 29–40.

92 Delephine N, Delephine G, Bacci G, et al. Influence of methotrexate pharmacokinetics on outcome for patients with high-grade osteogenic sarcoma. An analysis of the literature. Cancer 1996; 78: 2127–35.

93 Acquerreta I, Aldaz G, Girladaz J et al. Methotrexate pharmacokinetics and survival in osteosarcoma. Pediatr Blood Cancer 2004; 42: 52–8.

94 Bacci G, Ferrari S, Delephine N, et al. Predictive factors of histologic response to primary chemotherapy of osteogenic sarcoma of the extremities – a study of 272 patients preoperatively treated with high-dose methotrexate, doxorubicin, and cisplatin. J Clin Oncol 1998; 16: 658–63.

95 Graf N, Winkler K, Betlomevic N, et al. Methotrexate pharmacokinetics and prognosis in osteogenic sarcoma. J Clin Oncol 1994; 12: 1443–51.

96 Delephine N, Delephine G, Cornille H, et al. Dose escalation with pharmacokinetics monitoring in methotrexate chemotherapy of osteosarcoma. Anticancer Res 1995; 15: 489–94.

97 Zeicer S, Kellick M, Wexler LH, et al. Methotrextae levels and outcome in osteosarcoma. Pediatr Blood Cancer 2005; 44: 638–42.

98 Crews KR, Rodriguez-Gallindo C, Tan M, et al. High-dose methotrexate pharmacokinetics and outcome of children and young adults with osteosarcoma. Cancer 2004; 100: 1724–33.

99 Meyer WH, Loftin SK, Houghton PJ, et al. Accumulation, intracellular metabolism and antitumor activity of high- and low-dose methotrexate in human osteosarcoma xenografts. Cancer Commun 1990; 2: 219–29.

100 Guo W, Healy JH, Meyers PA, et al. Mechanisms of methotrexate resistance in osteosarcoma. Clin Cancer Res 1999; 5: 621–7.

101 Ifergan I, Meller I, Issakov J, et al. Reduced folate carrier protein expression in osteosarcoma: implications for the prediction of tumor chemosensitivity. Cancer 2003; 98: 1958–66.

102 Imanishi T, Abe Y, Suto R, et al. Expression of the human multidrug resistance gene (MDR1) and prognostic correlation in human osteogenic sarcoma. Tokai J Exp Clin Med 1994; 19: 39–46.

103 Wunder JS, Bull SB, Aneliunas V, et al. MDR1 gene expression and outcome in osteosarcoma: a prospective, multicentre study. J Clin Oncol 2000; 18: 2685–94.

104 Huang G, Mills L, Worth LL. Expression of human S-transferase P1 mediates the chemosensitivity of osteosarcoma cells. Mol Cancer Ther 2007; 6: 1610–9.

105 Aung L, Gorlick RG, Shi W, et al. Second malignant neoplasms in long-term survivors of osteosarcoma: Memorial Sloan-Kettering Cancer Center experience. Cancer 2002; 95: 1728–34.

106 Gorlick R,. Huvos AG, Heller G, et al. Expression of HER2/erbB-2 correlates with survival in osteosarcoma. J Clin Oncol 1999; 17: 2781–8.

107 Guo W, Healey JH, Meyers PA, et al. Mechanisms of methotrexate resistance in osteosarcoma. Clin Cancer Res 1999; 5: 621–7.

108 Baldini N, Scotlandi K, Barbanti-Brodano G, et al. Expression of P-glycoprotein in high-grade osteosarcomas in relation to clinical outcome. N Engl J Med 1995; 333: 1380–5.

109 Gebhardt MC, Lew RA, Bell RS, Baldini N, Litwak G, Mankin HJ. DNA ploidy as a prognostic indicator in human osteosarcoma. Chir Organi Mov 1990; 75: 18–21.

110 Imbriaco M, Yeh SD, Yeung H, et al. Thallium-201 scintigraphy for the evaluation of tumor response to preoperative chemotherapy in patients with osteosarcoma. Cancer 1997; 80: 1507–12.

111 Dyke JP, Panicek DM, Healey JH, et al. Fraction estimation of primary bone tumors undergoing induction chemotherapy using dynamic enhanced MRI. Radiology 2003; 228: 271–8.

112 Anderson PM, Wiseman GA, Dispenzeri A, et al. High-Dose samarium-153 ethylene diamine tetramethylene phosphonate: low toxicity of skeletal irradiation in patients with osteosarcoma and bone metastases. J Clin Oncol 2002; 20: 189–96.

113 Ko S– C, Cheon J, Kao C, et al. Osteocalcin promoter-based toxic gene therapy for the treatment of osteosarcoma in experimental models. Cancer Res 1996; 56: 4614–19.

114 Kaya M, Wada T, Kawaguchi S, et al. Increased pre- therapeutic serum vascular endothelial growth factor in patients with eary clinical relapse of osteoscaroma. Br J Cancer 2002; 86: 864–9.

115 Kaya M, Wada T, Akatsuka T, et al. Vascular endothelial growth factor expression in untreated osteosarcoma is predictive of pulmonary metastases and poor prognosis. Clin Cancer Res 2000; 6: 572–7.

116 Charity RM, Foukas AF, Deshmukh NS, et al. Vascular endothelial growth factor expression in osteosarcoma. Clin Orthop Relat Res 2006; 448: 193–8.

117 Glade– Bender J, Kandel JJ, Yamashiro DJ. VEGF bloking therapy in the treatment of cancer. Expert Opin Biol Ther; 2: 263–76.

118 Whang PJ, Triche TJ, Knutsen T, et al. Chromosome translocation in peripheral neuroepithelioma. N Engl J Med 1984; 311: 584–5.

119 McKeon C, Thiele CJ, Ross RA, et al. Indistinguishable patterns of protooncogene expression in two distinct but closely related tumors: Ewing's sarcoma and neuroepithelioma. Cancer Res 1988; 48: 4307–11.

120 Cotterill SJ, Ahrens S, Paulussen M, et al. Prognostic factors in Ewing's tumor of bone: analysis of 975 patients from the European Intergroup Cooperative Ewing's Sarcoma Study Group. J Clin Oncol 2000; 18: 3108–14.

121 Novakovic B, Goldstein AM, Wexler LH, Tucker MA. Increased risk of neuroectodermal tumors and stomach cancer in relatives of patients with Ewing's sarcoma family of tumors. J Natl Cancer Inst 1994; 86: 1702–6.

122 Buckley JD, Pendergrass TW, Buckley CM, et al. Epidemiology of osteosarcoma and Ewing's sarcoma in childhood: a study of 305 cases by the Children's Cancer Group. Cancer 1998; 83: 1440–8.

123 Aparicio J, Segura A, Montalar J, et al. Secondary cancers after Ewing sarcoma and Ewing sarcoma as second malignant neoplasm. Med Pediatr Oncol 1998; 30: 259–60.

124 Lipinski M, Braham K, Philip I, et al. Phenotypic characterization of Ewing sarcoma cell lines with monoclonal antibodies. J Cell Biochem 1986; 31: 289–96.

125 Delattre O, Zucman J, Melot T, et al. The Ewing family of tumors–a subgroup of small- round- cell tumors defined by specific chimeric transcripts. N Engl J Med 1994; 331: 294–9.

126 May WA, Lessnick SL, Braun BS, et al. The Ewing's sarcoma EWS/FLI-1 fusion gene encodes a more potent transcriptional activator and is a more powerful transforming gene than FLI-1. Mol Cell Biol 1993; 13: 7393–8.

127 Toretsky JA, Kalebic T, Blakesley V, et al. The insulin-like growth factor-I receptor is required for EWS/FLI-1 transformation of fibroblasts. J Biol Chem 1997; 272: 30822–7.

128 Deneen B, Denny CT. Loss of p16 pathways stabilizes EWS/FLI1 expression and complements EWS/FLI1 mediated transformation. Oncogene 2001; 20: 6731–41.

129 Paulussen M, Ahrens S, Burdach S, et al. Primary metastatic (stage IV) Ewing tumor: survival analysis of 171 patients from the EICESS studies. European Intergroup Cooperative Ewing Sarcoma Studies. Ann Oncol 1998; 9: 275–81.

130 Ferrari S, Bertoni F, Mercuri M, et al. Ewing's sarcoma of bone: relation between clinical characteristics and staging. Oncol Rep 2001; 8: 553–6.

131 Horowitz ME, Malawer MM, Shiao YW, et al. Ewing's Sarcoma Family of Tumours: Ewing's Sarcoma of Bone and Soft Tissue and the Peripheral Primitive Neuroectodermal Tumours. In: Pizzo PA, Poplack DG, (Eds). Principles and Practice of Pediatric Oncology, 3rd edn. Philadelphia, PA: Lippincott-Raven Publishers, 1997: 921–57.

132 Kovar H, Dworzak M, Strehl S, et al. Overexpression of the pseudo-autosomal gene MIC2 in Ewing's sarcoma and peripheral primitive neuroectodermal tumor. Oncogene 1990; 5: 1067–70.

133 Parham DM, Hijazi Y, Steinberg SM, et al. Neuroectodermal differentiation in Ewing's sarcoma family of tumors does not predict tumor behavior. Hum Pathol 1999; 30: 911–8.

134 Mugneret F, Lizard S, Aurias A, et al. Chromosomes in Ewing's sarcoma. II. Nonrandom additional changes, trisomy 8 and der(16) t(1; 16). Cancer Genet Cytogenet 1988; 32: 239–45.

135 Zoubek A, Pfleiderer C, Salzer KM, et al. Variability of EWS chimaeric transcripts in Ewing tumors: a comparison of clinical and molecular data. Br J Cancer 1994; 70: 908–13.

136 Miser JS, Kinsella TJ, Triche TJ, et al. Ifosfamide with mesna uroprotection and etoposide: an effective regimen in the treatment of recurrent sarcomas and other tumors of children and young adults. J Clin Oncol 1987; 5: 1191–8.

137 Nilbert M, Saeter G, Elomaa I, et al. Ewing's sarcoma treatment in Scandinavia 1984–1990. Ten-year results of the Scandinavian Sarcoma Group protocol SSG IV. Acta Oncol 1998; 37: 375–80.

138 Elomaa I, Blomqvist CP, Saeter G, et al. Five-year results in Ewing's sarcoma. The Scandinavian Sarcoma Group experience with the SSG IX protocol. Eur J Cancer, 2000; 36: 875–80.

139 Smeland S, Wiebe T, Brosjö O, et al. Chemotherapy in Ewing's sarcoma. The Scandinavian Sarcoma Group experience. Acta Orthop Scand 2004; 75(Suppl 311): 87–90.

140 Bacci G, Mercuri M, Longhi A, et al. Neoadjuvant chemotherapy for Ewing's tumor of bone: recent experience at the Rizzoli Orthopaedic Institute. Eur J Cancer 2002; 38: 2243–51.

141 Oberlin O, Le Deley MC, N'Guyen Bui B, et al. Prognostic factors in localised Ewing's tumors and peripheral neuroectodermal tumors: the third study of the French Society of Paediatric Oncology (EW 88 study). Br J Cancer 2001; 85: 1646–54.

142 Craft AW, Cotterill SJ, Bullimore JA, et al. Long-term results from the first UKCCSG Ewing's tumor study (ET-1). Eur J Cancer 1997; 33: 1061–9.

143 Craft A, Cotterill S, Malcom A, et al. Ifosfamide-containing chemotherapy in Ewing's sarcoma: the second United Kingdom Children's Cancer Study Group and the Medical Research Council Ewing's tumor study. J Clin Oncol 1998; 16: 3628–33.

144 Jürgens H, Exner U, Gardner H, et al. Multidisciplinary treatment of primary Ewing's sarcoma of bone. A 6-year experience of a European Cooperative trial. Cancer 1988; 61: 23–32.

145 Paulussen M, Ahrens S, Dunst J, et al. Localised Ewing tumor of bone: final results of the cooperative Ewing's Sarcoma Study CESS 86. J Clin Oncol, 2001; 19: 1818–29.

146 Paulussen M, Craft AW, Lewis I, et al. Results of the EICESS-92 Study: two randomized trials of Ewing's sarcoma treatment–cyclophosphamide compared with ifosfamide in standard-risk patients and assessment of benefit of etoposide added to standard treatment in high-risk patients, J Clin Oncol 2008; 26: 4385–93.

147 Nesbit ME, Gehan EA, Burgert EO, et al. Multimodal therapy for the management of primary, nonmetastatic Ewing's sarcoma of bone: a long-term follow-up of the First Intergroup study. J Clin Oncol 1990; 8: 1664–74.

148 Evans RG, Nesbit ME, Gehan EA, et al. Multimodal therapy for the management of localized Ewing's sarcoma of pelvic and sacral bones: a report from the second intergroup study. J Clin Oncol 1991; 9: 1173–80.

149 Grier H, Krailo M, Tarbell M, et al. Addition ifosfamide and etoposide to standard chemotherapy for Ewing's sarcoma and primitive neuroectodermal tumor of bone. N Engl J Med 2003; 348: 694–701.

150 Cangir A, Vietti TJ, Gehan EA, et al. Ewing's sarcoma metastatic at diagnosis. Results and comparisons of two intergroup Ewing's sarcoma studies. Cancer 1990; 66: 887–93.

151 Miser JS, Goldsby RE, Chen Z, et al. Treatment of metastatic Ewing sarcoma/primitive neuroectodermal tumor of bone: evaluation of increasing the dose intensity of chemotherapy – a report from the Children's Oncology Group. Pediatr Blood Cancer 2007; 49: 894–900.

152 Hawkins D, Barnett T, Bensinger W, Gooley T, Sanders J. Busulfan, melphalan, and thiotepa with or without total marrow irradiation with hematopoietic stem cell rescue for poor-risk Ewing-Sarcoma-Family tumors. Med Pediatr Oncol 2000; 34: 328–37.

153 Kushner BH, Meyers PA. How effective is dose-intensive/myeloablative therapy against Ewing's sarcoma/primitive neuroectodermal tumor metastatic to bone or bone marrow? The Memorial Sloan-Kettering experience and a literature review. J Clin Oncol 2001; 19: 870–80.

154 Pinkerton CR, Bataillard A, Guillo S, Oberlin O, Fervers B, Philip T. Treatment strategies for metastatic Ewing's sarcoma. Eur J Cancer 2001; 37: 1338–44.

155 Toretsky JA, Neckers L, Wexler LH. Detection of (11; 22)(q24; q12) translocation- bearing cells in peripheral blood progenitor cells of patients with Ewing's sarcoma family of tumors. J Natl Cancer Inst 1995; 87: 385–6.

156 Merino ME, Navid F, Christensen BL, et al. Immunomagnetic purging of Ewing's sarcoma from blood and bone marrow: quantitation by real-time polymerase chain reaction. J Clin Oncol 2001; 19: 3649–59.

157 Picci P, Rougraff BT, Bacci G, et al. Prognostic significance of histopathologic response to chemotherapy in nonmetastatic Ewing's sarcoma of the extremities. J Clin Oncol 1993; 11: 1763–9.

158 Brereton HD, Simon R, Pomeroy TC. Pre-treatment serum lactate dehydrogenase predicting metastatic spread in Ewing's sarcoma. Ann Intern Med 1975; 83: 352–4.

159 Bacci G, Ferrari S, Longhi A, et al. Prognostic significance of serum LDH in Ewing's sarcoma of bone. Oncol Rep 1999; 6: 807–11.

160 Zoubek A, Dockhorn-Dworniczak B, Delattre O, et al. Does expression of different EWS chimeric transcripts define clinically distinct risk groups of Ewing tumor patients? J Clin Oncol 1996; 14: 1245–51.

161 de Alava E, Kawai A, Healey JH, et al. EWS-FLI1 fusion transcript structure is an independent determinant of prognosis in Ewing's sarcoma. J Clin Oncol 1998; 16: 1248–55.

162 Kovar H, Jug G, Aryee DN, et al. Among genes involved in the RB dependent cell cycle regulatory cascade, the p16 tumor suppressor gene is frequently lost in the Ewing family of tumors. Oncogene 1997; 15: 2225–32.

163 Hattinger CM, Rumpler S, Strehl S, et al. Prognostic impact of deletions at 1p36 and numerical aberrations in Ewing tumors. Genes Chrom Cancer 1999; 24: 243–54.

164 Wei G, Antonescu CR, de Alava E, et al. Prognostic impact of INK4A deletion in Ewing sarcoma. Cancer 2000; 89: 793–9.

165 de Alava E, Antonescu CR, Panizo A, et al. Prognostic impact of P53 status in Ewing sarcoma. Cancer 2000; 89: 783–92.

166 Delephine H, Delephine G, Cornille H, et al. Prognostic factors in patients with localized Ewing's sarcoma: the effect on survival of actual received dose intensity and of histological response to induction therapy. J Chemother 1997; 9: 352–63.

167 Miser JS, Goldsby RE, Chen Z et al. Treatment of metastatic Ewing sarcoma/primitive neuroectodermal tumor of bone: evaluation of increasing the dose intensity of chemotherapy – a report form the Children's Oncology group. Pediatr Blood Cancer 2007; 49: 894–900

168 Perri T, Fogel M, Mor S et al. Effect of P – glycoprotein expression on outcome in the Ewing family of tumors. Pediatr Hematol Oncol 18: 325–34.

169 Wexler LH, Andrich MP, Venzon D, et al. Randomized trial of the cardioprotective agent ICRF – 187 in pediatric sarcoma patients treated with doxorubicin. J Clin Oncol 1996; 14: 362–72.

170 Granowetter L, Womer R, Devidas M. Comparison of dose intensified and standard dose chemotherapy for the treatment of non-metastatic Ewing's sarcoma and primitive neuroectodermal tumor of bone and soft tissue: a Pediatric Oncology Group – Children's Cancer Group phase III trial. Med Pediatr Oncol 2001; 37: O38.

171 Sweeney LE. Hypophosphataemic rickets after ifosfamide treatment in children. Clin Radiol 1993; 47: 345–7.

172 Kuttesch JF, Wexler LH, Marcus RB, et al. Second malignancies after Ewing's sarcoma: radiation dose-dependency of secondary sarcomas. J Clin Oncol 1996; 14: 2818–25.

173 Bhatia S, Krailo MD, Chen Z, et al. Therapy-related myelodysplasia and acute myeloid leukemia after Ewing sarcoma and primitive neuroectodermal tumor of bone: a report from the Children's Oncology Group. Blood 2007; 109: 46–51.

174 Saylors RL 3rd, Stine KC, Sullivan J, et al. Cyclophosphamide plus topotecan in children with recurrent or refractory solid tumors: a Pediatric Oncology Group phase II study. J Clin Oncol 2001; 19: 3463–9.

175 Bernstein M, Goorin A, Devidas M, et al. Topotecan and topotecan, cyclophosphamide window therapy in patients with Ewing sarcoma metastatic at diagnosis: an intergroup Pediatric Oncology Group study. In: SIOP, Brisbane 2001: O-51.

176 Landuzzi L, De Giovanni C, Nicoletti G, et al. The metastatic ability of Ewing's sarcoma cells is modulated by stem cell factor and by its receptor c-kit. Am J Pathol 2000; 157: 2123–31.

177 Mitsiades N, Poulaki V, Mitsiades C, Tsokos M. Ewing's sarcoma family tumors are sensitive to tumor necrosis factor-related apoptosis-inducing ligand and express death receptor 4 and death receptor 5. Cancer Res 2001; 61: 2704–12.

178 Zhou Z, Bolontrade MF, Reddy K, et al. Suppression of Ewing's sarcoma tumor growth, tumor vessel formation and vasculogenesis following anti vascular endothelial growth factor receptor-2 therapy. Clin Cancer Res 2007; 13: 4867–73.

179 Myatt SS, Burchill SA. The sensitivity of the Ewing's scarcoma family of tumors to fenretinide-induced cell death is increased by EWS-Fli1-dpendent modulation of p38(MAPK) activity. Oncogene 2008; 27: 985–96.

180 Bacci G, Ferrari, S, Bertoni F, et al. Neoadjuvant chemotherapy for peripheral malignant neuroectodermal tumor of bone: recent experience at the Instituto Rizzali. J Clin Oncol 2000; 18: 885–92.

181 Rosito P, Mancini AF, Rondelli R, et al. Italian Cooperative Study for the treatment of children and young adults with localised Ewing sarcoma of bone: a preliminary report of 6 years of experience. Cancer 1999; 86: 421–8.

182 Shankar AG, Pinkerton CR, Atra A, et al. Local therapy and other factors influencing site of relapse in patients with localised Ewing's sarcoma. United Kingdom Children's Cancer Study Group (UKCCSG). Eur J Cancer 1999; 35: 1698–704.

16 Hepatic Tumors

Penelope Brock[1], Derek J. Roebuck[2] and Jack Plaschkes[3]

[1] Great Ormond Street Hospital for Children NHS Trust, London, UK, [2] Department of Radiology, Great Ormond Street Hospital for Children NHS Trust, London, UK and [3] University Children's Hospital, Bern, Switzerland

Introduction

Malignant tumors

Primary malignant hepatic tumors are uncommon in children, representing about 1.3% of all pediatric cancer [1]. After the first few months of life (when various forms of liver hemangioma are common), malignant tumors are more common than benign [2]. Because they are unusual, malignant liver tumors have only recently been studied in clinical trials (see below).

• Ten distinct primary tumors and pseudotumors of the liver occur with some regularity, and a few others may be seen rarely, including leiomyosarcoma, rhabdoid tumor, and yolk sac tumor.
• Five of these neoplasms – hepatoblastoma (HB), infantile hemangioma, mesenchymal hamartoma, undifferentiated (embryonal) sarcoma, and embryonal rhabdomyosarcoma of the biliary tree – are mainly seen in children [3].

There are two main types of malignant tumor (Table 16.1), those of epithelial origin, comprising HB and hepatocellular carcinoma (HCC), and the mesenchymal tumors, e.g. rhabdomyosarcoma and undifferentiated sarcoma [4]. Epithelial liver malignancies are more common, and this chapter will focus mainly on HB and HCC.

Benign liver masses

The most common benign hepatic tumors in childhood are called hemangiomas. This term refers to at least three distinct tumors, with different biological behaviors [5]. Other commonly seen benign tumors are:
• Mesenchymal hamartoma.
• Focal nodular hyperplasia.
• Hepatic adenoma (almost exclusively a disease of older children).
• Primary hepatic teratoma (exceedingly rare).

Imaging techniques such as ultrasound, computed tomography (CT), and magnetic resonance imaging (MRI) are not always reliable in differentiating benign from malignant tumors.

The differential diagnosis of benign hepatic tumors includes non-neoplastic cystic masses (including choledochal and simple hepatic cysts), hematoma, parasitic cysts, and pyogenic and amebic liver abscesses [6].

The neonatal period

Primary liver tumors are very rare during the neonatal period; they are sometimes diagnosed by prenatal ultrasound [7]. A precise diagnosis is sometimes problematic because of non-specific clinical symptoms, misleading imaging and difficulties with histological interpretation.

• Infantile hemangioma is typically multifocal or diffuse. It grows in the first year of life, and then undergoes spontaneous regression. Treatment with corticosteroids, and more recently beta adrenergic receptor antagonists, is reserved for symptomatic patients. Further treatment with resection, embolization, or arterial ligation may be necessary.
• Rapidly-involuting congenital hemangiomas are usually solitary, and rarely require treatment.
• Mesenchymal hamartoma is usually mostly cystic, and should be resected whenever possible.
• Benign teratomas should be resected and if at all possible in the first 2 months of life before they can become malignant. Malignant choriocarcinomas should respond to chemotherapy and be amenable to delayed surgery [8].
• Malignant hepatoblastoma may occur in the newborn, and should be treated with chemotherapy to achieve resectability.

Historical perspective

Liver cancer was initially thought to be the unique domain of the surgeon. It was only in the 1980s, when cisplatin became known through its remarkable cure rate in testicular cancer, that doctors discovered that liver tumors in children could also be reduced in size by chemotherapy. It is the combination treatment of chemotherapy and surgery which has seen an extraordinary change in the outlook for children with HB over the last few decades. Nevertheless cure is only rarely achieved without ultimate complete resection – including, where necessary, liver transplantation.

Pediatric Hematology and Oncology, 1st edition. Edited by Edward J. Estlin, Richard J. Gilbertson, and Robert F. Wynn. © 2010 Blackwell Publishing Ltd.

Table 16.1 Differential diagnosis for liver tumors of childhood.

Malignant

Hepatoblastoma
Hepatocellular carcinoma
Undifferentiated (embryonal) sarcoma
Lymphoma
Rhabdomyosarcoma (biliary tract)
Germ-cell tumors
Rhabdoid tumors
Angiosarcoma

Benign

Vascular tumors (e.g. infantile hemangioma)
Mesenchmal hamartoma
Focal nodular hyperplasia
Hepatocellular adenoma

In HCC, chemotherapy has made little impact on survival and other strategies are being tried to increase the resection rate and decrease the recurrence rate.

The diagnosis is made by a combination of imaging, the serum tumor marker alpha-fetoprotein (AFP) and histopathology. Up to the 1980s, surgical resection was the mainstay of treatment and only patients with a resectable malignant tumor at diagnosis stood a chance of cure. Ultrasound (US) and MRI give a clear idea of the operability of the tumor at diagnosis.

There is a debate over initial surgery for resectable disease. The North Americans and associates still advocate primary surgery. Most of the rest of the world now treat with pre-operative chemotherapy, delayed surgery and post-operative chemotherapy.

Epidemiology

General considerations

The annual incidence of HB is approximately one per million children under the age of 15. HB presents mainly under the age of 5 years, with a median age of around 18 months.

• The incidence of HB is thought to be fairly constant worldwide.

• The major improvement in prognosis for children with HB has been achieved through worldwide collaboration in clinical trials. This type of collaboration is an example of how the treatment for rare diseases can be improved. In HB the 5-year overall survival rate has improved from 30 to 70%, and is over 80% for the majority of children who present with standard risk disease.

• No significant geographical variations have been found; those that exist are likely due to the different methods of registration. This would imply that environmental factors are not of great importance. In a case-control study of 75 children with HB in Los Angeles [9], case mothers were more likely to report occupational exposure to metals, petroleum products and paints or pigments,

and these associations were statistically significant. The only significant paternal exposure was to metals.

In contrast, the incidence of HCC varies around the world, depending mostly on the prevalence of hepatitis B (HBV) and more recently hepatitis C (HCV), which are both known to be predisposing factors. In Europe, data on 849 children diagnosed with malignant hepatic tumors (International Classification of Childhood Cancer, Group VII) before the age of 15 years during 1978–1997 were extracted from the ACCIS database with the following findings [10].

• Age-standardized incidence during 1988–1997 was 1.5 per million overall, 1.2 per million for HB and 0.2 per million for HCC.

• Over 90% of cases of HB occurred before age 5 years, whereas HCC had a fairly flat age distribution.

• Both tumors had an incidence in boys of 1.5–1.6 times those in girls.

• There were no significant time trends in incidence during 1978–1997.

In a population-based survey carried out in the UK [11] the incidence of malignant hepatic tumors in children from 1957 to 1986, was 1.20 per million person years and for HB was 0.77. In this study a congenital defect or related disorder was found in 21% of patients with a malignant liver tumor. The results suggest that HB is related to maldevelopment, whereas HCC is more usually a complication of metabolic and other disorders, which lead to cirrhosis.

Other national studies of the epidemiology of HB and HCC help define time trends and etiology. In a study of primary malignant hepatic tumors in children in the USA, the incidence of HB appears to have increased from 0.6 to 1.2 per million and HCC decreased from 0.45 to 0.29 per million from the 1970s to the 1990s [12]. The incidence of HB appears to be increasing slightly into the 2000s [13].

In South Africa there is a high incidence of HCC in children compared with the western world, but the link to HBV infection is not so clear. In a study of 194 children aged between 0 and 14 years with a malignant primary hepatic tumor between 1988 and 2003 in South Africa [14], there were 57% HB, 35% HCC, 5% sarcomas and 2% Burkitt's lymphoma. The incidence was 1.066 malignant liver tumors per year per 10 million children aged <14 years. Two thirds of the patients with HCC were positive for HBsAg and almost all were black. The mean age of onset was 1.47 years for HB and 10.48 years for HCC. AFP was raised in 100% of HB patients and 69% of those with HCC.

Hepatoblastoma and inherited conditions

Predisposition overgrowth syndromes are known to have an increased incidence of hepatoblastoma in young children. Abdominal ultrasound screening every 3–4 months until the age of 7 years is advised

Table 16.2 Constitutional genetic syndromes leading to hepatoblastoma.

Disease	Chromosome location	Gene
Familial adenomatous polyposis	5q21.22	*APC*
Beckwith-Wiedemann Syndrome	11p15.5	P57KiP2,Wnt,others
Li-Fraumeni syndrome	17p13	*TP53*, others
Trisomy 18	18	–
Glycogen storage diseases types I-IV	Several	–

(Adapted from Meuller BU, Lopez-Terrada D, Finegold MJ. Tumors of the liver. In: Pizzo PA, Poplack DG (Eds), Principles and Practices of Pediatric Oncology, 5th edn. Baltimore: Lippincott, Williams and Wilkins, 2005; permission pending.)

Most cases of HB are sporadic but there are clear associations with some familial conditions (Table 16.2). In the overgrowth syndromes, such as Beckwith-Weidemann syndrome and hemi-hypertrophy, screening for HB is advised with 3 monthly abdominal US until the age of 7 years [15]. Screening could be considered in children from families with familial adenomatous polyposis, who are also at increased risk of developing HB [16].

Hepatoblastoma and low birth weight

The association between HB and low birth weight was first noted by Ikeda *et al.* [17] and later confirmed by others. The role of possible treatment-related and other factors in premature infants weighing less than 1500 g has been examined in case-control studies [18–20]. There is no reason to believe that the outcome in congenital hepatoblastoma is worse than at an older age. Careful electrolyte and renal function monitoring and age- and weight-adapted chemotherapy dosing should be used [21]. Normal AFP levels are higher in infants [22].

Hepatocellular carcinoma

In some countries HCC is the third most common cause of death from cancer in adults. Because it is so rare in children there have been no specific pediatric trials until very recently (SIOPEL 5), and patients have often been treated with protocols designed for HB (e.g. SIOPEL 1 and INT-0098). Unfortunately, less than 30% are resectable at diagnosis. A small response to chemotherapy has been noted but the survival rate has remained about 20–30%.

Hepatic tumors and the link with hepatitis and the success of vaccination

The incidence of HCC is high in areas with endemic HBV infection. This is particularly true in Asia and Africa but also in the Inuit populations of Canada and Alaska [23]. The link between HCC in children and vertical transmission of HBV was made in the 1980s [24] and led to a pilot trial of universal immunization of newborns in an endemic area of rural China in 1983 [25].

> Since the introduction of mass hepatitis B vaccination programs in certain parts of the world the incidence of hepatocellular carcinoma has dramatically decreased. The most striking example of this has been in Taiwan

There has, however, been an extraordinary reduction in the incidence of this disease following the introduction of mass vaccination programs. The most remarkable of these was initiated in Taiwan.

• In the early 1980s, 15–20% of the population of Taiwan were estimated to be HBV carriers. A program of mass vaccination against hepatitis B was therefore launched in 1984. In the first 2 years, newborns of all hepatitis B surface antigen (HBsAg)-positive mothers were vaccinated. From 1986, all newborns, and then year-by-year pre-school children, primary school children, adolescents, young adults, and others have also been vaccinated.

• Vaccination coverage is over 90% for newborns, with 79% of pregnant women screened for HBsAg. The proportion of babies born to highly infectious carrier mothers who also became carriers, decreased from 86–96% to 12–14%; the decrease was from 10–12% to 3–4% for babies of less infectious mothers.

• Between 1989 and 1993, the prevalence of HBsAg in children aged 6 years fell from 10.5% to 1.7%.

The average annual incidence of HCC in children aged 6–14 years decreased significantly from 7 per million in 1981–1986 to 3.6 per million in 1990–1994. The incidence is now 1.3–2 per million [26]. The mass vaccination program has been highly effective in controlling chronic HBV infection and in preventing liver cancer in Taiwan. If a coverage rate of 90% of all newborns vaccinated against HBV can be maintained, by the year 2010 the carrier rate in Taiwan is expected to decline to <0.1% [27–30].

Following on from this success and that of China many countries are seeing the incidence of HCC decrease as the vaccinated population increases [23, 31–33]. In Alaska there are HCC screening programs, with twice yearly serum AFP monitoring in chronically HBV-infected individuals [34]. The program in Alaska has meant that 60% are detected early enough to be operable [23]. HBV vaccination is particularly relevant in sub-Saharan Africa where HCC is the most frequent malignancy in adult males [31] and where in both adults and children it carries a particularly poor prognosis due to a combination of co-morbidity and lack of resources [35].

HCC can occur in a child as young as 8 months following vertical transmission of HBV [36]. The child's serum and the tumor are usually positive for HBsAg [37].

HCV has recently become the cause of 75% of adult HCC in Japan. Treatment of HCV carriers with interferon reduces the incidence of HCC in this population [38]. Nationwide screening for HBV and HCV began in Japan in 2002. Primary liver cancer is the first human cancer largely amenable to prevention using hepatitis B vaccines and screening of blood and blood products for hepatitis B and C viruses [39].

Hepatic tumors and metabolic disorders

> Hepatitis B and certain rare familial metabolic disorders such as tyrosinemia and progressive familial intrahepatic cholestasis predispose to hepatocellular carcinoma

Many inherited diseases affect the liver. They can be considered primary (when the injury is from the cytopathic effect of an accumulated metabolite) or secondary (e.g. an infection caused by an immune deficiency). These disorders can lead to both benign and malignant neoplasms, of which HCC is the most common [40]. Most children with HCC, however, do not have cirrhosis.

Hepatic tumors and second malignancy

HCC has been reported to occur as a second malignancy following treatment with high-dose chemotherapy and irradiation [41], after acute lymphoblastic leukemia [42] and following HCV infection contracted during the treatment of childhood cancer [43]. (Table 16.3)

Clinical presentation

Hepatoblastoma

The infant or young child almost invariably presents with an abdominal mass, which can usually be shown on palpation to arise from the liver.

Table 16.3 Constitutional genetic syndromes leading to hepatocellular carcinoma.

Disease	Chromosome	Gene
Familial adenomatous polyposis	5q21.22	*APC*
Glycogen storage diseases types I–IV	Several	–
Hereditary tyrosinemia	15q23–25	*FAH*
Alagille syndrome	20p12	*JAG1*
Other familial cholestatic syndromes	18q21–22,2q24	*ABCB11*, others
Neurofibromatosis	17q11.2	*NF1*
Ataxia telangiectasia	11q22–23	*ATM*
Fanconi anemia	1q42, 3p, 20q13.2–13.3, others	*FANCC*, others

(Adapted from Meuller BU, Lopez-Terrada D, Finegold MJ. Tumors of the liver. In: Pizzo PA, Poplack DG (Eds), Principles and Practices of Pediatric Oncology, 5th edn. Baltimore: Lippincott, Williams and Wilkins, 2005; permission pending.)

- Patients in an advanced stage present with anorexia, fatigue, abdominal pain, and fever [44].
- It is helpful to watch the movement of the liver with the natural respirations of the child to show that the tumor is not arising from the kidneys or adrenal glands. This is usually made easy with US [45].
- Most children have normal liver function and are not jaundiced.
- Thrombocytosis is common. Infants with hepatomegaly from infection will usually be less well and febrile and may have a low platelet count.
- HB is usually localized to the liver, but when it does metastasize it is to the lung and only rarely to bone marrow, bone, or the brain.

Hepatocellular carcinoma

HCC presents later than HB, the mean age in children being 10 years. Most patients present with an abdominal mass and the following clinical characteristics can occur:
- The tumor may be large and may cause obstructive jaundice.
- In a Nigerian study [46] patients presented relatively late: 80% had weight loss, 50% had splenomegaly and 33% were jaundiced.
- Enzymatic liver function, however, is usually normal.
- Metastases are most frequently to the lung but are not uncommonly seen in bone.

Investigations and staging

Imaging

Accurate imaging is of prime importance for diagnosis and management [47]. The primary tumor must be assessed accurately, and metastatic disease detected when it exists. The best modalities for local extension are US, combined with CT or MRI (Figure 16.1), or occasionally both. Thoracic CT is mandatory to assess for pulmonary metastases. Skeletal scintigraphy (nuclear medicine bone scan) may be appropriate in children with HCC, but not HB where false-positive scans are apparently common [47].

Serum alpha-fetoprotein

In most cases of both HB and HCC serum AFP is raised above normal levels for age. More recently a category of high-risk patients with HB and a low serum AFP (<100 ng/ml) has been recognized [48]. Some of these tumors appear to be extrarenal rhabdoid tumors [49]. In view of the young age at diagnosis of most HB patients it is important to compare AFP values carefully with normal values seen in the first weeks and months of life. In one study mean serum AFP levels were 41 687 ng/ml in 256 term babies and 158 125 ng/ml in 90 premature babies born before the 37th gestational week, excluding samples from children with factors known to be associated with AFP elevation. In the first 4 weeks of life, AFP levels decreased by 50% in 5.1 days in term babies. Between days 180 and 720 of life, AFP levels up to

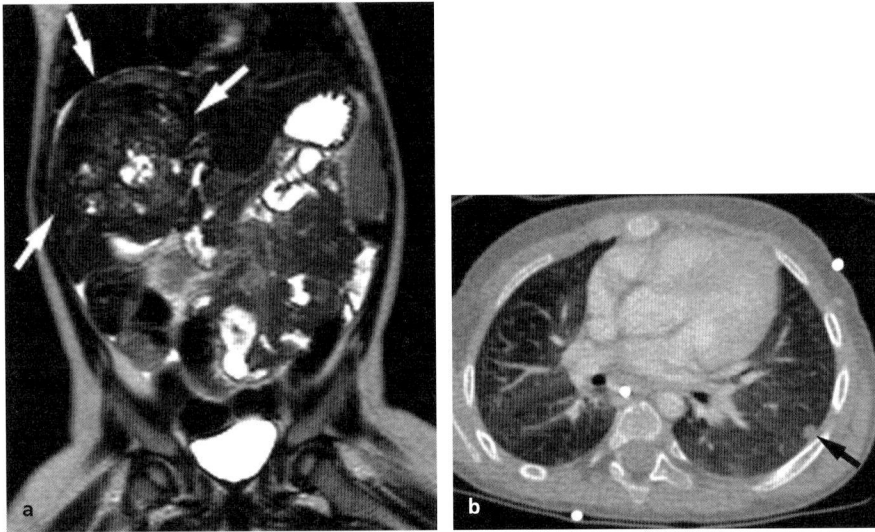

Figure 16.1 Cross-sectional imaging of hepatoblastoma. (a), Coronal magnetic resonance image of the abdomen shows a large heterogeneous liver tumor (arrows) arising from the right lobe. (b), Computed tomography shows a lung metastasis (arrow).

Table 16.4 Classic staging.

Stage I	No metastatic disease, tumor completely resected
Stage II	No metastatic disease, microscopic residual disease after resection of tumor, or tumor rupture (including tumor spill at the time of surgery)
Stage III	No distant metastases, tumor unresectable or resected with gross residual disease, or lymph node metastases
Stage IV	Distant metastases, irrespective of local extent of tumor

87 ng/ml were within the 95.5% interval (assumed logarithmic normal distribution). By the age of 2 years the infants in this study still had not reached adult serum AFP levels (0–6 ng/ml) [50].

Staging systems
The Children's Oncology Group staging of hepatoblastoma
This staging system includes treatment (resection) as one important criterion (Table 16.4).

PRETEXT
To compare results of different trials it is best to use a system which does not include any treatment variables. The TNM system avoids this pitfall but is not very suitable for HB since lymph nodes (N) at least in hepatoblastoma do not feature prominently or affect the prognosis, and there is no clear correlation between size (T) and outcome.

The PRETEXT (PRETreatment EXTent of disease) system was developed specifically for primary liver tumors. It is based on Couinaud's system of segmentation of the liver (Figure 16.2), because this best predicts the possibility of liver resection. The PRETEXT system was adopted by the SIOPEL group and found to be of prognostic significance when the results of the first SIOPEL trial were analyzed [51].

The system has needed refinements and for practical purposes clearer definitions to keep abreast of the great improvements in surgical techniques and imaging since it was originally conceived (Figure 16.2) [52]. In the 2005 revision the extent of liver involvement is graded from PRETEXT I to PRETEXT IV, and additional criteria are used to describe other potential risk factors for poor outcome (Table 16.5).

In children with HCC without cirrhosis, which is the majority, the PRETEXT staging can be applied because liver function is normal. In contrast, in adults with HCC the function of the liver is included in the predictive staging system.

Predictive staging systems for HCC in adults
There are a variety of predictive staging systems for HCC in use in adults. These are: 'Milan', 'BCLC-Barcelona Clinic Liver Cancer' [53], 'CLIP-Cancer of the Italian Liver Program', 'JIS-Japanese Integrated System', 'TNM', 'Okuda', as well as the original 'Childs-Pugh' system [54]. They all include some form of functional assessment of the liver which can restrict the indications for surgery and transplantation.

Recommendations for biopsy
The necessity for a biopsy in presumed HB is still controversial. The diagnosis of a solitary HB can, at the age of 6 months to 3 years, be confidently made on clinical, laboratory, and imaging findings alone. Rare exceptions do exist but since pre-operative chemotherapy is standard treatment most oncologists and a number of clinical trials require a firm diagnosis before commencing. Treating a benign or a different tumor with chemotherapy could be considered a serious error.

A laparoscopic or 'open' surgical biopsy is considered preferable by some, but the SIOPEL group currently recommends image-guided coaxial plugged needle biopsy (obtaining numerous cores), which appears to give equivalent results. Although

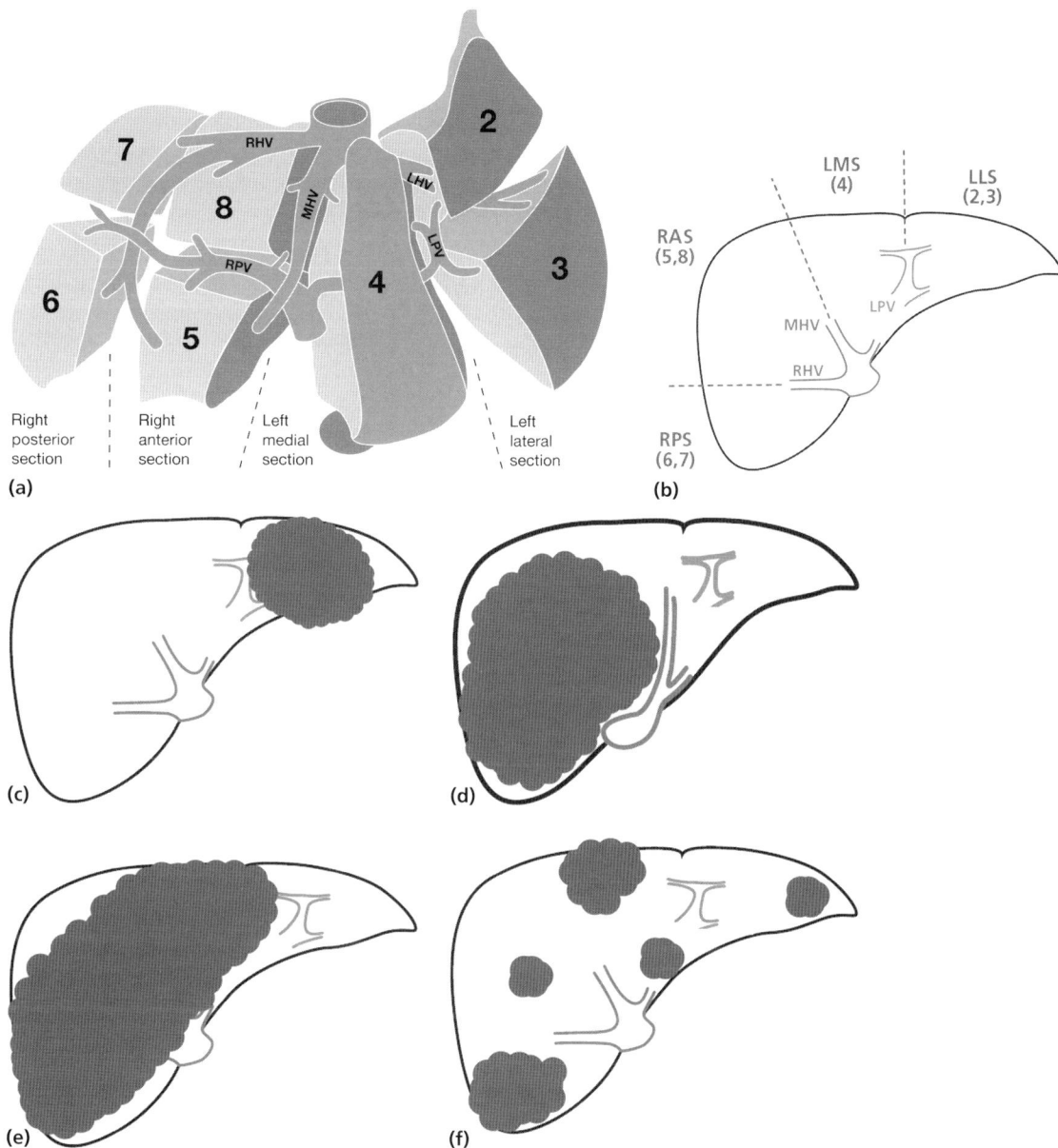

Figure 16.2 Couinaud's system of segmentation of the liver and PRETEXT grouping. (a), Exploded anterior view of the segmental anatomy of the liver. Couinaud's segments 2 to 8 are labeled. The umbilical portion of the left portal vein (LPV) separates the left medial section from the left lateral section. RPV, right portal vein. RHV, right hepatic vein. MHV, middle hepatic vein. LHV, left hepatic vein. (b), Transverse section of the liver showing the planes of the major venous structures used to assign a patient to a PRETEXT group. The hepatic and portal veins define the sections of the liver (segment numerals in parentheses). This schematic diagram shows how the RHV and MHV indicate the borders of the right posterior (RPS) and right anterior (RAS) sections and the left medial section (LMS). Note that the LPV actually lies caudal to the confluence of the hepatic veins and is not usually seen in the same transverse image. LLS, left lateral section. (c), PRETEXT I. This type is relatively unusual as liver tumors tend to be large at the time of presentation. (d), The most common form of PRETEXT II is a tumor arising in the right lobe of the liver. (e), The most common form of PRETEXT III is a large solitary mass. (f), Multifocal PRETEXT IV. (From Roebuck DJ, Aronson D, Clapuyt P, et al. 2005 PRETEXT: a revised staging system for primary malignant liver tumors of childhood developed by the SIOPEL group. Pediatr Radiol 2007; 37: 123–32.)

Table 16.5 2005 PRETEXT revision: summary of significant changes from the original PRETEXT system.

	Original PRETEXT	2005 PRETEXT
Involvement of segment 1 (caudate lobe) (C)	Segment 1 not considered	All tumors involving segment 1 are at least PRETEXT II by definition, involvement also coded as C1
Extrahepatic abdominal disease (E)	E+ included direct extension and abdominal lymph node involvement	Lymph node metastases not included
Metastatic disease (M)	M+ included distant lymph node metastasis	Lymph node metastases not included
Lymph node metastases (N)	Included in E+ and/or M+	Considered separately (N1, N2)
Tumour focality (F)	Not considered	Multifocal tumor = F1
Tumour rupture (H)	Not considered	Tumour rupture = H1

fine needle aspiration cytology (FNA) can be used, it is not accepted by most clinical trials.

Either surgical or needle biopsy may provide pre-treatment tumor tissue for biological studies. A protocol for the examination of hepatoblastoma tissue specimens has recently been published [55].

Histopathology and cytogenetics

Hepatoblastoma

The currently used histological classification is still based on morphology. However, with more results from clinical trials it will become necessary to elaborate the system and also to include biological criteria to allow for more refined treatment stratification.

• The present system is based on the epithelial components of hepatoblastoma (Table 16.6) although mesenchymal elements usually co-exist. The mesenchymal component may resemble osteoid. Hepatoblastomas arise from a precursor to the mature hepatocyte and therefore display many histological patterns [56].

• The small cell undifferentiated type is said to have a poor prognosis and the fetal type a good prognosis. The fetal type is reported in smaller series and only the 'pure fetal' subtype has an excellent prognosis and requires no chemotherapy. Only patients with completely resected tumors at diagnosis can fall into this category.

Aqcuired genetic changes in HB most commonly involve chromosome 20 or 8, sometimes in conjunction with complex structural changes and often in association with double-minute chromosomes [57–59]. Some changes are thought to be associated with poor outcome.

• The translocation t(1:4)(q12;q34) has been described in association with a trisomy in patients with high-risk HB.

• Amplification at 8q11.2-q13 (at the level for the *PLAG1* gene) has been found in poor prognosis HB, which could implicate insulin-like growth factor 2 (IGF2) in the pathogenesis of HB [60].

• Loss of heterozygosity at chromosome 11p15 is shared with other tumors including Wilms' tumor and rhabdomyosarcoma.

Table 16.6 Histopathological types of hepatoblastoma.

Embryonal

Relatively undifferentiated – primitive tubules formed by small epithelial cells with minimal cytoplasm are very similar to the liver of 6–8 week embryos.

Fetal

Relatively differentiated resembling mature hepatocytes – cords of uniform neoplastic hepatocytes smaller than normal cells of the fetal liver with a higher nuclear to cytoplasmic ratio.

Anaplastic

Small cell undifferentiated (SCUD) – these can be intermingled with epithelial tubules or form discrete nodules. These cells may be more resistant to chemotherapy. The small foci may be missed in small biopsies.

Macrotrabecular

Resembling hepatocellular carcinoma – when hepatoblastoma cells with either fetal or embryonal cytology grow in trabeculae of 20–100 or more cells rather than in the 2–4-cell thick cords of the fetal liver.

Mixed

This type contains diverse histological features. There may be nests of keratinizing squamous epithelium, or zones of elongated spindle cells having the cross striations of rhabdomyoblasts or contain clusters of hematopoietic cells as in normal fetal liver.

• Several studies have shown involvement of beta-catenin, which in tumors is localized in the nucleus whereas it is on the plasma membrane in normal hepatocytes. Mutation of *CTNNB1*, the beta-catenin gene, occurs in up to 48% of HBs [61], and this is associated with more aggressive tumors [62].

Hepatocellular carcinoma

Classification of HCC is based on the World Health Organization system, which includes four histological patterns and four cytological variants. There are three or four grades according to the degree of differentiation. The fibroamellar variant, which is etiologically and biologically distinct, occurs more commonly in adolescents and adults [63]. There is also a transitional type, recently described by Zimmermann's group, which is histologically intermediate between HB and HCC [64].

Principles for the treatment of hepatic tumors

Hepatoblastoma

> The SIOPEL strategy differs to the COG strategy in that it advocates preoperative chemotherapy for all patients, whereas COG use primary surgery for PRETEXT I and some PRETEXT II disease

Historically, two different approaches have been practised. In North America, primary surgery is still advocated, partly influenced by the fact that trials there began before the benefits of pre-operative chemotherapy were fully appreciated. In Europe, apart from Germany, most institutions advocate and practise neo-adjuvant therapy. It should be said that most surgeons now appreciate the advantages of pre-operative chemotherapy, not only because about 40% of tumors are unresectable at diagnosis and about half of these can be converted to become resectable, but also because the margins become clearer and the risk of intra-operative bleeding decreases.

Hepatocellular carcinoma

In HCC the situation is somewhat different, and primary surgery is the rule when feasible. Again many are unresectable at diagnosis, often due to the presence of multiple lesions as well as the size.

Surgery

As already stated both HB and HCC require surgical resection for cure. In general, only the standard anatomical resections are oncologically sound in surgery for malignant tumors (Figure 16.3).
• These are based on the classical eight segments described by Couinaud [65].
• The terms right and left lobectomy should be discarded in surgical descriptions. Right and left hepatectomy is more appropriate; also, extended right hepatectomy (right tri-segmentectomy) or extended left hepatectomy (left tri-segmentectomy).

Where liver function is normal and there is no underlying hepatic disorder, most children with a resectable tumor on imaging can be considered candidates for surgery. Radical resection can be obtained either conventionally by partial hepatectomy or with orthotopic liver transplant, but the surgical approach to hepatoblastoma differs considerably across the world. Good survival rates in hepatoblastoma patients who have received a primary transplant after a good response to chemotherapy support the strategy of avoiding partial hepatectomy in cases where radical resection appears difficult and doubtful [66].

Surgical techniques

> Surgery remains the mainstay of treatment for all liver tumors

In a chapter of this type it is not possible to go into the details, advances, and intricacies of surgical techniques. The resection techniques are similar to those used in adults (Figure 16.3). Depending on the preferences of the surgeon and the given anatomical conditions, either the hepatic veins are ligated and divided first, extrahepatically, followed by dissection and ligation of the hilar vessels and biliary structures of the corresponding part of the liver to be resected or vice versa. The parenchyma is divided using any of various techniques (Table 16.7).

Exposure of the liver and its ligaments is usually somewhat easier in young children, so that thoraco-abdominal incisions are rarely necessary. Vascular occlusion techniques, either total or partial, have been used more frequently in children. Resection techniques used range from finger fracture (Ton That Tung), US dissection, water jet dissection, laser beam hemostasis, and ligation of vessels, both centripetal and centrifugal (Lortat Jacob) [67].

Surgical margins and microscopic residual disease
Traditionally, a line of resection leaving a margin of healthy tissue of one to two centimetres has been recommended to minimize local recurrence (empirically and from retrospective studies).

It is now clear that a smaller margin is sometimes quite adequate in chemosensitive tumors which have 'shrunk' before surgery. SIOPEL and others have shown that even with evidence of microscopic residual disease (as determined by examination of the resected specimen), local recurrence rarely occurs after pre-operative chemotherapy [68].

Post-operative monitoring after resection
The functional reserve of the liver is extensive, and regeneration effective, so that up to four-fifths can be resected without serious side effects. Nevertheless careful monitoring of important functional metabolic parameters, e.g. prothrombin time, glucose, and biliribin are necessary in the early post-operative phase. Post-operative chemotherapy does not interfere to any great extent with wound healing or regeneration, and it is therefore advised to restart chemotherapy 10 to 15 days after surgery or liver transplant if there are no post-operative complications.

Liver transplantation
Hepatoblastoma
Liver transplantation is the most radical form of resection possible. The shortage of cadaver livers has in the past prevented more widespread use of this method in malignant disease. Living donor transplantation has to a large extent alleviated this problem. The risk involved to the healthy donor has been shown to be minimal.

Preliminary results in children transplanted for unresectable HB are surprisingly good so that this option can now be

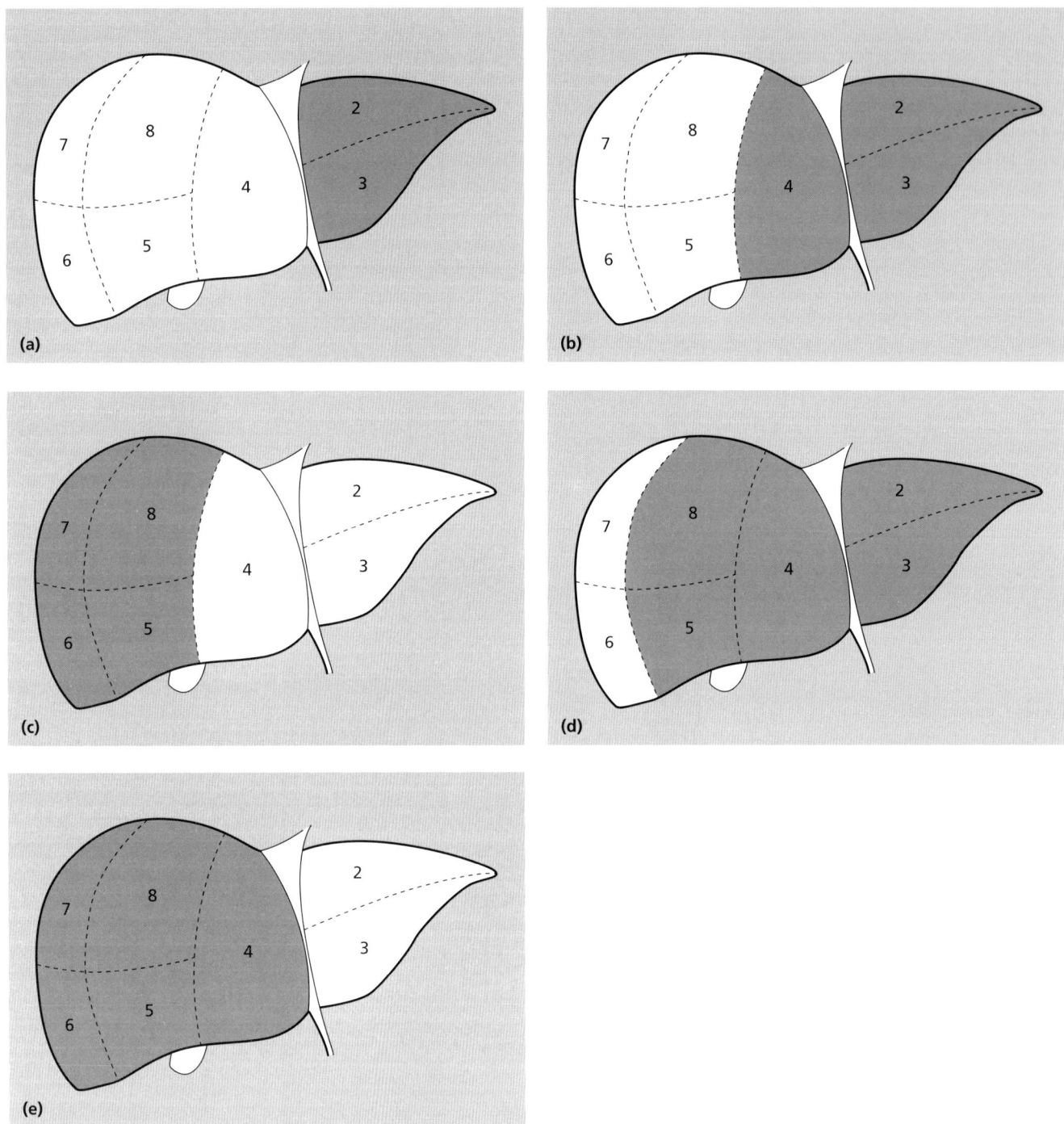

Figure 16.3 Options for partial hepatectomy. (a), Left lateral sectionectomy. (b), Left hemihepatectomy. (c), Right hemihepatectomy. (d), Extended left hemihepatectomy. (e), Extended right hemihepatectomy. (From Czauderna P, Otte JB, Roebuck DJ, et al. Surgical treatment of hepatoblastoma in children. Pediatr Radiol 2006; 36: 187–91.)

recommended in particular for chemosensitive tumors with an otherwise fatal outcome.

In multifocal (and solitary) HB invading all four liver sectors, and in centrally located tumors with close proximity to the major veins, the SIOPEL-1 study and an extensive review of the world experience have shown that primary transplantation provides a

long-term disease-free survival rate of about 80%. These children should be treated only in specialized centers [69, 70].

Hepatocellular carcinoma
The optimum selection criteria for liver transplant in HCC have still to be determined. However, patients with a good response to

chemotherapy who are in metastatic remission should not be refused liver transplant with a living donor.

Regional therapy

The dual blood supply of the liver from hepatic arteries and the portal vein makes hepatic tumors particularly suitable for arterial chemoembolization. The main indication in children has been as a bridge to transplantation, although unresectable tumors or recurrence may be successfully treated in this way [71]. An alternative technique, radioembolization with yttrium-90 microspheres, has been used in a few children. Both these techniques have a significant incidence of complications, and require equipment and expertise that is not available in all children's cancer centers. Other local therapies (e.g. percutaneous ethanol injection and radiofrequency ablation) are rarely used in children.

Summary of major findings of successive cooperative group studies in hepatoblastoma

The cooperative studies which have been carried out over the past two decades in various parts of the world have clearly shown that cisplatin combination chemotherapy together with surgery provides the best treatment outcome for HB. These studies have also revealed a number of prognostic factors in HB Tables (17.7–17.10).

Summary of major findings of successive cooperative group studies in hepatocellular carcinoma

The first study of the SIOPEL group (SIOPEL 1) [85] and the Intergroup Hepatoma Study (INT-0098) [84] included patients with HCC as well as HB. In SIOPEL 1 HCC was often advanced at the time of diagnosis; metastases were identified in 31% of the children and extrahepatic tumor extension, vascular invasion, or

Table 16.7 Major findings for successive North American trials for treatment of hepatoblastoma.

Study	Strategy	Patients (n)	Chemotherapy	Stage	Outcome	References
CCSG 1976–78	Primary surgery	62	Vincristine Cyclophosphamide 5FU Doxorubicin		3-year OS 30%	[72]
CCSG-823F 1986–89	Primary surgery	47	Cisplatin Doxorubicin		2-year EFS 66.6%	[73]
POG 8697 1986–89	Primary surgery	60	Cisplatin Vincristine 5FU	I(UH) and II III IV	3-year DFS 91% + −9.2% 67% + −10.8% 12.55% + −11.75%	[74]
INT-0098 Intergroup Hepatoma Study 1989–92	Primary surgery	173	Cisplatin Vincristine 5FU vs Cisplatin Doxorubicin		3 year OS 71% 3 year EFS 63%	[75]
P9645 Liver Tumor Study	Primary surgery	53	Cisplatin Vincristine 5FU vs	Stage III & IV	1 year EFS 57%	[76]
		56	Cisplatin Carboplatin		1 year EFS 37%	

OS, overall survival. EFS, event-free survival. DFS, disease-free survival.

Table 16.8 Major findings for successive German trials for treatment of hepatoblastoma.

Study	Strategy	Patients (n)	Chemotherapy	Stage	Outcome	References
CGP-HB89 1988–1993	Primary surgery	72	Ifosfamide Cisplatin Doxorubicin	I II III IV	DFS 75% median FU 64 months 100% 50% 71% 29%	[77]
CGP-HB94	Primary surgery	48	Ifosfamide Cisplatin Doxorubicin	Standard risk	Overall survival Median follow up 58 months 77%	[78]
		18	Etoposide Carboplatin	Advanced or recurrent		[79]

Table 16.9 Major findings for successive SIOPEL trials for treatment of hepatoblastoma.

Study	Strategy	Patients (*n*)	Chemotherapy	PRETEXT		Outcome	References
SIOPEL 1 1990–94	Primary chemotherapy*	154	Cisplatin Doxorubicin			3y OS 79% 3y EFS 67% 3y EFS by PRETEXT	[80] [81]
				I		100%	
				II		83%	
				III		59%	
				IV		44%	
				and metastases		28%	
SIOPEL 2 1995–98	Primary chemotherapy	Standard risk 77	Cisplatin			3y OS 91% PFS 89%	[82]
		High risk 58	Alternating cisplatin, carboplatin/doxorubicin			3y OS 53% PFS 48%	

* PRETEXT I were eligible for primary surgery > OS, overall survival. EFS, event-free survival. PFS, progression-free survival.

Table 16.10 Major findings for successive Japanese trials for treatment of hepatoblastoma.

Study [83]	Strategy	Patients (*n*)	Chemotherapy	Stage	Outcome
JPLT-1 1991–1999	Mixed	145 HB	Cisplatin THP Adriamycin		3/6 year OS 77.8%/73.4%
				I	100%/100%
				II	100%/95.7%
				III A	76.6%/73.8%
				III B	50.3%/50.3%
				IV	64.8%/38.9%

THP, tetrahydropyranil. OS, overall survival.

Table 16.11 Major findings of both North American and SIOPEL trials in hepatocellular carcinoma.

Study	Strategy	Patients (*n*)	Chemotherapy	Outcome	References
INT-0098 Intergroup Hepatoma Study 1989–92	Primary surgery	46	Cisplatin Vincristine 5FU vs Cisplatin Doxorubicin	5y EFS overall 19%	[84]
SIOPEL 1 1990–94	Primary chemotherapy	40	Cisplatin Doxorubicin	5y OS 28% EFS 17%	[85]

OS, overall survival. EFS, event-free survival.

both in 39%. Multifocal tumors were common (56%). Thirty-three per cent of tumors were associated with cirrhosis. Partial response to pre-operative cisplatin and doxorubicin (PLADO) chemotherapy was observed in 49% and complete tumor resection was achieved in 36%. Overall survival (OS) at 5 years was 28% and event-free survival (EFS) 17%.

In INT-0098 46 patients with HCC were enrolled and randomized to treatment with either cisplatin (CDDP), vincristine, and fluorouracil (regimen A) or CDDP and continuous-infusion doxorubicin (regimen B). For the entire cohort, the 5-year EFS estimate was 19% with no difference between regimen A and B.

Outcome was considerably worse in both studies for HCC compared with HB.

The current SIOPEL 5 trial, specifically designed for HCC, retained PLADO chemotherapy with the addition of thalidomide as an anti-angiogenic agent.

Early complications of treatment

The main complications are due to chemotherapy. In settings where full in-patient supportive care is not available, the mortality from intensive chemotherapy is still prohibitive. Fortunately, this is less of a risk when cisplatin is used as a single agent. This is why in resource-challenged nations cisplatin monotherapy for HB is being encouraged as a first-line therapy. Surgical morbidity has reduced with improved techniques and with the introduction of delayed surgery after pre-operative chemotherapy.

It has been claimed that complications of surgery for hepatoblastoma are not greater in primary surgery than in delayed post-chemotherapy surgery. This may apply to surgeons working in highly specialized liver surgery centers but in international trials the standard varies widely..

Determinants of prognosis

The 5-year survival from HB diagnosed during the period 1988–1997 was 63% overall, and ranged from 52% in Eastern Europe to 84% in the North. Survival from HCC was much lower (37%). Between 1978 and 1982 and 1993 and 1997, 5-year survival increased from 28% (95% confidence interval [95% CI] 18–39) to 66% (95% CI 55–74) for HB and from 17% (95% CI 6–33) to 50% (95% CI 26–70) for HCC. These increases reflect the impact of advances in treatment of childhood liver cancer at a population level [10]. For hepatoblastoma, a number of clinical trials have identified the following prognostic associations:
• Tumour resectability is the most important prognostic factor. This is reflected by stage III/IV or PRETEXT IV; involvement of hepatic veins or portal veins being poor prognostic factors.
• The presence of metastatic disease [51, 86].
• Low AFP, as noted above.

> Most hepatoblastomas are standard risk; high risk is defined as one of the following: metastases, PRETEXT IV involvement of the main portal vein or both its branches or all three hepatic veins, or serum AFP less than 100 ng/ml

In hepatocellular carcinoma the maximum diameter and number of nodules in the liver is also important as a determinant of prognosis, as an indicator of tumor resectability.

Strategies for follow up and overview of important late effects

Treatment for liver tumors relies on a combination of chemotherapy, surgery, and sometimes immunotherapy. In the case of HCC, antiangiogenic drug therapy may also be added. Follow up requires monitoring of the effects of the tumor and potential recurrence as well as the side effects of the treatment [87]. If liver transplant has been required then the follow up of the transplanted liver is the key component of continuing care.

Monitoring for recurrence

> Three-monthly monitoring of serum AFP and imaging, with US of the liver and chest radiography, is advisable for the first 3 years after stopping treatment

In the first year after stopping treatment regular monitoring of the serum tumor marker AFP, US of the liver and plain radiographs of the chest will be sufficient. If a patient is on a clinical trial then it is necessary to monitor according to the frequency requested in the trial. If the patient is not on a trial then 3-monthly follow up in the first year is probably adequate. It is wise, however, to follow the serum AFP more regularly until at least two consecutive normal values have been obtained. The rebound phenomenon, which occurs in the remaining liver in the weeks after surgery, can cause a rise in serum AFP. In general the serum AFP does not exceed 100 ng/ml after surgery unless tumor is still present. However, the serum AFP may not normalize for a number of weeks or even months after surgery. The trend should be towards normalization at 3 months post-surgery.

In the second and third year after stopping treatment monitoring can be less frequent. However, in a number of clinical trials 3-monthly serum AFP monitoring and imaging is maintained. In hepatoblastoma the likelihood of relapse after 3 years of follow up is less than 5%. In hepatocellular carcinoma this is less certain. Monitoring for recurrence up to 5 years is probably advisable in all patients.

Monitoring for side-effects of surgery

Side-effects of surgical resection are usually apparent early on in the post-operative period. These are commonly problems of bleeding or infection.

Monitoring for rejection and the side effects of liver transplant immunotherapy

Rejection and virally-induced lymphoproliferative disease (LPD) are the main concerns. The incidence of LPD varies according to the series and the type of immunotherapy used. Very close monitoring of patients post-transplant with early intervention should reduce this risk [88].

Monitoring for side-effects of chemotherapy

This is clearly related to the type, administration, and total cumulative dose of the chemotherapy administered.

Cisplatin

This is the most effective agent for the treatment of liver tumors but unfortunately carries a high risk of permanent renal and ototoxicity.

Monitor GFR, serum magnesium, and hearing

The renal toxicity has been relatively well controlled in liver tumor trials by reducing the total cumulative dose and by ensuring adequate chloride load in the administration fluid and a high rate of fluid throughput before and after the cisplatin infusion. Cisplatin toxicity affects both the glomerular filtration rate (GFR) and the tubular re-uptake of magnesium.

• The GFR following cisplatin treatment can, in young children, recover slightly within the first 2 years after stopping treatment [89]. This is not the case after treatment with ifosfamide when the GFR is likely to deteriorate further in the first year after stopping treatment.

• However, the proximal tubular function reflected by serum magnesium does not behave in the same way and can further deteriorate a number of years later. The simplest way of measuring the re-uptake of magnesium is by monitoring serum magnesium in a child who has not taken any magnesium supplements for a week.

Ototoxicity is bilateral and permanent and reflects the damage to the outer hair-cells of the cochlea. Although this does not improve with time there is slightly conflicting data in the literature on this, probably due to the fact that obtaining good audiometry in young children is difficult and concomitant middle ear infection or serous otitis media must be ruled out every time a child is tested. In North America, hearing is assessed according to the ASHA criteria. In Europe and many parts of the world cisplatin ototoxicity is graded by the Brock criteria. The Brock grading was designed for children receiving cisplatin chemotherapy for malignancy and assumed that baseline behavioral audiometry would be difficult to obtain accurately in a sick young child.

• The system assumes normal hearing at the time of starting treatment and allows for comparison of results between patients at the end or after the end of treatment when the child is well enough to cooperate with full pure-tone audiometry.

• The Brock grade correlates well with functional outcome although when grade 0 (minimal) is measured high-frequency hearing loss at the 30 dB range at 8000 Hz cannot be excluded. Therefore it is important when using the Brock grading not to assume that grade 0 equates to normal hearing [90].

The Germans have developed their own grading: again, however, this is a comparative system measuring hearing loss compared with baseline. It does, however, work well in older patients who can undergo baseline hearing testing prior to starting cisplatin chemotherapy. This is the case in most patients with medulloblastoma who get their surgery and radiotherapy prior to

starting chemotherapy and will also be the case for many patients with hepatocellular carcinoma who are older and more co-operative at the time of diagnosis.

Carboplatin

Monitor GFR, serum magnesium, and hearing

Carboplatin is less organ toxic than cisplatin. However, in combination with cisplatin it can give increased overall toxicity particularly to the ear. A number of treatment protocols for liver tumors advocate combined treatment and therefore toxicity monitoring in this situation is particularly important. In certain treatment protocols, at relapse or in high risk disease, high-dose carboplatin followed by peripheral blood stem cell rescue is used. High-dose carboplatin is in itself organ toxic and the follow up should then become similar to that of cisplatin [91].

Doxorubicin

Monitor cardiac function

Anthracyclines cause irreversible cardiomyocyte damage, and this is particularly serious in young children. If severe, compensatory ventricular hypertrophy will develop. The most important prognostic echocardiogram is that done at the end or 6 weeks after the end of treatment. However, life-long monitoring of cardiac function is advised for all patients who have received anthracyclines. Even if the echocardiogram is within normal limits this should be repeated every 5 years as a precaution, because early treatment of potential cardiac failure can be effective [92]

Vincristine

Monitor peripheral neuropathy

The neurotoxicity caused by vincristine is combined mesenteric and peripheral limb neurotoxicity. Vincristine can cause central nervous system toxicity but this is short term and will not present a problem at follow up if it has not been an issue during treatment. The constipation caused by the mesenteric toxicity is also mainly short term and needs to be actively counteracted during treatment. Normal bowel movements should be present again in the first few months after stopping treatment. The peripheral limb neuropathy, however, can take months to normalize. Most patients are not aware of their pathology until they realize that their mobility and balance has improved and are pleasantly surprised by their improved co-ordination and success in sport.

During treatment tendon reflexes are likely to be absent. These will gradually reappear over a period of months depending on the total cumulative dose of vincristine administered.

Fluorouracil

Fluorouracil is widely used in North American protocols and produces no known long-term problems.

Etoposide

Consider second cancers

Second cancers are the most serious potential long-term side effect of etoposide, but are rare after treatment of liver tumors. This is most likely due to the type of schedule administered and the low cumulative dose.

Novel therapeutic approaches

Novel therapeutic approaches are clearly required in both high-risk HB and in HCC.

High-risk hepatoblastoma

One approach in high-risk HR is dose-dense cisplatin (SIOPEL 4). Aggressive surgery to the lungs is also being more widely advocated, as with other malignancies. Hepatoblastoma is considered radio-sensitive and therefore this treatment modality may be useful for lung metastases, albeit at a limited dose as in Wilms' tumor. As the molecular biology of hepatoblastoma is better elucidated then more targeted therapy may become an option. AFP used for diagnosis and response monitoring might be used in future targeted antibody or vaccine-mediated therapy [93].

Hepatocellular carcinoma

This tumor is known to be highly angiogenic and is often large at the time of diagnosis. A new approach being currently tried is to combine standard chemotherapy with anti-angiogenic treatment. There are a number of potential anti-angiogenic agents, but not many have been sufficiently tested in children to be introduced immediately into the Phase III clinical trial setting. Further development of antiangiogenic therapy might even lead to antiangiogenic gene therapy [94].

Summary and future directions for management

Enormous strides have been made over the last two decades in the treatment of HB and in the eradication of endemic hepatitis B-related HCC. The introduction of combined cisplatin-containing chemotherapy together with aggressive surgery to both liver and lungs has improved the survival for HB worldwide. The introduction of combined chemotherapy and surgery has also improved the outcome in HCC, but to a much lesser degree.

Hepatoblastoma

Strategies for maintaining efficacy but reducing the long-term toxicity of cisplatin need to be sought. One such approach is the introduction of the chemoprotectant sodium thiosulfate [95–97] in a randomized clinical trial for standard risk hepatoblastoma (SIOPEL 6). Alternative platinum agents have not yet been found to be as effective; however, future agents might be. Alternative chemotherapy needs to be tested in both animal xenograft models and then in clinical trials. Because of the small numbers of relapsing patients worldwide collaboration will be necessary in order for this to be successful. In resource-challenged nations the use of cisplatin should be pursued. It is possible to give cisplatin in different ways – even in an outpatient setting in split doses, if this is the only resource available.

Hepatocellular carcinoma

Vaccination strategies for hepatitis B need to be sustained in areas where they have been successful and introduced in any areas where they are not yet completely distributed. In the future, endemic hepatitis B-related HCC should be eradicated. However, hepatitis C-related disease is more of a challenge. Treatment of hepatitis C carriers with interferon should be encouraged. Ultrasound screening programs for carriers of hepatitis C should reduce the mortality of HCC through early diagnosis of operable tumors. Enlarging the guidelines for liver transplant in this disease and the increasing experience in living-related liver transplant may also improve outcome.

Acknowledgement

Oliver Joris for tireless typing.

References

1 Miller RW, Young JL Jr, Novakovic B. Cancer 1995; 75: 395–405.
2 Perilongo G, Shafford EA. Liver tumors. Eur J Cancer 1999; 35: 953–8; discussion 958–9.
3 Stocker JT. Hepatic tumors in children. Clin Liver Dis 2001; 5: 259–81, viii–ix.
4 Weinberg AG, Finegold, MJ. Primary hepatic tumors of childhood. Hum Pathol 1983; 14: 512–32.
5 Christison-Lagay ER, Burrows PE, Alomari A, et al. Hepatic hemangiomas: subtype classification and development of a clinical practice algorithm and registry. J Pediatr Surg 2007; 42: 62–8.
6 Meyers RL, Scaife ER. Benign liver and biliary tract masses in infants and toddlers. Semin Pediatr Surg 2000; 9: 146–55.
7 Catanzarite V, Hilfiker M, Daneshmand S, et al. Prenatal diagnosis of fetal hepatoblastoma: case report and review of the literature. J Ultrasound Med 2008; 7: 1095–8.

8 von Schweinitz D. Neonatal liver tumors. Semin Neonatol 2003; 8: 403–10.

9 Buckley JD, Sather H, Ruccione K, et al. A case-control study of risk factors for hepatoblastoma. A report from the Childrens Cancer Study Group. Cancer 1989; 64: 1169–76.

10 Stiller CA, Pritchard J, Steliarova-Foucher E. Liver cancer in European children: incidence and survival, 1978–1997. Report from the Automated Childhood Cancer Information System project. Eur J Cancer 2006; 42: 2115–23.

11 Mann JR, Kasthuri N, Raafat F, et al. Malignant hepatic tumors in children: incidence, clinical features and aetiology. Paediatr Perinat Epidemiol 1990; 4: 276–89.

12 Darbari A, Sabin KM, Shapiro CN, et al. Epidemiology of primary hepatic malignancies in US children. Hepatology 2003; 38: 560–6.

13 Linabery AM, Ross JA. Trends in childhood cancer incidence in the US (1992–2004). Cancer 2008; 112: 416–32.

14 Moore SW, Millar AJ, Hadley GP, et al. Hepatocellular carcinoma and liver tumors in South African children: a case for increased prevalence. Cancer 2004; 101: 642–9.

15 Tan TY, Amor DJ. Tumour surveillance in Beckwith-Wiedemann syndrome and hemihyperplasia: a critical review of the evidence and suggested guidelines for local practice. J Paediatr Child Health 2006; 42: 486–90.

16 Aretz S, Koch A, Uhlhaas S, et al. Should children at risk for familial adenomatous polyposis be screened for hepatoblastoma and children with apparently sporadic hepatoblastoma be screened for APC germline mutations? Pediatr Blood Cancer 2006; 47: 811–8.

17 Ikeda M , Matsuyama S, Tanimura M. Association between hepatoblastoma and very low birth weight; a trend or a chance? J Pediatr 1997; 130: 557–60.

18 Trobaugh-Lotrario AD, Greffe B, Garza-Williams S, et al. Erythropoietin receptor presence in hepatoblastoma: a possible link to increased incidence of hepatoblastoma in very low birthweight infants. Pediatr Blood Cancer 2007; 49: 365–6.

19 Feusner J, Plaschkes J. Hepotablastoma and low birth weight: a trend or chance observation? Med Pediatr Oncol 2002; 39: 508–9.

20 Spector LG, Feusner JH, Ross JA. Hepatoblastoma and low birth weight. Pediatr Blood Cancer 2004; 43: 706.

21 Brock PR, Yeomans EC, Bellman SC, et al. Cisplatin therapy in infants: short and long-term morbidity. Br J Cancer Suppl 1992; 18: S36–40.

22 Kapfer SA, Petruzzi MJ, Caty MG. Hepatoblastoma in low birth weight infants: an institutional review. Pediatr Surg Int 2004; 20: 753–6.

23 McMahon BJ, Lanier AP, Wainwright RB. Hepatitis B and hepatocellular carcinoma in Eskimo/Inuit population. Int J Circumpolar Health 1998; 57 (Suppl 1): 414–9.

24 Coursaget P, Maupas P, Goudeau A, et al. Primary hepatocellular carcinoma in intertropical Africa: relationship between age and hepatitis B virus etiology. J Natl Cancer Inst 1980; 65: 687–90.

25 Sun TT, Chu YR, Ni ZQ, et al. A pilot study on universal immunization of newborn infants in an area of hepatitis B virus and primary hepatocellular carcinoma prevalence with a low dose of hepatitis B vaccine. J Cell Physiol Suppl 1986; 4: 83–90.

26 Chang MH. Cancer prevention by vaccination against hepatitis B. Recent results. Cancer Res 2009; 181: 85–94.

27 Chang MH, Chen CJ, Lai MS, et al. Universal hepatitis B vaccination in Taiwan and the incidence of hepatocellular carcinoma in children.

Taiwan Childhood Hepatoma Study Group. N Engl J Med 1997; 336: 1855–9.

28 Chang MH, Chen DS. Prospects for hepatitis B virus eradication and control of hepatocellular carcinoma. Baillieres Best Pract Res Clin Gastroenterol 1999; 13: 511–7.

29 Huang K, Lin S. Nationwide vaccination: a success story in Taiwan. Vaccine 2000; 18 (Suppl 1): S35–8.

30 Kane MA. Global control of primary hepatocellular carcinoma with hepatitis B vaccine: the contributions of research in Taiwan. Cancer Epidemiol Biomarkers Prev 2003; 12: 2–3.

31 Montesano R. Hepatitis B immunization and hepatocellular carcinoma: the Gambia Hepatitis Intervention. J Med Virol 2002; 67: 444–6.

32 Moore SW, Davidson A, Hadley GP, et al. Malignant liver tumors in South African children: a national audit. World J Surg 2008; 32: 1389–95.

33 Wichajarn K, Kosalaraksa P, Wiangnon S. Incidence of hepatocellular carcinoma in children in Khon Kaen before and after national hepatitis B vaccine program. Asian Pac J Cancer Prev 2008; 9: 507–10.

34 Heyward WL, Lanier AP, McMahon BJ, et al. Early detection of primary hepatocellular carcinoma. Screening for primary hepatocellular carcinoma among persons infected with hepatitis B virus. JAMA 1985; 254: 3052–4.

35 Hadley GP, Govender D, Landers G. Primary tumors of the liver in children: an African perspective. Pediatr Surg Int 2004; 20: 314–8.

36 Wu TC, Tong MJ, Hwang B, et al. Primary hepatocellular carcinoma and hepatitis B infection during childhood. Hepatology 1987; 7: 46–8.

37 Cheah PL, Looi LM, Lin HP, et al. Childhood primary hepatocellular carcinoma and hepatitis B virus infection. Cancer 1990; 65: 174–6.

38 Kiyosawa K, Umemura T, Ichijo T, et al. Hepatocellular carcinoma: recent trends in Japan. Gastroenterology 2004; 127(Suppl. 1): S17–26.

39 Bosch FX, Ribes J, Diaz M, et al. Primary liver cancer: worldwide incidence and trends. Gastroenterology 2004; 127(Suppl. 1): S5–S16.

40 Ishak KG. Inherited metabolic diseases of the liver. Clin Liver Dis 2002; 6: 455–79, viii.

41 Greten TF, Manns MP, Reinisch I, et al. Hepatocellular carcinoma occurring after successful treatment of childhood cancer with high dose chemotherapy and radiation. Gut 2005; 54: 732.

42 Kumari TP, Shanvas A, Mathews A, et al. Hepatocellular carcinoma: a rare late event in childhood acute lymphoblastic leukemia. J Pediatr Hematol Oncol 2000; 22: 289–90.

43 Strickland DK, Riely CA, Patrick CC, et al. Hepatitis C infection among survivors of childhood cancer. Blood 2000; 95: 3065–70.

44 Abbasoglu L, Gun F, Tansu Salman F, et al. Hepatoblastoma in children in Turkey. Acta Chir Belg 2004; 104: 318–21.

45 Roebuck D. Focal liver lesion in children. Pediatr Radiol 2008; 38(Suppl. 3): S518–22.

46 Akinyinka OO, Falade AG, Ogunbiyi O, et al. Hepatocellular carcinoma in Nigerian children. Ann Trop Paediatr 2001; 21: 165–8.

47 Roebuck DJ, Olsen O, Pariente D. Radiological staging in children with hepatoblastoma. Pediatr Radiol 2006; 36: 176–82.

48 De Ioris M, Brugieres L, Zimmermann A, et al. Hepatoblastoma with a low serum alpha-fetoprotein level at diagnosis: the SIOPEL group experience. Eur J Cancer 2008; 44: 545–50.

49 Trobaugh-Lotrario AD, Tomlinson GE, Finegold MJ, et al. Small cell undifferentiated variant of hepatoblastoma: adverse clinical and

molecular features similar to rhabdoid tumors. Pediatr Blood Cancer 2009; 52: 328–34.

50 Blohm ME, Vesterling-Horner D, Calaminus G, et al. Alpha 1-fetoprotein (AFP) reference values in infants up to 2 years of age. Pediatr Hematol Oncol 1998; 15: 135–42.

51 Brown J, Perilongo G, Shafford E, et al. Pretreatment prognostic factors for children with hepatoblastoma – results from the International Society of Paediatric Oncology (SIOP) study SIOPEL 1. Eur J Cancer 2000; 36: 1418–25.

52 Roebuck DJ, Aronson D, Clapuyt P, et al. 2005 PRETEXT: a revised staging system for primary malignant liver tumors of childhood developed by the SIOPEL group. Pediatr Radiol 2007; 37: 123–32.

53 Llovet JM. Updated treatment approach to hepatocellular carcinoma. J Gastroenterol 2005; 40: 225–35.

54 Huang JH, Chen CH, Chang TT, et al. Evaluation of predictive value of CLIP, Okuda, TNM and JIS staging systems for hepatocellular carcinoma patients undergoing surgery. J Gastroenterol Hepatol 2005; 20: 765–71.

55 Finegold MJ, Lopez-Terrada DH, Bowen J, et al. The College of American Pathologists. Protocol for the examination of specimens from pediatric patients with hepatoblastoma. Arch Pathol Lab Med 2007; 131 520–9.

56 Zimmermann A. The emerging family of hepatoblastoma tumors: from ontogenesis to oncogenesis. Eur J Cancer 2005 Jul; 41(11): 1503–14.

57 Mascarello JT, Jones MC, Kadota RP, et al. Hepatoblastoma characterized by trisomy 20 and double minutes. Cancer Genet Cytogenet 1990; 47: 243–7.

58 Sainati L, Leszl A, Stella M, et al. Cytogenetic analysis of hepatoblastoma: hypothesis of cytogenetic evolution in such tumors and results of a multicentric study. Cancer Genet Cytogenet 1998; 104: 39–44.

59 Ma SK, Cheung AN, Choy C, et al. Cytogenetic characterization of childhood hepatoblastoma. Cancer Genet Cytogenet 2000; 119: 32–6.

60 Weber RG, Pietsch T, von Schweinitz D, et al. Characterization of genomic alterations in hepatoblastomas. A role for gains on chromosomes 8q and 20 as predictors of poor outcome. Am J Pathol 2000; 157: 571–8.

61 Koch A, Denkhaus D, Albrecht S, et al. Childhood hepatoblastomas frequently carry a mutated degradation targeting box of the beta-catenin gene. Cancer Res 1999; 59: 269–73.

62 Park WS, Oh RR, Park JY, et al. Nuclear localization of beta-catenin is an important prognostic factor in hepatoblastoma. J Pathol 2001; 193: 483–90.

63 Katzenstein HM, Krailo MD, Malogolowkin MH, et al. Fibrolamellar hepatocellular carcinoma in children and adolescents. Cancer 2003; 97: 2006–12.

64 Prokurat A, Kluge P, Kościesza A, et al. Transitional liver cell tumors (TLCT) in older children and adolescents: a novel group of aggressive hepatic tumors expressing beta-catenin. Med Pediatr Oncol 2002; 39: 510–8.

65 Couinaud C. Etude anatomique et surgical. Mason 1957; 400–9.

66 Czauderna P, Otte JB, Aronson DC, et al. Childhood Liver Tumour Strategy Group of the International Society of Paediatric Oncology (SIOPEL). Guidelines for surgical treatment of hepatoblastoma in the modern era–recommendations from the Childhood Liver Tumour Strategy Group of the International Society of Paediatric Oncology (SIOPEL). Eur J Cancer 2005; 41: 1031–6.

67 Karpoff HM, Jamazin JR, Melandez J, Juman F, Blumgart LH. Techniques of hepatic resection. In: Blumgart LH, Juman F (Eds). Hepatobiliary cancer. American Cancer Society. BC Decker, 2000.

68 Schnater JM, Aronson DC, Plaschkes J, et al. Surgical view of the treatment of patients with hepatoblastoma: results from the first prospective trial of the International Society of Pediatric Oncology Liver Tumor Study Group. Cancer 2002; 94: 1111–20.

69 Otte JB, Pritchard J, Aronson DC, et al. International Society of Pediatric Oncology (SIOP). Liver transplantation for hepatoblastoma: results from the International Society of Pediatric Oncology (SIOP) study SIOPEL-1 and review of the world experience. Pediatr Blood Cancer 2004; 42: 74–83.

70 Otte JB, de Ville de Goyet J, Reding R. Liver transplantation for hepatoblastoma: indications and contraindications in the modern era. Pediatr Transplant 2005; 9: 557–65.

71 Czauderna P, Zbrzezniak G, Narozanski W, et al. Preliminary experience with arterial chemoembolization for hepatoblastoma and hepatocellular carcinoma in children. Pediatr Blood Cancer 2006; 46: 825–8.

72 Evans AE, Land VJ, Newton WA, et al. Combination chemotherapy in the treatment of children with malignant hepatoma. Cancer 1982; 50: 821–6.

73 Ortega JA, Krailo MD, Haas JE, et al. Effective treatment of unresectable or metastatic hepatoblastoma with cisplatin and continuous infusion doxorubicin chemotherapy: a report from the Childrens Cancer Study Group. J Clin Oncol 1991; 9: 2167–76.

74 Douglass EC, Finegold M, Reynolds M, et al. Cisplatin, vincristine and fluorouracil therapy for hepatoblastoma: a Pediatric Oncology Group Study. J Clin Oncol 1993; 11: 96–9.

75 Ortega JA, Douglass EC, Feusner JH, et al. Randomised comparison of cisplatin/vincristie/fluorouracil and cisplatin/continuous infusion doxorubicin for treatment of pediatric hepatoblastoma: a report from the Children Cancer Group and the Pediatric Oncology Group. J Clin Oncol 2000; 8: 2665–75.

76 Malogolowkin MH, Katzenstein H, et al. Intensified platinum therapy is an ineffective strategy for improving outcome in pediatric patients with advanced hepatoblastoma. J Clin Oncol 2006; 24: 2879–84.

77 Von Schweinitz D, Byrd DJ, Hecker H, et al. Efficiency and toxicity of ifosfamide, cisplatin and doxorubicin in the treatment of childhood hepatoblastoma. Study Committee of the Cooperative Paediatric Liver Tumour Study HB89 of the German Society for Peadiatric Oncology and Haematology. Eur J Cancer 1997; 33: 1243–9.

78 Fuchs J, Rydzynski J, Von Schweinitz D, et al. Study Committee of the Cooperative Pediatric Liver Tumor Study HB 94 for the German Society for Pediatric Oncology and Hematology. Pretreatment prognostic factors and treatment results in children with hepablastoma: a report from the German Cooperative Pediatric Liver Tumor Study HB 94. Cancer 2002; 95: 172–82.

79 Fuchs J, Bode U, von Schweinitz D, et al. Analysis of treatment efficiency of carboplatin and etoposide in combination with radical surgery in advanced and recurrent childhood hepatoblastoma: a report of the German Cooperative Pediatric Liver Tumor Study HB 89 and HB 94. Klin Padiatr 1999; 211: 305–9.

80 Pritchard J, Brown J, Shafford E, et al. Cisplatin, doxorubicin, and delayed surgery for childhood hepatoblastoma: a successful approach–results of the first prospective study of the International Society of Pediatric Oncology. J Clin Oncol 2000; 18: 3819–28.

81 Perilongo G, Brown J, Shafford E, Brock P, et al. Hepatoblastoma presenting with lung metastases: treatment results of the first

cooperative, prospective study of the International Society of Paediatric Oncology on childhood liver tumors. Cancer 2000; 89: 1845–53.

82 Perilongo G, Shafford E, Maibach R, et al. International Society of Paediatric Oncology-SIOPEL 2. Risk-adapted treatment for childhood hepatoblastoma. final report of the second study of the International Society of Paediatric Oncology–SIOPEL 2. Eur J Cancer 2004; 40: 411–21.

83 Sasaki F, Matsunaga T, Iwafuchi M, et al. (Japanese Study Group for Pediatric Liver Tumor). Outcome of hepatoblastoma treated with the JPLT-1 (Japanese Study Group for Pediatric Liver Tumor) Protocol-1: a report from the Japanese Study Group for Pediatric Liver Tumor. J Pediatr Surg 2002; 37: 851–6.

84 Katzenstein HM, Krailo MD, Malogolowkin MH, et al. Hepatocellular carcinoma in children and adolescents: results from the Pediatric Oncology Group and the Children's Cancer Group intergroup study. J Clin Oncol 2002; 20: 2789–97.

85 Czauderna P, Mackinlay G, Perilongo G, et al. Liver Tumors Study Group of the International Society of Pediatric Oncology. Hepatocellular carcinoma in children: results of the first prospective study of the International Society of Pediatric Oncology group. J Clin Oncol 2002; 20: 2798–804.

86 von Schweinitz D, Hecker H, Schmidt-von-Arndt G, et al. Prognostic factors and staging systems in childhood hepatoblastoma. Int J Cancer 1997; 74: 593–9.

87 Aslett H, Levitt G, Richardson A, et al. A review of long-term follow-up for survivors of childhood cancer. Eur J Cancer 2007; 43: 1781–90.

88 Ryckman FC, Alonso MH, Bucuvalas JC, et al. Long-term survival after liver transplantation. J Pediatr Surg 1999; 34: 845–9; discussion 849–50.

89 Brock PR, Koliouskas DE, Barratt TM, et al. Partial reversibility of cisplatin nephrotoxicity in children. J Pediatr 1991; 118: 531–4.

90 Brock PR, Bellman SC, Yeomans EC, et al. Cisplatin ototoxicity in children: a practical grading system. Med Pediatr Oncol 1991; 19: 295–300.

91 Kushner BH, Budnick A, Kramer K, et al. Ototoxicity from high-dose use of platinum compounds in patients with neuroblastoma. Cancer 2006; 107: 417–22.

92 Hudson MM, Rai SN, Nunez C, et al. Noninvasive evaluation of late anthracycline cardiac toxicity in childhood cancer survivors. J Clin Oncol 2007; 25: 3635–43.

93 Mizejewski GJ. Biological role of alpha-fetoprotein in cancer: prospects for anticancer therapy. Expert Rev Anticancer Ther 2002; 2: 709–35.

94 Ishikawa H, Nakao K, Matsumoto K, et al. Antiangiogenic gene therapy for hepatocellular carcinoma using angiostatin gene. Hepatology 2003; 37: 696–704.

95 Knight KR, Kraemer DF, Winter C, et al. Early changes in auditory function as a result of platinum chemotherapy: use of extended high-frequency audiometry and evoked distortion product otoacoustic emissions. J Clin Oncol 2007; 25: 1190–5.

96 Neuwelt EA, Gilmer-Knight K, Lacy C, et al. Toxicity profile of delayed high dose sodium thiosulfate in children treated with carboplatin in conjunction with blood-brain-barrier disruption. Pediatr Blood Cancer 2006; 47: 174–82.

97 Doolittle ND, Muldoon LL, Brummett RE, et al. Delayed sodium thiosulfate as an otoprotectant against carboplatin-induced hearing loss in patients with malignant brain tumors. Clin Cancer Res 2001; 7: 493–500.

17 Germ Cell Tumors

James Nicholson[1] and Roger Palmer[2]

[1] Addenbrooke's Hospital, Cambridge, UK and [2] MRC Cancer Cell Unit, Cambridge, UK

Introduction

Germ cell tumors (GCTs) comprise a rare and heterogeneous group of tumors with benign and malignant (MGCT) subtypes. They occur at many different anatomical sites from birth to adolescence and adulthood. The earliest record of a GCT is linked to an inscription on a Babylonian tablet from 625 to 539 BC and they have continued to fascinate researchers throughout history [1]. Teratomas, in particular, have attracted colourful descriptions by virtue of their tendency to contain mature somatic tissue such as hair and teeth. The first formal recognition of these tumors is attributed to LeBlanc, a veterinarian who removed a 'kyste dermoid' from the base of a horse's skull in 1831 [2]. It wasn't until Rudolf Virchow's first edition *Die Krankhaften Geschwülste* (The Pathological Tumors) in 1863 that the term teratoma was coined from the Greek *teras-atos* meaning monster and *–oma* denoting tumor [3].

The malignant tumors were initially described histopathologically according to the tissues in which they arise, resulting in the eponymous descriptions that are still used today. For instance, Schiller initially described the glomerulus-like structures within ovarian yolk-sac tumors [4], but misattributed this feature to a variety of tumors until Teilum linked this to the endodermal sinus of Duval seen in the rat placenta [5]. Histologically, the Schiller-Duval body is a pathognomonic feature of yolk-sac tumors (otherwise known as orchidoblastoma, endodermal sinus tumor, yolk sac carcinoma or Telium's tumor). However, the 'germ cell' origin of these tumors was not recognized until the 1960s [6], something that was initially viewed with great scepticism other than for seminoma (testicular germinoma) due to the multiple histologies and sites included in the classification [7].

GCTs are thought to arise from a common progenitor cell, the primordial germ cell (PGC) and are therefore totipotent, able to develop into any tissue along the three embryologic layers (mesoderm, ectoderm, and endoderm) as well as extraembryonic tissue (e.g. placenta). The result is a wide spectrum of tumors with diverse presentations, clinical behaviour, and response to therapy.

Pediatric Hematology and Oncology, 1st edition. Edited by Edward J. Estlin, Richard J. Gilbertson, and Robert F. Wynn. © 2010 Blackwell Publishing Ltd.

- GCT range from mature and immature teratoma to four different malignant subtypes (Figure 17.1), although more than one subtype can arise within the same tumor.
- Despite this heterogeneity, it has been possible to apply comparable surgical and chemotherapeutic strategies across the range of malignant extracranial tumor types.
- Treatment for intracranial tumors has evolved separately, combinations of chemotherapy and radiotherapy dominating modern treatment, with a limited role for surgery.

Prior to the introduction of platinum-based agents, survival of children with MGCTs was poor with event-free survival (EFS) <50%, despite combination chemotherapy [8]. The introduction of the 'Einhorn regimen' of cisPlatin in combination with Vinblastine and Bleomycin (PVB) in adult testicular MGCTs at Indiana University, USA, in 1974 was a turning point.[9]. This led to alternative combinations, of which Bleomycin, Etoposide and cisPlatin (BEP) led to an EFS approaching 78% for patients with greater than stage I disease [10]. When adapted for treatment of GCTs in children, BEP improved childhood survival rates from 47% to 89% [11]. These and similar platinum-based combinations of chemotherapy form the backbone of treatment of malignant GCTs to this day.

Abbreviations commonly used in descriptions of germ cell tumors

GCT	Germ cell tumor
MGCT	Malignant germ cell tumor
TGCT	Testicular germ cell tumor
SCT	Sacrococcygeal teratoma
CNS GCT	Central nervous system (intracranial) germ cell tumor
NGGCT	Non-germinomatous germ cell tumor
PGC	Primordial germ cell
YST	Yolk sac tumor (endodermal sinus tumor)
CHC	Choriocarcinoma
EC	Embryonal carcinoma
MT	Mature teratoma
IT	Immature teratoma
AFP	Alpha-fetoprotein
HCG or β-HCG	(Beta) human chorionic gonadotrophin
Conversion factors for units of AFP	
1 ng/ml = 0.83 IU/l	
1.205 ng/ml = 1 IU/l	

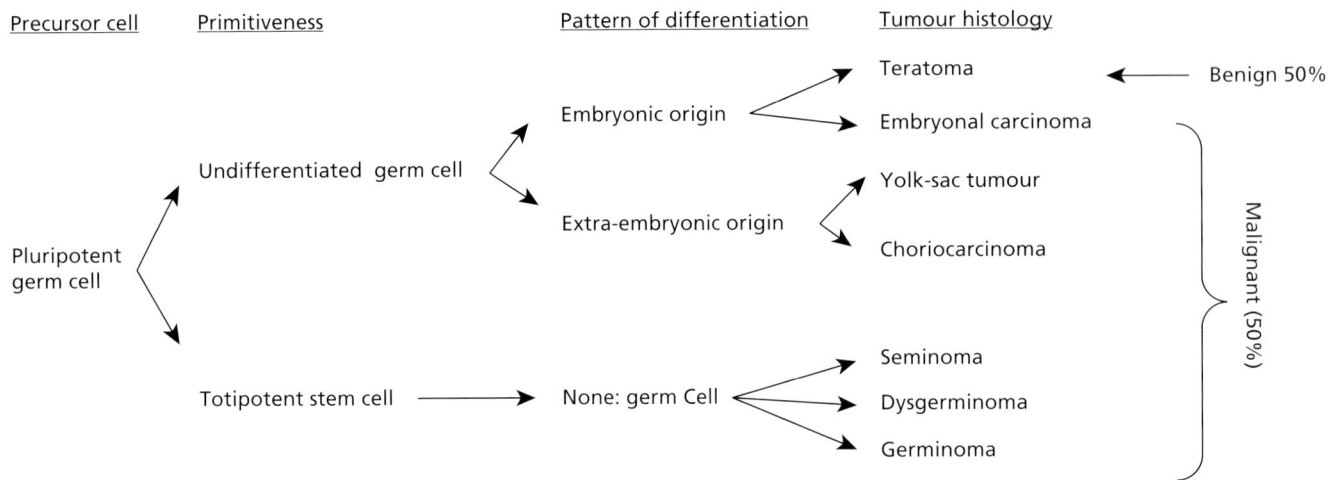

Figure 17.1 Germ cell tumor classification, based upon site (germinomatous tumors are histologically identical and termed seminomas if arising in the testis; dysgerminomas in the ovary and germinomas *per se* if extragonadal) and degree of primordial germ cell differentiation at time of deregulated growth.

Epidemiology and biology

Epidemiology of germ cell tumors

Malignant germ cell tumors account for 3–5% of childhood cancers and have an annual incidence of around 3–5 per million, under the age of 15 years [12].
• There is some geographical variation with MGCTs being more common in the USA and Japan and less frequent in the Middle East, particularly Egypt [13].
• Genetic factors play a part with children of Japanese and Southeast Asian descent at greatest risk [14], and black American males are considerably less likely to develop MGCTs than their white or female counterparts. In the UK 30–40 children are diagnosed with MGCTs each year and there is a slight female preponderance (0.87M:1F) [15].

Table 17.1 describes inherited syndromes associated with the development of GCTs.

There is a bimodal age distribution with a peak in incidence during infancy and early childhood, before the incidence drops to <0.1 per 100 000, when GCTs arise more frequently in girls than in boys (Figure 17.2). The annual incidence then increases during adolescence to 35 per million (male) and 25 per million (female) by the late teens. Accurate estimation of the incidence of all GCTs is confounded by the variable reporting of teratomas to registries and the inconsistency with which they are accorded malignant status, but the incidence of teratomas is thought to be at least equivalent to their malignant counterparts [16].

Gonadal tumors

Approximately 50% of all GCTs in childhood are gonadal (Figure 17.3) and, of these, testicular MGCTs are slightly more common than ovarian MGCTs [12, 17], although the precise ratio will depend on the age range studied. Testicular tumors occur predominantly in the first few years of life, with yolk sac tumor being the most common histology. They are rare in mid-childhood but the incidence rises again in adolescence, when seminomas (germinomas) and mixed malignant histologies predominate. Boys with testicular abnormalities, which range from dysgenetic gonads to maldescent, have a four- to 10-fold increase in the risk of malignancy in both ipsilateral and contralateral testis [18].

The incidence of ovarian germ cell tumors is very low before the age of 5 years and increases gradually to a peak in the early teens. Dysgerminomas and teratomas are more common than yolk sac tumors, whilst other malignant histologies are extremely rare. Bilateral ovarian GCTs, which are more likely in XY gonadal dysgenesis [19], are seen in about 5–10% of cases, and 10% of girls with MGCTs of the 'ovary' turn out to have an intersex state, with 2–3% having gonadoblastoma. Overall, childhood ovarian GCTs are reported to be 50% more frequent in the USA [20], whilst the rates across Europe are roughly equivalent to those reported in the UK [15]. The cause for this is unclear.

Extragonadal tumors

The incidence of extragonadal tumors varies with age and gender. They account for approximately 50% of all GCTs in childhood (Figure 17.3) but contribute only 5% of adult GCTs [7]. This may result from the increased propensity of mis-sited tissue to undergo malignant change and therefore become clinically evident at a younger age, as seen with undescended testes [21], or may reflect biological differences between pediatric and adult GCTs.
• They almost always arise in the midline, the central nervous system (CNS) and sacrococcygeal sites being the most common, each accounting for approximately 20% of all GCTs. Quoted incidences vary, with some reports suggesting up to 35% of all GCTs occurring in the coccyx, perhaps reflecting differences in reporting teratomas internationally [15, 17].
• Sacrococcygeal tumors are commoner in girls (3:1) and the majority present antenatally or in the neonatal period, occurring in 1:35–45 000 live births [22, 23], whilst intracranial and medi-

Table 17.1 Syndromes and clinical associations with germ cell tumors.

Syndrome	Characteristics	Chromosome or gene	Risk*	Link to OMIM†
Swyer Syndrome	Streak gonads, gonadoblastoma	XY gonadal dysgenesis	DG	http://www.ncbi.nlm.nih.gov/entrez/dispomim.cgi?id=306100
Klinefelter's syndrome	Hypogonadism, tall stature, language delay, gynaecomastia	XXY	ME	http://www.ncbi.nlm.nih.gov/entrez/dispomim.cgi?id=273300
Fraser syndrome	Renal agenesis, cryptophthalmos, cryptorchidism, male syndactyly	4q21 (*FRAS1*) or 13q13.3 (*FREM2*)	Gonadal GCT	http://www.ncbi.nlm.nih.gov/entrez/dispomim.cgi?id=219000
Turner syndrome	Short stature, streak gonad, aortic coarctation, horseshoe kidney	XO or mosaicism	DG	N/A
Russell-Silver syndrome (males only)	Dwarfism, triangular facies, learning difficulties	7p11.2 (*GRB10*) imprinting defect of 11p15 (*H19, IGF2*) ?17q23-q24	SE	http://www.ncbi.nlm.nih.gov/entrez/dispomim.cgi?id=180860
Schinzel-Giedion Syndrome	Midface retraction, coarse facies, skeletal abnormalities, mental retardation	?	Malignant SCT	http://www.ncbi.nlm.nih.gov/entrez/dispomim.cgi?id=269150
Down's syndrome	Dysmorphic features, CAVSD, mental retardation	Trisomy 21	Germinoma	http://www.ncbi.nlm.nih.gov/entrez/dispomim.cgi?id=190685
Ataxia telangiectasia	Cerebellar ataxia, telangiectasia, immune defects, predisposition to malignancy	11q22.3 *ATM*	Ovarian GCT	http://www.ncbi.nlm.nih.gov/entrez/dispomim.cgi?id=208900
Cowden disease	Multiple hamartomas (esp. skin, mucous membranes, breast & thyroid)	10q23.31, 10q22.3 *PTEN*	TGCT	http://www.ncbi.nlm.nih.gov/entrez/dispomim.cgi?id=158350
Currarino syndrome	Sacral agenesis	7q36 *MNX1*	SCT	http://www.ncbi.nlm.nih.gov/entrez/dispomim.cgi?id=176450
General associations				
Cryptorchidism	Undescended or maldescended testes	19p13.2, 13q13.1 *INSL3, RXFP2*	TGCT	http://www.ncbi.nlm.nih.gov/entrez/dispomim.cgi?id=219050
–	Monozygotic twins	N/A	SCT	http://www.ncbi.nlm.nih.gov/entrez/dispomim.cgi?id=276410
Pyloric stenosis	Vomiting, FTT, hypochloremic hypokalaemic metabolic alkalosis	12q24.2-q24.31 *NOS1*	4x↑ GCT	http://www.ncbi.nlm.nih.gov/entrez/dispomim.cgi?id=179010

* ME, mediastinal GCT, SE-seminoma. DG, dysgerminoma. TGCT, testicular germ cell tumor. SCT, sacrococcygeal teratoma. CAVSD, complete atrio-ventricular septal defect (endocardial cushion defect). FTT, failure to thrive. † Online Mendelian Inheritance in Man: http://www.ncbi.nlm.nih.gov/sites/entrez?db=omim

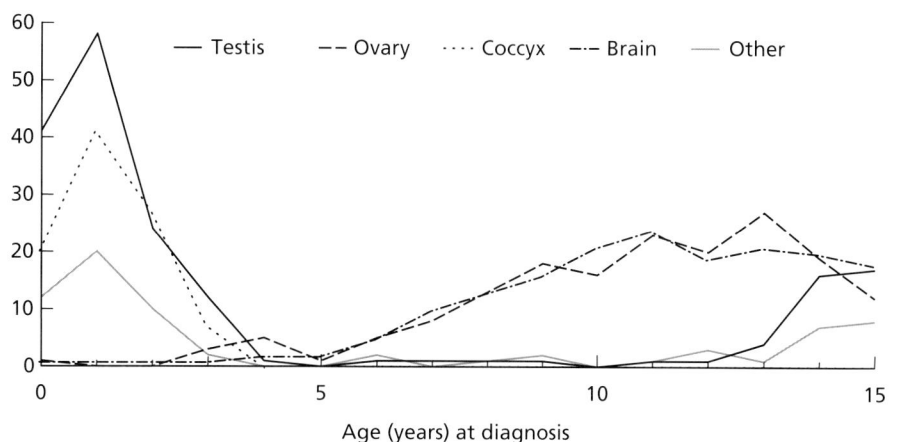

Figure 17.2 Age-related incidence by site of origin for 1548 malignant germ cell tumors enrolled onto the German MAKEI and MAHO trials (with kind permission of Dr G.Calaminus).

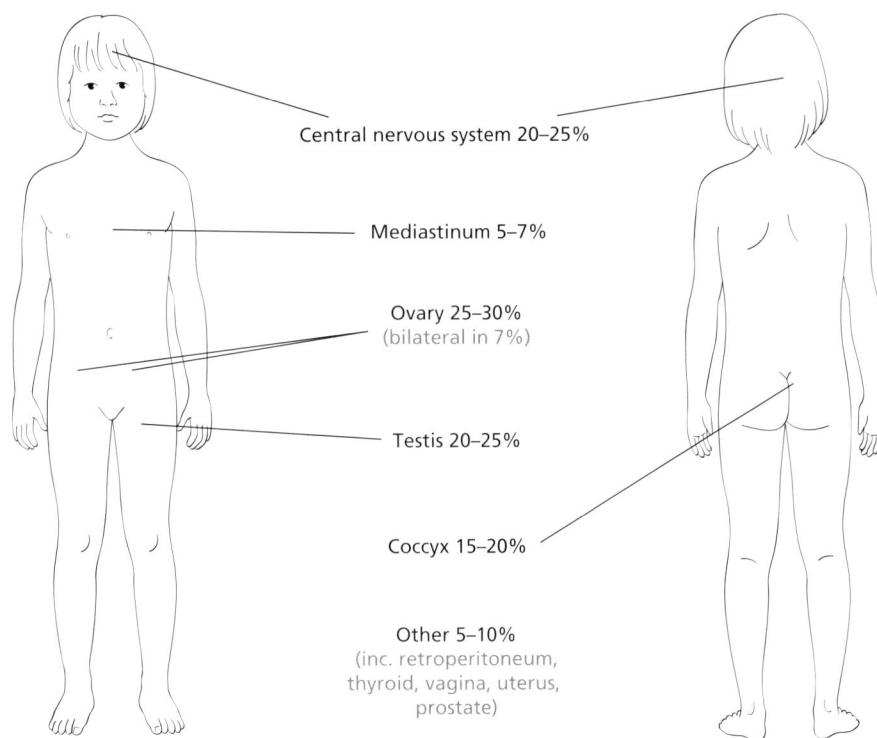

Figure 17.3 Site of origin for germ cell tumors in childhood.

astinal tumors are more common in boys (1.4:1) and occur in later childhood and adolescence.

• Mediastinal tumors account for approximately 7% of all GCTs, and retroperitoneal tumors for around 4%.

The overall incidence of childhood GCTs has been rising [24, 25]. This is mainly due to increases in CNS GCTs and gonadal tumors of late adolescence, but the cause for this is unclear and cannot be explained by the increasing incidence of cryptorchidism alone [26].

Histological subtypes of germ cell tumors

The number of histological types included under the umbrella of GCTs is a frequent source of confusion. These are listed in Table 17.2 and can be separated into:

• Germinomatous or seminomatous tumors (seminoma if testicular, dysgerminoma if ovarian, germinoma *per se* if extragonadal) and

• Non-germinomatous (NGGCT) or non-seminomatous tumors (including teratomas, embryonal carcinomas, yolk sac tumors, choriocarcinoma and polyembryona).

• Where the tumor is composed of more than one GCT histology, it is termed a mixed MGCT. Malignant teratoma now refers to teratoma containing malignant non-GCT components (e.g. primitive neuroectodermal tumor [PNET], neuroblastoma, squamous cell carcinoma).

Previously, the term malignant teratoma was used to describe a MGCT element admixed with teratoma, whilst teratocarcinoma described embryonal carcinoma admixed with teratoma, and

Table 17.2 Histological classification of pediatric germ cell tumors, modified from Dehner p. 282–312 [128] typically used in most countries at present.

Type	Histology	Subtypes
1	Germinoma	a Intratubular
		b Invasive
2	Teratoma	a Mature
		b Immature
		Grade 1 Immature tissue <1 low power(×4) Field (LPF)/slide
		Grade 2 Immature tissue 1–3 LPF/slide
		Grade 3 Immature tissue ≥4 LPF/slide +/– microfoci of probable yolk-sac tumor – Heifetz lesion [31]
		c Malignant teratoma (teratoma with non germ cell malignant component)
3	Embryonal carcinoma	
4	Yolk-sac tumor	
5	Choriocarcinoma	
6	Gonadoblastoma	
7	Mixed MGCT	Mixed malignant germ cell tumor (each GCT component listed)

mixed MGCT two or more MGCT elements (irrespective of the presence of teratoma).

Morphologically resembling the extra-embryonic yolk sac, yolk-sac tumors (YSTs) constitute the single largest histological

Table 17.3 Immunohistochemistry of germ cell tumors.

Histology	EMA	PLAP	L-CK	AFP	β-HCG	GPC3	Nanog	OCT-4	D2-40	AP-2γ	Sox2	c-Kit	CD30
Teratoma	−/(+)	−	+	−/+*	−	−	−	−	?	−/+	+	+	+
Embryonal carcinoma	−	+/−	+	−/(+)	−/(+)	−	+	+	−/(+)	+/−	+	−/+	+/(−)
Yolk-sac tumor	−	+/−	+	+	−	+	−	−	−	−	−	−	−
Choriocarcinoma	−	+/−	+	−	+	+/−	−	−	−	?	?	−	−
Germinoma	−	+	−/(+)	−	−/+†	−	+	+	+	+	−	+/−	−/(+)

* Immature enteral tissue can express alpha-fetoprotein. † Syncytiotrophoblastic cells giant cells can express ß-HCG.

Icons occurring first indicate the predominant staining pattern + or −, whilst icons in parentheses indicate that immunostaining is rarely and/or very weekly (+) or (−). EMA, epithelial membrane antigen. PLAP, placental alkaline phospatase. L-CK, low molecular weight cytokeratin. AFP, alpha-fetoprotein. ß-HCG, beta-human chorionic gonadotropin. GPC3, glypican-3. D2-40, oncofetal antigen podoplanin. GCTs are typically EMA negative, distinguishing them from adenocarcinomas.

subtype observed in pediatric GCTs. Typically composed of small pale cells with scant cytoplasm and oval nuclei, YSTs form a loose network of channels lines with microcysts and sparsely populated with the pathognomonic Schiller-Duval bodies in 75% of cases [27]. Periodic acid-Schiff (PAS) positive hyaline droplets are present in almost all YSTs, but in themselves are not diagnostic. Immunohistochemically, almost all YSTs stain positive for alpha-fetoprotein (AFP) and the cytokeratin, whilst placental alkaline phosphatase (PLAP) can be positive or negative, and they are typically negative for CD30 (Table 17.3).

Germinomas are morphologically identical to adult seminomas, composed of sheets of large polygonal cells with abundant cytoplasm, separated by fibrous bands, and typically with a striking lymphocytic reaction [28]. These tumors express PLAP and CD117 (c-KIT), and occasionally human chorionic gonadotrophin (HCG) from sparsely positioned syncytiotrophoblastic cells. New immunostains for Nanog, OCT-4, AP-2γ, and D2-40 have greatly assisted in the diagnosis [29].

Whilst rare in the pediatric age range, embryonal carcinomas (EC) form large epithelioid cells with prominent nucleoli. Syncytiotrophoblastic cells may also be sparsely present, permitting modest elevations in HCG, and weakly positive immunostains. Histological discrimination of these cells is usually possible since they are strongly CD30 positive, unlike germinomas (Table 17.3). Of exceptional rarity is the EC variant polyembryona, where the EC cells arrange into embryoid bodies that bear some resemblance to early embryos, positive for both AFP and HCG.

Choriocarcinoma, uncommon in childhood, comprises mononuclear multinucleated syncytiotrophoblastic and cytotrophoblastic cells which resemble chorionic villi, and appear to be highly invasive associated with extensive haemorrhage. They secrete abundant HCG.

Finally, gonadoblastoma is a benign but pre-malignant mixed stromal and GCT associated with dysgenetic gonads. It appears to arise only in the presence of the Y-chromosome, possibly as a result of *TSPY* expression, and whilst typically (if left untreated) these may develop into germinoma, non-germinoma and ITGCN (if testicular) is also possible.

Mature teratomas (MT) are regarded as benign and may contain tissue of any parenchymal cell type from more than one germ cell layer, typically all three, organized in a haphazard fashion. The status of immature teratomas (IT) is less clear, and they may contain neuroectodermal or blastemal tissues that may appear immature and aggressive (graded 1–3 on this basis), and consequently their treatment remains controversial. Both entities are frequently seen as components of mixed MGCTs and they are cytokeratin and occasionally epithelial membrane antigen (EMA) and AP-2γ positive (Table 17.3).

• ITs may produce low levels of AFP as a consequence of immature intestine or liver being present in the tumor, but this is not predictive of relapse.

• Marina et al. also noted that there was an increased frequency of microfoci of YST (21/73) or PNET (2/73) with increasing grade of immaturity, with more than half of grade 3 ITs containing YST microfoci (Heifetz lesions) compared with only 4% of grade 1 ITs [30]. These Heifetz lesions may be responsible for mildly elevated AFPs (observed in 45% of cases, with maximum AFP 1045 ng/ml) [30, 31].

• Around 25–30% of ovarian ITs are associated with mature glial deposits throughout the peritoneum and/or omentum (gliaomatosis peritonei). Gliomatosis is rarely seen at other sites, although has been reported with mediastinal and cervical teratomas [31].

Different histological subtypes of GCTs predominate at different ages. In neonates they are almost exclusively mature and immature teratoma, sometimes admixed with subtle foci of YCT. During infancy and early childhood, YSTs predominate, but later in childhood, germinomas are also seen, particularly in ovarian tumors, and the increase in incidence of GCTs seen from around the time of puberty is associated with the observation of all histological entities, especially in males [17].

Embryology

GCTs are thought to arise from PGCs, the embryonic precursors of gametes. PGCs form within the wall of an out-pouching of the extra-embryonic yolk sac at 3 weeks gestation, before they migrate towards the allantois and hindgut through the vitelline duct. Thereafter, the migrational path of the PGCs is along the wall of the hindgut and the dorsal mesentery into the genital ridge, which they reach at gestational week 5–6. Germ cell migration is complete by week 6–7 with subsequent obliteration of the vitelline duct and closure of the abdominal wall by week 11. The gonadal cords, later the mature gonads, appear as sex discernable organs from week 9. The migration process appears to be dependent upon SDF-1 [32]. Once in the gonadal ridge, PGCs undergo gender specific differentiation into oocytes or spermatogonia. Those that fail to reach the gonadal ridge typically apoptose in a *BAX*-dependent manner [33].

It is suggested that aberrant germ cell migration is responsible for the extragonadal sites at which GCTs arise. Recently, *BAX*-null mice, which permit the survival of ectopically sited PGCs, show a propensity to reside at the tail bud/sacral area with a 3:1 female predilection analogous to sacrococcygeal GCT (SCT) development in humans [34], suggesting that PGCs are indeed the precursors of GCTs, particularly those of early childhood. However, there was no mis-siting of PGCs outside of the abdominal cavity, leaving the origin of thymus/mediastinum or CNS GCTs open to question. Additionally, there is a suggestion that SCTs arise from Henson's node, a totipotent group of cells located at the tip of the coccyx as part of axis-formation during gastrulation, which might fit better with the observed epidemiology and malignant potential, which is at odds with that for pediatric teratomas at other sites [1].

Tumor markers

Tumor markers have been used routinely in the management of GCTs in childhood. Lactate dehydrogenase (LDH) is a non-specific marker of malignancy and whilst frequently measured at diagnosis, as a result of previous interest in its prognostic impact in non-seminomas of adulthood [35], it has little value in pediatric practice. Similarly, PLAP has been shown to be raised in germinoma, but is not sufficiently specific to have any diagnostic or prognostic value [36].

The secretion of AFP and HCG by GCTs is well recognized. Where levels are raised, markers are valuable in diagnosis, assessing response to treatment and surveillance once treatment is completed. AFP, an α-globulin, is the predominant serum binding protein in the fetus (later replaced by albumin) and is therefore very high at birth, usually falling to adult levels of <12 ng/ml (<10 IU/l; 1 ng/ml ≡ 0.84 IU/l) by 1 year of age.

However, at the extremes of the AFP range, a normal 2-year-old may have an AFP of 82 ng/ml, making interpretation of isolated AFP levels difficult in the neonate and infant [37]. As a tumor marker, AFP is produced by YSTs, yolk sac elements within mixed MGCTs and, at low levels, by some embryonal carcinomas and immature teratomas. It is also raised in primary liver tumors, particularly hepatoblastoma.

HCG is a glycoprotein composed of α and β subunits which is normally produced by syncytiotrophoblasts. Assay of the β subunit avoids cross-reactivity with other hormones (leuteinizing hormone [LH], follicle and thyroid stimulating hormones, and melatonin). Since relative levels of 'free β' and intact dimer

($\alpha + \beta$) vary between different tumor types, the most reliable measurement for detecting β-HCG secretion by tumor is 'total HCG', which includes both free β and dimer.

• Elevation of β-HCG levels implies the presence of syncytiotrophoblasts and is typically seen in choriocarcinoma or mixed MGCTs with choriocarcinoma as one component.

• Moderate elevation of β-HCG may be seen from syncytiotrophoblastic giant cells present within germinomas and occasionally in embryonal carcinoma.

In the presence of raised tumor markers, GCTs may be treated on the basis of radiological findings and raised tumor markers without tissue diagnosis, although histological confirmation is often available at diagnosis, especially for gonadal tumors, when primary excision is part of treatment. Where a biopsy is performed in a mixed tumor, particularly for extragonadal tumors, the GCT components in the tissue diagnosis may differ from the subtype suggested by marker estimation, or may under-report the range of histologies present as a result of sampling error [38]. The definitive histological diagnosis is less important in pediatric practice, since appropriately intensive treatment can be determined by the presence of raised markers in most cases.

Molecular biology

Current understanding of the biology of pediatric MGCTs is limited in comparison with hematological malignancies, other pediatric solid tumors and adult testicular GCTs (TGCTs).

• Genetic studies performed on adult TGCTs invariably demonstrate gain of the short arm of chromosome 12 (12p gain), irrespective of histology, usually resulting from isochromosome 12p [i(12p)] formation [39].

• This suggests that genes on 12p are essential in the pathogenesis of adult TGCTs. However, i(12p) is rare in pediatric MGCTs and is never seen in pure histology teratomas occurring in childhood.

• Despite this, 12p gain is not exclusive to adult MGCTs and a spectrum exists, where 12p gain is relatively less common in MGCTs of younger children (10–20% of cases <5 years old) and increases in frequency through to adulthood (50–60% of cases in adolescence) [40].

The biological and clinical relevance of 12p gain in childhood tumors has yet to be established, but it is notable that 12p gain was seen in both of the childhood MGCT relapses genetically assessed and reported to date [41, 42], and the only reported death from disease [40].

Numerical abnormalities of many other chromosomes are more frequently reported, although none as consistently as 12p gain in adult TGCTs [40]. Different histologies appear to show characteristic patterns of genomic imbalance irrespective of the site in which they occur [41], consistent with the hypothesis that they arise from the same progenitor cell:

• Pediatric YSTs commonly have loss on 1p36, 4q, 6q and gain on 3p.

• Pediatric germinomas are more likely to have gain on 12q, 19q and loss on 11q.

Biology may also help to explain the unusual behaviour of post-pubertal testicular or extra-gonadal MTs, which have demonstrated the ability to grow, undergo malignant change, and metastasize [43]. For instance truly benign teratomas do not demonstrate any cytogenetic aberrations, but post-pubertal non-ovarian teratomas may have i(12p) or genetic 12p gain. It has also been reported that malignant teratomas, containing non-GCT malignant components, retain the genetic abnormalities characteristic of GCTs (i.e. 12p gain), as well as acquiring the characteristic aberrations associated with the somatic malignancy present, suggesting that this malignancy arose from a malignant transformation within the GCT [44].

In addition, pediatric and adult MGCTs differ significantly in their global gene expression profiles supporting the suggestion that they differ biologically [45]. It is not possible to determine the timing of the potential biological shift between childhood and adult type patterns, although this appears to occur during puberty, and may be hormone driven. Furthermore, imprinting analysis is consistent between gonadal and extragonadal GCTs for a particular histological type (either pre- or post-puberty), supporting the hypothesis that GCTs, are all derived from the same progenitor cell [46].

Clinical presentation

The presentation of GCTs is determined by their site and occasionally by the presence of metastases.

Gonadal sites

Ovarian GCTs usually present as palpable masses with abdominal distension, typically with pain secondary to torsion or rupture and occasionally with symptoms secondary to hormonal disturbances. Those presenting with acute/sub-acute pain may frequently be misdiagnosed as acute appendicitis. The majority of pediatric ovarian masses are mature teratomas. Some are cystadenomas, whilst roughly 20% are malignant. In the neonatal period ovarian masses are invariably benign follicular cysts as a consequence of maternal oestrogen stimulation.

Testicular tumors present either in the first few years of life or in adolescence as painless scrotal swellings. Diagnostic error is common, with hydrocoele, inguinal hernia, and testicular torsion included in the differential diagnosis. If GCT is suspected then an inguinal surgical approach should be performed. In cases of testicular maldescent, orchidopexy makes testicular surveillance feasible, but there is little evidence that the risk of malignancy is reduced or fertility preserved. Testicular primaries in young children are much more likely to present at stage I (85% of cases in children compared with 35% in adults), and are typically teratomas and/or YSTs.

Extragonadal germ cell tumors

The majority of SCTs present antenatally or in the neonatal period, and can be extremely large, leading to hydrops fetalis or obstruction of labour. SCTs of the newborn are typically benign

(MT/IT). They are described according to the Altman classification for the American Academy of Pediatrics in 1974, which defines four types of SCT on the basis of predominant tumor location [47].
• Type I are predominantly external and comprise 45% of SCTs (Plate 17.1). They are readily identifiable at birth and are almost always benign.
• SCTs with tumor in both internal and external compartments are Type II (35%) or III (10%), with larger external or internal components respectively. These may present in later infancy, especially where the external component is small, or be misdiagnosed, for example as hemangiomas; but are associated with an increased risk of malignancy (21% and 34% respectively).
• Type IV SCTs (10%) are entirely internal, presacral or abdominal and more commonly have malignant elements (38%).

The increased incidence of malignancy with later presentations lends credence to the theory that they may have been primary teratomas, possibly benign at first, that escaped diagnosis [22, 47]. All types of SCT may extend intraspinally and be associated with neurological deficits at presentation, or following surgery. Outside the neonatal period they usually present with functional problems in bladder, bowels, and lower limbs.

Almost all mediastinal lesions are located in the anterior mediastinum. Frequently presenting with chest pain in older children, symptoms may also result from airway compression (commonly in younger children), heart failure or symptoms associated with aberrant hormone production (precocious puberty brought on by HCG mimicking LH). There is an increased incidence in boys with Klinefelter's syndrome (Table 17.1). Mediastinal tumors are less frequent in girls (typically ≤4 years of age), and tend to occur in boys in the adolescent years or adulthood.

Retroperitoneal GCTs present with abdominal symptoms, dependent on site and organs affected. They may form dumbbell tumors, similar to neuroblastoma, resulting in neurological compromise.

Other extragonadal sites at which GCTs occasionally arise include liver, bile duct, abdominal wall, head and neck, lip, pelvis, prostate, uterus, and vagina. Vaginal GCTs present with bleeding and should therefore be considered in cases of suspected sexual abuse. Teratomas may occur in the neck, oral cavity, or orbit. They are usually present at birth and are commonly benign.

Metastatic sites of disease

Distant metastases are seen at presentation in approximately 20% of extracranial GCTs [48]. The most common site is the lungs, but liver, bone, and bone marrow metastases are also seen [8]. Rarely, choriocarcinomas may metastasize to the brain, so this possibility should be borne in mind in tumors with high levels of β-HCG.

Central nervous system germ cell tumor presentation

GCTs should always be suspected in cases of midline intracranial tumors, particularly at suprasellar or pineal sites. Around 15% are bifocal, involving both sites.

• Most tumors involving the pineal and a minority of suprasellar tumors have raised intracranial pressure at diagnosis and may present as neurosurgical emergencies.

• Many present with neuroendocrine symptoms, of which diabetes insipidus is the most common and is seen in the majority of suprasellar tumors at diagnosis and a proportion of pineal tumors, whilst precocious puberty or panhypopituitarism may also be the first signs of disease in some cases.

• Visual disturbance is common at diagnosis, ranging from visual failure due to chiasmatic involvement to oculomotor palsies and, specifically for pineal tumors, paralysis of upward gaze (Parinaud's Syndrome). Intracranial GCTs may occasionally present with anorexia or other hypothalamic disturbance, change in behaviour, pyramidal tract signs, ataxia or seizures [49].

Metastases from intracranial germ cell tumors

Intracranial GCTs almost never spread to sites outside the CNS. The incidence of spinal or intracranial metastases is in the region of 20% [50].

Management of extracranial germ cell tumors

Investigation and staging of extracranial germ cell tumors

Imaging for germ cell tumors

Since GCTs can present in a multitude of extracranial sites, imaging and follow up will depend upon the site of the primary and initial stage, but may include any of the following:

• Plain X-ray may provide the first indication of a GCT, typically a mature teratoma, where calcification or aberrantly sited mature tissues (such as teeth) can be identified. It is typically employed, especially as a follow up screen, for the detection of pulmonary metastases.

• Ultrasound is frequently used as the initial examination of the primary site, particularly gonadal tumors. It is also an invaluable tool in the follow up of children, especially in marker negative GCTs, as a radiation-sparing modality.

• As with many tumors, CT is the mainstay of investigation of GCTs. It is typically used as a staging tool, to determine the presence of lung and liver metastases, but is also useful to determine local spread, such as regional lymph node involvement in gonadal GCTs.

• MRI is the preferred imaging modality in SCTs, to determine whether there is any intra-spinal component. It may replace CT as the original imaging modality and typically reveals a T1-weighted hypo-intense tumor. A hyper-intense T1 signal is highly suggestive of sebaceous fat within a teratoma, whilst other benign features include fluid levels within cysts and palm tree-like protrusions (Rokitansky protuberance) [51].

• [99m]Technetium Bone Scintigram – as part of the diagnostic work up a bone scan looking for distant skeletal metastases is typically performed. This need only be repeated in the event of relapse, or at the end of therapy if positive at diagnosis.

• ^{18}F-fluorodeoxyglucose (^{18}F-FDG) positron emission tomography (PET) is presently under evaluation in GCTs. Its role is likely to be in determining residual active disease following chemotherapy [52].

Staging

There are many staging systems presently in operation and this makes inter-study comparisons more difficult. The TNM classification has been adopted by most countries for testicular and extragonadal GCTs and is shown in Table 17.4. However, due to the rarity of ovarian GCTs, relative to adult epithelial cancer, these tumors may be staged according to the International Federation of Gynecologic Oncologists (FIGO) system (Table 17.5) [53].

On the basis of the staging, risk stratification is performed (Table 17.6). The treatment schedules used in the UK, France and USA include stratification on the basis of AFP level (for YSTs in children 6–12 months of age) which has been shown to have prognostic significance in children and adults [35, 48].

Treatment of extracranial germ cell tumors
Historical perspective

The treatment of GCTs has been one of the major successes in modern oncology. Historically, they were highly aggressive and rapidly fatal, with the exception of mature teratomas and gonadal germinomas. However, with the advent of effective combination chemotherapy malignant GCTs have come to epitomize the curable cancer. Advances in the treatment of this tumor group were largely led by adult TGCT trials. In children, early studies involved surgery, followed by adjuvant treatment in some cases

Table 17.4 TNM Classification for germ cell tumors.

Stage	Clinical	Post-surgical
I	Tumour <5 cm, no adenopathy, no metastasis	pS1: Tumour without loco-regional extension, completely removed, no metastasis
II	Tumour <greater or equal ≥5 cm, no adenopathy, no metastasis	pSII: Tumour with loco-regional extension, with or without lymph node involvement, completely removed, no metastasis
III	Tumour of any size, locoregional extension and/or lymph node involvement, no metastasis	pSIII: Tumour with loco-regional extension, with no metastasis, incompletely removed pSIIIa: Microscopic residue pSIIIb: Macroscopic residue
IV	Metastatic tumor, including distant lymph nodes (lumbar aortic are loco-regional for testicular tumor)	pSIV: Tumour with distant metastases

(Table 17.7a). For malignant tumors, where surgery, radiotherapy, and/or single agent chemotherapy was employed, the long-term survival was between 10 and 20% [62, 63].

For selected low-stage cases, aggressive surgical management alone, with orchidectomy and retroperitoneal lymph node dissection (RPLND), produced a durable long-term survival in a majority of adult TGCT patients [64], and was successfully adopted for childhood testicular GCTs [65]. Since active retroperitoneal lymph node involvement was rare in pre-pubertal testicular YSTs (only 4% reported by Brosman [66]) RPLND was largely abandoned in children. In addition, adjuvant chemotherapy for stage I TGCTs was also found to confer no survival advantage over orchidectomy alone [67].

Germinomatous tumors were recognized to be exquisitely radio-sensitive and this modality tended to be used in higher stage disease, but appeared ineffective at relapse [68]. The benefits of chemotherapy were initially less clear, partly because early reports did not differentiate between subtypes of GCTs. Pure germinomas appeared to respond as well to chemotherapy as radiotherapy, without the long-term fertility effects [63, 69]. However, chemotherapy alone was not considered to be curative in non-germinomatous GCTs, which were therefore subjected to extensive surgery, radiotherapy, and prolonged multi-drug chemotherapy in the search for a cure [57, 69]. This step-wise progression in treatment, adding radiotherapy and then chemotherapy to simple orchidectomy, resulted in improved outcome with each modality added [70].

For all GCTs, this intense combination therapy was associated with considerable morbidity, and treatment claimed as many lives as the disease itself [57].

• The combination of Vincristine, Actinomycin and Cyclophosphamide (VAC) was thought to be the most effective multi-drug schedule (Table 17.7a) and produced an overall survival in the region of 50–60% [71].

• The introduction of cis-diamminedichloroplatinum (cisplatin) revolutionized drug therapy for GCTs. In 1977, Einhorn and Donohue demonstrated the efficacy of cisplatin in disseminated adult TGCTs [9]. This was confirmed in larger trials and also in the pediatric age range where the most efficacious combination, in the treatment of extracranial MGCTs, was determined to be BEP [72].

Adult TGCT trials have since looked to refine the treatment strategies for both good and poor risk disease. For good risk TGCTs, BEP three-weekly for three courses is as effective as four courses, thereby reducing toxicity. The possibility of omitting bleomycin has also been explored, with mixed results [72]. In pediatric practice, concern regarding toxicity of high dose bleomycin led to the development of schedules with a substantially reduced dose [8].

Table 17.5 FIGO system of staging for ovarian tumors.

Stage I: tumor limited to the ovaries
• IA: one ovary, no ascites, intact capsule.
• IB: both ovaries, no ascites, intact capsule.
• IC: ruptured capsule, capsular involvement, positive peritoneal washings, or malignant ascites.

Stage II: ovarian tumor with pelvic extension
• IIA: pelvic extension to uterus or tubes.
• IIB: pelvic extension to other pelvic organs (bladder, rectum, or vagina).
• IIC: pelvic extension, plus findings indicated for stage IC.

Stage III: tumor outside the pelvis, or positive nodes
• IIIA: microscopic seeding outside the true pelvis.
• IIIB: gross deposits less than 2 cm.
• IIIC: gross deposits greater than 2 cm or positive nodes.

Stage IV: distant organ involvement, including liver parenchyma or pleural space

Table 17.6 Type of germ cell tumor by stage and by risk group [48, 54].

	Ovarian			Testicular			Extragonadal		
	USA	Germany*	UK	USA	Germany	UK	USA	Germany	UK
Stage I	Low	Low	Low	Low	Low[†]	Low	Intermediate	Low	Low[§]
Stage II	Intermediate	Intermediate	Intermediate[¶]	Intermediate	Intermediate	Intermediate	Intermediate	Intermediate	Intermediate**
Stage III	Intermediate	High	Intermediate[¶]	Intermediate	Intermediate[‡]	Intermediate	High	High	Intermediate**
Stage IV	Intermediate	High	High[††]	Intermediate	High	High[††]	High	High	High

* If yolk-sac tumor (YST) histology of the rare endometrioid/hepatoid morphology then upstaged to next category (i.e. low to intermediate risk). [†] If YST and confined to testis but not extending to scrotum or spermatic cord (non-YST or extension then intermediate risk). [‡] Unless locoregional nodes >5 cm or multiple nodal deposits (when high risk). [§] Surgery should avoid mutilation and complete resection may, therefore, rarely be achieved. [¶] Unless alpha-fetoprotein (AFP) ≥10 000 IU/l (when high risk). ** Unless AFP ≥10 000 IU/l or thoracic site (when high risk). [††] Except testicular stage IV in children <5 years, and/or pure germinoma/seminoma (when intermediate risk).

Table 17.7a Evolution of chemotherapeutic schedules for pediatric extracranial malignant germ cell tumors based largely on single institution experience. For abbreviations see Table 17.7c.

Study	Tumour type	Stage	Site	Chemotherapy	Irradiation	Reference
VAC (USA) Single institution 57 patients (1 week–18 years) 1962–1979	23 YST 15 EC 13 IT 4 Germinoma 2 CC 2 mixed	I/II (n = 22) III/IV (n = 35)	30 gonadal (20 ovary, 10 testis) 12 SCT 7 retroperitoneum 5 mediastinum 2 head/neck 1 vagina	Surgery alone (7 stage I, 2 stage II) Remainder predominantly VAC Overall outcome 42% 5y OS Risk factors – high stage (0% 2y OS), extragonadal site, <2y old at diagnosis.	Dysgerminomas exquisitely radiosensitive (n = 3)	[55]
T2 Protocol (USA) Single institution 22 patients (1–14 years) 1960–1974	8 YST 7 EC 2 DG 2 IT 3 mixed	I/II (n = 8) III/IV (n = 14) Incl. 10 cases of relapse, initially stage I	All ovarian	AdriaVAC (n = 10), 60% alive, Vs DOX alone or other combination (n = 8), 8% alive.		[56]
T2 Protocol (USA) Single institution 13 patients (1–22 years) 1971–1975	7 YST 2 DG 2 IT 2 mixed	III (n = 12) IV (n = 1)	All ovarian	Combination (surgery, XRT) and AdriaVAC every 8 weeks for 12–24 months (69% 2y EFS)		[57]
VAC + BP (France/Argentina) 35 patients (1–14 years) 1977–1982	Predominantly YST (raised AFP)	III (n = 16) IV (n = 19)	18 gonadal (12 ovary, 6 testis) 11 SCT 5 mediastinum 1 retroperitoneum	AC(M) + VPBD 6 = weekly (each combination 3-weekly) for 6 courses (63% 2y OS, 60% 2y EFS)		[58]
VAC vs PE (Brazil) Single institution 106 patients (0–18 years) 1983–1987	46 YST 20 EC 16 mixed 11 germinoma 8 'malignant teratoma' 5 IT	I/II (n = 42) III/IV (n = 64)	72 gonadal (37 ovary, 35 testis) 22 SCT 4 vagina 4 retroperitoneum 4 other	Surgery alone (n = 33) VAB-6 like (n = 21) 43% 5y OS EPO/VAC (n = 21) 54% 5y OS PE (n = 31) 81% 5y OS Significant improvement in outcome with cisplatin (high or standard dose)	XRT alone (n = 1) Inclusion of XRT as multimodal therapy in VAB-6 or EPO/VAC only (n = 16)	[59]
VAC vs PVB (Japan) 117 patients (0–17 years) 1975–2000	73 YST 16 EC 13 germinoma 4 CC 11 other	I (n = 54) II (n = 4) III (n = 14) IV (n = 33) NR (n = 12)	84 gonadal (53 testis, 31 ovary) 21 SCT 12 other 1 NR	Surgery alone (n = 29) Single agent/non-protocol combination (n = 50) 47% 5y OS VAC (n = 18) 67% 5y OS PVB (n = 20) 84% 5y OS		[60]
Carboplatin (USA) Single institution 23 patients (≤21 years) 1989–1998	N/R	I/II (n = 4) III (n = 11) IV (n = 8)	10 gonadal (6 ovary, 4 testis) 9 SCT 4 other	JEB (carboplatin 600 mg/m^2) every 3 weeks for 4–6 courses 91% 5y OS, 87% 5y EFS		[61]

Basis for current and future treatment strategies

Most of the experience on which current chemotherapeutic treatment strategies are based has been accumulated in predominantly national studies and the complexity and heterogeneity of GCTs makes comparisons between series difficult. However, there are clear patterns which emerge from the data published from across the world (Table 17.7b and 17.7c). For instance, a common theme which has evolved for all major groups is surgery only,

then watch and wait approach for stage 1 gonadal tumors (Table 17.6).

North America

In their most recent studies, the Americans achieved an EFS of 95% in their POG9048/CCG8881 study of low risk (gonadal) GCTs employing PEB chemotherapy. For high-risk MGCTs (stage I or II extragonadal and all stage III or IV), they compared

Table 17.7b Major findings of national extracranial germ cell tumor trials. For abbreviations see Table 17.7c.

Study	Tumour type	Stage	Site	Chemotherapy	Irradiation	Reference
CCG 861 (USA) 93 patients (0–21 years) 1978–1984	Non-seminomatous 41 YST 39 mixed 9 EC 4 CC	N/R	30 ovarian 63 extragonadal	VeBP + AC + DOX intensive induction, then less frequent maintenance for 2 years (54% 4 y OS, 49% 4 y EFS). Survival significantly better for ovarian than extragonadal (67% vs 48%)		[73]
IGR (France) Single institution 82 patients 1978–1984	Non-seminomatous (secreting GCTs) 63 histologically confirmed (34 YST, 7 IT, 3 CC, 1 EC, 18 mixed)	I (n = 25) III/IV (n = 57)	48 gonadal (28 ovary, 20 testis) 20 SCT 6 mediastinum 5 vagina 3 other	Surgery alone (n = 23) with 4 relapses requiring chemotherapy AC + VPBD (n = 61) 6-weekly for 6 courses For all patients 80% 2 y OS, 69% 2 y EFS		[63]
VAC/PVB (USA) Single institution 60 patients (3 months–17 years) 1979–1988	23 YST 13 mixed 9 germinoma 9 IT 3 EC 2 other 1 unreported	I (n = 18) II (n = 8) III (n = 25) IV (n = 9)	44 gonadal (32 ovary, 12 testis) 8 SCT 3 mediastinum 3 retroperitoneum 1 vagina 1 head/neck	Surgery alone for 17 stage 1 (all testis) & ovary (size <10 cm) VAC or PVB (80% 5 y OS). 5 y OS worse for higher stage (I-100%, II-87%, III-72%, IV-56%) PVB superior to VAC for high risk (extragonadal) and relapsed tumors. Cisplatin hearing loss in 8/22	XRT alone (n = 6, stage I-III germinoma) or in combination with chemotherapy (n = 12, stage IV). XRT highly effective, especially for germinoma (all alive).	[74]
SFOP TGM 85 (France) 67 patients (2 months–18 years) 1985–1989	Non-seminomatous	I/II (n = 49) III (n = 17) IV (n = 1)	48 gonadal (29 testis, 19 ovary) 9 SCT 5 mediastinum 4 retroperitoneum 1 neck	Surgery alone (complete resection), otherwise as stage III/IV AC + PVB (81% 2 y OS, 77% 3 y EFS) DOX omitted without adverse effects (esp. stage I/II) Higher stage did worse (39% 2 y EFS for stage III vs 87% for stage II chemotherapy), thus need to intensify treatment.		[75]
CCLG GC1 (UK) VAC/PVB/BEP 126 patients (0–15 years) 1979–1987	97 YST 13 mixed 11 IT 5 germinoma	I (n = 63) II (n = 18) III (n = 23) IV (n = 22)	89 gonadal (61 testis, 29 ovary) 21 SCT 5 mediastinum 4 vagina, uterus or prostate 2 retroperitoneum 4 other	Surgery alone (n = 44), all stage 1 (41 testis, 2 ovary, 1 SCT) Low-dose VAC (8% 5 y OS) High-dose VAC (±Dox) (87% 5 y OS) BEP (84% 5 y OS) PVB (67% 5 y OS) Bleomycin toxicity using PVB – 4 treatment related deaths. Frequent cisplatin induced renal impairment and deafness		[8]

Continued

Table 17.7b *Continued*

Study	Tumour type	Stage	Site	Chemotherapy	Irradiation	Reference
SFOP TGM 85 and 90 (France) 63 patients (0–18 years) 1985–1994	Non-seminomatous secreting GCTs AFP in 49 and HCG in 14 14 IT	I (n = 9) II (n = 21) III (n = 29) IV (n = 3) N/R (n = 1)	All ovarian	Surgery alone for 12 (pSI) secreting tumors and 10 ITs AC + PVB (TGM 85) 3-weekly for 3 courses, n = 23 JVB + AC (TGM 90) – Carboplatin 400 mg/m², 3-weekly for 3 courses or 2-courses beyond marker normalization, n = 40 85% 5 y OS, 74% 5 y EFS Greater number of relapses in TGM 90 (carboplatin)		[76]
SFOP TGM 85 and 90 (France) 81 patients (1–18 years) 1985–1994	Non-seminomatous Of 55 recorded (rest by markers): 37 YST 12 EC 4 IT 2 CC	I (n = 14) II (n = 28) III (n = 37) 2 bilateral	47 gonadal (36 ovary, 11 testis) 21 SCT 7 mediastinum 5 retroperitoneum 1 perineum	AC+PVB (TGM85) 3-weekly for 3 courses, n = 41 JVB + AC (TGM 90) – Carboplatin 400 mg/m², 3-weekly for 3 courses or 2-courses beyond marker normalization, n = 40 87% 3 y OS, 68% 3 y EFS Poor risk patients: AFP > 10 000 ng/ml, stage III and/or mediastinal/SCT site		[77]
Low risk strategy PEB (USA) POG9048/CCG8881 74 patients (8 months –16 years) 1990–1995	53 YST 15 mixed 3 NR 2 CC 1 EC	I (n = 41) II (n = 33)	All gonadal receiving chemotherapy (stage I/II ovary or stage II testis)	PEB 3-weekly for 4 courses 96% 6 y OS, 95% 6 y EFS 2 cases of AML (non 11q23) recorded Excellent survival figures – planned to treat stage I ovary with surgery alone approach (equivalent to testis stage I)		[78]
High risk strategy PEB (USA) POG9049/CCG8882 299 patients (1–20 years) 1990–1996	191 YST 60 mixed 31 germinoma 9 CC 3 EC 2 other 3 NR	I/II (n = 30) III (n = 136) IV (n = 133) Includes 16 surgery alone testis stage I relapses	134 gonadal (74 ovary, 60 testis) 87 SCT 39 mediastinum 26 retroperitoneum 12 vagina/uterus 1 penis	PEB/High-dose PEB 3-weekly for 4 courses (additional 2 courses if non-CR). 89% 6 y OS, 85% 6 y EFS High-dose PEB significantly improved EFS but not OS (more tumor related deaths with PEB, or toxic-treatment related deaths with high-dose PEB) High incidence of hearing loss with high-dose PEB		[11]
CCLG (UK) GC2 184 patients (0–16 years) 1989–1997	107 YST 55 'malignant teratoma' 20 germinoma 1 EC 1 CC	I (n = 69) II (n = 32) III (n = 35) IV (n = 42) NR (n = 6)	117 gonadal (63 testis, 54 ovary) 37 SCT 13 mediastinum 6 vagina/uterus 11 other	Surgery alone (40 testis, 6 ovary, 1 mediastinal) – all stage I JEB (n = 137), carboplatin 600 mg/m², 3-weekly until CR or for 2 courses beyond marker normalization. 93% 5 y OS (all), 91% 5 y OS (JEB), 88% 5 y EFS (JEB) AFP >10 000 ng/ml, mediastinal site and high stage of prognostic significance. Minimal long-term toxicity with carboplatin		[48]
TCG 91 (Italy) 95 patients (0–16 years) 1991–1998	73 Non-seminomatous 14 germinoma 8 mixed	I (n = 39) II (n = 5) III (n = 23) IV (n = 15)	59 gonadal (36 testis, 23 ovary) 30 SCT 2 mediastinum 5 others	Surgery alone (24 testis, 6 ovary) – all stage I JE/IVA (n = 64), carboplatin 800 mg/m²/ course (reduced dosing frequency) for 2–4 courses 83% OS, 72% EFS	XRT alone for stage 2 germinoma (n = 1)	[79]

Table 17.7c Site and histology specific findings.

Study	Tumour type	Stage	Site	Chemotherapy	Irradiation	Reference
Testicular site Surgery alone (USA) POG9048/CCG8891 63 patients (1 month – 5 years) 1990–1995	All YSTs	All stage I	All testicular	Surgery alone in all cases. 100% 6 y OS, 79 6 y EFS Excellent outcome, all relapses salvaged with chemotherapy. No need for RPLND in children 4 cases of trans-scrotal violation (with significantly greater relapse rate)		[80]
IGR – XRT therapy Study (France) Single institution 35 patients (4–18 years) 1978–1984	DG alone	I ($n = 14$) II ($n = 1$) III ($n = 17$) IV ($n = 3$)	All ovarian	Surgery alone for stage I ($n = 3$) ACPBD ($n = 1$) Demonstrated need for chemotherapy to reduce toxicity	94% 5 y OS 77.7% 5 y EFS 2 deaths – both stage IV. Very toxic (10 infertile and 1 late radiation death).	[63]
Ovarian site PEB (USA) POG9048/CCG8891 131 patients (1–20 years) 1990–1996	60 'malignant teratoma' (39 YST) 25 YST 23 DG 2 CC 10 mixed 2 gonadoblastoma 9 NR	I ($n = 41$) II ($n = 16$) III ($n = 58$) IV ($n = 16$)	All ovarian	PEB/High-dose PEB 3-weekly for 4 courses. >95% 6 y OS, >92% 6 y EFS Confirms that extensive surgery is not necessary for a successful outcome and that future advances should look at reduction in therapy (e.g. surgery alone for stage I)		[19]
Extragonadal site JEB (UK) CCLG GC1 and 2 98 patients (0–15 years) GC1 1979–1988 GC2 1989–1995	56 YST 34 'malignant teratoma' 2 germinoma 2 IT 4 N/R	I ($n = 10$) II ($n = 20$) III ($n = 18$) IV ($n = 48$) N/R ($n = 4$)	All extragonadal 59 SCT 15 mediastinum 11 retroperitoneum 7 vagina, uterus or prostate 3 head/neck 3 liver/bile duct	Surgery alone ($n = 3$, stage 1 SCTs) For all patients: GC1 (VAC ± DOX, PVB or BEP) 63% 10 y OS, 46% 5 y EFS GC2 (JEB, carboplatin 600 mg/m^2) 96% 5 y OS, 87% 5 y EFS Cisplatin (PVB or BEP) higher incidence of renal impairment and deafness. Carboplatin as effective as cisplatin with less morbidity		[81]
Extragonadal site PEB (USA) POG9049/CCG8882 165 patients (0–18 years) 1990–1996	136 YST 14 mixed 5 CC 4 germinoma 6 other	I/II ($n = 30$) III ($n = 61$) IV ($n = 74$)	All extragonadal 88 SCT 39 mediastinum 35 retroperitoneum 3 other	PEB/High-dose PEB 3-weekly for 4 courses. 83% 5 y OS, 79% 5 y EFS Worse prognosis with age ≥12 years High-dose PEB of borderline significant benefit to OS		[82]
SCT site PEB (USA) POG9049/CCG8882 74 patients 1990–1996	48 YST 24 'malignant teratoma' 2 NR	I ($n = 3$) II ($n = n = 10$) III ($n = 17$) IV ($n = 44$)	All SCT	PEB/High-dose PEB 3-weekly for 4 courses. 90% 4 y OS, 84% 4 y EFS Chemotherapy highly effective as: Outcome in primary or delayed resection, PEB or high-dose PEB, AND complete or partial resection equivalent		[22]
SCT site PEI/BEP/VIP (Germany) MAKEI 83/86 & 89 66 patients (7–119 months) 1983–995	45 YST 21 'malignant teratoma'	I/II/III ($n = 36$) IV ($n = 30$)	All SCT	81% 5 y OS, 76% 5 y EFS Prognostic factors – completeness of first surgical excision and stage IV (metastases not prognostically relevant if up front chemotherapy with delayed surgical excision)		[83]
Relapsed SCT site PEI ± XRT (Germany) MAKEI 83/86 and 89 22 patients 1983–1995	21 YST 1 mixed	All relapses 17 local 2 distant 3 combined	All Relapsed SCT	42% 5 y OS, 30% 5 y EFS Prognostically relevant: –Whether completely excised at salvage surgery –Whether first or subsequent relapse –If primary chemotherapy omitted etoposide (linked to metastatic rather than loco-regional relapse)		[84]

Continued

Table 17.7c *Continued*

Study	Tumour type	Stage	Site	Chemotherapy	Irradiation	Reference
Mediastinal site PEB (USA) POG9049/CCG8882 36 patients 1990–1996	14 YST 15 mixed 3 germinoma 2 CC	I/II (n = 8) III (n = 19) IV (n = 9)	All mediastinal	PEB/High-dose PEB 3-weekly for 4 courses. 71% 4y OS, 69% 4y EFS High rate of secondary cancer (2 AML, 1 erythrophagoctosis) Poor prognosis site, especially in boys (usually older ages). Bulky tumors appear to have worse outcome		[85]
Mediastinal site PEI/BEP/VIP (Germany) MAKEI 83/86/89 and 96 47 patients (0–17 years) 1983–1999	16 MT 15 YST 7 mixed 5 IT 3 germinoma 1 CC	I/II (n = 38) III/IV (n = 9)	All mediastinal	All MT/IT (n = 21) received surgery alone and germinomas (n = 3) XRT alone. Chemotherapy for MAKEI 83/86 -PVB/PEI, MAKEI 89 – BEP/VIP, MAKEI 96 – PEI (×4–8 courses). No difference in outcome despite different chemotherapy combinations. 87% 5y OS, 83% 5y EFS Complete resection imperative (whether primary, delayed or second look surgery) – EFS 94% vs 42%. Older age and high stage tended towards worse prognosis		[86]
Retroperitneal site PEB (USA) POG9049/CCG8882 25 patients (2 months – 18 years) 1990–1996	15 YST 3 CC 4 'malignant teratoma' 1 germinoma 2 mixed	I/II (n = 3) III (n = 5) IV (n = 17)	15 retroperitoneum 4 abdominal wall 3 liver 2 pelvis 1 small bowel	PEB/High-dose PEB 3-weekly for 4 courses. 88% 6y OS, 83% 6y EFS Initial compete excision uncommon and second look surgery merited to achieve complete resection		[87]
Genital tumors PEB (USA) POG9049/CCG8882 13 patients (5 months – 2 years) 1990–1996	All YST	All local disease	11 vagina 1 uterus 1 penis	PEB/High-dose PEB 3-weekly for 4 courses. 92% 4y OS, 76% 4y EFS Aim for conservative surgery (biopsy alone) and adjuvant chemotherapy		[88]
Immature teratomas (USA) POG9048/CCG8881 73 patients (0–17 years) 1990–1995	All IT	Grade I (23)* Grade II (29) Grade III (21)	51 gonadal (44 ovary, 7 testis) 7 retroperitoneum 7 head & neck 5 SCT 3 mediastinum	Surgery alone sufficient. Chemotherapy at relapse (7%) 100% 3y OS, 93% 3y EFS Presence of microfoci of YST (Heifetz lesions) more common with higher grade IT, yet rarely relapse.		[30]

XRT, radiotherapy. VAC, vincristine, actinomycin D, cyclophosphamide. AC(M), actinomycin D, cyclophosphamide, (methotrexate). VPBD, vincristine, cisPlatin, bleomycin, doxorubicin. VeBP, vinblastine, bleomycin, cisPlatin. AdriaVAC, adriamycin (doxorubicin – DOX) + VAC. BP, bleomycin + cisPlatin. PE, cisPlatin + etoposide. PEB (paediatric schedule BEP), cisPlatin, etoposide, bleomycin. BEP, bleomycin, etoposide, cisPlatin. ACPBD, actinomycin D, cyclophosphamide, cisPlatin, bleomycin, doxorubicin. VAB-6, vinblastine, actinomycin D, bleomycin, cyclophospamide, cisPlatin. P(J)VB, cisPlatin (J-carboplatin), vinblastine, bleomycin. YST, yolk sac tumor. EC, embryonal carcinoma. IT, immature teratoma. DG, dysgerminoma. SCT, sacrococcygeal teratoma, CC, choriocarcinoma. OS, overall Survival. EFS, event-free survival. N/R, not recorded. N/A, not applicable. SFOP, French Society of Paeditric Oncology. POG/CCG, Pediatric Oncology Group/Children's Cancer Group. CCLG, Children's Cancer and Leukaemia Group (formerly the United Kingdom Children's Cancer Study Group – UKCCSG). MAKEI, Maligne KEImzelltumoren. IGR, Insitut Gustave Roussy.
* Grading for immature teratomas, see Table 17.2. RPNLD, retroperitoneal lymph node dissection. Commonly used extracranial chemotherapy schedules: JEB (UK): carboplatin AUC 7.9 mg/ml.min or 600 mg/m^2 (D2), etoposide 120 mg/m^2 (D1–3), bleomycin 15 mg/m^2 (D3); PEB (USA): bleomycin 15 mg/m^2 (D1), etoposide 100 mg/m^2 (D1–5), cisplatin 20 mg/m^2 (D1–5); High-dose PEB (USA): bleomycin 15 mg/m^2 (D1), etoposide 100 mg/m^2 (D1–5), cisplatin 40 mg/m^2 (D1–5); BEP (Germany): bleomycin 15 mg/m^2 (D1–3), etoposide 80 mg/m^2 (D1–3), cisplatin 20 mg/m^2 (D4–8); PEI (Germany): cisplatin 20 mg/m^2 (D1–5), etoposide 100 mg/m^2 (D1–3), ifosfamide 1.5 g/m^2 (D1–5); PVB (Germany): cisplatin 20 mg/m^2 (D4–8), vinblastine 3 mg/m^2 [or 0.15 mg/kg] (D1–2), bleomycin 15 mg/m^2 (D1–3). NB, Drug or dose alterations required for infants <1 year of age and in presence of renal impairment.

high-dose (HD) cisplatin (200 mg/m^2) with standard cisplatin (100 mg/m^2) PEB in POG9049/CCG8882 [11]. Whilst they demonstrated an improved survival in this trial of 299 children compared with historical series, dose intensification of cisplatin did not lead to an increase in overall survival (OS), an increased EFS in the HD arm balanced by treatment-related fatal infections in the same group, and increased morbidity from renal impairment and hearing loss [89]. Attempts to reduce hearing loss with the chemical protection agent amifostine do not appear to protect against HDPEB-associated ototoxicity [90].

UK

Carboplatin, as part of JEB (with Etoposide and Bleomycin) has been the central plank of GCT treatment in the UK since 1989 [48], with results which compare favourably with cisplatin based strategies employed elsewhere in children. Even the survival for the highest risk patients were comparable with American figures (UK 5 year EFS of 85% ± 3.0% and USA 6year EFS of 84.4% ± 4.4%) [11]. The potential for less toxic treatment of MGCTs, at least in the younger patient, warrants further consideration. Attempts to identify a group of adult patients that could also benefit from substitution of carboplatin for cisplatin have been less successful. Lower survival rates were reported in adult TGCTs, treated with carboplatin [91–93], although the case for inferiority of carboplatin in lower risk adult patients was initially confounded by the use of lower doses than in the pediatric series. Carboplatin's role is therefore limited to single dose prophylactic treatment of stage I seminoma in adult TGCTs (where relapse can be reduced from ~20% in watch and wait, to <4% with carboplatin) [94].

Italy

The Italians employed a six-drug strategy using carboplatin, also to prevent cisplatin oto- and renal toxicity, and omitted bleomycin to avoid lung fibrosis. However, they encountered profound hematological toxicity including three reported septic deaths [79], for which the increased dose and frequency of carboplatin, with the addition of ifosfamide, may in part be responsible.

France

The French published their experience with various platinum-based regimens, and established high AFP (>10 000 ng/ml) as a risk factor for relapse [77]. They also explored the use of carboplatin but failed to demonstrate equivalent efficacy in a randomized study [76], although their conclusions were based on 400 mg/m^2 carboplatin rather than the 600 mg/m^2 employed in the UK GC2 study.

Germany

The German 'MAKEI' group have run studies in GCTs, in which the chemotherapy has moved towards combination of cisplatin and ifosfamide (PEI) with comparable outcomes to the bleomycin-containing regimens [83, 84].

The number of chemotherapy courses employed in treatment of GCTs varies by study and according to risk group, ranging from two or three in low risk cases to six courses in the highest risk cases. For secreting tumors, the number of courses has sometimes been determined by the rate of response, two additional courses being given after marker normalization and an additional two courses thereafter. Should there be residual disease after four cycles, second-look surgery could be performed. In the UK GC2 study, this strategy was employed but the median number of courses given was five (range 3–8) [48], which was more than given in alternative strategies for low and standard risk tumors.

Surgical management of extracranial germ cell tumors

Surgery was initially a diagnostic procedure before being shown to be a prognostic feature, with upfront complete surgical resection resulting in a better survival irrespective of effective adjuvant chemotherapy [73]. However, aggressive and mutilating surgery is not necessary, since GCTs (other than teratomas) are chemosensitive. Thus, delayed surgical excision, in particular for mediastinal GCTs but for any in which there is residual after chemotherapy, may be simpler and confirm treatment response. Indeed, the completeness of surgical resection, whether primary or delayed, appears to be prognostically significant [86].

Radiotherapy for extracranial germ cell tumors

Pure dysgerminoma is curable using radiotherapy alone. However, the late effects of radiotherapy, coupled with the exquisite chemosensitivity of these tumors has led to chemotherapy being preferred [69]. Radiotherapy is therefore avoided in primary treatment of extracranial GCTs, being reserved for intracranial GCTs, and used only occasionally for specific cases of extracranial GCT at the time of relapse and/or palliation.

Treatment of teratomas

Pure MT is cured by surgical excision and always behaves in a benign fashion if ovarian or testicular. Sacrococcygeal pure MTs on the other hand, may recur locally as malignant tumors in around 10% of cases, meriting careful post-operative follow up [16, 23]. Treatment of immature teratoma (IT) remains controversial, particularly in view of apparent differences between behaviour of these tumors in adults and children.
• There is good evidence that complete surgical excision is curative in children irrespective of grade [30], whilst incomplete removal is a risk factor for relapse [16].
• The evidence of benefit from adjuvant chemotherapy, advocated in adult practice for higher stage disease, is lacking in children [16, 95] and surgery remains the mainstay of treatment. Although malignant recurrences, salvageable with first line chemotherapy, have been particularly associated with the presence of either initial microfoci of YST or a raised AFP [31], the significance of moderately raised AFP levels in IT remains controversial; it may simply represent immature endodermal elements rather than a malignant element [30], and does not therefore necessarily justify chemotherapy.

• Where ovarian ITs are associated with abdominal deposits these may also be managed surgically, and resection of gliomatosis peritonei is not necessary.

Teratomas containing frank malignant germ cell elements are staged and treated as mixed MGCTs with surgery and chemotherapy as appropriate. If non-GCT malignant elements are present (typically neuroblastoma, PNET, sarcoma, myeloid leukemia, or carcinomas), adjuvant treatment of such malignant teratomas is based on the malignant component present, rather than on a MGCT strategy.

Management of extracranial germ cell tumors according to site

Testes

The recommended surgical approach for testicular GCTs is inguinal, to avoid scrotal contamination. Spermatic cord vascular mobilization and control, prior to testicular mobilization, is also recommended in most countries, but there is limited evidence to support this. Furthermore, there is no evidence that retroperitoneal lymph node biopsy carries any prognostic significance in childhood testicular GCTs, and treatment on the basis of imaging is therefore preferred. Management of the scenario of scrotal violation, in terms of staging and additional treatment required, is not clear. Hemiscrotectomy has been advocated to reduce the local relapse rate, through potential tumor seeding of the scrotal wound [80], but the value of such surgery in reducing relapse, and particularly in improving overall survival, is unproven.

The excellent salvage rate of relapses accounting for approximately 20% of cases following watch and wait for stage I tumors justifies this approach, with 100% cured in the UK series and comparable results reported elsewhere [79, 96]. The first sign of relapse in secreting tumors may be a rise in AFP and the various platinum-based strategies employed by different groups for GCTs produce similarly excellent outcomes for higher stage tumors and relapsed stage I cases.

Ovaries

Primary surgical excision, avoiding mutilation and preserving uninvolved structures and fertility, is standard management of ovarian MGCTs. At the same time ascitic fluid (or peritoneal washings) should be collected and the peritoneal surfaces, lymph nodes, omentum, and contralateral ovary should be examined and suspicious areas biopsied.

• Unresectable or bilateral tumors should be biopsied prior to possible fertility-conserving surgery following appropriate chemotherapy.

• However, bilateral gonadectomy is recommended for cases of gonadoblastoma.

• For completely excised stage I MGCT disease or teratoma, no further treatment is necessary and chemotherapy can be reserved for the minority who relapse [48, 19]. Careful attention to initial staging, and to surgical guidelines, including avoidance of tumor capsule rupture, is crucial if stage I tumors are to be treated safely

with a surgery and 'wait and watch' approach. Treatment of higher stage tumors and recurrences following wait and watch is given as for testicular GCTs.

Management of ovarian teratomas should be limited to surgery, even for ITs with abdominal deposits which should be removed if possible, and resection of associated gliomatosis peritonei is not usually considered necessary.

Genitourinary tract

These tumors, which are invariably YSTs and tend to occur in the very young (≤2 years of age), are chemosensitive and carry an excellent prognosis. They may occur in the vagina, uterus, prostate, perineum, or penis. Surgical biopsy may be required, but radical surgery is not necessary and should be avoided.

Mediastinum

Boys present earlier if associated with Klinefelter's syndrome (mean 16 years vs 27 years for all mediastinal GCTs [97]) and seem to do less well if ≥15 years of age, despite treatment, possibly suggesting that they are a particularly high-risk group [85]. There is a greater risk of associated hematological malignancies, particularly AML, with mediastinal GCTs, which may occur in 10–20% of cases. Of note, this association between mediastinal GCTs and AML may occur early following diagnosis or treatment and the leukemic clone typically displays i(12p). This suggests a GCT origin rather than treatment-induced rearrangements at 11q23, which is typical of etoposide therapy and occurs in <1% of GCTs treated with chemotherapy [98].

The potential risk of anesthesia at presentation in a tumor affecting the lower airways makes mediastinal GCTs, like lymphomas, challenging to investigate.

• The presence of raised tumor markers may make surgical diagnosis unnecessary; otherwise image guided biopsy can be considered.

• For most mediastinal tumors, chemotherapy is best given prior to attempting resection and has been shown to reduce the risk of capsule violation at the time of surgery as well as reducing phrenic nerve damage.

However, chemotherapy appears not to affect tumor adhesiveness to neighbouring structures (notably thymus and pericardium), so surgery remains challenging. The importance of complete resection, even of residual teratomatous tissue post-chemotherapy, is underlined by the tendency of these tumors to behave more like adult TGCTs and to develop 'Growing Teratoma Syndrome' which may undergo late malignant change, particularly in older boys [43]. Primary surgery is reserved for marker negative tumors (teratomas), although marker negative germinoma and/or EC will require subsequent chemotherapy followed by second look surgery [86].

Outcomes for mediastinal tumors are significantly worse than for their gonadal counterparts. The strongest prognostic indicator was completeness of tumor resection (5 year OS 100% vs 42%) followed by age <5 years and low stage [86].

Box 17.1 Treatment of malignant extracranial germ cell tumors: general principles.

- Primary surgery when possible

  Inguinal approach for testicular primaries

  Sampling of ascites for ovarian tumors
- Biopsy or diagnosis with raised markers in inoperable tumors
- Gonadal Stage I tumors: complete resection and 'watch and wait'
- All other stages: cisplatin-based chemotherapy, 2–4 courses*
- Extragonadal tumors: platinum-based chemotherapy

  High risk tumors: up to six courses*
- Surgery following chemotherapy for residual tumor
- Radiotherapy not part of routine first line treatment

*Depends on national practice and precise drug combination selected

Sacrococcygeal site (Plate 17.1)

As for pediatric teratomas at other sites, surgery is the mainstay of treatment for SCTs. Operative removal requires *en bloc* excision of the SCT along with the coccyx, and this was demonstrated to reduce the risk of relapse as early as 1951 [99]. SCTs comprising only MT or IT (i.e. without age-related marker elevation or radiological evidence of malignancy) are both treated with complete surgical excision alone, although microfoci of YST are more common the higher the IT grade and in turn increase the likelihood of relapse following surgery. Overall the recurrence rate is around 12.5% (MT 0–26%; IT 12–55%) with increased risk attributed to [38]:

- Incomplete resection or lack of *en bloc* removal of the coccyx.
- Pre-/peri-operative tumor spillage.
- Failure to appreciate malignancy within the original SCT specimen (likely sampling error).
- Presence of YST microfoci.

Fifty to 70% of all relapses contain MGCT (almost always YST), whilst the remainder are MT or IT. Relapse occasionally occurs with other somatic malignancies, particularly PNET. Repeated, often mutilating, surgical attempts to cure the children of their disease are a cause of considerable morbidity. SCTs with YST microfoci known to be incompletely excised are usually treated with primary chemotherapy. Despite treatment with chemotherapy, these tumors may later recur as IT rather than malignant tumors, and are fatal in a minority of cases [16].

SCT known to be malignant at diagnosis are considered high-risk tumors, and treated by chemotherapy and delayed resection, unless small and amenable to primary resection. This improves survival by facilitating complete surgical removal. This strategy should therefore be followed for marker positive disease or malignant SCT diagnosed by biopsy following radiological or clinical

suspicion. The presence of metastases has not been shown to influence survival where chemotherapy was given initially [83].

Treatment strategies for relapsed extracranial germ cell tumors

Chemotherapy naïve tumors that relapse following a watch and wait policy can undergo standard first line chemotherapy, according to national or institutional practice. Cases that progress on treatment or recur following chemotherapy present more difficulties, partly because of their rarity in childhood and the lack of trial data to direct treatment. Traditional second line therapy tends to involve more platinum-based agents in combination with other known active agents, including vinblastine, ifosfamide, and doxorubicin, schedules varying according to the first line combinations employed, with response rates in the region of 50% [48]. Whilst high-dose chemotherapy followed by autologous stem cell rescue has been employed successfully in adult TGCTs [100], the evidence for the benefit of this approach in children is limited, and based on small numbers [101].

Extracranial germ cell tumors: complications and follow up

Short-term complications of presentation and treatment of extracranial germ cell tumors

Chemotherapy side effects are mainly short term, including nausea and vomiting, alopecia, and myelosuppression. Complications of surgery for extracranial GCTs depend on the site involved and are relatively unusual, the highest risk of surgical morbidity associated with SCTs and mediastinal tumors.

Strategies for follow up of extracranial germ cell tumors and overview of important late effects

Most relapses occur within the first 2 years from diagnosis and therefore close monitoring of tumor markers through this period is essential. Most groups would advocate regular measurement until 3 years off treatment. Following surgery and/or during chemotherapy, markers are often measured weekly until normalization, then monthly for about 1 year with gradual reduction in frequency thereafter. Regular imaging of marker negative tumors should be undertaken, also for about 3 years.

Long-term toxicities of drugs commonly used in the treatment of intracranial MGCTs include the following:
- Etoposide: secondary AML, typically 3–5 years after treatment and associated with 11q23 clonal abnormalities, although this is low risk, occurring in ≤1% of childhood GCTs [98].
- Alkylating agents: renal toxicity (especially ifosfamide, usually manifest within a year of treatment), impaired fertility (especially cyclophosphamide, risk lower for ifosfamide but less evidence).
- Platinum drugs: hearing and renal impairment, greatest with cisplatin (usually manifest within a year of treatment). Hearing loss with cisplatin chemotherapy is common (44% at 2 years following a cumulative dose ≥400 mg/m^2 [102]) unlike carboplatin, and deteriorates beyond the time of finishing treatment, also exacerbated by extended field radiotherapy.

• Bleomycin: pulmonary toxicity; particularly in older patients and those with renal impairment [8]. Concerns that children may be more susceptible to bleomycin lung damage than adults, especially in those treated with cisplatin [8, 63], have led to dose reductions in pediatric protocols, without apparent compromise in terms of survival, and substitution of ifosfamide for bleomycin has also shown to be effective.

Management of intracranial germ cell tumors

Despite histological similarities with their extracranial counterparts, the anatomical locations of intracranial GCTs dictate a different approach in terms of investigation and treatment.

The main difference is that there is no demonstrated benefit of primary surgery for malignant tumors [103–105]. Of particular note is the:
• Importance of measuring markers in both CNS and serum for diagnosis.
• Requirement of radiotherapy for cure, either alone or in combination with chemotherapy.

In light of their rarity and the complexity of their management, patients with suspected intracranial GCTs should be referred to specialist centres for management by multidisciplinary teams.

Investigation and staging of intracranial GCTs
Given the importance of measurement of tumor markers in their diagnosis, it is important to consider the possibility of GCTs early in cases of intracranial tumors occurring in the midline, particularly at suprasellar or pineal sites. Diagnostic and staging investigations for intracranial GCTs include imaging, measurement of tumor markers and, in selected cases, histology.

Imaging
If the clinical presentation is suggestive of a GCT, radiological confirmation should be sought using MRI of the head and spine with contrast.
• MGCTs typically appear as solid masses on MRI that are hypo- or iso-intense on T1 and hyper- or iso-intense on T2-weighted images, with prominent enhancement following the administration of contrast.
• Germinomas are distinguished from other diagnoses by their homogeneous appearance and typical sites of involvement, with approximately 20% of cases being bifocal (pineal and suprasellar) and 20% metastatic, in which multifocal involvement is seen mainly within the ventricular system and spinal cord. Very small germinomas may be evident on MRI by the absence of the bright spot of the posterior pituitary in T1-weighted images together with thickening of the hypothalamus and infundibular stalk.
• Malignant NGGCTs present a more heterogenous texture compared with germinoma and bifocal disease is uncommon. CT scans show GCTs as iso- or hyperdense lesions, with occasional calcification; the presence of fat and calcification or intratumoral

cysts suggests the possibility of a mature teratomatous component [106, 107].
• Immature teratomas tend to have fewer or smaller cystic components and less calcification [106].

The differential diagnosis of small lesions in the suprasellar region includes Langerhans cell hystiocytosis, which can be difficult to differentiate due to loss of granules in the posterior pituitary, and sarcoidosis, which is extremely rare. With larger lesions, low grade glioma should be considered. In the pineal region, GCTs are the most likely diagnosis but the differential includes PNETs, low grade astrocytomas and pinealocytomas. Bifocal lesions are highly characteristic of germinoma, so these are often treated as germinoma without biopsy confirmation. MR Spectroscopy (MRS) may have a complementary role in differential diagnosis and a PET scan may also help to differentiate GCTs from low grade lesions, but neither technique is employed widely and both therefore need further evaluation [108].

Histology and tumor markers
Approximately half of CNS GCTs are pure germinoma and the remainder made up of non-germinomatous MGCTs (secreting tumors and EC), many of mixed histology, and a small number of mature and immature teratomas.

Since the management and prognosis is markedly different for germinomas and secreting GCTs, initial work-up must include the measurement of tumor markers in both the serum and cerebrospinal fluid (CSF) compartments, in addition to imaging of the head and spine, prior to any definitive surgical intervention.
• The marker levels regarded as significantly abnormal vary between groups and are controversial. This is particularly the case for β-HCG, which may be raised in germinoma due to syncytiotrophoblastic cells, in terms of the level at which this is regarded as indicative of a NGGCT, and the role a raised β-HCG has as a risk factor in germinoma.
• Levels of AFP >25 ng/ml and/or β-HCG >50 IU/l in either compartment are typically regarded as indicative of a secreting tumor, although in Japanese series much higher levels of β-HCG are allowed with germinomas. The importance of measuring markers in both compartments is underlined by the finding that around 10% of cases of secreting GCTs have elevated markers in one compartment only [109].

Diagnosis of pure germinoma is based on histology, but a positive biopsy alone is not sufficient to determine treatment since raised markers would imply mixed histology and dictate treatment as a secreting tumor (NGGCT).

Surgical intervention at presentation
Many patients with CNS GCTs present with hydrocephalus, requiring urgent surgery for control of intracranial pressure. CSF should be withdrawn as the first intervention in this procedure, prior to attempting biopsy or third ventriculostomy. In the absence of hydrocephalus, CSF should be obtained by lumbar puncture and levels of both serum and CSF markers obtained prior to any surgical intervention. If thresholds are reached for

the diagnosis of a secreting tumor, then histological confirmation is not necessary and should be avoided, because of the risks associated with surgery [103].

When serum and CSF markers are negative, a histological specimen will be necessary to establish the diagnosis. This may be obtained by stereotactic biopsy or via endoscopy in experienced hands. In some cases open biopsy may be considered appropriate, but it should be borne in mind that resection of CNS MGCTs does not confer any survival advantage and therefore the aim of the procedure should be to obtain diagnostic material. It is also important to remember that, although a small stereotactic biopsy may be insufficient to pick up all components of a mixed GCT, this lack of a complete histological profile will not influence management.

Staging of intracranial germ cell tumors

Metastatic disease is defined as the presence of visible deposits on cranial or spinal MRI, or positive CSF cytology. Lumbar puncture is the preferred technique for this purpose but CSF taken at the time of emergency surgery for raised pressure and/or acquisition of material for histology is acceptable if sampling is carried out prior to biopsy.

Bifocal tumors, involving both the suprasellar and pineal sites, constitute an entity peculiar to GCTs, and are more common in germinoma. The finding of diabetes insipidus (DI) in germinomas, which appear only to involve the pineal gland, raises the question as to whether the true incidence is greater than suggested by currently available imaging techniques. Practices vary in terms of the management of bifocal tumors, with European groups treating them as localized disease and the US as metastatic. However, the Canadian experience suggests that they can be considered as locoregional disease rather than metastatic entities [110].

Treatment of intracranial germ cell tumors
Historical perspective

Early treatment of intracranial GCTs was surgical and survival was poor, with no clear differentiation between different histologies at the pineal site. Despite the absence of effective three-dimensional imaging, prior to the advent of CT scan in the 1970s, germinomas were successfully treated from the 1950s with radiotherapy. At this time, they were diagnosed on the basis of clinical features, plain skull radiograph, and distortion of the posterior wall of the third ventricle on air studies.

• Jenkin et al. in Toronto (1978) reported treatment of pineal tumors without biopsy between 1958 and 1976, using radiotherapy in doses ranging from 35 to >50 Gy, with survival of 81% in patients under the age of 25. Patients over 25, who in hindsight were less likely to have GCTs, had only a 37% survival [111].
• At around the same time, Dearnaley's group in the UK reported the result of 34 cases treated between 1962 and 1987, using 50 Gy to the tumor bed and 30 Gy to the cranio-spinal axis [112]. The diagnosis of germinoma was based on initial response ('radiosensitivity test') and the 5-year overall survival was 82% with only

one local recurrence. There were 12 cases of 'malignant teratoma' (corresponding to mixed/secreting tumors or NGGCTs in current terminology) which responded poorly.

In the 1970s and 1980s, biopsy became more common to confirm diagnosis and secreting tumors were identified as requiring more treatment [113, 114]. During this time, cisplatin had been identified as an effective agent against TGCTs and was introduced into treatment strategies for childhood intracranial GCTs in the 1980s [115].

Basis for current and future treatment strategies

Since the 1980s, progress in development of treatment for intracranial GCTs has been made in the context of multi-centre national and international collaborative studies. However, the available evidence is based on Phase II and observational single arm studies rather than randomized controlled trials, and many of the published studies are based on small numbers of patients, compounded by the heterogeneity of pathologies represented. Direct comparisons are made more challenging by the variation between groups in terms of the criteria used for diagnosis, definitions used for risk groups, including the different interpretation of raised β-HCG in the presence of histologically confirmed germinoma, approach to primary surgery, detection of microscopic metastatic disease, and the difficulties of defining response. Results of some of the larger national and international collaborative published studies are summarized in Tables 17.8a and 17.8b.

Intracranial germinoma

Following the early studies demonstrating its efficacy, craniospinal radiotherapy became established as the 'Gold Standard' for treatment of intracranial germinoma in the 1980s [129, 130]. Since then, National and International studies have been designed to reduce the burden of treatment, given the potential for long-term side effects associated with radiotherapy (RT). Whilst well established as treatment for germinoma, optimal radiation treatment has been a matter for debate, most published studies being retrospective analyses with small numbers of patients. The German (MAKEI) group set out to investigate outcome for histologically proven germinoma in a multi-centre prospective trial using a dose reduction strategy in two consecutive protocols from 1983 (MAKEI 83/86 and MAKEI 89) [116].
• Reduction of the RT dose from 36 Gy CSI and a tumor boost of 14 Gy (MAKEI 83/86) to 30 Gy with a 15 Gy boost (MAKEI 89) was associated with relapse-free survival of 91% (median follow up 59.5 months), and demonstrated that the dose to both primary tumor and cranio-spinal axis could be reduced safely.
• These studies also drew attention to the importance of complete diagnostic work-up, since two relapsing patients showed elevation of markers at relapse, having been incompletely staged at diagnosis, and therefore suspected of having had previously undetected NGGCT at first diagnosis [116].

Attempts to cure intracranial germinoma with chemotherapy alone have been less successful. Two cooperative studies enrolled patients from the USA, Argentina, and Australia between 1989

Table 17.8a National and international series of treatment of intracranial germinoma.

Study	Tumour type	Chemotherapy	Radiotherapy	Conclusions	Reference
MAKEI (Germany) 60 patients 1983–1993	Germinoma	None	CSI – two different doses MAKEI 83/86 36 Gy CSI + 14 Gy boost MAKEI 89 30 Gy CSI + 15 Gy boost	5 year 91% RFS with CSI Scope for dose reduction	[116]
SFOP (France) 57 patients 1990–1996	Germinoma	CarboPEI (one cycle is one course each of Carboplatin/etoposide and ifosfamide/etoposide)	Focal 40 Gy	3 year EFS 96.4%	[117]
USA/Argentina/ Australia 45 patients 1989–1993	Germinoma	Carboplatin, etoposide and bleomycin (4 cycles). 2 further cycles with or without cyclophosphamide depending on response	None as part of primary treatment	Good initial response to chemotherapy 22/45 progressed or relapsed of which 19 salvaged	[118]
USA/Australia 19 patients 1995–1997	Germinoma	Cisplatin, etoposide, cyclophosphamide, bleomycin × 2 or 3 carboplatin, etoposide, bleomycin × 2–3. Number of courses dependent on response	None as part of primary treatment	5 year EFS 47% OS 68% Chemo alone good response but poor EFS	[119]
Japan 85 patients 1995–1999	Germinoma	Surgery 1st (8 complete resections) Carboplatin etoposide × 3 pre-RT Carboplatin etoposide × 3 post-RT (for HCG secreting only) NB *cisplatin used in place of carboplatin in some patients*	24 Gy extended local for 'good risk' (*n* = 75) 30 Gy extended local and 20 Gy focal for HCG secreting (*n* = 10)	9 (12%) relapses in good risk group No relapses in HCG secreting group	[120]
Japan 27 patients 1992–1999	Germinoma	Good risk (no HCG) Cisplatin/ etoposide x 3–4 courses HCG secreting or metastatic cisplatin/ etoposide/ifosfamide × 3–4	24 Gy focal or ventricular (localized good risk, *n* = 14) 24 Gy focal / ventricular + 6–10 Gy boost for HCG secreting (*n* = 11) 24 Gy CSI (+/– boost) for metastatic (*n* = 3)	5 year RFS/OS 86/93% pure germinoma 44/75% HCG secreting	[121]
Europe (SIOP CNS GCT 96) 170 patients 1996–2003	Germinoma	Two arms (non-randomized comparison): Option A: no chemotherapy Option B: CarboPEI × 2 cycles (one cycle is one course each of Carboplatin/etoposide and ifosfamide/etoposide)	Option A: 24 Gy CSI + 16 Gy boost Option B: 40 Gy focal	Option A (*n* = 113) EFS 93% Option B (*n* = 57) EFS 90% (interim analysis)	[122]

RFS, relapse-free survival. EFS, event-free survival. OS, overall survival. HCG, human choriogonadatrophin. RT, radiotherapy, CSI, cranio-spinal irradiation.

Table 17.8b National and international series of treatment of intracranial non-germinomatous germ cell tumors.

Study	Tumour type	Chemotherapy	Radiotherapy	Conclusions	Reference
MAKEI 89 (Germany) 28 patients 1989–1994	NGGCT	Bleomycin, etoposide, cisplatin × 2, vinblastine, ifosfamide, cisplatin × 2	30 Gy CSI + 20 Gy boost	EFS 57%	[123]
SFOP (France) 15 patients 1988–1992	NGGCT	6 cycles of chemotherapy, including vinblastine, bleomycin, carboplatin, etoposide, ifosfamide	Only if viable residual tumor	12/13 non-irradiated patients relapsed but OS 67%	[124]
SFOP (France) 38 patients 19–19	NGGCT	Alternating carboplatin/etoposide and ifosfamide/etoposide, 3–4 cycles	Focal 55 Gy	EFS 67%	[125]
USA 18 patients 1986–1994	NGGCT	Pre-radiation cisplatin/etoposide, 3–4 cycles Post-radiation vinblastine, bleomycin, carboplatin, etoposide, 4 cycles	Focal 55 Gy *or* CSI 36 Gy + 18 Gy boost	EFS 67% at 4 years	[126]
USA/Argentina/ Australia 26 patients 1989–1993	NGGCT	Carboplatin, etoposide and bleomycin (4 cycles) 2 further cycles with or without cyclophosphamide, depending on response	None as part of primary treatment	13/26 progressed or relapsed of which 6 survived	[118]
Europe (SIOP CNS GCT 96) 122 patients 1996–2003	NGGCT	Cisplatin, etoposide, ifosfamide × 4 courses	Localized disease 54 Gy focal 96 patients Metastatic 30 Gy CSI + 24 Gy boost 26 patients	Localized: EFS 68% Metastatic EFS 72% (interim analysis)	[127]

NGGCT, non-germinomatous germ cell tumor (includes tumors with components of yolk-sac tumor, choriocarcinoma and/or embryonal carcinoma). CSI, cranio-spinal irradiation. EFS, event-free survival. OS, overall survival.

Box 17.2 General principles of treatment for central nervous system germinoma.

Diagnosis requires biopsy (except bifocal disease)

Primary resection is not beneficial

Chemotherapy alone is insufficient

Curative treatment requires cranio-spinal radiotherapy or platinum-based chemotherapy followed by limited field radiotherapy to include ventricles

Radiotherapy dose (≥20 Gy) to the ventricles with total dose to tumor and metastatic deposits of up to 40 Gy (may be possible to reduce in combination therapy)

Small residuals following treatment (<2 cm) may be observed safely

Moderately raised human choriogonadotrophin (≤50 IU/l) consistent with diagnosis of germinoma

and 1993 [118] and 1995 and 1997 [131]. The first of these studies reported the outcomes of 45 patients receiving four cycles of carboplatin, etoposide, and bleomycin, followed by two additional cycles of the same drugs in complete responders, and two cycles intensified by cyclophosphamide in others. The same strategy was employed for NGGCTs in the same study. Although the response rate to chemotherapy was good, half of the germinomas relapsed, and seven patients died, three of disease and four of treatment-related toxicity. Kellie et al. [119] reported the results of 19 germinoma treated with a more intensive regimen of chemotherapy, but with no improvement in EFS, leading to the conclusion that a chemotherapy-only approach was an inadequate primary treatment for patients with intracranial germinoma, despite good initial responses.

A number of groups have set out to avoid cranio-spinal radiotherapy by treating localized germinoma with chemotherapy and limited field or focal RT.

• Buckner et al. described a series of nine patients with germinoma treated in the USA with four cycles of cisplatin and etoposide, followed by risk-adapted RT based on response and presence of spinal metastatic disease [132]. Eight of the nine patients remained in first continuous complete remission (CR) and one, with localized disease, relapsed in the spine. This study suggested that primary chemotherapy and irradiation, delivered according to extent of tumor and response to chemotherapy, was an effective treatment.

• Similar results were obtained in a larger French study (Societe Francaise d'Oncologie Pediatrique [SFOP], TGM-TC90-92) [117]. All patients with β-HCG <50 IU/l and AFP <12 ng/ml, and histologically proven germinoma received four alternating courses of etoposide/carboplatin and etoposide/ifosfamide, followed by 40 Gy to the tumor bed. A total of 60 biopsy proven cases were enrolled between 1990 and 1999 (Table 17.8a) [117] of which 10 relapsed, eight in the ventricles, either at the margins or outside the irradiation field [133]. It was concluded that, whilst the EFS of 83% and OS of 98% were comparable with radiotherapy alone reports, there was a need to increase the radiotherapy field to include the ventricles.

Comparison of Japanese studies with those from Europe and elsewhere is complicated by the differences in classification, and in particular the definition of an intermediate risk group in Japanese series [134]. In this classification, biopsy proven germinoma with high levels of HCG (>50 IU/l) are not classified with NGGCT or secreting tumors as mixed GCTs but as a higher risk group of germinoma. Nevertheless, their experiences in the treatment of pure germinoma, with and without raised HCG (Table 17.8a), support the use of limited field radiotherapy following complete response to cisplatin or carboplatin-based chemotherapy. They chose a total dose of only 24 Gy, based on protection of the pituitary [135] with promising EFS [134]. Approaches to primary surgery varied across this cohort, many undergoing primary resection and in eight cases complete removal prior to chemotherapy.

There have been no randomized studies for the treatment of germinoma. The largest international cooperative study reported to date, SIOP CNS GCT 96, sought to compare a strategy of cranio-spinal RT, at a reduced dose, as established in the preceding MAKEI study, with combined therapy similar to the SFOP group [136].

• Patients in the RT only group received 24 Gy to the craniospinal axis, with a further boost of 16 Gy to sites of disease; whereas those in the combined treatment group received four alternating courses of etoposide/carboplatin and etoposide/ifosfamide, followed by 40 Gy to the tumor bed.

• Treatment options were allocated in a non-randomized fashion, according to National preferences and those of treating institutions. The study recruited patients from 1997 to 2007 with interim results based on patients registered to the end of 2003.

• For germinoma, the EFS was 93% for patients receiving RT alone (n = 113) and 90% for the combined treatment arm (n = 57).

• As in the French series, relapses in the combined treatment group occurred predominantly in the ventricles. Metastatic disease at diagnosis was not a risk factor for recurrence, and there was no benefit of additional chemotherapy in this group, all of whom received cranio-spinal radiotherapy. Whilst the majority of patients successfully treated for germinoma had a radiological CR following treatment (Figure 17.4), small residual radiological abnormalities were found in 23% of cases with no adverse impact on survival [137].

Interest in the possibility of limited field (whole brain or ventricular field) radiotherapy alone for localized germinoma is increasing, and is the subject of ongoing trials. Promising results from a number of small reports suggest that it may be possible to spare the spine in fully staged germinoma treated with radiotherapy only [138]. Assessing the balance between toxicities from chemotherapy and radiotherapy is likely to be key to the direction of future trials and treatments for germinoma. Determination of the minimum effective treatment has been one of the major challenges for this tumor, since early studies of treatment [139] and is now more pertinent than ever with EFS in excess of 90%.

Intracranial non-germinomatous germ cell tumors
NGGCTs comprise a heterogeneous group of tumors, including YST (the most common component), choriocarcinoma and EC.

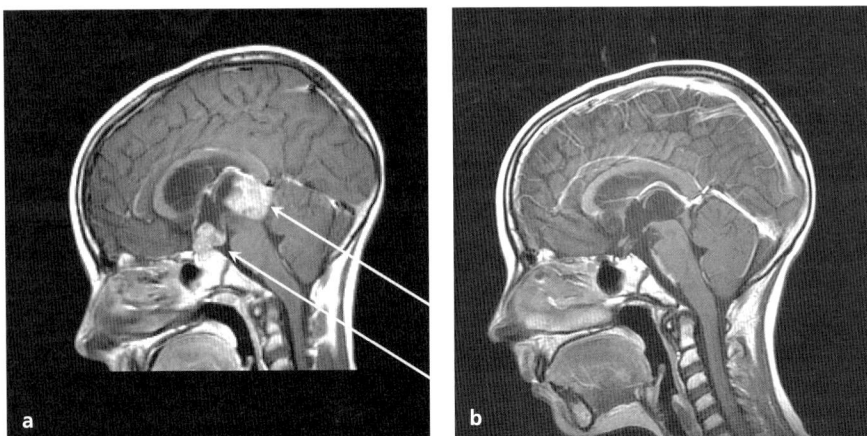

Figure 17.4 Bifocal germinoma-biopsy only, no resection, craniospinal radiotherapy. (a), Diagnosis. (b), Post-radiotherapy — 24 Gy CSI + 16 Gy boost.

• They are unified by a poorer prognosis than germinoma and have often been described generically as 'secreting GCTs' but this term is potentially misleading as EC, the least common subtype, is not associated with high AFP or HCG and, unlike the others, requires histological diagnosis [113, 114].

• Single histological subtypes are rarely seen and mixed MGCTs containing components of more than one of these, sometimes combined with germinoma, are most frequently found. Although past treatment of these tumors was similar to that given to germinoma, this started to diverge in the 1980s, with chemotherapy increasingly employed alongside radiotherapy to improve outcomes.

As with germinoma, attempts have been made to cure NGGCT with chemotherapy alone (Table 17.8b). Such an approach was employed by the French 'SFOP' group in the 1990s [124]. As with germinoma, response rates were good, but 12 of 13 patients treated with chemotherapy alone relapsed, demonstrating that sustained remission could only be achieved with additional RT. Similarly Balmaceda et al. reported a 50% relapse rate in 26 patients treated with chemotherapy alone, thereby suggesting that RT was necessary to achieve long-term remission [118].

Studies employing chemotherapy followed by RT have been more successful. Patte et al. reported a series of 38 patients with NGGCTs given three or four cycles of carboplatin/VP16 and VP16/Ifosfamide, followed by 55Gy focal RT, with EFS of 67% [125]. Similar results were reported from the German MAKEI group with BEP and VIP chemotherapy followed by cranio-spinal radiotherapy [136] and from the USA, where 18 patients received three or four cycles of cisplatin and etoposide followed by 55 Gy focal RT to localized disease and cranio-spinal irradiation in disseminated tumors, with 4-year EFS of 67% [126].

The largest series of NGGCT reported to date (also SIOP CNS GCT 96) produced interim results for 122 patients in 2005 [127] using four courses of 'PEI' chemotherapy (ifosfamide, etoposide and cisplatin) [140]. Following chemotherapy, 54Gy focal RT was delivered to localized tumors and cranio-spinal RT with

30 Gy and 24 Gy tumor boost for metastatic cases. EFS was similar for localized and metastatic cases (68% and 72% respectively), and relapses in the focal RT group almost always involved local failure, supporting the use of limited field RT [141]. AFP levels at diagnosis >1000 ng/ml and residual disease present at the end of treatment were the only significant adverse prognostic factors [142].

Central nervous system teratoma

The precise incidence of CNS teratomas is unclear because of variations in registration of this tumor entity, which is generally regarded as benign. They are undoubtedly rare and tend to occur in younger children than their malignant counterparts, with a small peak occurring in the first year of life. Information regarding their natural history, treatment, and outcome is also relatively sparse, and the impact of immature histology has not been systematically evaluated. Published evidence indicates that complete

---

Box 17.3 General principles of treatment for central nervous system non-germinoma.

Diagnosis by markers circumvents need for biopsy

Primary resection is not beneficial

Neither chemotherapy nor radiotherapy alone sufficient to cure

Treatment with cisplatin and alkylating agent-based chemotherapy, followed by focal radiotherapy for localized tumors or cranio-spinal radiotherapy for metastatic tumors

Recommended radiotherapy dose to tumor 54 Gy and 30 Gy to areas of subclinical disease in metastatic patients

Significant residuals following chemotherapy or radiotherapy should be removed

High alpha-fetoprotein (>10 000 ng/ml) at diagnosis confers poor prognosis.

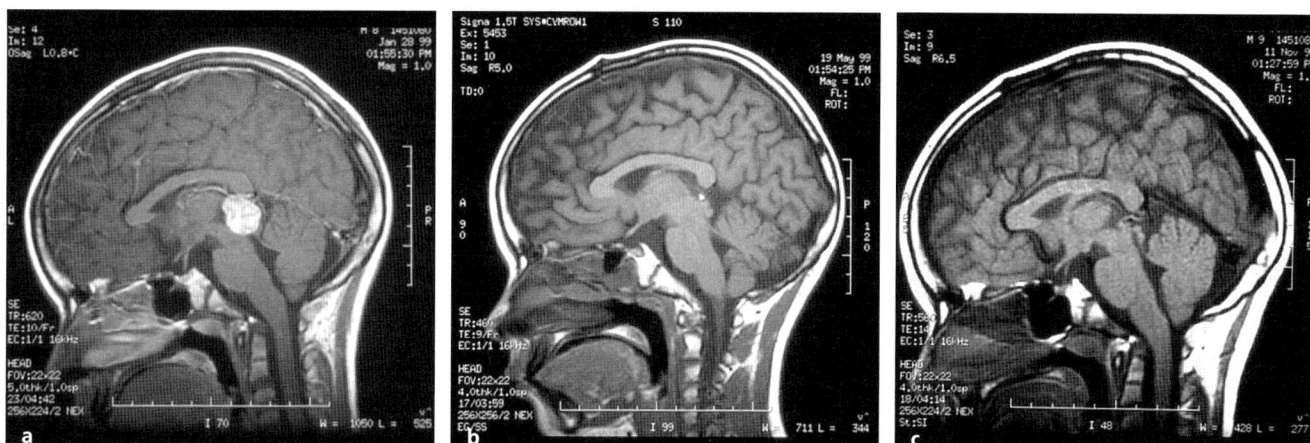

Figure 17.5 Non-germinoma (yolk sac tumor) raised AFP; no biopsy; no resection. (a), Diagnosis. (b), Post-chemotherapy. (c), Post-radiotherapy 54 Gy focal.

surgical resection is the best predictor of long-term survival, whilst there is some evidence of the benefit of radiotherapy in high dose, and anecdotal reports of responses of immature teratoma to chemotherapy [143–145].

The role of surgery in the treatment of intracranial germ cell tumors

Practices regarding primary surgery in malignant CNS GCTs have varied considerably, some groups opting to resect or debulk as a primary procedure in both germinoma and non-germinoma. However, the evidence for any benefit of primary surgery is lacking [105, 146] and the risks associated are very high [103].

• Primary surgical intervention in germinoma can therefore reasonably be limited to control of intracranial pressure and biopsy. Large residuals following chemotherapy are rarely reported, but second look surgery to unresponsive cases should be undertaken.

• Small residuals at end of treatment for germinoma may not require resection and may be observed [147].

For NGGCT, primary surgery is also of no benefit, and is rarely required for diagnostic purposes, but residuals at the end of treatment impact on outcome and resection should therefore be considered following chemotherapy or radiotherapy, unless tumor markers have not normalized, in which case surgery is unlikely to confer any survival benefit [104, 130]. Residual disease resected after treatment for malignant germ cell tumors has been found mainly to consist of teratoma, which is known to be resistant to radiotherapy, or necrotic or scar tissue [104, 132].

Treatment strategies for relapsed malignant central nervous system germ cell tumors

Treatment of relapsed intracranial GCTs may include combinations of platinum-based chemotherapy, surgery, and radiotherapy, depending on primary treatment received. High dose chemotherapy has been described, but the heterogeneity of primary treatments received, some introducing radiotherapy for the first time at relapse, suggests further work is needed to establish a role for this approach [148–150]. Salvage of NGGCT, which relapse following intensive platinum-based chemotherapy and radiotherapy, is unlikely to lead to long-term survival and salvage of patients who are resistant to primary treatment is unlikely to be successful [150].

Intracranial germ cell tumors: complications and follow up

Complications of presentation and treatment of intracranial germ cell tumors and overview of important late effects

The midline position of intracranial GCTs results in various combinations of raised intracranial pressure, pituitary and hypothalamic dysfunction, and effects on higher intellectual function, particularly involving memory and concentration, as a result of disruption of the limbic system. These may be exacerbated by effects of surgery, chemotherapy, and radiotherapy.

Endocrine deficits resulting from direct tumor effects, surgery, and radiotherapy to the pituitary area all contribute to loss of pituitary hormone function and are in general irreversible [129, 116]. The timing of the insult depends on the cause, tumor and surgical effects manifesting early with the impact of radiotherapy being delayed. The most common deficit seen at diagnosis is DI [49, 113, 151]. This leads to particular challenges for fluid management in cases receiving chemotherapy with platinum or alkylating agents accompanied by hyper-hydration [108]. Growth hormone deficiency is the next most common pituitary deficit seen and may be the presenting manifestation of a suprasellar tumor, a second peak of incidence occurring following treatment, as a result of radiotherapy damage to the pituitary. Other endocrine complications, seen less frequently, include delayed, arrested or precocious puberty, and disruption of the ACTH/cortisol and thyroid axes, the latter resulting either from pituitary or thyroid damage, following spinal radiotherapy. Early involvement of endocrinologists in the management of these patients is vital and needs to be ongoing through all stages of treatment and in follow up.

Toxicities of surgery include the following [103, 105]:
• Hemorrhage.
• Thrombotic complications.
• Ischemia.
• Infection.
• Hemiparesis.
• Seizures.
• DI.
• Cranial nerve palsies.

Toxicity from radiotherapy is dependent on dose and field but includes the following:
• Pituitary hormone failure (see above). Patients without panhypopituitarism caused by the tumor itself are likely to develop it as a result of treatment, particularly those with one hormonal deficit at diagnosis.
• Hair loss.
• Neuro-cognitive impairment. Concerns are based on the experience of severe cognitive sequelae seen in survivors of other, mostly posterior fossa, malignant brain tumors [152]. Evidence for significant neuro-cognitive deficits from the treatment of GCTs is limited but the dose of radiotherapy employed, patient age and sample size may be responsible for this variation [129, 153, 154].
• Reduced spinal growth in pre-pubertal children.
• Potential damage to organs close to spinal field (thyroid, mediastinum, ovaries).
• Second malignancies in radiotherapy field (particularly meningioma, glioma, sarcoma) akin to other tumor types but with some evidence specific to GCTs [155, 156]. The addition of chemotherapy (particularly alkylating agents) may increase the risk of second tumors [157].

Side effects of chemotherapy used to treat CNS GCTs were discussed in the section on complications of treatment of extracranial GCTs.

Quality of survival

Psychosocial and physical functioning is influenced by age, diagnosis, and treatment. Quality of life is worse for NGGCTs, leading to poorer functioning than germinoma, and tumors treated with radiotherapy. However, there is some evidence that emotional and psychological measures were not impaired compared with the normal population [154, 158, 159].

Strategies for follow up of central nervous system germ cell tumors

Most recurrences of CNS MGCTs occur within 2 years of finishing treatment, and surveillance with MRI scans and measurement of serum tumor markers, if raised at diagnosis, should be frequent during this time. MRI scans at lower frequency are usually recommended to a total of 5 years from end of treatment. Other follow-up interventions need to be focused on expected late effects of treatment, described above and should therefore include the following:

- Kidneys: both glomerular and tubular function monitored closely for the first year, and continued thereafter if abnormal.
- Hearing: deficits most likely to be picked up within a year of finishing treatment.
- Auxology.
- Pituitary hormone function.
- Neuropsychological assessments with appropriate support instigated as appropriate.
- Regular clinical review with focus on organ specific late effects as above and occurrence of second malignancies.

Novel therapeutic approaches

Whilst a plethora of anti-neoplastic drugs have been shown to be active against MGCTs, there remains a small proportion of MGCTs that do not respond to traditional chemotherapeutic schedules and progress or relapse despite first or second line therapy. In the quest for improved outcomes in this group of patients, there are many new, or re-invented, agents or approaches with potential promise.

- Topoisomerase I compounds (e.g. irinotecan, topotecan) in combination with paclitaxel and oxaliplatin have shown particular promise in phase II trials in heavily pre-treated multiply relapsed GCTs of adults [160].
- Thalidomide has displayed activity as a single agent in platinum unresponsive MGCTs [161].
- Anti-angiogenesis drugs have shown impressive *in vitro* activity in combination with carboplatin [162].
- High dose therapy and autologous stem cell rescue is impressive in multiply relapsed adult TGCTs [100], but was disappointing in a retrospective international review of childhood extragonadal MGCTs across Europe [101].
- Regional hyperthermia has been explored, in an attempt to increase the local effect of anti-neoplastic drugs for relapsed MGCTs, particularly in SCTs [163].

- Intrathecal chemotherapy using mafosfamide, with etoposide and cytarabine, have demonstrated promise in the treatment of a variety of brain tumors [164] and may be beneficial in treating leptomeningeal MGCT disease.
- Targeted therapy based on the molecular biology of GCTs, such as over-expression of c-Kit (CD117) in seminomatous tumors [165], targeted, unsuccessfully to date [166], using imatinib.

Summary and future directions

Overall, GCTs have been a success story with survival ever increasing [167]. For extracranial MGCTs, an overall survival in the region of 90% does not give the whole picture. In future, better risk stratification should allow exploration of new strategies for reducing intensity and toxicity of chemotherapeutic regimens, without adversely influencing outcomes, in good prognosis MGCTs, and increasing the cure rates for intermediate and poor prognosis MGCTs by adapting or intensifying treatment strategies [8, 11, 48, 59, 60, 63, 73, 77, 79, 81, 82]. Similarly, intracranial germinoma presently has a EFS in excess of 90%, and the future will focus on reduction of side effects and improvement in the quality-of-life outcomes. The balance between toxicities from chemotherapy and radiotherapy is likely to be the main influence on future CNS GCT treatment. Non-germinomatous CNS GCTs have a relatively inferior survival and clarification of risk groups requiring more intensive treatment is still required. Whilst the role of surgery is undoubtedly limited for CNS germ cell tumors, our understanding of the optimum timing of interventions and techniques used will continue to evolve, with the result that hazardous procedures are avoided for

---

Box 17.4 Recognized risk factors for recurrence of childhood non-central nervous system germ cell tumors (GCTs) [150–160].

High stage is associated with worse outcomes, and stage IV the worst.

Gonadal site has the best outcome, especially if completely excised. Stage IV gonadal GCTs are sometimes regarded as intermediate rather than high risk tumors.

Non-gonadal GCTs do less well, although are often higher stage at diagnosis. Of these vaginal, uterus, and prostate are favorable sites, whilst mediastinal and sacrococcygeal teratoma are unfavourable.

Increasing age (>11–12 years) is an adverse risk factor, particularly for extragonadal GCTs

Raised markers, alpha-fetoprotein >10 000 ng/ml and human chorionic gonadotrophin (>5000 IU/l are associated with significantly worse event-free survival

---

those who don't need them. However, due to the relative rarity of these tumors, progress on these fronts is only going to be possible through international collaborations and joint treatment trials.

Some of the other challenges in pediatric GCTs for the future include:

• Determination of the most effective relapse strategy following first line platinum-based chemotherapy.

• Prospective studies to identify the possible benefit of high-dose therapy and autologous stem cell rescue.

• Developing functional imaging (PET and functional MRI) and applying it to the management of GCTs, particularly in follow up of residual disease.

• Agreement on the management of teratoma with mildly raised AFP (≤1000 IU/l) and with microfoci of YST.

• Establishing the role of biological markers in disease prognosis and stratification of pediatric MGCTs, in particular 12p gain.

• Consideration of newer synthetic platinum compounds, e.g. oxaliplatin, satraplatin, picoplatin [168].

• Development of an internationally agreed and refined stratification system to facilitate international collaborative studies.

• Whether the addition of systemic chemotherapy in intracranial germinoma permits reduction in RT field or dose.

Related tumors (included in the differential diagnosis of gonadal germ cell tumors)

Sex-cord stromal tumors (SCSTs) are typically considered together with GCTs, because they occur in the gonads, although they are distinct tumors. They are much less common than GCTs and develop from the non-germ cell components of the gonad, occurring much more frequently in the ovary than testis. Around two-thirds of SCSTs are granulosa cell tumors (typically Juvenile type), 20% Sertoli-Leydig tumors, and the remainder thaecomas, fibromas, or 'other' sex-cord stromal tumors. They present in a similar way to GCTs, and are more likely to be associated with precocious puberty [169]. Curiously, these tumors may contain GCT-like cytogenetic features, but more typically trisomy 12 [170].

The diagnosis is suspected on raised serum inhibin levels and made on histology with expression of inhibin (A & B), calretinin and CD56 following surgical excision [171]. The majority are benign, of low stage, and cured by surgical excision. Those demonstrating malignant potential, based on high mitotic activity or high stage, are usually treated in a similar fashion to MGCTs, with platinum-based multi-agent chemotherapy [169].

Epithelial ovarian carcinomas are occasionally diagnosed in children, typically older girls with raised CA-125. These are best treated in the same way as the more common adult ovarian carcinoma [172]. Malignant enlargement of the testis may also been seen in leukemia, and para-testicular masses (such as rhabdomyosarcomas) may present as a suspected testicular GCT.

References

1 Exelby PR. Sacrococcygeal teratomas in children. CA Cancer J Clin 1972; 22: 202–8.

2 Comerci JT, Jr, Licciardi F, Bergh PA, et al. Mature cystic teratoma: a clinicopathologic evaluation of 517 cases and review of the literature. Obstet Gynecol 1994; 84; 22–8.

3 Virchow R. Die Krankhaften Geschwülste. 1863–1865. Berlin: Hirschwald.

4 Schiller W. Mesonephroma ovarii. Am J Cancer 1939; 35: 1–21.

5 Teilum G. Endodermal sinus tumors of the ovary and testis. Comparative morphogenesis of the so-called mesoephroma ovarii (Schiller) and extraembryonic (yolk sac-allantoic) structures of the rat's placenta. Cancer 1959; 12: 1092–105.

6 Teilum G. Classification of endodermal sinus tumor (mesoblatoma vitellinum) and so-called 'embryonal carcinoma' of the ovary. Acta Pathol Microbiol Scand 1965; 64: 407–29.

7 Collins DH, Pugh RC. Classification and frequency of testicular tumors. Br J Urol 1964; 36(supp l): 1–11.

8 Mann JR, Pearson D, Barrett A, et al. Results of the United Kingdom Children's Cancer Study Group's malignant germ cell tumor studies. Cancer 1989; 63: 1657–67.

9 Einhorn LH, Donohue J. Cis-diamminedichloroplatinum, vinblastine, and bleomycin combination chemotherapy in disseminated testicular cancer. Ann Intern Med 1977; 87: 293–8.

10 Williams SD, Birch R, Einhorn LH et al. Treatment of disseminated germ-cell tumors with cisplatin, bleomycin, and either vinblastine or etoposide. N Engl J Med 1987; 316: 1435–40.

11 Cushing B, Giller R, Cullen JW, et al. Randomized comparison of combination chemotherapy with etoposide, bleomycin, and either high-dose or standard-dose cisplatin in children and adolescents with high-risk malignant germ cell tumors: a pediatric intergroup study–Pediatric Oncology Group 9049 and Children's Cancer Group 8882. J Clin Oncol 2004; 22: 2691–700.

12 Palmer RD, Nicholson JC, Hale JP. Management of germ cell tumors in childhood. Curr Paediatr 2003; 13: 213–20.

13 Çavdar AO, Kutluk T. Childhood Cancer. In Freedman LS, et al. (Eds), Cancer Incidence in Four Member Countries (Cyprus, Egypt, Israel, and Jordan) of the Middle East Cancer Consortium (MECC) Compared with US SEER, Vol. NIH Pub. No. 06-5873. Bethesda, MD: National Cancer Institute, 2006.

14 Stiller CA, Parkin DM. Geographic and ethnic variations in the incidence of childhood cancer. Br Med Bull 1996; 52: 682–703.

15 Stiller C. Childhood Cancer in Britain: Incidence, Survival, Mortality. Oxford: Oxford University Press, 2007.

16 Gobel U, Calaminus G, Engert J, et al. Teratomas in infancy and childhood. Med Pediatr Oncol 1998; 31: 8–15.

17 Schneider DT, Calaminus G, Koch S, et al. Epidemiologic analysis of 1442 children and adolescents registered in the German germ cell tumor protocols. Pediatr Blood Cancer 2004; 42: 169–75.

18 Cools M, Drop SL, Wolffenbuttel KP, et al. Germ cell tumors in the intersex gonad: old paths, new directions, moving frontiers. Endocr Rev 2006; 27: 468–84.

19 Billmire D, Vinocur C, Rescorla F, et al. Outcome and staging evaluation in malignant germ cell tumors of the ovary in children and adolescents: an intergroup study. J Pediatr Surg 2004; 39: 424–9.

20 Bernstein L, Smith MA, Liu L. et al. Germ cell, trophoblastic and other gonadal neoplasms. In Gloeckler Ries LA, et al. (Eds), Cancer

Incidence and Survival among Children and Adolescents: United States SEER Program 1975–1995, Vol. Pub No 99-4649. Bethesda, MD: National Cancer Institute, 1999:125–37.

21 Docimo SG, Silver RI, Cromie W. The undescended testicle: diagnosis and management. Am Fam Physician 2000; 62: 2037–44, 2047–38.

22 Rescorla F, Billmire D, Stolar C, et al. The effect of cisplatin dose and surgical resection in children with malignant germ cell tumors at the sacrococcygeal region: a pediatric intergroup trial (POG 9049/CCG 8882). J Pediatr Surg 2001; 36: 12–17.

23 Huddart SN, Mann JR, Robinson K, et al. Sacrococcygeal teratomas: the UK Children's Cancer Study Group's experience. I. Neonatal. Pediatr Surg Int 2003; 19: 47–51.

24 Mann JR, Stiller CA. Changing pattern of incidence and survival in children with germ cell tumors (GCTs). Advances in Biosciences 1994; 91: 59–64.

25 Dreifaldt AC, Carlberg M, Hardell L. Increasing incidence rates of childhood malignant diseases in Sweden during the period 1960–1998. Eur J Cancer 2004; 40: 1351–60.

26 McGlynn KA, Graubard BI, Klebanoff MA, et al. Risk factors for cryptorchism among populations at differing risks of testicular cancer. Int J Epidemiol 2006; 35: 787–95.

27 Stocker JT, Askin FB. Pathology of Solid Tumors in Children. London: Chapman & Hall Medical, 1998.

28 Raghavan D. Germ Cell Tumors. Atlas of Clinical Oncology. London: BC Decker, 2003.

29 Iczkowski KA, Butler SL, Shanks JH, et al. Trials of new germ cell immunohistochemical stains in 93 extragonadal and metastatic germ cell tumors. Hum Pathol 2008; 39: 275–81.

30 Marina NM, Cushing B, Giller R, et al. Complete surgical excision is effective treatment for children with immature teratomas with or without malignant elements: a Pediatric Oncology Group/Children's Cancer Group Intergroup Study. J Clin Oncol 1999; 17: 2137–43.

31 Heifetz SA, Cushing B, Giller R, et al. Immature teratomas in children: pathologic considerations: a report from the combined Pediatric Oncology Group/Children's Cancer Group. Am J Surg Pathol 1998; 22: 1115–24.

32 Doitsidou M, Reichman-Fried M, Stebler J, et al. Guidance of primordial germ cell migration by the chemokine SDF-1. Cell 2002; 111: 647–59.

33 Stallock J, Molyneaux K, Schaible K, et al. The pro-apoptotic gene Bax is required for the death of ectopic primordial germ cells during their migration in the mouse embryo. Development 2003; 130: 6589–97.

34 Runyan C, Gu Y, Shoemaker A, et al. The distribution and behavior of extragonadal primordial germ cells in Bax mutant mice suggest a novel origin for sacrococcygeal germ cell tumors. Int J Dev Biol 2008; 52: 333–44.

35 International Germ Cell Consensus Classification: a prognostic factor-based staging system for metastatic germ cell cancers. International Germ Cell Cancer Collaborative Group. J Clin Oncol 1997; 15: 594–603.

36 Gadducci A, Cosio S, Carpi A, et al. Serum tumor markers in the management of ovarian, endometrial and cervical cancer. Biomed Pharmacother 2004; 58: 24–38.

37 Blohm ME, Vesterling-Horner D, Calaminus G, et al. Alpha 1-fetoprotein (AFP) reference values in infants up to 2 years of age. Pediatr Hematol Oncol 1998; 15:135–42.

38 De Backer A, Madern GC, Hakvoort-Cammel FG, et al. Study of the factors associated with recurrence in children with sacrococcygeal teratoma. J Pediatr Surg 2006; 41: 173–81.

39 Hoffner L, Deka R, Chakravarti A, et al. Cytogenetics and origins of pediatric germ cell tumors. Cancer Genet Cytogenet 1994; 74: 54–8.

40 Palmer RD, Foster NA, Vowler SL, et al. Malignant germ cell tumors of childhood: new associations of genomic imbalance. Br J Cancer 2007; 96: 667–76.

41 Rickert CH, Simon R, Bergmann M, et al. Comparative genomic hybridization in pineal germ cell tumors. J Neuropathol Exp Neurol 2000; 59: 815–21.

42 Riopel MA, Spellerberg A, Griffin CA, et al. Genetic analysis of ovarian germ cell tumors by comparative genomic hybridization. Cancer Res 1998; 58: 3105–10.

43 Logothetis CJ, Samuels ML, Trindade A, et al. The growing teratoma syndrome. Cancer 1982; 50: 1629–35.

44 Harms D, Zahn S, Gobel U, et al. Pathology and molecular biology of teratomas in childhood and adolescence. Klin Padiatr 2006; 218: 296–302.

45 Palmer RD, Barbosa-Morais NL, Gooding EL, et al. Pediatric malignant germ cell tumors show characteristic transcriptome profiles. Cancer Res 2008; 68: 4239–47.

46 Schneider DT, Schuster AE, Fritsch MK, et al. Multipoint imprinting analysis indicates a common precursor cell for gonadal and nongonadal pediatric germ cell tumors. Cancer Res 2001; 61: 7268–76.

47 Altman RP, Randolph JG, Lilly JR. Sacrococcygeal teratoma: American Academy of Pediatrics Surgical Section Survey – 1973. J Pediatr Surg 1974; 9: 389–98.

48 Mann JR, Raafat F, Robinson K, et al. The United Kingdom Children's Cancer Study Group's second germ cell tumor study: carboplatin, etoposide, and bleomycin are effective treatment for children with malignant extracranial germ cell tumors, with acceptable toxicity. J Clin Oncol 2000; 18: 3809–18.

49 Hoffman HJ, Otsubo H, Hendrick EB, et al. Intracranial germ-cell tumors in children. J Neurosurg 1991; 74: 545–51.

50 Calaminus G, Alapetite C, Frappaz D, et al. Update of protocol patients with CNS Germinoma treated according to SIOP CNS GCT 96. Neuro-oncology 2005; 7: 518.

51 Ueno T, Tanaka YO, Nagata M, et al. Spectrum of germ cell tumors: from head to toe. Radiographics 2004; 24: 387–404.

52 Johns Putra L, Lawrentschuk N, Ballok Z, et al. 18F-fluorodeoxyglucose positron emission tomography in evaluation of germ cell tumor after chemotherapy. Urology 2004; 64: 1202–7.

53 Cannistra SA. Cancer of the ovary. N Engl J Med 1993; 329: 1550–9.

54 Frazier AL, Rumcheva P, Olson T, et al. Application of the adult international germ cell classification system to pediatric malignant non-seminomatous germ cell tumors: a report from the Children's Oncology Group. Pediatr Blood Cancer 2008; 50: 746–51.

55 Brodeur GM, Howarth CB, Pratt CB, Caces J, Hustu HO. Malignant germ cell tumors in 57 children and adolescents. Cancer 1981; 48: 1890–8.

56 Wollner N, Exelby PR, Woodruff JM, Cham WC, Murphy ML, Lewis JL, Jr. Malignant ovarian tumors in childhood: prognosis in relation to initial therapy. Cancer 1976; 37: 1953–64.

57 Jereb B, Wollner N, Exelby P. Radiation in multidisciplinary treatment of children with malignant ovarian tumors. Cancer 1979; 43: 1037–42.

58 Flamant F, Schwartz L, Delons E, Caillaud JM, Hartmann O, Lemerle J. Nonseminomatous malignant germ cell tumors in children. Multidrug therapy in Stages III and IV. Cancer 1984; 54: 1687–91.

59 Lopes LF, Sonaglio V, Ribeiro KC, et al. Improvement in the outcome of children with germ cell tumors. Pediatr Blood Cancer 2008; 50: 250–3.

60 Suita S, Shono K, Tajiri T, et al. Malignant germ cell tumors: clinical characteristics, treatment, and outcome. A report from the study group for Pediatric Solid Malignant Tumors in the Kyushu Area, Japan. J Pediatr Surg 2002; 37: 1703–6.

61 Stern JW, Bunin N. Prospective study of carboplatin-based chemotherapy for pediatric germ cell tumors. Med Pediatr Oncol 2002; 39: 163–7.

62 Kurman RJ, Norris HJ. Endodermal sinus tumor of the ovary: a clinical and pathologic analysis of 71 cases. Cancer 1976; 38: 2404–19.

63 Flamant F, Baranzelli MC, Kalifa C, et al. Treatment of malignant germ cell tumors in children: experience of the Institut Gustave Roussy and the French Society of Pediatric Oncology. Crit Rev Oncol Hematol 1990; 10: 99–110.

64 Staubitz WJ, Magoss IV, Grace JT, et al. Surgical management of testis tumors. J Urol 1969; 101: 350–5.

65 Gangai MP. Testicular neoplasms in an infant. Cancer 1968; 22: 658–62.

66 Brosman SA. Testicular tumors in prepubertal children. Urology 1979; 13: 581–8.

67 Green DM. Testicular tumors in infants and children. Semin Surg Oncol 1986; 2: 156–62.

68 D'Angio GJ, Tefft M. Radiation therapy in the management of children with gynecologic cancers. Ann NY Acad Sci 1967; 142: 675–93.

69 Weinblatt ME, Ortega JA. Treatment of children with dysgerminoma of the ovary. Cancer 1982; 49: 2608–11.

70 Sabio H, Burgert EO Jr, Farrow GM, et al. Embryonal carcinoma of the testis in childhood. Cancer 1974; 34: 2118–21.

71 Slayton RE, Hreshchyshyn MM, Silverberg SC, et al. Treatment of malignant ovarian germ cell tumors: response to vincristine, dactinomycin, and cyclophosphamide (preliminary report). Cancer 1978; 42: 390–8.

72 Culine S, Kerbrat P, Kramar A, et al. Refining the optimal chemotherapy regimen for good-risk metastatic nonseminomatous germ-cell tumors: a randomized trial of the Genito-Urinary Group of the French Federation of Cancer Centers (GETUG T93BP). Ann Oncol 2007; 18: 917–24.

73 Ablin AR, Krailo MD, Ramsay NK, et al. Results of treatment of malignant germ cell tumors in 93 children: a report from the Childrens Cancer Study Group. J Clin Oncol 1991; 9: 1782–92.

74 Marina N, Fontanesi J, Kun L, et al. Treatment of childhood germ cell tumors. Review of the St Jude experience from 1979 to 1988. Cancer 1992; 70: 2568–75.

75 Baranzelli MC, Flamant F, De Lumley L, Le Gall E, Lejars O. Treatment of non-metastatic, non-seminomatous malignant germ-cell tumors in childhood: experience of the 'Societe Francaise d'Oncologie Pediatrique' MGCT 1985–1989 study. Med Pediatr Oncol 1993; 21: 395–401.

76 Baranzelli MC, Bouffet E, Quintana E, et al. Non-seminomatous ovarian germ cell tumors in children. Eur J Cancer 2000; 36: 376–83.

77 Baranzelli MC, Kramar A, Bouffet E, et al. Prognostic factors in children with localized malignant nonseminomatous germ cell tumors. J Clin Oncol 1999; 17: 1212.

78 Rogers PC, Olson TA, Cullen JW, et al. Treatment of children and adolescents with stage II testicular and stages I and II ovarian malignant germ cell tumors: a Pediatric Intergroup Study – Pediatric Oncology Group 9048 and Children's Cancer Group 8891. J Clin Oncol 2004; 22: 3563–9.

79 Lo Curto M, Lumia F, Alaggio R, et al. Malignant germ cell tumors in childhood: results of the first Italian cooperative study 'TCG 91'. Med Pediatr Oncol 2003; 41: 417–25.

80 Schlatter M, Rescorla F, Giller R, et al. Excellent outcome in patients with stage I germ cell tumors of the testes: a study of the Children's Cancer Group/Pediatric Oncology Group. J Pediatr Surg 2003; 38: 319–24.

81 Mann JR, Raafat F, Robinson K, et al. UKCCSGs germ cell tumor (GCT) studies: improving outcome for children with malignant extracranial non-gonadal tumors – carboplatin, etoposide, and bleomycin are effective and less toxic than previous regimens. United Kingdom Children's Cancer Study Group. Med Pediatr Oncol 1998; 30: 217–27.

82 Marina N, London WB, Frazier AL, et al. Prognostic factors in children with extragonadal malignant germ cell tumors: a pediatric intergroup study. J Clin Oncol 2006; 24: 2544–8.

83 Gobel U, Schneider DT, Calaminus G, et al. Multimodal treatment of malignant sacrococcygeal germ cell tumors: a prospective analysis of 66 patients of the German cooperative protocols MAKEI 83/86 and 89. J Clin Oncol 2001; 19: 1943–50.

84 Schneider DT, Wessalowski R, Calaminus G, et al. Treatment of recurrent malignant sacrococcygeal germ cell tumors: analysis of 22 patients registered in the German protocols MAKEI 83/86, 89, and 96. J Clin Oncol 2001; 19: 1951–60.

85 Billmire D, Vinocur C, Rescorla F, et al. Malignant mediastinal germ cell tumors: an intergroup study. J Pediatr Surg 2001; 36: 18–24.

86 Schneider DT, Calaminus G, Reinhard H, et al. Primary mediastinal germ cell tumors in children and adolescents: results of the German cooperative protocols MAKEI 83/86, 89, and 96. J Clin Oncol 2000; 18: 832–9.

87 Billmire D, Vinocur C, Rescorla F, et al. Malignant retroperitoneal and abdominal germ cell tumors: an intergroup study. J Pediatr Surg 2003; 38: 315–18; discussion 315–18.

88 Rescorla F, Billmire D, Vinocur C, et al. The effect of neoadjuvant chemotherapy and surgery in children with malignant germ cell tumors of the genital region: a pediatric intergroup trial. J Pediatr Surg 2003; 38: 910–12.

89 Li Y, Womer RB, Silber JH. Predicting cisplatin ototoxicity in children: the influence of age and the cumulative dose. Eur J Cancer 2004; 40: 2445–51.

90 Marina N, Chang KW, Malogolowkin M, et al. Amifostine does not protect against the ototoxicity of high-dose cisplatin combined with etoposide and bleomycin in pediatric germ-cell tumors: a Children's Oncology Group study. Cancer 2005; 104: 841–7.

91 Horwich A, Sleijfer DT, Fossa SD, et al. Randomized trial of bleomycin, etoposide, and cisplatin compared with bleomycin, etoposide, and carboplatin in good-prognosis metastatic nonseminomatous germ cell cancer: a Multiinstitutional Medical Research Council/European Organization for Research and Treatment of Cancer Trial. J Clin Oncol 1997; 15: 1844–52.

92 Bokemeyer C, Kohrmann O, Tischler J, et al. A randomized trial of cisplatin, etoposide and bleomycin (PEB) versus carboplatin, etoposide and bleomycin (CEB) for patients with 'good-risk' metastatic non-seminomatous germ cell tumors. Ann Oncol 1996; 7: 1015–21.

93 Shamash J, McLaren B, LeVay JH, et al. Carboplatin AUC8 in combination with etoposide and bleomycin in the treatment of intermediate and poor-risk metastatic germ cell tumors: a phase II study. Cancer Chemother Pharmacol 2001; 47: 370–2.

94 Horwich A, Shipley J, Huddart R. Testicular germ-cell cancer. Lancet 2006; 367: 754–65.

95 Mann JR, Gray ES, Thornton C, et al. Mature and immature extracranial teratomas in children: the UK Children's Cancer Study Group Experience. J Clin Oncol 2008; 26: 3590–7.

96 Schmidt P, Haas RJ, Gobel U, et al. [Results of the German studies (MAHO) for treatment of testicular germ cell tumors in children–an update]. Klin Padiatr 2002; 214: 167–72.

97 Dexeus FH, Logothetis CJ, Chong C, et al. Genetic abnormalities in men with germ cell tumors. J Urol 1988; 140: 80–4.

98 Schneider DT, Hilgenfeld E, Schwabe D, et al. Acute myelogenous leukemia after treatment for malignant germ cell tumors in children. J Clin Oncol 1999; 17: 3226–33.

99 Gross RW, Clatworthy HW Jr, Meeker IA Jr. Sacrococcygeal teratomas in infants and children; a report of 40 cases. Surg Gynecol Obstet 1951; 92: 341–54.

100 Einhorn LH, Williams SD, Chamness A, et al. High-dose chemotherapy and stem-cell rescue for metastatic germ-cell tumors. N Engl J Med 2007; 357: 340–8.

101 De Giorgi U, Rosti G, Slavin S., et al. Salvage high-dose chemotherapy for children with extragonadal germ-cell tumors. Br J Cancer 2005; 93: 412–17.

102 Bertolini P, Lassalle M, Mercier G, et al. Platinum compound-related ototoxicity in children: long-term follow-up reveals continuous worsening of hearing loss. J Pediatr Hematol Oncol 2004; 26: 649–55.

103 Nicholson JC, Punt J, Hale J, et al. Neurosurgical management of paediatric germ cell tumors of the central nervous system–a multidisciplinary team approach for the new millennium. Br J Neurosurg 2002; 16: 93–5.

104 Weiner HL, Lichtenbaum RA, Wisoff JH, et al. Delayed surgical resection of central nervous system germ cell tumors. Neurosurgery 2002; 50: 727–33.

105 Sawamura Y, de Tribolet N, Ishii N, et al. Management of primary intracranial germinomas: diagnostic surgery or radical resection? J Neurosurg 1997; 87: 262–6.

106 Fujimaki T, Matsutani M, Funada N, et al. CT and MRI features of intracranial germ cell tumors. J Neurooncol 1994; 19: 217–26.

107 Tien RD, Barkovich AJ, Edwards MS. MR imaging of pineal tumors. Am J Roentgenol 1990; 155: 143–51.

108 Janmohamed S, Grossman AB, Metcalfe K, et al. Suprasellar germ cell tumors: specific problems and the evolution of optimal management with a combined chemoradiotherapy regimen. Clin Endocrinol 2002; 57: 487–500.

109 Garré M, Alapetite C, Frappaz D, et al. Markers in serum/cerebrospinal fluid (CSF) in non-germinomatous CNS Germ cell tumors (GCT). Implication of site and Dissemination. Neuro-oncology 2005; 7: 526(Abstract).

110 Lafay-Cousin L, Millar BA, Mabbott D, et al. Limited-field radiation for bifocal germinoma. Int J Radiat Oncol Biol Phys 2006. 65: 486–92.

111 Jenkin RD, Simpson WJ, Keen CW. Pineal and suprasellar germinomas. Results of radiation treatment. J Neurosurg 1978; 48: 99–107.

112 Dearnaley DP, A'Hern RP, Whittaker S, et al. Pineal and CNS germ cell tumors: Royal Marsden Hospital experience 1962–1987. Int J Radiat Oncol Biol Phys 1990; 18: 773–81.

113 Jennings MT, Gelman R, Hochberg F. Intracranial germ-cell tumors: natural history and pathogenesis. J Neurosurg 1985; 63:155–67.

114 Rich TA, Cassady JR, Strand RD, et al. Radiation therapy for pineal and suprasellar germ cell tumors. Cancer 1985; 55: 932–40.

115 Allen JC, Kim JH, Packer RJ. Neoadjuvant chemotherapy for newly diagnosed germ-cell tumors of the central nervous system. J Neurosurg 1987; 67: 65–70.

116 Bamberg M, Kortmann RD, Calaminus G, et al. Radiation therapy for intracranial germinoma: results of the German cooperative prospective trials MAKEI 83/86/89. J Clin Oncol 1999; 17: 2585–92.

117 Bouffet E, Baranzelli MC, Patte C, et al. Combined treatment modality for intracranial germinomas: results of a multicentre SFOP experience. Societe Francaise d'Oncologie Pediatrique. Br J Cancer 1999; 79: 1199–204.

118 Balmaceda C, Heller G, Rosenblum M, et al. Chemotherapy without irradiation–a novel approach for newly diagnosed CNS germ cell tumors: results of an international cooperative trial. The First International Central Nervous System Germ Cell Tumor Study. J Clin Oncol 1996; 14: 2908–15.

119 Kellie SJ, Boyce H, Dunkel IJ, et al. Intensive cisplatin and cyclophosphamide-based chemotherapy without radiotherapy for intracranial germinomas: failure of a primary chemotherapy approach. Pediatr Blood Cancer 2004; 43: 126–33.

120 Matsutani M. Combined chemotherapy and radiation therapy for CNS germ cell tumors – the Japanese experience. J Neuro-oncol 2001; 54: 311–16.

121 Aoyama H, Shirato H, Ikeda J, Fujieda K, Miyasaka K, Sawamura Y. Induction chemotherapy followed by low-dose involved-field radiotherapy for intracranial germ cell tumors. J Clin Oncol 2002; 20: 857–65.

122 Calaminus G, Alapetite C, Frappaz D, et al. Update of protocol patients with CNS germinoma treated according to SIOP CNS GCT 96. Neuro-oncology 2005; 7: 518.

123 Calaminus G, Bamberg M, Harms D, et al. AFP/beta-HCG secreting CNS germ cell tumors: long-term outcome with respect to initial symptoms and primary tumor resection. Results of the cooperative trial MAKEI 89. Neuropediatrics 2005; 36: 71–7.

124 Baranzelli MC, Patte C, Bouffet E, et al. An attempt to treat pediatric intracranial alphaFP and betaHCG secreting germ cell tumors with chemotherapy alone. SFOP experience with 18 cases. Societe Francaise d'Oncologie Pediatrique. J Neurooncol 1998; 37: 229–39.

125 Patte C, Frappaz D, Raquin MA, et al. Treatment of Primary Intracranial Germ cell Tumours with Carboplatin-based Chemotherapy and Focal Irradiation. Germ Cell Tumours V. Vol. p131 (Abstract). Berlin: Springer, 2001.

126 Robertson PL, DaRosso RC, Allen JC. Improved prognosis of intracranial non-germinoma germ cell tumors with multimodality therapy. J Neurooncol 1997; 32: 71–80.

127 Calaminus G, Alapetite C, Frappaz D, et al. Update of protocol patients (pts) with CNS Non-Germinoma treated according to SIOP CNS GCT 96. Neuro-oncology, 2005; 7: 526(Abstract).

128 Finegold MJ, Bennington JL. Pathology of Neoplasia in Children and Adolescents. Saunders: Philadelphia, 1986.

129 Merchant TE, Sherwood SH, Mulhern RK, et al. CNS germinoma: disease control and long-term functional outcome for 12 children treated with craniospinal irradiation. Int J Radiat Oncol Biol Phys 2000; 46: 1171–6.

130 Shibamoto Y, Sasai K, Oya N, et al. Intracranial germinoma: radiation therapy with tumor volume-based dose selection. Radiology 2001; 218: 452–6.

131 Kellie SJ, Boyce H, Dunkel IJ, et al. Primary chemotherapy for intracranial nongerminomatous germ cell tumors: results of the second international CNS germ cell study group protocol. J Clin Oncol 2004; 22: 846–53.

132 Buckner JC, Peethambaram PP, Smithson WA, et al. Phase II trial of primary chemotherapy followed by reduced-dose radiation for CNS germ cell tumors. J Clin Oncol 1999; 17: 933–40.

133 Alapetite C, Patte C, Frappaz D, et al. Long term follow-up of intracranial germinoma treated with primary chemotherapy followed by focal radiation treatment: the SFOP-90 experience. Neuro-oncology 2005; 7: 517.

134 Matsutani M, Sano K, Takakura K, et al. Primary intracranial germ cell tumors: a clinical analysis of 153 histologically verified cases. J Neurosurg 1997; 86: 446–55.

135 Rappaport R, Brauner R. Growth and endocrine disorders secondary to cranial irradiation. Pediatr Res 1989; 25: 561–7.

136 Calaminus G, Alapetite C, Frappaz D, et al. Update of protocol patients with CNS Germinoma treated according to SIOP CNS GCT 96. Neuro-oncology 2005; 7: 518 (Abstract).

137 Eisert S, Nicholson J, Saran F, et al. Impact of Residual Lesions in Intracranial Germinoma – Interim Results from the SIOP CNS GCT 96 Study. Germ Cell Tumours V. Vol. p133 (Abstract). Berlin: Springer, 2001.

138 Rogers SJ, Mosleh-Shirazi MA, Saran FH. Radiotherapy of localised intracranial germinoma: time to sever historical ties? Lancet Oncol 2005; 6: 509–19.

139 Jenkin D, Berry M, Chan H, et al. Pineal region germinomas in childhood treatment considerations. Int J Radiat Oncol Biol Phys 1990; 18: 541–5.

140 Calaminus G, Andreussi L, Garre ML, et al. Secreting germ cell tumors of the central nervous system (CNS). First results of the cooperative German/Italian pilot study (CNS sGCT). Klin Padiatr 1997; 209: 222–7.

141 Brown JH, Saran FH. Defining the optimal radiation therapy for secreting CNS germ cell tumors: a critical review of the literature. Neuro-oncology 2005; 7: 531 (Abstract).

142 Nicholson JC, Alapetite C, Frappaz D, et al. Update on protocol patients with malignant non-germinomatous CNS germ cell tumors (NGGCT) treated according to SIOP CNS GCT 96 ; Impact of AFP level and residual tumor on outcome. Neuro-oncology 2005; 7: 527 (Abstract).

143 Im SH, Wang KC, Kim SK, et al. Congenital intracranial teratoma: prenatal diagnosis and postnatal successful resection. Med Pediatr Oncol 2003; 40: 57–61.

144 Calaminus G, Alapetite C, Frappaz D, et al. Intracranial teratoma (CNS TER) Experience collected in SIOP CNS GCT 96. Pediatr Blood Cancer 2006; 47: 427.

145 Garre ML, El-Hossainy MO, Fondelli P, et al. Is chemotherapy effective therapy for intracranial immature teratoma? A case report. Cancer 1996; 77: 977–82.

146 Weiner HL, Finlay JL. Surgery in the management of primary intracranial germ cell tumors. Childs Nerv Syst 1999; 15: 770–3.

147 Calaminus G, Eisert S, Nicholson J, et al. Are residual lesions in intracranial germinoma a risk factor for relapse? Analysis of patients treated within SIOP CNS GCT 96. Pediatr Blood Cancer 2004; 43: 350(Abstract).

148 Modak S, Gardner S, Dunkel IJ, et al. Thiotepa-based high-dose chemotherapy with autologous stem-cell rescue in patients with recurrent or progressive CNS germ cell tumors. J Clin Oncol 2004; 22: 1934–43.

149 Takayashi JA, Shirahata M, Kawabata Y, et al. Salvage treatment for repeatedly recurrent germinomas. Neuro-oncology 2005; 7: 522(Abstract).

150 Patte C, Frappaz D, Peciulyte V, et al. High dose VP16-Thiotepa (HD VP-TTP) with PBSC rescue in relapsing Intra Cranial Germinomas (ICG): the SFCE retrospective experience. In: Proceedings of the International Consensus Workshop for Myeloablative therapy for Malignant Brain Tumours of Childhood and Adolescence. Milan. 2006.

151 Corrias A, Alapetite C, Garre ML, et al. Endocrine disturbances and diabetes insipidus in patients with malignant cns germ cell tumors: clinical appearance and development under treatment in SIOP CNS GCT 96. Neuro-oncology 2005; 7: 523 (Abstract).

152 Spiegler BJ, Bouffet E, Greenberg ML, et al. Change in neurocognitive functioning after treatment with cranial radiation in childhood. J Clin Oncol 2004; 22: 706–13.

153 Ogawa K, Shikama N, Toita T, et al. Long-term results of radiotherapy for intracranial germinoma: a multi-institutional retrospective review of 126 patients. Int J Radiat Oncol Biol Phys 2004; 58: 705–13.

154 Sands SA, Kellie SJ, Davidow AL, et al. Long-term quality of life and neuropsychologic functioning for patients with CNS germ-cell tumors: from the First International CNS Germ-Cell Tumor Study. Neuro-Oncol 2001; 3: 174–83.

155 Sawamura Y, Ikeda J, Shirato H, et al. Germ cell tumors of the central nervous system: treatment consideration based on 111 cases and their long-term clinical outcomes. Eur J Cancer 1998; 34: 104–10.

156 Jabbour SK, Zhang Z, Wharam MD. Risk of second tumors in intracranial germinoma patients treated with radiation therapy. Neuro-oncology 2005; 7: 524 (Abstract).

157 Biti G, Cellai E, Magrini SM, et al. Second solid tumors and leukemia after treatment for Hodgkin's disease: an analysis of 1121 patients from a single institution. Int J Radiat Oncol Biol Phys 1994; 29: 25–31.

158 Wiener JA, Calaminus G, Teske C, et al. Quality of Survival in CNS Germinoma vs nongerminoma treated according to MAKEI 86/89. Neuro-oncology 2005; 7: 525 (Abstract).

159 Sutton LN, Radcliffe J, Goldwein JW, et al. Quality of life of adult survivors of germinomas treated with craniospinal irradiation. Neurosurgery 1999; 45: 1292–7; discussion 1297–8.

160 Shamash J, Powles T, Mutsvangwa K, et al. A phase II study using a topoisomerase I-based approach in patients with multiply relapsed germ-cell tumors. Ann Oncol 2007; 18: 925–30.

161 Rick O, Braun T, Siegert W, et al. Activity of thalidomide in patients with platinum-refractory germ-cell tumors. Eur J Cancer 2006; 42: 1775–9.

162 Abraham D, Abri S, Hofmann M, et al. Low dose carboplatin combined with angiostatic agents prevents metastasis in human testicular germ cell tumor xenografts. J Urol 2003; 170: 1388–93.

163 Wessalowski R, Schneider DT, Mils O, et al. An approach for cure: PEI-chemotherapy and regional deep hyperthermia in children and

adolescents with unresectable malignant tumors. Klin Padiatr 2003; 215: 303–9.

164 Slavc I, Peyrl A, Czech T, et al. Intrathecal chemotherapy for neoplastic meningitis: experience with mafosfamide, etoposide and depot cytarabine in 38 children with disseminated malignant intracranial tumors. Neuro-oncology 2005; 7: 523(Abstract).

165 McIntyre A, Summersgill B, Grygalewicz B, et al. Amplification and overexpression of the KIT gene is associated with progression in the seminoma subtype of testicular germ cell tumors of adolescents and adults. Cancer Res 2005; 65: 8085–9.

166 Einhorn LH, Brames MJ, Heinrich MC, et al. Phase II study of imatinib mesylate in chemotherapy refractory germ cell tumors expressing KIT. Am J Clin Oncol 2006; 29: 12–13.

167 Kramarova E, Mann JR, Magnani C, et al. Survival of children with malignant germ cell, trophoblastic and other gonadal tumors in Europe. Eur J Cancer 2001; 37: 750–9.

168 Kelland L. The resurgence of platinum-based cancer chemotherapy. Nat Rev Cancer 2007; 7: 573–84.

169 Schneider DT, Calaminus G, Wessalowski R, et al. Ovarian sex cord-stromal tumors in children and adolescents. J Clin Oncol 2003; 21: 2357–63.

170 Taruscio D, Carcangiu ML, Ward DC. Detection of trisomy 12 on ovarian sex cord stromal tumors by fluorescence in situ hybridization. Diagn Mol Pathol 1993; 2: 94–8.

171 McCluggage WG, McKenna M, McBride HA. CD56 is a sensitive and diagnostically useful immunohistochemical marker of ovarian sex cord-stromal tumors. Int J Gynecol Pathol 2007; 26: 322–7.

172 Schultz KA, Sencer SF, Messinger Y, et al. Pediatric ovarian tumors: a review of 67 cases. Pediatr Blood Cancer 2005; 44: 167–73.

18 Retinoblastoma

Edward J. Estlin[5], François Doz[3,4] and Michael Dyer[1,2]

[1] Department of Developmental Neurobiology, St Jude Children's Research Hospital, Memphis, TN, [2] Department of Ophthalmology, Howard Hughes Medical Institute, University of Tennessee Health Science Center, Memphis, TN, USA, [3] Department of Pediatric Oncology, Institute Curie, Paris, France, [4] University René Descartes, Paris, France and [5] Department of Paediatric Oncology, Royal Manchester Children's Hospital, Manchester, UK

Introduction and historical perspective

Retinoblastoma is a rare childhood cancer of the retina, and may have been one of the first diseases in which it was observed that excessive tissue growth led to death. Tumor growth in the anterior chamber of the eye and surrounding peri-ocular tissue could have been readily visualized in ancient times without specialized equipment, leading to the early understanding that this condition was virtually always fatal. Indeed, antiquities have been described that depict children with retinoblastoma [1]. Following the formal description of retinoblastoma in 1809 by James Wardrop [2], clinical experience with the therapy of retinoblastoma has highlighted important advances in therapy and the understanding of cancer etiology:

• Several of the earliest attempts to treat cancer were carried out on retinoblastoma patients, including the use of surgical enucleation [3, 4], radiation therapy [5] and chemotherapy with nitrogen mustard [6].

• The modern modalities of combination chemotherapy evolved from institutional experience of the treatment of this disease in the 1960s and 1970s [7,8].

As retinoblastoma survivors grew up to have their own families, it became clear that some were transmitting retinoblastoma susceptibility to their children in a Mendelian-dominant fashion. Based on this pattern of inheritance, the age of onset, and presentation of the disease (multifocal bilateral versus focal unilateral), Alfred Knudson proposed the existence of a recessive tumor suppressor gene in 1971 [9]. Specifically, he hypothesized that both copies of a putative tumor suppressor gene must be mutated for retinoblastoma to form. Knudson reasoned that children who inherit a defective copy of the putative tumor suppressor gene are much more likely to sustain a second mutation in their normal allele during retinal development and develop multifocal bilateral retinoblastoma at an early age. In contrast, children who develop sporadic retinoblastoma must sustain two inactivating mutations

Pediatric Hematology and Oncology, 1st edition. Edited by Edward J. Estlin, Richard J. Gilbertson, and Robert F. Wynn. © 2010 Blackwell Publishing Ltd.

to affect each allele in the same cellular lineage. The lower statistical probability of these combined events would result in fewer lesions (unilateral unifocal retinoblastoma) and a later age of onset that is precisely what is observed clinically.

Knudson's hypothesis was verified in 1986 with the identification and cloning of the first tumor suppressor gene, *RB1*, from families with retinoblastoma [10]. It was later discovered that the retinoblastoma (Rb) pathway is disrupted in virtually every human cancer [11] and this has led to a rapid increase in research on the *RB1* gene (located on chromosome 13q1.4) and protein over the past three decades. Despite these advances in our understanding of the Rb gene and pathway, only recently has laboratory research had an impact on the clinical management of retinoblastoma. In this chapter we will discuss our current understanding of the epidemiology, presentation and treatment of retinoblastoma along with recent developments for the modeling of retinoblastoma in mice and how those studies have led to novel therapeutic approaches. We will also discuss recent genetic studies to identify secondary genetic changes in retinoblastoma following *RB1* gene inactivation and new drugs that specifically target those genetic perturbations.

Epidemiology (Box 18.1)

Retinoblastoma is the most common pediatric cancer of the eye accounting for approximately 3% of all childhood cancers. There is no retinoblastoma predisposition by geographic origin or gender. Retinoblastoma affects very young children and is the third most common form of cancer in infants after neuroblastoma and leukemia [12].

• Overall, retinoblastoma is a rare cancer with an incidence between 1:14 000 and 1:34 000 live births for a total of approximately 300 cases per year in the United States, 115 cases per year in Western Europe and 5000–10 000 cases per year worldwide.

• The majority of retinoblastomas (90%) are diagnosed by 5 years of age with a median age of diagnosis of 18 months.

• There have been some reports of overlap of epidemiological risk factors for the development of retinoblastoma and papilloma

Box 18.1 Epidemiology of retinoblastoma.

- Incidence is between 1 in 14 000 and 1 in 34 000 live births
- 90% of cases diagnosed by the age of 5 years
- Median age of diagnosis 12 months for bilateral disease and 18 months for unilateral cases.
- 40% of cases hereditary with bilateral and multifocal features
- RB1 tumor suppressor gene mutations as a paradigm for understanding of cancer predisposition
- Genetic counselling is always proposed and screening offered where appropriate

Box 18.2 Presentation, investigation and grouping of retinoblastoma.

- Leucocoria and squint predominate as clinical findings
- Direct and indirect ophthalmoscopy under general anesthetic required for adequate examination
- Magnetic resonance imaging scans to define involvement of the optic nerve, anterior chamber, ocular fat and central nervous system extension
- Clinical risk grouping systems (Reese-Ellsworth and ABC Classification) help to predict success, in terms of ocular preservation, of conservative therapies

virus infection (HPV) [13]. Interestingly, human papillomavirus (HPV) genomic DNA has been detected in retinoblastomas from patients with these overlapping epidemiological risk factors in developing countries [13]. This has led to the hypothesis that HPV may contribute to retinoblastoma progression through the activity of the E7 and E6 viral oncoproteins. It is not known if this is due to the inactivation of the Rb pathway, the p53 pathway, or other pathways targeted by E7 and E6. Clearly, there may be some complex epidemiological factors that contribute to retinoblastoma progression and careful molecular, cellular, and biological studies are required to follow up on the significance of overlapping epidemiological risk factors.

• Recently, an elevated risk of retinoblastoma in children born after *in vitro* fertilization (IVF) [14] was reported in the Netherlands. However, subsequent analysis of retinoblastoma incidence in children born after IVF throughout the world has shown no increase relative to children born without IVF [15]. The mechanism underlying the increased retinoblastoma incidence in the children born by IVF in the Netherlands is not known but retinoblastoma predisposition should be closely monitored in children born by IVF to determine if there may be an epigenetic component to this increase as a result of current laboratory procedures used for assisted reproduction.

Clinical presentation and investigation (Box 18.2)

Presentation
In many cases, retinoblastoma is first detected by a parent or health professional as an abnormal pupillary reflex (leukocoria) or squint (strabismus). One of the major challenges with the clinical presentation of retinoblastoma is delayed diagnosis, and other clinical signs at presentation include iris rubeosis and orbital cellulitis [16]. Other non-malignant differential diagnoses need to be excluded by an expert team. There are two clinical forms of retinoblastoma:
• For approximately 40% of cases, the disease presents as a hereditary form that tends to be bilateral and multifocal. As mentioned

above, this reflects the inheritance of one defective copy of the *RB1* gene from an affected parent (15–25% of cases) or a new germ line mutation (75–85% of cases).
• The remaining 60% of retinoblastoma cases typically present as unifocal unilateral disease. In these cases, both copies of the *RB1* gene are mutated in a developing retinal cell. The lower statistical probability of inactivation of two alleles in a single cellular lineage is believed to account for the unifocal and unilateral disease presentation [9].
• The average age of diagnosis for bilateral retinoblastoma is around 12 months and for unilateral retinoblastoma it is 24 months. If there is a family history, the median age of diagnosis is younger because of more frequent genetic tests and monitoring to determine if the child inherited a defective copy of the *RB1* gene. When the disease is familial, the penetrance exceeds 90% in subsequent generations. Clinically and histologically, the heritable and sporadic forms of retinoblastoma are indistinguishable from one another. This is consistent with the common initiating genetic event in retinoblastoma, *RB1* gene inactivation [16].

Investigation and staging
Typically, examination under anesthesia (EUA), ultrasound scans, magnetic resonance imaging (MRI) and histological examination can all play a role in the diagnosis and staging of retinoblastoma [16]:
• Ophthalmosocopy (and in particular indirect ophthalmoscopy for the visualization of anterior lesions of the eye) reveals retinoblastoma to have a white appearance with angiomatoid dilatation of the associated blood vessels. In order to visualize the entire retina, an examination under anaesthetic is required, and the retina must be examined after maximal pupil dilatation with scleral indentation needed to determine the number of tumors, their size, and situation in the retina whether or not there are tumor foci in the peripheral retina and the presence or not of any sub-retinal fluid and vitreal seeds. In more advanced cases, hyphema, glaucoma, or inflammation may also be present.
• Ocular ultrasound demonstrates a tumor that has increased echogenicity in comparison to the vitreous, with fine calcification and retinal detachment observed in exophytic tumors.

• Computerized tomography describes an enhancing mass with a higher density than the vitreous.

• MRI scans are the investigation of choice to define the clinical extension to structures such as the optic nerve, anterior chamber of the eye or ocular fat, and also extension into the central nervous system (CNS) or the occurrence of the trilateral form of the disease as described below. Typically, retinoblastoma demonstrates higher signal intensity than the vitreous on T1-weighted imaging, and a relatively lower signal of T2-weighted sequences [17].

Retinoblastoma tumor growth has been classified into three patterns.

• Endophytic retinoblastoma tumor growth is characterized by a disruption in the retinal inner limiting membrane and the tumor appears as a white mass with small and disorganized tumor-associated blood vessels. Vitreous seeding often accompanies endophytic retinoblastoma and it is believed that these small fragments of tumor can initiate new foci if they become juxtaposed to the normal retinal vasculature.

• Exophytic retinoblastoma tumor growth is characterized by expansion in the sub-retinal space and is often associated with retinal detachment. In this type of retinoblastoma growth, tumor cells can invade the choroids through Bruch's membrane and invade the associated vasculature. The vasculature in the overlying retina appears abnormally patterned and may become larger. However, it is not uncommon for tumors to exhibit features of both endo- and exophytic growth.

• The third pattern of retinoblastoma growth is the diffuse infiltrating type. This is a rare form of retinoblastoma growth making up only 1–3% of tumors and is characterized by tumor infiltration of the retina without a discrete mass, often grows more slowly than exophytic or endophytic retinoblastoma growth, and the differential diagnosis of this condition is difficult also [18].

Classification, histopathological variants, and molecular oncology

Clinical risk grouping

There are currently two main grouping systems in use for retinoblastoma. The Reese-Ellsworth (Table 18.1) was developed in the 1960s at a time when most children received external beam radiotherapy as their conservative treatment [19], and is used to determine the likelihood of the success of preserving vision for children with intra-ocular disease. There are five groups in the Reese-Ellsworth system based on the number of lesions, the size of the lesions, and their location including the presence of vitreal seeds and the probability of success of conservative treatment through external beam radiotherapy.

Similarly, the ABC grouping system for Intraocular Retinoblastoma (Table 18.2) has been developed to predict the success of conservative approaches to modern treatments, in terms of the chances of ocular salvage and vision preservation in accordance with age, tumor location, vitreous seeding, and retinal

Table 18.1 Reese-Ellsworth Retinoblastoma Grouping System.

Group I (very favorable)
Ia Single tumor mass smaller than 4 dd, at or behind the equator
Ib Multiple independent tumors smaller than 4 dd, all at or behind equator

Group II (favorable)
IIa Single tumor 4–10 dd, at or behind equator
IIb Multiple tumors 4–10 dd, at or behind equator

Group III (doubtful)
IIIa Any tumor anterior to equator
IIIb Single tumor larger than 10 dd, behind equator

Group IV (unfavorable)
IVa Multiple tumors with some larger than 10 dd
IVb Any tumor extending anterior to the ora serrata

Group V (very unfavorable)
Va Massive tumors involving more than half the retina
Vb Vitreous seeding

dd, optic disc diameter.

Table 18.2 The ABC Grouping System.

Group A: small tumors away from the fovea and disc
• Tumors <3 mm in greatest dimension and confined to the retina and
• Located at least 3 mm from the foveola and 1.5 mm from the optic disc

Group B: all remaining tumors confined to the retina
• All other tumors confined to the retina and not in group A
• Subretinal fluid (without subretinal seeding) <3 mm from the base of the tumor

Group C: local subretinal fluid or vitreous seeding
• Subretinal fluid alone >3 mm and <6 mm from the tumor
• Vitreous or subretinal seeding >3 mm from the tumor

Group D: diffuse subretinal fluid or seeding
• Subretinal fluid >6 mm from the tumor
• Vitreous or subretinal seeding >3 mm from the tumor

Group E: presence of any one or more of these poor prognosis features
• More than two-thirds of the globe filled with tumor
• Tumor in the anterior segment or anterior to the vitreous
• Tumor in or on the ciliary body
• Iris neovascularization
• Neovascular glaucoma
• Opaque media from hemorrhage
• Tumor necrosis with aseptic orbital cellulitis
• Phthisis bulbi

Table 18.3 International Classification of Retinoblastoma (staging system).

Stage 0	Conservative treatment subject to pre-surgical ophthalmic classification
Stage I	Eye enucleated and resected histologically
Stage II	Eye enucleated with microscopic residual tumor (extrascleral disease and/or optic nerve margin and/or subarachnoid space involvement)
Stage III	Regional extension of retinoblastoma
	IIIa Overt orbital disease
	IIIb Pre-auricular and/or cervical lymph node extension
Stage IV	Metastatic disease
	IVa Hematogenous metastasis
	(1) Single lesion
	(2) Multiple lesion
	IVb Central nervous system metastasis
	(1) Pre-chiasmatic lesion
	(2) Central nervous system mass
	(3) Leptomeningeal disease

detachment [20]. Plate 18.1 illustrates examples of localized and extensive intraocular disease. Another recent classification (Table 18.3), as proposed by Chantada [21] relates directly to survival but not to ocular preservation.

Histopathology

Only a small number of histological features have been described in retinoblastoma including the Flexner-Wintersteiner and Homer-Wright rosettes [22]. Despite the classically better prognosis of the differentiated form of retinoblastoma, histological subtype has not been reproducibly found to relate to prognosis. More importantly, retinoblastoma is one of the few cancers for which there is a definitive diagnosis without histopathological review. This is because surgery is not performed for retinoblastoma due to the high risk of dissemination of the tumor outside of the eye as a result of surgical biopsy. Therefore, it is impossible to classify tumors by histopathological criteria and predict response to therapy. However, the following features can be discussed:
• For the largest tumors that require enucleation, the most important features of retinoblastomas that influence adjuvant treatment are the extent of optic nerve, choroidal/scleral and anterior segment invasion.
• When tumor size and location allow conservative approaches, the most important features that influence the success of these treatments are the presence of vitreal and sub-retinal seeds.

Vitreous seeding

Vitreal seeds are small clusters of retinoblastoma cells ranging from tens to hundreds of cell that are free-floating in the vitreous. The presence of extensive vitreal seeding in retinoblastoma is an important risk factor for conservative treatment outcome and is reflected in the retinoblastoma staging systems discussed above. Vitreal seeds are believed to be largely quiescent because they do not tend to get noticeably larger over time as visualized with the ophthalmoscope. As the seeds settle near the retinal vasculature it is believed that they re-enter the cell cycle and begin to form new tumor foci. Tumor cell seeds which grow in the sub-retinal space, when there is a localized or total retinal detachment in the exophytic forms of retinoblastoma, raise the same kind of challenges as vitreous seeds because of slower cell division and the lower access of the drugs.

Origin of retinoblastoma

A recent study has described some of the morphological changes that occur in mouse and human retinoblastomas as they progress and some hypotheses regarding the cell-of-origin for retinoblastoma have been discussed [23] .

It is believed that most human retinoblastomas are made up of undifferentiated tumor cells that have high mitotic indices and resemble retinal progenitor cells [23–25]. There is emerging consensus in the field that retinoblastomas arise from retinal progenitor cells during development of the retina [26]. There are several lines of evidence to support this hypothesis.
• Firstly, tumors clearly initiate *in utero* and premature babies have been delivered that have retinoblastoma already established [27].
• Secondly, the likely mechanism for mutations in the *RB1* gene is through errors in DNA replication that only occurs in retinal progenitor cells during fetal development [28].
• Thirdly, the retinoblastoma cells express markers of retinal progenitor cells and have many ultrastructural features of these cells [28].
• Finally, whereas tumors in the very young tend to affect the posterior pole of the retina, those found with follow up or for older children affect mainly the anterior part of the retina, a finding that may have a basis in the ontogeny of this structure [1].

However, even if retinoblastoma arises from a retinal progenitor cell, it does not preclude the possibility that the tumors may exhibit some morphological features of more differentiated retinal cells [28]. Thus, it is likely that Verhoeff's original proposal in the 1920s that retinoblastoma arose from embryonic retinal cells was correct and that any differentiated features of retinoblastoma cells are the consequence of the competence state of these progenitor cells, and the development of the first knock-out mouse model of retinoblastoma and subsequent studies on retinoblastoma differentiation have provided valuable insight into this process [29, 30].

Contemporary molecular biological techniques have allowed the characterization of the gross deletions and insertions in the RB1 gene for patients with retinoblastoma. For example, carriers of cytogenetic and submicroscopic whole *RB1* gene deletions mostly have unilateral tumors, and almost all patients with gross deletions with one breakpoint in RB1 have bilateral disease [31]. Furthermore, gain of chromosome 1q, 2p, 6p and 13q, and loss of 16q may play a part in retinoblastoma oncogenesis, and these observations are leading to further work to investigate candidate genes with oncogenic and tumor-suppressor function, and also their biological significance in terms of epigenetic phenomenon such as gene promoter methylation [32].

Trilateral retinoblastoma

The term trilateral retinoblastoma refers to a patient who has bilateral retinoblastoma and a second intracranial malignancy generally several months or years later, a phenomenon that has the following characteristics [33].

• The average time of diagnosis between retinoblastoma and the intracranial malignancy is 35 months.

• In most cases, the second tumor is a pinealoblastoma. This is not surprising because many of the genes and pathways that regulate retinal development also regulate pineal development.

• The pinealoblastomas have some histopathological features in common with retinoblastoma but detailed studies of human or mouse pinealoblastoma have not been carried out.

• Pinealoblastomas are highly invasive and usually fatal. Prior to the widespread use of systemic chemotherapy for the treatment of retinoblastoma, 3–6% of bilateral retinoblastoma patients went on to develop pinealoblastoma.

However, with the use of systemic broad-spectrum chemotherapy, pinealoblastoma and trilateral retinoblastoma incidence has decreased significantly. This is an important consideration as we move forward with locally delivered chemotherapy. It is likely that trilateral retinoblastoma may increase in bilateral retinoblastoma patients and will require at least some form of systemic chemotherapy. It is also likely that another factor that may have contributed to the reduction in incidence of pinealoblastoma in bilateral retinoblastoma patients is the reduction in external beam radiotherapy that coincided with the increased use of systemic chemotherapy. Long-term follow up in patients who receive ocular chemotherapy without radiotherapy will allow us to determine the relative contribution of these two mechanisms underlying the induction of trilateral retinoblastoma.

Metastatic retinoblastoma

The challenges, in terms of ocular salvage and patient survival for this poor prognosis disease, are well described in the face of metastatic retinoblastoma [16, 34]. Retinoblastoma can metastasize via several different routes depending on its pattern of growth in the eye, and extra-retinal involvement may increase the risk of extra-ocular disease.

• If the tumor invades the choroid, it often invades the extensive choroidal vasculature that may provide a route for distant metastases.

• In more advanced cases, the tumor can penetrate directly through the sclera into the peri-orbital tissue (as in localized disease also).

• Tumor cells that have invaded the anterior segment often metastasize to the regional lymph nodes.

• Optic nerve invasion can also lead to intracranial metastases, especially in cases undergoing enucleation where tumor involvement of the resection margin of the optic nerve and involvement of the subarachnoid space is demonstrated.

The most important features of retinoblastomas that predict metastatic progression are the extent of optic nerve, and invasion of the choroid and sclera, and anterior segment invasion is a less classic histological criteria, but also seems to be of value. At this time little is known about the genetic, molecular, or cellular changes that accompany metastatic retinoblastoma progression, although deletion of 1p and MYCN amplification is found more frequently in intraocular retinoblastoma [16]. Preventing metastatic retinoblastoma is highly important. This may be facilitated both by avoiding inappropriate and prolonged conservative attempts in the case of treatment failure, and by taking into account the histopathological risk factors that determine the need for adjuvant treatment. When metastatic disease occurs, the most successful approach for treating metastatic retinoblastoma currently involves intensified chemotherapy, and this will be discussed in more detail later in this chapter.

General principles of treatment for retinoblastoma (Box 18.3)

Many factors, in relation to tumor size, stage/grouping, age, and visual status need to be taken into account when deciding upon treatment for retinoblastoma, but:

• The first goal of retinoblastoma treatment is to preserve life, including performing enucleation when the intraocular tumors are not amenable to conservative approaches, and adjuvant treatment when this is indicated according to risk grouping and histology.

• If possible, the second aim is to preserve the eye, since enucleation is a radical procedure and should be avoided every time it is possible, even if no vision can be salvaged.

• Finally, the third aim is to preserve as much vision as possible, depending on the tumor site and size.

Box 18.3 Treatment and prognosis of retinoblastoma.

• Overall aim is to preserve vision and avoid enucleation where possible

• Chemoreduction with vincristine, carboplatin, and etoposide mainstay of initial therapy, with a variety of local techniques such as cryotherapy, photocoagulation and brachytherapy successful in international experience

• External beam radiotherapy utilized for more extensive disease

• Improving local delivery with subconjunctival and intra-arterial delivery is being evaluated

• Metastatic disease still carries a very poor prognosis

• Late effects relate to disease, genetic background and to therapy and include poor vision and eye damage (such as cataract) and second cancers

---

The recently published experience of conservative treatments for intraocular retinoblastoma from the Institute Curie in Paris highlights the contemporary approaches to treatment with chemoreduction, chemothermotherapy, cryotherapy, brachytherapy, and local therapy that are now achieving satisfactory rates of tumor control and a low need for external beam radiotherapy [35]. The general principles that guide the relative contribution of each of these treatment modalities is described below.

Chemotherapy for reduction of local disease and systemic control

Chemotherapy with combinations of the agents vincristine, carboplatin, and etoposide are the most commonly employed in contemporary treatment protocols for retinoblastoma, and in particular the chemoreduction of unilateral retinoblastoma in order to salvage the affected eyes and vision alongside local therapies. Chemotherapy has been found to lower the need for enucleation or external beam radiotherapy in institutional series, but this effect is greater for those patients with more localized disease with ocular salvage rates of 70–80% with localized compared with only 30–50% for more extensive intraocular disease [35–37].

Experience is also being reported for the use of subconjunctival carboplatin [16, 38] as a means for ocular salvage. In the setting of systemic administration, over 90% of tumors will respond to single agent carboplatin [39], and subconjunctival administration affords high vitreal concentrations of this agent than that achieved by systemic administration [38]. The utility of this subconjunctival therapy is currently being evaluated in the setting of therapy with systemic chemotherapy and local treatments for patients with vitreous seeding. In addition increased local delivery of chemotherapy with melphalan by the intra-arterial route is also being evaluated in an effort to reduce enucleation rates [40].

Surgery

For patients with advanced unilateral disease, if there is no chance of preserving vision in an eye with retinoblastoma, enucleation is performed, provided that there is no rupture of the ocular globe and the optic nerve is of sufficient length. Also, surgical procedures must take into account the requirement for careful pathological sampling for genetic analyses. Following enucleation, prosthetic implants, such as polymer-coated hydroxyapatite globes, are generally employed for cosmetic purposes, and also to promote bony growth of the residual socket [41].

External beam irradiation

Although the mainstay of conservative therapy for localized retinoblastoma before the advent of chemoreduction and other contemporary local treatments, external beam radiotherapy is now mainly employed for the therapy of advanced disease, especially when there is diffuse vitreous or subretinal seeding after failure of other methods of treatment and when preservation of vision is still a priority [16, 42]. Radiation is given to the entire retina as attempts to spare the anterior retina have met with a higher risk of anterior retinal relapse, and a dose of 45 Gy external beam radiotherapy appears to be sufficient for local control for tumors smaller than 10 disc diameters in size [43] or for Reese-Ellsworth Group I–II tumors [44], and larger or more extensive tumors may require higher doses of irradiation.

Focal therapies

Brachytherapy with ruthenium 106 or iodine125 plaque therapy has a long-established role as a focal therapy for anterior tumors with vitreous seeding [16], has been evaluated in the context of disease following failure of chemoreduction, and also for the control of extrascleral disease following enucleation. Although not entirely free of late sequelae, this modality may be expected to be associated with fewer late effects in terms of irradiation to surrounding tissues than external beam irradiation [45].

Chemotherapy and focal techniques such as cryotherapy can allow the successful treatment of retinoblastoma without the requirement for enucleation or external beam radiotherapy [46]. Cryotherapy is employed for small localized tumors without vitreous seeding and that are not in the vicinity of the macula and are anterior to the equator [47]. This approach can be repeated as necessary when the patient is undergoing an examination under anesthesia. However, for multiply recurrent tumors, other focal treatments should be envisaged (such as laser or brachytherapy); the key limiting factors for cryotherapy are the size and location of the tumor [16].

Laser photocoagulation is used to both kill tumor cells and to interrupt the blood supply to the tumor. This approach is only useful for smaller tumors, but allows repetitive application to tumors, including the foveal area of the retina, and alongside chemotherapy, can result in durable control of localized disease [48]. A further approach that is used in combination with carboplatin chemotherapy is chemo-thermotherapy. This technique relies upon transpupillary thermotherapy shortly after administration of systemic carboplatin and is most effective for small- or medium-sized tumors that are less than 12 mm in diameter [49].

Treatment of localized uniocular disease

The general approach to the treatment of localized retinoblastoma has changed over the past 10 years, with individual centers advocating an approach to therapy that has the dual aims of avoidance of enucleation and preservation of vision [16, 35, 46]. Current treatment strategies generally employ combinations of local therapies and systemic chemotherapy for this purpose, with the general principles of:
• Every effort is made to preserve sight, with initial chemoreduction to reduce tumor volume and enable the local therapies described above to consolidate the effects of chemotherapy.
• Radiotherapy for advanced disease.

Treatment of extensive uniocular disease

Even with contemporary treatment strategies, enucleation is still often required for extensive (e.g. Reese Ellworth Group V tumors), but the role of adjuvant chemotherapy with agents such as carboplatin-etoposide or vincristine-cyclophosphamide-doxorubicin is uncertain, although benefit is clearer for patients with stage II disease. External beam or interstitial radiotherapy can be employed in the case of microscopically-incomplete resection of tumor [16, 35].

Treatment of bilateral retinoblastoma

For children with bilateral retinoblastoma, conservative approaches aimed to preserve vision in at least one eye have been developed. The relative use of conservative measures depends on the number of tumors, their situation in relation to the optic disc and macula, the degree of retinal detachment, the extent of invasion of the vitreous and pre-retinal space, age at diagnosis, and family history of retinoblastoma [16].

Factors that relate to prognosis

The survival from a diagnosis of retinoblastoma in Western industrialized countries is excellent with more than 95% of children surviving their disease [50, 51]. Therefore, outcome measures for children with retinoblastoma are more related to considerations such as preservation of vision, ocular salvage, and the avoidance of enucleation and external beam irradiation than survival. The relative contribution of the various treatment modalities to eventual success or failure is obviously complex due to the different modalities of therapy employed, but certain inferences may be drawn from the literature with respect to prognosis:
• Treatments should be given in specialized onco-ophthalmological centres.
• For retinoblastoma treated with primary chemotherapy alone, the 72% of patients with disease that included the features of location in the macula, measuring greater than 2 mm in diameter or patient age older than 2 months was more likely not to require other therapies for control [52].
• For retinoblastoma treated with radiotherapy alone, the likelihood of control relates to the extent of disease as defined by the Reece-Ellsworth Group classification, with 79% of Group I–II eyes and 20% of Group III–V eyes being controlled by 45 Gy of external beam irradiation. A similar effect was also found for tumor size, with lesions larger than 15 mm less likely to be controlled than smaller lesions [44].

Contemporary institutional studies also highlight the factors that relate to ocular relapse, the need for external beam irradiation, and enucleation following treatment with chemoreduction and local therapies.
• The risk factors for ocular relapse include Reese-Ellsworth Group V and ABC Classification Group D eyes and the presence of subretinal seeds [35].

• The same factors plus vitreous seeding are risk factors for the eventual use of external beam irradiation [35]; female gender and greater number of chemoreduction treatments have also been reported [53].
• The risk factors for eventual enucleation (20–30% of cases) include advanced disease and sub-retinal seeds [35], tumor thickness, and tumor recurrence and older age at presentation have also been reported [53].
• The risk factors for extraocular relapse follow enucleation after failure of chemoreduction for retinoblastoma include scleral invasion and bilateral enucleation [54].

Although chemoreduction with agents such as vincristine, etoposide and carboplatin is an established practice for the treatment of retinoblastoma, there is a paucity of studies to relate patient outcomes with known cellular and molecular determinants of chemosensitivity for retinoblastoma. However, although *in vitro* drug sensitivity, as measured by means of the MTT assay, does not relate to tumor characteristics such as invasion and seeding, the relative chemosensitivity of undifferentiated tumors and lack of efficacy of cytosine arabinoside has been identified [55]. The efficacy of the chemotherapy agents vincristine, etoposide and anthracyclines could be impaired by the multi-drug resistance-associated protein MDR1, and although MDR1 positivity is more prevalent post-chemotherapy for patients with retinoblastoma, which may indicate MDR1 as a mechanism for resistance [56], MDR1 has not been found to relate to response [57] or histological invasiveness [58]. Therefore, the 60% response rate of retinoblastoma tumors to single agent idarubicin results may not relate to cellular factors such as MDR1, but to downstream determinants of cellular engagement of apoptosis [59].

Strategies for follow up and overview of important late effects

EUA is routinely performed at different time intervals after treatment is complete. The timing of the examinations depends on the age and particular presentation at diagnosis, the genetic counseling and the response to therapy. For children at risk of developing retinoblastoma, screening is typically carried out every month in the very young, and then at gradually increasing intervals of time thereafter, typically throughout childhood and increasingly, early adult life. However, it is recognized that institutional surveillance programs carry with them a significant impact on the patient, family, and hospital resources [60], and the late-effects burden for children with retinoblastoma is well characterized as follows:
• Chemoreduction and local control strategies result in over 80% vision salvage rates for Reese-Ellsworth Groups I–IV tumors, but only a 20% success for group V retinoblastoma [61]. The quality of preserved vision remains a function of tumor location and absence of subretinal fluid, with tumor margins at least 3 mm from the foveola predictive of eventual visual acuities of 20/40 or better [62]. Indeed, visual acuity for almost one-half of patients

with orbital preservation is near-normal, i.e. better than or equal to 6/12 [63].

• Complications of external beam radiotherapy include cataract and retinopathy, which can affect one-quarter of patients, and orbital deformities, although the later complication is less common [64]. Rarer complications of radiotherapy include retinal tears and detachment, sub-retinal fibrosis, vitreous traction bands, and pre-retinal fibrosis [65]. However, the evolution of techniques continues to allow a more accurate delivery of the 45–50 Gy treatment doses for retinoblastoma, and this may result in fewer ocular late effects and also reduce the risk of secondary cancers [66].

Genetic counseling and screening

One of the most important outcomes of the cloning of the *RB1* tumor suppressor gene was the ability to provide retinoblastoma survivors with genetic counseling. Point mutations and small deletions represent the vast majority of *RB1* germline mutations. Chromosomal aberrations have also been reported and these can be detected by cytogenetic analysis and/or molecular analyses [67–69]. The following features of genetic counseling for retinoblastoma include:

• It is essential to perform *RB1* gene analysis for every retinoblastoma patient because the absence of multiple bilateral tumors does not exclude the possibility of germline *RB1* mutations.

• The hereditary type of retinoblastoma shows an autosomal dominant pattern of inheritance with at least 90% penetrance on average. Long-term follow up is essential to educate retinoblastoma survivors of the risks of passing retinoblastoma susceptibility on to their children.

• The risk of developing retinoblastoma to survivors of inherited retinoblastoma is approximately 45% and it is 2.5% for survivors of unilateral retinoblastoma.

• The risk for passing on retinoblastoma susceptibility for unilateral retinoblastoma survivors (2.5%) is higher than in the general population (0.003%) because of the possibility of a low-penetrance *RB1* mutation or an individual with mosaic inactivation of *RB1*.

• Similarly, the risk of developing retinoblastoma for siblings of retinoblastoma patients with bilateral disease and a family history is 45%, and for the siblings of retinoblastoma patients with no family history and unilateral disease is 1%.

In the context of familial risk for retinoblastoma, surveillance investigations allow the detection of disease before the clinical sign of leucocoria is present, and this is associated with a higher ocular salvage rate [70]. However, it is also recognized that in patients in which retinoblastoma is detected early, at the time when tumors are smaller, actually do worse than in patients who are diagnosed later at a more advanced stage [71], a finding that may result in the posterior retinal location, often involving the macula, in very young children. However, screening is of benefit in terms of reduction of treatment burden and risk of enucleation.

Novel therapeutic approaches

In this section, we will discuss the role of experimental therapeutic approaches in helping to define novel combinations of chemotherapy agents for the treatment of retinoblastoma. For example, preclinical studies have revealed that the combination of topotecan and carboplatin is more effective than carboplatin and vincristine, or carboplatin, vincristine and etoposide in the xenograft setting for retinoblastoma [72], and this information may help promote the study of topotecan now that phase I evaluation of this agent in children is complete [73]. Other novel approaches to therapy has seen the encouraging response rates for refractory retinoblastoma found with the adenovirus vector/herpes simplex thymidine kinase gene activation of systemic acyclovir [74], and strategies to inhibit the VEGF-mediated growth and angiogenesis of retinoblastoma are being evaluated in the pre-clinical setting [75]. These strategies may eventually compliment therapeutic approaches based on the knowledge of cellular-adhesion molecules in the pathogenesis of retinoblastoma [76]. However, study of the functions of the retinoblastoma gene pathway interactions with p53 are the subject of preclinical developments that may soon translate into clinical practice.

Inactivation of the p53 pathway in retinoblastoma

Tumorigenesis involves sequential genetic lesions in pathways that regulate cell proliferation, cell survival, and other biological processes [11]. It has been proposed that both the p16^Ink4a-CycD/Cdk4-pRb and Arf-MDM2/MDMX-p53 pathways must be inactivated during cancer progression [77]. The primary role of the Rb pathway is to regulate cell division [77], and that of the p53 pathway is to regulate responses to cellular insults such as DNA damage or oncogenic stress [78]. The Rb and p53 pathways may be inactivated by mutations in the *RB1* and *p53* tumor suppressor genes themselves or through genetic alterations of other genes in the pathway. For example, some cancers have *MDM2* gene amplifications that functionally suppress the p53 pathway by reducing the steady-state levels of the p53 protein [79]. In relation to retinoblastoma, the following observations are emphasized:

• The first evidence that the p53 pathway may be important for retinoblastoma tumor progression came from studies on mouse models of retinoblastoma. In mouse models of retinoblastoma, tumor development is greatly enhanced when p53 is inactivated [80]; mice develop 100% penetrant bilateral retinoblastoma that invades the anterior chamber and surrounding tissue [81]. To determine if any previously overlooked mutations within the p53 pathway effectively block p53 activity and lead to a growth advantage for retinoblastoma cells, the Arf-MDM2/MDMX-p53 oncogenic stress response pathway was analyzed in detail.

• *MDMX* is amplified in 65% of human retinoblastomas, and *MDM2* is amplified in 10% of human retinoblastomas [82]. MDMX and MDM2 are similar in structure, but they inhibit p53 by distinct mechanisms [83]. MDM2 is a ubiquitin ligase that blocks p53 activity by binding to its transactivation domain and ubiquitinates p53 for degradation [84]. MDMX does not have ubiquitin ligase activity but effectively inhibits p53 activity by binding to its transactivation domain [84]. In retinoblastomas with *MDMX* gene amplifications, the levels of *MDMX* mRNA and protein were also increased [82]. This correlated with a decrease in p53 and p21 proteins, as previously shown in breast tumors with *MDMX* amplifications [84].

- These data suggest that amplification of MDMX and, to a lesser extent, MDM2 suppresses the p53 response to increased p14^{ARF} levels as a direct result of activation of the oncogenic stress pathway following *RB1* inactivation in retinoblastoma. Genetic analyses of human tumors have shown that disruption of one component of the p53 pathway relieves the selective pressure to inactivate other components of the same pathway [85]. For example, *p53* mutations and *MDM2* amplifications tend to be mutually exclusive [86]. Indeed, subsequent studies confirmed that p53 and many of the direct downstream effectors of the p53 pathway are intact in retinoblastoma cell lines [82]. By modulating the p53 and MDMX levels in retinoblastoma cells maintained in culture, predictable perturbation of p53-mediated cell death and cell cycle exit occurred [82].

On the basis of these data, it has been hypothesized that *RB1*-deficient retinoblasts sustain an *MDMX/MDM2* genetic amplification that allows them to suppress p53-mediated cell death and clonally expand to form retinoblastoma. To recapitulate this process *in vivo*, these changes have been engineered in a mouse model and in explants of human fetal retinae grown in cultures with the following findings.

- In the mouse model, the retinal cells that lacked *Rb* and *p107* but expressed *MDMX* had greater proliferation and survival than did cells lacking *Rb* and *p107* [96]. Importantly, invasive and aggressive retinoblastoma similar to that observed in *Chx10-Cre;Rb$^{Lox/-}$;p107$^{-/-}$;p53$^{Lox/-}$* mice now developed in the *Rb$^{Lox/Lox}$;p107$^{-/-}$* pups with ectopic expression of *MDMX* [82].
- In human fetal retinae, it was demonstrated that *MDMX* promotes human retinoblastoma by electroporating primary human fetal retinae (FW 14-15) with *RB1* siRNA, *MDMX* cDNA, and a green fluorescent protein (GFP) reporter gene. After 10 days in culture, these cells failed to differentiate, and the immature cells organized into rosettes similar to those seen in retinoblastoma [82]. Cells expressing *Rb1* siRNA alone induced p14^{ARF} and initiated p53-mediated apoptosis. Increased *MDMX* expression blocked cell death and increased proliferation by clonal expansion.
- The specificity of the MDMX effect on p53 was demonstrated by using an *MDMX* allele that has a single amino acid substitution (G57A) that blocks its ability to bind p53 [82, 84]. These data challenge the long-held belief that retinoblastoma is the exception to the principle that the Rb and p53 pathways must be inactivated for cancer progression, and demonstrate that inactivation of the p53 pathway is likely to be the second genetic perturbation that occurs in human retinoblastomas after the loss of *RB1*.

Targeted chemotherapy for retinoblastoma

Currently, no small-molecule inhibitors that bind MDMX and block its ability to bind p53 are available. It has been previously shown that the p53-binding domains of MDM2 and MDMX are highly conserved [87, 88]. Therefore, an inhibitor of the MDM2-p53 interaction may also inhibit the MDMX-p53 interaction [89]. A number of small molecule inhibitors of the MDM2-p53 interaction have been constructed [90]. However, the most widely utilized small molecule inhibitor of the MDM2-p53 interaction is nutlin-3.

- Nutlin-3 interacts with the p53-binding domain of MDM2, which is a hydrophobic pocket. The effects of nutlin-3A on retinoblastoma cells have been recently explored [90].
- Following treatment with nutlin-3A, a p53 response is induced inWeri1 and Y79 human retinoblastoma cell lines as indicated by an increase in p53 protein levels, and an increase in the protein levels of its downstream targets, MDM2 and p21. The authors also observed an induction of apoptosis following nutlin-3A treatment.
- In addition, the sensitivity of retinoblastoma cells to nutlin-3A was shown to be p53-dependent, because Y79 cells expressing a siRNA to p53 were less sensitive to nutlin-3A [90].

Furthermore, binding studies have shown that racemic nutlin-3 binds MDM2 and competes with fluorescently labeled p53 with an inhibition constant (K_i) of 0.7 μM; racemic nutlin-3 binds MDMX and competes with a K_i of 28 μM [82]. Racemic nutlin-3 also blocks MDMX-p53 binding in C33A cells, a cell line that expresses a mutant form of p53 (Cys273) [82]. Co-immunoprecipitation assays demonstrated that in cells treated with 10 μM racemic nutlin-3, the binding of MDM2 and MDMX to p53 was reduced. In *Mdm2*-deficient mouse embryonic fibroblasts (MEFs), we demonstrated that racemic nutlin-3 can block MDMX in the absence of MDM2. MEFs expressing MDMX only were sensitive to racemic nutlin-3, as demonstrated by reduced cell viability [82]. These studies demonstrate that racemic nutlin-3 can inhibit p53 binding by both MDM2 and MDMX.

Local drug delivery for retinoblastoma treatment

Systemic administration of nutlin-3 to treat tumors with *MDMX* amplification is not feasible due to its pharmacokinetics and toxicity in multiple organs; thus, there is a great need for specific, highly efficient MDMX antagonists. Retinoblastoma is ideal for local delivery of a targeted chemotherapeutic agent such as nutlin-3, because the eye is readily accessible for drug delivery. Subconjunctival administration of chemotherapies for retinoblastoma can also avoid the side effects of systemic administration and achieve higher intraocular concentrations.

Abramson *et al.* conducted a clinical study in which they injected as much as 2 ml carboplatin (10 mg/ml) subconjunctivally to treat intraocular retinoblastoma [91]. Some patients were also given cryotherapy to increase drug delivery. The mean number of injections was 2.8 per eye. Following treatment, regression of the solid retinal tumors and vitreous seeds was evaluated. Of the five eyes with solid retinal tumors that were treated, two responded, and three remained stable. Of the five eyes with vitreous disease, three responded. In the first eye, all vitreal seeds disappeared; in the second eye, disease regressed more than 50%; and in the third eye, all non-calcified seeds disappeared. The remaining two eyes with vitreal disease remained stable. The side effects were minimal; only one eye in one patient suffered a severe ocular side effect. The authors had previously addressed the question of systemic exposure to carboplatin following periocular injection in a primate model: the 2 hour mean blood level after periocular injection of carboplatin was 2.9% that of the mean peak level of carboplatin after intravenous injection. Therefore, systemic exposure to carboplatin was greatly reduced by local administration of the drug [92].

Testing of subconjunctival racemic nutlin-3 in the setting of a preclinical animal models, an orthotopic xenograft model for retinoblastoma, has been reported with the following findings [93].

- Racemic nutlin-3 alone significantly reduced tumor burden, as measured by luciferase activity [82].
- The combination of racemic nutlin-3 with the topoisomerase inhibitor topotecan (30–40 nM) induces a p53 response in retinoblastoma cells. Racemic nutlin-3 also induces a p53 response in retinoblastoma by inhibiting MDMX and MDM2 from binding to p53 [82].
- The combination of the two drugs resulted in a 20-fold synergistic killing of retinoblastoma cells *in vitro*. Subconjunctival administration of topotecan and racemic nutlin-3 in our orthotopic xenograft model resulted in an 82-fold reduction in tumor burden with no ocular or systemic side effects [82].

Previous studies for subconjunctival chemotherapeutic treatment for retinoblastoma have involved administration of 25 ml of drug in mice and up to 2 ml of drug in children [94–96]. The stock solution of racemic nutlin-3 used for these studies was 170 mM and showed no ocular toxicity. Thus, it is feasible to achieve the intraocular concentration of nutlin-3 needed to inactivate MDM2 and MDMX; this approach should prove effective in 75% of patients with retinoblastoma with either *MDM2* or *MDMX* gains or amplifications. Moreover, by combining MDM2/MDMX antagonists with drugs that induce a p53 response through DNA damage (i.e. topotecan), further enhancement of their antitumor effects may be gained. Retinoblastoma is not only a good model for studying the suppression of p53-mediated cell death by *MDMX* amplification, but it is also an ideal system in which to study local delivery of chemotherapy targeted to the Arf-MDM2/MDMX-p53 pathway. In addition, retinoblastoma would be easier to treat in developing countries if we could use local delivery of targeted therapy, because this approach would avoid the cost associated with managing the side effects of systemic broad-spectrum chemotherapy.

Summary and future directions (Box 18.4)

In industrialized Western countries, the survival following a diagnosis of retinoblastoma has improved from approximately 85%

Box 18.4 Future directions.

- p53 inactivation important in the pathogenesis of retinoblastoma
- Some of the novel therapeutic approaches include strategies based on inhibition of MDMX/MDM2 and p53 interactions
- Preclinical studies also exploring VEGF inhibition and adenoviral/herpes simplex thymidine kinase gene activation of systemic therapies such as acyclovir
- International collaborations to improve therapy of metastatic disease and vision/ocular salvage in localized disease
- Improving the outcomes for retinoblastoma in developing countries

---

in the 1970s to the present day success rates of over 95% [50, 51]. However, the treatment of metastatic disease and the preservation of vision and avoidance of enucleation for patients with more advanced or bilateral disease are continued challenges for the expert teams that treat children with retinoblastoma. This chapter has highlighted the novel approaches to therapy that are currently being developed, both in terms of local delivery of conventional chemotherapy agents and new therapies that target p53 interactions that appear to be important in the pathogenesis of retinoblastoma. Determining the feasibility of novel drugs will require systematic evaluation of ideal delivery techniques to maximize drug delivery allowing for efficacy, with every attempt made to minimize adverse effects and complications. Ease of the application will be essential if these techniques are to eventually be translated to widespread use outside of specialized academic centers. This is a promising field for the treatment of eye diseases in general and as more therapeutics becomes available, drug delivery will likely become the major hurdle to pass as the field progresses.

Indeed, an international consensus of the current state of retinoblastoma therapy world-wide recognizes that the excellent survival figures of the industrialized West reflect the complexity of multi-disciplinary care that is achievable, a situation that is seldom achievable in the developing world. The 'One World, One Vision' theme is leading to practical partnerships between academic treatment centers in Europe and North America and the developing countries, lay agencies and interest groups with the aim of bringing the success story that is the treatment of retinoblastoma to children around the world [97].

Acknowledgment

Many thanks to Dr Helen Jenkinson, Paediatric Oncologist at The Birmingham Children's Hospital, UK, for the provision of the images used for Plate 18.1, and for her advice and comments on the text of the chapter.

References

1 Munier F, Pescia G, Balmer A et al. Historical notes on retinoblastoma. Rev Med Suisse Romande 1987; 107: 591–7.

2 Wardrop J. Observations on the Fungus Hamatodes or Soft Cancer. Edinburgh: George Ramsay and Co, 1809.

3 Ferrall JM. Fungoid tumor of the orbit: operation. Dublin Med Press 1841; 5: 281.

4 Bonnet A. Cancer melanique de l'oeil; structure du cancer; disposition de ses vaisseaux. Bull Soc Anat Paris 1846; 21: 76.

5 Hilgartner HL. Report of a case of double glioma treated with x-ray. Medical Insurance 1902; 18: 322.

6 Kupfer C. Retinoblastoma treated with intravenous nitrogen mustard. Am J Opthalmol 1953; 36: 1721–3.

7 Lonsdale D, Berry DH, Holcomb TM, et al. Chemotherapeutic trials in patients with metastatic retinoblastoma. Cancer Chemother Rep 1968; 52: 631–4.

8 Pratt CB, Crom DB, Howarth C. The use of chemotherapy for extraocular retinoblastoma. Med Pediatr Oncol 1985; 13: 330–3.

9 Knudson A. Mutation and cancer: statistical study of retinoblastoma. Proc Natl Acad Sci USA 1971; 68: 820–3.

10 Friend S H, Bernard R, Rogelli S, et al. A human DNA segment with properties of the gene that predisposes to retinoblastoma and osteosarcoma. Nature 1986; 323: 643–6.

11 Hahn WC, Weinberg RA. Modelling the molecular circuitry of cancer. Nat Rev Cancer 2002; 2: 331–41.

12 Young J, Smith M, Roffers S et al. Retinoblastoma treatment. Bethesda: National Cancer Institute, 2003: 73–8.

13 Orjuela M, Castandea VP, Ridaura C et al. Presence of human papilloma virus in tumor tissue from children with retinoblastoma: an alternative mechanism for tumor development. Clin Cancer Res 2000; 6: 4010–6.

14 Moll AC, Imhof SM, Cruysberg JR et al. Incidence of retinoblastoma in children born after in-vitro fertilisation. Lancet 2003; 361: 309–10.

15 Bradbury BD, Jick H. In vitro fertilization and childhood retinoblastoma. Br J Clin Pharmacol 2004; 58: 209–11.

16 Aerts I, Lumbroso-Le Roic L, Gauthier-Villars M, et al. Retinoblastoma. Orphanet J Rare Diseases 2006; 1: 31.

17 Brisse H, Lumbroso L, Freneaux PC, et al. US, CT and MRI of diffuse infiltrative retinoblastoma: report of two cases with histological comparison. Am J Neuroradiol 2001; 22: 499–504.

18 Shields CL, Ghassemi F, Tuncer S, et al. Clinical spectrum of diffuse infiltrating retinoblastoma in 34 consecutive eyes. Ophthalmology 2008; 115: 2253–8.

19 Reese AB, Ellesworth RM. Management of retinoblastoma. Ann NY Acad Sci 1964; 114: 958–62.

20 Shields CL, Shields JA. Basic understanding of current classification and management of retinoblastoma. Curr Opin Ophthalmol 2006; 17: 228–34.

21 Chantada G, Doz F, Antoneli CB et al. A proposal for an international retinoblastoma staging system. Pediatr Blood Cancer 2006; 47: 801.

22 Flexner S. A peculiar glioma (neuroepithelioma?) of the retina. Bull Hopkins Hosp 1891; 2: 115–9.

23 Johnson DA, Zhang J, Frase S, et al. Neuronal differentiation and synaptogenesis in retinoblastoma. Cancer Res 2007; 67: 2101–11.

24 Zhang J, Gray J, Wu L et al. Rb regulates proliferation and rod photoreceptor development in the mouse retina. Nat Genet 2004; 36: 351–60.

25 Vooijs M, te Riele H, van der Valk M, et al. Tumor formation in mice with somatic inactivation of the retinoblastoma gene in interphotoreceptor retinol binding protein-expressing cells. Oncogene 2002; 21: 4635–45.

26 Cepko CL, Austin CP, Yang X, et al. Cell fate determination in the vertebrate retina. Proc Natl Acad Sci USA 1996; 93: 589–95.

27 Abramson DH, Schefler AC, Beaverson KL et al. Rapid growth of retinoblastoma in a premature twin. Arch Ophthalmol 2002; 120: 1232–3.

28 Dyer MA, Bremner R. The search for the retinoblastoma cell of origin. Nat Rev Cancer 2005; 5: 91–101.

29 Donovan SL, Schweers B, Martins R, Johnson D, Dyer MA. Compensation by tumor suppressor genes during retinal development in mice and humans. BMC Biol 2006; 4: 14.

30 Zhang J, Schweers B, Dyer MA. The first knockout mouse model of retinoblastoma. Cell Cycle 2004; 3: 952–9.

31 Albrecht P, Ansperger-Rescher B, Schüler A, et al. Spectrum of gross deletions and insertions in the RB1 gene in patients with retinoblastoma and association with phenotypic expression. Hum Mutat 2005; 26: 437–45.

32 Corson TW, Gallie BL. One hit, two hits, three hits, more? Genomic changes in the development of retinoblastoma. Genes Chromosomes Cancer 2007; 46: 617–34.

33 Antoneli CB, Ribeiro Kde C, Sakamato LH, et al. Trilateral retinoblastoma. Pediatr Blood Cancer 2007; 48: 306–10.

34 Dunkel IJ, Aledo A, Kernan NA, et al. Successful treatment of metastatic retinoblastoma. Cancer 2000; 89: 2117–21.

35 Lombroso-Le Rouic L, Aerts I, Vevy-Gabirel C, et al. Conservative treatments of intraocular retinoblastoma. Ophthalmology 2008; 115: 1405–10.

36 Shields CL, Honavar SG, Meadows AT, et al. Chemoreduction for unilateral retinoblastoma. Arch Ophthalmol 2002; 120: 1653–8.

37 Rodriguez-Galindo C, Wilson MW, Haik BG, et al. Treatment of intraocular retinoblastoma with vincristine and carboplatin. J Clin Oncol 2003; 21: 2019–25.

38 Mendelsohn ME, Abramson DH, Madden T, et al. Intraocular concentrations of chemotherapeutic agents after systemic or local administration. Arch Ophthalmol 1998; 116: 1209–12.

39 Dunkel IJ, Lee TC, Shi W, Beaverson KL, et al. A phase II trial of carboplatin for intraocular retinoblastoma. Pediatr Blood Cancer 2007; 49: 643–8.

40 Abrahamson DH, Dunkel IJ, Brodie ES, et al. Ophthalmology 2008; 115: 1398–404.

41 Shields CL, Uysal Y, Marr BP, et al. Experience with the polymer-coated hydroxyapatite implant after enucleation in 126 patients. Ophthalmology 2007; 114: 367–73.

42 Sheilds CL, Meadows AT, Leahey AM, et al. Continuing challenges in the management of retinoblastoma with chemotherapy. Retina 2004; 24: 849–62.

43 Foote RL, Garretson BR, Schomberg PJ, et al. External beam irradiation for retinoblastoma: patterns of failure and dose-response analysis. Int J Radiat Oncol Phys 1989; 16: 823–30.

44 Hernandez JC, Brady LW, Shields JA, et al. External beam irradiation for retinoblastoma: results, patterns of failure, and a proposal for treatment guidelines. Int J Radiat Oncol Biol Phys 1996; 35: 125–32.

45 Shields CL, Mashayekhi A, Sun H, et al. Iodine 125 plaque radiotherapy as salvage treatment for retinoblastoma recurrence after chemoreduction in 84 tumors. Ophthalmology 2006; 113: 2087–92.

46 Gallie BL, Budning A, DeBoer G, et al. Chemotherapy with focal therapy can cure intraocular retinoblastoma without radiotherapy. Arch Opthalmol 1996; 114: 1321–8.

47 Schefler AC, Cicciarelli N, Feuer W, et al. Macular retinoblastoma: evaluation of tumor control, local complications, and visual outcomes for eyes treated with chemotherapy and repetitive foveal laser ablation. Ophthalmology 2007; 114: 162–9.

48 Doz F, Khelfaoui F, Mosseri V, et al. The role of chemotherapy in orbital involvement of retinoblastoma. The experience of a single institution with 33 patients. Cancer 1994; 75: 722–32.

49 Schvartzman E, Chantada G, Fandino A, et al. Results of a stage-based protocol for the treatment of retinoblastoma. J Clin Oncol 1996; 14: 1532–6.

50 MacCarthy A, Birch JM, Draper GJ, et al. Retinoblastoma: treatment and survival in Great Britain 1963–2002. Br J Ophthalmol 2009; 93: 38–9.

51 Broaddus E, Topham A, Singh AD. Survival with retinoblastoma in the USA: 1975–2004. Br J Ophthalmol 2009; 93: 24–7.

52 Gombos DS, Kelly A, Coen PG, et al. Retinoblastoma treated with primary chemotherapy alone: the significance of tumor size, location and age. Br J Ophthalmol 2002; 86: 80–3.

53 Gunduz K, Gunlap I, Yalcindaq N, et al. Causes of chemoreduction failure in retinoblastoma and analysis of associated factors leading to eventual treatment with external beam radiotherapy ands enucleation. Ophthalmology 2004; 111: 1917–24.

54 Chantanda GL, Dunkel JJ, Antoneli CB, et al. Risk factors for extraocular relapse following enucleation after failure of chemoreduction in retinoblastoma. Pediatr Blood Cancer 2007; 49: 256–60.

55 Schouten-van Meeteren AYU, van der Valk P, et al. Histopathologic features of retinoblastoma and its relation with in vitro drug resistance measured by means of the MTT assay. Cancer 2001; 92: 2933–40.

56 Filho JP, Correa ZM, Odashiro AN, et al. Histopathological features and P-glycoprotein expression in retinoblastoma. Invest Ophthalmol Vis Sci 2005; 46; 3478–83.

57 Krishnakumar S, Mallikarjuna K, Desai N, et al. Multidrug resistant proteins: P-glycoprotein and lung resistance protein expression in retinoblastoma. Br J Ophthalmol 2004; 88: 1521–6.

58 Kamburoglu G, Kiratli H, Soylemezoglu F, et al. Clinicopathological parameters and expression of P-glycoprotein and MRP-1 in retinoblastoma. Ophthalmic Res 2007; 39: 191–7.

59 Chantanda GL, Fandino A, Mato G, et al. Phase II window of idarubicin in children with extraocular retinoblastoma. J Clin Oncol 1999; 17: 1847–50.

60 Wilson MW, Haik BG, Rodriguez-Galindo C. Socioeconomic impact of modern multidisciplinary management of retinoblastoma. Pediatrics 2006; 118: e331–6.

61 Zage PE, Reitman AJ, Seshadri R, et al. Outcomes of a two-drug chemotherapy regimen for intraocular retinoblastoma. Pediatr Blood Cancer 2008; 50: 567–72.

62 Demirci H, Shields CL, Meadows AT, et al. Long-term visual outcome following chemoreduction for retinoblastoma. Arch Ophthalmol 2005; 123: 1525–30.

63 Berman EL, Donaldson CE, Giblin M, et al. Outcomes in retinoblastoma, 1974–2005; the Children's Hospital, Westmead. Clin Experiment Ophthalmol 2007; 35: 5–12.

64 Pradhan DG, Sandridge AL, Mullaney P, et al. Radiation therapy for retinoblastoma: a retrospective review of 120 patients. Int J Radiat Oncol Biol Phys 1997; 39: 3–13.

65 Tawansy KA, Samuel MA, Shammas M, et al. Vitreoretinal complications of retinoblastoma treatment. Retina 2006; 26: S47–52.

66 Phillips C, Sexton M, Wheeler G, et al. Retinoblastoma: review of 30 years' experience with external beam radiotherapy. Australas Radiol 2003; 47: 226–30.

67 Dehainault, C, Lauge A, Caux-Moncoutier V. Multiplex PCR/ Liquid Chromatography assay for detection of gene rearrangements: application to RB1 gene. Nucleic Acids Res 2004; 32: e19.

68 Houdayer C, Gauthier-Villars M, Lauge A, et al. Comprehensive screening for constitutional RB1 mutations by DHPLC and QMPSF. Hum Mutat 2004; 23: 193–202.

69 Taylor M, Dehainault C, Desjardins L, et al. Genotype-phenotype correlations in hereditary familial retinoblastoma. Hum Mutat 2007; 28: 284–93.

70 Abramson DH, Beaverson K, Sangani P, et al. Screening for retinoblastoma: presenting signs as prognosticators of patient and ocular survival. Pediatrics 2003; 112: 1248–55.

71 Gombos D, Kelly A, Coen P, et al. Retinoblastoma treatment with primary chemotherapy alone: the significance of tumor size, location and age. Br J Ophthalmol 2002; 86: 80–3.

72 Laurie NA, Gray JK, Zhang J, et al. Topotecan combination chemotherapy in two new rodent modals of retinoblastoma. Clin Cancer Res 2005; 11: 7569–78.

73 Frangoul H, Ames MM, Mosher RB, et al. Phase I study of topotecan administered as a 21-day continuous infusion in children with recurrent solid tumors: a report from the Children's Cancer Group. Clin Cancer Res 1999; 5: 3956–62.

74 Chevez-Barrios P, Chintagumpala M, Mieler W, et al. Response of retinoblastoma with vitreous tumor seeding to adenovirus-mediated delivery of thymidine kinase followed by ganciclovir. J Clin Oncol 2005; 23: 7927–35.

75 Jia RB, Zhang P, Zhou YX, et al. VEGF-targeted RNA interference suppresses angiogenesis and tumor growth of retinoblastoma. Ophthalmic Res 2007; 39: 108–15.

76 Mohan A, Nalini V, Mallikarjuna K, et al. Expression of motility-related protein MRP1/CD9, N-cadherin, E-cadherin, alpha-catenin and beta-catenin in retinoblastoma. Exp Eye Res 2007; 84: 781–9.

77 Sherr C J, McCormick F. The RB and p53 pathways in cancer. Cancer Cell 2002; 2: 103–12.

78 Oren M. Decision making by p53: life, death and cancer. Cell Death Differ 2003; 10: 431–42.

79 Kubbutat MH, Jones SN, Vousden KH. Regulation of p53 stability by Mdm2. Nature 1997; 387: 299–303.

80 Howes KA, Ransom N, Papermaster DS, et al. Apoptosis or retinoblastoma: alternative fates of photoreceptors expressing the HPV-16 E7 gene in the presence or absence of p53. Genes Dev 1994; 8: 1300–10.

81 Dyer MA, Rodriguez-Galindo C, Wilson MW. Use of preclinical models to improve treatment of retinoblastoma. PLoS Med 2005; 2: e332.

82 Laurie NA, Donovan SL, Shih CS, et al. Inactivation of the p53 pathway in retinoblastoma. Nature 2006; 444: 61–6.

83 Toledo F, Krummel KA, Lee CJ, et al. A mouse p53 mutant lacking the proline-rich domain rescues Mdm4 deficiency and provides insight into the Mdm2-Mdm4-p53 regulatory network. Cancer Cell 2006; 9: 273–85.

84 Danovi D, Meulmeester E, Pasini D, et al. Amplification of Mdmx (or Mdm4) directly contributes to tumor formation by inhibiting p53 tumor suppressor activity. Mol Cell Biol 2004; 24: 5835–43.

85 Sherr CJ, McCormick F. The RB and p53 pathways in cancer. Cancer Cell 2002; 2: 103–12.

86 Kato MV, Shimizu T, Nagayoshi M et al. Loss of heterozygosity on chromosome 17 and mutation of the p53 gene in retinoblastoma. Cancer Lett 1996; 106: 75–82.

87 Shvarts A, Steegenga WT, Riteco N, et al. MDMX: a novel p53-binding protein with some functional properties of MDM2. Embo J 1996; 15: 5349–57.

88 Bottger V, Bottger A, Garcia-Echeverria C, et al. Comparative study of the p53-mdm2 and p53-MDMX interfaces. Oncogene 1999; 18: 189–99.

89 Marine JC, Jochemsen AG. MDMX as an essential regulator of p53 activity. Biochem Biophys Res Commun 2005; 331: 750–60.

90 Elison JR, Cobrinik D, Claros N, et al. Small molecule inhibition of HDM2 leads to p53-mediated cell death in retinoblastoma cells. Arch Ophthalmol 2006; 124: 1269–75.

91 Abramson DH, Frank CM, Dunkle IJ. A phase I/II study of subconjunctival carboplatin for intraocular retinoblastoma. Ophthalmology 1999; 106: 1947–50.

92 Mendelsohn ME, Abramson TH, Madden T, et al. Intraocular concentrations of chemotherapeutic agents after systemic or local administration. Arch Ophthalmol 1998; 116: 1209–12.

93 Laurie NA, Gray JK, Zhang J, et al. Topotecan combination chemotherapy in two new rodent models of retinoblastoma. Clin Cancer Res 2005; 11: 7569–78.

94 Abramson DH, Frank CM, Dunkle IJ. A phase I/II study of subconjunctival carboplatin for intraocular retinoblastoma. Ophthalmology 1999; 106: 1947–50.

95 Hayden BH, Murray TG, Scott IU, et al. Subconjunctival carboplatin in retinoblastoma: impact of tumor burden and dose schedule. Arch Ophthalmol 2000; 118: 1549–54.

96 Murray TG, Cicciarelli N, O'Brien JM, et al. Subconjunctival carboplatin therapy and cryotherapy in the treatment of transgenic murine retinoblastoma. Arch Ophthalmol 1997; 115: 1286–90.

97 Rodriguez-Galindo C, Wilson MW, Chantanda G, et al. Retinoblastoma: one world, one vision. Pediatrics 2008; 122: e763–70.

19 Rare Tumors

Bernadette Brennan[1] and Charles Stiller[2]

[1] Royal Manchester Children's Hospital, Manchester, UK and [2] Childhood Cancer Research Group, University of Oxford, Oxford, UK

Introduction

Cancer is rare in childhood compared with older age groups, affecting approximately 1 in 600 children during the first 15 years of life. However, some tumors are so rare that even pediatric oncologists may only encounter them once in their lifetime practice. Therefore, there are obvious advantages for pooling the experiences of the United Kingdom's Children's Cancer & Leukaemia Group (CCLG) with groups from other rare tumor registries and other national initiatives such as the Italian TREP project.

Any definition of 'rare' is bound to be arbitrary, but for this chapter we have defined rare childhood cancers as those categories in the International Classification of Childhood Cancer (Third edition [ICCC-3]), that have an age-standardized annual incidence of less than 1 per million children in the UK, excluding tumors of unspecified morphology [1]. Based on the UK National Registry of Childhood Tumors (NRCT), Table 19.1 describes the incidence rates and numbers of registrations in Britain during the period 1991–2000 for rare childhood cancers according to this definition, excluding leukemias, lymphomas and central nervous system (CNS) tumors which are either outside the scope of this chapter or dealt with in other sections of this book.

Histological subtypes of germ cell tumors which individually have an incidence below 1 per million have also been excluded on the grounds that clinically all malignant germ cell tumors in children are treated similarly. Overall, the tumors listed in Table 19.1 had:

- An incidence rate of 6.8 per million.
- Accounted for 16% of non-CNS malignant solid tumors.
- Accounted 5% of all childhood cancers.
- In both relative and absolute terms they were most frequent in the age group 10–14 years, where their incidence was 12.4 per million and where they accounted for 35% of non-CNS solid tumors and 11% of all cancers.

Carcinomas of all sites counted as rare tumors, and collectively formed 50% of the total. Soft tissue sarcomas were the next most frequent histological group, representing 36%. It is important to note that the same diagnostic groups are not necessarily rare in all populations. Most strikingly, Kaposi sarcoma is one of the most frequent childhood cancers in parts of central and east Africa most severely affected by the AIDS epidemic, whereas malignant melanoma is rare throughout most of Africa and Asia.

Despite their rarity, the tumors described in the chapter can cause much stress to both the families and the oncologist. However, rare tumors do not necessarily have a poor prognosis, and some tumor types may be easily treated and have very little chance of recurring. These include some tumors that are rare among children but occur more commonly in adults and we can learn a lot from their management in this setting so that this can be adapted for their treatment in childhood. A good example for this can be found for thyroid carcinoma (the follicular subtype is most commonly encountered in the pediatric population), where the 5-year survival for the 71 children diagnosed in Britain during 1991–2000 was 100% [2].

Other rare tumors, however, only occur in childhood or currently have a poor prognosis. This chapter will focus on a selection of these tumors that was the starting point for the Rare Tumor Guidelines that were produced by the Rare Tumor Working Group of the CCLG. In particular, we have included nasopharyngeal carcinoma, as this is one of the rare tumors frequently consulted about because of its challenging treatment, and as an example of a rare tumor where there has been a dramatic improvement in survival in recent years.

Nasopharyngeal carcinoma (Box 19.1)

Nasopharyngeal carcinoma (NPC) was first described as a separate entity by Regaud and Schmincke in 1921. Approximately one-third of nasopharyngeal carcinomas of the undifferentiated

Pediatric Hematology and Oncology, 1st edition. Edited by Edward J. Estlin, Richard J. Gilbertson, and Robert F. Wynn. © 2010 Blackwell Publishing Ltd.

Table 19.1 Rare childhood cancers in Great Britain, 1991–2000. Age standardized annual incidence per million children aged 0–14 years (ASR) and number of registrations (n). Leukemias, lymphomas and CNS tumors are excluded. Source: National Registry of Childhood Tumors [2].

ICCC-3	Definition	ASR	n
IV	Neuroblastoma and other peripheral nervous cell tumors		
IVb	Peripheral nervous cell tumors other than neuroblastoma	0.10	11
VI	Renal tumors		
VIa.2	Rhabdoid renal tumor	0.36	24
VIa.3	Kidney sarcomas	0.36	24
VIa.4	Peripheral primitive neuroectodermal tumor of the kidney	0.05	7
VIb	Renal carcinoma	0.16	19
VII	Hepatic tumors		
VIIb	Hepatic carcinoma	0.22	25
VIII	Malignant bone tumors		
VIIIb	Chondrosarcoma	0.10	12
VIIId	Other specified malignant bone tumors	0.14	16
IX	Soft tissue and other extraosseous sarcomas		
IXb.1	Fibroblastic and myoblastic tumors	0.35	37
IXb.2	Nerve sheath tumors	0.36	41
IXb.3	Other fibromatous neoplasms	0.02	2
IXc	Kaposi sarcoma	0.04	5
IXd.3	Extrarenal rhabdoid tumor	0.20	19
IXd.4	Liposarcomas	0.04	4
IXd.5	Fibrohistiocytic tumors	0.41	47
IXd.6	Leiomyosarcomas	0.10	12
IXd.7	Synovial sarcomas	0.49	58
IXd.8	Blood vessel tumors	0.11	11
IXd.9	Osseous and chondromatous neoplasms of soft tissue	0.08	9
IXd.10	Alveolar soft part sarcoma	0.09	10
IXd.11	Miscellaneous soft tissue sarcomas	0.18	19
X	Germ cell tumors, trophoblastic tumors and neoplasms of gonads		
Xd	Gonadal carcinomas	0.07	8
Xe	Other malignant non germ cell gonadal tumors	–	0
XI	Other malignant epithelial neoplasms and malignant melanomas		
XIa	Adrenocortical carcinoma	0.24	24
XIb	Thyroid carcinoma	0.60	71
XIc	Nasopharyngeal carcinoma	0.20	24
XIe	Skin carcinomas	0.70	82
XIf.1	Carcinomas of salivary glands	0.25	30
XIf.2	Carcinomas of colon and rectum	0.09	11
XIf.3	Carcinomas of appendix	0.12	15
XIf.4	Carcinomas of lung	0.08	10
XIf.5	Carcinomas of thymus	0.03	4
XIf.6	Carcinomas of breast	–	0
XIf.7	Carcinomas of cervix uteri	0.01	1
XIf.8	Carcinomas of bladder	0.05	6
XIf.9	Carcinomas of eye	–	0
XIf.10	Carcinomas of other specified sites	0.33	39
XIf.11	Carcinomas of unspecified site	0.11	12
XII	Other and unspecified malignant neoplasms		
XIIa.1	Gastrointestinal stromal tumor	0.02	2
XIIa.2	Pancreatoblastoma	0.04	4
XIIa.3	Pulmonary blastoma and pleuropulmonary blastoma	0.08	8
XIIa.4	Other complex mixed and stromal neoplasms	–	0
XIIa.5	Mesothelioma	0.03	3
XIIa.6	Other specified malignant tumors	–	0
	Total of non-central nervous system rare tumors	6.79	766
	Total of all non-central nervous system solid tumors	46.18	4770
	Total childhood cancers	139.19	14659

type are diagnosed in adolescents or young adults. Although rare in western populations, NPC accounts for one third of nasopharyngeal neoplasms of childhood. Presentation with lymphadenopathy implies the disease has spread beyond the primary site.

Epidemiology

During the years 1991–2000 there were 24 cases of NPC registered in the NRCT, with an annual incidence of 0.20 per million (age standardized, age 0–14 years); 83% of cases were in boys, and 88% in children aged 10–14 years [2]. The incidence of childhood NPC in western populations is generally low, but in parts of North Africa and the Middle East it can be as high as 2 per million.

Lo *et al.* showed that Epstein-Barr virus (EBV) DNA was detectable in the plasma samples of 96% of patients with non-keratinizing NPC compared with only 7% of controls [3]. The detection of nuclear antigen associated with Epstein-Barr virus (EBNA) has revealed that EBV can infect epithelial cells and is associated with their transformation [4].

Thus, the etiology of NPC (particularly the endemic form) seems to follow a multi-step process, in which EBV, ethnic background, and environmental carcinogens all seem to play an important role.

Clinical presentation

Cervical lymphadenopathy is the initial presentation in many patients. Symptoms related to the primary tumor include:
- Trismus, pain, otitis media, deafness, nasal regurgitation, and cranial nerve palsies.
- Larger growths may produce nasal obstruction or bleeding and a 'nasal twang' character for speech.
- Metastatic spread may result in bone pain or organ dysfunction.
- Rarely a paraneoplastic syndrome of osteoarthropathy may occur with widespread disease [5].

Investigation and staging

1 Computed tomography (CT)/magnetic resonance imagery (MRI) scan of head and neck – to below clavicles, assess base of skull erosion.
2 CT chest.
3 Bone isotope scan.
4 EBV viral capsid antigen and EBV-DNA.
5 Biopsy of either lymph nodes or primary tumor.

Staging

The tumor, node, metastasis (TNM) classification of the American Joint Committee on Cancer (6th Edition) [6], is usually used to determine the tumor staging.

Treatment and prognosis

Nasopharyngeal carcinoma is a very aggressive tumor and commonly metastasizes distally as well as to local lymph nodes, which are usually the supraclavicular, hilar, and mediastinal groups. Metastatic recurrence occurs early, usually within the first 2 years after the diagnosis is made. The prognosis of children in advanced stages with radiotherapy alone is poor, with the 5-year survival rate 20–30%.

Because of this poor prognosis NPC patients have been treated with various chemotherapy regimens, mainly administered in the adjuvant setting. However, there has been a paucity of larger-scale studies for the treatment of NPC of children and adolescents. In the last few years, several retrospective pediatric studies have been published. Most have been from regions where the incidence is appreciably higher than in western countries and have generally included fewer than 100 children and adolescents. Improvement in local control and overall survival has been consistently associated with chemoradiotherapy [7–9]. However, a randomized trial in children would not be possible without wide international collaboration and/or an increase in the upper age limit above 15 years. Examples of more contemporary treatment experiences for NPC include:

- Al-Sarraf et al. showed in a randomized study that chemoradiotherapy that included cisplatin and 5-fluorouracil (5-FU) was superior to radiotherapy alone for both survival and local control in adult NPC [10].
- The first multi-centre trial for the treatment of children and adolescents with NPC, the NPC-91-GPOH protocol in Germany, Austria, Belgium, and the Netherlands, was initiated in 1992. Of the 59 patients registered on the trial, 58 were high risk (stage III or IV) at the time of diagnosis and only one patient had stage II disease at diagnosis. The combined treatment of 5-FU and cisplatin before radiotherapy and adjuvant interferon therapy resulted in an event-free survival for stage III or IV patients of 91.37% with a medium follow up of 47.6 months. Furthermore these very good results were achieved with a total radiotherapy dose of only 60 Gy [5].

The prognosis for NPC has improved such that the 5-year survival has increased from 57% in the decade 1971–1980 to 83% in 1991–2000 [2]. However, although in childhood the presence of metastatic disease in cervical lymph nodes at diagnosis does not adversely affect prognosis, certain adverse characteristics for NPC have been identified, including:
- Factors associated with a poor prognosis are skull base involvement, extent of the primary tumor, and cranial nerve involvement [5].
- Plasma EBV DNA levels appears to correlate with treatment response [3] and may predict disease recurrence [11], suggesting that they may be an independent indicator of prognosis [12].

Strategies for follow up and expected late effects

Acute toxicity will depend on the chemotherapy regimen employed, but contributes to the known toxicity from radiotherapy, e.g. mucositis, weight loss, and xerostomia. Other important toxicities include:
• Cardiotoxicity following high-dose 5-FU combination with folinic acid, cisplatinum, and methotrexate [13].
• Ototoxicity is a significant risk following cisplatin with additional toxicity from radiotherapy. Therefore, long-term follow up with pure tone audiometry is essential.
• Nephropathy and tubulopathy associated with cisplatin is dose dependent but rarely causes renal failure.
• Regular clinical assessment of growth and pubertal stage with biochemical assessment as necessary in particular thyroid function.

Clinical examination for recurrence locally, in local lymph nodes and in metastatic sites is recommended with appropriate radiology.

Novel therapeutic approaches

Numerous investigations of the anti-tumor effect of the interferons (IFNs) in patients with malignant tumors have been published. For NPC, therapeutic effect has been observed in single cases, and in a patient with a recurrent EBV-associated NPC a response to the Type I-IFNs was demonstrated [14]. Subsequently IFN-β was piloted in seven young NPC patients [15]. Uniquely, the NPC-91-GPOH protocol includes immunotherapy with IFN-β after chemotherapy and radiotherapy, which may explain its superior results compared with regimens with similar chemoradiotherapy but without IFN [16].

Summary

Due to the anatomical position of NPC and the tendency to present with cervical lymph node metastases, NPC is not amenable to surgery for local control, and biopsy of involved lymph nodes is the usual surgical procedure. The event-free survival in most small chemotherapy series is comparable but usually achieved with relatively high doses of radiotherapy to the nasopharynx, i.e. 60–65Gy. However, the encouraging outcomes for therapy according to the NPC-91-GPOH protocol may be seen as representing the current best treatment [5]. Uniquely the NPC-91-GPOH protocol includes immunotherapy with IFN-β after chemotherapy and radiotherapy, which may explain its superior results compared with regimens without interferon [5].

Thus, the GPOH protocol could form the basis for an international protocol as most national groups are recommending a cisplatin/5-FU chemotherapy-based protocol for chemotherapy. It would be important to reproduce these superb results in a larger population, in order to gain experience of the true level of toxicity of this regimen (there have been anecdotal reports of death during treatment), and try to resolve what role IFN-β contributes to these results and whether the dose of radiotherapy in children could be reduced further.

Pleuropulmonary blastoma

Pleuropulmonary blastoma (PPB), an embryonal tumor of the thoraco-pulmonary mesenchyme, is a malignant tumor that occurs almost exclusively in children younger than 5 years of age. The origin of the tumor was first suggested by Spencer in 1961 as mesodermal blastema, because of histological similarities to the blastemal component seen in Wilms' tumor [17]. PPB was eventually described by Manivel as a pediatric entity distinct from the biphasic epithelial-stromal morphology seen in adult tumors [18]. Because of its rarity, the optimal management of PPB remains unclear and the prognosis is historically poor (Box 19.2).

Epidemiology

Between the years 1991 and 2005 there have been 13 cases of PPB registered in the NRCT, all but two of which were diagnosed at ages below 5 years [2]. Ten (77%) of these patients are alive but we have no way of knowing at present what type of PPB these patients have. It is probable that there is an under-reporting of cases, in particular type I which may be mistaken for benign congenital cysts, in particular congenital cystic adenomatoid malformations (CCAM).

A further distinctive feature of PPB is that 25% of cases occur in constitutional/familial settings in which PPB patients themselves or young family members have other dysplastic or neoplastic features [19], especially cystic nephroma and other renal tumors [20].

Clinical presentation

The most common presenting symptoms are respiratory distress, shortness of breath, cough, fever which can mimic chest infections, or pneumothorax. Patients may also present with nonspecific features with malaise, weight loss, and may complain of chest and abdominal pain. Symptoms of mestastatic disease such as pain, headache, and vomiting may also be apparent, depending on the extent and location of the disease. Cerebral metastasis is more frequent in PPB than in other childhood sarcomas and hence patients should be screened for this at diagnosis [21].

Box 19.2 Pleuropulmonaryblastoma.

• Complete surgical excision is crucial for treatment
• Chemotherapy has a role in achieving surgical excision in particular in type II and III
• The PPB International Registry is an important source of information and guidance for management
• Three histopathological subtypes – type I cystic, type II mixed and type III solid.
• Type II and III probably evolve from type I

Investigation, staging and histology

Investigations are performed to define the location, stage, and histology as follows:

1 CT/MRI scan of primary chest mass.
2 CT of the head.
3 Bone scintigraphy by ^{99}Tc-diphosphonate.

As PPB has commonly been treated on soft tissue sarcoma protocols in the past it is probably useful to use the Intergroup Rhabdomyosarcoma Study (IRS) staging system from both a management point of view and for comparison of outcome from the various previous small series:

Group I: Localized disease, completely resected.
Group II: Total gross resection with evidence of regional spread.
Group III: Incomplete resection with gross residual disease.
Group IV: Distant metastatic disease present at onset (lung, liver, bones, bone marrow, brain, and distant muscle and nodes)

Histologically, PPB typically contains a blastemal component and a malignant mesenchymal stroma that can show multiple sarcomatous (rhabdomyo-, chondro-, lipo-, fibro-sarcomatous) features [22]. The tumor can be classified into three main histopathological subtypes:

• Type 1 PPB is a cystic tumor occurring almost always in infants.
• Type III disease is purely solid in nature.
• Type II disease contains both solid and cystic areas within the tumor; both occur in older children compared with type I [23].

The histogenesis of different PPB types is probably linked, as patients previously treated for type I tumor have been shown to develop type II disease as recurrence [22] and progression from type I to type III PPB has also been reported [23]. Various reports have identified a history of thoracic or lung cysts in 25–40% of children with PPB several months before the definitive diagnosis, hypothesizing that PPB may arise in precursor developmental anomaly, similar to the relationship between nephrogenic rests and Wilms' tumor [17, 24].

Treatment

Total or radical surgery, with the aim to achieve maximum tumor resection if possible, remains important in the management of all types of PPB. This can be in the form of wedge excision, lobectomy, or pnemonectomy. Children with a total excision of tumor, or microscopic residual disease after initial surgery, were found to have an improved relapse-free survival [22, 25, 26]. Chemotherapy also appears to be more effective in preventing recurrence when used after total macroscopic tumor resection, but this observation will need to be verified in a larger cohort of patients. Other factors that relate to poorer survival include mediastinal and pleural involvement, when compared with patients with lung parenchymal involvement only [25].

Because the tumor is often extensive at diagnosis, delayed or second-look surgery is usually necessary after initial biopsy or debulking following neoadjuvant chemotherapy [22, 25]. However, there are reports of short-term survival (17 months on follow up) in patients with type I PPB receiving only complete resection without adjuvant treatment [25]. The role of surgery

alone in this subgroup of children is unconfirmed and there are other cases with disease recurrence following just initial surgery [27].

Priest *et al.* have published the largest series so far of type I PPB from the International PPB registry and cases from the literature, with an attempt to examine the role of chemotherapy in type I disease [27]. In a total series of 38 patients, 20 had surgery only with eight recurrences, whereas among 18 who had surgery upfront followed by various chemotherapy regimens (including vincristine, actinomycin, doxorubicin, ifosfamide, etoposide, and cyclophosphamide, which are agents typically employed for the therapy of soft tissue sarcoma), only one patient had a recurrence. This suggests a possible significant role for chemotherapy in type I PPB, but could reflect a bias to reporting or registering cases cured with chemotherapy, or indeed failure to recognize some surgically treated cystic cases as PPB.

The role of chemotherapy is more clearly defined in type II and III disease though this assumption is based on individual case reports demonstrating response to chemotherapy in patients with macroscopic disease, or better survival with adjuvant chemotherapy after upfront complete surgery. Three publications on this rare tumor are noteworthy as they include relatively high numbers of cases of type II and II PPB.

• An earlier report by Priest and colleagues describing 50 cases of PPB included 43 of types II and III, making it so far the largest series on outcome of these types [22]. Although the authors could not show a significant difference in survival between the different types of PPB, the 2-year event-free survival for types II and III , of 49% and 42 % respectively, was much lower than the 83% survival found for patients with type I disease. The chemotherapy received was diverse reflecting institutional choices but tended to be that used for soft tissue sarcomas and no conclusions could be made in this series in terms of response to treatment.

• The Italian Association for Pediatric Hematology and Oncology – Rare Tumors Pediatric Age (AIEOP-TREP) recently published the outcome in 11 cases of PPB, in particular 10 cases of type II and III disease [25]. All had received adjuvant chemotherapy; the early cases received CEVAIE (ifosfamide, vincristine, actinomycin, epirubicin, etoposide, carboplatin), later cases receiving VAIA (vincristine, actinomycin, ifosfamide, doxorubicin). After 9–10 weeks of chemotherapy three cases had a partial response, and one case a complete response where macroscopic tumor was left after initial surgery or biopsy. Furthermore in this small series those patients who had total surgery performed either before and/ or after chemotherapy, had significantly better survival. Factors for a poor outcome were extra-pulmonary disease in type II disease, as most of these cases relapsed. The role of radiotherapy was difficult to assess as only three patients received this treatment modality.

• A surprisingly good rate of survival is seen in the CWS (German Cooperative Soft Tissue sarcoma Group) series of 16 patients [25]. Chemotherapy was not dissimilar to the Italian group with IVA, VACA, VAIA, EVAIA or CEVAIE (combination of ifosfamide, vincristine, actinomycin, doxorubicin, etoposide, epirubicin, cyclophosphamide and carboplatin). The 5-year overall survival was 70% and in six out of eight patients with macroscopic disease, response to chemotherapy could be demonstrated. Again the role of radiotherapy remains unclear due to the small number of patients receiving it [26]. A similar conclusion can be drawn from the PPB Registry paper but there was a tendency to receive XRT in type III PPB [22].

Follow up and late effects

As the role of chemotherapy is not clearly defined in type I PPB (although recommended by the PPB Registry), an alternative strategy is rigorous monitoring for early detection of recurrence. This requires CT scans at least every 3 months, as infrequent plain radiographs will miss subtle early changes and there is known rapidity of recurrence. Salvage therapy may be unsuccessful if a solid, high grade sarcomatous tumor emerges, and follow up must continue for up to 36 months from diagnosis. It remains to be proven, however, that aggressive follow up alters outcome. The high incidence of CNS metastases at recurrence (44%) would encourage a low threshold for CNS imaging with symptoms.

For type II and III PPB, recurrence after multimodal aggressive upfront treatment heralds such a poor prognosis that detection of recurrence will not alter outcome. Therefore plain radiographs will usually suffice. The expected late effects for PPB reflect the initial treatment rather than PPB itself but the use of anthracycline-based chemotherapy protocols and radiation fields involving the chest/mediastinum will require careful follow up with echocardiograms.

Summary and future directions for management

The rarity of PPB has allowed only slow progress in the understanding of its clinical behaviour and management. The International PPB Registry has made huge advances recently in bringing together interested parties and with a future hope for international treatment guidelines and data analysis to improve our knowledge and ask further questions, and perhaps introduce novel therapies in type II and III which traditionally have a poor outcome. Furthermore, the International Registry allows the collection of biological material so that a better understanding of the biology and familial associations of PPB may drive novel therapies.

Pancreatoblastoma (Box 19.3)

Introduction and epidemiology

The term pancreatoblastoma was coined in 1977 by Horie *et al.* and has subsequently been employed to describe tumors previously known as 'infantile carcinoma of the pancreas' [28]. Pancreatoblastoma has several similarities to hepatoblastoma, a tumor found in an identical age group with a closely related morphological appearance. Both tumors occur in association with the Beckwith-Wiedemann syndrome [29, 30] and familial

---

Box 19.3 Pancreatoblastoma.

- Pancreatoblastoma has many similarities to hepatoblastoma
- Alph-fetoprotein levels are usually elevated
- Complete tumor excision is crucial for a good outcome
- Pancreatoblastoma is a chemosensitive tumor and in view of the similarities to hepatoblastoma, PLADO chemotherapy – cisplatin and doxorubicin – is recommended
- In the future SIOPEL hope to open an international protocol for pancreatoblastoma in particular to collect biological material

---

adenomatous polyposis [31], and often exhibit elevated plasma levels of alpha-fetoprotein [32, 33].

Six of the seven reported cases of pancreatoblastoma associated with Beckwith-Wiedemann syndrome has occurred in newborns and all but one were in males [34, 35]. This similarity may lead to diagnostic confusion as tumor origin cannot always be accurately determined on CT scanning.

Several reports indicate that surgical resection is more likely to be successful in pancreatoblastoma than in adult pancreatic carcinoma. Overall survival is at least 80% in children with completely resectable tumors at diagnosis [36]. By contrast the outlook for children with metastatic disease, usually hepatic or skeletal, is very poor [33, 37, 38]. Very limited biological studies have been done in this tumor. A single case report showed 11p15.5 LOH and overexpression of IGF2, typical of that found in other blastemal tumors such as Wilms' tumor and hepatoblastoma [30].

From 1971 to 2005, 48 cases of pancreatic tumor were reported to the NRCT (Table 19.2). Of this total, 28 were malignant of which 12 were pancreatoblastomas. In order of frequency these were pancreatoblastoma, islet cell tumors, papillary-cystic neoplasm and adenocarcinoma. Since ascertainment for non-malignant tumors is incomplete, it seems likely that over half of childhood pancreatic tumors are benign. Comparable information is not available from either the US (Giulio D'Angio, personal communication) or the International Society of Pediatric Oncology.

Clinical presentation

Children with pancreatoblastoma usually present late with upper abdominal pain and many have a palpable mass in the epigastrium. Mechanical obstruction of the upper duodenum and gastric outlet by tumor in the head of the pancreas may be associated with vomiting, jaundice, and gastrointestinal haemorrhaging. Poor nutritional intake and the resultant weight loss may also be found. Metastatic spread can be locally to regional lymph nodes, via the portal drainage system to the liver, and distally to the lungs.

Table 19.2 Pancreatic tumors reported to the NRCT, 1971–2005.

Histological classification	Number	% of total
Malignant		
Pancreatoblastoma	12	25
Islet cell carcinoma	4	8
Adenocarcinoma	2	4
Malignant carcinoid	1	2
Other (NHL, sarcoma, neuroblastoma, yolk sac tumor)	9	19
Non-malignant		
Papillary cystic neoplasm	11	23
Islet cell tumor	3	6
Insulinoma	2	4
Gastrinoma	2	4
Cystadenoma	1	2
Acinic cell tumor	1	2

Investigations

Investigation for pancreatoblastoma are detailed as follows:
1 Liver function tests.
2 Alpa-fetoprotein.
3 Lactate dehydrogenase (LDH).
4 CT or MRI scan of abdomen.
5 CT scan chest.
6 Isotope bone scan.
7 Bone marrow aspirate and trephine.

Staging

Stage 1 Localized primary tumor, completely resected.
Stage 2 Localized primary tumor, incompletely resected with microscopically residual disease, or biopsy only.
Stage 3 Primary tumor with infiltration of adjacent structures and or regional lymph nodes.
Stage 4 Metastatic disease to liver, lung, bones, or bone marrow.

Treatment

There is a paucity of data regarding the best treatment for pancreatoblastoma but as with hepatoblastoma, complete tumor excision appears to be crucial for a good outcome.

Pancreatoblastoma is a chemosensitive tumor and simple excision is associated with a high rate of local and metastatic recurrence, and the general principles for treatment are outlined as follows:
• Some localized tumors have been treated with surgery alone.
• Published case reports describe a varied response to chemotherapy, especially to cisplatin containing regimens that may be used pre-operatively to facilitate surgery [33, 39–43]. The latter paper contains a description of seven cases over a 20-year period in France. Cisplatin and doxorubicin was used in three of the four who were disease free at the time of publication and hence this regimen is suggested for unresectable tumors [43]. Vannier

describes a case which failed to respond to ifosfamide, vincristine, and actinomycin but responded to doxorubicin and cisplatin and remained disease free 40 months later at the time of publication [41].
• Responses to vincristine/ifosfamide/actinomycin-D and etoposide/ifosfamide/epirubicin have also been described [38, 44].
• Radiotherapy may have a role after local recurrence but this is based on a case report [45].

Follow up and late effects

Regular chest X-rays and ultrasound scans of the primary tumor site, together with AFP monitoring in AFP-secreting tumors, may detect recurrence before symptoms develop. Regular assessment of hearing, renal function, and echocardiograms in patients would be required following a cisplatin/doxorubicin chemotherapy regimen. The extent of the surgery will determine assessment of pancreatic exocrine and endocrine function.

Summary and future management

If the tumor is unresectable then in view of the many similarities between pancreablastoma and hepatoblastoma it is recommended that pancreatoblastoma is treated in accordance with SIOPEL 3, i.e. the PLADO chemotherapy arm (cisplatinum $80\,mg/m^2$ and doxorubicin $60\,mg^2$ infused over 48 hours) for a total of six courses. This approach is consistent with case reports described in the literature and incorporates a treatment plan which will be familiar to most pediatric oncology centres. Published evidence suggests that as in the case of hepatoblastoma, macroscopic surgical resection is important for cure and should be attempted after either two, three or four courses of PLADO depending on response. Radiotherapy may be indicated for either a persistently unresectable tumor or following grossly incomplete resection or microscopic disease. Primary surgery should not leave microscopic residue, so if this is likely to occur biopsy only should be performed.

Patients with pancreatoblastoma who are completely resected at presentation should have post-operative chemotherapy up to six courses of PLADO – cisplatin and doxorubicin. Under the auspices of the International Childhood Liver Tumor Strategy Group (SIOPEL) there is a plan to open an international protocol to examine the role of PLADO chemotherapy and, most importantly, to examine the biology of pancreatoblastoma in more detail.

Exracranial rhabdoid tumors (Box 19.4)

Extracranial malignant rhabdoid tumors comprise less than 1% of childhood malignancies but their poor prognosis results in significant relapses and death. They were first recognized as a separate pathological entity in the 1980s [46], and have now been reported widely at most anatomical sites in the body. To date the exact cell type of derivation remains unknown. Although there are many reports describing their lethal outcome [47, 48], there are no published series describing their management in a consistent manner on national or international protocols. The epidemiology, genetics and treatment of renal rhabdoid tumors are described in detail in Chapter 14, and the emphasis of this current description will be of non-renal extracranial malignant rhabdoid tumors. However, a comparison of the treatment philosophies of renal rhabdoid tumors is also undertaken as this builds on the description found in Chapter 14.

Epidemiology

Data from the UK National Registry of Childhood Tumors strongly suggest that rhabdoid tumors were incompletely diagnosed until quite recently, and that the date at which recorded incidence stabilized varied by primary site (Table 19.3). Approximate annual numbers of cases in the UK by primary site are: kidney, 2.3 (1981–2005); liver, 0.5 (1986–2005); other, 1.3 (1986–2005). Table 19.4 shows survival by site with no evidence of trends in survival over time.

Box 19.4 Exracranial rhabdoid tumors.

- Rhabdoid tumors have a poor prognosis
- Common sites are the kidney and liver but they occur at other sites
- Most patients are less than 2 years of age
- Characterized by a mutation in the *INI 1* gene which can be detected by immunohistochemial methods
- Surgery and chemotherapy – based on doxorubicin and alkylating agents – is recommended for treatment
- In Europe patients can be registered on the E*p*SSG non-rhabdomyosarcoma protocol

---

Table 19.3 Rhabdoid tumors by primary site and period of diagnosis reported to the NRCT, 1981–2005.

	Kidney	Liver	Other	Total
1981–1985	12	0	1	13
1986–1990	6	1	7	14
1991–1995	9	4	8	21
1996–2000	14	3	5	22
2001–2005	17	2	5	24

Clinical presentation

The commonest site of origin of malignant rhabdoid tumors is the kidney. The majority at this site present with either gross or microscopic hematuria. Another significant finding is fever, and probably about a quarter of renal rhabdoids will have hypercalcemia. The overall patterns of presentation are summarized as [49]:

- Malignant rhabdoids at other anatomical sites outside the CNS usually present as a mass, often associated with fever and cachexia in patients with large tumors or extensive metastases.
- Rhabdoid tumors of the kidney tend to metastasize to regional lymph nodes and lungs most frequently, but also to the liver, bone, and brain.
- In addition, there has been an association between rhabdoid tumors of the kidney and distinct secondary tumors of the brain.

Staging in extrarenal malignant rhabdoid tumor

In keeping with pediatric soft tissue sarcomas, staging should be defined according to both the clinical tumor-node-metastases (TNM) staging classification [6] and the IRS post-surgical grouping system.

TNM staging classification

The TNM T1 definition applies to tumors confined to the organ or tissue of origin, while T2 lesions invade contiguous structures:

- T1 and T2 groups are further classified as A or B according to tumor diameter, ≤ or >5 cm respectively.
- Regional node involvement is designated as N1 (no node involvement – N0).
- Distant metastases at onset as M1 (no metastases – M0).

IRS system

After initial surgery, patients will be classified according to the IRS system:

- Group I includes completely-excised tumors.
- Group II indicates grossly-resected tumors with microscopic residual disease and/or regional lymph nodal spread.
- Group III includes patients with gross residual disease after incomplete resection or biopsy.
- Group IV comprises patients with metastases at onset.

Treatment of malignant rhabdoid tumor of the kidney

In the UK, patients with malignant rhabdoid tumors of the kidney have historically been treated on two consecutive national

---

Table 19.4 Survival of children with rhabdoid tumors reported to the NRCT.

Primary site	Years of diagnosis	*n*	1 year (%)	2 year (%)	3 year (%)	4 year (%)
Kidney	1981–2005	58	33	26	24	24
Liver	1986–2005	10	20	10	10	10
Other	1986–2005	25	40	32	24	19

Wilms' tumor protocols (UKW2 and UKW3) with a combination of vincristine, actinomycin-D , and doxorubicin. In a recent audit of 21 patients with renal MRT treated on these protocols the overall survival was 35% (standard error 9%), with all the deaths occurring within 13 months of diagnosis. A more detailed analyisis of this experience shows that:

• Both Stage I patients survived, all three Stage II patients died and four of the nine Stage III patients survived.

• Only one of the (n = 7) Stage IV patients survived. Two of the four Stage III patients who survived had local radiotherapy. Anecdotally there is one Stage IV MRT patient alive in the UK who was diagnosed in 1996 and, following initial nephrectomy, was treated with an intensive regimen consisting of courses of vincristine 2 mg/m^2, carboplatin 500 mg/m^2, epirubicin 100 mg/m^2, and etoposide 300 mg/m^2, alternating with vincristine 2 mg/m^2, ifosfamide 7.5 g/m^2 and actinomycin-D 1.8 mg/m^2, and followed by a continuation regimen of oral etoposide [49].

In the United States patients with rhabdoid tumor of the kidney historically have been treated on the National Wilms' Tumor Study Group (NWTSG) trials with agents such as vincristine, actinomycin, and doxorubicin, with or without cyclophosphamide [50, 51]. The outcomes attained with these agents were poor (Table 19.4) [52, 53]. The International Society of Pediatric Oncology (SIOP) reported similarly unfavourable outcomes [54]. To try to improve upon these results, NWTS-5 adopted a different treatment strategy consisting of carboplatin/etoposide alternating with cyclophosphamide (Regimen RTK). Preliminary analysis of patients treated with this regimen revealed a survival percentage of 25.8%, implying that it was unlikely to demonstrate an improvement compared with previous studies, and this treatment arm was closed (Table 19.5).

Several case reports have documented the successful treatment of advanced or metastatic rhabdoid tumor of the kidney.

• Waldron et al. used ifosfamide/etoposide (IE) alternating with vincristine/doxorubicin/cyclophosphamide (VDCy) to cure a patient with Stage IV rhabdoid tumor of the kidney with metastases to the lung [50].

• Wagner et al. reported the successful treatment of two patients with distant metastatic rhabdoid tumor of the kidney using ifosfamide/carboplatin/etoposide (ICE) alternating with VDCy [51]. Of note, one of the patients described in this report had recurrent disease following treatment with Regimen RTK; he had a complete response to one cycle of ICE followed by one cycle of VDCy.

• Gururangan et al. reported encouraging, albeit transient, responses to ICE chemotherapy in patients with advanced-stage renal and extrarenal rhabdoid tumor [47].

Treatment of extrarenal malignant rhabdoid tumor

A retrospective review of patients with non-CNS extrarenal malignant rhabdoid tumor was reported by the IRS Group [56]. Twenty-six cases with features similar to MRT of the kidney were identified among 3000 cases of childhood soft tissue sarcoma treated on the IRS Studies I–III. The tumors originated in the soft tissues of the extremities, trunk, retroperitoneum, abdomen, and pelvis. Of the 26 patients, only five were alive, with survival times of 2–13 years. Hence, regardless of its tissue of origin, only 20–25% of patients with extrarenal malignant rhabdoid tumor survive.

During the same time period of UKW2 and UKW3, 22 children were added to the UK National Registry of Childhood Tumors with extracranial, extrarenal rhabdoid tumors. Only one patient is alive at the time of writing. The survivor was treated on SIOP MMT 95 protocol which includes vincristine, actinomycin--D, ifosfamide, etoposide, epirubicin and carboplatin.

Follow up and late effects

It is likely, despite more recent aggressive and multimodal therapy, that the majority of MRT will relapse commonly in the lungs but also locally and in the CNS. The outcome at relapse is extremely poor and therefore frequent imaging whilst on follow up other than regular chest X-rays probably has limited value. For those few survivors late effects screening should include renal and cardiac assessment depending on the primary site and therapy used, and regular examination of irradiated areas as most will have received therapy at a relatively young age.

Summary and future treatment

If feasible and safe, the tumor, whether renal or extrarenal, should be completely resected with good margins when first encountered. Failing complete surgical removal, open surgical biopsy is the preferred approach. Intensive chemotherapy, usually based around doxorubicin and alkylating agents alternating with ICE-based chemotherapy of carboplatin, etoposide, and ifosfamide is advocated. The later is often substituted with cyclophosphamide as most patients will have a single kidney. Early radiotherapy to all sites of disease is more controversial as the median age tends to be less than 1 year, but is recommended nonetheless. The current lack in consistent treatment warrants international cooperation for multimodal protocols and as such this has been recognized by the Children's Oncology Group (COG) in the USA and in Europe by the European paediatric Soft Tissue Sarcoma

Table 19.5 Percentage survival for patients with rhabdoid tumor of the kidney on NWTSG studies.

Stage	NWTS 1–3 (number of patients)	NWTS 1–5* (number of patients)	NWTS-5 Regimen RTK† (number of patients)
I	50% (6)	33.3% (15)	50.0% (2)
II	44% (9)	46.9% (25)	33.3% (3)
III	22% (37)	21.8% (58)	33.3% (9)
IV	0% (18)	8.4% (41)	21.4% (14)
V	–	–	0 % (3)

* [55]. † Preliminary analysis of NWTS-5, as of April, 2001.

Study Group (E*p*SSG). Both groups have similar multimodal protocols as above with the hope of future cooperation and data sharing of this rare but extremely poor prognostic tumor.

Adrenocortical carcinoma

Introduction and epidemiology (Box 19.5)

Adrenocortical carcinoma (ACC) is a cancer that arises from the adrenal cortex, the outer layer of the adrenal gland. And the epidemiological characteristics of this rare cancer of children are [57]:

• ACC comprises 0.2% of childhood malignancies with an international incidence of 0.5/1 million and occurs far more commonly in girls than boys (ratio 1.5:1).

• A bi-modal age distribution curve with a peak incidence at 3.5 and 57 years of age is seen.

• Predisposing genetic factors have been implicated in > 50 % of cases, probably > 95 % cases in Brazil.

• There is also an increased incidence of ACC in patients with isolated hemihypertrophy, Wiedemann-Beckwith syndrome, congenital adrenal hyperplasia (CAH) and Li-Fraumeni syndrome (LFS) [58–60]. Although a rare component of this later syndrome, ACC occurs 100 times more frequently than would be expected.

• Germline mutations of the *TP53* gene have been identified in most but not all of the families with classic LFS [61]. Molecular genetic analysis has shown that in most children with ACC, germline TP53 mutations are present [62, 63], suggesting that presentation with ACC in childhood may be the first manifestation of this familial cancer syndrome within a family. In the Brazilian cases, in contrast, the patient's family do not exhibit a high incidence of cancer and a single consistent mutation of the *TP53* gene is observed [64].

Data from The National Registry of Childhood Tumors (personal communication, Charles Stiller) demonstrates that incidence rates were 0.40 per million at age 0–4 years, 0.12 at age 5–9 years, 0.12 at age 10–4 years and 0.23 overall (age standardized). There was a marked excess of girls at all ages, with females accounting for 77% of registrations. Table 19.6 shows registra-

---

Box 19.5 Adrenocortical carcinoma (ACC).

• ACC often occurs in genetically susceptible individuals
• 50 % of children with ACC will have Li-Fraumeni syndrome
• Prognostic indicators include tumor size, extent of surgical resection and metastatic spread
• Extensive or unresectable disease may respond to chemotherapy usually cisplatin based and mitotane
• The IPACT registry is an important source of information for the management of ACC and the registration of patients

---

Table 19.6 Adrenocortical carcinoma in The National Registry of Childhood Tumors 1971–2002. Number of registrations by age (years) and sex (M = male; F = female).

	0–4	5–9	10–14	Total
M	12	3	3	18
F	36	12	12	60
Total	48	15	15	78

tions of adrenocortical carcinoma for 1971–2000 by age and sex, with females accounting for 76% of registrations. The incidence in the USA is similar at 0.2–0.3 cases per million, but internationally the incidence of ACC in southern Brazil, in particular the adjoining states of Sao Paulo and Parana, is 10–15 times that observed in the USA for reasons that are currently unclear.

Five-year survival in Britain increased from 25% in 1971–1980 to 50% in 1991–2000 [2]. Subsequent mortality from subsequent malignancies is notably high. Among the seventeen 10-year survivors among children diagnosed during 1971 onwards, there have been seven deaths, all from a second or later cancer.

Clinical presentation

A significant body of evidence on presentation has been collected and published from the International Paediatric Adrenocortical Tumor Registry (IPACTR) [62]. ACC typically presents during the first 5 years of life with a smaller peak during adolescence and in the later group a higher incidence of non-functioning tumors.

• Most ACC in children and adolescents are hormone secreting and the clinical presentation reflects the pattern of adrenocortical hormones secreted by that tumor. Less than 10% of adrenocortical tumors are non-secreting.

• Signs and symptoms of virilization are present in over 90% of cases. Hirsuitism, acne, and deepening of the voice may be apparent in both sexes.

• Girls may also present with cliteromegaly and facial hair while boys present with phallomegaly and virilization.

• Cushing's syndrome occurs in a third of cases with moon facies, centripetal fat distribution and plethora being the most common sign.

• Hypertension is often present and children may present in hypertensive crisis.

• Generally, ACC are inefficient in producing active hormones such as cortisol and about half will be large enough to palpate at diagnosis.

Investigations and staging

The following clinical, biochemical, and histological investigations contribute towards the diagnosis of ACC:

1 24-hour urinary collection to measure steroid profile: free cortisol, 17-hydroxycorticosteroids (17-OH), and androgens.

2 24 hour urinary catecholamines to exclude phaeochromocytoma.

Table 19.7 IPACTR staging for adrenal tumors.

Stage	
I	Total excision of tumor, small tumor (100 g or <100 cm³) Absence of metastases and normal hormone levels after surgery
II	Completely resected, large tumors (>200 cm³ or >100 g) with normal post-operative hormone levels, tumor spillage during surgery
III	Gross or microscopic residual or inoperable tumor
	Patients with retroperitoneal lymph node involvement
IV	Distant metastases

3 Plasma samples for: electrolytes, glucose, calcium, cortisol, dehydroepiandrosterone sulfate (DHEA-S), testosterone, androstenedione, 11-deoxycortisol, oestradiol, renin and 17-hydroxyprogesterone.
4 ACTH at 08.00 and 24.00 h.
5 CT/MRI scan of abdomen.
6 CT scan of chest.
7 Bone isotope scan.

The distinction between benign (adenomas) and malignant (carcinomas) tumors may not be easy although mitotic rate, venous, capsular or adjacent organ invasion, tumor necrosis and atypical mitosis determine aggressive behaviour and hence malignancy. Tumor weight, and hence size and volume, and mitotic activity are usually the best discriminators and form part of the staging system as below (Table 19.7) used by the IPACTR [65].

At the time of diagnosis two-thirds will have limited disease (completely resected tumors), and the remaining patients have either unresectable or metastatic disease. Outcome is predicted by stage with excellent outcome for Stage I, (>90%) and very poor outcome for Stage IV, (<10%). In between it is more difficult but local recurrence probably occurs in 30–50% of Stage II disease

Treatment
Surgery
• Complete, radical surgical resection is the treatment of choice and may be curative, especially in small tumors.
• Patients achieving complete resection at Stage I survive significantly longer than those with residual disease [66]. In one recent series, survival rate reached 70% if resection was complete, but was a dismal 7% if complete resection was not achieved [67].
• Surgical resection of isolated recurrence and metastatic disease is also indicated where possible.
• Because of tumor friability, rupture of the capsule and tumor spillage can be frequent; up to 20% of cases in Sandrini's series and is associated with a worse outcome [68]. Infiltration of the vena cava makes radical surgery difficult but resection in this clinical scenario has been reported in patients undergoing cardiopulmonary bypass [66].

Chemotherapy
In patients with incomplete resection or metastatic spread, i.e. stage II and above, treatment options include chemotherapy and

or mitotane. Due to the rarity of this condition no randomized or controlled studies have been performed. It is not completely clear whether chemotherapy or mitotane should be the initial treatment of choice, although an International Registry of Adrenocortical Tumors co-ordinated at St Jude's Hospital recommends the use of both.
• Mitotane, the ortho-prime derivative of an insecticide, dichlorodiphenyl-dichloroethane (DDD), was serendipitously noted to cause adrenal necrosis, leading to its use in ACC [69].
• Mitotane is usually effective in controlling the endocrine symptoms and may cause tumor regression but is not an antineoplastic agent.
• A recent large retrospective study in adults concluded that mitotane did not have a significant effect on survival [70].
• There is, however, some evidence that mitotane is more effective in children than adults [71–73], particularly if the neoplasm is hormonally active [74].
• Studies have shown that mitotane exhibits a clear dose response curve, being most effective when the serum level is >14 mg/l [75].

Unpleasant side effects, including gastrointestinal, neurological, dermal, and miscellaneous, are common and very careful monitoring is essential. Side effects can be minimized by keeping the serum mitotane level between 14 and 20 mg/l and measuring it monthly [75]. It is possible that the equivocal results achieved with mitotane reflect the administration of sub-therapeutic levels of this drug, particularly as it has a narrow therapeutic window [70, 76]. It is also important to recognize that higher than normal doses of mineralocoticoid and glucocorticoid therapy are required due to an increased serum steroid-binding capacity during mitotane therapy [77].

Effective chemotherapeutic agents include cisplatinum, etoposide, doxorubicin, 5-FU and cyclophosphamide. However, they have been less well evaluated than mitotane [67, 78–83].
• The combination of cisplatin, etoposide, and mitotane, whilst tolerable, may confer a survival advantage over chemotherapy alone in one adult study. However, no randomized trials have been performed with this combination [79].
• The combination of mitotane with cisplatin, etoposide, and doxorubicin has been extensively used in children with ACT by the investigators of IPACTR with responses [65, 84].

Radiotherapy
Radiotherapy has been used but the use of this modality of treatment in the presence of a high risk of genetic predisposition to cancer is not advised, indeed secondary tumors have been reported within the radiation field [85].

Follow up and late effects
Since 50–80% of ACTs in childhood have a genetic basis, referral to a local cancer geneticist is recommended for appropriate genetic counselling, testing and family follow up. Associated syndromes and genetic conditions include:
• Li-Fraumeni syndrome.
• Isolated hemi-hypertrophy.

- Beckwith-Wiedemann syndrome.
- MEN I.
- Carney complex.

Follow up should involve regular surveillance with clinical examination, ultrasound examination of the abdomen, chest X-rays and estimations of urinary steroid profiles which were raised pre-operatively. It is also important to recognize that higher than normal doses of mineralocoticoid and glucocorticoid therapy are required due to an increased serum steroid-binding capacity during mitotane therapy. Patients need regular endocrine review during therapy and once therapies have finished, and have a lower threshold for adrenal gland crises, in particular during infection [71–73].

Summary

There is still much to be learned concerning the biology of ACC, in particular the relationship between genetic predisposition and environmental factors. For stage I patients, in the absence of entry into a phase III study, surgery only is recommended. The current COG study recommends retroperitoneal lymph node sampling to assess early metastatic spread which if detected and aggressively resected may reduce further local recurrence. In patients with stage II disease, the COG study recommends extended lymph node dissection, hopefully at the time of initial resection. For stage III and IV disease, eight cycles of chemotherapy, cisplatin-based with 8 months of mitotane concurrently, is recommended. This usually includes etoposide and more recently doxorubicin, the later combination being the chemotherapy in the COG study. Surgery to remove all measurable disease and retroperitoneal lymph nodes is recommended, usually after two to four cycles of chemotherapy.

The optimum treatment is still unclear, and enrolment of patients in the International Paediatric Adrenocortical Tumor Registry which COG has now adopted as a formal phase III study, is recommended if we are to make further progress in the management of this tumor. The emergence of the proposed COG study should encourage international cooperation to discover the optimal therapy for this rare tumor.

Acknowledgments

We would like to acknowledge members of the Children's Cancer and Leukaemia Group (CCLG) Rare Tumor Committee who wrote and contributed to the CCLG guidelines – Murray Yule, Ross Pinkerton, Hamish Wallace, Richard Grundy, Rob Wheeler, Anthony Ng and Julia Chisholm.

References

1 Steliarova-Foucher E. International Classification of Childhood Cancer (3rd Edition [ICCC-3]). 2006.

2 Stiller C. Childhood Cancer in Britain: Incidence, Survival, Mortality. Oxford: Oxford University Press, 2007.

3 Lo YM, Chay LYS, Lo K-W, et al. Quantitative analysis of cell-free Epstein-Barr virus DNA in plasma of patients with nasopharyngeal carcinoma. Cancer Res 1999; 59: 1188–91.

4 Wolf H, zur Hausen H, Becker V. EB viral genomes in epithelial nasopharyngeal carcinoma cells. Nature (NEW), Biol 1973; 244: 245–57.

5 Mertens R, Granzen B, Lassay L, et al. Treatment of nasopharyngeal carcinoma in children and adolescents. Cancer 2005; 104: 1083–9.

6 Greene FL, Page DL, Fleming ID, et al. (Eds). American Joint Committee on Cancer: Manual for Staging Cancer, 6th Edition. New York: Springer-Verlag, 2002.

7 Daoud J, Toumi N, Bouaziz M, et al. Nasopharyngeal carcinoma in childhood and adolescence: analysis of a series of 32 patients treated with combined chemotherapy and radiotherapy. Eur J Cancer 2003; 39: 2349–54.

8 Küpeli S, Varan A, Özyar E, et al. Treatment results of 84 patients with nasopharyngeal carcinoma in childhood. Pediatr Blood Cancer 2006; 46: 454–8.

9 Laskar S, Sanghavi V, Muchaden MA, et al. Nasopharyngeal carcinoma in children: ten years' experience at the Tata Memorial Hospital, Mumbai. Int J Radiat Oncol Biol Phys 2004; 58: 189–95.

10 Al Sarraf M, Le Blanc M, Giri PG, et al. Chemoradiotherapy versus radio-therapy in patients with advanced nasopharyngeal cancer: Phase III randomized Intergroup study 0099. J Clin Oncol 1998; 16: 1310–7.

11 Lo YM, Chan LY, Chan AT, et al. Quantitative and temporal correlation between circulating cell-free Epstein-Barr virus DNA and tumor recurrence in nasopharyngeal carcinoma. Cancer Res 1999; 59: 5452–5.

12 Lin J-C, Wang WY, Chen KY, et al. Quantification of plasma Epstein-Barr virus DNA in patients with advanced nasopharyngeal carcinoma. N Engl J Med 2004; 350: 2461–70.

13 Blutters-Sawatzki R, Grathwohl J, Mertens R, et al. Severe cardiotoxicity of high-dose 5-Fluorouracil in combination with folinic acid, cisplatin and methotrexate in a 14-year-old boy with nasopharyngeal carcinoma (Schminck tumor). Oncology 1995; 52: 291–4.

14 Treuner J, Niethammer D, Dannecker G, et al. Successful treatment of nasopharyngeal carcinoma with interferon. Lancet 1980; 12: 817–8.

15 Mertens R, Karstens JH, Ammon J, et al. Bisherige Erfahrungen der Interferontherapie an 7 Patienten mit NPC. In: Wannenmacher M (Ed.), Nasopharynxtumoren. München: Urban & Schwarzenberg, 1984: 188–93.

16 Rodriguez-Galindo C, Wofford M, Castleberry RP, et al. Preradiation chemotherapy with methotrexate, cisplatin, 5-fluorouracil, and leucovorin for pediatric nasopharyngeal carcinoma. Cancer 2005; 103: 850–7.

17 Spencer H. Pulmonary blastoma. J Pathol Bacteriol 1961; 82: 161–5.

18 Manivel JC, Priest JR, Watterson J, et al. Pleuropulmonary blastoma: the so-called pulmonary blastoma of childhood. Cancer 1988; 62: 1516–26.

19 Priest JR, Watterson J, Strong L, et al. Pleuropulmonary blastoma: a marker for familial disease. J Pediatr 1996; 128: 220–4.

20 Boman F, Hill DA, Williams GM, et al. Familial association of pleuropulmonary blastoma with cystic nephroma and other renal tumors: a report from the International Pleuropulmonary Blastoma Registry. J Pediatr 2006; 149: 850–4.

21 Priest JR, Magnuson J, Williams GM et al. Cerebral metastases and other central nervous system complications of pleuropulmonary blastoma. Pediatr Blood Cancer 2007; 49: 266–73.

22 Priest JR, McDermott MB, Bhatia S, et al. Pleuropulmonary blastoma. A clinicopathologic study of 50 cases. Cancer 1997; 80: 147–61.

23 Wright JR Jr. Pleuropulmonary blastoma. A case report documenting transition from type 1 (cystic) to type III (solid). Cancer 2000; 88: 2853–8.

24 Murphy JJ, Blair GK, Fraser GC. Rhabdomyosarcoma arising within congenital pulmonary cysts: report of three cases. J Pediatr Surg 1992; 27: 1364–7.

25 Indolfi P, Casale F, Carli M, et al. Pleuropulmonary blastoma, management and prognosis of 11 cases. Cancer 2000; 89: 1396–401.

26 Kirsh S, Leuschner I, Int-Veen C, et al. Sixteen children with pleuropulmonary blastoma – results of the German Cooperative Soft Tissue Sarcoma Group. Poster presented at Pan European Sarcoma Trials Meeting, Stuttgart, 2006.

27 Priest JR, Hill DA, Williams GM, et al. Type I pleuropulmonary blastoma: a report from the international pleuropulmonary registry. J Clin Onc 2006; 24: 4492–8.

28 Horie A, Yano Y, Kotoo Y, et al. Morphogenesis of pancreatoblastoma, infantile carcinoma of the pancreas. Cancer 1977; 39: 247–54.

29 Drut R, Jones MC. Congenital pancreatoblastoma in Wiedemann-Beckwith syndrome: an emerging association. Pediatr Pathol 1988; 8: 331–9.

30 Kerr N-J, Fukazawa R, Reeve AE, Sullivan MJ. Wiedemann-Beckwith Syndrome, pancreatoblastoma and the WNT signalling pathway. AMJ Pathol 2002; 60: 154.

31 Abraham SC, Wu T-T, Klimstra DS, et al. Distinctive molecular genetic alterations in sporadic and familial adenomatous polyposis-associated pancreatoblastomas. Frequent alterations in the APC/ß-catenin pathway and chromosome 11p. Am J Pathol 2001; 159: 1619–27.

32 Morohoshi T, Sagawa F, Mitsuya T, et al. Pancreatoblastoma with marked elevation of serum alpha-fetoprotein. Virchows Arch A Pathol Anat 1990; 416: 265–70.

33 Morgan ER, Perryman JH, Reynolds M, et al. Pancreatic blastomatous tumor in a child responding to therapy used in hepatoblastoma: case report and review of the literature. Med Pediatr Oncol 1996; 26: 284–92.

34 Pelizzo G, Consocenti G, Kalache KD, et al. Antenatal manifestation of congenital pancreatoblastoma in a fetus with Beckwith Weidemann syndrome. Prenat Diagn 2003; 23: 292–4.

35 Muguerza R, Rodriguez A, Formigo E, et al. Pancreatoblastoma associated with incomplete Beckwith-Wiedemann syndrome: case report and review of the literature. J Pediatr Surg 2005; 40: 1341–4.

36 Camprodon R, Quintanilla E. Successful long-term results with resection of pancreatic carcinoma in children. Favourable prognosis for an uncommon neoplasm. Surgery 1984; 95: 420–6.

37 Hord JD, Janco RL. Letter to the Editor: Chemotherapy for unresectable pancreatoblastoma. Med Pediatr Oncol 1996; 26: 432–3.

38 Lee AC, Wong AW, Cheng MY, et al. Letter to the Editor: Response to Hord and Janco re chemotherapy for unresectable pancreatoblastoma. Med Pediatr Oncol 1997; 29: 237.

39 Iseki M, Suzuki T, Koizumi Y, et al. Alpha-fetoprotein producing pancreatoblastoma. Cancer 1986; 57: 1833–5.

40 Inomata Y, Nishizowa T, Takasoan H, et al. Pancreatoblastoma resected by delayed primary operation after effective chemotherapy. J Pediatr Surg 1992; 27: 1570–1572.

41 Vannier JP, Flamant F, Hernet J, et al. Pancreatoblastoma: response to chemotherapy. Med Pediatr Oncol 1991; 19: 187–91.

42 Eden OB, Shaw MP. Letter to the Editor: Chemotherapy for Pancreatoblastoma. Med Pediatr Oncol 1992; 20: 357–9.

43 Defachelles AS, de Lassalle EM, Boutard P, Nelken B, Schneider P, Patte C. Pancreatoblastoma in childhood: clinical course and therapeutic management of seven patients. Med Ped Onc 2001: 37: 47–52.

44 Bergstraesser E, Ohnacker H, Stamm B, et al. Pancreatoblastoma in childhood. The role of alpha-fetoprotein. Med Padiatr Oncol 1998; 30: 126–7.

45 Griffin BR, Wisbeck WM, Schaller RT, et al. Radiotherapy for locally recurrent infantile pancreatic carcinoma (pancreatoblastoma). Cancer 1987; 60: 1734–6.

46 Haas JE, Palmer NF, Weinberg AG. Ultrastructure of malignant rhabdoid tumor of the kidney: a distinctive renal tumor of children. Hum Pathol 1981; 12: 646.

47 Gururangan S, Bowman LC, Parham DM, et al. Primary extracranial rhabdoid tumors. Cancer 1993; 71: 2653–9.

48 Hirose M, Yamada T, Toyasaka T, et al. Rhabdoid tumor of the kidney: a report of two cases with respective tumor markers and a specific chromosomal abnormality, del(11p130. Med Pediatr Oncol 1996; 27: 174–8.

49 Brennan BMD, Foot ABM, et al. Where to next with extracranial rhabdoid tumors in children. Eur J Cancer 2004; 40: 624–6.

50 Waldron PE, Rodgers BM, Kelly MD, Womer RB. Successful treatment of a patient with stage IV rhabdoid tumor of the kidney: case report and review. J Pediatr Hematol/Oncol 1999; 21: 53–7.

51 Wagner L, Hill DA, Fuller C, et al. Treatment of metastatic rhabdoid tumor of the kidney, J Pediatr Hematol Oncol 2002; 24: 385–8.

52 D'Angio GJ, Breslow N, Beckwith JB, et al. Treatment of Wilms' tumor. Results of the Third National Wilms' Tumor Study. Cancer 1989; 64: 349–60.

53 Dome JS, Hill DA, McCarville MB. Rhabdoid tumor of the kidney. eMedicine Journal 3, http://www.emedicine.com/ped/topic3012.htm, 2002. Boston Medical Publishing.

54 Vujanic GM, Sandstedt B, Harms D, et al. Rhabdoid tumor of the kidney: a clinicopathological study of 22 patients from the International Society of Paediatric Oncology (SIOP) nephroblastoma file. Histopathology 1996; 28: 333–40.

55 Tomlinson GE, Breslow NE, Dome J, et al. Rhabdoid tumor of the kidney in The National Wilms' Tumor Study: age at diagnosis as a prognostic factor. J Clin Oncol 2005; 23: 7641–5.

56 Kodet R, Newton WA, Jr, Sachs N, et al. Rhabdoid tumors of soft tissues: a clinicopathologic study of 26 cases enrolled on the Intergroup Rhabdomyosarcoma Study. Hum Pathol 1991; 22: 674–84.

57 Stiller CA. International variations in the incidence of childhood carcinomas. Cancer Epidemiol Biomarkers Prev 1984; 3: 305–10.

58 Wiedemann HR. Tumors and hemihypertrophy associated with Wiedemann-Beckwith syndrome. Eur J Pediatr 1983; 141: 129.

59 Hanwi GJ, Serbin RA, Kruger FA. Does adrenocortical hyperplasia result in adrenocortical carcinoma. New Engl J Med 1957; 257: 1153–7.

60 Li FP, Fraumeni JF, Mulvihill JJ, et al. A cancer family syndrome in twenty-four kindreds. Cancer Res 1988; 48: 5358–62.

61 Malkin D, Li FP, Strong LC, et al. Germ line p53 mutations in a familial syndrome of breast cancer, sarcomas, and other neoplasms. Science 1990; 250: 1233–8.

62 Varley JM, McGown G, Thorncroft M, et al. Are there low-penetrance TP53 alleles? Evidence from childhood adrenocortical tumors. Am J Hum Genet 1999; 65: 995–1006.

63 Wagner J, Portwine C, Rabin K, Leclerc J-M, Narod SA, Malkin D. High frequency of germline p53 mutations in childhood adrenocortical cancer. J Natl Cancer Inst 1994; 86: 1707–10.

64 Ribeiro RC, Sandrini F, Figueiredo B, et al. An inherited p53 mutation that contributes in a tissue-specific manner to pediatric adrenal cortical carcinoma. Proc Natl Acad Sci USA 2001; 98: 9330–5.

65 Michalkiewicz E, Sandrini R, Figueiredo B, et al. Clinical and outcome characteristics of children with adrenocortical tumors: a report from the International Pediatric Adrenocortical Tumor Registry. J Clin Oncol 2004; 22: 838–45.

66 Michalkiewicz EL, Sandrini R, Bugg MF, et al. Clinical characteristics of small functioning adrenocortical tumors in children. Med Pediatr Oncol 1997; 28: 175–8.

67 Teinturier C, Paychard MS, Brugieres L, et al. Clinical and prognostic aspects of adrenocortical neoplasms in childhood. Med Ped Onc 1999; 32: 106–11.

68 Sandrini R, Ribeiro RC, DeLacerda L. Extensive personal experience: childhood adrenocortical tumors. J Clin Endo Metab 1997; 82: 2027–31.

69 Wood AA, Woodward G. Severe adrenal cortical atrophy (cytotoxic) and hepatic damage produced in dogs by feeding 2,2-bis (parachlorophenyl)=1,1 dichloroethane (DDD or TDE). Arch Pathol 1949; 48: 387–94.

70 van Slooten HV, Moolenaar AJ, van Seters AP, et al. The treatment of adrenocortical carcinoma with o,p'-DDD: the prognostic implications of serum monitoring. Eur J Clin Oncol 1984; 20: 47–53.

71 Greig F, Oberfield SE, Levine LS, et al. Recovery of adrenal function after treatment of adrenocortical carcinoma with o,p'-DDD. Clin Endocrinol 1984; 20: 389–99.

72 Korth-Schutz S, Levine LS, Roth JA, et al. Virilizing adrenal tumor in a child suppressed with dexamethasone for 3 years. Effect of o,p'-DDD on seruma nd urinary androgens. J Clin Endocrinol Metab 1977; 44: 433–9.

73 Helson L, Wollner M, Murphy ML, et al. Metastatic adrenal cortical carcinoma: biochemical changes accompanying clinical regression. Clin Chem 1971; 17: 1191–3.

74 Hogan TF, Gilchrist KW, Westring DW, et al. A clinical and pathological study of adrenocortical carcinoma. Cancer 1980; 45: 2880–3.

75 Moolenaar AJ, van Slooten H, van Seters AP, et al. Blood levels of o,p'-DDD following administration in various vehicles after a single dose and in long treatment. Cancer Chemother Pharmacol 1981; 7: 51–4.

76 Haak HR, Hermans J, van de Velde CJ, et al. Optimal treatment of adrenocortical carcinoma with mitotane: results in a consecutive series of 96 patients. Br J Cancer 1994; 69: 947–51.

77 van Seters AP, Moolenaar AJ. Mitotane increases the blood level of hormone-binding proteins. Acta Endocrinol 1991; 124: 526–33.

78 van Slooten H, van Oosterom AT. CAP (cyclophosphamide, doxorubicin and cisplatin) regimen in adrenal cortical carcinoma. Cancer Treat Rep 1983; 67: 377–9.

79 Bonacci R, Gigliotti A, Baudin E, et al. Cytotoxic therapy with etoposide and cisplatin in advanced adrenocortical carcinoma. Br J Cancer 1998; 78: 546–9.

80 Ayass M, Gross S, Harper J, et al. High-dose carboplatinum and VP-16 in the treatment of metastatic adrenal carcinoma. Am J Ped Hem Onc 1991; 13: 470–2.

81 Crock PA, Clark AC. Combination chemotherapy for adrenal carcinoma: response in a 51/2 year old male. Med Pediatr Oncol 1989; 17: 62–5.

82 Johnson DH, Greco FA. Treatment of metastatic adrenal cortical carcinoma with cisplatin and etoposide. Cancer 1986; 58: 2198–202.

83 Schlumberger M, Brugiers L, Gicquel C, et al. 5-Fluouracil, doxorubicin and cisplatin for the treatment of adrenal cortical carcinoma. Cancer 1991; 67: 2997–3000.

84 Zancanella P, Pianovski MA, Oliveira BH, et al. Mitotane associated with cisplatin, etoposide, and doxorubicin in advanced childhood adrenocortical carcinoma: mitotane monitoring and tumor regression. J Pediatr Hematol Oncol 2006; 28: 513–24.

85 Squire RA, Bianchi A, Jakate SM. Radiation induced sarcoma of the breast in a female adolescent. Cancer 1988; 60: 2444–7.

IV Supportive Care, Long-Term Issues, and Palliative Care

20 Supportive Care: Physical Consequences of Cancer and its Therapies

Bob Phillips[1] and Roderick Skinner[2]

[1] Leeds Teaching Hospitals Trust, Leeds, UK and [2] Department of Paediatric and Adolescent Oncology, Royal Victoria Infirmary, Newcastle upon Tyne, UK

Introduction

This chapter presents a series of summaries relating to common and important physical problems which arise as a consequence of cancer or its therapies. It covers:

- Oncological emergencies.
- Central venous access devices.
- Symptom control (in relation to pain, gastrointestinal toxicity and nutrition).
- The consequences of marrow suppression.
- Venous thromboembolism.
- Multidisciplinary team working.

Oncological emergencies

Spinal cord compression

This may be defined as external compression of the spinal cord by malignant disease or its complications causing disruption of normal neurological functioning.

How common is it?

Spinal cord compression is a feature of many different malignancies in childhood (see 'What causes it?').

How is it diagnosed?

The symptoms of spinal cord compression vary with the level of the lesion. In almost all cases, pain and/or motor disability are present (see Table 20.1) The differential diagnosis includes vascular accident or transverse myelitis.

A complete neurological examination should be undertaken as indicated by symptoms, to both confirm signs which suggest cord compression and to provide a baseline for evaluating response to therapy. The imaging modality of choice is spinal MRI (Figure 20.1) [3].

Pediatric Hematology and Oncology, 1st edition. Edited by Edward J. Estlin, Richard J. Gilbertson, and Robert F. Wynn. © 2010 Blackwell Publishing Ltd.

What causes it?

Almost all malignant conditions (including leukemia) have been associated with spinal cord compression in children (see Table 20.2).

How should it be managed?

Initial treatment with dexamethasone is used as a holding measure [7]. Definitive treatment may be successfully undertaken with chemotherapy where rapid response is expected (e.g. neuroblastoma, lymphoma/leukemia) and this produces fewer long-term side effects than surgery and/or radiotherapy [1, 6]. For other tumors these modalities remain essential.

What is the outcome?

The neurological outcome of spinal cord compression relates to the severity of impairment rather than the duration between symptoms and diagnosis [1]. Those initially paraplegic may recover full function (estimates from 0% to 66%), but those with less severe symptoms have a greater chance (50%->90%) [1, 2, 5, 6].

Acute biochemical derangements
How common are they, when do they occur and what causes them?

Several acute biochemical derangements may complicate childhood malignancy or its treatment. Although the prevalence of the individual disorders is variable and in some cases poorly documented, collectively they are common. Those most frequently observed in children with malignancy include derangements of phosphate and potassium due to tumor lysis syndrome (TLS), hyper- or hyponatremia, hypercalcemia, and the consequences of acute nephrotoxicity. Numerous other biochemical abnormalities, with a wide variety of causes, may occur less frequently.

Tumor lysis syndrome
What is tumor lysis syndrome?

TLS is the constellation of biochemical and consequent clinical abnormalities due to tumor cell necrosis occurring before or within the first few days after initiation of therapy for malignancies, especially leukemia [8].

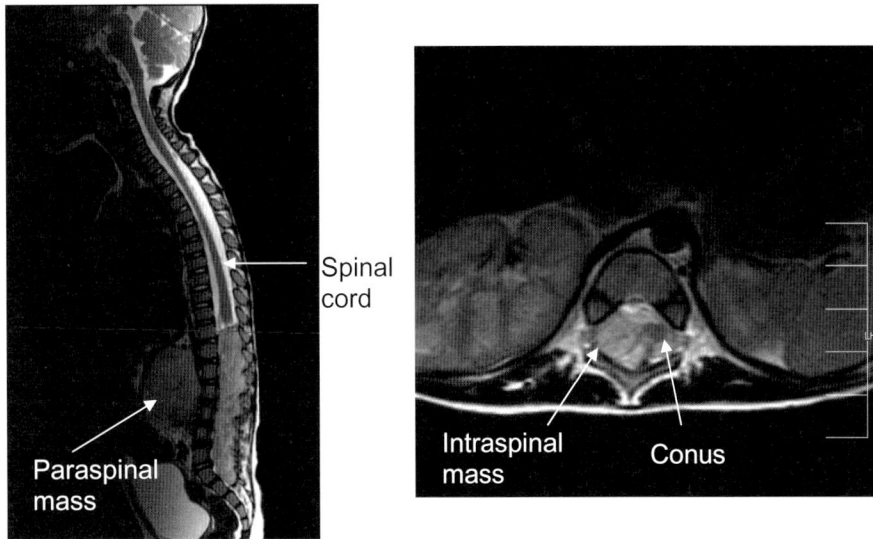

Figure 20.1 Compressed cord on MRI (with thanks to Dr Simon Bailey).

Table 20.1 Frequency of symptoms of spinal cord compression [1, 2].

Symptom	Proportion of patients (%)
Motor dysfunction	>90
Radicular or back pain	55–95
Sensation change	12–56
Sphincter dysfunction	8.5–34
Asymptomatic	2–3

Table 20.2 Frequency of spinal cord dysfunction in childhood malignancies (includes presentation, relapse and progressive disease) [1, 2, 4–6].

Tumour type	Overall % of tumor type with cord compression (%) ($n = 3771$)
Ewing's sarcoma	19
CNS PNET	11
Retinoblastoma	8
Langerhans cell histiocytosis	7
Osteosarcoma	7
Neuroblastoma	6
Soft tissue sarcomas	5
Germ cell tumors	5
Non- Hodgkin lymphoma	2
Hodgkin lymphoma	2
Others	1
Wilms' tumor	1

CNS PNET, central nervous system primitive neuroectodermal tumor.

How common is it and when does it occur?

Most cases of TLS occur in hematological malignancy, especially:

- Burkitt's lymphoma and other 'bulky' non-Hodgkin lymphomas (NHL).
- Acute lymphoblastic leukemia (ALL), especially with bulky organomegaly, large nodal masses, high white counts (>50×10^9/l) or mature B-cell ALL.
- Acute myeloid leukemia (AML), especially if WCC >100×10^9/l).

Biochemical evidence of TLS has been reported in up to ~25% of mixed series of children and adults with acute leukemia and NHL, whilst clinically significant TLS occurs in ~5% [8, 9]. TLS may occur, albeit very rarely, in solid tumors.

Patients with hematological malignancy and a high disease burden (judged by white cell count or disease bulk), and those with a high pre-treatment urate concentration, are at high risk of developing TLS [8, 10].

What causes it?

TLS is due to malignant cell death with rapid release of intracellular contents into the circulation. High risk malignancies are those with a high proliferative rate and sensitivity to chemotherapy [8].

How is it diagnosed?

The characteristic clinical/biochemical findings are:
- Hyperuricemia, leading to renal colic and arthralgia.
- Hyperphosphatemia, resulting in tissue calcium phosphate deposition.
- Hyperkalemia, resulting in muscle weakness, arrythmias, paresthesia.
- Acute renal failure (ARF) due to hyperuricemia and acute nephrocalcinosis, which may cause fluid overload and cardiac failure. Dialysis/hemofiltration may be necessary.
- Hypocalcemia (usually secondary to hyperphosphatemia), leading to paresthesia, tetany, carpopedal spasm, seizures and arrhythmias.

How should it be managed?

Prevention is easier than treatment.

• Intravenous hydration ($3\,l/m^2$/day, without added potassium or alkali) is given for ≥12 hours pre-chemotherapy, along with allopurinol (xanthine oxidase inhibitor) or, in high risk patients, rasburicase (urate oxidase).

• Identification of high-risk patients allows pre-treatment placement of a central venous catheter that will enable hemodialysis/hemofiltration and careful monitoring of biochemistry and renal function.

• Fluid balance should be managed carefully (give frusemide to maintain urine output), and blood pressure monitored and treated if elevated.

• Treat electrolyte abnormalities (eg hyperkalemia) aggressively, and maintain close liaison with nephrologists.

• Hyperuricemia (>0.5 mmol/l) should be treated with rasburicase.

• Dialysis necessary in 2–3% of high-risk patients for renal failure, hyperkalemia or hyperphosphatemia [10, 11].

What is the outcome?

Improvements in identification and management of high-risk patients have reduced the frequency of acute renal failure in TLS greatly. However, once established, TLS is a medical emergency, with high reported risks of ARF (45%) and death (15%) in one retrospective multicenter international study [9].

Other acute biochemical derangements

Hypernatremia

Uncontrolled central diabetes insipidus (CDI) causes polyuria, polydipsia, and a risk of severe hypernatremic dehydration. The causes of CDI in pediatric oncology include:

• Suprasellar/chiasmatic tumors (or complicating their surgical treatment) – responsible for 23–55% of cases of CDI in two longitudinal series from pediatric endocrinology units [12, 13].
  • Craniopharyngioma
  • Pineal tumors
  • Intracranial germinoma
  • More rarely, optic tract (visual pathway) glioma
• Langerhans cell histiocytosis (LCH) – CDI is an uncommon feature of LCH (~1% in recent British Paediatric Surveillance Unit nationwide cohort study [14]), but still accounts for 10–15% of childhood CDI [12, 13].

Hyponatremia

The potential causes include:

• Syndrome of inappropriate antidiuretic hormone secretion (SIADH) – ADH secretion and hence urine osmolality and sodium inappropriately high (urine sodium >50 mmol/l) in relation to low/normal serum osmolality and sodium concentrations, leading to increased water reabsorption with dilutional hyponatremia. SIADH may complicate [15, 16]:
  • Chemotherapy – vincristine, vinblastine, cyclophosphamide, ifosfamide, cisplatin, melphalan

  • Other drugs – e.g. morphine, carbamazepine, thiazide diuretics
  • CNS tumors
  • Rarely Hodgkin disease (HD), NHL
  • Pulmonary infection
• Iatrogenic (overhydration with hypotonic fluids) [17].
• Renal tubular sodium leakage:
  • Chemotherapy – especially platinum drugs (cisplatin, carboplatin) [18, 19]
  • Cerebral salt wasting (especially post-neurosurgery) [20]
• Failure to give stress doses of corticosteroids.

Hypercalcemia

Although hypercalcemia may occur at diagnosis, relapse, or during disease progression, it is reported in only 0.4% of children with malignancy (25 of 3239 children treated at a single centre over 29 years) [21], compared with 5–20% in adults. Hypercalcemia may occur due to reduced renal calcium loss or increased bone resorption, often due to humoral factors (especially PTH-related peptide) [22]. Many childhood malignancies may cause hypercalcemia [21]:

• Acute leukemia – 44% (predominantly ALL), usually at initial presentation, responded well to therapy of malignancy and specific treatment of hypercalcemia.

• Solid tumors – 56% (variety of diagnoses, but rhabdomyosarcoma largest single group), often later in disease course, less responsive.
  • Other reports have noted an association with infantile renal tumors [23]

Nephrotoxicity

Several cytotoxic and anti-infective drugs may cause acute renal toxicity [24]. The acute presentation is usually due to:

• Acute renal (glomerular) impairment, which may be subclinical (revealed only by an elevated serum creatinine concentration), or may lead to clinical manifestations including hypertension, fluid retention, and the consequences of hyperkalemia.

• Reduced renal tubular electrolyte reabsorption, with a number of patterns typical of individual drugs:
  • Platinum drugs (cisplatin, and to much lesser extent carboplatin) – hypomagnesemia (very common), hypocalcemia
  • Ifosfamide – hypophosphatemia (common), renal tubular acidosis, other electrolyte deficiencies, very rarely nephrogenic diabetes insipidus
  • Amphotericin B – hypokalemia (very common, but may be reduced by use of amiloride [25]), hypomagnesemia (common); amphotericin nephrotoxicity is less common and severe with liposomal preparations [26]
  • Aminoglycosides – electrolyte deficiencies, especially hypomagnesaemia (usually after prolonged treatment) [27]
  • Ciclosporin, tacrolimus – hypomagnesemia (common) [28, 29]

How are they diagnosed?

Usually by biochemical monitoring, but sometimes present with characteristic clinical manifestations, e.g.:

• Hypernatremia – anorexia, nausea, weakness, altered mental status, irritability, progressing to stupor, fits, and coma; signs of dehydration and volume depletion may be present if treatment delayed or inadequate.

• Hyponatremia – nausea, lethargy, progressing to confusion, fits, coma.

• Hypokalemia – muscle weakness, cardiac arrhythmias.

• Hyperkalemia – cardiac arrhythymias.

• Hypocalcemia or hypomagnesaemia – tetany, convulsions, cardiac arrhythmias.

• Hypercalcemia – nausea, constipation, abdominal pain, anorexia, irritability, muscle weakness, polyuria leading to dehydration, renal damage (risk of nephrocalcinosis).

• Hypophosphatemia – muscle weakness, rickets.

• Renal tubular acidosis – acidotic breathing.

How should they be managed?

If possible, the underlying cause should be treated or removed. It is seldom justifiable to stop potentially curative chemotherapy, but the regimen may be modified (e.g. dose reduction, substituting cylophosphamide for ifosfamide). Specific treatment strategies include:

• Excessively rapid correction of hyper- and hyponatremia should be avoided since it may cause irreversible neurological damage [30, 31].

• Hypernatremia in CDI [31] should be corrected carefully and slowly (≤12 mmol/l per 24 hours), usually with intravenous (i.v.) 0.45% saline. May need initial resuscitation with i.v. isotonic fluid if hypovolemic at presentation. DDAVP (desmopressin) may be needed acutely, especially in immediate post-neurosurgical CDI [32]. Endocrine input ± intensive care essential.

• SIADH [15] – fluid restriction, with nephrology input ± intensive care if neurological symptoms present; serum sodium concentration should be raised slowly (<2 mmol/l/hour).

• Hypercalcemia [21, 22] – vigorous hydration with intravenous saline, ± frusemide (given with care to avoid hypovolemia), to improve renal calcium clearance. Additional specific strategies may include:

• Bisphosphonates (e.g. pamidronate) – reduce bone resorption and osteoclast activity

• Calcitonin – inhibits bone resorption and renal tubular calcium reabsorption

• Renal tubular electrolyte leakage – regular oral electrolyte supplementation (dose titrated as necessary) usually sufficient for prevention of complications, but intravenous treatment often necessary in acutely ill children.

What is the outcome?

Most acute biochemical derangements can be readily treated, although hypercalcemia may be refractory in the presence of progressive solid tumors. Chemotherapy-induced nephrotoxicity may persist long after treatment withdrawal.

Superior vena cava obstruction
What is it and when does it occur?

Superior vena cava (SVC) syndrome (SVCS) describes the clinical picture due to compression or complete obstruction of the SVC by a mediastinal mass. The term superior mediastinal syndrome (SMS) describes the association of SVCS with tracheal compression.

How common is it?

SVCS is rare, occurring in <1% of newly diagnosed pediatric malignancies [33].

What causes it?

Several pediatric malignancies may present, relapse, or progress with mediastinal masses leading to SVCS (Box 20.1).

Most cases of SVCS presenting at initial diagnosis are due to hematological malignancies, whereas SVCS at disease relapse is often due to solid tumors [33].

In addition, CVAD-associated thrombosis may cause SVCS [34], and disseminated infection (e.g. candidiasis) is a rare cause [33].

How is it diagnosed?

SVCS has a characteristic clinical presentation, often with rapid onset and progression (especially in NHL or T-ALL):

• Ill patient.

• Facial, neck and upper thoracic plethora, edema, cyanosis.

• Distended jugular and collateral chest wall veins.

• Anxious, impaired conscious level (cerebral edema).

• Occasionally – dysphagia, hoarse voice (vocal cord paralysis), Horner's syndrome.

Some features are due to compression of the trachea or main bronchi (SMS):

Box 20.1 The commonest causes of superior cava vena obstruction [33].

Classically anterior superior mediastinal mass

• Non-Hodgkin lymphoma (approximately 30%)

• Acute lymphocytic leukemia (especially T-cell) (25%)

• Hodgkin disease (10–20%)

Posterior mediastinal mass

• Germ cell tumor (teratoma) (<10%)

• Neuroblastoma (<10%)

Sarcoma (<10%) – often middle mediastinal mass (heart, great vessels)

Thymoma (rare) – anterior superior mediastinal mass

• Dyspnea, tachypnea, cough, wheezing, stridor.
• Orthopnea – avoid placing patients in supine position (may precipitate complete tracheal obstruction).

Chest X-ray reveals the mediastinal mass, sometimes with associated pulmonary collapse/consolidation, pleural or pericardial effusion. CT scan reveals the extent of tracheal compression more accurately. Suspected CVAD-associated thrombosis may be demonstrated by echocardiography or Doppler ultrasound.

The effects of SMS in younger children are exacerbated by the relatively smaller tracheal diameter.

How should it be managed?

Ideally, urgent biopsy should be sought to permit tissue diagnosis, but not at the cost of catastrophic respiratory collapse precipitated by general anesthetic (GA) in patients with incipient large airways obstruction. Such patients should be managed in an upright position. Important diagnostic information may be obtained by other means without GA, e.g.:
• Blood count.
• Bone marrow aspirate/biopsy or lymph node biopsy under local anesthetic.
• Pleural aspirate.

Definitive treatment is required urgently. Chemotherapy, guided by the underlying diagnosis, is usually rapidly effective. Occasionally, presumptive treatment (e.g. with steroids) may need to be commenced to reduce the mediastinal mass in the absence of a definite diagnosis. If so, definitive investigations, based on the likely differential diagnosis (e.g. including lumbar puncture for suspected ALL), should be performed as soon as deemed safe, although histology may have been rendered uninterpretable. Radiotherapy is effective, but may cause initial increased respiratory distress due to tumor swelling, and is now seldom employed. Rarely, surgery may be required in less chemo- or radiosensitive malignancies.

Central venous access device (CVAD)-associated thrombosis should be treated by thrombolytic therapy (which may be delivered via the CVAD), which is usually followed by systemic anticoagulation (often with low molecular weight heparin).

Patients with mediastinal masses due to T-cell ALL or NHL are at high risk of TLS, and should be managed accordingly (see above). Although central venous access should ideally be placed before commencing treatment, this is not always feasible. Since these malignancies are usually very chemosensitive, most contemporary treatment protocols incorporate a 'gentler' cytoreductive prephase of prednisolone ± low dose cyclophosphamide for a few days [35] in an effort to reduce the size of the mediastinal mass whilst avoiding significant TLS. This is then followed by full dose combination 'induction' chemotherapy.

What is the outcome?

SVCS/SMS is potentially life threatening, but most of the underlying malignancies have a good prognosis.

Hyperleucocytosis

Hyperleucocytosis is usually defined as the presence of a peripheral white cell count (WCC) >100 × 10⁹/l. This has a risk of potentially fatal clinical sequelae.

How common is it and when does it occur?

Hyperleucocytosis is present in:
• Most children with chronic phase, and nearly all with accelerated phase or blast crisis, chronic myeloid leukemia (CML) [36].
• Up to ~20% children with AML, especially those with infantile AML.
• Up to ~10% children with ALL, especially those with infantile, T-cell or Philadelphia positive ALL [37].

The threshold for developing clinical symptoms is variable: lower in AML (typically >200 × 10⁹/l) due to larger size of myeloblasts, and higher in ALL and CML (typically >300 × 10⁹/l).

What causes it?

The clinical features of hyperleucocytosis are caused by increased blood viscosity, blast cell aggregation and endothelial damage, which promote leucostasis and thrombosis.

How is it diagnosed?

In the presence of hyperleucocytosis (i.e. WCC >100 × 10⁹/l), symptoms/signs of clinically significant sequelae include:
• Central nervous system (CNS) – altered mental status / consciousness, headache, visual disturbance, retinal hemorrhage, cranial nerve palsies.
• Pulmonary – tachypnea, hypoxia, respiratory failure, pulmonary infiltrates on chest X-ray.
• Cardiovascular – congestive cardiac failure.
• Hematological – coagulopathy, bleeding (CNS, pulmonary, mouth, epistaxis, gastrointestinal, uterine).
• Renal – acute renal failure.
Children with hyperleucocytosis are also at high risk of developing TLS.

How should it be managed?

Prevention is preferable to treatment. Therefore, it is important to start anti-leukemic treatment as soon as possible, as well as taking steps to prevent TLS (see Tumor Lysis Syndrome).
• Avoid blood transfusion (which may increase blood viscosity) if at all possible, but;
• Give platelet transfusion to decrease risk of CNS hemorrhage if platelets <20 × 10⁹/l (this will not increase blood viscosity significantly).
• Consider leucopheresis or exchange transfusion in patients with very high WCC (>200 × 10⁹/l), especially in the presence of symptoms/signs of hyperleucocytosis, but the benefit is only temporary.

What is the outcome?

Historically, the reported mortality rate of hyperleucocytosis in children was higher in AML (23%) than in ALL (5%) [38], most

Box 20.2 Seizure key facts.

- Seizures are common in pediatric oncology patients
- Most seizures have a definable cause:
  Drug-related
  Thrombosis or bleed involving the central nervous system
  Metabolic disturbance
  Tumor or infiltration
  Infection
  Hypoxia
- Status epilepticus is a medical emergency and needs rapid, intensive management

Table 20.3 Causes of seizures (data from [48, 50, 51])

Cause	Overall %
Unknown	17
Drugs	14
Leukoencephalopathy	12
Metastasis / infiltration	11
Stroke	11
Metabolic	9
Hypertension	7
Central nervous system infection	7
Multiple causes	4
Systemic sepsis	3
2nd tumor/relapse	3
Venous sinus thrombosis	2
Other defined cause	3

commonly due to CNS hemorrhage or thrombosis, pulmonary leucostasis or the consequences of TLS. Although more recent series describe lower mortality rates of approximately 2% in hyperleucocytosis associated with ALL [39], recent analyses of BFM and Dutch AML trials demonstrate that 2.5–4% of children died within 15 days of starting treatment due to leucostasis or bleeding [40, 41].

Seizures

Seizures are defined by the International League Against Epilepsy (ILE) as the 'manifestation of excessive hypersynchronous, usually self limited, activity of neurones in the brain' [42]. They may have motor, non-motor and dyscognitive elements.

How common are they?

Seizures are a relatively common occurrence in children being treated for malignancy. Around 10% of patients with primary brain tumors may have seizures [43]. In solid tumors, the proportion is about 5% [44, 45] and in acute lymphoblastic leukemia, it is even lower (~2%) (Box 20.2).

How is it diagnosed?

Seizures are diagnosed clinically. *Status epilepticus* is defined as an epileptic seizure (or recurrent seizures without full recovery) lasting longer than 30 minutes [46].

After emergency management, further investigations should include neurological examination, a septic screen, full blood count, electrolytes, calcium, magnesium, and serum glucose estimation [47]. An urgent CT scan should be undertaken and if this reveals no cause, an MRI of the brain may be helpful. One- to two-thirds of patients have been shown to have abnormal brain imaging [48–51].

What causes it?

The general causes of seizures in pediatric oncology patients are listed in Table 20.3.

L-asparaginase produces intracranial thrombosis, vincristine may cause hyponatremia [52] (or act directly [53]), intrathecal and high-dose methotrexate, and ifosfamide cause seizure and encephalopathy [50, 54] and many other medications lower the seizure threshold. Neurosurgery [55] and radiotherapy [56] also produce risks of seizures.

How should it be managed?

Convulsive status epilepticus is a medical emergency, and requires treatment (see Figure 20.2).

Non-convulsive status epilepticus is significantly more difficult to diagnose. It should be treated as convulsive status epilepticus, but with less urgency [47].

What is the outcome?

Most children who do not have a primary brain tumor will only have a single seizure. [49, 57]. It is uncommon for a chronic seizure disorder to develop, and if it does, it is often related to a structural brain abnormality [48, 57]. For those who have a primary brain tumor, a higher proportion develops epilepsy, including late-onset seizures [55, 56, 58].

Hypertension

Hypertension is defined as persistently raised systolic (SBP) or diastolic blood pressure (DBP) (see Box 20.3) [59].

How common is it?

Hypertension as a presenting feature varies according to disease type and may develop during treatment (see 'What causes it?').

How is it diagnosed?

Hypertension should be diagnosed by comparing three separate blood pressure measurements using a validated and calibrated device against age/sex/height normalized values [59].

In cases of severe hypertension, the symptoms of headache and lethargy may be present, developing into visual disturbance,

Airway   Breathing   Circulation

Give high flow oxygen
Measure blood glucose
Confirm epileptic seizure

IMMEDIATE i.v. ACCESS   NO i.v. ACCESS

1. LORAZEPAM   0.1 mg/kg i.v.   1. DIAZEPAM   0.5 mg/kg PR

(give over 30–60 seconds)

Seizure continuing at   i.v. ACCESS   seizure continuing at
10 minutes   10 minutes

2. LORAZEPAM   0.1 mg/kg i.v.   2. PARALDEHYDE   0.4 mg/kg PR
(give over 30–60 seconds)   (give with the same volume of olive oil)

Seizure continuing at 10 minutes   Seizure continuing at 10 minutes

CALL FOR SENIOR HELP

3. PHENYTOIN 18 mg/kg i.v. OVER 20 MINUTES
or
IF ALREADY ON PHENYTOIN GIVE PHENOBARBITONE 20 mg/kg i.v. OVER 10 MINUTES

(Use intraosseous route if still no i.v. access)

AND

PARALDEHYDE 0.4 ml/kg PR + SAME VOLUME OF OLIVE OIL IF NOT
ALREADY GIVEN

AND

CALL ON-CALL ANESTHETIST OR INTENSIVE CARE MEDIC

Seizure continues 20 minutes after commencing step 3

4. RAPID SEQUENCE INDUCTION OF ANESTHESIA USING THIOPENTONE
4 mg/kg i.v.

TRANSFER TO INTENSIVE CARE UNIT

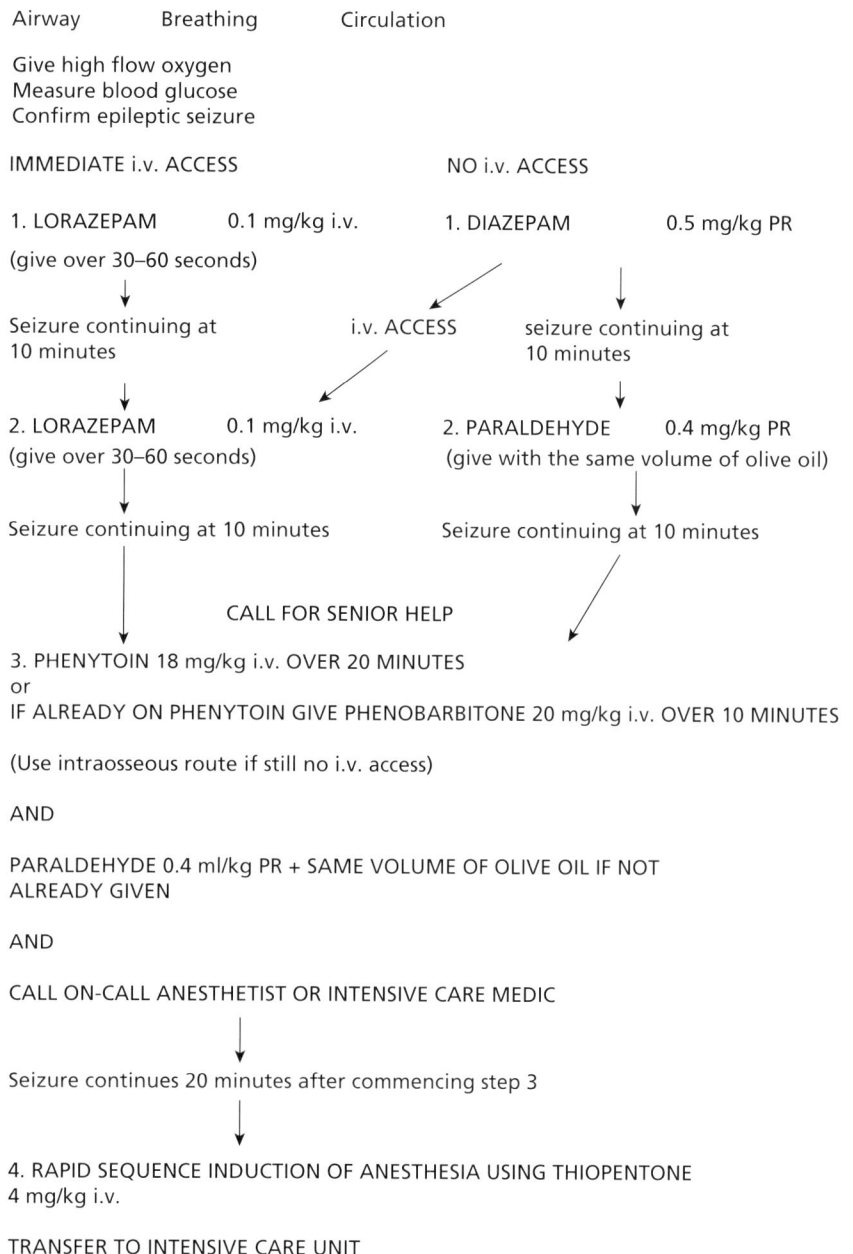

Figure 20.2 Management of convulsive status epilepticus ([46] with permission).

Box 20.3 Hypertension – key facts.

- Hypertension is systolic or diastolic blood pressure >95th percentile for age, sex and height
- Severe hypertension is systolic or diastolic blood pressure >99th percentile + 5 mmHg
- Investigation and treatment should be undertaken urgently in symptomatic or severe hypertension
- Wilm's tumor, neurogenic tumors (e.g. neuroblastoma) and lymphoma/leukemia are frequently associated with hypertension

altered mental status, and finally seizure and coma. Imaging of the renal tract is warranted to rule out immediately remediable causes.

What causes it?
A variety of tumor types have been associated with hypertension at diagnosis (Table 20.4). Treatment may induce hypertension: by pain, medication (e.g. steroids or ciclosporin), renal impairment (e.g. cisplatin-induced), thrombosis or surgical/radiation-induced renal vascular damage. The pathophysiology varies; Wilms' tumor may produce renin [60], leukemia/lymphoma may have renal infiltration [61] and neurogenic tumors produce vasoactive peptides [62].

Table 20.4 Frequency of hypertension at diagnosis of malignancy (data from references [60–63]).

Tumour type	Proportion with hypertension (%)
Phaeochromocytoma	~100
Wilms' tumor	40–55
Neuroblastoma	10–30
Acute lymphoblastic leukemia	~25

How should it be managed?

Symptomatic severe hypertension requires closely monitored intravenous anti-hypertensive treatment. The aim should be to reduce the BP by 25% or less in 8 hours, then to the 95th percentile gently over 48 hours [59]. Hydralazine, labetalol, and sodium nitroprusside may be used.

Anti-hypertensive treatment is recommended for all children with an underlying cause for their hypertension. Investigations with urine and plasma catecholamines and renin levels, abdominal ultrasound, or brain imaging may be appropriate. The general principle of starting at a low dose of antihypertensive and increasing incrementally is widely accepted [59].

What is the outcome?

Severe hypertension in childhood is associated with acute adverse events (such as hypertensive encephalopathy, seizures, cerebrovascular accident and congestive cardiac failure) [59, 61, 64, 65].

There is a strong presumption that hypertension in childhood and young adult life will lead to cardiovascular problems [59] though the evidence is weaker than for adult hypertension. Many survivors of childhood cancer have ongoing problems with hypertension [66].

Raised intracranial pressure

Significantly raised intracranial pressure is defined as cerebrospinal fluid (CSF) pressure >20 mmHg [67].

How common is it?

Raised intracranial pressure (ICP) is a common presenting feature of CNS tumors [43]. About 60% have some features of raised ICP at diagnosis, ranging from 80% in posterior fossa masses to <10% of spinal cord primaries. Raised ICP is an occasionally noted presenting feature of non-CNS tumors [68, 69] (Box 20.4).

How is it diagnosed?

The key clinical features vary with age (see Table 20.5) and may be difficult to detect, except in retrospect. Emergency CT scan is indicated to confirm the diagnosis and identify any remediable cause [71].

What causes it?

Raised ICP is caused by imbalance in CSF production and absorption within the CNS. In primary presentations it is commonly the

---

> **Box 20.4 Raised intracranial pressure – key facts.**
>
> - Raised intracranial pressure presents differently at different ages, but headache (or irritability), vomiting with/without nausea and drowsiness are important early symptoms
> - Central nervous system tumors, medication, infection and bleeding are all potential causes
> - Changes in conscious level denote an emergency situation – urgent stabilization and neurosurgical advice are required

Table 20.5 Signs and symptoms of raised intracranial pressure [43, 70].

Infants	Older children
Irritability	Change in personality
Lethargy/drowsiness	Lethargy/drowsiness
Head banging/holding	Headache (especially 'early morning')
Vomiting	Vomiting +/– nausea
Macrocephaly	
Bulging fontanelle	
Developmental regression	Ataxia (late)
Squint	Diplopia
Papilloedema (late)	Papilloedema (late)

effect of a mass lesion. It is also reported with ATRA [72], ciclosporin [73], hemorrhage [74], and infection [48]. Failure of ventricular shunts is a common cause of raised ICP [70, 75].

How should it be managed?

The management of severe raised ICP requires emergency treatment and neurosurgical input. Treatment should maintain cerebral perfusion pressure, remove any identifiable cause, or divert the flow of CSF. The patient may benefit from dexamethasone (although supportive data are scanty [76]). Intracranial pressure monitoring, sedation, intubation, mild hypercapnea, and osmotic diuretics may be required [77].

Less severe raised ICP can be managed symptomatically with dexamethasone while investigations are underway. Towards the end of life, it may be inappropriate to treat raised ICP [76].

What is the outcome?

In extreme cases, raised ICP leads to seizures, coma and death by tonsillar herniation. In most cases, the outcome relates to the underlying cause.

Septic shock

Septic shock is the extreme end of a continuum of inflammatory responses to an infectious stimulus. 'Sepsis' is the syndrome of infection-induced systemic inflammatory response. 'Severe sepsis' adds organ dysfunction and/or hypoperfusion abnormalities. 'Septic shock' is hypotension unresponsive to 40 ml/kg fluid, with organ dysfunction and/or hypoperfusion [78].

How common is it?
Septic shock is uncommon (severe sepsis requiring intensive care occurs in less than 5% of episodes of febrile neutropenia [79]).

How is it diagnosed?
Sepsis is defined by clinical and laboratory findings (abnormal serum glucose, lactate or acute phase reactants) that demonstrate an inflammatory response to a presumed infectious source [78].

What causes it?
The pathophysiology of the sepsis syndrome is complex. It occurs when the initial inflammatory response to infection becomes amplified, then dysregulated [80]. It includes factors related to the infectious organism and also the host response [81]. The most common infectious organisms in immunocompromised oncology/hematology patients can be summarized as in Table 20.6.

It is notable that Gram positive organisms account for 33–50% of admissions to intensive care units (ICUs), despite the prevailing wisdom that Gram negative bacteremia is the cause of most severe septic episodes.

Table 20.6 Common bacterial causes of sepsis from [79, 82, 83].

Gram positive	Gram negative
Coagulase negative staphylococci	E. Coli
Streptococci	Klebsiella
Staphlycoccus aureus	Enterobacter spp
	Stenotrophomonas

Box 20.5 Septic shock – key facts.

- Sepsis is characterized by significant clinical signs in response to infection:

  Tachycardia

  Tachypnea

  Poor peripheral perfusion

  Altered mental status

  Raised serum lactate

- Severe sepsis is sepsis with hypotension or end-organ dysfunction

- Septic shock is severe sepsis which does not respond to 40 ml/kg fluid

---

How should it be managed?
An international consensus and systematic review produced the 'Surviving Sepsis' guidelines in 2004 [78]. Prompt recognition and treatment of sepsis is emphasized, before progression to severe sepsis. Early resuscitation with fluid, use of inotropes, early mechanical ventilation and consideration of steroids are all important.

A bolus of fluid is 20 ml/kg given over 5–10 minutes, capped at 500–1000 ml. It is uncertain whether saline or albumin is the preferable resuscitation fluid for children [84]. In critically ill adults, 4.5% albumin is no better than 0.9% saline in fluid resuscitation [85]. Fluid refractory shock requires inotropes and intensive care therapy [78].

What is the outcome?
Septic shock remains potentially fatal – up to 50% of patients who are admitted to pediatric ICU with three organ dysfunction die [86]. Severe septic shock outcomes may be improved if we can achieve more rapid recognition and effective treatment of hypotensive, hypovolemic, and hypoxic patients before they decompensate [78].

Pleural and pericardial effusions
Pleural or pericardial effusions result from abnormal accumulation of fluid into the pleural or pericardial sacs, and may be due to local or systemic neoplastic disease, or complications of its treatment. Those effusions due to malignancy itself usually occur at diagnosis or relapse, and may become persistent in the context of progressive disease.

How common are they, and what causes them?
Although pleural effusions are relatively common presentations of malignancy or complications of its treatment in children, pericardial effusions are rarer. There are no published data concerning their overall frequency, but the commoner causes of effusions in children with malignancy include:
- The malignancy itself [87]:
  - Leukemia – pleural (commoner) and/or pericardial effusions may occur in ALL (especially T-cell), and rarely in AML (especially M5) [88, 89]
  - Lymphoma – predominantly pleural effusions, commoner in NHL (especially T-cell) than Hodgkin disease
  - Wide variety of solid tumors, including sarcomas (rhabdomyosarcoma, soft tissue, Ewing, osteosarcoma), neuroblastoma, medulloblastoma (pleural and/or pericardial) [87]
- Treatment:
  - Radiotherapy – pericardial and/or (less commonly) pleural
  - Colony stimulating factors (CSFs) [90] – pericardial and/or (less commonly) pleural
  - Drugs – a few case reports or small case series have described pleural effusions associated with chemotherapy (rare, e.g. cyclophosphamide, methotrexate) [91] or tyrosine kinase inhibitors (e.g. dasatinib) [92]

• Infection – tuberculosis, pneumococcal, aspergillus (pleural and/or pericardial)
• Graft-versus-host disease (GvHD) – pleural and/or pericardial (rare) [93].

How are they diagnosed?

Both pleural and pericardial effusions may present with:
• Dyspnea
• Orthopnea
• Chest pain
• Irritable cough.

Clinical signs, although usually obvious in larger effusions, may be difficult to elicit, especially in younger children, and small effusions may only be detected radiologically (including echocardiography). Large pericardial effusions may lead to cardiac tamponade.

Diagnostic evaluation depends on the clinical context (the cause may be obvious in progressive disease) and includes fluid aspiration and measurement of protein concentration, cell count, microscopy, culture, cytology, and immunophenotyping. Effusions due to malignancy or infection are typically exudates (fluid protein >25 g/l, or >50% of serum protein concentration [94]). A chylous pleural effusion implies obstructed lymphatic drainage.

How should they be managed?

Management of pleural and pericardial effusions includes:
• Treatment of the underlying cause with e.g. cytotoxic or anti-infective treatment, but this may not be feasible for advanced and progressive malignancy.
• Relief of the consequences of the effusion(s) – may not be necessary if rapid and effective treatment of the cause is possible.

Although 'emergency' fluid aspiration may be necessary to relieve severe symptoms or in the presence of cardiac tamponade [90], the rapid institution of effective chemotherapy leads to rapid improvement in most pleural and pericardial effusions occurring at initial presentation of malignancy, and avoids the potential complications of invasive procedures [89]. However, effusions may be persistent or recurrent and cause severe symptoms in progressive disease, and may necessitate repeated aspiration procedures or continuous catheter drainage. Most information about chemical pleurodesis or intrapleural chemotherapy is derived from adult literature [95], but the potential effectiveness of doxycycline or cisplatin in malignant effusions in children has been demonstrated in small series [96, 97]. Rarely, surgical pleurectomy or pericardiectomy may be required.

What is the outcome?

The acute presentation of an effusion is usually amenable to medical or surgical treatment, but the long-term prognosis depends on the underlying cause.

Hemorrhage and bleeding

Acute thrombocytopenic hemorrhage was a common cause of death in leukemic patients prior to the development of effective platelet transfusion support in the early 1960s, accounting for 63% of deaths in one autopsy study [98].

Life-threatening bleeding is now rare in children with malignancy, but high-risk clinical scenarios include:
• Leukemia – at initial presentation, relapse or during progression [99]:
  • Especially acute promyelocytic leukemia (APL, M3 AML), and (to a lesser extent) M5 AML
  • Associated risk factors include hyperleukocytosis, thrombocytopenia and infection
• Severe thrombocytopenia following intensive chemotherapy or hemopoietic stem cell transplantation (HSCT) [100]:
  • Frequently associated with mucosal damage, e.g. mucositis, hemorrhagic cystitis
• Rarer causes of bone marrow failure – e.g. aplastic anemia [101].
• Disseminated intravascular coagulation (DIC), usually complicating newly diagnosed acute leukemia (especially APL) or severe infection [102].
• Invasive solid malignancies – may complicate progressive disease [103].
• Severe invasive infection, especially moulds (e.g. aspergillosis) – uncommon [104, 105].

What causes it?

Severe thrombocytopenia is the commonest underlying factor, but clotting factor deficiency may complicate APL or DIC. Although major vascular invasion by tumor or infection is rare, it is often life-threatening. Many episodes of severe hemorrhage are multifactorial.

How is it diagnosed?

The diagnosis of major hemorrhage is usually clinically obvious:
• Site of overt blood loss, especially gastrointestinal, hemorrhagic cystitis, respiratory.
• Hypovolemic shock.

However, especially in the appropriate clinical context, it is important to maintain a high index of suspicion of more subtle presentations of incipient major bleeding, e.g. unexplained tachycardia and/or hypotension and/or falling hemoglobin.

How should it be managed?

The management of major hemorrhage includes:
• Urgent volume replacement (crystalloid and/or colloid) followed by red cell transfusion [106] – there is no consistent evidence for superiority of colloids over crystalloids in hypovolemic shock [107]
• Optimizing hemostasis:
  • Thrombocytopenia – platelet transfusion(s)
  • Coagulopathy – clotting factor support, especially in DIC and APL [102, 108]

• Identification and management of a bleeding source may occasionally involve [103]:
  • Endoscopy, cystoscopy (with bladder irrigation) – may allow local measures to control bleeding
  • Interventional radiology – may permit embolization
  • Surgery – arterial ligation or resection of bleeding tissue
  • Local or systemic hemostatic agents

In addition, underlying cause(s) should be treated (e.g. the malignancy, infection, or mucosal damage).

Prevention is preferable to treatment, e.g. by H_2-receptor or proton-pump inhibition for upper gastrointestinal protection, or prophylactic platelet transfusions in severe thrombocytopenia (see Thrombocytopenia).

What is the outcome?

In most cases, the outcome depends on the underlying cause(s), and how easily this can be corrected. However, despite modern supportive care, severe hemorrhage may still lead to death (albeit fortunately rarely).

Central venous access devices

What is a central venous access device?

A central venous access device (CVAD) is an indwelling intravascular device used for medium/long-term central venous access. There are two main types of CVAD (Figure 20.3):
• Tunnelled external (usually cuffed) central venous catheter (CVC) – e.g. Hickman line. Single, double or (occasionally) triple lumen versions are used, depending on anticipated intensity of usage,
• Implantable subcutaneous port – e.g. Port-a-cath (single or double lumen).

A cross-sectional audit of UK pediatric oncology centres published in 1997 found that 84% of CVAD insertions were for external CVCs (36% single lumen, 62% double, 2% triple), and 16% subcutaneous ports [109].

Why and when are CVADs used?

CVADs allow blood samples to be taken and intravenous fluids, drugs, blood products and parenteral nutrition to be given without frequent venepuncture thereby reducing pain and distress for the child. They reduce greatly the frequency of potentially devastating extravasation of vesicant chemotherapy (e.g. vincristine, anthracyclines). Therefore, they are inserted at diagnosis, or soon after, in most children receiving chemotherapy.

However, many centres avoid CVAD placement during induction treatment for ALL since it may be associated with an increased risk of venous thrombosis at the site of, or adjacent to, the CVAD (although this is not conclusively proven). Some children receiving protocols that involve no or only infrequent use of vesicant chemotherapy do not require CVADs, e.g. some children during maintenance ALL treatment.

What are the complications of CVADs, and how are these managed?

A large prospective observational study of CVCs inserted in two Italian pediatric oncology centres [110] recorded:
• Complication rate (CR) 2.2 per 1000 CVC days at risk; at least one CVC-related complication occurred in 40% of patients.
• Complications commoner in patients with leukemia or lymphoma.
• Infection (CVC-related bacteraemia, or less commonly tunnel or exit site; most commonly with coagulase negative staphylococci, occasionally other Gram-positive or Gram-negative bacteria, or fungi) – 40% of all complications. Commoner in double-lumen (CR 1.4) than single-lumen (CR 0.5) CVCs ($P < 0.0001$).
• Malfunction (failure to sample blood or allow infusion despite flushing) – 36%.
• Mechanical (malposition, cuff migration, rupture, dislodgement) – 20%.
• Thrombosis (right atrial, deep venous, pulmonary embolism) – 4%.

Although no death was reported in this study, fatal CVAD complications (principally overwhelming sepsis or venous thromboembolism) are well described, if rare.

Infectious and mechanical problems are commoner in external (especially multiple lumen) CVCs than in ports [111, 112].

CVAD-related infection is usually (but not always) manifest by fever temporally associated with accessing the CVAD, without another identified source.
• CVAD-related infection should be investigated with central and (ideally) peripheral cultures followed by appropriate intravenous antibiotics, delivered via the CVAD. *Staphylococcus aureus,*

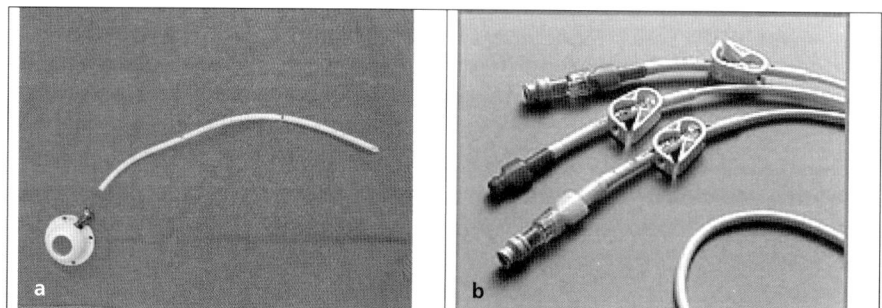

Figure 20.3 (a), Subcutaneous port. (b), Triple-lumen external central venous catheter.

Pseudomonal and Candidal infection are highly unlikely to be cured, and line removal is strongly advised [113].
• Adjuvant treatments such as antibiotic, taurolidine (an antibacterial and antifungal), or urokinase (to disrupt CVAD-related clots and biofilm) locks instilled into the CVAD lumens are used sometimes, but their efficacy is unproven.

CVAD-related thrombosis should be suspected in the presence of poor CVAD function or suspicious clinical signs, investigated and treated promptly (see Venous Thrombosis).

Prevention of complications is preferable to treating them:
• Scrupulous attention should be paid to sterile technique when accessing or flushing CVADs, whilst infections should be suspected and treated vigorously.
• Regular flushing with heparinized saline reduces failure and infection rates. There is no clear evidence of superiority of any one specific method [113].

Symptom care

Pain
Pain can be nociceptive pain (the sensation of tissue injury) or neuropathic pain (arising from the abnormal excitability of damaged nervous tissue) [114].

How common is it?
Pain is a common problem. Estimates of prevalence vary between 33% and 78% (at diagnosis) [43, 115, 116] and 25% to 50% (during treatment) [116, 117].

How is it diagnosed?
Pain is assessed, and reassessed, by asking and observing the patient, supplemented with information from their caregiver. Different tools have been validated for assessing pain in children of different ages [114] (Box 20.6).

What causes it?
The cancer-related causes of pain are varied, and can include infiltration, obstruction, fracture, mucositis, and radiation dermatitis.

How should it be managed?
Pain management begins with a comprehensive assessment of the pain and potential underlying factors (e.g. fracture) [114].

Box 20.6 Pain key facts.

• Pain is a distressing experience, and should be evaluated thoroughly
• Regular assessment and appropriate analgesia, in addition to treatment directed at the primary cause, are essential
• Refractory pain may be amenable to direct intervention with nerve blocks, vertebroplasty or similar procedures

---

Step 4 – Interventional approaches
Step 3 – Parenteral strong opioids
Step 2 – Weak opioids
Step 1 – Non-opioid analgesics

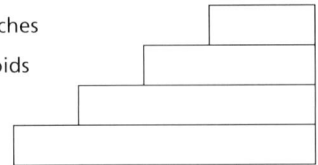

Figure 20.4 Pain ladder.

For painful procedures, prophylaxis is essential, especially in children who undergo multiple procedures (as the pain experience is enhanced by repetition [118]) Topical anesthetics (amethocaine is better than EMLA [119]) and psychological therapies (distraction, hypnosis, and cognitive behavioural therapy) [120] are effective.

Relief of pain should be based on the World Health Organization approach: provided regularly, increasing in intensity as required, oral wherever possible but tailored to the child (e.g. using i.v. opiate in severe mucositis and *not* oral codeine) [114]. Specific analgesic procedures (such as nerve blocks and vertebroplasties) may be required in refractory pain [114]. Psychological adjuncts may help chronic/recurrent pain [121, 122] (see Figure 20.4).

When using non-opioids, the risk of their antipyretic properties needs considering. Non-steroidal anti-inflammatories have risks of bleeding and renal impairment. Neuropathic pain is treated with the addition of anti-depressant (e.g. amitriptiyline [123]) or anti-epileptic (e.g. gabapentin [124]) medications.

What is the outcome?
Most children will achieve significant reductions in pain to minimal or zero levels, with strong collaborations between doctors and nurses being of paramount importance in achieving this aim [117].

Treatment-induced nausea and vomiting
The experience of nausea and act of vomiting are common side effects of treatment.

How common is it and what causes it?
The incidence varies with the type of treatment received (see Tables 20.7 and 20.8) (Box 20.7).

How should it be managed?
Prevention is the aim of treatment (see Table 20.9) If a patient vomits more than twice in 12 hours, or experiences nausea which interferes with normal activity, additional anti-emetics should be considered.

There is a paucity of data from randomized trials in children and teenagers [127, 128]. A new anti-emetic (NK1 receptor antagonist; aprepitant) has been used in adults. It adds significantly to $5HT_3$ antagonist and corticosteroid treatment [126]. In patients who experience anticipatory nausea and vomiting, psychological techniques [129] may be effective. The addition of low-dose benzodiazepine may be beneficial [126].

Table 20.7 Emetogenicity of chemotherapy agents [125, 126]. Risk = chance of vomiting if left untreated.

High risk (>90%)
Cisplatin
Cyclophosphamide >1500 mg/m^2
Carmustine
Dacarbazine
Procarbazine
High dose methotrexate >3 g/m^2

Moderate (30–90%)
Carboplatin
Cytarabine >1 g/m^2
Ifosfamide
Cyclophosphamide <1500 mg/m^2
Doxorubicin
Daunorubicin
Epirubicin
Idarubicin
Irinotecan
Imatinib

Low (10–30%)
Topotecan
Etoposide
Mitoxantrone
Mitomycin
Cytarabine <100 mg/m^2
5-Fluorouracil

Minimal (<10%)
Bleomycin
Busulfan
2-Chlorodeoxyadenosine
Fludarabine
Low dose methotrexate <50 mg/m^2
6-mercaptopurine
Vinblastine
Vincristine
Vinorelbine

Table 20.8 Emetogenicity of radiotherapy regimes [126].

High (>90%)	Total body irradiation
Moderate (60–90%)	Upper abdomen
Low (30–59%)	Cranium (radiosurgery) and craniospinal
Minimal (<30%)	Head and neck, extremities, cranium and breast

What is the outcome?

Nausea and vomiting rarely produce long-term physical problems, but can be psychologically debilitating [129, 130]. In around 90% of patients vomiting can be controlled [127, 128].

Box 20.7 Nausea and vomiting key facts.

- Nausea and vomiting remain the most distressing side effects of treatment for malignant disease
- Nausea and vomiting are manageable side effects in the vast majority of patients undergoing chemotherapy and/or radiotherapy
- Prophylactic antiemetics should be prescribed based on the risk of emesis
- Psychological therapies should be available for the treatment of anticipatory nausea and vomiting

---

Table 20.9 Suggestions for prophylaxis of treatment induced nausea and vomiting.

Risk rank	First line	Second line
High	5HT$_3$ antagonist + corticosteroid *In teenagers add aprepitant*	Add metoclopramide
Moderate	5HT$_3$ antagonist	Add corticosteroid
Low	None	5HT$_3$ antagonist
Minimal	None	Metoclopramide

Box 20.8 Gastrointestinal mucositis key facts.

- Mucositis is a triad of gastro-intestinal tract pain, mucosal ulceration and diarrhoea
- It is one of the commonest complications of the treatment of malignant disease in childhood
- Treatment is symptomatic, addressing pain, hydration/nutrition, and gastrointestinal disturbance
- Severe gastrointestinal mucositis (neutropenic enterocolitis, typhlitis) can be life threatening

---

Gastrointestinal mucositis

Mucositis is a triad of gastro-intestinal pain, mucosal ulceration, and diarrhoea (Box 20.8) [131].

How common is it?

Mucositis occurs in up to 75% of patients (depending on treatment) [131]. Severe mucositis (neutropenic enterocolitis, typhlitis) occurs in 2–3% of patients [132, 133].

How is it diagnosed?

Assessing pain, oral health [131], nutritional status, and diarrhoeal loss is required. Mucositis scales are poorly validated in pediatrics [134]. Neutropenic enterocolitis is characterized by extreme abdominal pain and tenderness, often with fever and ileus. Abdominal ultrasound or CT can help rule out other abdominal pathology (e.g. appendicitis) [133, 135] (Box 20.8).

What causes it?

Mucositis occurs after chemotherapy (especially with doxorubicin, 5-fluorouracil, high-dose methotrexate, etoposide, high-dose alkylating agents) and radiotherapy (head and neck, total body irradiation, and abdominal) [132].

The pathogenesis of mucositis consists of an inflammatory phase (hours) followed by an epithelial phase (days), degrading into an ulcerative phase, followed by healing [136]. The usual cellular, mucosal, and bacterial barriers are disrupted and translocation of bacteria, yeasts, and viruses into the bloodstream occurs [136].

How should it be managed?

The management of mucositis is analgesia and maintenance of hydration/nutrition [131]. No specific treatment prevents or cures mucositis. Maintenance of hydration and nutrition is important, but whether enteral or parenteral nutrition is best is debatable [137, 138]. A Cochrane review is underway [139]. Anti-diarrhoeal agents are infrequently used in children, unlike adults [132], but may be useful [140, 141]. Mucosal superinfections should be treated aggressively; candidiasis with a systemically absorbed antifungal [131] and herpetic gingivostomatitis with aciclovir [131].

Neutropenic enterocolitis is usually successfully managed using a similar approach, reserving operations for the unstable child with evidence of perforation or necrosis [135].

What is the outcome?

Mucositis causes pain, diarrhoea, weight loss and impaired quality of life [131, 137]. It carries the risk of severe infection [142]. Non-operative management of neutropenic enterocolitis is effective, but has a small mortality rate (~5%) [133, 135]. Long-term side effects are rare.

Constipation

Constipation is the delayed or painful passage of hard stools [143]. Plain abdominal X-rays are poor at excluding or confirming constipation [144].

How common is it?

Constipation is extremely common, affecting about half of oncology patients [145].

What causes it?

The etiology is multi-factorial. These factors include gender (women worse [146]), tumor effects, and poor mobility, diet and hydration [145, 147]. Problem medications include opiates, vinca alkaloids, carboplatin, and ondansetron [145, 147].

Box 20.9 Treating constipation.

Start simple:
diet, hydration and comfortable toilet facilities
Add softeners:
lactulose, docusate or Movicol
Add stimulants (to evacuate):
senna, docusate or bisacodyl. Consider picosulphate
Remember Maintenance:
Only slowly reduce laxatives, think about prophylaxis

How should it be managed?

There are no good data on which to base the management of constipation in children and young people with cancer. A suggested approach is detailed in Box 20.9.

What is the outcome?

Constipation causes pain, discomfort, and reduced quality of life [145, 148]. Severe constipation may necessitate a reduction in the intensity of anti-cancer treatment.

Anorexia and malnutrition

Protein energy malnutrition (PEM) is present when protein, carbohydrate and fat (macronutrient) intake is insufficient to meet metabolic requirements.

Cachexia is a state of severe malnutrition with anorexia, weight loss, muscle wasting, anemia and a range of metabolic derangements including hypoalbuminemia, hypoglycemia, lactic acidosis, glucose intolerance, and insulin resistance.

What causes malnutrition in children with malignancy and how common is it?

Reduced oral intake is very common in children with malignancy due to:
• Physical factors, e.g. mucositis, nausea/vomiting, constipation, lethargy, pain.
• Psychological factors, e.g. loss of appetite, impaired taste, psychological dysfunction.
• Social factors, e.g. lack of opportunity ('nil by mouth'), lack of consistency due to repeated hospitalization.

Cachexia is usually multifactorial, due to effects of:
• The malignancy itself (which may be mediated in part by cytokines, e.g. TNFα).
• Treatment (including complications such as febrile neutropenia which may increase metabolic rate).
• Reduced intake (see above).

The prevalence of PEM at diagnosis is low (6–8%) in children with ALL [149], but higher in those with solid tumors [150, 151]. PEM is commoner during treatment [152].

Why is it important?

Effective management of PEM may:

- Restore lost weight.
- Allow cytotoxic treatment to be delivered with fewer delays and complications [152, 153].
- Improve immune response, although it has not been proven that this reduces the risk of infection [152].

How is it evaluated?

Initial evaluation should include assessment of baseline nutritional status, which may itself indicate the need for nutritional supplementation, and identification of those patients whose future treatment will place them at greater risk of developing PEM. Assessment of baseline nutritional status should include:

- Dietary history.
- Anthropometric measurements.
- Biochemical measurements.

Anthropometric assessment includes [152]: weight, height (plotted on centile charts) and (if trained personnel can measure them) mid upper arm circumference and triceps skin- fold thickness.

Ideally, lean body mass should be measured with DEXA (dual-energy X-ray absorptiometry) scanning or bioelectrical impedance, but this is very rarely achieved in clinical practice.

Biochemical evaluation is often based on serum albumin concentration, which is well suited to evaluation of long-term malnutrition (due to its long half-life), but insensitive to acute malnutrition. Hypoalbuminemia may also be caused by reduced hepatic synthesis or increased renal loss. Serum pre-albumin concentration may be preferable for early detection of acute malnutrition due to its much shorter half-life [154].

How and when is nutritional supplementation given?

Nutritional interventions are performed in a stepwise manner, but a lack of clear evidence [155] to guide these steps leads to marked inter-centre variation in practice (Box 20.10) [156].

Immunity and infections

What is immunosupression?

Immunosupression in children with cancer is the result of reduced innate and adaptive immunity. Innate defences are the non-specific barriers to infection (e.g. mucosal integrity, natural killer cells and cytokines). Adaptive immunity is pathogen-specific.

How common is it?

Immunosupression is an almost universal complication of intensive chemotherapy, and a presenting feature of many malignant hematological conditions.

Box 20.10 Nutritional support.

1 General nutritional advice for all

2 When predefined anthropometric criteria are reached (e.g. <90% weight for height, ≥5% weight loss from baseline) or nutritional intake significantly reduced for prolonged period (e.g. <75% of required intake for >1 week) [157] (actual criteria used vary greatly between centres [156]):

- Improve nutritional content of regular intake with high calorie foods
- Add calorie or nutritionally complete supplements (but compliance is often poor)
- Role of specific nutritional supplements (e.g. glutamine) is not well established

3 If further weight loss or intake still poor use enteral nurition:

- nasogastric
- gastrostomy (often inserted by percutanaeous endoscopic method, PEG)
- jejunostomy (rarely used)

4 Parenteral nutrition (PN) – indicated for severe weight loss or if gastrointestinal symptoms prevent effective enteral feeding (e.g. in severe enteritis, post-HSCT). PN may be complicated by CVAD-associated infection, electrolyte imbalance or hepatic dysfunction

---

How is it diagnosed?

The degree of neutropenia is used as an indicator of risk of infection (but monocytopenia is stronger [158]). Lymphopenia also increases the risk of infection [159].

How should it be managed?

Leukopenia may be reduced by the use of colony-stimulating factors. This has no demonstrable effect on mortality, but may reduce the duration of neutropenia, the number of admissions and length of hospitalization [160]. Reducing the risk of infectious complications involves prevention, early recognition, and prompt treatment of complications.

Bacterial infection

Fully implanted CVADs reduce the risk of line infection (see CVAD section) [161]. Prophylactic quinolones probably reduce mortality (relative risk ~ 0.6) [162]. Centerwide use has increased antibiotic resistance but reduced mortality rates [163]. Early recognition and prompt treatment of presumed infection has led to the tremendous decrease in mortality rates in pediatric febrile neutropenia [142]. There is now a move towards risk-stratified therapy with reduced intensity treatment in lower risk groups.

Antibiotic treatment needs to be tailored to local antibiotic resistance patterns. Addition of an aminoglycoside is common although many randomized trials show it only increases harm (nephrotoxicity) [164]. Glycopeptides as first-line therapy are unnecessary [165].

Fungal infection

Invasive fungal infections by both molds and yeasts have a high mortality, morbidity, and cost. Invasive mold infections (e.g. aspergillosis) can present as a persistent fever during profound and prolonged neutropenia, sometimes with chest, sinus, skin, or soft tissue signs. Diagnosis is difficult, with microbiological isolation or histological identification of fungus rare [166]. The European Organisation for Research and Treatment of Cancer (EORTC) criteria categorize episodes as possible, probable, and proven [167].

Prevention with anti-fungals in select populations (e.g. stem cell transplants, relapsed ALL) is effective [168]. Such prophylaxis may be undertaken with oral (e.g. itraconazole) or parenteral (e.g. amphotericin B) agents. High-efficiency particulate air (HEPA) filtration may be useful [169].

Antifungal treatment for patients with persistent neutropenic fever should be commenced [167]. The removal of central venous access should be strongly considered in candidaemia [170]. The choice of therapeutic agents is guided largely by the adult literature [171] with more specific agents being used for yeasts (e.g. fluconazole) than molds (e.g. amphotericin B).

Pneumocystis infection

Pneumocystis jiroveci (previously PCP) pneumonia is rare and classically presents as a severe, acute respiratory infection with fever, tachypnea, hypoxia, and exercise-induced dyspnea [172]. The risk of infection is increased in lymphopenia [173]. Trimethoprim/sulfamethoxazole is effective at reducing the risk with infrequent significant side effects [174]. Alternative agents for prophylaxis include pentamadine, oral dapsone, or atovaquone.

Treatment requires high-dose trimethoprim-sulfamethoxazole (or alternative agent). Using adjuvant corticosteroids has strong evidence of benefit for patients with HIV [175] but little evidence in oncology [173, 176].

Viral infection

A wide range of viral infections cause significant disease. Of particular note are the herpes viruses, some respiratory viruses (influenza, parainfluenza, adenovirus, and respiratory syncytial virus [RSV]), and polyoma viruses.

Prevention of viral diseases can be attempted in particular situations (e.g. aciclovir post-transplant [177]). Immunization may be effective with influenza [178], family vaccination for varicella [179] or passive immunization for disease contacts who are varicella zoster virus (VZV)-seronegative [179].

Treatment of viral disease is sometimes possible (e.g. herpes simplex vires [HSV] and VZV with aciclovir [180], cytomegalovirus (CMV) with ganciclovir [181], influenza with oseltamivir [182]).

What is the outcome?

The overall outcome for febrile neutropenic episodes is good (with appropriate management), with mortality rates of ~1% [79], Invasive fungal infections have 60–80% short-term mortality rates [171]. Candidemia has a lower, but still substantial, mortality rate of ~25% [170]. Estimates of mortality in PCP are approximately 25% [174, 183]. Most viral infections are self limiting but mortality rates following transplant are considerably higher [177, 181].

Anemia

Anemia may be defined broadly as a reduction in the blood hemoglobin (Hb) concentration, or red cell mass, below the age-related normal range. The precise hemoglobin concentration distinguishing anemia from normal is often taken to be two standard deviations below the normal population's mean (see Table 20.10) [184].

How common is it?

Anemia, defined as above, is extremely common both at diagnosis and during treatment in children with malignancy. A large European survey reported that anemia occurred in over 80% of children with cancer, including 97% of those with leukemia [185].

What causes it?

Anaemia in children with malignancy is usually multifactorial. The commonest factor is reduced red cell production, which may be due to:
• Bone marrow infiltration:
  • Leukemia
  • Disseminated solid tumors (e.g. stage 4 neuroblastoma)
• Treatment:
  • Chemotherapy
  • Radiotherapy, especially to red marrow-rich bones (e.g. pelvis, spine, cranium)
  • HSCT (may be prolonged in presence of GvHD)
• Chronic disease.

Table 20.10 Diagnosis of anemia (lower limit of normal blood haemoglobin) (adapted from [184]).

Age (years), sex	Lower limit of normal blood hemoglobin (g/dl)
0.5–4.9	11.0
5.0–7.9	11.5
8.0–11.9	12.0
12.0–17.9 (female)	12.0
12.0–14.9 (male)	12.5
15.0–17.9 (male)	13.0

• Hematinic deficiency (iron, folate), especially in context of increased red cell turnover.
• Red cell aplasia (especially parvovirus B19 infection).
Less commonly, other factors may cause or contribute to anemia:
• Bleeding (including repeated blood sampling, especially in infants).
• Hemolysis:
  • Immune-mediated (e.g. transfusion reaction, mycoplasma infection)
  • Non-immune-mediated (sepsis, DIC)
• Other infections, especially viral (e.g. CMV, EBV)
• Intravenous fluid therapy (dilutional).

How is it diagnosed?
Anemia should be suspected in the presence of typical symptoms/signs, especially:
• Lethargy, weakness, increased need for sleep.
• Dyspnea on exertion (e.g. climbing stairs).
• Headache, irritability, poor school performance.
• Poor feeding/appetite.
• Pallor (skin, conjunctivae).
• Tachycardia.

How should it be managed?
Children and adolescents vary greatly in their ability to tolerate anemia. Although a useful rule of thumb is to consider red cell concentrate transfusion when the hemoglobin falls below approximately 8 g/dl (Box 20.11), the final decision will be influenced by several factors including:
• General condition.
• Presence or absence of symptoms.
• Presence or absence of bleeding.
• Speed of fall in hemoglobin.
• Stage of treatment (which influences likelihood of marrow recovery and hence improvement in hemoglobin without transfusion).
• Underlying diagnosis (e.g. lower hemoglobin threshold of 7 g/dl recommended in aplastic anemia to minimize number of transfusions required).

Box 20.11 The formula recommended in the UK to calculate the volume of red cell concentrate required.

Volume (ml) = (desired Hb [g/dl] − actual Hb) × weight (kg) × 3 [106, 186]

given at 5 ml/kg/h (maximum 150 ml/h) [106]

The transfusion rate should be reduced in patients with severe chronic anemia to reduce the risk of fluid overload and cardiac decompensation

There are several potentially serious risks of transfusion [187]:
• Patient identification errors (wrong unit of blood or wrong patient) – occurs in about 1 in 25 000 units transfused; fortunately serious harm is rare but transfusion of ABO-incompatible blood still causes approximately one death per year (all ages) in the UK.
• Transmission of blood-borne infection has been reduced greatly by modern transfusion techniques, especially viral screening of donors and/or donated products:
  • CMV – although this risk has been reduced (but not eliminated) by leukodepletion (see below), some pediatric oncology and many HSCT units still adopt a precautionary policy of using CMV-negative blood products for all patients (some do so selectively for CMV-negative recipients)
  • Hepatitis B – risk is 1 in 900 000 transfusions
  • Hepatitis C – risk is <1 in 30 million transfusions
  • HIV – risk is <1 in 8 million transfusions
  • Bacterial infection – very rare, but responsible for about one death per year (all ages) in the UK
  • Prion disease (variant Creutzfeld-Jakob disease [vCJD]) – risk not yet quantifiable, but a major potential concern; leukodepletion of all blood products (to $<5 \times 10^6$ leukocytes per unit) was introduced in 1999 in an attempt to combat this risk
• Transfusion-associated graft-versus-host disease – this frequently lethal complication may be prevented by using irradiated blood products in susceptible patients (HSCT patients and donors [to avoid subsequent transmission to patient], immunodeficiency, Hodgkin disease, patients treated with purine analogues, e.g. fludarabine, cladribine [186]), although many units adopt a precautionary policy of using irradiated products in all patients receiving chemotherapy or undergoing treatment for aplastic anemia.

What is the outcome?
The benefits of contemporary blood product transfusion far exceed the risks, but care is still required to evaluate the relative merits or otherwise of transfusion in each individual clinical scenario.

Thrombocytopenia

Thrombocytopenia is defined by a platelet count below the normal range ($150–400 \times 10^9$/l). However, in the absence of other coagulation disturbances or impaired platelet function, severe hemorrhagic complications are rare at platelet counts $>10 \times 10^9$/l [188].

How common is it?
Like anemia, thrombocytopenia is very common at diagnosis or during treatment of malignancy. At diagnosis, approximately 75% of children with ALL [189] or AML [190] have platelet counts $<100 \times 10^9$/l, whilst >90% with severe aplastic anemia

have counts <40 × 10⁹/l [191]. Less commonly, children with disseminated solid tumors (e.g. stage 4 neuroblastoma) are thrombocytopenic at presentation or relapse [192]. The frequency and severity of chemotherapy-induced thrombocytopenia usually mirrors that of anemia and leucopenia, but it may be greater and more protracted with some drugs, e.g. carboplatin, temozolomide.

What causes it?

Thrombocytopenia in children with malignancy is often multifactorial. The commonest factor is reduced megakaryocyte (and hence platelet) production, which may be due to:
• Bone marrow infiltration (leukemia, disseminated solid tumors).
• Treatment (chemotherapy, radiotherapy, HSCT [may be prolonged in presence of GvHD or viral infection]).

Thrombocytopenia may also be due to increased platelet consumption occurring as a result of several disease or treatment-related factors:
• Non-immune-mediated (severe infection, bleeding, DIC, heparin).
• Post-HSCT (thrombotic thrombocytopenic purpura (TTP)/microangiopathy).
• Immune-mediated (uncommon in children with malignancy) – drugs (e.g. heparin, cotrimoxazole); anti-HLA antibodies; anti-platelet antibodies.
Less commonly, other factors may cause or contribute to thrombocytopenia:
• Splenic sequestration.
• Massive blood transfusion (dilutional).

Artefactual thrombocytopenia may occur due to technical problems (e.g. clots in sample).

How is it diagnosed?

Thrombocytopenia is common in oncological practice and should be suspected in the presence of typical symptoms/signs, especially:
• Increased frequency/severity of bruising (often spontaneous).
• Petechiae, purpura.
• Spontaneous bleeding (typically mucosal – oral, nasal, rectal), which may be severe and difficult to control.
• Increased bleeding with minimal trauma.

How should it be managed?

A blood count should be performed to evaluate both the severity (platelet count) and the effect (hemoglobin) of thrombocytopenia. In some circumstances, a clotting profile may be necessary to exclude coagulopathy. Platelet transfusions are provided in two forms [193]:
• Random platelet pool (usually from up to six donors) or single donor apheresis pack – both providing standard adult therapeutic dose (ATD) of >240 × 10⁹ platelets in 150–350 ml.
• Pediatric split unit (single donor) – providing 0.25 ATD (>55 × 10⁹ platelets) in 50–70 ml.

Platelet transfusions may be given for (adapted and extended from [193]):
• Prophylaxis – criteria for transfusion vary with clinical scenarios and between centres, but generally accepted thresholds are:
  • Aplastic anemia (well patient, i.e. no current infection or bleeding) – <5 × 10⁹/l
  • Well patient after conventional chemotherapy – <10 × 10⁹/l
  • Unwell patient after conventional chemotherapy, or brain tumor with residual disease, or in presence of additional coagulopathy – <20 × 10⁹/l
  • Allogeneic HSCT recipients – <20 × 10⁹/l
  • Procedures – to raise platelet count >50 × 10⁹/l (or >100 × 10⁹/l for high risk procedures, e.g. neurosurgery) pre- and for at least 24 hours post-procedure
• Treatment – to raise platelet count >50 × 10⁹/l in presence of active or recent bleeding (or >100 × 10⁹/l in high risk scenarios, e.g. CNS or retinal bleeding).

Dose is age/size-dependent (adapted from [193]):
• Infants – one pediatric split unit or 50 ml of an adult random donor pool or single donor apheresis pack (scale dose down for smaller infants).
• Children >12 months age – 10–15 ml/kg from adult random donor pool or single donor apheresis pack (use whole pool/pack if >20 kg).
• Consider using whole pool/pack if fluid overload is not a concern (this may be a better use of a valuable resource).

Conventionally, platelet transfusion refractoriness is defined as poor platelet increments (measured 1 hour post-transfusion) after at least two ABO-compatible fresh (<72 hours old) transfusions, and should trigger investigation for HLA-alloimmunization, platelet consumption (e.g. DIC, veno-occlusive disease) and consideration of active bleeding or infection. Management may include use of:
• Double dose of fresh platelets.
• HLA-matched platelets.

What is the outcome?

Severe morbidity or mortality due to hemorrhage are now very rare (see Bleeding).

Venous thromboembolism

What is it?

Thrombosis is characterized by the pathological presence of intravascular coagulation, whilst embolism describes vascular obstruction due to dislodgement of a thrombus. Venous thromboembolism (VTE) in children with malignancy occurs in two main clinical scenarios [194]:
• CVAD-associated (occurring in ~1.5% of CVADs) [110] – arising at the CVAD tip or within its lumen.
• Tumor-related (rare) – due to large vein obstruction, e.g. by mediastinal, pelvic or extremity tumors.

Arterial thromboembolism is rare in childhood malignancy, but may occasionally complicate asparaginase treatment [195].

How common is venous thromboembolism and why does it occur?
CVAD-associated VTE is most prevalent in children with ALL, especially during induction therapy [196], occurring in an average of 3–5% of patients (but with a wide range of 1–37% in published studies) [196, 197], as a consequence of [198, 199]:
• Increased thrombin generation due to ALL itself.
• Suppression of endogenous anticoagulants (especially antithrombin) by asparaginase.
• Promotion of factor VIII /von Willebrand factor complexes and increased plasminogen activator inhibitor levels due to steroids.
• Use of CVADs.

Individual studies of the relevance of inherited prothrombotic disorders in the pathogenesis of VTE in ALL have given conflicting findings. However, a large prospective study [200], and a subsequent meta-analysis of five studies [196], suggest a relationship between the presence of at least one prothrombotic factor and the development of VTE, although this risk may itself be modulated by the treatment regimen used (particularly the dose, exact type, and timing of steroid and asparaginase treatments) [196, 201].

How is venous thromboembolism diagnosed?
• CVAD-associated thrombosis may be asymptomatic or may lead to characteristic clinical symptoms and signs (e.g. edema, warmth, collateral circulation, impaired venous return).
• Although several imaging modalities may reveal venous thrombosis at the site of, or adjacent to, a CVAD (e.g. linogram, venogram, Doppler ultrasound, echocardiogram), there is little published evidence to guide the optimum investigation strategy in children.
Major CVAD-related thromboembolic events include CNS venous thrombosis, SVC thrombosis, right atrial thrombosis and pulmonary embolism.

How and when is it treated?
Prevention is preferable to treatment. Most CVADs in children with malignancy are placed in the upper venous system; in this context, the risk of thrombosis may be lower when the device is placed on the right side and in the jugular (rather than subclavian) vein [202]. In ALL, the importance of the timing of CVAD insertion is uncertain, and may be modulated by the type, dose and scheduling of asparaginase and steroid treatment [201]. Many UK centres delay insertion until after induction therapy in an effort to reduce the risk of thrombosis.

The treatment of established CVAD-associated VTE varies greatly between centers. Most centres remove the CVAD unless this is impractical (e.g. if alternative venous access is very difficult), but there is less agreement and little published

pediatric literature about the need for and nature of additional strategies, including systemic anticoagulation (low molecular weight heparin and warfarin have both been used) and less often thrombolysis (often delivered via the CVAD itself) [203].

There is particular uncertainty about the optimum management of asymptomatic CVAD-associated thrombosis, which has been found in nearly 40% of children undergoing elective removal of vascular ports [198, 204].

What is the outcome?
The consequences of CVAD-associated thrombosis include:
• Distress to patient / family due to CVAD malfunction.
• Inconvenience to staff due to CVAD malfunction.
• Requirement to remove (± replace) CVAD.
• Delay or impairment in ability to deliver planned and optimum chemotherapy.
• Risk of:
  • Deep venous thrombosis (may be recurrent)
  • SVC syndrome
  • Pulmonary embolism
  • Post-thrombotic syndrome (pain, swelling, ulceration of affected limb)
  • Death (the average reported case fatality of symptomatic VTE in ALL is 15% [197])

Multidisciplinary team working and supportive care

What is multidisciplinary care?
Multidisciplinary, multiprofessional care is the coordinated provision of care between different professions (e.g. nurses, doctors, psychologists, pharmacists, educationalists, and play therapists) and disciplines (e.g. surgery, hematology, oncology, radiology, and histopathology). It is felt to enhance the delivery of holistic and effective treatment of the child and family who have a malignant disease (205).

How common is it?
Multidisciplinary team (MDT) working is an essential part of principle treatment centers in pediatric oncology and hematology [205]. The composition of MDTs varies with local service provision [206].

How should it be undertaken?
Good MDT working relies on excellent communication of roles and responsibilities to enable each member to provide the service that they are best placed to deliver, with respect to their professional skills and the individual family concerned (Box 20.12 and 20.13). The philosophy of MDT working should be of mutual respect and valuing unique aspects of each team members' contribution to care.

Box 20.12 Example: 'needle phobic' children.

Two different 11-year-old children with profound procedural distress surrounding venupuncture were treated by the same multidisciplinary team in different ways. One child proceeded through a formal programme of psychological support and therapy, remaining distant from medical staff except during periods of venupuncture, and significantly reduced their distress. The child and their family were supported by liaison nursing staff (community-working, hospital-centered) through this time. Another child used a close relationship with a play therapist and restricted, specific members of medical and nursing staff to increase their confidence. Through clear provision of information and choice, a person-centered solution was found.

Box 20.13 Example: growing up in pediatric oncology.

The transition of care from pediatric to adult settings is a challenge. Young people who have been diagnosed with an oncological disease when school age, but relapse later, find this problematic. The provision of skilled nursing support to ensure coordination of information and facilitating negotiations between the adult oncology team and the young adult enhances the quality of the treatment experience.

What is the outcome?

Very few robust pieces of research are found on MDT working, with only one RCT and two small cohort studies examining their effects [205]. It appears that quality of care is improved. Strict adherence to role-separation and team working has prevented the accidental administration of vincristine in the UK, though there is no room for complacency [207].

References

1 De Bernardi B, Pianca C, Pistamiglio P, et al. Neuroblastoma with symptomatic spinal cord compression at diagnosis: treatment and results with 76 cases. J Clin Oncol 2001; 19: 183–90.

2 Pollono D, Tomarchia S, Drut R, et al. Spinal cord compression: a review of 70 pediatric patients. Ped Hematol Oncol 2003; 20: 457–66.

3 Carmody RF, Yang PJ, Seeley GW, et al. Spinal cord compression due to metastatic disease: diagnosis with MR imaging versus myelography. Radiology 1989; 173: 225–9.

4 Bouffet E, Marec-Berard P, Thiesse P, et al. Spinal cord compression by secondary epi- and intradural metastases in childhood. Childs Nerv Syst 1997; 13: 383–7.

5 Jaume Mora NW. Primary epidural non-Hodgkin lymphoma: spinal cord compression syndrome as the initial form of presentation in childhood non-Hodgkin lymphoma. Medical and Pediatric Oncology 1999; 32: 102–5.

6 Plantaz D, Rubie H, Michon J, et al. The treatment of neuroblastoma with intraspinal extension with chemotherapy followed by surgical removal of residual disease. A prospective study of 42 patients – results of the NBL 90 Study of the French Society of Pediatric Oncology. Cancer 1996; 78: 311–9.

7 Loblaw DA, Perry J, Chambers A, Laperriere NJ. Systematic review of the diagnosis and management of malignant extradural spinal cord compression: the Cancer Care Ontario Practice Guidelines Initiative's Neuro-Oncology Disease Site Group. J Clin Oncol 2005 Mar 20; 23: 2028–37.

8 Cairo MS, Bishop M. Tumour lysis syndrome: new therapeutic strategies and classification. Br J Haematol 2004; 127: 3–11.

9 Annemans L, Moeremans K, Lamotte M, et al. Incidence, medical resource utilisation and costs of hyperuricemia and tumor lysis syndrome in patients with acute leukaemia and Non-Hodgkin's lymphoma in four European countries. Leuk Lymphoma 2003; 44: 77–83.

10 Goldman SC, Holcenberg JS, Finklestein JZ, et al. A randomized comparison between rasburicase and allopurinol in children with lymphoma or leukemia at high risk for tumor lysis. Blood 2001; 97: 2998–3003.

11 Jeha S, Kantarjian H, Irwin D, et al. Efficacy and safety of rasburicase, a recombinant urate oxidase (Elitek™), in the management of malignancy-associated hyperuricemia in pediatric and adult patients: final results of a multicenter compassionate use trial. Leukemia 2005; 19: 34–8.

12 Maghnie M, Cosi G, Genevese E, et al. Central diabetes insipidus in children and young adults. New Engl J Med 2000; 343: 998–1007.

13 De Buyst J, Massa G, Christophe C, Tenoutasse S, Heinrichs C. Clinical, hormonal and imaging findings in 27 children with central diabetes insipidus. Eur J Pediatr 2007; 166: 43–9.

14 Salotti J, Nanduri V, Windebank K, et al. Langerhans cell histiocytosis (LCH) in children in the UK and Eire: an epidemiological survey. Pediatr Blood Cancer 2006; 48: 754.

15 Sorensen JB, Andersen MK, Hansen HH. Syndrome of inappropriate secretion of antidiuretic hormone (SIADH) in malignant disease. J Intern Med 1995; 238: 97–110.

16 Kirch C, Gachot B, Germann N, et al. Recurrent ifosfamide-induced hyponatraemia. Eur J Cancer 1997; 33: 2438–9.

17 Duke T, Kinney S, Waters K. Hyponatraemia and seizures in oncology patients asscoiated with hypotonic intravenous fluids. J Paediatr Child Health 2005; 41: 685–6.

18 Kurtzberg J, Dennis VW, Kinney TR. Cisplatinum-induced renal salt wasting. Med Pediatr Oncol 1984; 12: 150–4.

19 Tscherning C, Rubie H, Chancholle A, et al. Recurrent renal salt wasting in a child treated with carboplatin and etoposide. Cancer 1994; 73: 1761–3.

20 Jimenez R, Casado-Flores J, Nieto M, et al. Cerebral salt wasting syndrome in children with acute central nervous system injury. Pediatr Neurol 2006; 35: 261–3.

21 McKay C, Furman WL. Hypercalcemia complicating childhood malignancies. Cancer 1993; 72: 256–60.

22 Esbrit P. Hypercalcemia of malignancy – new insights into an old syndrome. Clin Lab 2001; 47: 67–71.

23 Jayabose S, Iqbal K, Newman L, et al. Hypercalcemia in childhood renal tumors. Cancer 1988; 61: 788–91.

24 Rossi R, Kleta R, Ehrich JHH. Renal involvement in children with malignancies. Pediatr Nephrol 1999; 13: 153–62.

25 Smith SR, Galloway MJ, Reilly JT, Davies JM. Amiloride prevents amphotericin B related hypokalaemia in neutropenic patients. J Clin Pathol 1988; 41: 494–7.

26 Prentice HG, Hann IM, Herbrecht R, et al. A randomized comparison of liposomal versus conventional amphotericin B for the treatment of pyrexia of unknown origin in neutropenic patients. Br J Haematol 1997; 98: 711–8.

27 Akbar A, Rees JHM, Nyamugunduru G, et al. Aminoglycoside-associated hypomagnesaemia in children with cystic fibrosis. Acta Paediatr 1999; 88: 783–5.

28 Barton CH, Varizi ND, Martin DC, Choi S, Alikhani S. Hypomagnesemia and renal magnesium wasting in renal transplant recipients receiving cyclosporine. Am J Med 1987; 83: 693–9.

29 Navaneethan SD, Sankarasubbaiyan S, Gross MD, Jeevanantham V, Monk RD. Tacrolimus-associated hypomagnesemia in renal transplant recipients. Transplant Proc 2006; 38: 1320–2.

30 Reynolds RM, Padfield PL, Seckl JR. Disorders of sodium balance. BMJ 2006; 332: 702–5.

31 Haycock GB. Hypernatraemia: diagnosis and management. Arch Dis Child Ed Pract 2006; 91: ep8–13.

32 Cheetham T, Baylis PH. Diabetes insipidus in children: pathophysiology, diagnosis and management. Paediatr Drugs 2002; 4: 785–96.

33 Ingram L, Rivera G, Shapiro DDN. Superior vena cava syndrome associated with childhood malignancy. Analysis of 24 cases. Med Pediatr Oncol 1990; 18: 476–81.

34 Wilson LD, Detterbeck FC, Yahalom J. Superior vena cava syndrome with malignant causes. New Engl J Med 2007; 356: 1862–9.

35 Reiter A, Schrappe M, Tiemann M, et al. Improved treatment results in childhood B-cell neoplasms with tailored intensification of therapy: a report of the Berlin-Frankfurt-Munster Group Trial NHL-BFM 90. Blood 1999; 94: 3294–306.

36 Rowe JM, Lichtman MA. Hyperleukocytosis and leuokostasis: common features of childhood chronic myelogenous leukemia. Blood 1984; 63: 1230–4.

37 Eguiguren JM, Schell MJ, Crist WM, et al. Complications and outcome in childhood acute lymphoblastic leukemia with hyperleukocytosis. Blood 1992; 79: 871–5.

38 Bunin NJ, Pui CH. Differing complications of hyperleukocytosis in children with acute lymphoblastic or acute nonlymphoblastic leukemia. J Clin Oncol 1985; 3: 1590–5.

39 Lowe EJ, Pui CH, Hancock ML, et al. Early complications in children with acute lymphoblastic leukemia presenting with hyperleukocytosis. Pediatr Blood Cancer 2005; 45: 10–5.

40 Slats AM, Egeler RM, van der Does-van den Berg A, et al. Causes of death – other than progressive leukemia – in childhood acute lymphoblastic (ALL) and myeloid leukemia (AML): the Dutch Childhood Oncology Group experience. Leukemia 2005; 19: 537–44.

41 Creutzig U, Zimmermann M, Reinhardt D, et al. Early deaths and treatment-related mortality in children undergoing therapy for acute myeloid leukemia: analysis of the multicenter clinical trials AML-BFM 93 and Aml-bfm 98. J Clin Oncol 2004; 22: 4384–93.

42 Blume WT, Lüders HO, Mizrahi E, et al. Glossary from A Proposed Diagnostic Schema for People with Epileptic Seizures and with Epilepsy: Report of the ILAE Task Force on Classification and Terminology; 2007 Contract No.: Document Number.

43 Wilne S, Collier J, Kennedy C, et al. Presentation of childhood CNS tumors: a systematic review and meta-analysis. Lancet Oncol 2007; 8: 685–95.

44 Kramer ED, Lewis D, Raney B, Womer R, Packer RJ. Neurologic complications in children with soft tissue and osseous sarcoma. Cancer 1989; 64: 2600–3.

45 Weyl-Ben Arush M, Stein M, et al. Neurologic complications in pediatric solid tumors. Oncology 1995; 52: 89–92.

46 The Status Epilepticus Working Party MotSEWP, Appleton R, Choonara I, Martland T, Phillips B, et al. The treatment of convulsive status epilepticus in children. Arch Dis Child 2000; 83: 415–9.

47 Meierkord H, Boon P, Engelsen B, et al. EFNS guideline on the management of status epilepticus. Eur J Neurol 2006; 13: 445–50.

48 Antunes NL, De Angelis LM. Neurologic consultations in children with systemic cancer. Pediatr Neurol 1999; 20: 121–4.

49 Dufourg MN, Landman-Parker J, Auclerc MF, et al. Age and high-dose methotrexate are associated to clinical acute encephalopathy in FRALLE 93 trial for acute lymphoblastic leukemia in children. Leukemia 2006; 21: 238–47.

50 Kuskonmaz B, Unal S, Gumruk F, Cetin M, Tuncer AM, Gurgey A. The neurologic complications in pediatric acute lymphoblastic leukemia patients excluding leukemic infiltration. Leuk Res 2006; 30: 537–41.

51 Antunes NL. Seizures in children with systemic cancer. Pediatr Neurol 2003; 28: 190–3.

52 Duke T, Kinney S, Waters K. Hyponatraemia and seizures in oncology patients associated with hypotonic intravenous fluids. J Paediatr Child Health 2005; 41: 685–6.

53 Hurwitz RL, Mahoney DH, Jr, Armstrong DL, Browder TM. Reversible encephalopathy and seizures as a result of conventional vincristine administration. Med Pediatr Oncol 1988; 16: 216–9.

54 Pratt CB, Green AA, Horowitz ME, et al. Central nervous system toxicity following the treatment of pediatric patients with ifosfamide/mesna. J Clin Oncol 1986; 4: 1253–61.

55 Khan RB, Boop FA, Onar A, Sanford RA. Seizures in children with low-grade tumors: outcome after tumor resection and risk factors for uncontrolled seizures. J Neurosurg 2006; 104: 377–82.

56 Packer RJ, Gurney JG, Punyko JA, et al. Long-term neurologic and neurosensory sequelae in adult survivors of a childhood brain tumor: childhood cancer survivor study. J Clin Oncol 2003; 21: 3255–61.

57 Maytal J, Grossman R, Yusuf FH, et al. Prognosis and treatment of seizures in children with acute lymphoblastic leukemia. Epilepsia 1995; 36: 831–6.

58 Khan RB, Hunt DL, Boop FA, et al. Seizures in children with primary brain tumors: incidence and long-term outcome. Epilepsy Res 2005; 64: 85–91.

59 National High Blood Pressure Education Program Working Group on High Blood Pressure in Children and A. The Fourth Report on the Diagnosis, Evaluation, and Treatment of High Blood Pressure in Children and Adolescents. Pediatrics 2004; 114: 555–76.

60 Maas MH, Cransberg K, Grotel Mv, Pieters R, Heuvel-Eibrink Mvd. Renin-induced hypertension in Wilms tumor patients. Pediatr Blood Cancer 2007; 48: 500–3.

61 Attard-Montalto SP, Saha V, Ng YY, et al. High incidence of hypertension in children presenting with acute lymphoblastic leukemia. Pediatr Hematol Oncol 1994; 11: 519–25.

62 Sullivan J, Groshong T, Tobias JD. Presenting signs and symptoms of pheochromocytoma in pediatric-aged patients. Clin Pediatr (Phila) 2005; 44: 715–9.

63 Madre C, Orbach D, Baudouin V, et al. Hypertension in childhood cancer: a frequent complication of certain tumor sites. J Pediatr Hematol Oncol 2006; 28: 659–64.

64 Pavlakis SG, Frank Y, Kalina P, Chandra M, Lu D. Occipital-parietal encephalopathy: a new name for an old syndrome. Pediatr Neurol 1997; 16: 145–8.

65 Agarwala B, Mehrotra N, Waldman JD. Congestive heart failure caused by wilms' tumor. Pediatr Cardiol 1997; 18: 43–4.

66 Haddy TB, Mosher RB, Reaman GH. Hypertension and prehypertension in long-term survivors of childhood and adolescent cancer. Pediatr Blood Cancer 2007; 49: 79–83.

67 Adelson PD, Bratton SL, Carney NA, et al. Guidelines for the acute medical management of severe traumatic brain injury in infants, children, and adolescents. Chapter 7. Intracranial pressure monitoring technology. Crit Care Med 2003; 4(3 Suppl): S28–30.

68 Fisher PG, Chiello C. Meningeal leukemia with cerebrospinal fluid block. Med Pediatr Oncol 2000; 34: 281–3.

69 Russell NH, Lewis IJ, Martin J. Acute lymphoblastic leukaemia presenting with raised intracranial pressure. Arch Dis Child 1985; 60: 575–7.

70 Barnes NP, Jones SJ, Hayward RD, Harkness WJ, Thompson D. Ventriculoperitoneal shunt block: what are the best predictive clinical indicators. Arch Dis Child 2002; 87: 198–201.

71 Chu WCW, Lee V, Howard RG, Roebuck DJ, Chik KW, Li CK. Imaging findings of paediatric oncology patients presenting with acute neurological symptoms. Clin Radiol 2003; 58: 589–603.

72 Visani G, Manfroi S, Tosi P, Martinelli G. All-trans-retinoic acid and pseudotumor cerebri. Leuk Lymph 1996; 23: 437–42.

73 Somech R, Doyle J. Pseudotumor cerebri after allogeneic bone marrow transplant associated with cyclosporine a use for graft-versus-host disease prophylaxis. J Pediatr Hematol/Oncol 2007; 29: 66–8.

74 Kyrnetskiy EE, Kun LE, Boop FA, et al. Types, causes, and outcome of intracranial hemorrhage in children with cancer. J Neurosurg 2005; 102(1 Suppl): 31–5.

75 Heinsbergen INA, Rotteveel JAN, Roeleveld NEL, Grotenhuis A. Outcome in shunted hydrocephalic children. Eur J Paediatr Neurol 2002; 6: 99–107.

76 Glaser AW, Buxton N, Walker D. Corticosteroids in the management of central nervous system tumors. Arch Dis Child 1997; 76: 76–8.

77 Guidelines for the acute medical management of severe traumatic brain injury in infants, children, and adolescents. J Trauma 2003; 54(6 Suppl): S235–310.

78 Dellinger RP, Carlet JM, Masur H, et al. Surviving Sepsis Campaign guidelines for management of severe sepsis and septic shock. Crit Care Med 2004; 32: 858–73.

79 Duncan C, Chisholm JC, Freeman S, et al. A prospective study of admissions for febrile neutropenia in secondary paediatric units in South East England. Pediatr Blood Cancer 2007; 49: 678–81.

80 Cohen J. The immunopathogenesis of sepsis. Nature 2002; 420: 885–91.

81 Klein NJ. Mannose-binding lectin: do we need it? Mol Immunol 2005; 42: 919–24.

82 Frakking FN, van de Wetering MD, Brouwer N, et al. The role of mannose-binding lectin (MBL) in paediatric oncology patients with febrile neutropenia. Eur J Cancer 2006; 42: 909–16.

83 Parson S, Tomas K, Wensley D. Outcome and predictors of mortality in paaediatric oncology patients requiring intensive care. J Intensive Care Med 2001; 16: 29–35.

84 The Albumin Reviewers. Human albumin solution for resuscitation and volume expansion in critically ill patients. Cochrane Database of Systematic Reviews: Reviews 2004 Issue 4. Chichester: John Wiley & Sons. DOI: 101002/14651858CD001208pub2. 2004.

85 Investigators SS. Effect of baseline serum albumin concentration on outcome of resuscitation with albumin or saline in patients in intensive care units: analysis of data from the saline versus albumin fluid evaluation (SAFE) study. BMJ 2006; 333: 1044.

86 Hallahan AR, Shaw PJ, Rowell G, O'Connell A, Schell D, Gillis J. Improved outcomes of children with malignancy admitted to a pediatric intensive care unit. Crit Care Med 2000; 28: 3718–21.

87 Wong JW, Pitlik D, Abdul-Karim FW. Cytology of pleural, peritoneal and pericardial fluids in children. Acta Cytol 1997; 41: 467–73.

88 da Costa CML, de Camargo B, Lamelas RGy, et al. Cardiac tamponade complicating hyperleukocytosis in a child with leukemia. Med Pediatr Oncol 1999; 32: 120–3.

89 Arya LS, Narain S, Thavaraj V, Saxena A, Bhargava M. Leukemic pericardial effusion causing cardiac tamponade. Med Pediatr Oncol 2002; 38: 282–4.

90 Medary I, Steinherz LJ, Aronson DC, La Quaglia MP. Cardiac tamponade in the pediatric oncology population: treatment by percutaneous catheter drainage. J Pediatr Surg 1996; 31: 197–200.

91 Morelock SY, Sahn SA. Drugs and the pleura. Chest 1999; 116: 212–21.

92 Quintas-Cardama A, Kantarjian H, O'Brien S, et al. Pleural effusion in patients with chronic myelogenous leukemia treated with dasatinib after imatinib failure. J Clin Oncol 2007; 25: 3908–14.

93 Seber A, Khan SP, Kersey JH. Unexplained effusions: association with allogeneic bone marrow transplantation and acute or chronic graft-versus-host disease. Bone Marrow Transplant 1996; 17: 207–11.

94 Beers SL, Abramo TJ. Pleural effusions. Pediatr Emerg Care 2007; 23: 330–4.

95 Walker-Renard PB, Vaughan LM, Sahn SA. Chemical pleurodesis for malignant pleural effusions. Ann Intern Med 1994; 120: 56–64.

96 Boyer MW, Moertel CL, Priest JR, Woods WG. Use of intracavitary cisplatin for the treatment of childhood solid tumors in the chest or abdominal cavity. J Clin Oncol 1995; 13: 631–6.

97 Hoffer FA, Hancock ML, Hinds PS, Oigbokie N, Rai SN, Rao B. Pleurodesis for effusions in pediatric oncology patients at end of life. Pediatr Radiol 2007; 37: 269–73.

98 Han T, Stutzman L, Cohen E, Kim U. Effect of platelet transfusion on hemorrhage in patients with acute leukemia. An autopsy study. Cancer 1966; 19: 1937–42.

99 Athale UH, Chan AK. Hemorrhagic complications in pediatric hematological malignancies. Semin Thromb Hemost 2007; 33: 408–15.

100 Nevo S, Enger C, Hartley E, et al. Acute bleeding and thrombocytopenia after bone marrow transplantation. Bone Marrow Transplant 2001; 27: 65–72.

101 Chen RL, Lin KH, Chen BW, et al. Long-term observation of pediatric aplastic anemia. J Formos Med Assoc 1992; 91: 390–5.

102 Bick RL. Disseminated intravascular coagulation: a review of etiology, pathophysiology, diagnosis, and management: guidelines for care. Clin Appl Thromb Hemost 2002; 8: 1–31.

103 Pereira J, Phan T. Management of bleeding in patients with advanced cancer. Oncologist 2004; 9: 561–70.

104 Gorelik O, Cohen N, Shpirer I, et al. Fatal haemoptysis induced by invasive pulmonary aspergillosis in patients with acute leukaemia during bone marrow and clinical remission: report of two cases and review of the literature. J Infect 2000; 41: 277–82.

105 Coplin WM, Cochran MS, Levine SR, Crawford SW. Stroke after bone marrow transplantation. Frequency, aetiology and outcome. Brain 2001; 124: 1043–51.

106 McLelland DBL (Ed.). Handbook of Transfusion Medicine. 4th edn. London: The Stationery Office; 2007.

107 Investigators. TSS. A comparison of albumin and saline for fluid resuscitation in the intensive care unit. New Engl J Med 2004; 350: 2247–56.

108 Sanz MA, Tallman MS, Lo-Coco F. Tricks of the trade for the appropriate management of newly diagnosed acute promyelocytic leukemia. Blood 2005; 105: 3019–25.

109 Tweddle DA, Windebank KP, Barrett AM, Leese DC, Gowing R. Central venous catheter use in UKCCSG oncology centres. Arch Dis Child 1997; 77: 58–9.

110 Fratino G, Molinari AC, Parodi S, et al. Central venous catheter-related complications in children with oncological/hematological diseases: an observational study of 418 devices. Ann Oncol 2005; 16: 648–54.

111 La Quaglia MP, Lucas A, Thaler HT, et al. A prospective analysis of vascular access device-related infections in children. J Pediatr Surg 1992; 27: 840–2.

112 Schwarz RE, Groeger JS, Coit DG. Subcutaneously implanted central venous access devices in cancer patients. Cancer 1997; 79: 1635–40.

113 Simon A, Bode U, Beutel K. Diagnosis and treatment of catheter-related infections in paediatric oncology: an update. Clin Microbiol Infect 2006; 12: 606–20.

114 Angheleshu DL, NCCN Pediatric Cancer Pain Panel. Pediatric cancer pain. Memphis: St Jude Children's Reseearch Hospital, 2007. Report No.: v1.2007 Contract No: ocument Number.

115 Miser AW, McCalla J, Dothage JA, Wesley M, Miser JS. Pain as a presenting symptom in children and young adults with newly diagnosed malignancy. Pain 1987; 29: 85–90.

116 Ljungman G, Gordh T, Sorensen S, Kreuger A. Pain variations during cancer treatment in children: a descriptive survey. Pediatr Hematol Oncol 2000; 17: 211–21.

117 Miser AW, Dothage JA, Wesley RA, Miser JS. The prevalence of pain in a pediatric and young adult cancer population. Pain 1987; 29: 73–83.

118 Hockenberry-Eaton M, Barrera P, Brown M, et al. Pain management in children with cancer. Texas: Texas Children's Hospital, 1999 Contract No: Document Number.

119 Lander J, Weltman B, So S. EMLA and Amethocaine for reduction of children's pain associated with needle insertion. Cochrane Database of Systematic Reviews: Reviews 2006 Issue 3. Chichester: John Wiley & Sons. DOI: 01002/14651858CD004236pub2. 2006.

120 Uman L, Chambers C, McGrath P, Kisely S. Psychological interventions for needle-related procedural pain and distress in children and adolescents. Cochrane Database of Systematic Reviews: Reviews 2006 Issue 4. Chichester: John Wiley & Sons.

121 Eccleston C, Yorke L, Morley S, Williams A, Mastroyannopoulou K. Psychological therapies for the management of chronic and recurrent pain in children and adolescents. Cochrane Database of Systematic Reviews: Reviews 2003 Issue 1. Chichester: John Wiley & Sons. DOI: 101002/14651858CD003968.

122 Richardson J, Smith JE, McCall G, Pilkington K. Hypnosis for procedure-related pain and distress in pediatric cancer patients: a systematic review of effectiveness and methodology related to hypnosis interventions. J Pain Symptom Management 2006; 31: 70–84.

123 Saarto T, Wiffen PJ. Antidepressants for neuropathic pain. Cochrane Database Syst Rev 2005; 20: CD005454.

124 Wiffen PJ, McQuay HJ, Edwards JE, Moore RA. Gabapentin for acute and chronic pain. Cochrane Database Syst Rev 2005; 20: CD005452.

125 Hesketh PJ, Kris MG, Grunberg SM, et al. Proposal for classifying the acute emetogenicity of cancer chemotherapy. J Clin Oncol 1997; 15: 103–9.

126 The Antiemetic Subcommittee of the Multinational Association of Supportive Care in Cancer. Prevention of chemotherapy- and radiotherapy-induced emesis: results of the 2004 Perugia International Antiemetic Consensus Conference. Ann Oncol 2006; 17: 20–8.

127 Roila F, Feyer P, Maranzano E, et al. Antiemetics in children receiving chemotherapy. Supp Care Cancer 2005; 13: 129–31.

128 Antonarakis ES, Evans JL, Heard GF, Noonan LM, Pizer BL, Hain RDW. Prophylaxis of acute chemotherapy-induced nausea and vomiting in children with cancer: what is the evidence? Pediatr Blood Cancer 2004; 43: 651–8.

129 Richardson J, Smith JE, McCall G, et al. Hypnosis for nausea and vomiting in cancer chemotherapy: a systematic review of the research evidence. Eur J Cancer Care 2007; 16: 402–12.

130 de Boer-Dennert M, de Wit R, et al. Patient perceptions of the side-effects of chemotherapy: the influence of 5HT3 antagonists. Br J Cancer 1997; 76: 1055–61.

131 Glenny A-M. Mouth Care for Children and Young People with Cancer: Guideline. London: CCLG; 2006 Feb 2006. Report No: 1 Contract No.: Document Number.

132 Keefe DM, Schubert MM. Updated clinical practice guidelines for the prevention and treatment of mucositis. Cancer 2007; 109: 820–31.

133 McCarville MB, Adelman CS, Li C, et al. Typhlitis in childhood cancer. Cancer 2005; 104: 380–7.

134 Tomlinson D, Judd P, Hendershot E, Maloney A-M, Sung L. Measurement of oral mucositis in children: a review of the literature. Support Care Cancer 2007.

135 Schlatter M, Snyder K, Freyer D. Successful nonoperative management of typhlitis in pediatric oncology patients. J Pediatr Surg 2002; 37: 1151–5.

136 Blijlevens NM, Donnelly JP, De Pauw BE. Mucosal barrier injury: biology, pathology, clinical counterparts and consequences of intensive treatment for haematological malignancy: an overview. Bone Marrow Transplant 2000; 25: 1269–78.

137 Schmid I, Schmitt M, Streiter M, et al. Parenteral nutrition is not superior to replacement fluid therapy for the supportive treatment of chemotherapy induced oral mucositis in children. Eur J Cancer 2006; 42: 205–11.

138 Christensen ML, Hancock ML. Parenteral nutrition associated with increased infection rate in children with cancer. Cancer 1993; 72: 2732–8.

139 Jones LV, Davey T, Pizer B, Smyth R. Nutritional support in children with cancer undergoing chemotherapy Cochrane Database of Systematic Reviews: Protocols 2001 Issue 4. Chichester: John Wiley & Sons. DOI: 101002/14651858CD003298. 2001.

140 Vassal G, Couanet D, Stockdale E, et al. Phase II trial of irinotecan in children with relapsed or refractory rhabdomyosarcoma: a joint study of the French Society of Pediatric Oncology and the United Kingdom Children's Cancer Study Group. J Clin Oncol 2007; 25: 356–61.

141 Beckman RA, Siden R, Yanik GA, Levine JE. Continuous octreotide infusion for the treatment of secretory diarrhea caused by acute intestinal graft-versus-host disease in a child. J Pediatr Hematol Oncol 2000; 22: 344–50.

142 Chisholm JC, Dommett R. The evolution towards ambulatory and day-case management of febrile neutropenia. Br J Haematol 2006; 135: 3–16.

143 Benninga M, Candy DC, Catto-Smith AG, et al. The Paris Consensus on Childhood Constipation Terminology (PACCT) Group. J Pediatr Gastroenterol Nutr 2005; 40: 273–5.

144 Reuchlin-Vroklage LM, Bierma-Zeinstra S, Benninga MA, Berger MY. Diagnostic value of abdominal radiography in constipated children: a systematic review. Arch Pediatr Adolesc Med 2005; 159: 671–8.

145 Smith S. Evidence-based management of constipation in the oncology patient. Eur J Oncol Nurs 2001; 5: 18–25.

146 Chitkara DK, Talley NJ, Locke GR, 3rd, et al. Medical presentation of constipation from childhood to early adulthood: a population-based cohort study. Clin Gastroenterol Hepatol 2007; 5: 1059–64.

147 Selwood K. Constipation in paediatric oncology. Eur J Oncol Nursing 2006; 10: 68–70.

148 Voskuijl WP, van der Zaag-Loonen HJ, Ketel IJG, Grootenhuis MA, Derkx BHF, Benninga MA. Health related quality of life in disorders of defecation: the Defecation Disorder List. Arch Dis Child 2004; 89: 1124–7.

149 Reilly JJ, Weir J, McColl JH, Gibson BES. Prevalence of protein-energy malnutrition at diagnosis in children with acute lymphoblastic leukemia. J Pediatr Gastroenterol Nutr 1999; 29: 194–7.

150 Tyc VL, Vallelunga L, Mahoney S, Smith BF, Mulhern RK. Nutritional and treatment-related characteristics of pediatric oncology patients referred or not referred for nutritional support. Med Pediatr Oncol 1995; 25: 379–88.

151 Carter P, Carr D, van Eys J, Coody D. Nutritional parameters in children with cancer. J Am Diet Ass 1983; 82: 616–22.

152 Sala A, Pencharz P, Barr RD. Children, cancer, and nutrition – a dynamic triangle in review. Cancer 2004; 100: 677–87.

153 Mauer AM, Burgess JB, Donaldson SS, et al. Special nutritional needs of children with malignancies: a review. J Parenter Enteral Nutr 1990; 14: 315–24.

154 Elhasid R, Laor A, Lischinsky S, Postovsky S, Arush MWB. Nutritional status of children with solid tumors. Cancer 1999; 86: 119–25.

155 Jones LV, Davey T, Pizer B, Smyth R. Nutritional support in children with cancer undergoing chemotherapy. (Protocol). Cochrane Database of Systematic Reviews. 2001; Issue 4: Art. No.: CD003298. Chichester: John Wiley & Sons. DOI: 10.1002/14651858.CD003298.

156 Ladas EJ, Sacks N, Brophy P, Rogers PC. Standards of nutritional care in pediatric oncology: results from a nationwide survey on the standards of practice in pediatric oncology. A Children's Oncology Group study. Pediatr Blood Cancer 2006; 46: 339–44.

157 Andrassy RJ, Chwals WJ. Nutritional support of the pediatric oncology patient. Nutrition 1998; 14: 124–9.

158 Ammann RA, Hirt A, Luthy AR, Aebi C. Predicting bacteremia in children with fever and chemotherapy-induced neutropenia. Pediatr Infect Dis J 2004; 23: 61–7.

159 Roblot F, Imbert S, Godet C, et al. Risk factors analysis for pneumocystis jiroveci pneumonia (PCP) in patients with haematological malignancies and pneumonia. Scand J Infect Dis 2004; 36: 848–54.

160 Wittman B, Horan J, Lyman GH. Prophylactic colony-stimulating factors in children receiving myelosuppressive chemotherapy: a meta-analysis of randomized controlled trials. Cancer Treat Rev 2006; 32: 289–303.

161 Ingram J, Weitzman S, Greenberg ML, et al. Complications of indwelling venous access lines in the pediatric hematology patient: a prospective comparison of external venous catheters and subcutaneous ports. Am J Pediatr Hematol Oncol 1991; 13: 130–6.

162 Gafter-Gvili A, Fraser A, Paul M, van de Wetering M, Kremer L, Leibovici L. Antibiotic prophylaxis for bacterial infections in afebrile neutropenic patients following chemotherapy. Cochrane Database Syst Rev 2005; 19: CD004386.

163 Reuter S, Kern WV, Sigge A, et al. Impact of fluoroquinolone prophylaxis on reduced infection-related mortality among patients with neutropenia and hematologic malignancies. Clin Infect Dis 2005; 40: 1087–93.

164 Paul M, Soares-Weiser K, Grozinsky S, Leibovici L. Beta-lactam versus beta-lactam-aminoglycoside combination therapy in cancer patients with neutropenia. Cochrane Database of Systematic Reviews: Reviews 2003 Issue 3. Chichester: John Wiley & Sons. DOI: 101002/14651858CD003038. 2003.

165 Vancomycin added to empirical combination antibiotic therapy for fever in granulocytopenic cancer patients. European Organization for Research and Treatment of Cancer (EORTC) International Antimicrobial Therapy Cooperative Group and the National Cancer Institute of Canada-Clinical Trials Group. J Infect Dis 1991; 163: 951–8.

166 Castagnola E, Cesaro S, Giacchino M, et al. Fungal infections in children with cancer: a prospective, multicenter surveillance study. Pediatr Infect Dis J 2006; 25: 634–9.

167 Empiric antifungal therapy in febrile granulocytopenic patients. EORTC International Antimicrobial Therapy Cooperative Group. Am J Med 1989; 86: 668–72.

168 Groll AH, Just-Nuebling G, Kurz M, et al. Fluconazole versus nystatin in the prevention of candida infections in children and adolescents undergoing remission induction or consolidation chemotherapy for cancer. J Antimicrob Chemother 1997; 40: 855–62.

169 Eckmanns T, Ruden H, Gastmeier P. The influence of high-efficiency particulate air filtration on mortality and fungal infection among highly immunosuppressed patients: a systematic review. J Infect Dis 2006; 193: 1408–18.

170 Kibbler CC, Seaton S, Barnes RA, et al. Management and outcome of bloodstream infections due to Candida species in England and Wales. J Hosp Infect 2003; 54: 18–24.

171 Blyth CC, Palasanthiran P, O'Brien TA. Antifungal therapy in children with invasive fungal infections: a systematic review. Pediatrics 2007; 119: 772–84.

172 Pagano L, Fianchi L, Mele L, et al. Pneumocystis carinii pneumonia in patients with malignant haematological diseases: 10 years' experience of infection in GIMEMA centres. Br J Haematol 2002; 117: 379–86.

173 Roblot F, Le Moal G, Godet C, et al. Pneumocystis carinii pneumonia in patients with hematologic malignancies: a descriptive study. J Infect 2003; 47: 19–27.

174 Green H, Paul M, Vidal L, Leibovici L. Prophylaxis for Pneumocystis pneumonia (PCP) in non-HIV immunocompromised patients. Cochrane Database Syst Rev 2007; 18: CD005590.

175 Briel M, Bucher M, Boscacci R, Furrer H. Adjunctive corticosteroids for Pneumocystis jiroveci pneumonia in patients with HIV-infection. Cochrane Database of Systematic Reviews: Reviews 2006 Issue 3. Chichester: John Wiley & Sons. DOI: 101002/14651858CD006150. 2006.

176 Pareja JG, Garland R, Koziel H. Use of adjunctive corticosteroids in severe adult non-HIV Pneumocystis carinii pneumonia. Chest 1998; 113: 1215–24.

177 Selby PJ, Powles RL, Easton D, et al. The prophylactic role of intravenous and long-term oral acyclovir after allogeneic bone marrow transplantation. Br J Cancer 1989; 59: 434–8.

178 Chief Medical Officer. Influenza Immunisation Programme 2007/2008. London: Department of Health, 2007: 10.

179 Health Protection Agency. General Information – Chickenpox (Varicella). London: Department of Health, 2006 [updated 2006; cited 2007 1 October]; http://www.hpa.org.uk/infections/topics_az/chickenpox/gen_info.htm.

180 Balfour HH, Jr, Bean B, Laskin OL, et al. Acyclovir halts progression of herpes zoster in immunocompromised patients. N Engl J Med 1983; 308: 1448–53.

181 Goodrich JM, Mori M, Gleaves CA, et al. Early treatment with ganciclovir to prevent cytomegalovirus disease after allogeneic bone marrow transplantation. N Engl J Med 1991; 325: 1601–7.

182 Flu treatment – Zanamivir (Review), Amantadine and Oseltamivir: Guidance. London: National Insitute of Clinical Excellence, 2003, 23 February. Report No.: 58 Contract No.: Document Number.

183 Poulsen A, Demeny AK, Bang C, Kim P, Nielsen G, Schmiegelow K. Pneumocystis carinii pneumonia during maintenance treatment of childhood acute lymphoblastic leukemia. Med Pediatr Oncol 2001; 37: 20–3.

184 Oski FA, Brugnara C, Nathan DG. A diagnostic approach to the anemic patient. In: Nathan DG, Orkin SH, Ginsburg D, Look AT (Eds), Hematology of Infancy and Childhood, 6th edn. Philadelphia: Saunders, 2003: 409–18.

185 Michon J. Incidence of anemia in pediatric cancer patients in Europe: results of a large, international survey. Med Pediatr Oncol 2002; 39: 448–50.

186 Force. BCfSiHTT. Transfusion guidelines for neonates and older children. Br J Haematol 2004; 124: 433–53.

187 Bolton-Maggs PHB, Murphy MF. Blood transfusion. Arch Dis Child 2004; 89: 4–7.

188 Norfolk DR, Ancliffe PJ, Contreras M, et al. Consensus conference on platelet transfusion, Royal College of Physicians of Edinburgh, 27–28 November 1997. Synopsis of background papers. Br J Haematol 1998; 101: 609–17.

189 Margolin JF, Steuber CP, Poplack DG. Acute lymphoblastic leukemia. In: Pizzo PA, Poplack DG (Eds). Principles and Practice of Pediatric Oncology, 5th edn. Philadelphia: Lippincott Williams & Wilkins, 2006: 538–90.

190 Choi SI, Simone JV. Acute nonlymphocytic leukemia in 171 children. Med Pediatr Oncol 1976; 2: 119–46.

191 Li FP, Alter BP, Nathan DG. The mortality of acquired aplastic anemia in children. Blood 1972; 40: 153–62.

192 Quinn JJ, Altman AJ. The multiple hematologic manifestations of neuroblastoma. Am J Pediatr Hematol Oncol 1979; 1: 201–5.

193 British Committee for Standards in Haematology BTTF. Guidelines for the use of platelet transfusions. Br J Haematol 2003; 122: 10–23.

194 Payne JH, Vora AJ. Thrombosis and acute lymphoblastic leukaemia. Br J Haematol 2007; 138: 430–45.

195 Packer RJ, Rorke LB, Lange BJ, Siegel KR, Evans AE. Cerebrovascular accidents in children with cancer. Pediatrics 1985; 76: 194–201.

196 Caruso V, Iacoviello L, Di Castelnuovo A, et al. Thrombotic complications in childhood acute lymphoblastic leukemia: a meta-analysis of 17 prospective studies comprising 1752 pediatric patients. Blood 2006; 108: 2216–22.

197 Athale UH, Chan AKC. Thrombosis in children with acute lymphoblastic leukemia. Part I. Epidemiology of thrombosis in children with acute lymphoblastic leukemia. Thromb Res 2003; 111: 125–31.

198 Journeycake JM, Buchanan GR. Thrombotic complications of central venous catheters in children. Curr Opin Hematol 2003; 10: 369–74.

199 Athale UH, Chan AKC. Thrombosis in children with acute lymphoblastic leukemia. Part II. Pathogenesis of thrombosis in children with acute lymphoblastic leukemia: effects of the disease and therapy. Thromb Res 2003; 111: 199–212.

200 Nowak-Gottl U, Wermes C, Junker R, et al. Prospective evaluation of the thrombotic risk in children with acute lymphoblastic leukemia carrying the MTHFR TT 677 genotype, the prothrombin G20210A variant, and further prothrombotic risk factors. Blood 1999; 93: 1595–9.

201 Athale UH, Siciliano SA, Crowther M, et al. Thromboembolism in children with acute lymphoblastic leukaemia treated on Dana-Farber Cancer Institute protocols: effect of age and risk stratification of disease. Br J Haematol 2005; 129: 803–10.

202 Male C, Chait P, Andrew M, et al. Central venous line-related thrombosis in children: association with central venous line location and insertion technique. Blood 2003; 101: 4273–8.

203 Skinner R, Koller K, McIntosh N, McCarthy A, Pizer B. Prevention and management of central venous catheter occlusion and thrombosis. Pediatr Blood Cancer: in press.

204 Glaser DW, Medeiros D, Rollins N, Buchanan GR. Catheter-related thrombosis in children with cancer. J Pediatr 2001; 138: 255–9.

205 National Insitute of Clinical Excellence. Improving outcomes guidance for children and young people with cancer. London: NCCC, 2005.

206 Mitchell W, Clarke S, Sloper P. Survey of psychosocial support provided by UK paediatric oncology centres. Arch Dis Child 2005; 90: 796–800.

207 Department of Health. Updated national guidance on the safe administration of intrathecal chemotherapy; 2003, 2 October. Report No.: HSC 2003/010.

21 Psychosocial Needs of Children with Cancer and Their Families

Ged Lalor[1] and Louise Talbot[2]

[1] Department of Paediatric Oncology and Haematology, Royal Manchester Children's Hospital, Manchester, UK and

[2] Paediatric Psychosocial Department, Royal Manchester Children's Hospital, Manchester, UK

Introduction

Since most childhood cancers do not discriminate on grounds of gender, ethnicity, religion, or social class, the psychosocial issues confronting multi-disciplinary (MDT) members during treatment of the child are as diverse as the communities they serve. However, there are a number of issues of psychosocial need that arise frequently at the beginning of treatment while others become more apparent as it progresses.

Practical adjustments

After the initial shock of diagnosis and the start of treatment have been absorbed, most households are confronted by very different financial circumstances (Box 21.1).

Early assessment of financial circumstances is essential; however, the timing and sensitivity of such interventions is crucial and has an enormous influence upon the relationship between the family and MDT members during and after treatment. Good communication within the MDT will enable the social worker to discuss matters such as employment, debt, benefits and additional expenses when the family is ready.

Family competence – strengths and needs

Assessment of the family's ability to cope with the practical, emotional, and psychological aspects of cancer treatment demands an extraordinary range of skills and a commitment to sharing them with colleagues from other disciplines. This will include:
- Family history before diagnosis.
- Parental roles.
- Needs of the siblings.
- Role of extended family members.
- Physical and mental health within the family.

Pediatric Hematology and Oncology, 1st edition. Edited by Edward J. Estlin, Richard J. Gilbertson, and Robert F. Wynn. © 2010 Blackwell Publishing Ltd.

- Peer groups.
- Community support/community pressures.
- Housing.
- Education.
- Employment/finances.

While examination of a family's functioning may never be an exact science, there are studies of patterns of adjustment and adaptation and the extent to which they are subject to stress. When accurate and comprehensive assessments are available to all members of the MDT at an early stage of the treatment journey, the advantages in terms of minimizing such stressors appear unarguable. While elements of unpredictability over an individual's ability to cope with treatment will always be present, assessment information enables physicians, nurses, and other treatment providers to tailor their input to gain maximum benefit. By contrast, when we overlook information that may not be immediately apparent around the time of diagnosis – for example, a history of debt, earlier post-natal depression, or conflict with the extended family – successful clinical outcomes are subject to avoidable risk.

Changing relationships

One way to attempt an exploration of this highly complex process lies in an examination of the effect of a cancer diagnosis upon roles within the family and friendship networks of the patient.
- Side effects of treatment can drastically alter the child or young person's self image and role within the family. This, along with the demands of the treatment regime, has profound implications for the roles of others.
- Two parent households commonly experience a polarization in the roles of parents as one assumes greater responsibility for care of the child with cancer and the other's role as breadwinner is more pronounced.

The number of households headed by single parents and those with step-parents and -siblings has multiplied in many societies in recent decades. This has been accompanied by massive changes to the ethnic, religious, and cultural compositions of those societies. Such demographic changes strengthen the argument for

---

Box 21.1 Financial considerations of families of children with cancer.

- In recent years employment levels in the UK among two parent and single parent families have risen.
- The 'traditional' family of the male breadwinner and female home maker has become less common as patterns of home ownership and consumption have changed.
- The demands of most treatment regimes make it impossible for both parents (or a single parent) to continue in employment.
- Household income frequently declines as expenditure increases due to hospital travel and subsistence costs.

---

sensitive and accurate assessments by health care professionals from the moment of diagnosis.
- The needs of siblings add to the pressure upon parents and can alter their roles and relationships with members of the extended family.
- Adolescent peer relationships, where issues such as self-image, physical appearance, self-confidence or sporting prowess are so important, face inevitable changes.

Much of the work on behavior problems in children with cancer has focused on differences between groups of children with cancer and matched or non-matched controls. Whilst research would suggest that children with cancer do not exhibit higher levels of behavior problems than controls [1], research investigating the parenting practices and beliefs held by parents of children with cancer is still somewhat scarce.

Prevalence

Reported prevalence rates of behavioral problems in children with cancer or brain tumors vary from study to study as a function of the specific behavioral dimensions studied and the measurement tools used.
- Nonetheless, prevalence rates of between 39% [2] and 62% [3] have been reported.
- These figures are considerably higher than those reported in the general population, where the reported prevalence of conduct disorders and oppositional defiant disorders vary between 4 and 14% depending upon the criteria used and population studied [4].

However, even when using a conservative estimate based upon population norms, a significant number of children who have received treatment for a CNS tumor will exhibit behavior problems.

Parental reports

Rearing a child with a chronic illness such as cancer puts extra demands on parenting skills, especially regarding discipline issues [5]. Results of studies which investigated how parental distress affects psychosocial outcome in children who have been treated for cancer, suggest that parents are concerned about the impact of the cancer diagnosis and treatment on their parenting behavior [6].
- In terms of short-term impact of childhood cancer on parenting behavior, parental consistency has been seen to fluctuate over the 6 month initial period of diagnosis and treatment, with consistency increasing over time, and other parenting strategies (i.e. control, nurturance, and responsiveness) remaining stable [6].
- Where research has asked families of children with brain tumors to report the most important problem by phase of illness, the 'availability of help in dealing with my child's personality or moods' was one of the two most frequently endorsed items during the hospital discharge, adjuvant treatment, and recurrence phases of their illness [7].

However, where parenting styles of parents of children with cancer were compared with parents of healthy children, parents of children with cancer rated the item 'I tend to spoil my child' as fairly descriptive of them, whereas the item 'I have strict, well-established rules for my child' they rated as less descriptive of them [8]. This finding also varied as a function of time since diagnosis. Very little research has been conducted which has specifically looked at the impact of childhood cancer on parenting strategies in the long term.

Theoretical rationale

Existing literature on parenting a child with cancer has generally been related to issues of discipline and permissiveness [9]. As reinforced by the literature, parents of children with chronic illness are often depleted of energy, coping skills, and effective parenting techniques due to the fear, distress, anxiety, and crisis that overcomes them [10, 11].
- As a consequence, usual parenting and disciplinary strategies have been reported to be destabilized during treatment for cancer and in the immediate aftermath [12].
- Parents reported difficulties in regaining a balance between applying normal rules, where the risk is to be seen as harsh or unfeeling, and 'spoiling' the child, particularly when family members and friends so often give the child gifts [12].

Research by Van Dongen-Melman, Van Zuuren and Verhulst [13] indicated that parents of children who have had cancer perceive their child as extremely vulnerable. As a result the parents felt the need to restrict the child's daily activities on a physical level, and were concerned about the effects that the illness had had on the child on a psychological level. Also, many tried to compensate for the difficult or distressing events that the child had experienced by trying to protect the child from more potentially unhappy or stressful events and as a consequence, parents were reported to over-indulge the children in a material and psychological respect.

Parents were also thought to reduce the demands and expectations placed upon the child resulting in the subordination of the parent's expectations and happiness, trying not to upset the child unnecessarily and reducing conflicts by reducing demands. Setting limits was reported to be particularly difficult.

Mothers of children with cancer have been found to find it both difficult and time-consuming to manage behavioral problems in their children (e.g. aggressive behavior, crying, and mood change) [14].

Relationship to outcome

Research on the impact of parenting strategies used upon short- and long-term outcome is still in its infancy. However, in the immediate aftermath of diagnosis and during active treatment, parents who reported that their child (aged 2–7 years) was very anxious before medical procedures, set fewer rules and used less consistent, less organized and more permissive discipline practices [15].

• Parents who used vague rather than specific instructions also reported higher levels of child distress during medical procedures [16]; highly permissive parents have been found to experience more difficulties obtaining cooperation with medical procedures [17].

• Parents who were responsive and nurturing had fewer adherence problems with their children [18].

• Adolescents who were found to have difficulties adhering to treatment regimes were also found to have higher levels of depression, lower self-esteem, and higher levels of parent–child incongruence [19].

With regards to longer term outcome, externalizing behaviors reported shortly after diagnosis showed a significant association with externalizing behaviors 2–3 years later [20]. In addition to behavior problems, research has also looked at the relationship between parenting practices and children's' quality of life.

• Parents of children with cancer frequently report heightened perceptions of their child's vulnerability and as a consequence feel over-protective and find it very difficult to allow their child to make age-appropriate developmental transitions.

• Quality of life in children with cancer has been found to be compromised by prevention-focused parenting (focus on avoiding negative outcomes) rather than promotion focused parenting (focus on approaching positive outcomes) [21].

• Parents of children who have been treated for cancer of the central nervous system have reported use of more prevention-focused parenting than parents of children from other cancer groups [22].

A further dimension of parenting that has been found to be affected by the cancer experience is the relationship between the parent and the child with cancer. In a qualitative study by Patterson, Holm and Gurney [23], 40% of the parents in the study reported that they experienced strains in their relationship with their child with cancer. Four sub-themes were identified: concern that the parent was over-protective; uncertainty or conflict with the child over how much independence to allow; and conflict over taking medications. Furthermore, some parents report a lack of positive experiences with their child with cancer [8] which has important implications for all who work with these families.

Existing literature on parent interventions for children with cancer

On the whole, interventions with parents of children with cancer has focused on ameliorating the distress experienced by the parents and improving coping skills, as poor parental coping has been associated with poor outcomes in young patients including anxiety, hopelessness, and externalizing behaviors [24]. A further intervention which has been evaluated is problem-solving training for parents. Mothers of children with cancer who received problem-solving training were able to reduce significantly their emotional distress compared with mothers in a control group [25]. However, to date, no studies have evaluated the use of behavioral parent training in dealing with behavioral issues in children with cancer.

Education

Apprehension and uncertainty about the child's education during and after treatment are characteristic responses to the cancer diagnosis. Teaching staff in mainstream schools rarely have personal or professional experience of childhood cancer; this can leave them open to many of the myths and inaccuracies which are prevalent in the wider community. Specialist social workers and outreach nurses can correct such misconceptions by providing information and practical advice to education professionals when invited to the patient's school. Information and training courses for teachers delivered by health professionals may be more efficient methods of reaching the target audience.

The aim for all children undergoing treatment for cancer is to cause as little disruption as possible to the normal educational routines; however, most treatment regimes lead to lengthy absences from school for a number of reasons; physical side effects, emotional or behavioral reactions, or extended in-patient stays. Local education authorities in the United Kingdom have a legal duty to provide home tuition for children unable to attend their usual schools. Hospital schools with staff skilled in tailoring the demands of a national curriculum to the abilities of all children receiving treatment for cancer are an invaluable resource. The tension between an educational environment characterized by pressure to achieve and a child experiencing demotivation or intellectual impairment presents an enormous challenge.

Family finances

Few families come through childhood cancer treatment financially unscathed. The double blow of increased expenses and diminished income experienced by many (if not most) families is well-documented [26]. Social workers with a good understanding of sickness and disability benefit systems can have an

Table 21.1 Website resources for Australia and New Zealand.

Name of organization	Web address	Features
Challenge	http://www.challenge.org.au	• Non-profit organization established in 1983 to provide children living with cancer and other life-threatening blood disorders with the opportunity to put their illness aside and interact with other children in similar circumstances • Offers services that include camps, family activities, hospital and parent support, art and music therapy, financial support, holiday accommodation and an extensive ticketing program
Childhood Cancer Support	http://ccs.org.au	• Relies on donations and sponsorship • Provides free accommodation, counselling, financial assistance, and recreational activities
Cancer Society Of New Zealand	http://www.cancernz.org.nz/	• Devoted to providing support, education, and funding of cancer research in New Zealand
Children's Cancer Institute Australia	http://www.ccia.org.au/	• Australian research institute devoted to childhood cancer
Childhood Cancer Foundation Canada- Candlelighters	http://www.candlelighters.ca/	• National support and information network enhancing the quality of life of children with cancer

Table 21.2 Website resources for Africa.

Name of organization	Web address	Features
South African Myeloma Foundation	http://www.geocities.com/HotSprings/5137/	• Research into myeloma
CHOC Childhood Cancer Foundation	http://www.chocpmb.org.za/	• Voluntary group • Brings parents of sufferers together

Table 21.3 Website resources for Asia.

Name of organization	Web address	Features
Children's Cancer Foundation	http://www.ccf.org.hk	• Supplement services provided by the Hospital authority • Enhance children's quality of life
Children's Cancer Foundation: Singapore	http://www.ccf.org.sg	• Improve children's quality of life • Promoting awareness • Providing counselling etc.

enormous impact upon the daily lives of families of a child with cancer.

The benefits systems in many countries are unwieldy and vary in their generosity. The United Kingdom has a number of non-governmental grant-making bodies able to respond quickly to requests on behalf of families experiencing financial hardship [27].

Support and information sources: international resources for families and health professionals

Information and support for children, families and health professionals is becoming ever important in clinical practice. Some selected examples of the range of website-based resources in relation to children with cancer are described in Tables 21.1–21.8.

Summary

The social and psychological care of children with cancer is an important, but as yet relatively under-researched, area of practice in the clinical setting. Studies that integrate the principles of health sciences such a sociology, psychology, informatics and economics will require a unique collaboration between patients, families, and health professionals and would be a major challenge to design, fund, and conduct with national and international outcomes in mind.

Acknowledgements

Thanks are given to Miss Rachel Estlin for her help in researching the various website addresses and functionalities that are described in this chapter.

Table 21.4 Website resources for Europe (non-UK) – patients and families.

Name of organization	Web address	Features
Barretstown Gang Camp	http://www.barretstowngc.ie/	• Specially designed camp for children with serious illnesses – primarily cancer and serious blood diseases – from Ireland, Britain and throughout Europe, and their families
International Society of Paediatric Oncology (SIOP)	http://www.siop.nl/	• Annual scientific meeting meeting on all aspects of pediatric oncology • Also sponsors regional/continental meetings to promote the exchange of information and good practice in pediatric oncology
Innovative Therapies For Childhood Cancer	http://www.itcc-consortium.org/	• It is an academic European Consortium, comprising a pre-clinical network of nine research laboratories specializing in pediatric tumor biology and pharmacology, and a clinical network of 34 pediatric oncology centres, with specific expertise in early drug development and clinical trials • ITCC runs clinical and translational research connecting new drugs, biology and the unmet needs of children with cancer
International Union Against Cancer (UICC)	http://www.uicc.org	• World Cancer Day • Raise awareness
Childhood Cancer Foundation Of Sweden	http://www.barncancerfonden.se	• Raising funds
Cancer Society Of Finland	http://www.cancer.fi/	• National Public Health Organization
Danish Cancer Society	http://www.cancer.dk	• Research • Patient support • Prevention
Gesellschaft fur Padiatrische Onkologie und Hamatologie (GPOH)	http://www.kinderkrebsinfo.de/	• Running clinical trials
Netherlands Cancer Institute	http://www.nki.nl/	• Research and services
Neuroblastoma Infantil	http://www.neuroblastomainfantil.info/	• Childhood neuroblastoma information for parents and public
Dutch Childhood Cancer Parent Organisation (VOKK)	http://www.vokk.nl	• National organization of parents of children of cancer • Support of parents and families • Information • Advocacy
Swiss Cancer League	http://www.swisscancer.ch	• Research and fundraising

Table 21.5 European website resources for health professionals (non-UK).

Name of organization	Web address	Features
International Society of Paediatric Oncology (SIOP)	http://www.siop.nl/	• Annual scientific meeting meeting on all aspects of pediatric oncology • Also sponsors regional/continental meetings to promote the exchange of information and good practice in pediatric oncology
Innovative Therapies For Childhood Cancer	http://www.itcc-consortium.org/	• It is an academic European Consortium, comprising a pre-clinical network of nine research laboratories specializing in pediatric tumor biology and pharmacology, and a clinical network of 34 pediatric oncology centres, with specific expertise in early drug development and clinical trials. • ITCC runs clinical and translational research connecting new drugs, biology and the unmet needs of children with cancer.
Gesellschaft fur Padiatrische Onkologie und Hamatologie (GPOH)	http://www.kinderkrebsinfo.de/	• Running clinical trials
German Childhood Cancer Registry	http://info.imsd.uni-mainz.de/K_Krebsregister/english/	• This registry, based in Mainz, covers a population of 13.2 million children with cases for Western Germany from 1980 and for Eastern Germany since 1991. The Web site includes details of research studies and publications. English and German language.

Table 21.6 Selected websites for North America.

Name of organization	Web address	Features
Children's Oncology Group (COG)	http://www.childrensoncologygroup.org/	• Children's Oncology Group (COG) researchers work together to identify cancer causes and pioneer new treatments and cures
Pediatric Brain Tumour Consortium (PBTC)	http://www.pbtc.org/	• Identify through laboratory and clinical science superior treatment strategies for children with brain cancers • Working within institutions and communities to improve support services and follow up care for these patients and their families.
NIH- National Institutes Of Health	http://www.nih.gov/index.html	• NIH scientists investigate ways to prevent disease as well as the causes, treatments, and even cures for common and rare diseases
St Jude's Children's Research Hospital	http://www.stjude.org	• Research efforts are directed at understanding the molecular, genetic and chemical bases of catastrophic diseases in children • Identifying cures for such diseases and promoting their prevention • Research is focused specifically on cancers, acquired and inherited immunodeficiencies, infectious diseases and genetic disorders
American Brain Tumor Association	http://www.abta.org/	• American Brain Tumor Association exists to eliminate brain tumors through research and to meet the needs of brain tumor patients and their families
National Brain Tumor Foundation	http://www.braintumor.org	• NBTF has funded cutting edge research into new treatments, improving traditional treatments and enhancing the quality of life of all brain tumor patients
Have A Heart Children's Cancer Society	http://www.haveaheartcharity.org/	• Raising funds to provide aid to families struggling to manage financially
Candlelighters Childhood Cancer Foundation	http://www.candlelighters.org/	• Support research • Raise awareness and provide information about cancer to patients' families
Alex's Lemonade Stand	http://www.alexslemonade.org/	• Hold lemonade stands to raise funds for children's cancer research

Table 21.7 Website resources for the United Kingdom.

Name of organization	Web address	Features
Charlie's Challenge	http://www.charlieschallenge.com	• Raises money to finance research into brain tumors
CLIC Sargent	http://www.clicsargent.org.uk	• Information about childhood cancer diagnosis, conditions and treatment
CCLG- Children's Cancer And Leukaemia Group	http://www.ukccsg.org/	• National professional body responsible for the organization of the treatment and management of children with cancer in the UK • Coordination of national and international clinical trials, including biological studies • Other areas of activity include national cancer registration and provision of information for patients and families
CR-UK- Cancer Research UK	http://www.cancerresearchuk.org/	• UKs leading charity dedicated to cancer research
Cancerbackup	http://www.cancerbackup.org.uk	• UKs leading cancer information charity, with over 6500 pages of up-to-date cancer information, practical advice and support for cancer patients, their families and carers
Macmillan Cancer Support	http://www.macmillan.org.uk/	• Provide practical, medical, emotional and financial support, and campaign for better cancer care
Leukaemia Research Fund	http://www.lrf.org.uk/	• Dedicated exclusively to researching blood cancers and disorders including leukemia, Hodgkin's and other lymphomas, and myeloma
Samantha Dickson Brain Tumour Trust	http://www.braintumortrust.co.uk	• Largest dedicated brain tumor charity in the UK with the highest level of laboratory based brain tumor research in the country • Offers support to patients diagnosed with a brain tumor as well as their families and/or carers.
Ali's Dream	http://alisdream.f2s.com/right.htm	• Raising funds for research into childhood brain tumors • Fund scientific, medical and patient/carer qualitative/quantitative research in pursuit of their objectives • Established a pediatric focused scientific and medical advisory board and invite applications for funding via leaflet distribution at relevant conferences and contacting known research units
The Neuroblastoma Society	http://www.nsoc.co.uk/index.htm	• Raises funds for British research into the disease
Lennox Children's Cancer Fund	http://www.lennoxccf.org.uk/	• Provide emotional, practical and financial help to sufferers and their families • Formed with the intention of providing help to hospitals' specialist children's cancer wards by supplying funds for refurbishment, toys etc.

Table 21.8 Website resources for South America.

Name of organization	Web address	Features
Cancer Society of Brazil	http://www.sbcancer.org.br	• Research and fund raising
Fundacion Nuestros Hijo	http://www.fundacionnuestroshijos.cl/index2.htm	• Improving quality of life for low income children with cancer

References

1 Noll RB, Gartstein MA, Vannatta K, Correll J, Bukowski WM, Davies WH. Social, emotional, and behavioral functioning of children with cancer. Pediatrics 1999; 103: 71–8.

2 Danoff BF, Cowchock S, Marquette C, Mulgrew L, Kramer S. Assessment of long term effects of primary radiation therapy for brain tumors in children Cancer 1982; 49: 1580–6.

3 Kun LE, Mulhern RK, Crisco JJ. Quality of life in children treated for brain tumors. Intellectual, emotional, and academic function. J Neurosurg 1983; 58: 1–6.

4 Cohen P, Cohen J, Kasen S, et al. An epidemiological study of disorders in late childhood and adolescence–I. Age- and gender-specific prevalence. J Child Psychol Psych 1993; 34: 851–67.

5 Van Dongen-Melman JE, Sanders-Woudstra JA. Psychosocial aspects of childhood cancer: a review of the literature. J Child Psychol Psych 1986; 27: 145–80.

6 Steele RG, Long A, Reddy KA, Luhr M, Phipps S. Changes in maternal distress and child-rearing strategies across treatment for pediatric cancer. J Pediatr Psychol 2003 ; 28: 447–52.

7 Freeman K, O DC, Meola C. Childhood brain tumors: parental concerns and stressors by phase of illness. J Pediatr Oncol Nurs 2004; 21: 87–97.

8 Hillman KA. Comparing child-rearing practices in parents of children with cancer and parents of healthy children. J Pediatr Oncol Nurs 1997; 14: 53–67.

9 Eiser C, Richard Eiser J, Greco V. Parenting a child with cancer: promotion and prevention-focused parenting. Pediatr Rehabil 2002; 5: 215–21.

10 Goldberg S, Morris P, Simmons RJ, Fowler RS, Levison H. Chronic illness in infancy and parenting stress: a comparison of three groups of parents. J Pediatr Psychol 1990; 15: 347–58.

11 Speechley KN, Noh S. Surviving childhood cancer, social support, and parents' psychological adjustment. J Pediatr Psychol 1992; 17: 15–31.

12 Young B, Dixon-Woods M, Findlay M, Heney D. Parenting in a crisis: conceptualising mothers of children with cancer. Soc Sci Med 2002; 55: 1835–47.

13 Van Dongen-Melman JE, Van Zuuren FJ, Verhulst FC. Experiences of parents of childhood cancer survivors: a qualitative analysis. Patient Educ Couns 1998; 34: 185–200.

14 Svavarsdottir EK. Caring for a child with cancer: a longitudinal perspective. J Adv Nurs 2005; 50: 153–61.

15 Davies WH, Noll RB, DeStefano L, Bukowski WM, Kulkarni R. Differences in the child-rearing practices of parents of children with cancer and controls: the perspectives of parents and professionals. J Pediatr Psychol 1991; 16: 295–306.

16 Dolgin MJ, Katz ER. Conditioned aversions in pediatric cancer patients receiving chemotherapy. J Pediatr Psychol 1998; 8: 82–5.

17 Manne SL, Bakeman R, Jacobsen PB, Gorfinkle K, Bernstein D, Redd WH. Adult-child interaction during invasive medical procedures. Health Psychol 1992; 11: 241–9.

18 Manne SL, Jacobsen PB, Gorfinkle K, Gerstein F, Redd WH. Treatment adherence difficulties among children with cancer: the role of parenting style. J Pediatr Psychol 1993; 18: 47–62.

19 Kennard BD, Stewart SM, Olvera R, et al. Nonadherence in adolescent oncology patients: preliminary data on psychological risk factors and relationship to outcome. J Clin Psychol Med Set 2004; 11: 30–9.

20 Carpentieri SC, Mulhern RK, Douglas S, Hanna S, et al. Behavioral resiliency among children surviving brain tumors: a longitudinal study. J Clin Child Psychol 1993; 22: 236–46.

21 Eiser C, Eiser JR, Greco V. Surviving childhood cancer: quality of life and parental regulatory focus. Pers Soc Psychol Bull 2004; 30: 123–33.

22 Eiser C, Richard Eiser J, Greco V. Parenting a child with cancer: promotion and prevention-focused parenting. Pediatr Rehabil 2002; 5: 215–21.

23 Patterson J, Holm K, Gurney J. The impact of childhood cancer on the family: a qualitative analysis of strain, resources, and coping behaviours. Psycho-oncology 2004; 13: 390–407.

24 Frank NC, Blount RL, Brown RT. Attributions, coping, and adjustment in children with cancer. J Pediatr Psychol 1997; 22: 563–76.

25 Sahler OJ, Varni JW, Fairclough DL, et al. Problem-solving skills training for mothers of children with newly diagnosed cancer: a randomized trial. J Dev Behav Pediatr 2002 ; 23: 77–86.

26 www.macmillan.org.uk – Access to benefits.

27 A comprehensive list of grant-giving organizations can be found in the Guide to Grants for Individuals in Need, published and updated annually by the Directory of Social Change (24 Stephenson Way, London, NW1 2DP).

22 Late Effects in Relation to Childhood Cancer

Louise Talbot[1] and Helen Spoudeas[2]

[1] Paediatric Psychosocial Department, Royal Manchester Children's Hospital, Manchester, UK

[2] London Centre for Paediatric and Adolescent Endocrinology, Neuroendocrine Division, University College London and Great Ormond Street Hospitals, London, UK

Introduction

Defining late effects of childhood cancer therapy

Approximately 1:1000 children (20% more boys than girls) are diagnosed with a malignancy (most commonly, leukemia (32%), lymphomas (10%) or tumors of the CNS (24%) before their 15th birthday, this until recently, being second only to accidents as a major cause of mortality in childhood [1]. In the last three decades, with more intensive and centralized therapies and enhanced supportive care increasing 5-year survival from 25% to 75% (Figure. 22.1(a)), the term 'late effects' has been coined to describe the increasingly recognized medical and psychosocial consequences affecting up to 60–85% survivors – the 'price' of cure [2, 3].

Traditionally these 'late effects' (and the services being developed to support them) are equated with the treatment-related (radiation or chemotherapy) organ toxicities and psychological morbidity experienced by those surviving more than 5 years from diagnosis, namely growth impairment, hypothalamo-pituitary, endocrine and reproductive dysfunction, abnormalities of cardiac and pulmonary function, renal and hepatic impairment, secondary malignancies, cognitive and psychosocial complications and even premature death. Arguably, however, this rather narrow view fails to recognize the potential contribution of the disease/tumor itself – as well as any tumor-related or surgery-induced complications – to the late outcome, particularly where the disease affects a vital organ such as the brain, cardio-respiratory or reproductive organs, or causes obvious disfigurement.

This is important because delaying late effects surveillance and support until this late stage after cure, potentially reduces the positive impact that early preventative and rehabilitative strategies, especially targeted endocrine and psychological support, may have on reducing late morbidities which have their origins at the time of diagnosis.

For the first time, there now exists a cohort of young adult cancer survivors (0.1–0.25% aged 20–30 years) facing a future

with significant morbidity (Figure 22.1b). The average adult cured of cancer survives 10 years. The average child cured of this disease can look forward to a further survival, but with a potentially reduced quality of life (QoL) [4]. Since the latter results from the substantial health burden caused by treatment-induced, late, multi-organ and neuro-psychological toxicity, and impacts widely on public health, any intervention proven to enhance well-being, functional independence and QoL is now an important and necessary therapeutic goal.

Furthermore, with childhood cancer survival rates now so high (80%), an ethical re-evaluation between cure at any price vs its personal cost and quality of future survival is arguably urgently warranted. To put this in perspective, a modern high-dose intensive treatment burden which improves the cancer cure rate from 70% to 80%, whilst admirably curing 10% more children, in so doing diverts rehabilitative resources from, and puts at risk, the larger 90% majority who experience unnecessary treatment toxicity, prolonged hospitalization and illness experience, 20% of whom will still die and 70% of whom would have been cured by older less costly and probably less toxic therapies. We have recently published the first and largest cross-sectional evidence that the addition of chemotherapy to craniospinal irradiation for standard risk medulloblastoma reduces health status in 7-year PNET 3 trial survivors in the UK [5], whilst conferring a significant benefit only in 5-year event-free (74.2% vs 59.8%), but not overall (76.7% vs 64.9%) survival. It is now time to discard assumptions as to the relative toxicities of co-administered surgical, radiotherapeutic, and chemotherapeutic strategies in childhood cancers (statistically classified as rare), based on cross-sectional and retrospective studies of survivors, and give equal priority to the careful prospective evaluation of health-related quality of survival in future randomized trials at diagnosis and before and after diverse treatments, as well as into the very long term.

Eighty-five percent of childhood cancer survivors, particularly those treated youngest, most intensively, or for central nervous system (CNS) tumors, face cognitive, neuropsychological, and endocrine impairment. Future challenges include the prevention of premature mortality from treatment-induced second tumors, cardiac, pulmonary and renal toxicity, and morbidity from

Pediatric Hematology and Oncology, 1st edition. Edited by Edward J. Estlin, Richard J. Gilbertson, and Robert F. Wynn. © 2010 Blackwell Publishing Ltd.

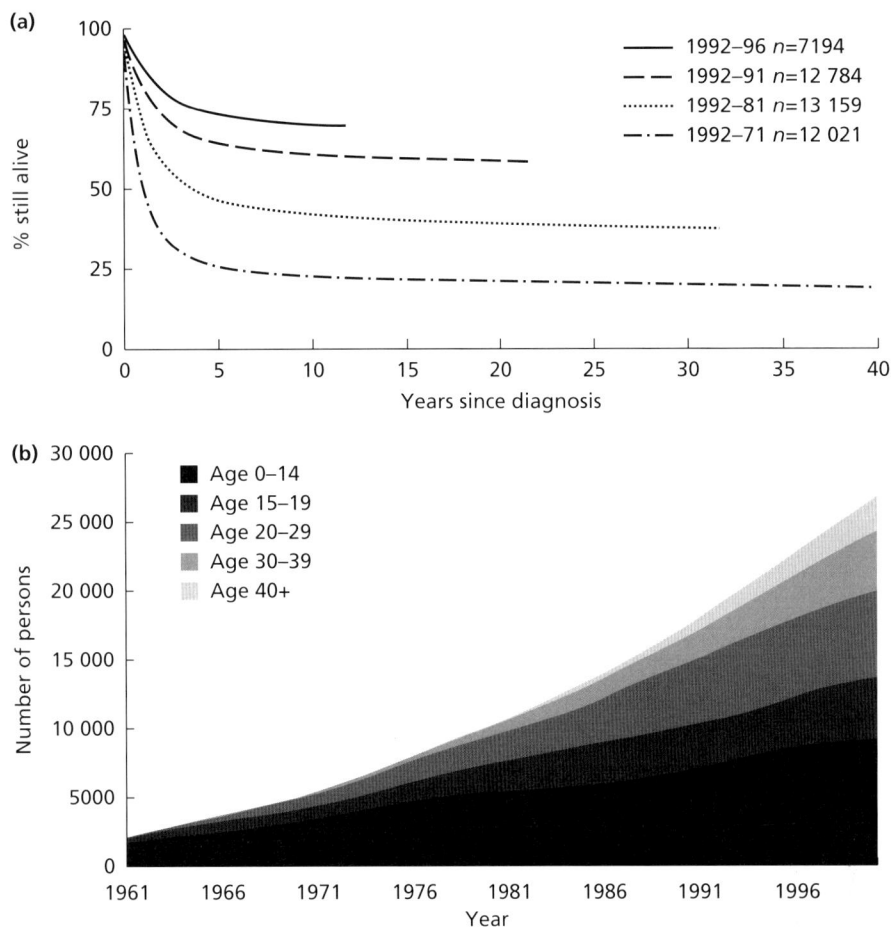

(a)

(b)

Figure 22.1 (a), Five-year survival rates of childhood cancer patients diagnosed in successive periods, Great Britain 1962–96. (b), Number alive in specified age group at the end of each calendar year with prior diagnosis of childhood cancer, Great Britain, 1961–2000. Data reproduced with permission from the National Registry of Childhood Tumours (2004) [6].

hypopituitarism, obesity and their metabolic consequences. Improving quality of life (QoL) by early hormone replacement, preservation of fertility and neuropsychological rehabilitation will enable these young people to achieve employment, independence, and successful peer relationships.

The changing therapeutic baseline (see Box 22.1)

Cranial and total body irradiation (TBI), both responsible for late neurocognitive and endocrine toxicity [7–9], are increasingly being substituted by more aggressive chemotherapy and/or the reduction, hyperfractionation, or more focal (stereotactic) application of the cranial irradiation dose. However, it is unclear whether these strategies compromise cure or the quality of survival. Chemotherapy may cause neural and endocrine toxicity [7], whilst the pre-existing disease and its peri-operative course must also contribute, particularly where the CNS tumor site is 'central' [10–12], i.e. close to the thalamic, suprasellar, and hypothalamo-pituitary areas (HPA), rather than more lateral or inferior. The few available longitudinal studies suggest that:
• Irradiation compounds an already pre-existing neurosecretory dysfunction [13].
• That chemotherapy is additively toxic, to both the CNS [13] and peripheral target glands [14, 15].

Box 22.1 Difficulties in determining etiopathology of late effects.

• Assumptions as to causation based on retrospective, cross-sectional survivor studies in mixed diagnostic and treatment groups
• Lack of prospective detailed long-term health-related outcomes in all patients entering randomized cancer treatment trials (i.e. intention to treat analysis)
• Quality (as opposed to quantity) of survival not a primary outcome measure in cancer trials
• Multimodality therapy with potentially multiple, diverse and additive neural, systemic and local effects
• Changing treatment and disease baseline over time – increasingly intensive therapies and increasingly severe disease
• The long evolutionary trajectory of late effects
• The plasticity/adaptability of the developing young person/organ
• The age-dependent effects
• The inconsistent application and availability of targeted rehabilitative or protective interventions

• Endocrinopathies, skeletal irradiation, chemotherapy and glucocorticoids, malnutrition and prolonged ill-health all independently influence sexual maturation and bone mineral accretion, thereby confounding data on infertility or osteopenia in survivors [16].

The picture has also been confused by discrepancies between 24-hour physiological and pharmacological hormone secretion in longitudinal [13, 17], and cross-sectional survivor studies [18, 19] of cranial irradiation, the long evolutionary time course, the largely retrospective, cross-sectional studies, and the changing multimodal and individually tailored therapy baseline.

Although final height and fertility are important endocrine end-points, current data often relate to already outdated treatment regimens, whilst better surgical, supportive, and rehabilitative opportunities, including new assisted reproduction techniques and better school awareness of individual needs, will surely alter outcome, hopefully for the better, for those undergoing treatment today. Before the balance between cure and late morbidity can be truly evaluated, the toxicity of new cancer treatments must be critically appraised over many years.

Late effects of CNS directed treatments

Cranial irradiation therapy or radiotherapy (CRT) is seen as the most important treatment for many childhood CNS tumors, including medulloblastoma/primitive neuroectodermal tumor (PNET), glioma and ependymoma [20]. The indications for radiotherapy, the dose administered, and the extent of irradiation to the neuroaxis, vary with cancer or tumor type and patients age. In children with CNS tumors, the goal of CRT is the selective destruction of neoplastic cells. Typically, CRT is delivered once daily, 5 days a week for up to 6 weeks. The total dose delivered to the brain in the context of CNS tumors, can be more than twice that given in the treatment of acute lymphoblastic leukemia (ALL) [21].

CRT, in combination with a variety of chemotherapeutic regimens, has been widely used in the treatment of ALL for over 25 years [22], and is cited as one of the most important factors in improving survivorship and life expectancy for children in this group. Traditionally, CRT was used to destroy cancer cells which had seeded through the blood or cerebrospinal tissue to the brain. However, with the resultant improved survival rates, reports began to emerge in the 1970s and 1980s of adverse neurocognitive sequelae.

The late effects of CRT include neurocognitive deficits, endocrine dysfunction, secondary tumors, hair loss, hearing loss and risk of other neurological sequelae, such as cerebrovascular accidents and epilepsy, all of which will be discussed later.

Changes in treatment protocols to manage the risk of mortality and morbidity following treatment have followed. As a result, children with standard risk ALL are no longer routinely administered CRT unless they experience relapse. Similarly, the role of CRT for treatment in childhood CNS tumors is central to national and international trials in order to manage the associated morbidity.

Neurocognitive late effects of irradiation

General intellectual abilities

Early studies of neurocognitive outcome relied heavily on measures of intelligence and academic achievement scores. Whilst useful as an indicator of overall function, these summary scores serve only as distant markers of more specific core cognitive functions [23], and the emphasis upon such scores as reliable indicators of the presence or absence of deficit is likely to mask more subtle underlying difficulties. In addition, these summary measures do not provide adequate explanation on the exact deficits that underlie changes in IQ and achievement seen in survivors of childhood cancer.

Reviews of the long-term cognitive effects of CRT in both CNS tumors and ALL agree that children in both groups are at risk of significant cognitive morbidity [23–25], and that therapy was often associated with significantly lower Full Scale IQ (FSIQ) than comparison groups.

Summary scores of intellectual or cognitive function are typically expressed as standardized scores with a mean of 100 and a standard deviation of 15. In relation to children with CNS tumors:
• Retrospective studies of children irradiated for brain tumors have found that only 10% of children achieved FSIQ scores >90 and 30–50% of children actually had FSIQ scores <70 [24–26].
• Children treated for medulloblastoma with CRT, with or without adjuvant chemotherapy, have demonstrated a mean estimated FSIQ more than one standard deviation below the population mean [27].
• Longitudinal studies of IQ have shown declines in IQ over time [28], and declines in academic achievements such as literacy and arithmetic abilities [29]. However, this is thought to represent a failure to learn and acquire skills rather than an absolute decline in abilities [27, 29].

Similar results have been observed in children treated for ALL with CRT. A study of 104 children treated via a variety of chemotherapy modalities, some with adjuvant CRT, found that significantly fewer children treated with CRT exceeded average IQ scores when compared with those treated with chemotherapy alone [30]. Later studies have indicated that although performance on measures of intelligence and achievement may be worse for children treated for ALL with CRT than those treated with chemotherapy alone [31], and worse than sibling controls [32], the degree of impairment is frequently mild at initial evaluation [31] but is progressive over time [22]. Reviews would suggest that intellectual declines are usually more severe among children who are younger at the time of treatment and those who receive more aggressive therapy [33].

Mental processing deficits

In order to identify the early cognitive changes that predict later IQ loss, research has increasingly focused on specific cognitive deficits that are thought to contribute to the general neurocognitive late effects. Memory and attention are the fundamental processes by which information or knowledge is acquired. Attention and memory deficits are hypothesized to limit the information base available to the child, which then makes the acquisition of new information more difficult. Effective attention and memory systems allow for the accumulations of knowledge that are reflected later in intelligence and achievement scores such as the FSIQ [34]. The possibility that IQ deficits following CRT may be due to the interruption of the normal development of processing speed and working memory has also been proposed [35]. Separation of mental processing deficits into those associated with 'attention' and those involving 'working memory' is a useful approach used in recent reviews (e.g. [33, 36]), although it is acknowledged that the two constructs are not independent from each other.

Attention

Attention is not seen as being a unitary construct and may be operationalized in tasks which require particular attentional skills or processes such as alertness, sustained attention, divided attention, focused attention and selective attention [34]. Unfortunately, within oncology research, the construct of attention is often poorly defined and measures lack specificity. As a result, global difficulties within the domain of attention may be reported, when actually only specific deficits may be present or studies may fail to report poorer 'attentional abilities' following CRT, as the actual skill or deficit may be too specific to be captured by the generic measure employed in the study. This of course leads to the risk of type I (false positive) and type II (false negative) errors. Despite this, there does seem to be general agreement that treatment with CRT for both ALL and CNS tumors leads to a variety of difficulties in the domain of attention (e.g. [22, 31, 36]), particularly selective or focused attention [36–38].

Working memory

It has been proposed that differences in IQ scores between children treated with CRT for ALL and healthy controls are mediated by differences in working memory [35]. Working memory has been described as 'the 'online' maintenance of information while it is being processed: the constant updating of incoming information so that processing can be accomplished and decisions can be made' [34, p.27]. Examples of day-to-day tasks which use working memory, are solving mathematical problems without pen and paper or holding a telephone number in mind whilst dialling it.

The working memory abilities of children who have received CRT for ALL [39] and CNS tumors [40] are reported to be poorer than healthy controls and this is thought to mediate poorer FSIQ scores as indicators of overall intelligence [35]. In children with CNS tumors, CRT and tumor site have been associated with severe working memory deficits, especially for tumors in the thalamic region [41].

As noted above, difficulties in attentional or working memory abilities can have a very significant impact upon a child or adolescent's ability to achieve academically. Some research has been conducted into attentional remediation using pharmacology

---

Box 22.2 Factors associated with less favourable neurocognitive outcome in pediatric central nervous system (CNS) tumors [52].

- Hydrocephalus
- Site of tumor
- Peri-operative surgical complications
- Volume of cranial irradiation therapy
- Methotrexate – especially with cranial irradiation therapy
- Young age at diagnosis and treatment
- Time since treatment
- Moya-moya syndrome

---

typically used in the treatment of attention deficit hyperactivity disorder, which has reported mixed but tentatively positive results [42]. Similarly, attentional retraining programs have also begun to emerge which have reported positive results [43].

Variables associated with outcome

A number of child, tumor and treatment-related factors have been consistently investigated in research regarding their influence upon neurocognitive outcome. These factors are discussed below and summarized in Box 22.2.

Cranial irradiation therapy dose

The impact of total dose and dose fraction are variables frequently investigated with regard to their influence on neurocognitive outcome in both CNS and non-CNS cancer treatment. The following issues have been reported:
- Data on reduced dose irradiation are contradictory:

  i A number of studies investigating the impact of reducing CRT dose from 2400 to 1800 cGy in prophylactic treatment for leukemia, found no difference in cognitive outcome data [21, 41].

  ii However, other studies (e.g. [44]) have reported that IQ and memory scores were at the expected mean for age 7 years following treatment with 1800 cGy and chemotherapy, with only 25% of patients achieving IQ scores below 90.
- In children receiving CRT for brain tumors, reduction in CRT dose has been shown to be beneficial for younger (4–7 years old at treatment) but not older children[8], although other studies have demonstrated a benefit of a lower dose across the group [27, 45].
- There does, however, appear to be agreement that outcome in children who have had a second course of CRT following relapse is poorer, with studies demonstrating significantly greater declines in IQ over time [46, 47].

The role of volume of radiation to the brain appears to be somewhat less controversial. When whole brain irradiation is compared with posterior fossa irradiation alone or other focal

CRT, irradiation of larger areas is associated with more severe cognitive sequelae [48, 49], although the effects of risk-adapted CRT on reading, spelling, and IQ is thought to be moderated by age, with the greatest declines seen in children less that 7 years old at diagnosis [50].

Age at treatment
Young age at treatment is one of the most important risk factors for neuro-toxicity in both children with acute lymphoblastic leukemia and children with brain tumors [48, 51]. A number of factors have been suggested to contribute to the poorer cognitive outcome seen in children diagnosed and treated in infancy:
• Deficient development of white matter, or white matter loss following CRT, might provide a neuroanatomical explanation for the severe impact of CRT on cognition in the very young [52].
• Since intellectual ability at diagnosis is thought to be more predictive of IQ later than is age per se, younger children may be more vulnerable to decline prior to CRT due to the interaction of their tumor with their brain development [53].

Questions have been raised as to whether epidemiological factors may largely explain poorer outcome in children diagnosed and treated in infancy. Namely, children under the age of 2 years have the worst survival rates [54], possibly because a disproportionately high number of children in the age group are diagnosed with supratentorial tumors, which are associated with worse outcome [53]. However, Moore et al. [55] concluded that even when tumor diagnosis, tumor location, and demographic factors are matched, infants are at greater risk than older children for significant and long-term neuropsychological morbidity. Gender has not been found to influence outcome in CNS tumors [56].

Hydrocephalus
Presence of a shunt has been shown to be significantly associated with reduced FSIQ; the effect of which has been estimated at 11 FSIQ points [56], and also with difficulties in sustained attention [38], and lower arithmetic abilities [29]. However, other studies have not replicated this effect consistently [57].

Tumor location
Tumor location has been thought to play a role in the long-term outcome for children with CNS tumors. Supratentorial tumors are associated with greater cognitive impairment than infratentorial tumors, even when whole brain CRT was not used in treatment [58]. In addition, hemispheric tumors have been reported to be associated with greater cognitive impairment than tumors of the third or fourth ventricles [48, 56].

Late effects of CNS chemotherapy

Neurological late effects
Epilepsy
Seizures are common neurological complications of cancer and may occur at various points in the disease history. The causality

---

Box 22.3 Neuroprotection summary.

• Many children with brain tumors have significant central nervous system late effects, which are difficult to predict or prevent at the present time
• Modifications to the treatment regime to reduce the direct side effects can only be justified if the cure rate is equivalent
• Strategies for prevention of central nervous system late effects might be targeted at vascular risk factors if these prove to be part of the pathophysiology
• Early recognition of cerebrovascular disease, e.g. when children present with transient ischaemic attacks rather than stroke, and of the specific cognitive and behavioural problems may allow targeted management of the individual
• The long term risks of cerebrovascular disease in survivors during adolescence and early adulthood are unknown
• Due consideration will need to be given to clinical priorities for screening for risks, stratify preventative and therapeutic intervention for cerebrovascular disease in this patient group

---

for seizures is thought to be multifactorial including the presence of space-occupying tumors in the cranial cavity, metabolic disorders, and the direct effect of medications on the CNS [59]. Epilepsy is rarely associated with non-CNS cancers. The highest prevalence has been found in children with supratentorial tumors and lowest rates were associated with hematopoietic cancers [60]. Treatment is largely with anticonvulsant drugs but is problematic during treatment phases due to interactions with chemotherapeutic drugs, and epilepsy is a significant long-term sequelae in these patients.

The incidence of seizures in children with ALL ranges from 4 to 13% [61] and may be associated with metabolic disorders which are often resolvable with treatment, intracranial hemorrhage and stroke, infection and chemotherapy-induced adverse drug reactions [61], which are also often resolvable. Issues around the need for neuroprotective strategies are summarized in Box 22.3.

Ototoxicity
The chemotherapy agent cisplatin is most likely to be associated with longer-term hearing sequelae for children who receive therapy for cancer. In particular, cisplatin affects higher frequencies of hearing, i.e. 4000–8000 Hz, but also the more normal conversational frequencies of 500–2000 Hz, in a manner that depends on cumulative dose up to a total of 600 mg/m^2 [62].
• Although the cisplatin analogue carboplatin is well tolerated in the longer term and causes little or no ototoxicity at standard doses, cisplatin causes a sensorineural hearing deficit that deteriorates over time, especially when cumulative doses exceed 400 mg/m^2 [63].
• Cisplatin ototoxicity may relate to higher free platinum concentrations in the plasma during the time of infusion, and in

keeping with this, schedules that recommend a longer infusion time per given dose tend to be better tolerated [64].

However, in the context of children with CNS tumors, then the combination of cisplatin and posterior fossa radiotherapy may lower the tolerance of either agent in terms of ototoxicity. For example, although when given after cisplatin, radiotherapy has no deleterious effects on hearing [65], younger age and prior irradiation each contribute to the severity of hearing loss at a given cisplatin exposure level [66].

Late neuroendocrine toxicity
Radiobiology
The radiosensitivity of a tissue is directly proportional to its mitotic activity and inversely proportional to its degree of differentiation [67]. All organs are damaged by irradiation but the late effects on specialized, slowly- or non-proliferating cell populations (such as the brain) are manifest only with time. Fractionation of the dose generally improves the therapeutic margin, but there is evidence to suggest the gonads are an exception to this rule [67, 68]. Other long-term consequences include life-shortening mutagenicity and carcinogenesis [67, 69]. With conventional external beam radiotherapy, late neuroendocrine effects depend upon [12, 67]:
- The volume of the brain irradiated.
- The fraction size and interfraction interval.
- The age of the child.
- The total dose delivered.
- The time elapsed since injury.

The irradiation field for most infratentorial childhood brain tumors is demarcated by the pituitary margins and the pituitary dose is at least 40–45 Gy. The highest hypothalamo-pituitary doses (up to 70 Gy) occur after treatment for nasopharyngeal tumors, with consequent multiple pituitary deficits [70]. Yttrium-90 implants and the newer stereotactic irradiation techniques, although more focused, currently have limited application in childhood cancer.

Chemotherapy, radiation, and toxicity
Additive effects from combined drugs and radiation may cause cumulative toxicity in late-responding tissues, without time for regeneration between the two treatment modalities. Toxicity to the thyroid [15], gonad [14], and skeleton [71], as well as to central pituitary hormone secretion [13], is greater when adjuvant chemotherapy and irradiation are combined. Thus, using chemotherapy to delay, but not necessarily avoid, potentially curative cranial irradiation in the youngest children [9, 67] may cause additive injury that is evident only in the longer term.

Neuroendocrine consequences of cranial irradiation
Panhypopituitarism (Box 22.4)
After surgery for pituitary tumors, the few adults (37/165 in one series) with more than one intact pituitary hormone, suffer an evolving 'post-irradiation' (20–45 Gy) endocrine deficit which is dose- and fractionation-dependent and hierarchical in nature

---

> **Box 22.4 Neuroendocrine consequences of cranial irradiation.**
>
> - Panhypopituitarism
> - Growth failure and growth hormone deficiency
> - Precocious puberty
> - Hypothalamo-pituitary adrenal integrity
> - Obesity

[12, 72] (Figure 22.2(a)). However, delayed tumor- or surgery-induced neuronal injury may also play a part.

- Experimental pituitary irradiation in rats [73] causes the characteristic growth hormone (GH) deficit seen in humans [12] but not the adrenocorticotrophic hormone (ACTH) and gonadotropin deficiency seen in man.
- Furthermore, the relative radioresistance of thyroid stimulating hormone (TSH) and prolactin secretion noted in the human subjects [12] was absent in rats, these hormones and GH being affected early [73] – perhaps a reflection of their common developmental origin [74].
- Post-irradiation pituitary deficiencies are also noted in children after high doses (>50 Gy) for orbital and middle ear tumors [75].
- However, after lower cranial doses for brain tumors (30–50 Gy) or leukemia (18–24 Gy) [76], the high prevalence of deficiencies other than GH noted in the adult pituitary studies [12] have not been confirmed in childhood survivors of posterior fossa or laterally placed tumors [11, 13–15, 77, 78], despite similar pituitary doses and 10-year follow-up. GH deficiency is the earliest and often the only abnormality and the deficit is usually permanent [77, 78] (Figure 22.2(b)).

Given the clear-cut time- and dose-dependency, pituitary deficiencies are likely to be multiple and to manifest quickly and most completely in the youngest children receiving the highest irradiation doses or where tumors are close to the HPA, i.e. 'central' [12, 70]. By contrast, they may be single, evolve more slowly or be qualitative rather than quantitative in nature after irradiation to more laterally sited tumors [13, 72] or after the lower cranial doses used in leukemia prophylaxis [17, 76, 79] and TBI [19, 80, 81], particularly if fraction size is also reduced (Table 22.1). This may well result in a cohort of survivors who need hormone replacement therapy as adults rather than as children [82].

Nature and site of the neuro-endocrine defect
The neuroendocrine consequences of cranial irradiation are summarised in Box 22.5. Whether the post-irradiation endocrinopathy is neural or vascular, hypothalamic or pituitary, is still hotly debated. The few available studies do not suggest that either hypothalamic [79] or hypophyseal-portal blood flow [83] are compromised. The hypothalamus or its portal connections are perceived to be more radio-sensitive than the pituitary; evidence sited includes hyperprolactinaemia after >50 Gy [73], for

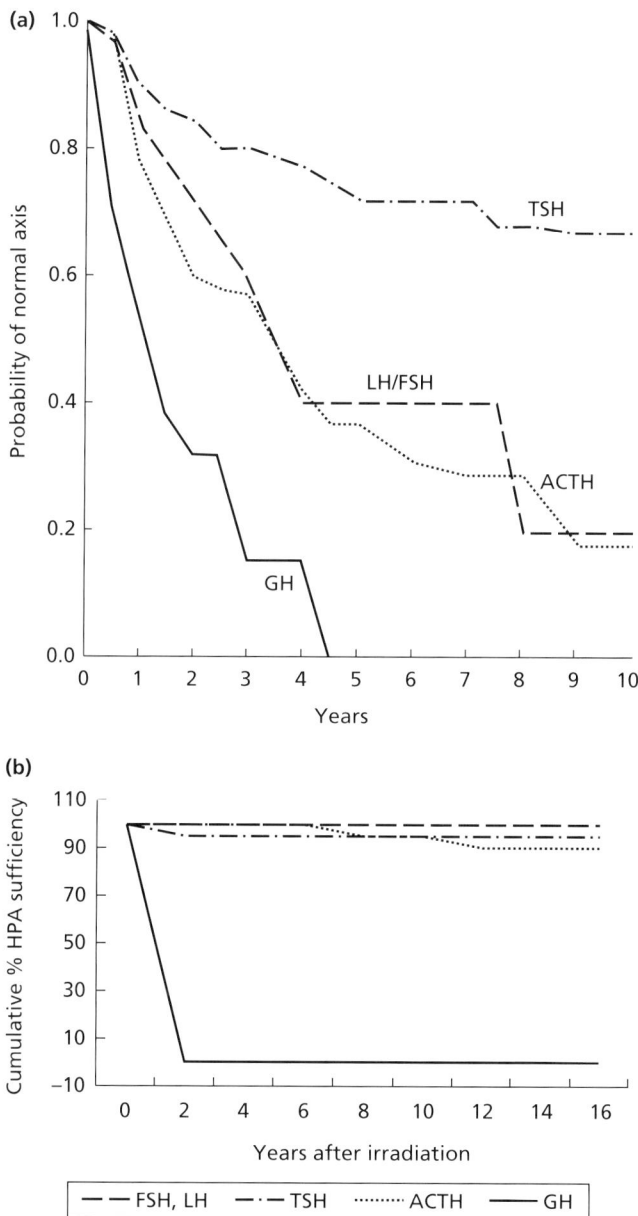

Table 22.1 Likely endocrine deficit according to cranial irradiation dose (brain tumors distant from pituitary area).

Dose	Endocrinopathy	
>55–70 Gy	Hyperprolactinaemia, panhypopituitarism	
30–55 Gy	GH insufficiency, evolving endocrinopathy	
18–24 Gy	Neurosecretory disturbance	Pubertal GH insuffiency,early puberty, adult GHD
10–15 Gy	Neurosecretory disturbance	Adult GHD

GH, growth hormone. GHD, growth hormone deficiency.

Box 22.5 Etiologies of hypothalamo-pituitary dysfunction after central nervous system directed therapy.

- Growth hormone deficiency affects all cranially irradiated survivors eventually, but adrenocorticotrophin hormone deficiency is rare if there has been no hypothalamic-pituitary area disease.

- The hypothalamic and/or pituitary nature of the post-irradiation endocrinopathy needs clarification.

- Cranial irradiation is not the only culprit, surgery and disease being significant in its causation.

- Systemic chemotherapy also crosses the disrupted blood–brain barrier and results in additive central toxicity

- The differentiation of hypothalamic from pituitary disease has important therapeutic and etiological implications

Figure 22.2 (a), Ten-year life-table analysis in 37 of 165 adults with intrasellar or anatomically adjacent tumors, and normal post-operative hypothalamo-pituitary function, indicating the likelihood of an evolving endocrinopathy after 37.5–42.5 Gy pituitary irradiation in 15 fractions over 20–22 days. GH is most sensitive, all adults being GH deficient within 5 years, whilst ACTH and gonadotrophins (LH and FSH) are increasingly affected over time (80% at 10 years). TSH is most resistant. (Redrawn with permission from [12].) (b), Ten-year probability of an evolving endocrinopathy, occurring after a median estimated hypothalamo-pituitary irradiation dose (DXR) of at least 40 Gy in 1.8 Gy fractions, in 20 young adult survivors of resected posterior fossa brain tumors tested twice – at the onset of growth failure and at completion of growth – who were otherwise asymptomaticGH deficiency was present in all patients tested at first assessment and was permanent. ACTH (10%) and TSH (5%) deficiencies were comparatively rare and there was no case of gonadotrophin deficiency or hyperprolactinaemia over the duration of follow-up. (Redrawn with permission [28].)

nasopharyngeal or pituitary tumors, attributed to disrupted hypothalamic inhibitory dopaminergic tone [70, 73]. However, hyperprolactinaemia is not seen after treatment for extrasellar tumors in childhood [70, 77, 84, 88], nor has diabetes insipidus, a typical hypothalamic disorder, been reported [70]. Selective damage to hypothalamic control centers is suggested by discordant suppression of insulin-mediated and spontaneous GH release in irradiated rhesus monkeys [85], children with leukemia [19, 86] and brain tumors [13] and paradoxically preserved GH responses to other centrally-acting agents or hypothalamic releasing factors [83, 88]. Since GH secretion [13, 18, 77] and pituitary GHRH responses [77, 87, 88] decline with time, direct pituitary damage is a possibility.

Spontaneous GH secretory profiles *before* low (10 Gy) [19] or high (30–50Gy) [13] cranial irradiation doses already reveal disturbed GH pulsatility, with suppressed insulin-induced and paradoxically-preserved physiological GH peaks. We proposed [13] that the disease (cerebellar tumor) and/or its surgery, somehow disrupt afferent or efferent GH chemoreceptor responses to hypoglycemia and suppress hypothalamic somatostatin secretory tone, important in regulating GH pulsatility. Superimposing cranial irradiation also suppresses physiological GH peak generation, suggesting eventual hypothalamic GH-releasing factor (GHRH) deficiency [13], and possible consequent dysfunction or atrophy of the pituitary somatotroph [77, 88]. Chemotherapy plays an important contributory part in this evolving neural dysregulation at the HPA [13].

The distinction between hypothalamic and pituitary dysfunction has therapeutic relevance. Hypothalamic gonadotrophin- and growth hormone-releasing factors restore fertility [89] and growth [90], respectively, but only if the pituitary is intact. Because the response to GHRH also depends on hypothalamic somatostatin secretion which is disturbed by cranial irradiation [13, 19], GH-releasing factor therapy is less effective than recombinant human GH (*r-h*GH) in enhancing growth [90]. If the etiology and site of the damage are accurately determined, protective strategies can be attempted before irradiation commences [91].

Growth failure and growth hormone deficiency
Growth failure, disturbed physiological GH secretion and/or attenuated stimulated peak GH responses, affect 60–100% of children within 2–5 years of fractionated (<2 Gy) cranial irradiation doses of >30 Gy [10, 11, 13].
• The speed of onset is dose-dependent [72] but there is unlikely to be a lowest 'safe' dose. The few studies of physiological 24-hour GH secretion before and after TBI (10 Gy) [19], cranial irradiation (24Gy) for leukemia [10] or brain tumors distant from the HPA (>30 Gy) [13] suggest a steadily evolving picture of neurosecretory disturbance with time and irradiation dose-intensity [13, 19, 92], which is eventually severe and permanent [77, 82, 88].
• Abnormalities in GH pulsatility after 10 Gy of slow dose-rate TBI [19], or fractionated (2 Gy) cranial doses of 18 Gy [92] and 24 Gy [93] are particularly evident in puberty [79, 93]. More favourable reports [92] have assessed mean or peak GH secretion only and may miss the early qualitative, subtle disturbances in GH pulsatility and failure to augment pubertal GH secretion adequately [79, 93].

Diagnosing GH deficiency
After treatment for brain tumor and cranial irradiation for leukemia, GH deficiency is common, its prevalence increasing with time and affecting almost all cranially irradiated survivors within 5 years [11, 94]. To the untrained observer the diagnosis is masked by early puberty, obesity, and the confounding effects of spinal irradiation. Accurate diagnosis requires a high index of suspicion and careful growth and development surveillance by trained endocrine personnel. In a recent multicenter report, the prevalence of GH replacement therapy among 545 children treated for medulloblastoma before 15 years of age, varied from 5% to 73%, and was commenced on average only 4 years after diagnosis [95], presumably accounting for the short adult statures reported.

Discrepancies between growth velocities, stimulated GH responses and 24 hour endogenous GH secretion [17, 19, 86], complicate the diagnosis of GH deficiency in survivors of lower cranial irradiation doses as used in acute leukemia. By contrast, these discrepancies are rare after the higher cranial irradiation doses used to treat brain tumors, except when studied within 2 years of diagnosis [13], presumably due both to the greater speed with which GH deficiency develops and the degree of the deficiency (Figure 22.3).

Serum insulin-like growth factor-1 (IGF-1) and its binding protein (IGF-BP3), are also unreliable estimates of 24 hour [77, 88] or stimulated [88, 96] GH secretion in cranially irradiated children. Possible reasons include disrupted hypothalamic feedback [88], nutritional influences early in the disease [96], pubertal hormonal changes and increased IGF-BP3 protease activity in malignancy. However, as the severity of GH deficiency evolves with time, the accuracy of the tests improves to 83% and 71% for IGF-1 and IGF-BP3 respectively [77]. The lack of a 'gold standard' for assessing GH secretory status makes it imperative that all slowly growing children have a full endocrinological assessment.

Growth hormone therapy and tumor relapse
The risk that *r-h*GH may predispose to malignancy or relapse [97, 98] is only theoretical [99, 100], at least when used in replacement doses, though very large numbers of GH-treated individuals would have to be studied to achieve statistical certainty. There are reports of acute leukemia in GH-treated children but half had predisposing conditions, and leukemia has also been reported in *un*treated patients with idiopathic GH deficiency [101]. Although lymphocyte subsets are normal in GH-deficient patients, consistent with the absence of clinical immunodeficiency, lymphocyte natural killer activity is reduced in some individuals [102]. GH receptors are present on lymphocytes. If leukemic transformation has already taken place, GH might accelerate the process, but the concentrations needed are 10 times higher than those used therapeutically [98].
• Amongst 6284 GH-treated individuals in the USA with 59 736 patient years of follow-up, just three cases of leukemia occurred (RR 1.8, 95% CI, 0.8–7.5).
• This figure increased to six cases at 83 917 patient years of follow-up (RR 2.6, 95% CI 1.2–5.2), but five of these patients had previous cranial tumors and all except one had been pre-treated with cranial irradiation [99].
Further reassuring evidence comes from a rodent tumor-bearing model, whose GH-induced improvement in nitrogen-wasting and cachexia was not at the expense of an increase in primary tumor size; there was a surprising reduction in the size and number of pulmonary metastases compared with placebo-treated animals [103]. Nevertheless, supraphysiological doses should be used rarely and only with extreme caution in the clinic.

To achieve a maximum response to therapy, *r-h*GH should be substituted early, before (an age-appropriate) puberty. However, most centers are cautious about introducing this therapy within

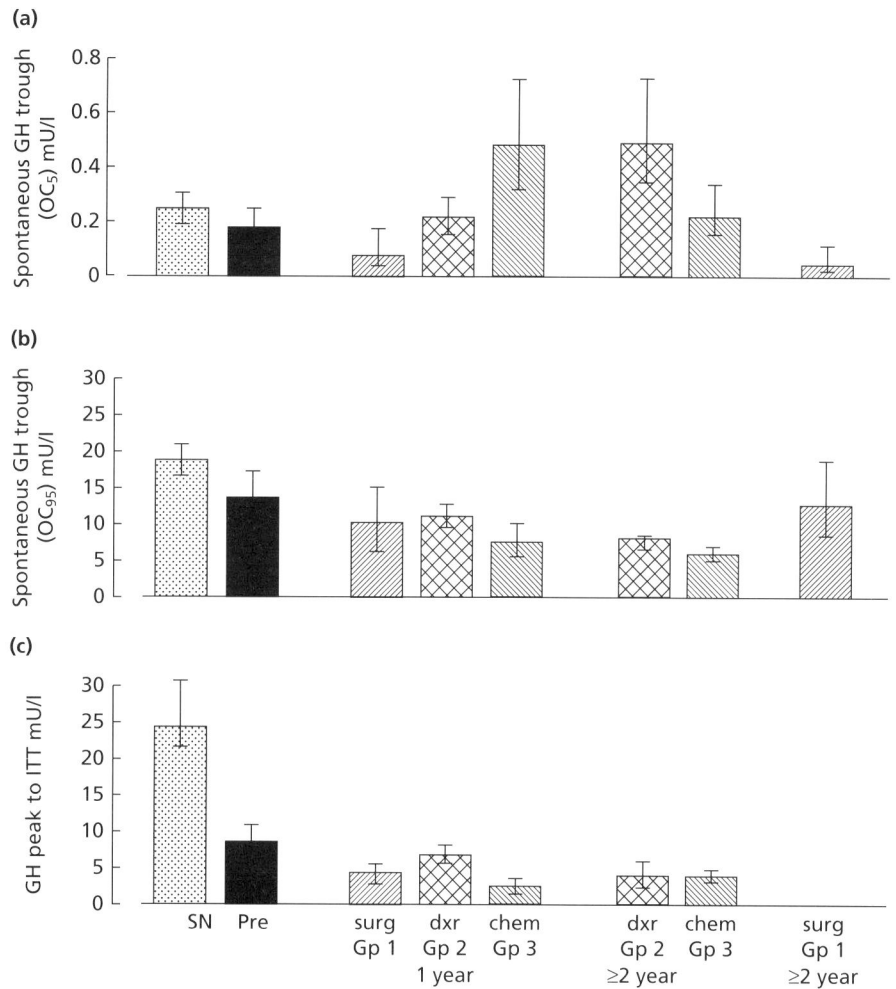

Figure 22.3 Relationship of (a), spontaneous GH troughs (OC$_5$), (b), spontaneous GH peaks (OC$_{95}$), and (c), stimulated peak GH responses to hypoglycaemia (ITT), with increasing therapeutic intensity and time in short normal (SN) controls, and children with brain tumors before (pre) radiotherapy and at 1 and 2–5 years after neurosurgery alone (surg, Gp1), or with additional >30 Gy cranial irradiation (dxr, Gp 2), and >30 Gy cranial irradiation with adjuvant chemotherapy (chem, Gp 3). Note the wide variation in trough secretion across groups compared with controls, and the marked early discrepancy between spontaneous (preserved) and stimulated (attenuated) peaks, even in children treated with surgery only (Gp 1). This discrepancy becomes concordant with time and intensity of therapy as spontaneous GH secretion fails. (Redrawn with permission [13].)

the first 1–2 years after cancer treatment, as this is the time of highest relapse rate. By pharmacological testing, most children treated for brain tumors will be deficient within that time. However, the diagnosis may be delayed or difficult in children treated with lower cranial irradiation doses for leukemia because of the discrepancies discussed previously. It is therefore paramount to carefully document growth (sitting and standing height), weight and pubertal status 3–6 monthly from cancer diagnosis until adult height, and also to measure parental heights. Growth and growth velocity must be carefully interpreted in the light of mid-parental target height, the tendency to early puberty, advanced skeletal maturity, inexorable weight gain, and previous therapy (e.g. spinal irradiation with/without chemotherapy). The smallest, youngest and most intensively treated children are particularly at risk of failing to achieve an adequate adult height even with r-hGH replacement. Supportive evidence of GH deficiency, from pharmacological (glucagon or insulin-hypoglycemia) or physiological tests, is invariably required for licensing purposes, especially as radiation treatments become more focused and refined. Nevertheless, there may be instances where tests are not

confirmatory and further physiological assessment or even a therapeutic trial of r-hGH may be necessary.

GH deficiency in adulthood

Adult survivors of low cranial irradiation doses are at real risk of adult GH deficiency with its attendant implications for reduced bone mineralization, altered body composition (increased fat mass), decreased cardiac performance and atherogenic lipid profile, and reduced quality of life due to the adult GH deficiency syndrome [104]. Cardiac contractility may be further reduced by significant (30%) irradiation scatter to the mediastinum from the spinal dose [105], and the adjuvant toxicity of potentially cardiotoxic chemotherapeutic agents needs to be considered in this context and also in relation to the potential for lung fibrosis [105].

Although GH replacement appears safe in these patients from the point of view of disease relapse [106, 107], there have been concerns that supraphysiological doses of GH may promote tissue overgrowth, which could enhance risks for tumor recurrence or second tumor development . However, there is as yet no evidence for this in childhood.

Precocious puberty

Precocious (early) puberty is a recognized presentation of optic, hypothalamic, and other 'central' tumors but has also been detected after treatment for more laterally or inferiorly placed tumors [11, 108]. Possible co-existent gonadotoxicity induced by chemotherapy [109, 110] or spinal irradiation [14] confounds the true prevalence. Gonadotrophin deficiency arresting pubertal development is also possible [14], although more likely after high dose irradiation of pituitary or closely-located tumors [72].

Early puberty, directly related to the age at irradiation [108], occurs particularly in girls, whose hypothalamic gonadotrophin pulse generator is known to be more sensitive, but also in boys, and is more evident after lower (24 or 18 Gy), rather than higher, cranial irradiation doses.

• This finding has become more evident since spinal irradiation was omitted from neuraxial prophylaxis [108, 111].
• The increased prevalence of early puberty in females treated with 18 Gy rather than 24 Gy cranial irradiation [111], suggests that damage to higher puberty-inhibitory centers may occur after low cranial irradiation doses, whilst higher doses may ablate hypothalamic GnRH or pituitary gonadotrophin release; the absence of this phenomenon after lower (7.5–15 Gy) TBI doses is explained by its severe gonadotoxicity [110].
• Cranially-irradiated female leukemia survivors are also at risk of obesity [112], raising the possibility that neuroregulatory changes in leptin secretion may contribute to the early puberty [113].

Hypothalmo-pituitary adrenal integrity

After estimated hypothalamo-pituitary (HPA) irradiation doses up to 50–55 Gy given to treat laterally- or inferiorly-placed brain tumors, symptomatic ACTH deficiency has not been reported. Two–13 years after HPA doses far in excess of 50 Gy to adults with nasopharyngeal tumors, an 18–35% dose-related prevalence of asymptomatic, subnormal cortisol response to metyrapone was reported. By contrast, pituitary responses to hypothalamic corticotropin-releasing factor were normal [70].

In a series of 20 cranially-irradiated childhood survivors of posterior fossa tumors, 10 years after estimated pituitary doses of 40–45 Gy at our institution, all but two demonstrated adequate (>500 nmol/l) cortisol responses to hypoglycaemia, despite persistently suboptimal growth hormone responses [88] (Figure 22.2(b)). The two exceptional patients were asymptomatic with normal responses to low dose ACTH stimulation; in one of them late onset 21-hydroxylase deficiency was diagnosed. This experience contrasts with the high (80%) prevalence of ACTH insufficiency observed in adults [12], suggesting earlier surgery- or tumor-related contributions to the latter. The etiologies of hypothalamo-pituitary dysfunction after CNS-directed therapy are summarized in Box 22.5. Twenty-four hour physiological secretion profiles in children with leukemia who had received 18 Gy or 24 Gy cranial irradiation 3.5–10 years previously, showed no disruption in the amount or pattern of ACTH and cortisol secretion compared with normal controls [114].

Obesity

Excessive weight gain is a recognized complication of suprasellar, but not intrasellar, tumors and their treatment. For some time, growth may be maintained in the face of GH deficiency by increased IGF-bioavailability, modulated in turn by hyperinsulinemia, which further drives the obesity [115]. There is some evidence to suggest that obesity in these circumstances results from ventromedial hypothalamic lesions causing disinhibition of vagal tone at the level of the pancreatic β cell; in extreme cases truncal vagotomy has alleviated the obesity [116].

The tendency to obesity observed in cranially-irradiated youngsters without hypothalamic lesions is harder to explain [112, 117], and just as difficult to treat. Whether the eventual insulin resistance is also primarily the result of increased vagal tone or secondary to hyperphagia involving central satiety centers is unknown.
• Recent work suggests that survivors of leukemia have decreased metabolic expenditure, rather than increased metabolic intake, entirely due to reduced physical activity [118].
• Corticosteroid use may also be an important contributory factor. In studies so far, cortisol secretion appears normal in childhood [114] but in adults with prolonged GH deficiency syndrome, there may be a change in the bioavailability of cortisol through 11β-hydroxy-steroid dehydrogenase and the cortisol-cortisone shuttle [119].

Obesity and insulin resistance pose a real risk of premature death from diabetes and cardiovascular disease. GH deficiency aggravates obesity, whilst GH therapy decreases fat mass, increases lean mass through direct actions on adipocytes and suppresses leptin in parallel [113]. Both insulin and leptin are suppressed by somatostatin which paradoxically, may improve short-term insulin resistance in this situation [118]. Leptin signalling modulates energy balance via effects on the hypothalamus and other tissues, maintaining adipose tissue mass within a finite physiological range. Any role that disturbances in this pathway might play in the evolution of obesity (or early puberty) after cranial irradiation remains still has to be elucidated, but 'healthy lifestyle' measures and adult GH replacement therapy need to be considered in these circumstances, even if there are no other significant endocrinopathies.

Neurocognitive late effects of CNS chemotherapy

Most studies compare neuropsychological outcome between children treated with CRT and chemotherapy as CNS prophylaxis, and conclude that children treated with CRT experience less favourable cognitive outcome, as discussed above. Prospective longitudinal studies on cognitive functions in children treated for ALL with chemotherapy only are scarce and have shown mixed results.

Kingma *et al.* [120] found that children surviving ALL have no major cognitive impairment after chemotherapy, including intrathecal and high-dose intravenous methotrexate. Similarly, Schatz *et al.* [35] found that children treated with intrathecal methotrexate showed similar working memory and processing speed as their demographically matched control group.

However, other studies have shown poorer performance IQ scores following chemotherapy with intrathecal methotrexate [121]. Modest declines in academic arithmetic [122, 123], verbal fluency and visual-motor abilities [123], perceptual motor skills [122], poorer auditory memory and fine motor functioning have also been found relative to healthy controls [120]. Specific information processing deficits have been shown, with slower speed of information processing especially in focused attention tasks and situations where large amounts of information are presented [124].

Variables associated with outcome

The influence of dose and demographic factors on outcome appears somewhat less severe in relation to chemotherapy than in CRT treatment regimens (see Box 22.6 for summary). Whereas younger age at treatment with CRT is seen as being predictive of poorer cognitive outcome, this is not thought to be the case in chemotherapeutic treatment. Studies have demonstrated:
• Infants treated for ALL whose diagnosis was before the age of 12 months showed no increased risk of neurodevelopmental sequelae [125].
• The dose of intrathecal methotrexate for CNS prophylaxis for ALL was not found to relate to neuropsychological performance [39].
• Gender is important in specific cognitive domains in that girls treated with chemotherapy only as CNS prophylactic therapy, performed more poorly than normative samples for non-verbal tasks, whereas boys did not show any differences [126].
• In relation to actual drugs used, comparison between patients who received dexamethasone during the intensification and maintenance phase of therapy and those who received prednisone as the corticosteriod component of therapy, showed that children treated with dexamethasone performed less well on cognitive testing [127] and are at increased risk of neurocognitive side effects [128].

Box 22.6 Risk factors for decreasing cognition in children with acute lymphocytic anaemia [52].

• Cranial irradiation
• Young age at time of irradiation
• Central nervous system relapse
• Female gender
• Methotrexate therapy
   In combination with cranial irradiation therapy
   Leptomenigeal disease
   High dose with frequent administration
• Time since irradiation

Quality of life studies
Health-related quality of life

As more children survive childhood cancer, the quality of the life saved has become an important area of research [129, 130]. This is particularly relevant in clinical trials where the short- and long-term morbidity associated with a treatment regimen and mortality risks need to be carefully balanced. Assessment of health-related quality of life (HRQoL) may also be useful in identifying patients at risk for adjustment problems [131], but is associated with a number of challenges (Box 22.7).

Measurement issues

Despite the increasing number of publications relating to HRQoL, few studies clearly specify what it is that is being measured [132]. The definition put forward by the World Health Organization (WHO) Quality of Life Group, encompasses a number of domains including physical, mental, and social wellbeing and states that HRQoL is 'the state of complete physical, mental and social wellbeing and not merely the absence of disease or infirmity' and that furthermore, it is the 'individual's perception of their position in life, the context of culture and value systems in which they live and in relation to their goals, expectations, standards and concerns' [133] which determines their quality of life.

Whilst mortality and morbidity may be relatively easy to quantify, measurement of the HRQoL in the child presents a number of challenges as detailed in a number of reviews in the area (e.g. [130, 134]). In summary:
• The relatively high prevalence of cognitive impairment in the childhood cancer population, particularly in children with CNS tumors, raises questions regarding the reliability of child reports, and as a result there has been an over-reliance on proxy-ratings of HRQoL.
• The presence of cognitive impairment and the sometimes poor health status of the child with cancer, has led many researchers to rely on proxy ratings. Inconsistent proxy-reports between self-report by children with cancer and their parents have been reported frequently in the literature [4] and the use of multi-source data collection has been suggested [135].
• Although patient self-report is considered the standard for measuring perceived HRQoL, it is the parents' perception of their child's HRQoL that may influence health care utilization [136].

Box 22.7 Key challenges in HRQoL research to date.

• Presence of cognitive impairment in population
• Over-reliance on proxy-ratings
• Small sample sizes and heterogeneous samples
• Variation in measurement tools used
• Lack of disease specific measures
• Applicability of measures to UK population

• Reviews which have examined the agreement between self- and proxy report in children with cancer, overall suggest that there is a consistent bias for parent-proxies to underestimate the negative impact of the disease and treatment for the children [137].
• As a result parent-proxy reports are more valid for children who are younger than 12 years of age but less so for adolescents.
• In studies of children with CNS tumors, parent and child reports have shown reasonable agreement [138] and agreement between children and teachers, and parents and teachers on the domains of cognition, pain, self esteem, and hearing were good. Discrepancies have been noted between children and parents on reports of confidence for the future and self esteem [139].

In addition, the small sample sizes of many studies, and heterogeneous samples employed in other studies raises questions over the generalizability of study findings within and between groups. The variation in measurement instruments employed has made comparison between studies difficult, and the lack of disease-specific measures makes identification of specific areas of burden for individual patient groups difficult. Finally, the cultural appropriateness of measures developed outside of the UK may be questionable for use within the UK, without specific research into the applicability of the measure to the UK population.

Much research has focused on the differences in reported HRQoL between children with cancer and healthy controls, and between children with cancers involving the CNS and those which do not. Overall, it would seem that:
• A considerable proportion of children who have experienced cancer in childhood report HRQoL scores at least one standard deviation below reported norms for healthy children [140].
• Children whose cancer involves the CNS typically report poorer HRQoL than children with non-CNS cancers [140].

Health-related quality of life in children with central nervous system tumors
Research into HRQoL in children with CNS tumors has indicated that 66% of children show dysfunction on some level of QoL, [129] with the greatest burden of morbidity being associated with cognition [129, 141] and emotion, with each affecting more than 50% of children with CNS tumors [141]. Pain [141] and fatigue [140] are surprisingly prevalent, and fatigue is inversely related to overall HRQoL in children with CNS and non-CNS cancers [140]. Assessment of HRQoL using multi-attribute measures, such as the Health Utilities Index [142], has indicated the complex nature of the morbidity burden experienced by survivors of CNS tumors through the large number of unique health states reported [141].

Predictors of health-related quality of life in children with central nervous system tumors
The relationship between tumor location and HRQoL remains equivocal. Some research has suggested that supratentorial tumors may be associated with poorer HRQoL [143], whereas others have found no such association [138]. Tumor pathology has been associated with differences in parent reports of physical and emotional functioning, but not child reports, in that parents of children with low grade glioma reported higher HRQoL [138] and unsurprisingly, children with demonstrable disease have been shown to report poorer HRQoL than those without [129].

Whilst some research has reported that treatment received is not a predictor of HRQoL [143], others found that treatment received was consistently associated with overall HRQoL, with CRT being consistently associated to lower total HRQoL scores [138] and that specifically:
• Craniospinal CRT is associated with lower HRQoL [129].
• Insertion of shunts has been associated with lower reports of overall HRQoL and social functioning in parent and child reports, and with lower reports of physical and psychological functioning in child reports [138].
• CRT before the age of 5 years old has also been associated with poorer HRQoL [129]. However, two studies have suggested that age at treatment is not a predictor of overall HRQoL [138, 143], which is somewhat surprising given the established links between age at treatment and neurocognitive deficits and further, the links between poorer cognition and overall HRQoL.

The physical and psychological HRQoL scores of children with brain tumors has been found to show a quadratic or inverted U shape, with those who are undergoing treatment reporting lower HRQoL followed by a sharp increase in those who have completed treatment less than 12 months previously and sharp declines in those for whom more than 12 months had elapsed since their treatment [140].

Health-related quality of life in children with non-central nervous system cancer
HRQoL in children with non-CNS cancers is considerably more variable, and the most common approach to measurement has involved the use of measures developed to assess domains of physical or emotional functioning assumed to be related to quality of life [144]. In many studies, no major differences have been found between the HRQoL of children with non-CNS cancer and healthy controls [144], indeed some research has indicated that survivors reported better levels of vitality, stress, depression, discomfort, and sleeping dimensions than controls [145]. However, in studies of children who had received treatment for ALL it would seem that subsets of children do experience impaired HRQoL.

Feeny et al. [146] reported that 25% of patients had deficits in multiple domains of HRQoL and 30% had deficits in the domain of emotion. Similarly, Meeske et al. [140] reported that 37% of children with ALL had scores more than one standard deviation below the mean overall QoL score reported for healthy children. The research into predictors of poor HRQoL in non-CNS cancers is less extensive than for children with CNS cancers. However, with regards to treatment received, Moe et al. [147] followed up a matched control group of children treated with methotrexate rather than CRT as CNS prophylaxis. No difference was found

---

Box 22.8 Long-term outcomes – childhood and adolescence.

- Require special educational needs programs
- Experienced grade retention or repetition
- Experience difficulties in maths, English and science
- Less likely to have close friends
- Those who received treatment including cranial irradiation therapy have greatest reported difficulties
- Acute lymphoblasic anemia and cranial irradiation therapy tumors associated with poorer outcomes than other cancers
- Higher self-esteem and parental education are protective factors

---

Box 22.9 Long-term outcome – adulthood.

- Lower likelihood of post-secondary education
- Lower rates of employment and higher rates of unemployment
- Impaired close relationships
- Lower rates or marriage and cohabitation
- Lower rates of parenthood

---

between survivors and controls in physical, mental health, or HRQoL.

Long-term outcome

As noted earlier, with improved survival rates came the need to investigate the educational, social, and economic outcome of childhood cancer survivors both in childhood and adolescence (Box 22.8) and further into adulthood (Box 22.9).

Outcome in childhood/adolescence

Barrera et al. [148] conducted a large-scale multi-center retrospective study of 800 survivors of childhood cancers who were aged 17 years or younger at assessment. This study investigated the educational and social outcomes of survivors compared with control participants.

- Survivors were more likely to receive special educational programs or to have failed or repeated a grade.
- Survivors were more likely to obtain below average or failing grades in all curriculum subjects, with the greatest differences observed in mathematics followed by English and science.
- Parents of children with CNS tumors and ALL reported poorer outcomes than parents of survivors of other childhood cancer types, with survivors of CNS tumors most likely to have reported difficulties in maths and English.

- Children treated with CRT were more likely to attend learning difficulty or special educational need provisions within the educational setting, to have failed a grade or experienced other academic difficulties compared with those whose treatment excluded CRT or intrathecal methotrexate.
- In the Barrera et al. [148] study, age at diagnosis, age at evaluation and gender were not related to survivor's educational difficulties.

In the same study, parental reports of social and emotional competence indicated that survivors of childhood cancer were more likely than controls to have no close friends, with parents of survivors of CNS tumors, leukemia and neuroblastoma reporting highest odds ratios. Factors associated with lower likelihood of social and educational difficulties included higher rated self-esteem and parental educational achievement.

Outcomes in adulthood

Only a small number of studies have evaluated the long-term outcome of survivors of childhood cancer with respect to social and emotional factors in adulthood. These studies found that although many survivors function well and lead comparable lives to people who have not experienced cancer in childhood, a number of important differences repeatedly emerge.

Given the reported risk of adverse cognitive outcomes in children treated for cancer, it is perhaps not surprising that a proportion of cancer survivors report poorer educational outcomes relative to their peers. Individuals, particularly females [149], who have received cancer diagnoses were significantly less likely to have completed secondary education beyond high school or 11th grade [149, 150], with survivors of CNS tumors achieving a lower educational level than leukemia survivors, and radiotherapy being the strongest independent prognostic factor of educational achievement [149].

The employment outcomes of survivors show a similar pattern, with survivors being less likely to be employed than controls [149] and more likely to be unemployed [151, 152], or to have never been employed at all [153]. When cancer types are considered separately, whilst the employment rates of survivors of blood cancers and bone cancers were found to be lower than controls, this result was not statistically significant, whereas survivors of CNS tumors were found to be five times more likely to be unemployed [152]. Factors associated with higher rates of unemployment in cancer survivors include:
- Female gender [153–155].
- CRT [153, 156].
- Lower IQ.
- Motor impairment and epilepsy [157].
- Tumor location was significant in survivors of CNS tumors (supratentorial vs infratentorial tumors) [153].

When examining long-term outcomes associated with living situations and interpersonal relationships, survivors were more likely than controls to have impaired close relationships [158], consistently less likely to be married or living as married than controls [149, 150, 153], less likely to have children [149, 150], and men were more likely to still be living with their parents [149]. In survivors of CNS tumors, the odds ratios of not being married were higher for men than women, for those who had received CRT than those who had not, and for people who had diagnoses of supratentorial rather than infratentorial tumors, [153] with the overall risk of not being married being 4.5 times greater for survivors of CNS tumors than survivors of leukemia who did not receive CRT [149].

Late effects of non CNS-directed radiotherapy and chemotherapy

A prospective evaluation of the late effects of childhood cancer therapy indicates that for 223 consecutive survivors of childhood cancer, 75% had at least one medical problem, and the organ systems most frequently affected were [159]:

- The nervous system in 39%.
- The endocrine system in 32%.
- The ears/eyes in 22%.
- The kidneys in 17%.
- The liver in 12%.

These late effects do influence physical performance and daily activities, especially for survivors of CNS tumors and cancers involving the bone [160] (Box 22.10).

Endocrine late effects
Growth
The influence of chemotherapy on growth: leukemia

Growth retardation during treatment for acute leukemia is partially counteracted by 'catch-up' after cessation of 'maintenance' chemotherapy. However, depending on the intensity of chemotherapy, significant height loss can be detected in 40–70% [127, 161] patients at 6-year follow-up. Chemotherapy also aggravates the growth failure of children with brain tumors given craniospinal irradiation [71], and deficient short-term growth has also been described in children given only chemotherapy, without

---

Box 22.10 Late effects of non-central nervous system-directed treatment.

- Endocrine dysfunction
  Growth
  Thyroid dysfunction
  Fertility
  Adrenal dysfunction
- Impaired bone mineralization
- Cardiotoxicity
- Nephrotoxicity

---

cranial irradiation [162, 163] or TBI [164]. However, irradiation probably causes the long-term deceleration which is not so evident in the chemotherapy-only group [163].

Studies *in vitro* [165] and *in vivo* [162] have shown that chemotherapeutic agents suppress human osteoblast proliferation and enhance osteoclast activity. Glucocorticoids modify these actions [166] and have their own negative effects on growth and bone mineralization. The disease induces a low bone turnover and GH-resistant state aggravated by chemotherapy. Disease control, weight gain, and glucocorticoid withdrawal all increase bone and soft tissue turnover and growth velocity. This effect is reduced by methotrexate [162], whilst alkylating agents and anitimetabolites also cross the disrupted blood–brain barrier and perturb central GH secretion [13].

Not all patients with leukemia require growth-directed investigation or therapy. Nevertheless, despite temporary 'catch-up', 90% of 115 children aged <12 years at irradiation (24 Gy) suffered mean adult height deficits of one (5 cm) (67%) or two (10 cm) standard deviations (SD) (33%) from pre-treatment scores, with spinal irradiation aggravating the problem [167]. In those treated before the age of 7 years, attenuated pubertal growth is evident [163] and accords with failure to augment pubertal GH secretion [79, 93] as described in the previous section. Asymmetric body proportions (longer legs) of adult survivors [168] pre-treated with cranial, but not spinal, irradiation is also suggestive of compromised pubertal spinal growth from undiagnosed pubertal GH insufficiency. Similar disproportion is evident in a cohort of brain tumor survivors, even those not given spinal irradiation [11], (Figure 22.4) stressing the importance of specialist endocrine input, both before and during puberty, before the 'window of opportunity' for treatment is lost.

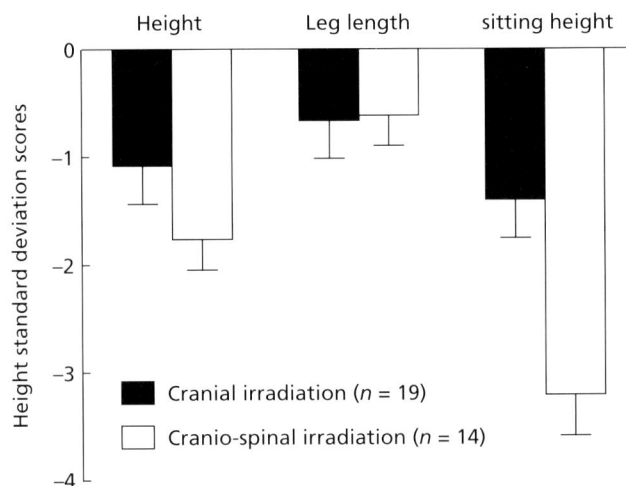

Figure 22.4 Adult height without endocrine therapy of 33 patients irradiated in childhood for brain tumors. All patients are short, but the greatest deficit is seen in the spine, even in those not receiving spinal irradiation, although less severe, suggesting a subtle GH disturbance affecting pubertal (and hence) spinal growth. (Redrawn from [7].)

The influence of spinal irradiation on growth
Hodgkin's disease
Spinal growth impairment and skeletal disproportion were first described after 18 fractionated doses of 44 Gy to the midplane in both mantle and 'inverted Y' fields [169]. Estimated vertebral scatter ranged from 40 to 100% despite shielding. The height deficit was worse in children irradiated under the age of 6 years or during puberty [169].

Brain tumors
Craniospinal irradiation (27–35 Gy in 22–27 days) impairs spinal growth [16, 170] (Figure 22.4). The younger the child the greater the deficit, which is estimated at 9 cm if irradiation is administered at 1 year, 7 cm at 5 years and 5.5 cm at 10 years [170]. Spinal growth is a major component of the pubertal growth spurt so the disproportionate deficit, compounded by pubertal GH deficiency, may only then become apparent, at a time when growth promotion is limited. Hyperfractionation may decrease the deleterious effects [171] if the overall treatment time is simultaneously accelerated.

Leukemia
Almost 50% of those receiving craniospinal irradiation (24 Gy) suffered height loss of >2 SD from pre-treatment values, as compared with 32% of their peers receiving only cranial irradiation (24 Gy) and intrathecal methotrexate. Furthermore, no 'catch-up' growth was observed in the craniospinal group, presumably due to the absence of a significant spinal pubertal spurt [167]. Chemotherapy and steroids are contributory [162, 166, 167].

Total body irradiation
Both single (7.5–10 Gy) and fractionated (12–15.75 Gy) TBI regimens cause progressive growth failure [172–174], 33% of patients being >2 SD below the mean at 5 years [173].
• This is partly due to GH deficiency, which increases with time and irradiation dose (42% and 87% of those transplanted in first and second remission, respectively), and is not observed after chemotherapy alone [172], but is also due to growth plate and bony matrix damage [169].
• Disruption of bone matrix integrity must account for the poor growth response to r-hGH [173], the lack of correlation between GH secretion and height loss [175] or growth rate [164], and the accrual of further height deficits despite r-hGH therapy [176].
• Other endocrinopathies, steroid and cytotoxic therapy [165, 166], and graft versus host disease may also be involved. Patients should be warned that, at best, pre-treatment centile positions can only be maintained by r-hGH therapy, and that at worst, additional pubertal and thus adult height deficits are likely (Figure 22.5).

Thyroid dysfunction
Radiation damage to the thyroid gland causes hypothyroidism, usually compensated by increased TSH production, and thyroid tumors (see Box 22.11 for summary). Hypothyroidism is dose-

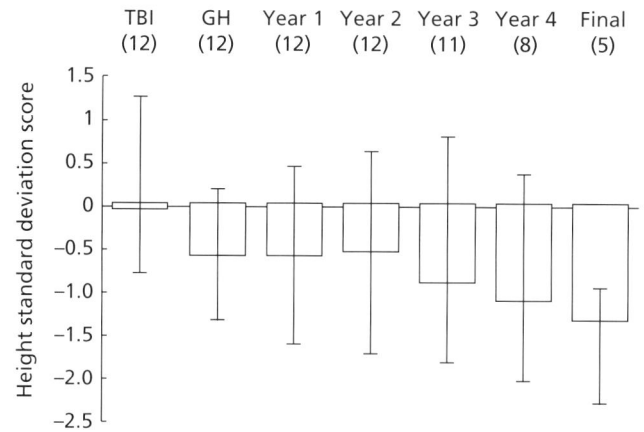

Figure 22.5 Stature (expressed as height standard deviation scores [SDS]) of 12 leukemic children at our center who were prepubertal at the time of total body irradiation (TBI), followed longitudinally to adult height from the time of growth hormone replacement (GH) for confirmed GH deficiency. The numbers of subjects are shown in parantheses. Note that institution of GH therapy initially only maintains the height position without 'catch-up growth', and subsequently fails to prevent an ongoing pubertal deficit to adult height.

Box 22.11 Thyroid dysfunction.

• After cranio-spinal irradiation +/− additively toxic chemotherapy, primary thyroid (and gonadal) dysfunction may co-exist with (and mask) thyrotropin-releasing hormone (or gonadotrophin-releasing hormone) hypothalamo-pituitary disturbance

• The loss of the nocturnal thyrotropin surge and the possible 'recovery' of compensated hypothyroidism after cranial irradiation, may indicate higher hypothalamic disturbance

• Compensated primary hypothyroidism after cranial or craniospinal irradiation deserves treatment to suppress thyrotropin-releasing hormone because of the risk of malignancy in the irradiated thyroid gland

• Thyroid swellings should be carefully assessed with scans, needle biopsy, and a low threshold for thyroidectomy

and time-dependent and has been well documented after fractionated doses to the neck in excess of 25 Gy [177]. The suggestion that its incidence is greater in the youngest patients has not been confirmed [178].

Hodgkin's disease
In those under 16 years, the prevalence of hypothyroidism within 2 years of 36–44 Gy mantle irradiation (1.5–2 Gy fractions) vary between 37% and 88% [178, 179], with 25–53% 'compensated' and 0–58% 'overt'. The use of posterior spinal and laryngeal blocks at 30 Gy and 20 Gy, respectively, did not reduce the overall incidence of hypothyroidism (57%), though it was overt in fewer cases (5%) at a median follow-up of 65 months [180].

Transient hyperthyroidism has been reported after adjuvant MOPP chemotherapy [178] treated without neck irradiation, and just one report documents primary thyroid dysfunction in 24 of 54 adults with advanced Hodgkin's disease who received chemotherapy but not radiotherapy [181].

Craniospinal and total body irradiation

Compensated or less commonly frank hypothyroidism, occurred in 30–40% of children with brain tumors treated with cranio-spinal (30–35 Gy) irradiation but not chemotherapy, most within 4 years of treatment.

• Chemotherapy increased this risk [15, 182].

• A similar proportion developed hypothyroidism, compensated at first and progressing to overt hypothyroidism 5–10 years later, after TBI [174].

• After 7.5–10 Gy single fraction TBI, 28% and 13% developed compensated and overt hypothyroidism respectively.

• After 12–15.75 Gy fractionated TBI, these figures were 12% and 3%, respectively, though the overtly hypothyroid group were followed for only half the number of years [174, 183].

• These figures have proved overestimates so far as the long-term is concerned, since recovery occurred in 33% at a median of 60 months and no overt cases of hypothyroidism developed [184].

Elevations in TSH have been attributed to primary thyroid gland damage. Because of the carcinogenic potential of prolonged stimulation in the irradiated gland, annual thyroid palpation (with repeated ultrasound examinations, and needle biopsy and thyroidectomy as necessary), and thyroid function tests (with thyroxine replacement if TSH is persistently elevated), are often recommended. However, documented recovery after mantle [178] and spinal irradiation [182] and after TBI [184], raises the possibility that elevations in TSH may be evidence of hypothalamic irradiation damage, disturbing the normal day-to-night TSH variation by obliterating the nocturnal TSH surge [88] (Figure 22.6).

Whilst chemotherapy is apparently additive to the effects of irradiation [15, 182], the independent role of the drugs used is probably slight, since thyroid dysfunction was not observed in a large series of 105 children transplanted for thalassaemia, and in only one of 50 transplanted for aplastic anemia with 'conditioning' chemotherapy, without TBI [183].

Fertility

Reproductive capacity

It is difficult to forecast the growth, pubertal progress, and ultimate reproductive potential of a prepubertal child receiving both cranial irradiation (with its potential effects on pituitary hormone secretion, both activating and depleting), and potentially gonadotoxic therapy, since many sites on the hypothalamo-pituitary target-gland axis may be affected simultaneously by multimodal therapies and/or disease. Sub-clinical target gland toxicity (such as might occur after lower or scattered irradiation doses to the gonad) [14] may carry important implications for

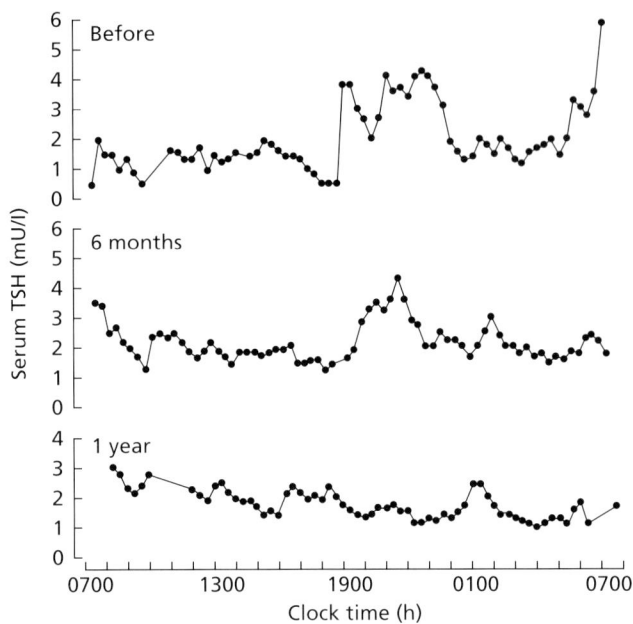

Figure 22.6 Twenty-four-hour TSH pulsatility profiles in the same child with a posterior fossa brain tumor before, 6 months and 12 months after cranial irradiation. Note the gradual loss of the normal nocturnal TSH surge with time after irradiation within the normal TSH range. (Redrawn from [88].)

future reproductive capacity, which may not be detectable for many years. Indeed the observation that early puberty is evident, despite gonadotoxic chemotherapy and scattered gonadal irradiation [182], suggests that disrupted hypothalamic control predominates over peripheral target gland toxicity, at least at these low estimated scattered irradiation doses to the ovary (approximately 4 Gy) [110] or testis (<2 Gy) [109]. For such reasons, it is important to ascertain, if possible, longitudinal growth, puberty and hormonal data before treatment, and at intervals thereafter until growth and puberty are complete. They are ideally performed together with questionnaire-derived Quality of Life (QoL) outcomes. Despite the long follow-up required, final height data and long-term reproductive outcome are important outcome measures impacting on QoL, which are being addressed in the newest UKCCSG and SIOP protocols for PNET tumors.

Factors influencing fertility

All girls are born with a fixed ovarian pool of oocytes which undergo progressive atresia from before birth until the menopause.

• Given the larger residual ovarian pool in younger (as opposed to older) girls and the greater radiosensitivity of the testicular (sperm producing) Sertoli cells as compared with the (hormone secreting) Leydig cells [185, 186], it is likely that most children will experience a spontaneous puberty, often earlier than expected, despite scattered spinal irradiation and gonadotoxic chemotherapy [11].

• However, this does not exclude the co-existent possibility of male subfertility or a premature menopause [187] at some time in the future, nor of bone demineralization due to sub-clinical sex steroid deficiency.

• In addition, there is evidence for dose-dependent recovery of sperm counts with time, after graded irradiation doses to the testis [68], and after gonadotoxic chemotherapy, the speed of recovery can be hormonally modulated [188] provided the doses are not ablative [189].

Therefore, in the youngest patients there may be a window for the application of assisted reproductive technology which has revolutionized male infertility. Early referral to an endocrine or reproductive center for both males and females is recommended for detailed counseling about future reproductive and sexual health.

Adrenal dysfunction

Clinical signs of cortisol deficiency may be vague and the diagnosis missed by conventional tests such as insulin-induced hypoglycaemia [190] or standard (250μg) ACTH (synacthen) stimulation [191], which lack sensitivity due to their pharmacological nature. Low doses of ACTH (500 ng/1.73 m²) have been proposed as a more physiological test of adrenal reserve [191]. The 24% prevalence of subnormal adrenal responses to metyrapone after TBI [174], suggest that subclinical adrenal damage may develop as time passes.

Impaired bone mineralization

Osteoporosis has been blamed on the adult GH deficiency syndrome [82], but skeletal changes observed in cancer survivors may be also be attributable to other hormonal (sex steroid) deficiencies (Box 22.12). Skeletal irradiation [169], corticosteroids and antineoplastic agents [162, 165, 166] may also impair mineralization directly or indirectly by inducing renal tubulopathies. Disease (e.g. leukemia), prolonged bed rest, and changes in Vitamin D metabolism may also influence bone mineral density. Concern that a lower peak bone mass in adolescence will cause osteoporosis later in adult life, is therefore valid. However, the interpretation of surrogate markers of bone mineral density (BMD), such as DEXA measurements at the lumbar spine, needs to be undertaken with care. Sex- and age-standardized reference charts may be misleading in a population that is short because of GH deficiency and spinal irradiation, and with pubertal maturation delay. [16] In adults, other femoral and distal radial sites may be used but corrections should still be made for size [16]. Volumetric densities, independent of bone size and measured with quantitative computed tomography, are the current 'gold standard' [192].

In children with newly diagnosed cancer [193] or leukemia [162], two longitudinal studies documented negative bone turnover at diagnosis, decreases in Vitamin D metabolites [193] and GH resistance [162]. The resulting impaired accrual of

---

Box 22.12 Assessment and prevention of bone demineralization.

• Size correction factors for size are needed when assessing bone mineral density in the cancer survivor

• Hormone and dietary replacement therapies should be optimized to aid peak bone mineral accretion, age-appropriate puberty, uterine enlargement, hair re-growth, and prevent obesity

• Weight bearing, aerobic exercise and a healthy calcium-containing diet should be encouraged to prevent osteopenia, obesity and insulin resistance

• Growth hormone replacement therapy should be considered in adult life for those with severe and multiple pituitary deficiencies

• The benefit of growth hormone replacement in the adult with isolated growth hormone deficiency is not proven

---

cortical (femoral neck) but not trabecular (lumbar spine) bone [193] recovered with disease remission. Prospective studies like these help delineate the multifactorial etiology of peak bone mass impairment and encourage appropriate intervention strategies.

Cardiotoxicity

The anthracycline class of chemotherapy agents has long been recognized as a cause of late cardiac insufficiency for children surviving childhood cancer [194].

The major concerns for the long term relate to abnormalities of left ventricular performance [195], and although the incidence of such findings is low for children who receive a cumulative dose of 90–270 mg/m² of anthracycline, there may be no safe dose to avoid late cardiac toxicity [195]. In particular, depressed cardiac function is found after many years of observation for the survivors of childhood ALL who receive between 224 and 550 mg/m² cumulative dose of anthracyclines.

The clinical significance of anthracycline-related cardiac toxicity is emphasized by the incidence of clinical heart failure, which shows:

• A cumulative incidence of 2.8%.

• A much higher relative risk of almost 12 was found for the population of patients who receive a cumulative anthracycline dose of greater than 300 mg/m² [196], which means that 1 in 10 who receive this cumulative dose of anthracycline will develop heart failure [197].

However, the actual impact of this finding remains to be evaluated, as peripartum worsening of heart failure has not been described as a clinically important phenomenon in a recent study [198].

Nephrotoxicity

Mild-to-moderate sub-clinical glomerular and tubular damage can be identified in many childhood cancer survivors [199], and abnormalities of magnesium absorption from the kidney may have important long-term consequences for bony health and integrity [200].

In pediatric clinical oncology practice, therapy with cisplatin and ifosfamide is most related to nephrotoxicity in the long term. As with ototoxicity, the pharmacokinetic profile of long-duration infusion is associated with less nephrotoxicity in terms of glomerular and tubular function [15]. Similarly, extensive study of ifosfamide nephrotoxicity in children has identified that although cumulative ifosfamide doses of >199 g/m^2 are associated with a very high risk of severe toxicity, a reduction of cumulative dose to <84 g/m^2 will reduce, but not abolish the risk of this complication [201]. In the longer term, considerable nephrotoxicity with concomitant need for replacement therapies with magnesium, phosphate and potassium etc., can be present many years after completion of chemotherapy, and show little signs of recovery [202].

Conclusion and summary

Neuropsychological late effects

The impact of cancer upon the child's psychological and cognitive development and outcome vary according to:

- Type of cancer (CNS vs non-CNS)
- Age at diagnosis and treatment (under 7 years vs older)
- Treatment received (radiotherapy vs surgery only, chemotherapy or combinations)
- Post-operative complications and sequelae.

The main domains in which difficulties have been identified include:

- Attention, concentration and working memory. This impacts upon global measures such as IQ.
- Speed of information processing, which with the above may impair performance in a variety of academic areas.

For many children, social and educational impairments may only become fully apparent some years following treatment. The varied and complex needs of children following diagnosis and treatment for cancer do not easily fit within the special educational needs support system. This requires a significant level of global cognitive impairment (with abilities below the 1st centile in many cases) before a Statement of Special Educational Need is issued. Furthermore, a considerable amount of longitudinal data is also frequently required, detailing interventions put in place by the school from within their own resources to ameliorate the problem. This is problematic for a number of reasons:

- Many children 'mask' their failure to learn and acquire new skills at the same rate as their peers through use of pre-morbid skills.
- Children may show deficits in specific areas (e.g. attention) which are unlikely to be specifically assessed by non-specialist educational or clinical psychologists.

- Difficulties may be misinterpreted as behavioural rather than cognitive in origin.
- All of the above require an element of recognition of difficulty from both the parent and teacher, which may not be forthcoming without specific information and advice.
- Because of the specific nature of difficulties and preservation of some skills, children may not be prioritized for assessment and support within their peer group in the context of a stretched and pressurized education system.

The efficacy of psychological and neuropsychological intervention in improving the medium and long-term outcomes of children who have received cancer diagnoses in childhood, is an emergent area of research. Some interesting pilot work is ongoing with children diagnosed with CNS tumors, and is awaiting evaluation [203–205].

Reduced HRQoL is also frequently reported by childhood cancer survivors following diagnosis, and in the medium and longer term following treatment. This is seen to be especially true if the cancer originated in the CNS or if only parental reports are considered.

It is hoped that as services for children with cancer continue to develop, long-term surveillance for late effects is included and is considered in the early stages following treatment. At present the funding for, and availability of, clinical psychology sessions to oncology services remain variable and frequently inadequate [206]. The availability of specialist neuropsychological assessment and intervention is even scarcer. In order for difficulties to be identified early, involvement of clinical and neuropsychology services within the oncology MDT is essential, as recognized in recent National Institute for Clinical Excellence (NICE) guidance [207].

Assessment for all children at key transition points would appear vital in informing educational services regarding the needs of children diagnosed with cancer in childhood, and to advise on children who may need additional funding for school to meet their needs. Suggested transition points would include:

- Approximately 12 months following treatment, especially if radiotherapy was included.
- Prior to standardized examination and assessment points to inform application for special consideration in exams (SATS and GCSEs).
- At transition between primary and secondary education.

Neuroendocrine assessment

Cranial irradiation to the HPA usually results in dysfunction. Its incidence, time course, and severity as indicated by the number of affected anterior pituitary hormones, are dependent not only on the dose, fractionation, and time elapsed since irradiation, but also on the innate hierarchical sensitivity of each hormone and the site of any disease.

- Irradiation is not the only culprit. Tumor position, surgery, and chemotherapy also contribute to late toxicity at all levels of the hypothalamo-pituitary-target gland axis.

• If tumors have not involved the 'central' pituitary area, the GH axis is the most sensitive and the adrenal axis the most resistant to the effects of direct irradiation.

• Since endocrinopathies may evolve over many years, lifelong endocrine follow-up, in an age-appropriate multidisciplinary setting, is necessary after cranial irradiation.

Difficulties in interpreting growth rates of children with radiation-induced skeletal lesions, and in evaluating the GH and ACTH responses to pharmacological stimuli, make it important to define the pathophysiology of post-irradiation endocrinopathies. With better understanding of the neuroregulatory control of hormonal secretion, this is now a priority, because it will help target potential protective strategies as well as the most appropriate replacement therapy. Instituting therapy early, before clinical symptoms, may be of especial benefit in terms of normal pubertal and social adjustment, growth, fertility, and bone mineralization.

GH replacement therapy has been traditionally discontinued after the end of adolescence. However, an increasing number of reports suggest an important role for GH on atherogenic lipid profiles, body mass and bone density as well as QoL. Replacement therapy may have to be continued indefinitely at lower doses for longer, particularly in older patients and those with multiple endocrinopathies.

• Because of the potential hazards of indiscriminate replacement therapy and real concerns about GH mitogenicity, it becomes all the more important to establish accurate normal ranges for pharmacological and physiological tests of GH release at all ages and to understand the factors implicated in their action.

• More resources need to be allocated to encouraging a healthy, active life-style and increased metabolic expenditure, perhaps delaying the need for adult GH replacement in those with isolated GH deficiency.

Recognition of the precise causes and evolutionary changes leading to neuro-endocrine sequelae, will greatly assist oncologists and radiotherapists in planning their treatment protocols to reduce morbidity and prolong survival. The new challenge of addressing the causes of obesity and hyperinsulinemia, defining the etiology of premature puberty, attempts to preserve fertility, as well as directly improving psychosocial and neuro-rehabilitation, will ensure that pediatric endocrinologists and oncologists continue to work closely together in a multidisciplinary setting for the foreseeable future. Oncologists and radiotherapists must plan the timing of treatment protocols with the intention of reducing neuroendocrine morbidity and prolonging survival. Reducing the neuro-endocrine burden of morbidity, whether it is due to treatment or damage, will lighten the load for the brain tumor survivor, who may also be struggling with the neurological or cognitive consequences of brain injury.

Current NICE Guidance on the long-term follow-up of childhood cancer survivors emphasizes the importance of specialist MDTs to aid effective communication. If clinicians with expertise in the management of late effects are available at every center, appropriate referrals can be made at the right time and links are formed with adult services for appropriate transitional arrangements [207].

References

1 Hewitt M, Weiner SJ, Simone JV. Childhood cancer survivorship: improving care and quality of life. National Cancer Policy Board, editor. Washington DC: National Academy of Sciences, 2003.

2 Oeffinger KC, Mertens AC, Sklar CA, et al. Chronic health conditions in adult survivors of childhood cancer. N Engl J Med 2006; 355: 1572–82.

3 Stevens MC, Mahler H, Parkes S. The health status of adult survivors of cancer in childhood. Eur J Cancer 1998; 34: 694–8.

4 Calaminus G, Kiebert G. Studies on health-related quality of life in childhood cancer in the European setting: an overview. Int J Cancer Suppl 1999; 12: 83–6.

5 Bull KS, Spoudeas HA, Yadegarfar G, Kennedy CR. Reduction of health status 7 years after addition of chemotherapy to craniospinal irradiation for medulloblastoma: a follow-up study in PNET 3 trial survivors on behalf of the CCLG (formerly UKCCSG). J Clin Oncol 2007; 25: 4239–45.

6 Cancer Research UK. Childhood Cancer – UK. Journal [serial on the Internet]. 2004 Date: Available from: http://publications.cancerresearchuk.org/WebRoot/crukstoredb/CRUK_PDFs/CSCHILD04.pdf.

7 Mahoney DH, Jr, Shuster JJ, Nitschke R, et al. Acute neurotoxicity in children with B-precursor acute lymphoid leukemia: an association with intermediate-dose intravenous methotrexate and intrathecal triple therapy – a Pediatric Oncology Group study. J Clin Oncol 1998; 16: 1712–22.

8 Mulhern R, Kepner J, Thomas P, et al. Neuropsychological functioning of survivors of childhood medulloblastoma randomised to receive conventional or reduced dose craniospinal irradiation: a pediatric oncology group study. J Clin Oncol 1998; 16: 1723–8.

9 Ris MD, Packer R, Goldwein J, Jones-Wallace D, Boyett JM. Intellectual outcome after reduced-dose radiation therapy plus adjuvant chemotherapy for medulloblastoma: a Children's Cancer Group study. J Clin Oncol 2001; 19: 3470–6.

10 Brauner R, Rappaport R, Prevot C, et al. A prospective study of the development of growth hormone deficiency in children given cranial irradiation, and its relation to statural growth. J Clin Endocrinol Metab 1989; 68: 346–51.

11 Darendeliler F, Livesey EA, Hindmarsh PC, Brook CG. Growth and growth hormone secretion in children following treatment of brain tumors with radiotherapy. Acta Paediatr Scand 1990; 79: 950–6.

12 Littley MD, Shalet SM, Beardwell CG, Ahmed SR, Applegate G, Sutton ML. Hypopituitarism following external radiotherapy for pituitary tumors in adults. Q J Med 1989 Feb; 70: 145–60.

13 Spoudeas HA, Hindmarsh PC, Matthews DR, Brook CG. Evolution of growth hormone neurosecretory disturbance after cranial irradiation for childhood brain tumors: a prospective study. J Endocrinol 1996; 150: 329–42.

14 Livesey EA, Brook CG. Gonadal dysfunction after treatment of intracranial tumors. Arch Dis Child 1988; 63: 495–500.

15 Livesey EA, Brook CG. Thyroid dysfunction after radiotherapy and chemotherapy of brain tumors. Arch Dis Child 1989; 64: 593–5.

16 Prentice A, Parsons TJ, Cole TJ. Uncritical use of bone mineral density in absorptiometry may lead to size-related artifacts in the identification of bone mineral determinants. Am J Clin Nutr 1994; 60: 837–42.

17 Spiliotis BE, August GP, Hung W, Sonis W, Mendelson W, Bercu BB. Growth hormone neurosecretory dysfunction. A treatable cause of short stature. JAMA. 1984; 251: 2223–30.

18 Jorgensen EV, Schwartz ID, Hvizdala E, et al. Neurotransmitter control of growth hormone secretion in children after cranial radiation therapy. J Pediatr Endocrinol 1993; 6: 131–42.

19 Ryalls M, Spoudeas HA, Hindmarsh PC, et al. Short-term endocrine consequences of total body irradiation and bone marrow transplantation in children treated for leukemia. J Endocrinol 1993; 136: 331–8.

20 Estlin E, Lowis S. General principles of radiotherapy. In: Estlin E, Lowis S (Eds), Central Nervous System Tumours of Childhood. London: MacKeith Press, 2005: 163–77.

21 Mulhern R, Fairclough D, Ochs D. A prospective comparison of neuropsychological performance in children surviving leukemia who received 18-Gy, 24-Gy or no cranial irradiation. J Clin Oncol 1991; 9: 1348–56.

22 Anderson V, Godber T, Smilbert E, Weiskop S, Ekert H. Cognitive and academic outcome following cranial irradiation and chemotherapy in children: a longitudinal study. Br J Cancer 2000; 82: 255–62.

23 Butler R, Haser J. Neurocognitive treatment effects of treatment for childhood cancer. Mental Retard Dev Dis Res Rev 2006; 12: 184–91.

24 Duffner PK, Cohen M, Thomas P. Late effects of treatment on the intelligence of children with posterior fossa tumors. Cancer 1983; 51: 233–7.

25 Hirsch J, Reiner D, Czernichow P, et al. Medulloblastoma in childhood: survival and functional results. Acta Neurochir 1978; 48: 1–15.

26 Spunberg JJ, Chang CH, Goldman M, Auricchio E, Bell JJ. Quality of long-term survival following irradiation for intracranial tumors in children under the age of two. Int J Radiat Oncol Biol Phys 1981; 7: 727–36.

27 Palmer S, Goloubeva O, Reddick W, et al. Patterns of intellectual development among survivors of pediatric medulloblastoma: a longitudinal analysis. J Clin Oncol 2001; 19: 2302–8.

28 Mulhern RK, Merchant TE, Gajjar A, Reddick WE, Kun LE. Late neurocognitive sequelae in survivors of brain tumors in childhood. Lancet Oncol 2004; 5: 399–408.

29 Mabbott D, Spiegler B, Greenberg M, Rutka J, Hyder D. Serial evaluation of academic and behavioral outcome after treatment with cranial radiation in childhood. J Clin Oncol 2005; 23: 2256–63.

30 Rowland J, Glidewell O, Sibley R. Effects of different forms of central nervous system prophylaxis on neuropsychological function in childhood leukemia. J Clin Oncol 1984; 2: 1327–35.

31 Anderson V, Smibert E, Ekert H, Godber T. Intellectual, educational and behavioural sequelae after cranial irradiation and chemotherapy. Arch Dis Child 1994; 70: 476–83.

32 Goff J, Anderson H, Cooper P. Distractability and memory deficits in long-term survivors of acute lymphoblastic leukemia. Dev Beh Pediatr 1980; 1: 153–63.

33 Mulhern R, White H, Phipps S. Neuropsychological aspects of medical treatments in children with cancer. In: Kreitler S, Ben-Arush M (Eds),. Psychosocial Aspects of Pediatric Oncology. Chichester: Wiley; 2004: 9–41.

34 Dennis M, Hetherington CR, Spiegler BJ. Memory and attention after childhood brain tumors. Med Pediatr Oncol 1998; 1(Suppl 1): 25–33.

35 Schatz J, Kramer J, Ablin A, Matthay K. Processing speed, working memory, and IQ: a developmental model of cognitive deficits following cranial radiation therapy. Neuropsychology 2000; 14: 189–200.

36 Mulhern RK, White H, Phipps S. Neuropsychological outcomes. In Wallace H, Green D (Eds), Late Effects of Childhood Cancer. London: Arnold, 2004: 18–36.

37 Rodgers J, Horrocks J, Britton P, Kernahan J. Attentional ability among survivors of leukaemia. Arch Dis Child 1999; 80: 318–23.

38 Shortman R, McCarter R, Penn A, Lowis S, Stevens M, Sharples P. Attentional performance and its determinants in children with brain tumors and normal controls during the first year after diagnosis. Arch Dis Child 2007; 92 (Suppl I): A95.

39 Langer T, Martus P, Ottensmeier H, Hertzberg H, Beck J, Meier W. CNS late effects after ALL therapy in childhood. Part III: neuropsychological performance in long-term survivors of childhood ALL: impairments if concentration, attention and memory. Med Pediatr Oncol 2002; 38: 320–8.

40 Dennis M, Spiegler BJ, Fitz CR, et al. Brain tumors in children and adolescents–I. Effects on working, associative and serial order memory of IQ, age at tumor onset and age of tumor. Neuropsychologia 1991; 29: 813–27.

41 Rodgers J, Britton P, Kernahan J, et al. Cognitive function after two doses of cranial irradiation for acute lymphoblastic leukaemia. Arch Dis Child 1991; 66: 1245–6.

42 Butler RW, Mulhern RK. Neurocognitive interventions for children and adolescents surviving cancer. J Pediatr Psychol 2005; 30: 65–78.

43 Butler RW. Attentional processes and their remediation in childhood cancer. Med Pediatr Oncol 1998; Suppl 1: 75–8.

44 Waber D, Shapiro B, Carpentieri S, et al.. Excellent therapeutic efficacy and minimal late neurotoxicity in children treated with 18 grays of cranial radiation therapy for high-risk acute lymphoblastic leukemia. Cancer 2001; 92: 15–22.

45 Grill J, Kieffer V, Bulteau C, et al. Long-term intellectual outcome in children with posterior fossa tumors according to radiation doses and volumes. Int J Rad Oncol, Biol Phys 1999; 45: 137–45.

46 Longeway K, Mulhern R, Crisco J, et al. Treatment of meningeal relapse in acute lymphoblastic leukemia, II: a prospective study of intellectual loss specific to CNS relapse and therapy. Am J Ped Hematol Oncol 1990; 12: 45–50.

47 Mulhern RK, Ochs D, Fairclough D. Intellectual and academic achievement status after CNS relapse: a retrospective analysis of 40 children treated for acute lymphoblastic leukemia. J Clin Oncol 1987; 5: 933–40.

48 Ellenberg L, McComb J, Siegel S. Factors affecting outcome in pediatric brain tumor patients. Neurosurgery 1987; 21: 638–44.

49 Jannoun L, Bloom H. Long-term psychological effects in children treated for intracranial tumors. Int J Rad Oncol Biol Phys 1989; 18: 747–53.

50 Mulhern R, Palmer S, Merchant T, et al. Neurocognitive consequences of risk-adapted therapy for childhood medulloblastoma. J Clin Oncol 2005; 23: 5511–9.

51 Radcliffe J, Packer R, Atkins T, et al. Three and four year cognitive outcome in children with non-cortical brain tumors treated with whole-brain radiotherapy. Ann Neurol 1992; 32: 551–4.

52 Duffner PK. Long-term effects of radiation therapy on cognitive and endocrine function in children with leukemia and brain tumors. The Neurologist 2004; 10: 293–310.

53 Armstrong CL, Gyato K, Awadalla AW, Lustig R, Tochner ZA. A critical review of the clinical effects of therapeutic irradiation damage to the brain: the roots of controversy. Neuropsychol Rev 2004; 14: 65–86.

54 Duffner PK, Cohen ME, Myers MH, Heise HW. Survival of children with brain tumors: SEER Program, 1973–1980. Neurology. 1986 Date created: 1986/05/23/ Date completed: 1986/05/23/ Date revised: 2004/11/17/; 36: 597–601.

55 Moore BD, Ater JL, Copeland DR. Improved neuropsychological outcome in children with brain tumors diagnosed during infancy and treated without cranial irradiation. J Child Neurol 1992; 7: 281–90.

56 Reimers TS, Ehrenfels S, Mortensen EL, et al. Cognitive deficits in long-term survivors of childhood brain tumors: identification of predictive factors. Med Pediatr Oncol 2003; 40: 26–34.

57 Rønning C, Sundet K, Due-Tønnessen B, Lundar T, Helseth E. Persistent cognitive dysfunction secondary to cerebellar injury in patients treated for posterior fossa tumors in childhood. Pediatr Neurosurg 2005; 41: 15–21.

58 Kun LE, Mulhern RK, Crisco JJ. Quality of life in children treated for brain tumors. Intellectual, emotional, and academic function. J Neurosurg 1983; 58: 1–6.

59 Armstrong TS, Kanusky JT, Gilbert MR. Seize the moment to learn about epilepsy in people with cancer. Clin J Oncol Nurs 2003; 7: 163–9.

60 Recht LD, Glanz M. Neoplastic diseases. In: Engle J, Pedly TA (Eds), Epilepsy: A Comprehensive Textbook. Philadelphia: Lippincott-Raven Publishers, 1997: 2579–80.

61 Duffner P. Long-term neurologic consequences of CNS therapy. In: Wallace H, Green D (Eds), Late Effects of Childhood Cancer. London: Arnold, 2004: 5–17.

62 Skinner R, Pearson AD, Amineddine HA, et al. Ototoxicity of cis-platinum in children and adolescents. Br J Cancer 1990; 61: 927–31.

63 Bertolini P, Lassalle M, Mercier G, et al. Platinum compound-related ototoxicity in children: long-term follow-up reveals continuous worsening of hearing loss. J Pediatr Hematol Oncol 2004; 26: 649–55.

64 Lanvers-Kaminsky C, Krefeld B, Dinnesen AG, et al. Continuous or repeated prolonged cisplatin infusions in children: a prospective study on ototoxicity, platinum concentrations, and standard serum parameters. Pediatr Blood Cancer 2006; 47: 183–93.

65 Kretschmar CS, Warren MP, Lavally BL, et al. Ototoxicity of preradiation cisplatin for children with central nervous system tumors. J Clin Oncol 1990; 8: 1191–8.

66 Schell MJ, McHaney VA, Green AA, et al. Hearing loss in children and young adults receiving cisplatin with or without prior cranial irradiation. J Clin Oncol 1989; 7: 754–60.

67 Coggle JE. Biological Effects of Radiation, 2nd edn. London: Taylor and Francis, 1983.

68 Ash P. The influence of radiation on fertility in man. Br J Radiol 1980; 53: 271–8.

69 Hawkins MM, Draper GJ, Kingston JE. Incidence of second primary tumors among childhood cancer survivors. Br J Cancer 1987; 56: 339–47.

70 Constine LS, Woolf PD, Cann D, et al. Hypothalamic-pituitary dysfunction after radiation for brain tumors. N Engl J Med 1993; 328: 87–94.

71 Olshan JS, Gubernick J, Packer RJ, et al. The effects of adjuvant chemotherapy on growth in children with medulloblastoma. Cancer 1992 Oct 1; 70: 2013–7.

72 Clayton PE, Shalet SM. Dose dependency of time of onset of radiation-induced growth hormone deficiency. J Pediatr 1991; 118: 226–8.

73 Shalet S, Fairhall K, Sparks E, Hendry J, Robinson I. Radiosensitivity of hypothalamo-pituitary (HP) function in the rat is time and dose dependent. Horm Res [Abstr] 1999; 51(Suppl 2): P103.

74 Dattani MT, Robinson IC. The molecular basis for developmental disorders of the pituitary gland in man. Clin Genet 2000; 57: 337–46.

75 Richards GE, Wara WM, Grumbach MM, Kaplan SL, Sheline GE, Conte FA. Delayed onset of hypopituitarism: sequelae of therapeutic irradiation of central nervous system, eye, and middle ear tumors. J Pediatr 1976; 89: 553–9.

76 Shalet SM, Beardwell CG, Jones PH, Pearson D. Growth hormone deficiency after treatment of acute leukaemia in children. Arch Dis Child 1976; 51: 489–93.

77 Achermann JC, Hindmarsh PC, Brook CG. The relationship between the growth hormone and insulin-like growth factor axis in long-term survivors of childhood brain tumors. Clin Endocrinol (Oxf) 1998; 49: 639–45.

78 Spoudeas HA, Wallace WH, Walker D. Is germ cell harvest and storage justified in minors treated for cancer? BMJ 2000; 320: 316.

79 Crowne EC, Moore C, Wallace WH, et al. A novel variant of growth hormone (GH) insufficiency following low dose cranial irradiation. Clin Endocrinol 1992; 36: 59–68.

80 Littley MD, Shalet SM, Morgenstern GR, Deakin DP. Endocrine and reproductive dysfunction following fractionated total body irradiation in adults. Q J Med 1991; 78: 265–74.

81 Ogilvy-Stuart AL, Clark DJ, Wallace WH, et al. Endocrine deficit after fractionated total body irradiation. Arch Dis Child 1992; 67: 1107–10.

82 Brennan BM, Rahim A, Mackie EM, Eden OB, Shalet SM. Growth hormone status in adults treated for acute lymphoblastic leukaemia in childhood. Clin Endocrinol 1998; 48: 777–83.

83 Achermann JC. The pathophysiology of post-irradiation growth hormone insufficiency [MD Thesis]. London: University of London,1997.

84 Spoudeas HA, Charmandari E, Brook CGD. Hypothalamo-pituitary-adrenal axis integrity after cranial irradiation for childhood posterior fossa tumors . Med Paediatr Oncol 2003; 40: 224–9.

85 Chrousos GP, Poplack D, Brown T, et al. Effects of cranial radiation on hypothalamic-adenohypophyseal function: abnormal growth hormone secretory dynamics. J Clin Endocrinol Metab 1982; 54: 1135–9.

86 Dickinson WP, Berry DH, Dickinson L, et al. Differential effects of cranial radiation on growth hormone response to arginine and insulin infusion. J Pediatr 1978; 92: 754–7.

87 Lustig RH, Schriock EA, Kaplan SL, Grumbach MM. Effect of growth hormone-releasing factor on growth hormone release in children with radiation-induced growth hormone deficiency. Pediatrics 1985; 76: 274–9.

88 Spoudeas HA. The evolution of growth hormone neurosecretory disturbance during high dose cranial irradiation and chemotherapy for childhood brain tumors [MD Thesis]. London: University of London, 1995.

89 Hall JE, Martin KA, Whitney HA, et al. Potential for fertility with replacement of hypothalamic gonadotropin-releasing hormone in

long term female survivors of cranial tumors. J Clin Endocrinol Metab 1994; 79: 1166–72.

90 Ogilvy-Stuart AL, Stirling HF, Kelnar CJ, et al. Treatment of radiation-induced growth hormone deficiency with growth hormone-releasing hormone. Clin Endocrinol 1997; 46: 571–8.

91 Chiarenza A, Lempereur L, Palmucci T, et al. Responsiveness of irradiated rat anterior pituitary cells to hypothalamic releasing hormones is restored by treatment with growth hormone. Neuroendocrinology 2000; 72: 392–9.

92 Marky I, Mellander L, Lannering B, Albertsson-Wikland K. A longitudinal study of growth and growth hormone secretion in children during treatment for acute lymphoblastic leukemia. Med Pediatr Oncol 1991; 19: 258–64.

93 Moell C, Garwicz S, Westgren U, Wiebe T, Albertsson-Wikland K. Suppressed spontaneous secretion of growth hormone in girls after treatment for acute lymphoblastic leukaemia. Arch Dis Child 1989 Feb; 64: 252–8.

94 Livesey EA, Hindmarsh PC, Brook CG, et al. Endocrine disorders following treatment of childhood brain tumors. Br J Cancer 1990; 61: 622–5.

95 Packer RJ. Clinical Trials Report. Curr Neurol Neurosci Rep 2001; 1: 135–6.

96 Nivot S, Benelli C, Clot JP, et al. Nonparallel changes of growth hormone (GH) and insulin-like growth factor-I, insulin-like growth factor binding protein-3, and GH-binding protein, after craniospinal irradiation and chemotherapy. J Clin Endocrinol Metab 1994; 78: 597–601.

97 Tedeschi B, Spadoni GL, Sanna ML, et al. Increased chromosome fragility in lymphocytes of short normal children treated with recombinant human growth hormone. Hum Genet 1993; 91: 459–63.

98 Zadik Z, Estrov Z, Karov Y, Hahn T, Barak Y. The effect of growth hormone and IGF-I on clonogenic growth of hematopoietic cells in leukemic patients during active disease and during remission–a preliminary report. J Pediatr Endocrinol 1993; 6: 79–83.

99 Fradkin JE, Mills JL, Schonberger LB, et al. Risk of leukemia after treatment with pituitary growth hormone. JAMA 1993; 270: 2829–32.

100 Swerdlow AJ, Reddingius RE, Higgins CD, et al. Growth hormone treatment of children with brain tumors and risk of tumor recurrence. J Clin Endocrinol Metab 2000; 85: 4444–9.

101 Redman GP, Shu S, Norris D. Leukaemia and growth hormone. Lancet 1988; 331: 1314.

102 Kiess W, Doerr H, Eisl E, Butenandt O, Belohradsky BH. Lymphocyte subsets and natural-killer activity in growth hormone deficiency. N Engl J Med 1986; 314: 321.

103 Torosian MH, Donoway RB. Growth hormone inhibits tumor metastasis. Cancer 1991; 67: 2280–3.

104 ter Maaten JC. Should we start and continue growth hormone (GH) replacement therapy in adults with GH deficiency? Ann Med 2000; 32: 452–61.

105 Jakacki RI, Goldwein JW, Larsen RL, et al. Cardiac dysfunction following spinal irradiation during childhood. J Clin Oncol 1993; 11: 1033–8.

106 Swerdlow AJ, Higgins CD, Adlard P, Preece MA. Risk of cancer in patients treated with human pituitary growth hormone in the UK, 1959–85: a cohort study. Lancet 2002; 360: 273–7.

107 Packer RJ, Boyett JM, Janss AJ, et al. Growth hormone replacement therapy in children with medulloblastoma: use and effect on tumor control. J Clin Oncol 2001 19: 480–7.

108 Ogilvy-Stuart AL, Clayton PE, Shalet SM. Cranial irradiation and early puberty. J Clin Endocrinol Metab 1994; 78: 1282–6.

109 Clayton PE, Shalet SM, Price DA, Campbell RH. Testicular damage after chemotherapy for childhood brain tumors. J Pediatr 1988; 112: 922–6.

110 Clayton PE, Shalet SM, Price DA, Jones PH. Ovarian function following chemotherapy for childhood brain tumors. Med Pediatr Oncol 1989; 17: 92–6.

111 Mills JL, Fears TR, Robison LL, Nicholson HS, Sklar CA, Byrne J. Menarche in a cohort of 188 long-term survivors of acute lymphoblastic leukemia. J Pediatr 1997; 131: 598–602.

112 Odame I, Reilly JJ, Gibson BE, Donaldson MD. Patterns of obesity in boys and girls after treatment for acute lymphoblastic leukaemia. Arch Dis Child 1994; 71: 147–9.

113 Randeva HS, Murray RD, Lewandowski K, O'Hare P, Brabant G, Hillhouse EW, et al. Effects of growth hormone on parts of the leptin system. J Endocrinol 2000; 164(Suppl): P135.

114 Crowne EC, Wallace WH, Gibson S, Moore CM, White A, Shalet SM. Adrenocorticotrophin and cortisol secretion in children after low dose cranial irradiation. Clin Endocrinol 1993; 39: 297–305.

115 Tiulpakov AN, Mazerkina NA, Brook CG, Hindmarsh PC, Peterkova VA, Gorelyshev SK. Growth in children with craniopharyngioma following surgery. Clin Endocrinol 1998; 49: 733–8.

116 Smith DK, Sarfeh J, Howard L. Truncal vagotomy in hypothalamic obesity. Lancet 1983; 1: 1330–1.

117 Lustig RH, Rose SR, Burghen GA, et al. Hypothalamic obesity caused by cranial insult in children: altered glucose and insulin dynamics and reversal by a somatostatin agonist. J Pediatr 1999; 135: 162–8.

118 Reilly JJ, Ventham JC, Ralston JM, Donaldson M, Gibson B. Reduced energy expenditure in preobese children treated for acute lymphoblastic leukemia. Pediatr Res 1998; 44: 557–62.

119 Gelding SV, Taylor NF, Wood PJ, et al. The effect of growth hormone replacement therapy on cortisol-cortisone interconversion in hypopituitary adults: evidence for growth hormone modulation of extrarenal 11 beta-hydroxysteroid dehydrogenase activity. Clin Endocrinol 1998; 48: 153–62.

120 Kingma A, Van Dommelen R, Mooyaart E, Wlimink J, Deelman B, Kamps WA. No major cognitive impairment in young children with acute lymphoblastic leukemia using chemotherapy only: a prospective longitudinal study. J Pediatr Hematol Oncol 2002; 24: 106–14.

121 Montour P, Kuehn S, Keene D, et al. Cognitive changes in children treated for acute lymphoblastic leukemia with chemotherapy only according to the pediatric oncology group 9605 protocol. J Child Neurol 2005; 20: 129–33.

122 Copeland D, Moore B, Francis D, Jaffe N, Culbert S. Neuropsychologic effects of chemotherapy on children with cancer: a longitudinal study. J Clin Oncol 1996; 14: 2826–35.

123 Espy K, Moore I, Kaufmann P, et al. Chemotherapeutic CNS prophylaxis and neuropsychologic change in children with acute lymphoblastic leukemia: a prospective study. J Pediatr Psychol 2001; 26: 1–9.

124 Mennes M, Stiers P, Vandenbussche E, et al. Attention and information processing in survivors of childhood acute lymphoblastic leukemia treated with chemotherapy only. Pediatr Blood Cancer 2005; 44: 478–86.

125 Kaleita T, Reaman G, MacLean W, Sather H, Whitt J. Neurodevelopmental outcome of infants with acute lymphoblastic leukemia: a children's cancer group report. Cancer 1999; 85: 1859–65.

126 Brown RT, Madan S, Walco GA, et al. Cognitive and academic late effects among children previously treated for acute lymphoblastic leukemia receiving chemotherapy and CNS prophylaxis. J Pediatr Psychol 1998; 23: 333–40.

127 Kirk JA, Raghupathy P, Stevens MM, et al. Growth failure and growth-hormone deficiency after treatment for acute lymphoblastic leukaemia. Lancet 1987; 1: 190–3.

128 Waber D, Carpentieri S, Klar Nea. Cognitive sequelae in children treated for acute lymphoblastic leukaemia with dexamethasone or prednisone. J Ped Hematol Oncol 2000; 22: 206–13.

129 Barr RD, Simpson T, Whitton A, Rush B, Furlong W, Feeny DH. Health-related quality of life in survivors of tumors of the central nervous system in childhood – a preference-based approach to measurement in a cross-sectional study. Eur J Cancer 1999; 35: 248–55.

130 Eiser C, Morse R. A review of measures of quality of life for children with chronic illness. Arch Dis Child 2001; 84: 205–11.

131 Varni J, Burwinkle T, Seid M, Skarr D. The PedsQL 4.0 as a pediatric population health measure: feasibility, reliability and validity. Ambul Pediatr 2003; 3: 329–41.

132 Gill T, Feinstein A. A critical appraisal of the quality of life measurements. JAMA. 1994; 272: 619–26.

133 World Health Organization. World Health Organization Constitution. Geneva: World Health Organization, 1947.

134 Tao ML, Parsons SK. Quality-of-life assessment in pediatric brain tumor patients and survivors: lessons learned and challenges to face. J Clin Oncol 2005; 23: 5424–6.

135 Holmbeck G, Li S, Schurman J, Friedman D, Coakley R. Collecting and managing multisource and multimethod data in studies of pediatric populations. J Pediatr Psychol 2002; 27: 5–18.

136 Varni JW, Setoguchi Y. Screening for behavioral and emotional disorders in children and adolescents with congenital or acquired limb deficiencies. Am J Dis Child 1992; 146: 103–7.

137 Chang P, Yeh C. Agreement between child self-report and parent proxy-report to evaluate quality of life in children with cancer. Psycho-oncology 2005; 14: 125–34.

138 Bhat SR, Goodwin TL, Burwinkle TM, et al. Profile of daily life in children with brain tumors: an assessment of health-related quality of life. J Clin Oncol 2005; 23: 5493–500.

139 Glaser A, Rashid N, Chin Lynn U, Walker D. School behaviour and health status after central nervous system tumors. Br J Cancer 1997; 67: 643–50.

140 Meeske K, Katz ER, Palmer SN, Burwinkle T, Varni JW. Parent proxy-reported health-related quality of life and fatigue in pediatric patients diagnosed with brain tumors and acute lymphoblastic leukemia. Cancer 2004; 101: 2116–25.

141 Glaser A, Kennedy C, Punt J, Walker D. Standardized quantitative assessment of brain tumor survivors treated within clinical trials in childhood. Int J Cancer Suppl 1999; 12: 77–82.

142 Feeny D, Torrance G, Furlong W. Health Utilities Index. In: Spilker B, (Ed.), Quality of Life and Pharmacoeconomics in Clinical Trials. 2nd edn. Philadelphia: Lippincott-Raven Press, 1996: 239–52.

143 Foreman NK, Faestel PM, Pearson J, Disabato J, Poole M, Wilkening G, et al. Health status in 52 long-term survivors of pediatric brain tumors. J Neurooncol 1999; 41: 47–53.

144 Eiser C. Quality of life. In Wallace H, Green D (Eds), Late Effects of Childhood Cancer. London: Arnold, 2004: 335–49.

145 Apajasalo M, Sintonen H, Simes M, et al. Health related quality of life of adults surviving malignancies in childhood. Eur J Cancer 1996; 32A: 1354–8.

146 Feeny D, Leiper A, Barr R, et al. The comprehensive assessment of health status in survivors of childhood cancer: application to high-risk acute lymphoblastic leukaemia. Br J Cancer 1993; 67: 1047–52.

147 Moe P, Holen A, Glomstein A, Madsen B, et al. Long term survival and quality of life in patients treated with a national ALL protocol 15–20 years later: IDM/HDM and late effects? Pediatr Hematol Oncol 1997; 14: 54–62.

148 Barrera M, Shaw A, Speechley K, Maunsell E, Pogany L. Educational and social late effects of childhood cancer and related clinical, personal and familial characteristics. Cancer 2005; 15: 1751–60.

149 Langeveld N, Ubbink M, Last B, Grootenhuis M, Voûte P, De Haan R. Educational achievement, employment and living situation in long-term young adult survivors of childhood cancer in the Netherlands. Psycho-Oncology 2003; 12: 213–25.

150 Lannering B, Marky I, Lundberg A, Olsson E. Long term sequelae after pediatric brain tumors: their effect on disability and quality of life. Med Pediatr Oncol 1990; 18: 304–10.

151 Tebbi C, Bromberg C, Piedmonte M. Long-term vocational adjustment of cancer patients diagnosed during adolescence. Cancer 1989; 63: 213–8.

152 De Boer AGEM, Verbeek JHAM, Van Dijk FJH. Adult survivors of childhood cancer and unemployment: a meta-analysis. Cancer 2006; 107: 1–11.

153 Mostow E, Bryne J, Connolly R, Mulvihill J. Quality of life in long term survivors of CNS tumors of childhood and adolescence. J Clin Oncol 1991; 9: 592–9.

154 Green D, Zevon M, Hall B. Achievement of life goals by adult survivors of modern treatment for childhood cancer. Cancer 1991; 67: 206–13.

155 Nagarajan R, Neglia J, Clohisy D, et al. Education, employment, insurance, and marital status among 694 survivors of pediatric lower extremity bone tumors: a report from the childhood cancer survivors survey. Cancer 2003; 97: 2554–64.

156 Hays D, Landsverk J, Sallan S, et al. Educational, occupational, and insurance status of childhood cancer survivors in their fourth and fifth decades of life. J Clin Oncol 1992; 10: 1397–406.

157 Macedoni LM, Jereb B, Todorovski L. Long-term sequelae in children treated for brain tumors: impairments, disability, and handicap. Pediatr Hematol Oncol 2003; 20: 89–101.

158 Hill J, Kodryn H, Mackie E, McNally R, Eden T. Adult psychosocial functioning following childhood cancer: the different roles of sons' and daughters' relationships with their fathers and mothers. J Child Psychol Psychiatry 2003; 44: 752–62.

159 Lackner H, Benesch M, Schagerl S, Kerbl R, Schwinger W, Urban C. Prospective evaluation of late effects after childhood cancer therapy with a follow-up over 9 years. Eur J Pediatr 2000; 159: 750–8.

160 Ness KK, Mertens AC, Hudson MM, et al. Limitations on physical performance and daily activities among long-term survivors of childhood cancer. Ann Intern Med 2005; 143: 639–47.

161 Clayton PE, Shalet SM, Morris-Jones PH, Price DA. Growth in children treated for acute lymphoblastic leukaemia. Lancet 1988; 1: 460–2.

162 Crofton PM, Ahmed SF, Wade JC, et al. Effects of intensive chemotherapy on bone and collagen turnover and the growth hormone axis in children with acute lymphoblastic leukemia. J Clin Endocrinol Metab 1998; 83: 3121–9.

163 Hokken-Koelega AC, van Doorn JW, Hahlen K, Stijnen T, de Muinck Keizer-Schrama SM, Drop SL. Long-term effects of

treatment for acute lymphoblastic leukemia with and without cranial irradiation on growth and puberty: a comparative study. Pediatr Res 1993; 33: 577–82.

164 Wingard JR, Plotnick LP, Freemer CS, et al. Growth in children after bone marrow transplantation: busulfan plus cyclophosphamide versus cyclophosphamide plus total body irradiation. Blood 1992; 79: 1068–73.

165 Robson H, Anderson E, Eden OB, et al. Chemotherapeutic agents used in the treatment of childhood malignancies have direct effects on growth plate chondrocyte proliferation. J Endocrinol 1998; 157: 225–35.

166 Robson H, Anderson E, Eden O, et al. Glucocorticoid pretreatment reduces the cytotoxic effects of a variety of DNA-damaging agents on rat tibial growth-plate chondrocytes in vitro. Cancer Chemother Pharmacol 1998; 42: 171–6.

167 Schriock EA, Schell MJ, Carter M, Hustu O, Ochs JJ. Abnormal growth patterns and adult short stature in 115 long-term survivors of childhood leukemia. J Clin Oncol 1991; 9: 400–5.

168 Davies HA, Didcock E, Didi M, Ogilvy-Stuart A, Wales JK, Shalet SM. Disproportionate short stature after cranial irradiation and combination chemotherapy for leukaemia. Arch Dis Child 1994; 70: 472–5.

169 Probert JC, Parker BR, Kaplan HS. Growth retardation in children after megavoltage irradiation of the spine. Cancer 1973; 32: 634–9.

170 Shalet SM, Gibson B, Swindell R, Pearson D. Effect of spinal irradiation on growth. Arch Dis Child 1987; 62: 461–4.

171 Hartsell WF, Hanson WR, Conterato DJ, Hendrickson FR. Hyperfractionation decreases the deleterious effects of conventional radiation fractionation on vertebral growth in animals. Cancer 1989; 63: 2452–5.

172 Bushhouse S, Ramsay NK, Pescovitz OH, et al. Growth in children following irradiation for bone marrow transplantation. Am J Pediatr Hematol Oncol 1989; 11: 134–40.

173 Papadimitriou A, Urena M, Hamill G, Stanhope R, Leiper AD. Growth hormone treatment of growth failure secondary to total body irradiation and bone marrow transplantation. Arch Dis Child 1991; 66: 689–92.

174 Sanders JE, Pritchard S, Mahoney P, et al. Growth and development following marrow transplantation for leukemia. Blood 1986; 68: 1129–35.

175 Brauner R, Fontoura M, Zucker JM, et al. Growth and growth hormone secretion after bone marrow transplantation. Arch Dis Child 1993; 68: 458–63.

176 Milikic V, Spoudeas HA, Achermann JC, et al. Growth after total body irradiation (TBI): response to growth hormone (GH) therapy. Horm Res 1995; 44(Suppl): 217.

177 Samaan NA, Vieto R, Schultz PN, et al. Hypothalamic, pituitary and thyroid dysfunction after radiotherapy to the head and neck. Int J Radiat Oncol Biol Phys 1982; 8: 1857–67.

178 Devney RB, Sklar CA, Nesbit ME, Jr, et al. Serial thyroid function measurements in children with Hodgkin disease. J Pediatr 1984; 105: 223–7.

179 Green DM, Brecher ML, Yakar D, et al. Thyroid function in pediatric patients after neck irradiation for Hodgkin disease. Med Pediatr Oncol 1980; 8: 127–36.

180 Mauch PM, Weinstein H, Botnick L, et al. An evaluation of long-term survival and treatment complications in children with Hodgkin's disease. Cancer 1983; 51: 925–32.

181 Sutcliffe SB, Chapman R, Wrigley PF. Cyclical combination chemotherapy and thyroid function in patients with advanced Hodgkin's disease. Med Pediatr Oncol 1981; 9: 439–48.

182 Ogilvy-Stuart AL, Shalet SM, Gattamaneni HR. Thyroid function after treatment of brain tumors in children. J Pediatr 1991; 119: 733–7.

183 Sanders JE. The impact of marrow transplant preparative regimens on subsequent growth and development. The Seattle Marrow Transplant Team. Semin Hematol 1991; 28: 244–9.

184 Katsanis E, Shapiro RS, Robison LL, et al. Thyroid dysfunction following bone marrow transplantation: long-term follow-up of 80 pediatric patients. Bone Marrow Transplant 1990; 5: 335–40.

185 Castillo LA, Craft AW, Kernahan J, et al. Gonadal function after 12-Gy testicular irradiation in childhood acute lymphoblastic leukaemia. Med Pediatr Oncol 1990; 18: 185–9.

186 Shalet SM, Tsatsoulis A, Whitehead E, Read G. Vulnerability of the human Leydig cell to radiation damage is dependent upon age. J Endocrinol 1989; 120: 161–5.

187 Wallace WH, Shalet SM, Crowne EC, Morris-Jones PH, Gattamaneni HR. Ovarian failure following abdominal irradiation in childhood: natural history and prognosis. Clin Oncol (R Coll Radiol) 1989; 1: 75–9.

188 Masala A, Faedda R, Alagna S, et al. Use of testosterone to prevent cyclophosphamide-induced azoospermia. Ann Intern Med 1997; 126: 292–5.

189 Thomson AB, Critchley HO, Kelnar CJ, Wallace WH. Late reproductive sequelae following treatment of childhood cancer and options for fertility preservation. Best Pract Res Clin Endocrinol Metab 2002; 16: 311–34.

190 Tsatsoulis A, Shalet SM, Harrison J, Ratcliffe WA, Beardwell CG, Robinson EL. Adrenocorticotrophin (ACTH) deficiency undetected by standard dynamic tests of the hypothalamic-pituitary-adrenal axis. Clin Endocrinol 1988; 28: 225–32.

191 Crowley S, Hindmarsh PC, Holownia P, Honour JW, Brook CG. The use of low doses of ACTH in the investigation of adrenal function in man. J Endocrinol 1991; 130: 475–9.

192 Gilsanz V, Carlson ME, Roe TF, Ortega JA. Osteoporosis after cranial irradiation for acute lymphoblastic leukemia. J Pediatr 1990; 117(2 Pt 1): 238–44.

193 Arikoski P, Komulainen J, Riikonen P, Voutilainen R, Knip M, Kroger H. Alterations in bone turnover and impaired development of bone mineral density in newly diagnosed children with cancer: a 1-year prospective study. J Clin Endocrinol Metab 1999; 84: 3174–81.

194 Sorensen K, Levitt GA, Bull C, Dorup I, Sullivan ID. Late anthracycline cardiotoxicity after childhood cancer: a prospective longitudinal study. Cancer 2003; 97: 1991–8.

195 Sorensen K, Levitt G, Bull C, Chessells J, Sullivan I. Anthracycline dose in childhood acute lymphoblastic leukemia: issues of early survival versus late cardiotoxicity. J Clin Oncol 1997; 15: 61–8.

196 Kremer LC, van Dalen EC, Offringa M, Ottenkamp J, Voute PA. Anthracycline-induced clinical heart failure in a cohort of 607 children: long-term follow-up study. J Clin Oncol 2001; 19: 191–6.

197 van Dalen EC, van der Pal HJ, Kok WE, Caron HN, Kremer LC. Clinical heart failure in a cohort of children treated with anthracyclines: a long-term follow-up study. Eur J Cancer 2006; 42: 3191–8.

198 van Dalen EC, van der Pal HJ, van den Bos C, Kok WE, Caron HN, Kremer LC. Clinical heart failure during pregnancy and delivery in

a cohort of female childhood cancer survivors treated with anthracyclines. Eur J Cancer 2006; 42: 2549–53.

199 Bardi E, Olah AV, Bartyik K, et al. Late effects on renal glomerular and tubular function in childhood cancer survivors. Pediatr Blood Cancer 2004; 43: 668–73.

200 Goren MP. Cisplatin nephrotoxicity affects magnesium and calcium metabolism. Med Pediatr Oncol 2003; 41: 186–9.

201 Skinner R, Cotterill SJ, Stevens MC. Risk factors for nephrotoxicity after ifosfamide treatment in children: a UKCCSG Late Effects Group study. United Kingdom Children's Cancer Study Group. Br J Cancer 2000; 82: 1636–45.

202 Skinner R. Chronic ifosfamide nephrotoxicity in children. Med Pediatr Oncol 2003; 41: 190–7.

203 Talbot L, Howie E, Verduyn C, Gattamaneni HR, Kamaly I, Estlin E. Psychological interventions for children with CNS tumors. Neuro-oncol 2008; 10: 459.

204 Talbot L, Verduyn C, Estlin E. Neuropsychology, education and psychological interventions for children with central nervous system tumors. Arch Dis Child 2007; 92(Suppl I): A94–A5.

205 Talbot L, Verduyn C, Howie E, Estlin E. Neuropsychological interventions in relation to the education of children of children following diagnosis of a tumor of the central nervous system. Childs Nerv Syst 2007; 23: 1074.

206 Mitchell W, Clarke S, Sloper P. Survey of psychosocial support provided by UK paediatric oncology centres. Arch Dis Child 2005; 90: 796–800.

207 NICE. Guidance on Cancer Services: Improving Outcomes in Children and Young People with Cancer: The Manual. London: National Institute for Clinical Excellence, 2005.

23 Palliative Care

Lynda Brook

Department of Pediatric Oncology, Alder Hey Children's Hospital, Liverpool, UK

Introduction

This chapter provides a comprehensive overview of the physical and emotional needs of children with incurable malignancy and their families. The principles of palliative care are discussed and correlated with the needs of the child and family from the point of diagnosis through to cure or end of life. We consider assessment and management of the common physical symptoms and review changes as the child moves towards end of life including planning for end-of-life care, and ensuring optimum symptom management when the enteral route is no longer available. We also consider psychosocial support for the child and family with specific emphasis on end-of-life care (Box 23.1).

Epidemiology

Although approximately 75% of children with malignancy can now be cured, cancer remains the leading cause of death, after trauma, for children in resource-rich countries. An increasing proportion of these children are now dying during active disease-directed therapy [2]. The impact of a child dying during active treatment is no less than when a child dies of progressive incurable disease [3]. But discussions regarding withholding cardiopulmonary resuscitation and hospice care are likely to be held earlier when a child dies of progressive disease than when death is related to a complication of treatment [4].

Reported duration of palliative care varies widely due to differences in definition of the start of palliative care. The shortest duration of palliative care is generally reported in hematological malignancies and the longest with central nervous system (CNS) tumors [5–9].

Children with malignancy represent the single largest diagnostic group of children receiving end-of-life care at home [12, 13]. In areas with an active homecare program between 80% and 88% of children with progressive disease are reported as being cared for at home in the last month of life [5, 11, 14, 15] (Tables 23.1 and 23.2).

Pediatric Hematology and Oncology, 1st edition. Edited by Edward J. Estlin, Richard J. Gilbertson, and Robert F. Wynn. © 2010 Blackwell Publishing Ltd.

Symptoms and their effect on quality of life

Reported incidence of symptoms and suffering may be affected significantly by the type and timing of questioning and the meaning that the child and family attach to the symptoms [11]. Whilst cancer symptoms result in suffering by the children and families they are accepted as an integral part of overcoming cancer and complete symptom relief is never expected [16].

Symptoms in different types of malignancy

Severity of pain and hence requirements for higher doses of analgesia is seen in solid tumors, particularly when there is central or peripheral neuropathic pain [8, 20, 21]. Neurological symptoms, particularly headache, are experienced by almost all children with primary CNS tumors [5, 7]. Children with leukemia and lymphoma are more likely to have problems with bleeding than those with CNS tumors (Tables 23.3 and 23.4).

Principles of palliative care

When does palliative care start?

The scope of palliative care extends from the point of diagnosis [22]. Even if cure is likely, the child and family have to adjust to an uncertain future and the loss of hopes and expectations for the child or young person's life and health [23].

If death is likely or quality of life is poor, the balance between benefits and potential harm from ongoing treatment aimed at cure or prolongation of life will alter. Families may vary in how strongly they wish to pursue treatments aimed at cure or significantly prolonging life. It is imperative that the family and child where possible are helped, through open and honest communication, to make a realistic and informed choice focusing on quality of life, the wishes of child themselves and those of the family [24].

At all times from diagnosis through to end of life, management of distressing symptoms particularly pain, is essential [25].

Introducing the concept of palliative care

Clinicians cite unrealistic expectations of cure by parents (and patients) and family denial as the biggest single barrier to high quality end-of-life care [26], and where both professionals and parents recognize the child's prognosis earlier, discussion of

Box 23.1 What is palliative care for children? [1].

- Palliative care for children is the active total care of the child's body, mind, and spirit and also involves giving support to the family
- It begins when illness is diagnosed and continues regardless of whether or not a child receives treatment directed at the disease
- Healthcare providers must evaluate and alleviate a child's physical, psychological, and social distress
- Effective palliative care requires a broad multidisciplinary approach that includes the family and makes use of available community resources; it can be successfully implemented even if resources are limited
- It can be provided in tertiary care facilities, in community health centres, and even in children's homes
- Life-limiting illness is defined as a condition where premature death is usual.
- Life-threatening illness is one where there is a high probability of premature death due to severe illness but there is a chance of long-term survival to adulthood and would include children receiving treatment for cancer

Table 23.1 Age and place of death for 0–24 year olds dying of cancer in the UK 1995–9 [10].

Place of death	Number of deaths (%)		Total
	0–15 years	16–24 years	
Home	901 (52.2)	448 (30.4)	1349
Hospice	54 (3.1)	139 (9.4)	193
Hospital	747 (43.3)	849 (57.7)	1596
Other	23 (1.3)	36 (2.4)	59

Table 23.2 Factors influencing setting for end-of-life care and place of death in children and young adults with cancer [5, 9–12].

Hospital	Home	Hospice
• Death during active treatment*	• Death following cessation of active treatment	• Death following cessation of active treatment
• Shorter interval between cessation of active treatment and death	• Longer interval between cessation of active treatment and death	• Longer interval between cessation of active treatment and death
• No active home-care or hospice program	• Active home-care program	• Local age-appropriate hospice facilities
		• Hospice facilities that accept patients on chemotherapy
• Leukemia or lymphoma	• Solid tumor	• Primary central nervous system tumor
• Bone marrow transplant patients		
• Older age at time of death	• Younger age at time of death	• Older age at time of death
• Lower social class of area or high childhood poverty		
• Late or absent realization and acceptance of end of life	• Early realization and acceptance of end of life	• Early realization and acceptance of end of life

*Defined at treatment aimed at cure or prolonging life.

Table 23.3 Cumulative incidence of physical symptoms in children with malignancy receiving palliative care [5, 7, 11, 16–19].

Rank	Incidence	%	Suffering	%
1	Weakness	91	Fatigue	80
2	Fatigue	88	Lack of mobility	76
3	Pain	88	Pain	69
4	Poor appetite	74	Poor appetite	61
5	Weight loss	67	Dyspnea	48
6	Lack of mobility	62	Problems with swallowing	44
7	Dyspnea	58	Problems with speech	34
8	Nausea and vomiting	56	Problems with micturition	32
9	Sadness/ depression	53	Paralysis	29
10	Constipation	52	Nausea and vomiting	23
11	Drowsiness	46	Constipation or diarrhea	20
12	Problems with speech	42		
13	Headache	40		
14	Excess respiratory tract secretions	40		
15	Anemia	39		

Table 23.4 Treatment of symptoms and response to treatment [5, 7, 11].

Rank	Most likely to be treated	%	Rank	Most likely to respond	%
1	Bleeding	91.7	1	Itch	83.3
2	Pain	90.8	2	Pain	58.4
3	Itch	85.7	3	Vomiting	36.5
4	Constipation	85.2	4	Nausea	36.3
5	Dyspnea	79.1	5	Constipation	36.1
6	Vomiting	77.0	6	Fatigue	24.9
7	Nausea	76.8	7	Dyspnea	18.7
8	Poor mobility	76.2	8	Weakness	18
9	Insomnia	75	9	Bleeding	16.7
10	Incontinence of urine/ feces	75	10	Poor appetite	14.9
11	Drowsiness	72.7	11	Problems with swallowing	13
12	Poor appetite	52.2	12	Diarrhea	12.0
13	Diarrhea	48.9	13	Weight loss	10
14	Fatigue	26.4	14	Insomnia	9.1
			15	Poor mobility	7.7

palliative care is easier [4]. However, physicians' own death-anxiety is also a factor [27]. Parents may construe palliative care negatively as an independent process at the end of their child's lives rather than as a component of a wider and continuous process [28]. Accordingly, an integrated care model is required [29], incorporating open and honest communication throughout [30] and providing cancer directed, symptom directed, and supportive care throughout the child's illness [31].

Role of palliative chemotherapy and radiotherapy

Some children and families may wish to explore the possibility of phase 1 or 2 trials in the hope of response to treatment, altruism, or symptom relief [32]. However, children dying of treatment-related complications not infrequently have refractory or relapsed disease, usually die in hospital and have a poorer quality of life in the last month before death than those who die of progressive disease [11, 15]. Palliative chemotherapy must not be an opportunity for collusion between professional and family, delaying access to essential symptom management, psychosocial and hospice [33], and a decision that families later regret [15].

Principles of symptom management (Boxes 23.2 and 23.3 and Figure 23.1)

1 *Assessment* of problems and their impact on quality of life including self report from the child wherever possible, supported by information from parents and nursing staff. Specific questioning to identify the 'most troublesome' symptom reveals additional information in up to one-third of cancer patients and assists in developing shared priorities for symptom management [34].

Box 23.2 Specific issues in pediatric palliative care.

- Small number of children
- Spread over a large geographical area
- Social, educational, and developmental needs of the child or young person
- Few professionals have significant experience in pediatric palliative care; many will never have looked after a dying child before
- Most UK General Practitioners (family doctors) will only look after a child dying at home once or twice in their entire career
- On average a nurse on a UK children's ward will look after a dying child once every 3–5 years
- Large fluctuations in demand for services particularly for end-of-life care at home

---

Box 23.3 Priorities for effective symptom management.

- Symptoms controlled to allow restful sleep
- Symptoms controlled during daytime waking hours
- Symptoms controlled on movement/during activity

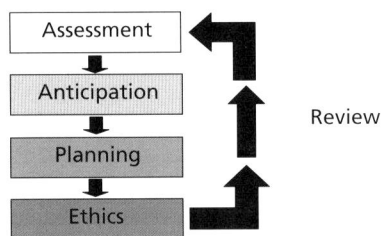

Figure 23.1 A model for assessment and decision making in palliative care.

2 *Anticipation* of recurrence of previously treated symptom and problems or development of new problems: often these can be predicted from known pathology and previous symptoms.

3 *Planning* for managing an increase in severity of current symptoms and occurrence of new problems.

4 *Ethics:* to evaluate carefully the potential risks and benefits of any treatment proposed ensuring that the primary aim is achieving quality of life rather than prolonging life at all costs; the need to evaluate carefully the potential risks and benefits of any treatment option is paramount.

5 *Review:* regularly and up to several times a day to evaluate the effects of symptom management, identify new problems and build the family's trust and confidence in supporting professionals.

Teamwork and co-ordination of care

Caring for a dying child is stressful for the multidisciplinary team as well as the family. In the hospital setting professionals will have established significant relationships with the child and family whereas in the primary care setting the family doctor may have had little contact with the child or family since diagnosis [35]. Professionals frequently report feeling unskilled and unsupported when providing palliative care for children [36] (Box 23.4).

Box 23.4 Effective team working in pediatric oncology palliative care [37–41].

- Ensure that each member of the team is aware of other professionals in the extended team and how to contact them
- Clear but flexible delineation of roles, responsibilities, and lines of accountability
- Knowledge of and adherence to professional boundaries
- Frequent reciprocal communication at all levels
- Regular team meetings for reflection, planning of care, and sharing of experiences
- Clear team leadership
- Meetings with doctors, nurses, and other professionals after the death
- Identify an appropriate resource for specialist palliative care advice before a crisis is reached

---

Pain (Box 23.5)

Classification of pain
- Etiology and pathophysiology.
- Timing (incident pain).
- Psychological distress (and other factors that influence pain threshold).

Etiology and pathophysiology
Nociceptive pain
Nociceptive pain due to activation of sensory nerve endings by noxious stimuli.

Box 23.5 Definitions of pain.

'Pain is whatever the patient says hurts'
  'Pain is an unpleasant sensory and emotional experience associated with actual or potential tissue damage or described in terms of such damage' (International Association for the Study of Pain)

Visceral pain:
- Characterized by deep aching sensations.
- Commonly referred, poorly localized and associated with nausea.

Muscle spasm:
- Spasmodic cramping pain.
- Often associated with tenderness, stiffness, or limitation of movement.

Bony pain:
- Well localized aching pain.
- Generally corresponding to underlying bone.
- Exacerbated by moving or weight bearing.

Neuropathic pain
Pain due to abnormal function of peripheral or central neurons. This may be due to compression, for example by tumor or damage to the nerve itself, for example following amputation.
- Described as burning, stabbing, lancinating or tingling.
- Maybe associated with:
    Allodynia (exacerbation by light touch).
    Abnormal sensation (pain in an area of altered or absent sensation is always neuropathic).

Timing
Acute pain: brief short-lived pain extending over hours to days. Other features:
- Variable intensity.
- May recur.
- Acute concomitants: the child looks pale, clammy, distressed and 'in pain'.

Persistent pain: is persistent over time and extending over days to weeks. Other features:
- Variable intensity.
- No autonomic concomitants.
- Psychomotor inertia [42]: the child appears withdrawn, listless and subdued.

Breakthrough pain (Figure 23.2): transitory exacerbation of pain, often lasting from seconds to minutes, three or four times a day and occurring on a background of otherwise stable chronic pain [43].
- Incident pain: associated with specific precipitating factors.
- End of dose pain: occurring at the end of the dosing interval due to decreasing analgesic levels.
- Idiopathic: no clear precipitant.

Assessment
Pain is multidimensional, having physical psychological social and spiritual aspects. Thorough assessment and regular re-assessment is the key to effective pain management.

History (Table 23.5)
- Talk to the child's parents or carers but remember to question the child where possible.
- Remember there may be multiple pains.

Background pain

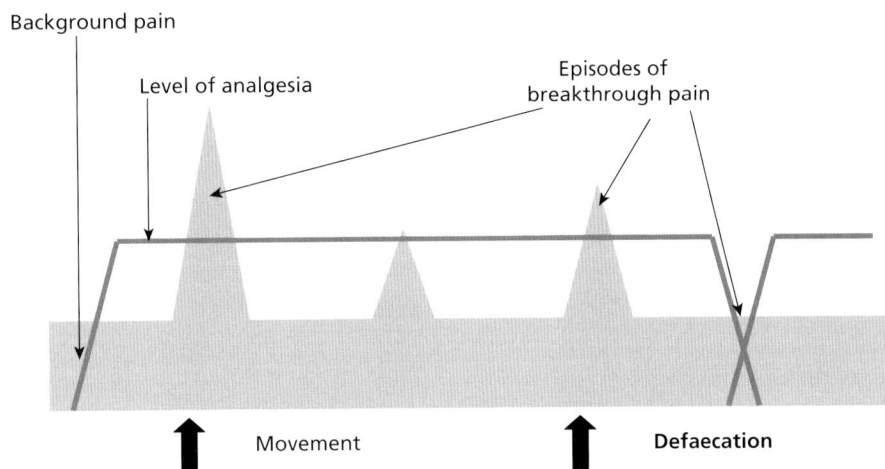

Figure 23.2 Classification of breakthrough pain.

Table 23.5 Factors that influence pain threshold.

Decreased pain threshold	Increased pain threshold
Discomfort	Relief of other symptoms
Insomnia	Sleep
Fatigue	Sympathy
Anxiety	Understanding
Fear	Companionship
Anger	Relaxation
Sadness	Creative activity
Boredom	Reduction in anxiety
Social isolation	Happiness

Table 23.6 Specific aspects of paediatric pain.

Child	Parent	Nurse
Can locate their pain and use self report tools from 3 years	Ratings correspond more closely to patient ratings	Consistently underestimate pain compared with patient or parent
Under-report pain if previous negative consequences	Under-report their child's pain if they are stressed or have not seen their child in severe pain before	Document less than 50% of the pain their patients describe
Evidence of pain experience from neonate onwards: pain tolerance increases with age	May identify non-verbal clues to pain in their child: best source of information on pain in their child	Perception of a child's pain is related to professional background, personal pain experience and physical pathology

• Identify the cause of the pain (if possible).
• Additional information that will also assist in pain management:
  • Location of the pain and radiation
  • Timing of the pain
  • Nature of the pain, e.g. burning, aching, shooting. If necessary use a list of words and ask the patient to choose
  • Effect of analgesia, particularly strong opioids
  • Other factors predisposing, precipitating, or maintaining pain
  • Factors that may alter pain threshold, including other symptoms, psychological, cultural, and social factors (Table 23.5)
  • Coping style
  • Severity of the pain, using a validated pain rating scale wherever possible, and the effect of pain on quality of life

Examination
• Careful observation can reveal a lot about a child's pain: a child may be playing, active, or asleep and still be in pain.
• Look, feel, move.
• Signs of pathology.
• Sensory changes.
• Atrophy or muscle wasting.

Response to analgesia
• *Opioid responsive pain:* somatic visceral pain, e.g. hepatic capsule pain.
• *Opioid semi-responsive pain:* relieved by a combination of opioid and co-analgesic, e.g. neuropathic pain, pain of raised intracranial pressure, bone pain, local inflammation.
• *Opioid resistant pain:* little or no analgesic effect despite opioids in appropriate doses, e.g. muscle spasm, some neuropathic pain.

Pain rating scales

Pain rating scales provide quantitative information to evaluate the severity of pain and the response to treatment [44] but must be used in conjunction with a detailed pain history and examination.

Self report should be used wherever possible:
• Pictorial rating scales in children over 4 or 5 years, e.g. The Oucher [45]

• Numerical rating scales, a visual analogue scale, or a colour rating scale in older children

When self report is not possible the DEGR [42] has been designed and specifically validated for use in children aged 2–6 years with persistent cancer pain.

Pain management (Box 23.6)

As pain is a complex multidimensional entity a combination of pharmacological and non-pharmacological approaches are required for optimum pain management.

Pharmacological management of pain (Box 23.7)

The WHO analgesic ladder provides useful guidance on the selection of analgesics according to efficacy and severity of pain [46] (Figure 23.3). If the pain is not adequately controlled, an appro-priate analgesic from the next 'step' should be substituted. Although it is usual to start with 'step 1' analgesics, severe cancer pain may sometimes require immediate use of a strong opioid.

Analgesics

Step 1:

• Paracetamol: enteral, intravenous and rectal preparations.
• Non steroidal anti-inflamatory drugs: wide range of drugs with varying potency and routes of administration.

Box 23.6 Six steps to effective pain management in palliative care.

1 Take a detailed pain history and undertake appropriate physical examination

2 Identify specific problems in the assessment of pain in children

3 Classify the cause of pain according to the mechanism, timing, and psychological factors

4 Implement appropriate management strategy for pain including treating the pain itself and where possible the underlying cause

5 Assess the response to pain management at regular intervals

6 Anticipate and plan for future changes over time

Box 23.7 Principles of prescription and administration of analgesia in palliative care.

1 By the WHO analgesic ladder (Figure 23.3)
  • Appropriate use of co-analgesia

2 By the clock
  • Regular analgesia preferably using a sustained-release preparation to facilitate once or twice daily dosing
  • As required immediate release analgesia available for breakthrough pain

3 By the most appropriate route
  • The most simple, effective, and least painful route
  • Consider rectal, transdermal, or subcutaneous routes if the enteral route is unavailable or unreliable

4 By the child
  • Doses individualized according to the child's symptoms and pathology
  • Re-assessed regularly
  • There is no ceiling dose for strong opioids in palliative care

---

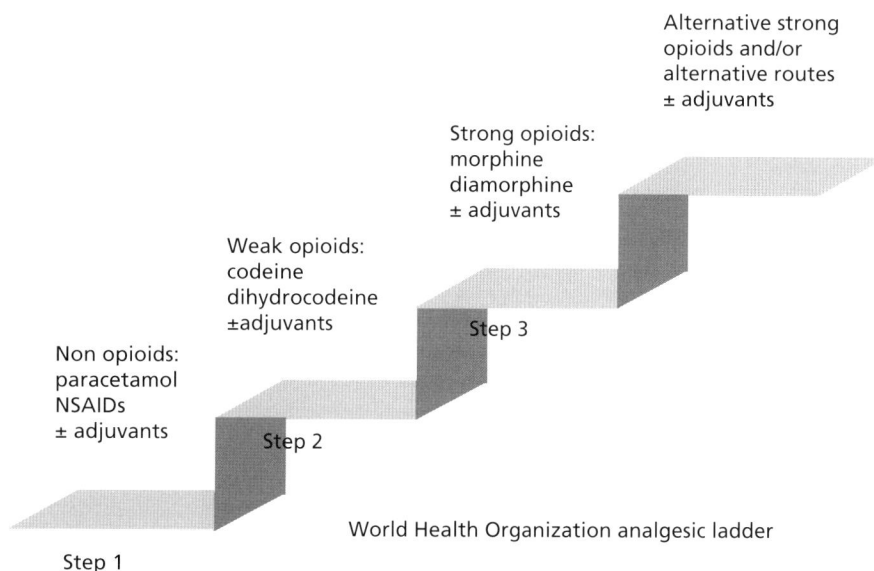

Non opioids:
paracetamol
NSAIDs
± adjuvants

Step 1

Weak opioids:
codeine
dihydrocodeine
±adjuvants

Step 2

Strong opioids:
morphine
diamorphine
± adjuvants

Step 3

Alternative strong
opioids and/or
alternative routes
± adjuvants

World Health Organization analgesic ladder

Figure 23.3 World Health Organization analgesic ladder.

• Cox-2 inhibitors: can be used in thrombocytopenia due to lack of anti-platelet effects.

Step 2:

• Constipation is inevitable with regular weak opioids: a prophylactic stimulant laxative is required.

• Dihydrocodeine: enteral, immediate release, and sustained release preparations; injection for subcutaneous administration.

• Ceiling effect with codeine and dihydrocodeine: additional analgesia is not achieved by increasing the dose above the normal maximum

• Ten percent of Caucasians are poor metabolizers of codeine with corresponding lack of efficacy [47].

Step 3 – strong opioids:

• Frequently required alone or in combination with non-opioid analgesics and adjuvant drugs to provide effective pain relief [48].

• No analgesic ceiling effect.

• No absolute maximum dose.

• Six to 10% of children will require very large doses of strong opioids to obtain good analgesia [8, 20, 21].

• No evidence to suggest that starting or increasing doses of opioids or very high doses of opioids hastens death [49] despite theoretical concerns.

Morphine

Strong opioid of choice for pediatric palliative care due to:

• Extensive experience of this drug [50].

• Range of available preparations including oral immediate and sustained relief, rectal preparations and injection for intravenous or subcutaneous use.

• Availability of pharmacokinetic data: young children (<2 years) eliminate morphine metabolites more slowly but children between 2 and 9 years may eliminate morphine more rapidly than adults [51].

Starting a regular sustained-release preparation and titrating with immediate-release morphine at one-sixth of the total daily dose of sustained-release preparation may achieve pain control more quickly than titrating with immediate-release preparation alone [52]. Use of a sustained-release strong opioid preparation reduces fluctuation in drug levels, reduces the number of doses, improves concordance and minimizes the need for night-time dosing [53]. Immediate-release morphine should be available as required for breakthrough pain.

If breakthrough analgesia is required on average more than twice in a 24-hour period the background sustained release opioid dose and the immediate release opioid dose should be increased in an increment of 30–50% of the previous total daily dose.

Opioid side effects [54]

• *Constipation* is inevitable and prophylactic stimulant laxatives should always be prescribed. Peripherally acting opioid receptor antagonists may provide a specific antidote to opioid-induced constipation [55].

• *Nausea and vomiting* are less common than in adults and routine anti-emetics are not commonly required.

• *Drowsiness and mental clouding* can occur at the start of treatment and sometimes following a dose increase. This almost always resolves within a few days.

• *Itching* is fairly common, particularly in older children [53]. This is a central phenomenon and antihistamines are not effective. Simple emollients or a 5-HT3 antagonist such as ondanestron may be indicated [56].

• *Respiratory depression* is very uncommon in the conscious patient with severe pain and an appropriate dose and rate of increase of strong opioid [57].

• *Nightmares and hallucinations.*

• *Urinary retention* may be a problem particularly after rapid dose escalation. Bethanecol or a peripherally acting opioid receptor antagonist [58] may avoid the need for catheterization.

• *Psychological addiction and tolerance* are not a problem when opioids are used correctly in palliative care.

• *Myoclonus* is an occasional problem particularly with high doses or rapid dose escalation. If dose reduction is not effective or possible, introduction of a low dose benzodiazepine may be effective [59].

Opioid rotation (Box 23.8)

If pain cannot be controlled by morphine and appropriate co-analgesics without unacceptable toxicity it may be necessary to consider rotation to an alternative opioid [60] (Table 23.7). Opioid rotation is a widely practiced method of reducing opioid side effects, increasing efficacy, and reducing the effects of long-term administration of opioids and is thought to be effective because of incomplete cross-tolerance. It is unclear whether the improved outcome following opioid rotation is a true drug effect, or merely improved tolerability as a result of dose reduction [61].

Alternative opioids for breakthrough pain

Immediate-release morphine is the standard for breakthrough pain, the onset of action is 20–30 minutes, and the peak not reached until 1 hour. For some episodes of breakthrough pain, the severity of pain will have significantly subsided before peak

---

Box 23.8 Indications for opioid rotation.

• Intolerable side effects not responsive to dose reduction or treatment of side effect

• Dose-limiting side effects

• Dose escalation or NMDA wind-up pain

• Loss or reduced reliability of the enteral route may also necessitate rotating to an alternative opioid as well as an alternative route

Table 23.7 Options for opioid rotation [62–65].

	Specific indications	Available routes	Approximate potency ratio	Notes
Alfentanil	Renal impairment	Continuous subcutaneous or intravenous infusion only	Potency approximately 30 × that of morphine	Elimination not significantly affected by renal failure. Ultra short acting
Fentanyl	Renal impairment. Loss of the enteral route. Severe constipation with other opioids not responsive to appropriate laxative therapy	Transdermal patch Intravenous infusion	25 µg transdermal fentanyl = 90 mg enteral morphine/24 h	Elimination not significantly affected by renal failure. Transdermal patch not suitable for titration of unstable pain. Time to reach steady state may be longer in children and elimination half life shorter
Methadone	Pain only partially responsive to opioids particularly neuropathic pain. Intolerable adverse effects of morphine	Long half life (12–150 hours) Risk of accumulation and toxicity	Potency ratio varies by up to 50 × depending on dose of morphine or other opioid	Careful titration in a unit familiar with this drug is strongly recommended

analgesic effect, resulting in excess sedation and poor analgesia. Alternative opioids with a more rapid onset of action include fentanyl administered via the oral transmucosal or sublingual routes [66], intranasal diamorphine [67], and sublingual morphine [68].

Co-analgesics and adjuvant approaches
Neuropathic pain
Neuropathic pain is commonly only partially responsive to opioid analgesia [69] and a combination of an opioid, a non-opioid analgesic such as a non-steroidal anti-inflammatory drug (NSAID) [70], and additional co-analgesics are required for optimum pain management [71].
• NSAIDs have demonstrable efficacy in reducing pain and opioid doses, although not specifically in patients with neuropathic pain [70] or in children.
• Tricyclic antidepressants such as amitryptiline have demonstrable analgesic and opioid sparing effects in neuropathic pain [72] including in children [73, 74]. However, up to 20% of patients may experience significant adverse effects.
• Anticonvulsants, specifically gabapentin or carbamazepine, have demonstrable analgesic effects in neuropathic pain [75] including in children [76].

Other adjuvant drugs
Corticosteroids reduce the headache of raised intracranial pressure and neuropathic pain by reduction in peritumor edema [77].
Ketamine is an analgesic at sub-anesthetic doses and the most potent N-methyl D-asparate (NMDA) receptor channel antagonist available for clinical use. Opioid-sparing effects and overall improvement in pain control have been demonstrated in case series of low dose ketamine in children and young adults with cancer [78], but there is currently insufficient randomized controlled trial evidence to confirm these findings [79].

Bone pain
• NSAIDs have theoretical advantage in bone pain due to their peripheral anti-inflammatory effect. Efficacy in reducing pain and opioid doses has been demonstrated, although not specifically in patients with bony metastases [70] or in children.
• Bisphosphonates such as pamidronate and zoledronic acid are effective in reducing pain and risk of fractures from bone metastases in adults [80], but may be less effective than radiotherapy [81].
• Radiotherapy is effective in palliation of pain due to isolated bony metastases [82, 83].

Non-pharmacological approaches to pain management
Psychological factors can exacerbate physical symptoms and reduce effectiveness of coping mechanisms with an adverse effect on quality of life. Non-drug therapies should be an integral part of the management of children's pain, complementing, but not replacing appropriate drug therapy.

Gastrointestinal symptoms

Nausea and vomiting (Table 23.8)
Pathophysiology
Two separate areas in the brain, the chemoreceptor trigger zone (CTZ) and the vomiting center are responsible for vomiting and associated symptoms [84].

Table 23.8 Mechanism of action, etiology, and diagnostic features of nausea and vomiting [84].

Mechanism of action	Etiology	Diagnostic features
Chemical trigger zone (CTZ) stimulation D2, 5HT3 receptors	Chemicals: • Drugs (e.g. opioids, metronidazole) • Metabolites (hypercalcemia, uremia) • Toxins	• Presence of one or more emetogenic drugs or biochemical disturbance • Frequent small volume vomits, nausea, and retching. • Little relief from nausea following vomiting
Vomiting centre (VC) stimulation H1, AChm, 5HT2 receptors	Autonomic afferents: • Stretch receptors in serosae and viscera • Irritated GI mucosa: drugs, infection, RXT Direct stimulation: • Head and neck radiotherapy • Brainstem metastases • Raised intracranial pressure	• Presence of one or more etiological factors • Frequent small volume vomits, variable nausea, and retching. • Raised intracranial pressure also associated with vomiting particularly first thing in the morning often with little associated nausea
Higher centre stimulation 5HT GABA receptors	• Pain • Fear • Anxiety • Memory	• Presence of one or more etiological factors • May include anticipatory nausea and vomiting or nausea and vomiting associated with a particular situation or occurrence
Mechanical causes Gastric stasis May not be mediated by VC (less nausea)	• Reduced motility from drugs (amitriptyline, hyoscine, opioids) • Local tumor causing (partial) outflow obstruction	• Infrequent large volume vomiting • Most frequently in the evenings • Significant relief from nausea following vomit
Intrinsic GI mucosal damage 5HT3 receptors	GI inflammation: • Palliative chemotherapy • Radiotherapy • Gastritis	• Presence of one or more etiological factors • Frequent small volume vomits, nausea, and retching • Little relief from nausea following vomiting

Management (Tables 23.9 and 23.10)

Pharmacological management based on knowledge of the most important pathophysiological mechanisms for emetogenesis and the relevant neurotransmitters is suggested [84–86] but the evidence to support this approach has been questioned [87]. Evidence to support the use of anti-emetics in children is almost exclusively limited to post-operative nausea and vomiting, or nausea and vomiting associated with cancer chemotherapy.

Constipation

There is a wide range in normal bowel habit and constipation cannot simply be defined in terms of stool frequency.

Pathophysiology (Table 23.11)

Assessment involves identifying any potentially treatable underlying cause(s) and baseline assessment of the child's normal pattern of bowel action. There is insufficient evidence to support the preferential administration of one laxative above another in

cancer palliative care [90]; a regime based on underlying pathophysiological mechanisms is recommended.

Anorexia and cachexia

Cancer cachexia is a complex syndrome characterized by progressive tissue nutritional depletion and decreased nutrient intake manifest as anorexia (loss of appetite) and profound weight loss.

Pathophysiology

The syndrome is a complex interaction between host and the tumor resulting in [91, 92]:
• Tumor production of catabolic mediator.
• An aberrant inflammatory response.
• Alterations in the neuroendocrine axis: release of cortisol and catecholamines.
• Weight loss arises equally from loss of muscle and fat (unlike starvation).

Table 23.9 Management of nausea and vomiting according to underlying pathophysiological mechanism(s) [84, 87].

Mechanism of action	Management
Chemical trigger zone (CTZ) stimulation D2, 5HT3 receptors	Treat any reversible underlying cause; review medication Haloperidol or droperidol • Blocks D2 receptors • Once daily, low dose required • Caution in movement disorders • Contraindicated with metoclopramide or levomepromazine Levomepromazine • (2nd line – stop haloperidol) • Low dose
Vomiting centre (VC) stimulation H1, AChm, 5HT2 receptors	Treat any reversible underlying cause; review medication Cyclizine • Blocks H1 and AChm receptors • S/E site irritation if given subcutaneously, poor solubility, anticholinergic effects: drownsiness, constipation, dry mouth Levomepromazine • (2nd line – stop cyclizine) • Low dose
Higher centre stimulation 5HT GABA receptors	Non-pharmacological interventions: • Communication: explore triggers and anxieties with patient and carers • Relaxation • Massage • Acupressure ('sea bands') • Hypnosis • Behavioural therapy • Aromatherapy Benzodiazepines • Lorazepam (sublingual) • Midazolam • S/E: Drowsiness
Mechanical causes Gastric stasis May not be mediated by VC (less nausea)	Treat any reversible underlying cause; review medication Domperidone • Blocks D2 receptors Metoclopramide • Blocks D2 and stimulates 5HT4 receptors Erythromycin • Prokinetic • Dose lower than anti-infective dose • S/E nausea (stearate > maleate form) Other • PPI or H2 antagonist • Small meals • Drainage, e.g. gastrostomy on free drainage • Minimize gastric irritation (antibiotics, chemo, NSAIDs) • Octreotide: reduces secretions, and therefore colic and nausea, in small bowel obstruction [88]
Intrinsic GI mucosal damage 5HT3 receptors	Treat any reversible underlying cause; review medication Ondansetron • Blocks 5-HT3 receptors • Probably inhibits vagal afferents to VC • Trusted by carers during active treatment, less useful in other situations. • More effective combined with dexamethasone or haloperidol • S/E constipation

Table 23.10 Second line management of nausea and vomiting.

Reason for poor efficacy	Action
Insufficient drug delivery • Poor compliance • Dose not being absorbed • Dose too low Additional causes not previously identified • Is this the most appropriate drug for the likely cause(s)? • Other receptors may be involved.	• Ensure compliance through education, reinforcement or changing preparation or route • Consider increased dose or alternative route before changing antiemetic Consider broadening therapy or an alternative drug Levomepromazine • Broad spectrum: mainly blocks 5-HT2 and to some extent D2, H1, AChm • Anti-emetic effects at low doses • S/E: significant sedation, hypotension, lower convulsive threshold Dexamethasone [89] • For N and V in brain tumors, liver infiltration and possibly gastrointestinal obstruction • Consider pulsed therapy (3–5 days) whilst establishing alternative anti-emetic Careful consideration needed of: • Duration of treatment • Cushingoid side effects • Patient and carer choices

Table 23.11 Pathophysiology and management of constipation in palliative care.

Mechanism	Features	Management
Reduced stool volume • Decreased enteral intake • Decreased fluid content of stool • Decreased fibre content of diet	• Presence of one or more etiological factors • Small volume hard stool passed infrequently	• Treat any reversible underlying cause; consider increased fluids, dietary intake or dietary fibre • Osmotic or bulk forming laxative • Lactulose • Glycols (movicol)

Decreased gastrointestinal mobility
• Drugs:
  ○ Opioids
  ○ Anticholinegics (hyoscine, levomepromazine, cyclizine)
  ○ 5-HT3 antagonists
  ○ Partial or total obstruction
  ○ Reduced volume stool
	• Presence of one or more etiological factors
	• Soft or hard stool passed infrequently
		• Treat any reversible underlying cause
		• Peripheral opioid antagonists for opioid induced constipation [55]
		• Stimulant laxative
		• Senna
		• Dantron
		• Rectal route
		  ○ Glycerine suppository
		  ○ Bisacodyl suppository
		  ○ Micralax enema
		  ○ Phosphate enema (caution risk of electrolyte disturbance if used frequently)

• Increased lipolysis.
• Increased catabolism of skeletal muscle.
• Decrease in protein synthesis.
• Overall decrease in energy expenditure due to decreased physical activity.

Assessment

A specific tool for assessment of anorexia-cachexia related quality of life [93] has been described. The effect of anorexia, cachexia, and weight loss may be particularly significant for young adults with a strong sense of self image and also for parents whose instinct is to nurture and feed their child.

Management

Management of anorexia, cachexia, and weight loss is undertaken with the aim of improving quality of life, not empirical changes in weight or body mass index. Trials of nutritional interventions in adults with cancer cachexia have failed to demonstrate consistent benefits [92]. Benefits of intensive nutritional thereapy in children with cancer during intensive chemotherapy may be due to antitumor effect and not necessarily applicable to palliative care. The anabolic steroid megestrol acetate has been demonstrated to have beneficial effects on appetite and weight gain in adult palliative care but the effects on quality of life are less well established [94] and adverse effects may preclude use in children [95].

Other symptoms

Breathlessness
Pathophysiology
The sensation of breathlessness appears to arise from a complex interaction between abnormalities of respiratory function and perception of respiratory effort related to the activity of mechanoreceptors, chemoreceptors, and efferent activity from the respiratory center by direct ascending stimulation [96].

Assessment
Dyspnea is a complex multidimensional symptom. Effective management of dyspnea requires assessment of:
• Severity of the dyspnea itself.
• Precipitating and relieving factors.
• Impact on quality of life.
• Associated psychological impact.
Breathlessness is usually associated with the increased work of breathing but does not correlate with objective measures such as respiratory rate, oxygen saturation arterial blood gas measurements [97], or spirometry [98].

Management of breathlessness
Effective management of breathlessness requires pharmacological symptom management as well as non-pharmacological approaches to reduce associated anxiety and distress and the impact of breathlessness on quality of life [99] (Box 23.9).

Box 23.9 Management of breathlessness.

Non-pharmacological approaches
• Reduce and manage anxiety
  • Relaxation and breathing techniques
  • Explanation and reassurance
• Reduction in physical activity, e.g. wheelchair, stair-lift etc.
• Increase sensation of moving air, e.g. fan
Pharmacological approaches
• *Pro re nata* (PRN) enteral strong opioids at 25–50% analgesic doses
• Regular enteral strong opioids at 25–50% analgesic doses
• PRN buccal or enteral benzodiazepines, e.g. buccal midazolam
• Supplemental oxygen if hypoxemic

Opioids
Endogenous opioids appear to modify respiratory output in healthy adults possibly via action on the brainstem respiratory center. In a systematic review and meta-analysis enteral or subcutaneous strong opioids, at 25–50% of the usual analgesic dose, have been shown to improve significantly the sensation of dyspnea in adults with advanced disease [100]. When administered at appropriate doses opioids reduce the rate of breathing and sensation of dyspnea without measurable changes in oxygen saturation or $pCO2$ [101].

Benzodiazepines
Benzodiazepines may reduce the anxiety associated with dyspnea but randomized controlled trial evidence to support this approach is limited [102]. Randomized controlled trials of supplemental oxygen in adults with cancer demonstrate improvement in dyspnea only when there is associated hypoxia [103].

Non-pharmacological approaches
Randomized controlled-trial evidence suggests that psychological approaches such as relaxation techniques may be helpful in reducing the severity of dyspnea, improving quality of life [104].

Neurological symptoms

Fatigue (asthenia)
Pathophysiology
The pathophysiology of fatigue is not fully understood [105]. The relative contribution of primary and secondary causes of fatigue is likely to fluctuate throughout the disease trajectory (Box 23.10).

Pathophysiology of primary tumor related fatigue: peripheral energy depletion.
1 Dysregulation of central mechanisms:
  • Hypothalamic-pituitary-adrenal axis.
  • Serotonin metabolism.
2 High levels of pro-inflammatory cytokines.

Assessment
Fatigue is a multidimensional construct with physical, cognitive and affective dimensions [105]. Children appear to experience fatigue differently to adults and are more aware of the physical sensation of tiredness [106]. Fatigue may be fundamentally different from other symptoms in that it may be an inevitable part of end of life itself [105] (Box 23.11).

Where self report is not possible proxy measures may be used. However, professionals tend to underestimate and families overestimate severity of fatigue and the impact on quality of life. Hockenberry *et al.* [107] have demonstrated validity and reliability of childhood fatigue scales for self and proxy reporting.

Management
Fatigue is under-reported and under-treated in adults [105] and children [5, 11, 108].

Box 23.10 Secondary causes of fatigue.

Hematological/ circulatory
- Anemia
- Cardiac failure

Infection
- Fever

Metabolic
- Dehydration
- Electrolyte imbalance
- Hypomagnesaemia, hypercalcaemia
- Hepatic failure
- Renal failure
- Cachexia

Endocrine

Psychological
- Depression
- Sleep disturbance
- Anxiety
- Emotional distress

Sedative medication
- Benzodiazepines
- Strong opioids
- Antidepressants
- Anti-convulsants
- Phenothiazines

Musculoskeletal
- Local weakness
- Myopathy

Box 23.11 Assessment of fatigue.

- Physical, cognitive and affective dimensions
- Severity
- Impact of the symptom on quality of life
- Sleep pattern
- Medication
- Identify any treatable underlying causes; consider laboratory investigations

---

Treatment of primary fatigue

Pharmacological and non-pharmacological approaches may be considered. However, in the final stage of life, fatigue may provide protection and shielding from suffering, and treatment may be detrimental [105].

The natural response to fatigue is to rest and this is often reinforced by healthcare professionals [109]. However, strong evidence from meta-analysis [105, 110] suggests that aerobic exercise will reduce fatigue in cancer survivors and patients receiving cancer treatment. The introduction of a sleep program, psychotherapy, and relaxation therapy may also improve quality of life and severity of fatigue [105].

The psychostimulants methyphenedate and modafinil may reduce fatigue, but although there is randomized controlled-trial evidence to support routine use of these drugs in palliative care in adults, their use is still considered as controversial [105]. There are no published reports of pharmacological treatment of cancer-related fatigue in children.

Treating secondary causes of fatigue may be considered but efficacy may be limited at end of life and outcomes of treatment need to be carefully evaluated.

Communication and psychological symptoms

Anxiety and depression

Symptoms of anxiety and low mood are frequently considered to be inevitable and justifiable consequences of incurable malignancy and end of life [111]. Consequently, pathological anxiety states and significant depressive illness are frequently under-recognized and under-treated [5, 112] (Box 23.12).

Etiology and predisposing factors

Prevalence and expression of psychological distress related to anticipatory grief in palliative care will be influenced by the child's developmental understanding of death. The child's developmental understanding of death is also related to age, anxiety, cognitive ability, serration ability, and death experience [117].

Assessment (Table 23.12)

Recognition of anxiety and depression requires effective communication with the child and family. Children older than 12 years of age relate more directly to adults outside the family and are more likely to report psychological symptoms than those less than 7 years of age.

A number of depressive and anxiety disorders are associated with palliative care in children and young adults [118]:
- Major depressive disorder.
- Dysthymia.
- Generalized anxiety disorder.
- Anxiety disorder due to a general medical condition.
- Adjustment disorder with anxiety or depressed mood.

A number of measures have been designed for recognition of anxiety or depression in children but none have been specifically evaluated in pediatric palliative care.

Management of anxiety and depression

Both psychotherapeutic and pharmacological approaches have been advocated for the management of anxiety and depression in

Box 23.12 Factors associated with increased psychological distress in children receiving palliative care [113–116] and their families.

Child
- Inability to complete appropriate developmental tasks
- Teenage or young adult rather than younger child
- Female sex
- Anxious and/or depressive personality type
- Presence of associated family distress
- Higher levels of anticipatory grief
- Ineffective communication with family and professionals
- Loss of interpersonal relationships
- Loss of sense of identity and 'self'

Symptoms
- Poorly controlled especially:

  Pain

  Sleep disturbance

  Appetite and weight loss
- Poor quality of life and low performance status
- Change in appearance
- Loss of control over bodily functions

Disease-related
- Higher levels of anxiety associated with disease relapse than at diagnosis
- Intricate or protracted pre-diagnostic phase
- Continued uncertainty about prognosis

Professionals
- Poor team communication
- Lack of coherent leadership
- Different perspectives regarding aims of treatment or palliation
- Poor communication between the healthcare team and the family

Family
- Poor experience of pain and discomfort in their child; inability to tolerate the child's discomfort
- Religious or spiritual uncertainty
- High risk for complicated grief
- Lack of pro-active parenting and coping style
- Role alteration and inability to use pro-active coping style, e.g. inpatient environment, intensive care
- Siblings being cared for by substitute caregiver
- Poor social circumstances including financial difficulties, lack of appropriate accommodation, and poor social support networks
- Ineffective communication within the family
- Family history of major psychiatric disorder particularly depression
- Child abuse or neglect
- Previous stressful life events
- The effectiveness of complex communication channels within the family

Table 23.12 Differentiation of anticipatory grief from depression [112].

Characteristics of grief	Characteristics of depression
Feelings, emotions, and behaviors relate to a specific actual or anticipated loss	Feelings, emotions, and behaviors fulfil criteria for a major psychiatric disorder
	Distress is usually generalized to all aspects of life
Affects almost all terminally ill adults (and probably children)	Affects up to 50% terminally ill adults (prevalence in children unknown but likely to be similar)
Somatic distress, loss of usual patterns of behaviour, agitation, sleep and appetite disturbances, decreased concentration, social withdrawal	Symptoms of hopelessness, helplessness, worthlessness, guilt and suicidal ideation in addition to symptoms of grief
Patients retain the capacity for pleasure	Patients enjoy nothing
Grief comes in waves	Depression is constant and unremitting
Patients express passive wishes for death to come quickly	Patients express intense and persistant suicidal ideation
Patients are able to look forward to the future	Patients have no sense of a positive future

children. However, evidence for the management of anxiety and depression in cancer and palliative care is largely limited to adults.

Talking about facts and feelings
There have been no randomized controlled trials of psychosocial support, counselling or more formalized psychotherapy in anxiety or depression in palliative care in adults [112] or children [118].

During palliative and end-of-life care children and families need to manage anxiety related to great uncertainty and anticipatory grief. Higher parental ratings of physician care are associated with physicians giving clear information about what to expect in the end-of-life period, communicating with care and sensitivity, and preparing the parent for circumstances around the child's death [24, 119].

Children know much more than is often perceived and are very skilled at hearing unspoken feelings [120]. More mature death understanding is associated with lower levels of death fear when age and general anxiety are controlled [121]. However, it is unclear how directly these findings can be translated to dying children.

Parents vary in their confidence when sharing prognosis with their dying child. However, a higher proportion of parents regret not discussing end of life with their child if they sense that their child was aware of their impending death [122]. Parents also value direct communiction between physician and child [24] and involvement of the child in decision making [28] during end-of-life care as long as parents consider the child old enough for such communication.

Enhancing positive coping styles

Parents and siblings experience similar losses to the child but from a different perspective. Parents and siblings responses can affect the child directly and shape how the family is able to respond to and support the child. Better family coping and greater resilience is associated with [123]:

• Care of the child at home.
• Keeping the disruption of everyday family life to a minimum.
• Helping the child and family to maintain some sense of being in control.
• Good social networks.
• Strong family and interpersonal relationships.
• Seeking social support in times of crisis.
• Families that are able to communicate openly and honestly.

Psychotherapy

A number of different psychotherapeutic approaches are appropriate for anxiety and depression in palliative care. Due to the child's deteriorating condition, protracted interventions or therapy to mediate longstanding dysfunction in families or individuals is unlikely to be appropriate or effective in palliative and end-of-life care.

Systematic review evidence suggests that psychotherapy using supportive, cognitive behavioural and problem solving approaches appears to be effective in the management of adults with depressive symptoms [124]. Meta-analysis of psychotherapy (cognitive and non-cognitive) in the management of depression in healthy children and adults [125] suggests a moderate benefit.

Systematic review evidence suggests that cognitive behavioural therapy is effective in children with anxiety disorders [126, 127]. However, these studies were not undertaken in children with cancer or children receiving palliative care.

Pharmacological management of anxiety and depression

Pharmacotherapy for anxiety and depression in children and young adults, outside the palliative care setting, is generally reserved for use in severe symptoms in combination with psychotherapy. However, in palliative care, use of pharmacotherapy may be appropriate where psychotherapeutic approaches are unavailable [115], or their use is limited due to the child's deteriorating clinical condition reducing the ability of the child to participate.

Fluoxetine is the only selective serotonin re-uptake inhibitor for which there is consistent evidence from clinical trials that it is effective in reducing depression symptoms in both children and adolescents who are not medically ill. However, use of selective serotonin re-uptake inhibitors in children and adolescents with depression has been associated with an increased risk of suicidal ideation and behaviour [128].

Although not specific to palliative care, data from a good quality systematic review suggests tricyclic antidepressant agents are not useful in treating depression in pre-pubertal children. There is marginal evidence to support the use of tricyclic antidepressants in the treatment of depression in adolescents although

the magnitude of this effect is likely to be moderate at best [129].

There is some evidence in adult palliative care that, in the short-term, psychostimulants can reduce the symptoms of depression in palliative care specifically when a rapid onset of action is required for short-term use [130].

Use of benzodiazepines in anxiety states in palliative care in children is based on expert opinion. There are no good quality studies on the role of benzodiazepines (or other drugs) in the treatment of anxiety associated with terminal illness to draw a conclusion about their efficacy [131].

The last few hours and days

The last few hours and days of life represent a period of rapid symptom escalation together with progressive deterioration in the child's overall condition and frequently loss of the enteral route for symptom management. Considerations include the choice of setting for end-of-life care, a proactive response to escalating symptoms and loss of the oral route for medication [132], and management of new symptoms including pressure area problems, noisy breathing due to retained secretions (death rattle), terminal agitation, and delirium.

Recognition of end of life

Recognition of the last few hours and days of life, and diagnosing 'dying', can be difficult [133], but features suggestive of the last few hours and days of life in adults with cancer may be relevant (Box 23.13).

Discussing resuscitation and advance care planning

Ideally, the aims of treatment and advance care planning are discussed with the child and family throughout the child's illness, with the focus of discussions changing as the aims of treatment change and cure becomes increasingly unlikely. Advance care planning, including documentation of a Do Not Attempt Resuscitation (DNAR) order, is likely to reduce parental and medical staff stress accompanying the death of a child, optimize management of the terminal phase of the disease, and improve family satisfaction with communication and end-of-life care [134]. However, professionals, families, and children vary in their ability and willingness to take part in such advance discussions

---

Box 23.13 Features strongly suggestive of the last few hours and days of life in adults with cancer.

• Bed bound
• No longer able to take tablets
• Taking only sips of fluid
• Comatose or semi-comatose

[135]. Involvement of children in discussions regarding end-of-life care including location of death and limitation of treatment has been reported [9].

Practical considerations around choice of place of care and place death

Where a choice is available, the majority of families will elect for end-of-life care at home [5, 11, 14, 15]. There is considerable evidence to suggest that families of children who die at home have less difficulty in adjusting and cope better in the medium to long term [136], but studies in adults have shown home death to be more stressful for families of the deceased [137]. A more recent study [3] in children failed to show any significant difference in short-term outcome between parents of children with malignancy dying an acute hospital death and those dying a palliative death, predominantly at home. However, a greater proportion of the siblings of the child dying an acute death reported problems compared with those of children who died a palliative death.

End-of-life care at home allows the child and family greater control over their environment with involvement of fewer professionals and increased opportunities for privacy and time together [138].

If the intention is for the child to be cared for at home during end of life, then anticipatory planning is essential. End-of-life care at home is likely to be difficult, if not impossible, without adequate support, but if this is available it is not usually necessary to move a child. If adequate professional support is not available families are more likely to report a difficult moment of death [139].

Occasionally, difficulties with symptom control, psychological distress, or family wishes mean that the child is transferred to a pediatric hospice or hospital [19]. This should not necessarily be seen as a failure but a choice ensuring the best care for the child and family.

Care in hospital and intensive care

Much can be done to bring the 'home from home' environment to the child and family in hospital. This may include attention to privacy, involvement in care and decision making [114, 140], stopping intrusive and inappropriate monitoring and keeping the family together, for example by the provision of family accommodation. However, it is often difficult for siblings to spend much time with their brother or sister in hospital [141]. A number of studies have shown that families of children with cancer who die in hospital experience greater guilt, anxiety, depression, and interpersonal problems than those of children who die at home [3]. End-of-life care in a children's hospice is an alternative that may be available but is infrequently chosen for children dying of malignancy and their families

Loss of the oral route

Loss of the oral (enteral) route may be relative or absolute and related to an overall deterioration in the child's condition together with an increasing need for medication to control distressing symptoms (Box 23.14).

In all cases medication should be reviewed and consideration given to:
• Simplifying the medication regime: discontinuing non-essential medications.
• Optimizing the route of administration.
The choice of route for medication will depend on the the child's requirement for symptom management, available routes, and preference of the child and family. Medication given for breakthrough symptoms such as pain or agitation must be available to be administered immediately, should symptoms arise (Table 23.13).

Box 23.14 Causes of loss of the oral (enteral) route in end of life care.

• Child too unwell to take medication due to generalized debility or decreasing conscious level
• Child too un-cooperative to take medication (including due to poorly controlled symptoms)
• Excessive numbers or volume of medication
• Nausea or vomiting
• Poor absorption of medication due to obstruction or ileus

Table 23.13 Alternative routes for administration of medication.

Route	Examples
Buccal or sublingual	Diamorphine [F. Craig, personal communication] Fentanyl [66] Morphine [68] Midazolam [142] Lorazepam
Gastrostomy	All liquid preparations Most tablets (other than sustained release preparations) can also be crushed and administered down a gastrostomy
Transdermal	Fentanyl* Hyoscine hydrobromide
Subcutaneous (or intravenous if long- term central venous access)	Antiemetics: haloperidol, levomepromazine, cyclizine Opioid analgesics: morphine, diamorphine, fentanyl, alfentanyl, hydromorphone Antisecretory agents: hyoscine hydrobromide, hyoscine butylbromide, glycorronium bromide Benzodiazepines: Midazolam, clonazepam

*Not suitable for titration of rapidly deteriorating pain.

Buccal or sublingual route

Expert opinion strongly supports the use of the buccal and sub-cutaneous routes in administration of medication for symptom control in pediatric oncology palliative care.

Subcutaneous or intravenous infusions

Use of subcutaneous or intravenous infusions is frequently required when the oral route is no longer available and during periods of rapid symptom escalation. It is common practice to administer multiple drugs as a single infusion run over 24 hours [143]. Compatibility tables are available to indicate which drugs can be mixed together in this way and the most appropriate diluent [144]. Breakthrough medication is given via the oral route if possible or via subcutaneous, intravenous buccal or sublingual routes as appropriate.

Palliative care drug boxes

Palliative care drug boxes, containing medication for symptom management to be administered via continuous intravenous or subcutaneous infusion have been advocated [145, 146] as a method for ensuring prompt and effective symptom management and avoiding unnecessary hospital admission during end-of-life care at home.

Retrostopective review of the contents and use of palliative care drug boxes in pediatric palliative care [146] suggests that the majority of symptoms can be controlled with a combination of six medication(s) suitable for subcutaneous or intravenous administration:

• A strong opiate: morphine or diamorphine.
• A combination of antiemetics, e.g. cyclizine, haloperidol, levomepromazine.
• A sedative and non-sedative antipsychotic: haloperidol and levomepromazine.
• A benzodiazepine, e.g.midazolam.
• An antisecretory agent, e.g. hyoscine hydrobromide.

Decreased fluid intake, and the possibility of suffering through thirst, is a frequently voiced parental concern. However, it is unclear whether decreased oral intake and thirst are as much of a problem for the child. It is helpful to consider that the child is dying from a disease process of which decreased oral intake, and possibly dehydration, is a part, rather than dehydration being the cause of death [147]. A low prevalence of hunger and thirst is reported in adults dying of cancer despite decreased oral intake. The relationship between symptoms of dry mouth, thirst, and fluid intake at end of life is unclear [148]. Benefits of artificial hydration at end of life are unclear [149].

Noisy breathing due to retained respiratory tract secretions (death rattle)

In the last few hours of life a child's breathing may become noisy, with the characteristic sound of retained secretions in the oropharynx in a child too weak to swallow. Prevalence of noisy breathing increases as death approaches with reported median onset at 16 hours before death [150]. Increased risk of noisy

breathing is associated with a prolonged dying phase, CNS tumor, lung tumors, pulmonary edema and lower respiratory tract infection [150, 151].

Prevention and prompt management are important as treatment measures are more effective at reducing the severity of the problem than in stopping it altogether. There are three components to effective management of noisy breathing at the end of life:

• Explanation and reassurance for the family: the child is not drowning or choking.
• Positioning of the patient; flat or slightly head down with the head turned to the side.
• Consider oropharyngeal suction.

Pharmacological management

Antimuscarinic drugs (hyoscine hydrobromide, hyoscine butyl-bromide, and glycopyrronium) can be effective in drying of respiratory secretions but there is no substantial evidence from systematic review, that any intervention, be it pharmacological or non-pharmacological, is superior to placebo in the treatment of death rattle [152].

Terminal delirium (Box 23.15)

Assessment

Diagnostic Statistic Manual (DSM) criteria for acute confusion can be considered as applicable to children. Reports of difference in prevalence of individual features of acute confusional states in children compared with adults are conflicting [156]. Acute confusional states are likely to be significantly under-recognized [157].

Management

Effective management of acute confusion at the end of life involves:

• Identification and treatment of any reversible underlying cause.
• Pharmacological management of resistant symptoms or where no reversible underlying cause has been identified.
• Support and explanation for the family.

Acute confusional states due to hypercalcemia or medication are most likely to be reversible whilst those due to hepatic failure, hypoxia, and disseminated intravascular coagulation are most likely to be resistant to treatment [155]. Intravenous hydration has not been shown to improve symptoms of acute confusion and may worsen fluid retention symptoms [158].

Haloperidol is considered as first choice therapy in the management of confusion at the end of life in adult patients with cancer [159] and critically ill children [160]. As monotherapy, benzodiazepines may aggravate rather than alleviate delirium at end of life but may be beneficial when haloperidol is insufficient to control agitated delirium [161].

Care of the child after death

In the immediate period after the death of the child, the over-whelming need for the family is privacy and time in order to

---

Box 23.15 Etiology and predisposing factors for acute confusional states at the end of life [153–155].

Type of malignancy
• Hematological malignancy or central nervous system tumor

Poorly controlled symptoms
• Pain
• Psychological distress
• Spiritual distress
• Urinary or fecal retention

Drugs
• Opioids
• Anticholinergic antisecretory
• Anxiolytic
• Antidepressants
• Antipsychotics
• Antiepelipetics
• Steroids
• Non-steroidal anti-inflammatory drugs

Metabolic disturbance
• Dehydration
• Hypercalcemia
• Hepatic failure
• Renal failure
• Hypoxia
• Hypotension and circulatory shock

Infection

Disturbance of hemostasis
• Disseminated intravascular coagulation

---

begin to adjust to their loss. Mothers describe the specific need to be with their child's body [162, 163]. The family may also value advice and support regarding practical arrangements to be made after the child has died [164].

The memory of the child and their last illness will not be forgotten [139]. The family needs time and space to work through their loss and reframe it as part of who they are and their future as a family.

Families particularly value when health professionals make contact after bereavement [135, 165]. Parents of deceased children value the opportunity to discuss issues such as the chronology of events, events surrounding the death, ways to help others, bereavement support and what to tell others [166]. They seek reassurance and the opportunity to voice gratitude and voice complaints. Consistency of bereavement follow up is valued [167]. However, although loss of a child is associated with a

higher prevalence of complicated grief, most families do not experience long-term problems [3].

Conclusion and future directions

Despite significant advances in curative treatment for pediatric malignancy, approximately 25% children will ultimately die from their malignancy, or from complications of treatment aimed at cure. The scope of palliative care starts from the diagnosis of a life-threatening malignancy and extends through to end-of-life care and bereavement. The aim of palliative care is to provide support for the child and family, throughout their journey from diagnosis to end of life, to control distressing symptoms and to optimize quality of life.

Effective communication with the child and family, and between healthcare professionals, is the foundation of successful palliative care. This means sharing distressing news sensitively but honestly and working together to share the burden of life-threatening illness and ultimately the loss of a child to cancer.

Much can be done to reduce the burden of symptoms of children with incurable malignancy and improve their quality of life. Three symptoms: fatigue, weight loss, and pain are consistently reported as the most prevalent and causing the highest level of suffering for children with cancer. Sadly, at the current time although much can be done to alleviate suffering due to pain, therapeutic options for cancer-related fatigue and cachexia are extremely limited and more research is particularly needed in this area.

Psychological distress, anxiety, and depression remain significantly under-recognized and under-treated. However, much of the psychological stress of caring for a child with incurable malignancy can be eased by facilitating pro-active coping mechanisms. These include helping the family to retain some sense of control, involving them in the care of their child, ensuring privacy and time for family members to be together, keeping disruption to a minimum, and encouraging support from the family's own social networks. Caring for the child at home is one way of ensuring that the child and family are able to utilize many of these coping strategies but there is much that can be done to facilitate their use in other care settings.

The research evidence underpinning the practice of pediatric palliative care is rapidly expanding. Research in pediatric palliative care is immensely challenging from both practical and ethical perspectives. The wealth of systematic reviews almost universally demonstrates that there is insufficient evidence to guide clinical practice in pediatric oncology palliative care. The first priority is the development of robust outcome measures which can then be used in randomized controlled clinical trials to evaluate interventions for the most prevalent symptoms and problems. We owe it to children with incurable malignancy and their families to develop a collaborative international program of research, as has been done with curative treatment for malignancy, in order ensure the optimum treatment for distressing symptoms and improving quality of life.

References

1 European Association for Palliative Care Taskforce on Palliative Care for Children and Adolescents. IMPaCCT standards for paediatric palliative care in Europe. Eur J Pall Care 2007; 14: 109–114.

2 Magnani C, Patore G, Coebergh JW, Viscomi S, Spix C, Steliarova-Foucher E. Trends in survival after childhood cancer in Europe, 1978–1997; report from the automatic childhood cancer information system project (ACCIS). Eur J Cancer 2006; 42: 1981–35

3 Sirkia K, Saarinen-Pihkala UM, Hovi L. Coping of parents and siblings with the death of a child with cancer: death after terminal care compared with death during active anticancer therapy. Acta Paediatr 2000; 89: 717–29.

4 Wolfe J, Klar N, Grier HE, et al. Understanding of prognosis among parents of children who died of cancer: impact on treatment goals and integration of palliative care. JAMA 2000; 284: 2469–75.

5 Theunissen JMJ, Hoogerbrugge PM, van Achterberg T, et al. Symptoms in the palliative phase of children with cancer. Paediatr Blood Cancer 2007; 49: 160–5.

6 Mallinson J, Jones PD. A 7 year review of deaths on the general paediatric wards at John Hunter Children's hospital 1991–97. J Paediatr Child Health 2000; 36: 252–5.

7 Goldman A, Hewitt M, Collins GS, et al. Symptoms in children/young people with progressive malignant disease: United Kingdom Children's Cancer Study Group/ Paediatric Oncology Nurses Forum survey. Pediatrics 2006; 117: e1179–86.

8 Sirkia K, Hovi L, Pouttu J, et al. Pain medication during terminal care of children with cancer. J Pain Symptom Manage 1998; 15: 220–26.

9 Bradshaw G, Hinds PS, Lensihng MS, et al. Cancer related deaths in children and adolescents. J Palliat Med 2005; 8: 86–95.

10 Higginson IJ, Thompson M. Children and young people who die from cancer: epidemiology and place of death in England (1995–9). BMJ 2003; 327: 478–9.

11 Wolfe J, Grier HE, Klar N, et al. Symptoms and suffering at the end of life in children with cancer. N Eng J Med 2000; 342: 326–33.

12 Feudtner C, Silveira MJ, Christakis DA. Where do children with complex chronic conditions die? Patterns in Washington State 1980–1998. Pediatrics 2002; 109: 656–60.

13 Jones R, Trenholme A, Horsburgh M, et al. The need for paediatric palliative care in New Zealand. NZ Med J 2002; 115: U198.

14 Vickers J, Thompson G, Collins GS, et al. Place and provision of palliative care for children with progressive cancer: a study by the Paediatric Oncology Nurses Forum/United Kingdom Children's Cancer Study Group Palliative Care Working Group. J Clin Oncol 2007; 25: 4472–6.

15 Hechler T, Blankenburg M, Friedrischdorf SJ, et al. Parents' perspective on symptoms, quality of life characteristics of death and end of life decisions for children dying from cancer. Klin Padiatr 2008; 220:166–74.

16 Woodgate RL, Degner LF. Expectations and beliefs about children's cancer symptoms; perspectives of children with cancer and their families. Oncol Nurs Forum 2003; 30: 479–91.

17 Jalmsell L, Kreicbergs U, Onelöv E, et al. Symptoms affecting children with malignancies during the last month of life: a nationwide follow-up. Pediatrics 2006; 117: 1314–20.

18 Hongo T, Watanabe C, Okada S, et al. Analysis of the circumstances at the end of life in children with cancer: symptom suffering and acceptance. Pediatr Int 2003; 45: 60–4.

19 McCallum D, Byrne P, Bruera E. How children die in hospital. J Pain Symptom Manage 2000; 20: 417–23.

20 Collins JJ, Grier HE, Kinney HC, Berde CB. Control of severe pain in children with terminal malignancy. J Pediatr 1995; 126: 653–7.

21 Dougherty M, DeBaun MR. Rapid increase of morphine and benzodiazepine usage in the last three days of life in children with cancer is related to neuropathic pain. J Pediatr 2003; 142: 373–6.

22 Mack JW, Wolfe W. Early integration of paediatric palliative care; for some children palliative care starts at diagnosis. Curr Opin Paediatr 2006; 18: 10–14.

23 Woodgate RL. Life is never the same: childhood cancer narratives. Eur J Cancer Care 2006; 15: 8–18.

24 Mack JW, Wolfe J, Grier HE, et al. Communication about prognosis between parents and physicians of children with cancer: parent preferences and the impact of prognostic information. J Clin Oncol 2006; 24: 5265–70.

25 Harris MB. Palliative care in children with cancer. Which child and when? J Natl Cancer Inst Monogr 2004; 32: 144–9.

26 Hilden J, Emanual EJ, Fairclough DL, et al. Attitudes and practices among paediatric oncologist regarding end of life care: results of the 1998 American Society of Oncology Survey. J Clin Oncol 2001; 19: 205–12.

27 Barr P. Relationship of neonatologists end of life decisions to their personal fear of death. Arch Dis Child Fetal Neonat Ed 2007; 92: F104–7.

28 Monterosso L, Krisjanson LJ. Supportive and palliative care needs of families of children who die from cancer: an Australian Study. Palliat Med 2008; 22: 59–69.

29 Docherty SL, Miles MS, Brandon D. Searching for the 'dying point': providers' experiences with palliative care in pediatric acute care. Pediatr Nurs 2007; 33: 335–41.

30 Valdimarsdottir U, Kreicbergs U, Hauksdottire A, et al. Parents intellectual and emotional awareness of their child's impending death due to cancer: a population based long-term follow-up study. Lancet Oncol 2007; 8: 706–14.

31 Bluebond-Langner M, Belasco JB, Goldman A, et al. Understanding parents' approaches to care and treatment of children with cancer when standard therapy has failed. J Clin Oncol 2007; 25: 2414–9.

32 Archer VR, Billingham LJ, Cullen MH. Palliative chemotherapy: no longer a contradiction in terms. Oncologist 1999; 4: 470–7.

33 Fowler K, Poehling K, Billheimer D, et al. Hospice referral practices for children with cancer: a survey of paediatric oncologists. J Clin Oncol 2006; 24: 1099–104.

34 Hoekstra J, Vernooij-Dassen MJ, de Vos R, et al. The added value of assessing the 'most troublesome' symptom among patients with cancer in the palliative phase. Patient Educ Couns 2007; 65: 223–9.

35 Anonymous. Doctor–patient relationships in primary care. Doctor help! My child has cancer. BMJ 1999; 319: 554–6.

36 Contro NA, Larson J, Scofield S, et al. Hospital staff and family perspectives regarding quality of pediatric palliative care. Pediatrics 2004; 114: 1248–52.

37 Perilongo G Rigon L, Sianati L, et al. Palliative care for dying children; proposals for better care. Med Pediatr Oncol 2001; 37: 59–61.

38 Shipman C, Addington Hall J, Barclay S, et al. How and why do GPs use specialist palliative care services. Palliat Med 2002; 16 ; 241–6.

39 Baverstock A, Finlay F. Specialist registrars' emotional response to a patient's death. Arch Dis Child 2006; 91; 774–6.

40 Baverstock AC, Finlay FO. A study of staff support mechanisms within children's hospices. In J Palliat Nurs 2006; 12: 506–8.

41 Rourke MT. Compassion fatigue in pediatric palliative care providers. Pediatr Clin North Am 2007; 54: 631–44.

42 Gauvin-Piquard A, Rodary C, Rezvani A, et al. The development of the DEGR(R): a scale to assess pain in young children with cancer. Eur J Pain 1999: 3: 165–76.

43 Friedrischsdorf SJ, Finney D, Begin M, et al. Breakthrough pain in children with cancer. J Pain Symptom Manage 2007; 34: 209–16.

44 Hain RD. Pain scales in children a review. Palliat Med 1997; 11:341–50.

45 Beyer JE, Denyes MJ, Villarruel AM. The creation, validation and continuing development of the Oucher: a measure of pain intensity in children. J Pediatr Nurse 1992; 7: 335–46.

46 Zernikow B, Smale H, Michel E, et al. Paediatric cancer pain management using the WHO analgesic ladder – results of a prospective analysis from 2265 treatment days during a quality improvement study. Eur J Pain 2006; 10: 587–95.

47 Lurcott G. The effects of the genetic absence and inhibition of CYP2D6 on the metabolism of codeine and its derivatives, hyroxycodone and oxycodone. Anaesth Prog 1999; 45: 154–6.

48 Monteiro Caran EM, Dias CG, Serber A, et al. Clinical aspects and treatment of pain in children and adolescents with cancer. Pediatr Blood Cancer 2005; 45: 925–32.

49 Portenoy RK, Sibirceva U, Smout R, et al. Opioid use and survival at the end of life: a survey of a hospice population. J Pain Symptom Manage 2006; 32: 532–40.

50 Wiffen PJ, Edwards JE, Barden J, et al. Oral morphine for cancer pain. Cochrane Database of Systematic Reviews 2003 issue 4 Art No: CD 003868. DOI10.1002/14651858.CD003868.

51 Hain RD, Miser A, Devins M, Wallace WH. Strong opioids in paediatric palliative medicine. Paediatr Drugs 2005; 7: 1–9.

52 Klepstad P, Kaasa S, Jystad A, et al. Immediate or sustained release morphine for dose finding during start of morphine to cancer patients: a randomised controlled trial. Pain 2003; 101: 193–8.

53 Zernikow B, Linena G. Long acting morphine for pain control in paediatric oncology. Med Pediatr Oncol 2001; 36: 451–8.

54 Siden H, Nalewajek G. High dose opioids in paediatric palliative care. J Pain Symptom Manage 2003; 25: 397–9.

55 Becker G, Galandi D, Blum HE. Peripherally acting opioid antagonists in the treatment of opiate-related constipation: a systematic review. J Pain Symptom Manage 2007; 34: 547–65.

56 Twycross R, Greaves MW, Handwerker H, et al. Itch: scratching more than the surface. Q J Med 2003; 96: 7–26.

57 Gill AM, Cousins A, Nunn AJ, et al. Opioid induced respiratory depression in pediatric patients. Ann Pharmacother 1996; 30: 125–9.

58 Roscow CE, Gomery R, Chen TY, et al. Reversal of opioid-induced bladder dysfunction by intravenous naloxone and methylnaltrexone. Clin Pharmacol Ther 2007; 82: 48–53.

59 Vella-Brincat J, Macleod AD. Adverse effects of opioids on the central nervous systems of palliative care patients. J Pain Palliat Care Pharmacother 2007; 21: 15–25.

60 Hanks GW, De Conno F, Cherny N, et al. Morphine and alternative opioids in cancer pain: the EAPC recommendations. Br J Cancer 2001; 84: 587–93.

61 Quigley C. Opioid switching to improve pain relief and drug tolerability. Cochrane Database Syst Rev 2004; CD004847.

62 Zernikow B, Michel E, Anderson B. Transdermal fentanyl in childhood and adolescence: a comprehensive literature review. J Pain 2007; 8: 187–207.

63 Nicholson AB. Methadone for cancer pain. Cochrane Database of Systematic Reviews 2004. Issue 1. Art No: CD003971. DOI: 10:1002/14651858.CD003971.pub2.

64 Davies D, DeVlamming D, Haines C. Methadone analgesia for children with advanced cancer. Pediatr Blood Cancer 2008; 51: 393–7.

65 Drake R, Longowrd J, Collins JJ. Opioid rotaion in children with cancer. J Palliat Med 2004; 7: 419–22.

66 Zeppetella G, Ribeiro MD. Opioids for the management of breakthrough (episodic) pain in cancer patients. Cochrane Database Syst Rev 2006; (1): CD004311.

67 Kendall JM, Reeves BC, Latter VS. Nasal diamorphine trial group. Multicentre randomised controlled trial of nasal diamorphine for analgesia in children and teenagers with clinical fractures. BMJ 2001; 322: 261–5.

68 Engelhart T, Crawford M. Sublingual morphine may be a suitable alternative for pain control in children in the postoperative period. Pediatr Anaesth 2001; 11: 81–3.

69 Eisenberg E, McNichol E, Carr DB. Opioids for neuropathic pain. Cochrane Database of Systematic Reviews 2006, Issue 3. Art No: CD006146. DOI 10.1002/14651858.CD006146.

70 McNichol E, Strassels SA, Goudas L, et al. NSAIDS or paracetamol alone or in combination with opioids for cancer pain. Cochrane Database of Systematic Reviews 2005. Issue 2. Art No: CD005160. DOI 10.1002/1465858.CD005180.

71 Keskinbora K, Pekel AF, Aydinli I. Gabapentin and an opioid combination versus opioid along for the management of neuropathic cancer pain: a randomised open trial. J Pain Symptom Manage 2007; 34: 183–9.

72 Saarto T, Wiffen PJ. Antidepressants for neuropathic pain. Cochrane Database of Systematic Reviews 2005, Issue 3. Art No CD005454. DOI: 10.1002/14651858.CD005454.

73 Collins JJ, Kerner J, Sentivany S, et al. Intravenous amitryptiline in pediatrics. J Pain Symptom Manage 1995; 10: 471–5.

74 Rogers AG. Use of amitryptiline (Elavil) for phantom limb pain in younger children. J Pain Symptom Manage 1989; 4: 96.

75 Wiffen P, Collins S, McQuay H, et al. Anticonvulsant drugs for acute and chronic pain. Cochrane Database of Systematic Reviews 2005; Issue 3. Art No: CD001133. DOI: 10.1002/14651858.CD001133.pub2.

76 Butkovic D, Toljan S, Mihovilovic-Novak B. Experience with gabapentin for neuropathic pain in adolescents: a report of five cases. Pediatr Anaesth 2006; 16: 325–9.

77 Glaser AW, Buxton N, Walker D Steroids in the management of central nervous system tumors. Arch Dis Chil 1997; 76: 76–8.

78 Finkel JC, Pestieau SR, Quezado ZM. Ketamine as an adjuvant for treatment of cancer pain in children and adolescents. J Pain 2007; 8: 515–21.

79 Bell R Eccleston C, Kalso E. Ketamine as an adjuvant to opioids for cancer pain. Cochrane database of systematic reviews 2003 Issue 1. Art No: CD003351. DOI: 10.1002/14651858.CD003351.

80 Ross JR, Saunders Y, Edmonds PM, et al. Systematic review of role of bisphosphoates on skeletal morbidity in metastatic cancer. BMJ 2003; 327: 469–72.

81 Wong R, Wiffen PJ. Bisphosphonates for the relief of pain secondary to bone metastases. Cochrane Database of Systematic Reviews 2002, Issue 2. Art No.: CD002068.DOI: 10.1002/14651858.XCD002068.

82 McQuay HJ, Collins SL, Carroll D, et al. Radiotherapy for the palliation of painful bone metastases. Cochrane Database of Systematic Reviews 1999, Issue 3. Art No.: CD001793. DOI:10.1002/14651858. CD001793.

83 Paulino AC. Palliative radiotherapy in children with neuroblastoma. Pediatr Hematol Oncol 2003; 20: 111–7.

84 Mannix K. Palliation of nausea and vomiting in malignancy. Clin Med 2006; 6: 144–7.

85 McVey P. Nausea and vomiting in the patient with advanced cancer: an overview of pharmacological and non-pharmacological management. Collegian 2001; 8: 41–2.

86 Bentley A, Boyd K. Use of clinical pictures in the management of nausea and vomiting: a prospective audit. Palliat Med 2001; 15: 247–53.

87 Glare P, Periera G, Krsithanson LJ, et al. Systematic review of the efficacy of antiemetics in the treatment of nausea in patients with far-advanced cancer. Support Care Cancer 2004; 12: 432–40.

88 Mercadente S, Casuccio A, Mangione S. Medical treatment for inoperable malignant bowel obstruction: a qualitative systematic review. J Pain Symptom Manage 2007; 33: 217–23.

89 Feuer DJ, Broadley KE. Corticosteroids for the resolution of malignant bowel obstruction in advanced gynaecological and gastrointestinal cancer. Cochrane Database of Systematic Reviews 1999; Issue 3. Art No: CD 001219. DOI: 10.1002/14651858.CD001219.

90 Miles CL, Fellowes D, Goodman ML, et al. Laxatives for the management of constipation in palliative care patients. Cochrane Database of Systematic Reviews 2006; Issue 4. Art No: CD 003448. DOI: 10.1002/14651858.CD003448.pub2.

91 Morley JE, Thomas DR, Wilson MM. Cachexia: pathophysiology and clinical relevance. Am J Clin Nutr 2006; 83: 735–43.

92 Good P, Cavenagh J, Mather M, et al. Medically assisted nutrition for palliative care in adult patients. Cochrane Database Syst Rev 2008; 8: CD006274.

93 Lai JS, Celia D, Peterman A, et al. Anorexia/cachexia-related quality of life for children with cancer. Cancer 2005; 104: 1531–9.

94 Berenstein EG, Ortiz Z. Megestrol acetate for treatment of anorexia-cachexia syndrome. Cochrane Database of Systematic Reviews 2005; Issue 2. Art No: CD 004310. DOI: 10.1002/14651858.CD004310.pub2.

95 Orme LM, Bond JD, Humphreys MS, et al. Megastrol acetate in pediatric oncology patients may lead to severe symptomatic adrenal suppression. Cancer 2003; 98: 397–405.

96 Ripamonti C, Bruera E. Dyspnoea pathophysiology and assessment. J Pain Symptom Manage 1997; 13: 220–32.

97 Thomas JR, Von Gunten CF. Treatment of dyspnoea in cancer patients. Oncology (Williston Park) 2002; 16: 745–50.

98 Heyse-Moore L, Beynon T, Ross V. Does spirometry predict dyspnoea in advanced cancer? Palliat Med 2000; 14: 189–95.

99 Henoch I, Bergman B, Danielson E. Dyspnoea experience and management strategies in patients with lung cancer. Psychooncology 2008; 17: 709–15.

100 Jennings AL, Davies AN, Higgins JPT, et al. Opioids for the palliation of breathlessness in terminal illness. Cochrane Database of Systematic Reviews 2001, Issue 4. Art No:CD002066. DOI: 101002/14651858.CD002066.

101 Clemens KE, Klaschik E. Symptomatic therapy of dyspnoea with strong opioids and its effect on ventilation in palliative care patients. J Pain Symptom Manage 2007; 33: 473–81.

102 Navigante AN, Cerchiettie LC, Castro MA, et al. Midazolam as an adjunct therapy to morphine in the alleviation of severe dyspnoea perception in patients with advanced cancer. J Pain Symptom Manage 2006; 31: 38–47.

103 Bruera E, Sweeney C, Willey J, et al. A randomized controlled trial of supplemental oxygen versus air in cancer patients with dyspnoea. Palliat Med 2003; 17: 659–63.

104 Hately J, Luarence V, Scott A, et al. Breathlessness clinics within specialist palliative care settings can improve the quality of life and functional capacity of patients with lung cancer. Palliat Med 2003; 17: 410–7.

105 Radbruch L, Elsner F, et al. Fatigue in palliative care patients – an EAPC approach. Palliat Med 2008; 22: 13–32.

106 Hinds PS, Hockenberry-Eaton M, Gilger E, et al. Comparing patient, parent and staff descriptions of fatigue in pediatric oncology patients. Cancer Nurs 1999; 22: 277–88.

107 Hockenberry MJ, Hinds PS, Barrera P, et al. Three instruments to assess fatigue in children with cancer: the child, parent and staff perspectives. J Pain Symptom Manage 2003; 25: 319–28.

108 Gibson F, Garnett M, Richardson A, Edwards J, Sepion B. Heavy to carry: a survey of parents' and healthcare professionals' perceptions of cancer related fatigue in children and young people. Cancer Nurs 2005; 28: 27–35.

109 Stone P, Ream E, Reichardson A, et al. Cancer-related fatigue – a difference of opinion? Results of a multicentre survey of health professionals, patients and caregivers. Eur J Cancer Care (Engl) 2003; 12: 20–7.

110 Schmitz KH, Hotzmn J, Courneya KS, et al. Controlled physical activity trials in cancer survivors; a systematic review and meta-analysis. Cancer Epidemiol Biomarkers Prev 2005; 14; 1588–95.

111 Burroughs H, Lovell K, Orley M, et al. 'Justifiable depression': how primary care professionals and patients view late-life depression? A qualitative study. Fam Pract 2006; 23: 369–77.

112 Block SD. Assessing and managing depressionin the terminally ill patients. ACP-ASIM End of Life Care Consensus Panel. American College of Physicians-American Society of Internal Medicine. Ann Intern Med 2000; 132: 209–18.

113 McSherry M, Kehoe K, Carroll JM, et al. Psychosocial and spiritual needs of children living with a life limiting illness. Pediatr Clin North Am 2007; 45: 609–29.

114 Shudy M, de Almeida ML, Ly S, et al. Impact of pediatric critical illness and injury on families: a systematic literature review. Pediatrics 2006; 118 (Suppl 3): S203–18.

115 Bhatia SK, Bhatia SC. Childhood and adolescent depression. Am Fam Phys 2007; 75: 73–80.

116 Hoven E, Anclaire M, Samuelsson U, et al. The influence of pediatric cancer diagnosis and illness complication factors on parental distress. J Pediatr Haematol Oncol 2008; 30: 807–14.

117 Hunter SB, Smith DE. Predictors of children's understandings of death: age, cognitive ability, death experience and maternal communicative competence. Omega (Westport) 2008; 57: 143–62.

118 Kersun LS, Shemesh E. Depression and anxiety in children at the end of life. Pediatr Clin N Am 2007; 54: 691–708.

119 Hsiao JL, Evan EE, Zeltzer LK. Parent and child perspectives on physician communication in pediatric palliative care. Palliat Support Care 2007; 5: 355–65.

120 Gottlieb D. Voices of conflict; voices of healing. Lincoln, NE: People with Disabilities Press, 2001.

121 Slaughter V, Griffiths M. Death understanding and fear of death in young children. Clin Child Psychol Psych 2007; 12: 525–35.

122 Kreicbergs U, Valdimarsdottir U, Onelov E, et al. Talking about death with children who have severe malignant disease. N Eng J Med 2004; 351: 1175–86.

123 Brook L, Vickers J, Barber M. The place of care – planning what is needed. In Goldman A, Hain R, Lieben S (Eds), Oxford Textbook of Palliative Care for Children. Oxford: Oxford University Press, 2006.

124 Akechi T, Okuyama T, Onishi J, et al. Psychotherapy for depression among incurable patients. Cochrane Database Syst Rev 2008; 16: CD005537.

125 Weisz JR, McCarty CA, Valeri SM. Effects of psychotherapy for depression in children and adolescents: a meta-analysis. Psychol Bull 2006; 132; 132–49.

126 James A, Soler A, Weatherall R. Cognitive behavioural therapy for anxiety disorders in children and adolescents. Cochrane Database Syst Rev 2005; 19: CD004690.

127 Compton SN, March JS, Brent D, et al. Congitive behavioural psychotherapy for anxiety and depressive disorders in the children and adolescents: an evidence based medicine review. J Am Acad Child Adolesc Psychaitr 2004; 43; 930–59.

128 Hetrick SE, Merry SN, McKenzie J, et al. Selective serotonin reuptake inhibitors (SSRIs) for depressive disorders in children and adolescents. Cochrane Database of Systematic Reviews 2007, Issue 3. Art. No.: CD004851. DOI: 10.1002/14651858.CD004851.pub2.

129 Hazell P, O'Connell D, Heathcote D, et al. Tricyclic drugs for depression in children and adolescents. Cochrane Database of Systematic Reviews 2002, Issue 2. Art. No.: CD002317. DOI: 10.1002/14651858. CD002317.

130 Candy M, Jones L, Williams R, et al. Psychostimulants for depression. Cochrane Database Syst Rev 2008; 16: CD006722.

131 Jackson KC, Lipman AG. Drug therapy for anxiety in adult palliative care patients. Cochrane Database of Systematic Reviews 2004, Issue 1. Art. No.: CD004596. DOI: 10.1002/14651858.CD004596.

132 Houlahan KE, Branowicki PA, Mack JW, et al. Can end of life care for the pediatric patient suffering with escalating and intractable symptoms be improved? J Pediatr Oncol Nurs 2006; 23: 45–51.

133 Brook L, Hain R. Predicting death in children. Arch Dis Child 2008; 93: 1067–70.

134 Postovsky S, Levenzon A, Ofir R, et al. 'Do not resuscitate orders' among children with solid tumors at the end of life. Pediatr Hematol Oncol 2004; 21: 661–8.

135 Neergard MA, Olesen F, Jensen AB, et al. Palliative care for cancer patients in a primary health care setting: Bereaved relatives' experience, a qualitative group interview study. BMC Palliat Care 2008; 15; 7.

136 Papadatou D, Yfantopoulous J, Kosmidis HV. Death of a child at home or in hospital: experiences of Greek mothers. Death Studies 1996; 20: 215–35.

137 Addington-Hall J, Karlsen S. Do home deaths increase distress in bereavement? Palliat Med 2000; 14 : 161–1.

138 Vickers J, Carlisle C. Choices and control: parental experiences in pediatric terminal home care. J Paediatr Oncol Nurs 2000; 17: 12–21.

139 Kreicbergs U, Valdimarsdottir U, Onelov E, Bjork O, Steineck G. Care related distress: a nationwide study of parents who lost their child to cancer. J Clin Oncol 2005; 23: 9162–71.

140 Corlett J, Twycross A. Negotiation of parental roles within family-centred care: a review of the research. J Clin Nurs 2006; 15: 1308–16.

141 Nolbris M, Hellstrom AL. Siblings' needs and issues when a brother or sister dies of cancer. J Pediatr Oncol Nurs 2005; 22: 227–33.

142 McIntyre J, Robertson S, Norris E, et al. Safety and efficacy of buccal midazolam versus rectal diazepam for emergency treatment of seizures in children: a randomized controlled trial. Lancet 2005; 366: 205–10.

143 O'Doherty CA, Hall EJ, Schofield L, et al. Drugs and syringe drivers: a survey of adult specialist palliative care practice in the United Kingdom and Eire. Palliat Med 2001; 12: 149–54.

144 Dickman A, Schneider J, Vargra J. The Syringe Driver. Continuous Subcutaneous Infusions in Palliative Care. Oxford: Oxford University Press, 2005.

145 Amass C, Allen M. How a 'just in case' approach can improve out of hours palliative care. Pharm J 2005; 275: 22–3.

146 Brook L, Vickers J, Osbourne C. Paediatric palliative care drug boxes: facilitating safe and effective symptom management at home at end of life. Arch Dis Child 2007; 92 (Suppl 1): A58.

147 Bavin L. Artificial rehydration in the last days of life: is it beneficial? Int J Palliat Nurs 2007; 13: 445–9.

148 Morita T, Tey Y, Tsunoda J, et al. Determinants of the sensation of thirst in terminally ill cancer patients. Support Care Cancer 2001; 9: 177–86.

149 Good P, Cavenagh J, Mather M, et al. Medically assisted hydration for palliative care patients. Cochrane Database Syst Rev 2008; 16: CD006273.

150 Kass RM, Ellershaw J. Respiratory tract secretions in the dying patient: a retrospective study. J Pain Symptom Manage 2003; 26: 897–902.

151 Morita T, Tsunoda J, Inoue S, et al. Risk factors for death rattle in terminally ill cancer patients: a prospective exploratory study. Palliat Med 2000; 14: 19–23.

152 Wee B, Hillier R. Interventions for noisy breathing in patients near to death. Cochrane Database of Systematic Reviews 2008, Issue 1. Art. No.: CD005177. DOI: 10.1002/14651858.CD005177.pub2.

153 Leonard M, Raju B, Conroy M, et al. Reversibility of delirium in terminally ill patients and predictors of mortality. Palliat Med 2008; 22: 848–54.

154 White C, McCann MA, Jackson N. First do no harm… Terminal restlessness or drug induced delirium. J Palliat Med 2007; 10:345–51.

155 Morita T, Tey Y, Tsunoda J, et al. Underlying pathologies and their associations with clinical features in terminal delirium in cancer patients. J Pain Symptom Manage 2001; 22: 997–1006.

156 Leentjens AF, Schieveld JN, Leonard M, et al. A comparison of the phenomenology of pediatric, adult and geriatric delirium. J Psychosom Res 2008; 64: 219–23.

157 Morita T, Shima Y, Miyashita M, et al. Physician and nurse-reported effects of intravenous hydration therapy on symptoms in terminally ill patients with cancer. J Palliat Med 2004; 7: 683–93.

158 Fang CK, Chen HW, Lui SI. Prevalence detection and treatment of delirium in terminal cancer inpatients: a prospective study. Jpn J Clin Oncol 2008; 38: 56–63.

159 Jackson KC, Lipman AG. Drug therapy for delirium in terminally ill adult patients. Cochrane Database of Systematic Reviews 2004, Issue 2. Art. No.: CD004770. DOI: 10.1002/14651858.CD004770.

160 Scheiveld JN, Leroy PL, van Os J, et al. Pediatric delirium in critical illness: phenomenology, clinical correlates and treatment response in 40 cases in the pediatric intensive unit. Intensive Care Med 2007; 33: 1033–40.

161 Kehl KA. Treatment of terminal restlessness: a review of the evidence. J Pain Palliat Care Pharmacother 2004; 18: 5–30.

162 Laakso H. Paunonen-Ilmonen M. Mothers' grief following the death of a child. J Adv Nurs 2001; 36: 69–77.

163 Davies R. Mothers' stories of loss: their need to be with their dying child and their child's body after death. J Child Health Care 2005; 9: 288–300.

164 Laakso H, Paunonen-Ilmonen M. Mothers' experience of social support following the death of a child. J Clin Nurse 2002; 11: 176–85.

165 De Cinque N, Monterosso L, Dadd G, et al. Bereavement support for familes following the death of a child from cancer. J Psychosoc Oncol 2006; 24: 65–83.

166 Jankovic M, Masera G, Uderzo C, et al. Meetings with parents after the death of their child from leukaemia. Pediatr Hematol Oncol 1989; 6: 155–60.

167 Contro N, Larrson J, Scofield S, Sourkes B, Cohen H. Family perspectives on the quality of paediatric palliative care. Arch Paediatr Adolesc Med 2002; 156: 14–19.

24 Clinical Trials Involving Children with Cancer – Organizational and Ethical Issues

Sue Ablett[1] and Edward J. Estlin[2]

[1] Children's Cancer and Leukaemia Group (CCLG), Leicester, UK and [2] Department of Pediatric Oncology, Royal Manchester Children's Hospital, Manchester, UK

In this chapter, an overview of the factors that relate to the conduct and organization of clinical trials involving children with cancer at the national and international level will be given. These considerations will be related to the logistical and ethical issues that can act as important challenges for the various types of clinical trial, but with particular reference to the relatively recent advent of the European clinical trials legislature.

National models for the conduct of clinical trials for children with cancer

Given the relative rarity of childhood cancer, national collaboration in multi-center studies has long been the norm. There are a number of different permutations, which mainly reflect historical development [1].
• In the United Kingdom, as elsewhere, the coordination of clinical trials has traditionally been divided into leukemia (under the auspices of the UK Childhood Leukaemia Working Party) and solid tumors (under the UK Children's Cancer Study Group [UKCCSG}). In August 2006 those two groups merged to form the Children's Cancer and Leukaemia Group (CCLG).
• The UK model has recently evolved from a purely centralised one, with all activities co-ordinated by a central data centre to the separation of activity into clinical trial development which is overseen by the relevant National Cancer Research Institute Clinical Studies Development Groups and trial conduct and monitoring which is overseen by a single clinical trials unit for the majority of studies. Issues that relate to standards and governance will be overseen by research networks with the professional body of the CCLG taking a co-ordinating overview.

Within Europe, a number of national groups exist but a different model has largely developed, with clinical trials being hosted in a range of institutions determined in the main by the presence of an eminent clinician with a key interest in a particular tumor type. The concept of a single coordinating center is less common.

Within North America, four separate groups – Children's Cancer Group, Pediatric Oncology Group (POG) and the disease specific Intergroup Rhabdomyosarcoma Study Group and National Wilms' Tumor Study Group, came together in 2001 to form a single collaborative group – the Children's Oncology Group (COG). COG now represents 215 centers across the United States and Canada, as well as Australia, New Zealand, and a number of other countries.

By comparison with the dispersed European coordination model, establishment of a central coordination center does have significant implications for overhead costs of staffing and accommodation. The mechanism of funding differs between Europe and North America.
• In the UK the main source of funding is from competitive grants, both core and project, awarded from a number of grant awarding charitable organizations, primarily Cancer Research UK, supplemented by some other charitable funding.
• There has traditionally been little or no government funding to support children's cancer research.
• Similar funding mechanisms apply throughout Europe. Participation in an international trial represents considerable challenges, as each participating group has to obtain its own national funding.
• For the Children's Oncology Group the main source of funding is the National Cancer Institute, again awarded on the basis of a competitive funding bid.
• There has hitherto been little pharmaceutical company support and very few pharma led trials.

The long and varied history of development of clinical trials within Europe, and the lack of a single funding source, has prevented development of a unified approach and unified processes. Different national legislation governing the regulation of clinical trials is also a factor. Thus there is a range of protocol templates and widely differing views on Case Report Form design and content, and a number of different electronic trial reporting and management facilities in use. Although there is ongoing discussion about a more unified approach within the International

Pediatric Hematology and Oncology, 1st edition. Edited by Edward J. Estlin, Richard J. Gilbertson, and Robert F. Wynn. © 2010 Blackwell Publishing Ltd.

Society of Paediatric Oncology (SIOP) in Europe in relation to clinical trials, it is hard to see, in the short term, how this situation will change. While the Children's Oncology Group undoubtedly has its management challenges because of its size, and potential conflict of varying legislation between the United States and Canada and federal versus state and provincial legislation, as a single cooperative group covering the whole of North America it does have the advantages of a single protocol template and protocol development process and single remote data entry system, thus facilitating greatly training and use by participating sites.

Whatever the size and structure, all participating in clinical trials are now subject to increasing levels of bureaucracy and legislation. Many national groups face similar problems of overstretched resources, insecure funding, and the challenges of taking forward trials in the rarer tumors of childhood. Further collaboration will be essential to ensure that progress can be made and that maximum use is made of resources, experience, and expertise [1].

International collaborations

For the vast majority of tumor types, international collaboration is essential in order to ensure sufficient numbers of patients are available for the completion of a clinical trial in a timely manner. In the United Kingdom, for instance, the only disease where there are sufficient patients for the relatively rapid conduct of a national randomized clinical trial is acute lymphoblastic leukemia (ALL).

International collaboration is, however, complex, takes time and effort to establish and maintain, and is expensive. Potential barriers to international collaboration, which must be overcome, include issues of culture and language, history, and entrenched practice. Compromise is essential. There is currently no international funding stream, and funding must be obtained at a national level by all participating groups/countries [1].

There is no single model of international collaboration. Within Europe, the norm is for a number of participating national groups/countries to collaborate with one taking the lead coordination role – a role which is both a privilege and a responsibility. The studies may be conducted under the auspices of SIOP or as Intergroup studies, such as the Ewing's studies. Early phase trials within Europe are now largely coordinated through ITCC (Innovative Therapies for Childhood Cancer), a cooperative representing 34 centers in six countries. Within North America, the formation of a single group (Children's Oncology Group) has been important in streamlining and harmonizing processes across all aspects of trial activity. Electronic data capture is being used increasingly and is seen as the way forward for international trials. While there is a single system in use within COG trials, this is not the case within Europe [1].

Perhaps the biggest barrier to international collaboration is now the legislation governing the conduct of clinical trials.

Within Europe, the introduction in May 2004 of the Clinical Trials Directive [2] was designed to harmonize the conduct of clinical trials across the growing European Community. The varying implementation of the Directive into national legislation by each of the member states has, however, done little to harmonize and certainly added to the complexity of conducting clinical trials across Europe.

Legislation involving data storage, protection and transfer

Data relating to patients on clinical trials is by its very nature both confidential and sensitive. A range of legislation, which will vary across countries, but is likely to cover both aspects of data protection and freedom of information, covers handling of personal data.

• The legislation covers data held manually and electronically, including X-rays and scans, and all aspects of the processing of such data. There is both organizational and individual responsibility for compliance [3].

• Although the legislation will vary from country to country, it is likely that the basic principles of data protection will apply universally, i.e. that data are held and processed fairly and lawfully, with appropriate consent having been given, are maintained accurately, and are only disclosed appropriately.

For any organization conducting clinical trials there will be a requirement for compliance with whatever national legislation applies. This may involve a registration process. Locally for participating sites there will also be data protection issues, relating primarily to release of patient data to a third party. The same rules apply whether data are being transferred on paper Case Report Forms or electronically via remote data entry.

The requirements for confidentiality of sensitive patient data may prohibit the use of full names and fully identifiable information. This does, however, raise the issue of potential conflict of confidentiality versus patient safety. In any situation where there is a danger of patient data being confused with that of another patient then full identification should be used, though always with a clear explanation of that fact in the Patient Information Sheet, and explicit consent obtained.

The national ethics committees are charged with ensuring that patients or their parents are fully informed within the Parent/Patient Information Sheets about any data processing, including details about any data transfer arrangements and assurances about confidentiality. This will also include assurances that no individual will be named in any publication arising from the trial, or in any conference presentation. In the event of withdrawal of consent during the course of a trial, it must be made clear to the participant that data held to that point will be retained but will not be used for analysis. Integral to this process is the informed consent of the participant or their parent to participate in a trial on the basis of the information provided.

Data transfer issues become more complex within international trials, particularly where the same levels of data protection legislation cannot be guaranteed across national boundaries. It is important that individuals are made aware if this is likely to apply to their data [4].

Ethical considerations

The application of general ethical principles such as respect for a person's self-determination, the balance of risk and benefit, and informed consent apply to all areas of clinical study in pediatric oncology. Indeed, informed consent is currently and most commonly viewed as a means of protection of a potentially vulnerable research subject from harm [5]. However, in adult oncology practice the development of increasingly lengthy and unreadable consent sheets has had little or no impact on patient understanding or decision making in early clinical trials [6]. Moreover, the issue of consent in all aspects of medical research is becoming increasingly complex for pediatric oncology. This has led to a great emphasis on the Parent/Patient Information Sheets in protocols, usually with demands for a range of age-specific sheets. Changes in data protection regulations within the UK [3] are very specific about the need for explicit consent.

Conduct of Phase I trials

Although the majority of children with cancer are now cured of their disease, a significant number have either disease resistant to current therapy, or are unable to tolerate the short- and long-term complications of their treatment. Therefore, Phase I trials are needed for both the rational introduction of new therapies into pediatric oncology practice, and the evaluation of combinations of new and established agents.

• However, adult Phase I experience with new agents is not an adequate predictor of the tolerability of a new agent in children [7].

• Indeed, internationally agreed guidelines for the conduct of Phase I trials in children with cancer have been reported, which describe the determination of the maximum tolerated dose (MTD) which can be taken forward to a Phase II efficacy study, and dose limiting toxicity (DLT) of a new agent or combination [8].

• The strict methodology required for Phase I studies may serve to highlight the ethical and practical difficulties associated with this stage of clinical development.

The common practice in pediatric Phase I trials is to commence with a starting dose that is 80% of the adult maximum tolerated dose. The dose level is generally raised by increments of 25–30%, with children being evaluated in cohorts of three at each dose level for toxicity.

• A critical aspect of the design of Phase I studies is the definition of DLT and MTD, and strict criteria are applied for toxicity evaluation and eligibility whereby children are required to complete a defined period (usually one month) of observation during the first treatment cycle.

• Indeed, although over 90% of children who have been entered into phase I trials in recent years have been eligible for the evaluation of toxicity [9], this requirement may be more difficult to fulfill for children with leukemia when compared with children with solid tumors [10].

• The severity of toxicities is graded according to the National Cancer Institute Common Toxicity Criteria [11], and the MTD is determined as that dose level in which 0 or 1 children in a cohort of six experiences DLT.

In addition, standard criteria for disease response are applied in this clinical setting, and almost all pediatric Phase I studies should investigate the pharmacokinetic behavior of new agents. Pharmacological studies may identify subgroups of children who are especially susceptible to toxicity by virtue of altered metabolism or elimination, and allow the rational selection of schedules of administration that can be taken forward for Phase II study [8].

Since the eligibility criteria for entry of children into Phase I trials usually demand that they have failed all recognized conventional treatments, this may create difficulty in reconciling the often natural desire of parents and children themselves to proceed with treatment at any cost, and the need to provide good quality palliative care to children who will in most cases die.

A survey of the perceptions of pediatricians from the UKCCSG and POG with regard to Phase I trials in pediatric oncology sought to identify ethical and other considerations inherent in the conduct of these studies, perceived parental and children's motivations, and physician expectations with regard toxicity and benefit [9].

• Overall, respondents felt that parents entered their children for medical benefit, altruism, and hope of cure.

• Medical coercion was not felt to be important. Furthermore, although many respondents felt that children could benefit from medical improvement, feelings of altruism and maintenance of hope, respectively, the chance of cure, or complete remission, was felt to be very small.

• Similarly, parents were felt to potentially benefit through altruism and maintenance of hope. Whereas 83% of UKCCSG respondents indicated Phase I trials were associated with ethical difficulties, this was a concern for only 48% of POG respondents. The main ethical concerns of respondents were risk of toxicity, consent of the child, unrealistic hope, and coercion. However, although the majority of respondents expected a child to have at least a 50% chance of toxicity, the likelihood of life- threatening toxicity was felt to be very small.

Thus, pediatricians from the UKCCSG and POG had largely realistic expectations for toxicity and benefit in relation to Phase I studies in pediatric oncology, where literature reviews have identified a 7.9–10% objective response rate compared with a 0.56–0.7% drug-related toxicity for children participating in these studies [9, 12]. Although pediatricians identified altruism, the expectation of medical benefit, and psychological factors such as the maintenance of hope as reasons that parents enter their children into phase I studies [9], there have been no studies of the perceptions of children or their parents in this area.

In contrast, several adult studies have identified that patients who participate in phase I trials are almost exclusively motivated by the hope of therapeutic benefit [13, 14]. Furthermore, the majority of patients were unable to state the research purposes of the trial in which they were participating [13], or whether alternatives to clinical trial participation, including palliative care or non-experimental therapies had been discussed with them [4]. However, cohort-specific consent methodologies are being developed for adult phase I studies, in which an interactive consent process by which patients can become directly involved in decisions of dose escalation may reduce some of the ethical dilemmas in this area [15]. Therefore, studies are needed to investigate the motivation and perceptions for parents and children with regard to the consent process for phase I trials in pediatric oncology.

In addition to improvements in the understanding of the consent process for phase I trials, future phase I studies in pediatric oncology may be required to embrace methodologies based on the pharmacokinetics and pharmacodynamics of the agents under study. For example, significant antitumor activity has been demonstrated for a phase I study of ifosfamide, carboplatin, and etoposide, where a pharmacologically-guided dose escalation for carboplatin has been employed [16]. In addition, continual reassessment methodologies for phase I studies are being developed in an adult cancer setting, and it is hoped that these will minimize the number of patients treated at sub-optimal dose levels [17]. Finally, an action-based methodology may prove an important innovation in phase I trial design, where an end-point of a study may be defined by the biochemical evidence of maximal inhibition of the target enzyme [18].

Conduct of Phase II trials

Phase II studies are required to determine whether or not a new agent or treatment strategy appears sufficiently active to warrant further study, as determined by objective response rates of 20–30%, but may also further define the toxicity profile and pharmacokinetics of new agents. As with phase I studies, phase II studies in pediatric oncology are conducted on a multi-institutional or group collaborative basis [19]. Phase II trials in pediatric oncology usually follow a two-stage design that allows early termination of studies if the activity level is too low or is adequately high [20].

Many of the ethical issues related to phase II trials of new agents are similar to those discussed above for the conduct of phase I trials. However, the nature of Phase II studies may translate into greater therapeutic intent on behalf of an investigator, with the consequence of raising patient or parental expectations. Although this aspect of consent has not been formally studied in the adult or pediatric setting, the overall response rates within the phase II setting is very low for many types of pediatric cancer, which may be an important ethical consideration in obtaining informed parental consent [19].

Conduct of Phase III trials

Phase III trials compare the efficacy of an experimental therapy with that of a standard or control therapy, and as with earlier clinical studies in pediatric cancer are usually only feasible in a collaborative group or multicenter setting. Phase III clinical trials may usually include a randomization between treatment arms, and are commonly based on sequential or factorial designs [21]. As with earlier clinical studies in pediatric oncology, Phase III clinical trials face several logistical difficulties. This may be exemplified by the example of central pathological review, where misclassification of tumors can result in a reduction in statistical power and inaccurate estimates of median survival [22].

Much of the debate about ethical issues in phase III trials has focused on the issue of equipoise, i.e. the state of genuine uncertainty on the part of a clinical investigator or treating physician toward the comparative merits of different treatments for cancer. However, the work of the Rainbow Center for Pediatric Ethics in Cleveland, North America, has done much to inform the pediatric community of the many challenges that are faced if consent is to be truly optimized and informed. For a major study of randomization into childhood leukemia trials at six treatment centers in the USA, several themes have been identified as follows:

• Parents are often in shock at the time of diagnosis of leukemia for their children, but found that discussions with medical staff to be more helpful than information sheets [23].
• In keeping with this, the clinicians involved were concerned about information overload and increased anxiety for parents in this setting [24].
• Clinicians tend not to involve children in discussions about randomization [25].
• Consent forms tend not to indicate that research participants have a right to receive information or summaries of the outcomes of the studies they are involved in [26].
• Problems of consent-related communication and understanding were more frequently found for parents of lower socioeconomic status or where little or no English was spoken [27].
• Only 50% of parents understood the concepts involved in the randomization for their child's clinical trials, and this was particularly true for ethnic minority families and those of lower socioeconomic status [28].
• A staged approach to consent improves parental comprehension [29], which is more of a problem in comparison to similar situations in adult oncological practice, where a more full engagement between physician and patient has been observed [30].
• Physician rapport and partnership building related to parent participation in the informed consent process, but information giving did not [31].
• The understanding of the consent process tends to deteriorate over time [32].
• The effect of altruistic considerations on the consent process is marginal [33].
• The parents themselves have suggested improvements for timing, sequence, checking for understanding, anticipatory guid-

ance, segues into randomized clinical trials, discussion with historical perspective, and choice [34].

Although pediatric oncology represents a remarkable model of organization and cooperation, there are many areas of difficulty in the conduct of clinical trials in pediatric oncology. Due to the relatively small numbers of patients involved, clinical trials in pediatric oncology must maximize the clinical and scientific information gained from their conduct. The ethical considerations for the conduct of clinical trials in pediatric oncology need further study, especially in the areas of parental and patient consent in the early clinical trial setting. However, running clinical trials across national boundaries is not easy: it requires considerable understanding of other cultures, tact, and diplomacy and, at times, willingness to compromise.

References

1 Ablett S, Pinkerton CR. Recruiting children into cancer trials – the role of the United Kingdom Children's Cancer Study Group (UKCCSG). Br J Cancer 2003; 88: 1661–5.

2 EU GCP Directive: Proposal for a European Parliament and Council Directive on the Approximation of the laws, regulations and administrative provisions of the member states relating to the implementation of good clinical practice in the conduct of clinical trials on medicinal products for human use. COM (97) 0369-c4-0446/97.97/0197(COD): Official Journal of the European Communities, 1997, C379, 27.

3 Data Protection Act 1998.

4 CPMP Working Party on the Efficacy of Medicinal Products. European Community Commission notes for guidance: Good Clinical Practice for Trials of Medicinal Products in the European Community. J Pharmacol Toxicol 1990; 67: 361–72.

5 Daugherty CK. Ethical issues in the development of new agents. Invest New Drugs 1999; 17: 145–53.

6 Daugherty CK. Impact of therapeutic research on informed consent and the ethics of clinical trials: a medical oncology perspective. J Clin Oncol 1999; 17: 1601–17.

7 Marsoni S, Ungerleider R, Hurson S, Hammershaimb L. Tolerance to antineoplastic agents in children and adults. Cancer Treat Rep 1985; 69: 1263–9.

8 Smith M, Bernstein M, Bleyer WA, et al. Conduct of Phase I trials in children with cancer. J Clin Oncol 1998; 16: 966–78.

9 Estlin EJ, Cotterill S, Pratt CB, Pearson ADJ, Bernstein M. Phase I trials in pediatric oncology: perceptions of pediatricians from the United Kingdom Children's Cancer Study Group and the Pediatric Oncology Group. J Clin Oncol 2000; 18: 1900–5.

10 Estlin EJ, Pinkerton CR, Lewis IJ, et al. A Phase I study of nolatrexed dihydrochloride in children patients with advanced cancer. A United Kingdom Children's cancer Study group Investigation. Br J Cancer 2001; 84: 11–18.

11 MacDonald J, Haller D, Mayer R. Grading of toxicity. In MacDonald J, Haller D, Mayer R (Eds), Manual of Oncologic Therapeutics, 3rd Edn. Philadelphia, PA: Lippincott, 1995: 519–23.

12 Shah, S, Weitman S, Langevin A-M, et al. Phase I therapy trials in children with cancer. J Ped Haematol Oncol 1998; 20: 431–8.

13 Daugherty C, Ratain MJ, Grochowski E, et al. Perceptions of cancer patients and their physicians in Phase I trials. J Clin Oncol 1995; 13: 1062–72.

14 Itoh K, Sasaki Y, Fuji H, et al. Patients in phase trials of anti-cancer agents in Japan: motivation, comprehension and expectations. Br J Cancer 1997; 76: 107–13.

15 Daugherty CK, Ratain MJ, Minami H, et al. Study of cohort-specific consent and patient control in phase I cancer trials. J Clin Oncol 1998; 16: 2305–12.

16 Marina, NM, Rodman, JH, Murray, DJ, et al. Phase I study of escalating targeted doses of carboplatin combined with ifosfamide and etoposide in treatment of newly diagnosed pediatric solid tumors. J Natl Cancer Inst 1994; 86: 544–8.

17 Kramar A, Lebecq A, Candalh E. Continual reassessment methods in phase I trials of the combination of two drugs in oncology. Stat Med 1999; 18: 1849–64.

18 Kerr, DJ. Phase I clinical trials: adapting methodology to face new challenges. Ann Oncol 1994; 5 (Suppl. 4): S67–S70.

19 Weitman S, Ochoa, S, Sullivan J, et al. Pediatric Phase II cancer chemotherapy trials, a Pediatric Oncology Group study. J Pediatr Hematol Oncol 1997; 19: 187–91.

20 Fleming TR. One-sided multiple testing procedure for Phase II clinical trials. Biometrics 1982; 38: 143–51.

21 Ungerleider, RS, Ellenberg, SS. Cancer clinical trials: design, conduct, analysis and reporting. In Pizzo PA, Poplack DG (Eds), Principles and Practice of Pediatric Oncology, 3rd edn. Philadelphia: Lippincott-Raven Publishers, 1997, 385–406.

22 Scott CB, Nelson JS, Farnan NC, et al. Central pathology review in clinical trials for patients with malignant glioma. A report of Radiation Therapy Oncology Group 83-02. Cancer 1995; 76; 307–13.

23 Kodish ED, Pentz RD, Noll RB, Ruccione K, Buckley J, Lange BJ. Informed consent in the Children's Cancer Group: results of preliminary research. Cancer 1998; 82: 2467–81.

24 Simon C, Eder M, Raiz P, Zyzanski S, Pentz R, Kodish ED. Informed consent for pediatric leukaemia research: clinician perspectives. Cancer 2001; 92: 691–700.

25 Olechnowicz JQ, Eder M, Simon C, Zyzanski S, Kodish E. Assent observed: children's involvement in leukaemia treatment and research discussions. Pediatrics 2002; 109: 806–14.

26 Fernandez CV, Kodish E, Taweel S, Shurin S, Weijer C. Children's Oncology Group. Disclosure of the right of research participants to receive research results: an analysis of consent forms in the Children's Oncology Group. Cancer 2003; 97: 2904–9.

27 Simon C, Zyzanski SJ, Eder M, Raiz P, Kodish ED, Siminoff LA. Groups potentially at risk for making poorly informed decisions about entry into clinical trials for childhood cancer. J Clin Oncol 2003; 21: 2173–8.

28 Kodish E, Eder M, Noll RB, et al. Communication of randomization in childhood leukaemia trials. JAMA 2004; 291: 470–5.

29 Angiolillo AL, Simon C, Kodish E, et al. Staged informed consent for a randomized clinical trial in childhood leukaemia: impact on the consent process. Pediatr Blood Cancer 2004; 42: 433–7.

30 Simon CM, Siminoff LA, Kodish ED, Burant C. Comparison of the informed consent process for randomized clinical trials in pediatric and adult oncology. J Clin Oncol 2004; 22: 2708–17.

31 Drotar D, Miller V, Willard V, Anthony K, Kodish E. Correlates of parental participation during informed consent for randomized clini-

cal trials in the treatment of childhood leukaemia. Ethics Behav 2004; 14: 1–15.

32 Greenley RN, Drotar D, Zyzanksi SJ, Kodish E. Stability of parental undertstanding of random assignment in childhood leukaemia trials: an empirical examination of informed consent. J Clin Oncol 2006; 24: 891–7.

33 Simon C, Eder M, Kodish E, Siminoff L. Altruistic discourse in the informed consent process for childhood cancer clinical trials. Am J Bioeth 2006; 6: 40–7.

34 Eder ML, Yamokoski AD, Wittmann PW, Kodish ED. Improving informed consent; suggestions from parents of children with leukaemia. Pediatrics 2007; 119: e849–59.

Index

Index

Index